FIRST AID FOR THE® USMLE STEP 1 2016

TAO LE, MD, MHS
Associate Clinical Professor
Chief, Section of Allergy and Immunology
Department of Medicine
University of Louisville

VIKAS BHUSHAN, MD
Diagnostic Radiologist
Los Angeles

MATTHEW SOCHAT, MD
Resident, Department of Internal Medicine
Temple University Hospital

MEHBOOB KALANI, MD
Resident, Department of Internal Medicine
Allegheny Health Network Medical Education Consortium

YASH CHAVDA, DO
Resident, Department of Emergency Medicine
St. Barnabas Hospital, Bronx

KIMBERLY KALLIANOS, MD
Resident, Department of Radiology and Biomedical Imaging
University of California, San Francisco

FRANCIS DENG
Washington University School of Medicine in St. Louis
Class of 2016

PATRICK SYLVESTER, MD
Resident, Department of Emergency Medicine
The Ohio State University

Mc Graw Hill Education

New York / Chicago / San Francisco / Athens / London / Madrid / Mexico City
Milan / New Delhi / Singapore / Sydney / Toronto

First Aid for the® USMLE Step 1 2016: A Student-to-Student Guide

1 2 3 4 5 6 7 8 9 0 RMN/RMN 19 18 17 16 15

ISBN 978-1-25-958737-5
MHID 1-25-958737-1
ISSN 1532-6020

Notice

Medicine is an ever-changing science. As new research and clinical experience broaden our knowledge, changes in treatment and drug therapy are required. The authors and the publisher of this work have checked with sources believed to be reliable in their efforts to provide information that is complete and generally in accord with the standards accepted at the time of publication. However, in view of the possibility of human error or changes in medical sciences, neither the authors nor the publisher nor any other party who has been involved in the preparation or publication of this work warrants that the information contained herein is in every respect accurate or complete, and they disclaim all responsibility for any errors or omissions or for the results obtained from use of the information contained in this work. Readers are encouraged to confirm the information contained herein with other sources. For example and in particular, readers are advised to check the product information sheet included in the package of each drug they plan to administer to be certain that the information contained in this work is accurate and that changes have not been made in the recommended dose or in the contraindications for administration. This recommendation is of particular importance in connection with new or infrequently used drugs.

This book was set in Electra LT Std by Rainbow Graphics.
The editors were Catherine A. Johnson and Christina M. Thomas.
Project management was provided by Rainbow Graphics.
The production supervisor was Jeffrey Herzich.
RR Donnelley was printer and binder.

This book is printed on acid-free paper.

International Edition ISBN 978-12-5925099-6, MHID 1-25-925099-7.

Dedication

To the contributors to this and past editions, who took time to share their knowledge, insight, and humor for the benefit of students and physicians everywhere.

Contents

Contributing Authors

RAM BABOO, MBBS, MS (Surgery)
Post Graduate Institute of Medical Education and Research

EMILIA CALVARESI, PhD
University of Illinois at Urbana-Champaign College of Medicine
Class of 2017

ANGELA GAUTHIER
Yale School of Medicine
Class of 2017

BENJAMIN GOUGH
Lake Erie College of Osteopathic Medicine
Class of 2016

JAN ANDRE GRAUMAN, MA
Adjunct Assistant Professor
University of Victoria School of Nursing

JACQUELINE HAIRSTON
Icahn School of Medicine at Mount Sinai
Class of 2016

DAVID HUANG
The Warren Alpert Medical School of Brown University
Class of 2017

M. SCOTT MOORE, DO
Resident, Department of Pathology
University of Arizona

CAROLINE MURRELL
Wake Forest School of Medicine
Class of 2017

JUN YEN NG
The University of Queensland
Class of 2015

SARAH SCHIMANSKY, MB BCh BAO
Foundation Doctor
North Bristol NHS Trust

JARED SHENSON
Vanderbilt University School of Medicine
Class of 2016

NINO SIKHARULIDZE, MD
Department of Endocrinology
Tbilisi State Medical University

ANDREW ZUREICK
University of Michigan Medical School
Class of 2017

Image and Illustration Team

JOCELYN COMPTON, MD
Resident, Department of Orthopedic Surgery
University of Iowa Hospitals and Clinics

RYAN W. HADDEN
UAB School of Medicine
Class of 2017

PRAMOD THEETHA KARIYANNA, MD
Resident, Department of Internal Medicine
SUNY Downstate Medical Center

RICHARD P. USATINE, MD
Professor, Dermatology and Cutaneous Surgery
Professor, Family and Community Medicine
University of Texas Health Science Center San Antonio

RENATA VELAPATIÑO, MD
San Martín de Porres University

Associate Authors

MARIA BAKKAL
University of Aleppo School of Medicine

PRIYANKA CHILAKAMARRI
University of Vermont College of Medicine
Class of 2016

PRITHA CHITAGI, MD
Resident, Department of Internal Medicine
Wayne State University

PATRICK HUDSON, MD
Oregon Health & Science University
Class of 2015

KRISHAN JETHWA, MD
Resident, Department of Radiation Oncology
Mayo Clinic

YIANNIS KOULLIAS, MD
Resident, Department of Internal Medicine
Brigham and Women's Hospital

SHAWN VERMA
The Warren Alpert Medical School of Brown University
Class of 2018

Image and Illustration Team

WENDY ABBOTT
Kentucky College of Osteopathic Medicine
Class of 2015

KEVIN AU, MD
Resident, Department of Vascular Surgery
Louisiana State University

Faculty Advisors

MARIA ANTONELLI, MD
Rheumatology Fellow, Department of Medicine
Case Western Reserve University School of Medicine

HERMAN BAGGA, MD
Fellow, Department of Urology
Cleveland Clinic

ADITYA BARDIA, MBBS, MPH
Attending Physician, Massachusetts General Hospital
Harvard Medical School

SHASHANK BEHERE, MD
Fellow, Nemours Cardiac Center
Nemours/Alfred I duPont Hospital for Children

PAULETTE BERND, PhD
Professor, Department of Pathology and Cell Biology
Columbia University College of Physicians and Surgeons

J. PETER CAMPBELL, MD, MPH
Assistant Professor, Department of Ophthalmology
Oregon Health & Science University

BROOKS D. CASH, MD
Professor of Medicine, Division of Gastroenterology
University of South Alabama School of Medicine

PETER V. CHIN-HONG, MD
Professor, Department of Medicine
University of California, San Francisco

SHIVANI VERMA CHMURA, MD
Adjunct Clinical Faculty, Department of Psychiatry
Stanford University School of Medicine

LINDA S. COSTANZO, PhD
Professor, Physiology & Biophysics
Virginia Commonwealth University School of Medicine

ANTHONY L. DeFRANCO, PhD
Professor, Department of Microbiology and Immunology
University of California, San Francisco School of Medicine

CHARLES S. DELA CRUZ, MD, PhD
Assistant Professor, Department of Pulmonary and Critical Care Medicine
Yale School of Medicine

RICHARD S. FINKEL, PharmD
Clinical Assistant Professor, Department of Pharmaceutical Sciences
Nova Southeastern University College of Pharmacy

CONRAD FISCHER, MD
Residency Program Director, Brookdale University Hospital
Brooklyn, New York
Associate Professor, Medicine, Physiology, and Pharmacology
Touro College of Medicine

JEFFREY J. GOLD, MD
Associate Professor, Department of Neurology
University of California, San Diego School of Medicine

RYAN C.W. HALL, MD
Assistant Professor, Department of Psychiatry
University of South Florida

LOUISE HAWLEY, PhD
Immediate Past Professor and Chair, Department of Microbiology
Ross University School of Medicine

MARGARET HAYES, MD
Fellow, Department of Pulmonary and Critical Care
Johns Hopkins Hospital

JEFFREY W. HOFMANN, PhD
The Warren Alpert Medical School of Brown University
MD Candidate

DEEPALI JAIN, MD
Assistant Professor, Department of Pathology
All India Institute of Medical Sciences

BRIAN C. JENSEN, MD
Assistant Professor, Division of Child and Adolescent Psychiatry
University of Louisville School of Medicine

KRISTINE KRAFTS, MD
Assistant Professor, Department of Basic Sciences
University of Minnesota School of Medicine

GERALD LEE, MD
Assistant Professor, Department of Pediatrics
University of Louisville School of Medicine

KACHIU LEE, MD, MPH
Department of Dermatology
Harvard Medical School

WARREN LEVINSON, MD, PhD
Professor, Department of Microbiology and Immunology
University of California, San Francisco School of Medicine

PETER MARKS, MD, PhD
Associate Professor, Department of Internal Medicine
Yale School of Medicine

J. RYAN MARTIN, MD
Assistant Professor of Obstetrics, Gynecology, and Reproductive Sciences
Yale School of Medicine

THOMAS A. PANAVELIL, PhD
Professor of Pharmacology
Nova Southeastern University College of Pharmacy

JEANNINE RAHIMIAN, MD, MBA
Associate Professor, Obstetrics and Gynecology
David Geffen School of Medicine at UCLA

SOROUSH RAIS-BAHRAMI, MD
Assistant Professor, Urology and Radiology
The University of Alabama at Birmingham School of Medicine

SASAN SAKIANI, MD
Fellow, Division of Gastroenterology and Hepatology
Case Western Reserve University School of Medicine

JOSEPH L. SCHINDLER, MD
Assistant Professor, Neurology and Neurosurgery
Yale School of Medicine

MELANIE SCHORR, MD
Research Fellow, Department of Medicine
Massachusetts General Hospital

NATHAN W. SKELLEY, MD
Sports Medicine Fellow, Department of Orthopedic Surgery
Massachusetts General Hospital, Harvard Medical School

HOWARD M. STEINMAN, PhD
Assistant Dean, Biomedical Science Education
Professor, Department of Biochemistry
Albert Einstein College of Medicine

STEPHEN F. THUNG, MD
Associate Professor, Department of Obstetrics and Gynecology
The Ohio State University College of Medicine

PRASHANT VAISHNAVA, MD
Assistant Professor, Department of Medicine
Mount Sinai Hospital and Icahn School of Medicine

J. MATTHEW VELKEY, PhD
Assistant Dean, Basic Science Education
Duke University School of Medicine

HILARY J. VERNON, MD, PhD
Assistant Professor, McKusick Nathans Institute of Genetic Medicine
Johns Hopkins University

BRIAN WALCOTT, MD
Clinical Instructor, Department of Neurological Surgery
University of California, San Francisco

TISHA SHIH-YUN WANG, MD
Assistant Clinical Professor, Department of Pulmonary and Critical Care
University of California, Los Angeles

SYLVIA WASSERTHEIL-SMOLLER, PhD
Distinguished University Professor Emerita
Department of Epidemiology and Population Health
Albert Einstein College of Medicine

ADAM WEINSTEIN, MD
Assistant Professor, Section of Pediatric Nephrology
Geisel School of Medicine at Dartmouth

KAREN L. WHALEN, PharmD
Clinical Professor, Department of Pharmacotherapy and Translational Research
University of Florida College of Pharmacy

Preface

With the 26th edition of *First Aid for the USMLE Step 1,* we continue our commitment to providing students with the most useful and up-to-date preparation guide for the USMLE Step 1. This edition represents an outstanding revision in many ways, including:

- 50+ entirely new facts, including a new section on quality improvement principles and safety science.
- Hundreds of major fact updates culled from more than 100,000 comments and suggestions.
- Extensive text revisions, new mnemonics, clarifications, and corrections curated by a team of more than 30 student authors who excelled on their Step 1 examinations and verified by a team of expert faculty advisors and nationally recognized USMLE instructors.
- Updated with more than 250 new or revised full-color photos to help visualize various disorders, descriptive findings, and basic science concepts. Labeled and captioned photographs have been optimized to aid retention by engaging visual memory in a manner complementary to mnemonics.
- Updated with dozens of new and revised diagrams. We continue to expand our collaboration with USMLE-Rx (MedIQ Learning, LLC) to develop and enhance illustrations with improved information design to help students integrate pathophysiology, therapeutics, and diseases into memorable frameworks for annotation and personalization.
- Thicker, embossed cover and heavy-duty binding for increased durability and longevity.
- A revised exam preparation guide with updated data from the NBME and NRMP. The guide also features new high-yield techniques for efficient and effective test preparation. The updated supplemental guide for IMGs, osteopathic and podiatry students, and students with a disability can be found at our blog, **www.firstaidteam.com**.
- An updated summary guide to student-recommended USMLE Step 1 review resources, including mobile apps for iOS and Android. The full resource guide with detailed descriptions can be found at our blog, **www.firstaidteam.com**.
- Real-time Step 1 updates and corrections can also be found exclusively on our blog.

We invite students and faculty to share their thoughts and ideas to help us continually improve *First Aid for the USMLE Step 1* through our blog and collaborative editorial platform. (See How to Contribute, p. xvii.)

Louisville	Tao Le
Los Angeles	Vikas Bhushan
Philadelphia	Matthew Sochat
New York City	Yash Chavda
St. Louis	Francis Deng
Pittsburgh	Mehboob Kalani
San Francisco	Kimberly Kallianos
Athens, Ohio	Patrick Sylvester

Special Acknowledgments

This has been a collaborative project from the start. We gratefully acknowledge the thousands of thoughtful comments, corrections, and advice of the many medical students, international medical graduates, and faculty who have supported the authors in our continuing development of *First Aid for the USMLE Step 1*.

We provide special acknowledgment and thanks to the following students who made exemplary contributions to this edition through our voting, proofreading, and crowdsourcing platform: Nicolas Austin, Kashif Badar, Stefan Campbell, Anup Chalise, Wendy Chen, Crosby Culp, Helen Dainton, Katy Demitruk, Okubit Gebreyonas, Gino Giannone, Richard Godby, Christina Govas, Bharath Guntupalli, Isaiah Hammonds, Cinthia Marie Gonzalez Hernandez, Joyce Ho, M Ho, Benjamin Hans Jeuk, Nikhar Kinger, Vladimer Kitiashvili, Martin Ma, Micah Mathai, James McCoy, Melissa Meghpara, Theresa Meloche, Ryan Meyer, Sarah Michelson, Joseph Mininni, JB Moses, Natia Murvelashvili, Thomas Nienaber, Michael Nguygen, Ishan Patel, Iqra Patoli, Eric Pease, Jimmy Tam Huy Pham, Anthony Purgianto, Mohsin Raza, Moshe Roberts, Casey Joseph Rosenthal, Anna Sevilla, Avinainder Singh, Feba Sunny, Amelia St. Ange, Angela Taeschner, Nkechi Ukeekwe, Vaishnavi Vaidyanathan, Paul Walden, Matthew Wallace, Isabella Wu, and Xuebao Zhang.

For help on the First Aid Team blog, thanks to Mark Ard (Editor), Edison Cano, Tim Durso, Luke Murray, Ryan Nguyen, and Joe Savarese. For support and encouragement throughout the process, we are grateful to Thao Pham and Jonathan Kirsch, Esq. Thanks to Louise Petersen for organizing and supporting the project. Thanks to our publisher, McGraw-Hill, for the valuable assistance of its staff, including Midge Haramis and Jeffrey Herzich. For enthusiasm, support, and commitment for this ongoing and ever-challenging project, thanks to our editor, Catherine Johnson.

We are also very grateful to Dr. Fred Howell and Dr. Robert Cannon of Textensor Ltd for providing us extensive customization and support for their powerful A.nnotate collaborative editing platform, which allows us to efficiently manage thousands of contributions. Thanks to Dr. Richard Usatine for his outstanding dermatologic and clinical image contributions. Thanks also to Jean-Christophe Fournet (www.humpath.com), Dr. Ed Uthman, and Dr. Frank Gaillard (www.radiopaedia.org) for generously allowing us to access some of their striking photographs. We especially thank Dr. Kristine Krafts for many insightful text and image contributions throughout the extensive revision.

For exceptional editorial support, enormous thanks to our tireless senior editor, Emma D. Underdown, and her team of editors, Christine Diedrich, Allison Battista, Linda Davoli, Janene Matragrano, Isabel Nogueira, Rebecca Stigall, and Hannah Warnshuis. Many thanks to Tara Price for page design and all-around InDesign expertise. Special thanks to Jan Bednarczuk for a greatly improved index. We are also grateful to our medical illustrators, Hans Neuhart and Diana Kryski, for their creative work on the new and updated illustrations. In particular, we thank Diana and Dr. Krafts for optimizing all of our photographs. Lastly, tremendous thanks to Rainbow Graphics, especially David Hommel and Donna Campbell, for remarkable ongoing editorial and production support under time pressure.

Louisville	Tao Le
Los Angeles	Vikas Bhushan
Philadelphia	Matthew Sochat
New York City	Yash Chavda
St. Louis	Francis Deng
Pittsburgh	Mehboob Kalani
San Francisco	Kimberly Kallianos
Athens, Ohio	Patrick Sylvester

General Acknowledgments

Each year we are fortunate to receive the input of thousands of medical students and graduates who provide new material, clarifications, and potential corrections through our website and our collaborative editing platform. This has been a tremendous help in clarifying difficult concepts, correcting errata from the previous edition, and minimizing new errata during the revision of the current edition. This reflects our long-standing vision of a true, student-to-student publication. We have done our best to thank each person individually below, but we recognize that errors and omissions are likely. Therefore, we will post an updated list of acknowledgments at our website, www.firstaidteam.com/bonus/. We will gladly make corrections if they are brought to our attention.

For submitting contributions and corrections, many thanks to Aaiza Malik, Stephanie Aaron, Abdul Muqtadir Abbasi, Mashya Abbassi, Ibrahim Abdelfattah, Ahmad Abdelhady, Andrew Abdelsayed, Khaled Abdulla, Alissa Aboff, Scott R. Abrahamson, Omar Abu Slieh, Naief AbuDaff, Noor Abu-Farsakh, Ra'ed Abujajeh, Bernardo Acevedo, Ian Ackers, David Adams, Cameron Adler, Neda Afshar, Vivian Agumadu, Masood Ahmad, Anosh Ahmed, Ayesha Ahmed, Muhammad Ahsan Ahsan, Himanshu Ajrawat, Zoey Akah, Marib Akanda, Adam Akbar, Anas Alabkaa, Ameen Al-Aghil, Mohammad Alam, Maryam Alaradi, Jemma Alarcon, Lourdes Alberty, Yeisel Alfonso, Mohammed Alhaidar, Mohamed Al-Hajji, Albert Alhatem, Muneer Al-Husseini, Daniel Alicea Delgado, Khalid Al-Kharraz, Rami Alkhoury, Yasser Almalky, Hussein Al-Mohamad, Ahmed Alnajar, Ahmad Al-Shyoukh, Morgan Altinok, Priscilla Alvarez, Abdullah Mohammed Alwadai, Frank Javier Amiama, Omid Amidi, Yajie An, Anna Anderson, David Anderson, Luke Andrea, Mehdi Ansari, Norin Ansari, Saeed Arefanian, Muhammad Mustafa Arif, Hassaan Arshad, Abdul Aziz Asbeutah, Syed Faaz Ashraf, Saira Aslam, Rizwan Attiq, Audrey Avila, Divya Ayyala, Katelynn Bachman, Marcus Badgeley, Denis Balaban, Vyshnavy Balendra, Muhammad Sher Khoh Qaisrani Baloch, Debdeep Banerjee, Behnoud Baradaran Noveiry, Eric Barbarite, Carlos Barbosa, Gauri Barlingay, Allison Basel, Jasper Bash, Mohammad Bashir, Jason Batey, Suraj Batish, Gabriel Batistuta, Richard Baylis, Andy Beck, Eric Behar, Amin Bemanian, Alex Benedick, Amanda Bennett, Kenechukwu Ben-Okafor, Ekta Bery, Abhinandan Bhagat, Shea Bielby, Vinoth Birabaharan, Brian Birnbaum, Malla Bishal, Aaron Blackshaw, Allison Blake, Stephanie Borinsky, Sminu Bose, Jeff Brady, Hemal Brahmbhat, Shay Brikman, Kenneth Brock, Carl Brophy, Sareena Brown, Alyssa Bruehlman, Kristin Bubel, Tapan Buch, Abraham Burshan, Katherine Butler, Kaitlyn Buzard, Trevor Cabrera, Cecilia Cai, Sunny Cai, Katharine Caldwell, Linelle Campbell, Edison Cano, Sean Cantwell, Justin Cappuzzo, Paul Cartwright, Marianne Casilla-Lennon, Nicole Castagno, Colombe Castellucci, Kenan Celtik, Abdelkader Chaar, Aron Chacko, Mac Chamberlin, Cindy Chang, Jodie Chang, Sherry Chao, Muhammad Chatha, Hafsa Chaudhry, Lakshpaul Chauhan, Sumir Chawla, Jenny Chen, Adam Cheng, Carling Cheung, Chideraa Chibuezeoke, Doug Chieffe, Priyanka Chilakamarri, Edward Cho, Joanne Cho, Jessica M. Cho, Ujval Choksi, Renee Cholyway, Andrew Chomchuensawat, Manita Choudhary, Nicholas Choy, Robert Chris, Bill Christian, La Nyka Christian, Alice Chuang, Hyun Bae Chun, Benjamin Chung, Jonathan Chung, Hyunsoo Chung, Angelo Ciliberti, Beth Clymer, Michael Lawrenz Co, Sam Cochran, Chen Cohen, Lauren Coleman, Jensyn Cone, Michael Conte, Rafael Contreras, Alejandro Cortes, Eliana Costantino Burgazzi, Erica Couzens, Ian Cox, Ronald Crandall, Daniel Crespo Artunduaga, John Cummins, Jennifer Cushman, Farah Dadabhoy, Chelsea Dahl, Amulya Dakka, Patrick Steven Damaso, Kathryn Davis, Korbin Davis, Solomon Dawson, Felice De Stefano, James Deardorff, Andrew DeCrescenzo, Carina Dehner, David DeMik, Daniel Denis, Jacqueline Joanna Denysiak, Margaret DeOliveira, Tricia Derges, Vaibhav Desai, Sagar Deshpande, Divya Dethier, Michael Dever, Jessie Dhaliwal, Gurpreet Dhanda, Ashley Dickens, Katherine Dittman, Isaac Dodd, Ricardo Domingo, Florence Doo, Atbin Doroodchi, Saman Doroodgar Jorshery, Irena Doubelt, Thomas Drzymala, Stephanie Dudzinski, Parikshit Duriseti, Sara Dusing, Marco Duverseau, Jeremy eckes, Susannah Eckman, Hamid Ehsani-Nia, Ian Eisenhauer, Alexander El Sehamy, Abdelkhalek Elagamy, Abd El-Hameed Elmestarihi, Ghassan Elwanni, David Epstein, Jonathan Erdman, Semih Eren, Lee Eschenroeder, Pedro Mario Espino-Grosso, Maria Espiridion, Cynthia Estrada, Daniel Ezidiegwu, Emmanuel Fadiora, Matthew Fadus, Giselle Falconi, Tyler Fanning, Joseph Farahany, Shimon Farber, David Farchadi, Saba Farooqi,

Sohail Farshadsefat, Saul Feierstein, Timothy Feliciano, Yuan Feng, Charles Fennie, Laviel Fernandez, Renae R. Fisher, Matthew Fishman, Natalie Foertmeyer, Sandra Fong, Daniel Franco, Matthew Franklin, Peter Fredericks, Eli Fredman, Mohamed Gad, Anita Gade, Abdulaziz Ahmad Galadari, Avi Gandhi, Himali Gandhi, Sangeetha Gandhi, Jared Gans, Jacqueline Garavito, Russell Garcia, Anna Garza, Nicholas Geiger, Marianne Gelter, Alejandro Gener, Tobin George, Maikel Ragaei Ramzi Fahmi Gerges, Rupendra Ghatak, Pashmeena Gilani, Arshpal Gill, Zachary Gillooly, Christin Giordano, Aaron Goldberg, Monica Gonzalez, Jennipher Gonzalez, Andres Javier Gonzalez Salazar, Jose Manuel Gonzalez-Boffill, Jared Goodman, George Gorgy, Gavin Gorrell, Powell Graham, Sarah Grajower, Nathaniel Greenbaum, Brian Grice, Laura Groomes, Xavier Guell, Evin Guilliams, Sadaf Gulzar, Marcus Gunner, Chuner Guo, Prerna Gupta, Nita Gupta, Olga Guzovsky, Varan Haghshenas, Brandon Haghverdian, Jeremiah Haines, Zakary Hambsch, Sheiva Hamidi, Nicola Hampel, Arielle Hancu, Adeena Haque, Adam Harari, Noah Haroian, Jamison Harvey, Hunaid Hasan, Hassan J. Hashm, Asmaa Ibrahim Hassan Abd El Rehim, Fadi Hawa, Maham Hayat, Mona Hdeib, Sarah He, Richard Hickman, Kelsi Hirai, Erika Ho, Luqman Hodgkinson, Dana Holiday, Tyler Holliday, Kenneth Holton, Evan Horn, Katherine Hounshell, Jonathan Hourmozdi, Levi Howard, Ann Hua, Stephanie Huang, Eleanor Huber, Allyson Hughes, Steven Hull, Faisal Hussain, Catalina Hwang, Ibrahim Hyder, David Ianacone, Raafe Islam, Monica Jain, Sakshi Jain, Aditi Jalla, Nadia Jamil, Varendra Jamwant, James Jarvis, Jake Jasinski, Anam Javed, Majdoline Jayoushe, Seyed Behzad Jazayeri, Manana Jikurashvili, Rowen Jin, Adam Johnson, Aaron Johnson, Joel Johnson, Kyle Johnson, Christine Jokisch, Katherine Joltikov, Mitchell Jomsky, Sumeeth Jonathan, Jeletta Jose, Abhijeet Joshi, Shirley Ju, Lindsay Juarez, Jai Jung, Anis Kadado, Andrew Kaddis, Michael Kagan, Alyssa Kahn, Samantha Kaiser, Aaron Kala, Sumatt Kamal, Suthasenthuran Kanagalingam, Priyanka Kancherla, Melissa Kander, Kylie Kang, Edward Kanive, Agata Kantorowska, Neil Kapil, Kamran Karim, Nabin Raj Karki, Reema Kashif, Neil Kataria, LaDonna Kearse, Eytan Keidar, Nikhil Keny, Tamer Khashab, Nasir Khatri, Dae Kim, Erica Kim, Wi Jin Kim, Yoo Jung Kim, Brandon Kimbrel, Michael Kingberg, Ken Kitayama, Eleanore Knox, Gary Kocharian, Christine Koh, Mary Kombazdjian, Katerina Konstantinoff, Logan Konty, Efthymios Kostaras, Conrad Kozlowski, Casey Kramer, Andrew Krause, Rahul Krishna, Manjula Krishnamurthy, Nithya Krishnan, Elaine Kuhn, Anila Kumar, Matthew Kurian, Jason Kushner, Marcin Kuzma, Myoung Kwan Kwak, Frank Lacy, Jimmy Lam, Barbara Lam, Richa Lamba, Mary Lan, Rachel Landgren, Paul Lapis, Michael Larson, Daniel Layon, Duc Le, Jeremy Le, Stephenie Le, Aaron A. Lebron Burgos, Hyonju Lee, Paul Lee, Christopher Lee, Clement Lee, James Lee, Johanna Lee, Chewang Lee, Jenny Lee, William Lee, Michelle T. Lee, Eric Lepkowsky, Kenneth Less, Nathaniel Leu, Ori Levi, Rebecca Levin-Epstein, Edgar Miles Leviste, Alvin Li, Jonathan Li, Yedda Li, Jonathan Lim, Peter Lin, Stephanie Linscheid, Matthew Lippmann, Wen Liu, Kelvin Lo, Tony Logli, Tiffany Loh, Gregory Lohr, Shamelia Loiseau, Jerica Lomax, Paola Lopomo, Alnardo Lora, Luis Gerald Lora Garcla, Dexter Louie, Sean Love, Michael Lovelace, Casey Luce, Jesus-Mario Luevano Jr., Benjamin Lurvey, Terrance Lynn, James (Trey) Lyons, Julianne Macaulay, Adrian Maciejewski, Ashwini Mahadev, Satish Maharaj, Gajendra Maharjan, Mohammed Mahdi, Mahmoud Mahfouz, Zunair Thomas Nienaber a Mahmood, Nodari Maisuradze, Naomi Malam, Lydia Maleknia, Melody Malig, Aaiza Malik, Harsh Malik, Rohail Malik, Bishal Malla, Sandra-Jane Mancini, Evan Mannion, Bryan Manzana, Simon Martin, Beatriz Martinez, Jorge Martinez Bencosme, Chris Massey, Abraham Mathai, Gurneet Matharoo, Monica Mattes, Patrick Ryan Mayock, Brian Mayrsohn, Alex McDonald, Bailey McGuinness, Robert McKenna, Drew Mehta, Nehali Mehta, Matthew Meier, Stephanie Mejia, Janet Melnyk, Nicholaus Memphis, Deveer Menchaca, Joseph Mendez, Mohammed Meraj, John Mercke, Andrew Mergl, Paul Mergo, Yanet Merlo, Mohammad Mertaban, Jie Min, Sara Mitchell, Eric Mlodzinski, Saad Al-Deen Mohammad, Fatemeh Mohammadpour, Raghav Mohan, Guarina Molina Vargas, Rajat Moman, Grant Moody, John Moon, Sarah Morrison, Christopher Moutos, Lana Moy, Mudassar Mudassar, Harsha Musunuru, Syed Muzzammiluddin, Annamalai Nadarajan, Shehni Nadeem, Muhammad Luqman Farrukh Nagi, Nadav Nahumi, Alireza Najafian, Farnaz Najmi Varzaneh, Fabian Nalichowski, Aneesh Nandam, Andrew Napier, Anand Narayanan, Brenton Nash, Iraj Nasrabadi, Abdullah Nasser, Jared Nathanson, Arash Nazeri, Derek Nelsen, Jacob Nelson, Nancy Ngo, Rejoice Ngongoni, Andrew Nguyen, Daniel Nguyen, Jenny Kim Nguyen, Mai-Trang Nguyen, Rio Nomoto, Salem Noureldine, Chigozie Michael Nwalozie, McEdwin Obi, Fernando Alekos Ocampo Gonzalez, Alejandro Ochoa, Olaitan Omole, Erin Ong, Chinasa Onuoha, Brenda Ortiz, Jordan Owens, Michael Owyong, Caitlin Pacheco, Preetinder Padda, Jayapriya Palaniappan, Laura Palmer, Khang Wen Pang, Lloyd Panjikaran, Aneta Pariaszevski, Andrew Park, Andrew Park, Shagufta Parveen, Michael Pasyk, Aashish Patel, Anuj Patel, Bhavin Bharat Patel, Karnav Patel, Mehul Patel, Pranav Patel, Shalvi Patel, Suhag Patel, Vinita Patel, Ravi Pathak, Saikrishna Patibandla, David Patterson, Melissa Pavelack, Kevin Pearson, Alexander Pennekamp, Brent Penque, Steven Perry, Christine Pham, Andrew S. Phan, Christina Pindar, Lauren Pioppo, Keyhan Piran, Stephen Pittman, Andryus Planutis, Andrew Plaska, Peter Plumeri,

Bella Plumptre, Vivek Podder, Utsav Pokharel, Tymon Pol, Eduardo Polanco Olio, Jason Polder, Stephanie Popofsky, Samuel Potter, Arun Prashar, Gina Provenzano, Preston Pugh, Audrey Pulitzer, Maria Punchak, Juozas Pundzius, Tyler Putnam, Ryan Qasawa, Nabeel Qureshi, Mohamad Raad, Leen Raddaoui, Saad Rahmat, Aara Raja, Vinaya Rajan, Arun Rajaratnam, Josean Ramos, Randy Ramsaywak, Maria Ramzi, Shobha Ranaweera, Harjot Randhawa, Karandeep Randhawa, Dhakshitha Rao, Huma Rasheed, Krishna Ravella, Bibi S Razack, Maheen Razi, Shazli Razi, Sushma Reddy, Quint Reid, Jon Reimer, Tong Ren, Mobeen Reza, Felix Richter, Chad Rieck, Joshua Ring, Julia Ringel, José Rios Russo, Taylor Rising, Reynolds Risseeuw, Kenny Rivera, Maria Eugenia Rivera Hernandez, Carlos Rivera Reyes, Miriam Rivera-Mendoza, Rhonda Robeel, Mark Robertshaw, Terrance Rodrigues, Catalina Rodriguez, Juliana D. Rodriguez, Nicole Rodriguez, Michael Rodriguez Tirado, Austin Rohl, Gregory Roloff, Gina Rong, Anthony Rooney, Holly Rose, Samuel Rose, Talal Roshan, Matthew Rossi, Vanessa Rota, Julietta Rubin, Martin Runnström, Jonathan Runyon, Nicholas Russo, Paul Rutkowski, Yazan Saba, Mohamed Sabra, Stuart Sacks, Rorita Sadhu, Nick Saggese, Nitin Sajankila, Carolina Salazar, Mohamad Saleh, Sumeet Salhotra, Tareq Salous, Iliana Sanchez, Jacqueline Sanchez, Gurmanpal Sandhu, Hasanin Zafar Sheikh Sanim, Melodie Sarebanha, Darya Savel, Mossum Sawhney, Stephen Schaeffer, Lance Schell, Collin Schenk, Christian Schuetz, Noah Schwartz, Adeeb Sebai, Natalya Sebastian, Eric Secrist, Siavash Sedghi, Manjinder Singh Sekhon, Roopak Sekhon, Jesse Sengillo, Debashree Sengupta, Angie Seo, Nicolas Seranio, Eric Seronick, Christina Serret, Anand Sewak, Lorenzo Sewanan, Mij Sha, Nadine Shabeeb, Anna Shah, Bindiya Shah, Harsh Shah, Muneeb Shah, Neil V. Shah, Neal Shah, Omer Shahab, Salma Shakh, Alan Shamrock, Saber Shamspour, Bryan Shapiro, Dolly Sharma, Darshan Shastri, Ling Shen, Mina Shenouda, Nomi Sherwin, Prajwal Shetty, Yue Shi, Benjamin Shin, Corey Shy, Haley Sibley, Tarik Silk, Jenna Silverstein, Silvia Simione, Brittany Simpson, Kiran Singh, Nainwant Singh, Vir Singh, Vikal Singh, Ann Skariya, Colby Smith, Christopher M. Smith, Wesley Smith, Tom Soker, Mohamed Soliman, Wilbur Song, Mihir Soparkar, Vlasios Sotirchos, Wilfredo Soto-Fuentes, Katherine Specht, Menachem Spira, Nicholas Squires, Anandhasayanan Sriramalu, Joseph D. Steffens, Jesintha Stephenson, Kristen Stevens, Florian Stroie, Benjamin Stuart, Nicholas Stukel, David Sukhai, Lishi Sun, Kiran Sury, Kriti Suwal, Alexa Swailes, Erica Swenson, Andrew Swiergosz, Adam Swiger, Ben Switzer, Mark Anthony Sy, Sarah Syeda, Omar Taani, Dawood Tafti, Mohamed Taha, Omar Taibah, Khandokar Talib, Wasif Talpur, Michael Tanael, Bashar Tanous, Syeda Taranum, David Taylor, Abiolah Telesford, Parker Thompson, Sandra Tomlinson-Hansen, Ileana A. Torres-Burgos, Ryan Town, Marie-Alexandria Tremis, Anuragh Trikha, Jefferson Triozzi, Marcelo Troya Maldonado, Michael Tseng, Harika Reddy Tula, John S. Underwood, Dhaval Upadhyay, Eva Urrechaga, Arthur Uyesugi, Akash Vadhavana, Spencer Vale, Devan Van Lanen-Wanek, Garrett Van Ostran, Leah Vance, Anu Varghese, Ilan Vashurin, Photios Frank Vassilyadi, Andrew Vaughan, Aleks Vayntraub, Erick Candido Velasquez Centellas, M.C. Viali, Josue Villegas Galaviz, Hongphuc Vo, Shaan Wadhawan, Gregory Wai, Sara Walker, Gary Walker, Xiamo Wang, Charles Wang, David Wang, Junjie Wang, Ezekiel Wang, Leonard Washington, Bradley Wasser, Alyssa Watkins, Josh Waytz, Corinne Webb, William Weber, Melanie Weinstein, Gong Weng, Winsor Wesson, Benjamin Westerhaus, Kendrick White, Raymond Whitham, Bettina Wiener-Fererhofer, James Wilhite, Augustine Wilson, Blake Young Wilson, Michael Wilson, Lindsey Winer, Amanda Witte, Zachary Wolner, Jeff Wong, Matthew Woodward, John Worth, Jonathan Wright, Michael Wyderko, Grace Xiong, Antonio Yaghy, Xiaofeng Yan, Daniel Yanes, Derek Yang, Linlin Yang, Samuel Yap, Kevin Yen, Isaac Yeung, Emily Yin, Peter You, Ann Young, Christopher Young, Steven Young, Elliot Yu, Guo Yu, Helena Yu, Alice Yu, Alex Yuan, James Yuan, Shuai Yuan, Mohammad Zahid, Rachil Zaia, Mohammad Zaidi, Theodore Zaki, Alan Zats, Bartosz Zawada, Michelle Zeidan, Pamela Zelnick, Ehud Zeltzer, Steven Qian Zhang, Bill Zhang, Zhihang Zhang, Jennifer Zhao, Xiao Zheng, Xiya Zhu, Hairan Zhu, Rhushi Ziradkar, Mark Zivney, Marcin Zuberek, Omry Zuckerman, Kathleen Zuniga, and Frank Zurfley.

How to Contribute

This version of *First Aid for the USMLE Step 1* incorporates thousands of contributions and improvements suggested by student and faculty advisors. We invite you to participate in this process. Please send us your suggestions for:

- Study and test-taking strategies for the USMLE Step 1
- New facts, mnemonics, diagrams, and clinical images
- High-yield topics that may appear on future Step 1 exams
- Personal ratings and comments on review books, question banks, apps, videos, and courses

For each new entry incorporated into the next edition, you will receive up to a **$20 Amazon.com gift card** as well as personal acknowledgment in the next edition. Significant contributions will be compensated at the discretion of the authors. Also, let us know about material in this edition that you feel is low yield and should be deleted.

All submissions including potential errata should ideally be supported with hyperlinks to a dynamically updated Web resource such as UpToDate, AccessMedicine, and ClinicalKey.

We welcome potential errata on grammar and style if the change improves readability. Please note that *First Aid* style is somewhat unique; for example, we have fully adopted the AMA *Manual of Style* recommendations on eponyms ("We recommend that the possessive form be omitted in eponymous terms") and on abbreviations (no periods with eg, ie, etc).

The preferred way to submit new entries, clarifications, mnemonics, or potential corrections with a valid, authoritative reference is via our website: **www.firstaidteam.com**.

This website will be continuously updated with validated errata, new high-yield content, and a new online platform to contribute suggestions, mnemonics, diagrams, clinical images, and potential errata.

Alternatively, you can email us at: **firstaidteam@yahoo.com**.

Contributions submitted by **May 15, 2016**, receive priority consideration for the 2017 edition of *First Aid for the USMLE Step 1*. We thank you for taking the time to share your experience and apologize in advance that we cannot individually respond to all contributors as we receive thousands of contributions each year.

▶ NOTE TO CONTRIBUTORS

All contributions become property of the authors and are subject to editing and reviewing. Please verify all data and spellings carefully. Contributions should be supported by at least two high-quality references.

Check our website first to avoid duplicate submissions. In the event that similar or duplicate entries are received, only the first complete entry received with valid, authoritative references will be credited. Please follow the style, punctuation, and format of this edition as much as possible.

▶ JOIN THE FIRST AID TEAM

The *First Aid* author team is pleased to offer part-time and full-time paid internships in medical education and publishing to motivated medical students and physicians. Internships range from a few months (eg, a summer) up to a full year. Participants will have an opportunity to author, edit, and earn academic credit on a wide variety of projects, including the popular *First Aid* series.

For 2016, we are actively seeking passionate medical students and graduates with a specific interest in improving our medical illustrations, expanding our database of medical photographs, and developing the software that supports our crowdsourcing platform. We welcome people with prior experience and talent in these areas. Relevant skills include clinical imaging, digital photography, digital asset management, information design, medical illustration, graphic design, and software development.

Please email us at **firstaidteam@yahoo.com** with a CV and summary of your interest or sample work.

How to Use This Book

CONGRATULATIONS: You now possess the book that has guided nearly two million students to USMLE success for over 25 years. With appropriate care, the binding should last the useful life of the book. Keep in mind that putting excessive flattening pressure on any binding will accelerate its failure. If you purchased a book that you believe is defective, please **immediately** return it to the place of purchase. If you encounter ongoing issues, you can also contact Customer Service at our publisher, McGraw-Hill Education, at https://www.mheducation.com/contact.html.

START EARLY: Use this book as early as possible while learning the basic medical sciences. The first semester of your first year is not too early! Devise a study plan by reading Section I: Guide to Efficient Exam Preparation, and make an early decision on resources to use by checking Section IV: Top-Rated Review Resources. Note that *First Aid* is neither a textbook nor a comprehensive review book, and it is not a panacea for inadequate preparation.

LET *FIRST AID* BE YOUR GUIDE: Annotate material from other resources, such as class notes or comprehensive textbooks, into your book. This will keep all the high-yield information you need in one place. Other tips on keeping yourself organized:

- For best results, use fine-tipped ballpoint pens (eg, BIC Pro+, Uni-Ball Jetstream Sports, Pilot Drawing Pen, Zebra F-301). If you like gel pens, try Pentel Slicci, and for markers that dry almost immediately, consider Staedtler Triplus Fineliner, Pilot Drawing Pen, and Sharpies.
- Consider using pens with different colors of ink to indicate different sources of information (eg, green for UWorld Step 1 Qbank, blue for USMLE-Rx Step 1 Qmax).
- Choose highlighters that are bright and dry quickly to minimize smudging and bleeding through the page (eg, Tombow Kei Coat, Sharpie Gel).
- Many students de-spine their book and get it 3-hole-punched. This will allow you to insert materials from other sources, such as course syllabi.

INTEGRATE STUDY WITH CASES, FLASH CARDS, AND QUESTIONS: To broaden your learning strategy, consider integrating your *First Aid* study with case-based reviews (eg, *First Aid Cases for the USMLE Step 1*), flash cards (eg, First Aid Flash Facts), and practice questions (eg, the USMLE-Rx Step 1 Qmax). Read the chapter in the book, then test your comprehension by using cases, flash cards, and questions that cover the same topics. Maintain access to more comprehensive resources (eg, *First Aid for the Basic Sciences: General Principles* and *Organ Systems* and First Aid Express videos) for deeper review as needed.

PRIME YOUR MEMORY: Return to your annotated Sections II and III several days before taking the USMLE Step 1. The book can serve as a useful way of retaining key associations and keeping high-yield facts fresh in your memory just prior to the exam. The Rapid Review section includes high-yield topics to help guide your studying.

CONTRIBUTE TO FIRST AID: Reviewing the book immediately after your exam can help us improve the next edition. Decide what was truly high and low yield and send us your comments. Feel free to send us scanned images from your annotated *First Aid* book as additional support. Of course, always remember that **all examinees are under agreement with the NBME to not disclose the specific details of copyrighted test material.**

Selected USMLE Laboratory Values

* = Included in the Biochemical Profile (SMA-12)

Blood, Plasma, Serum	Reference Range	SI Reference Intervals
*Alanine aminotransferase (ALT, GPT at 30°C)	8–20 U/L	8–20 U/L
Amylase, serum	25–125 U/L	25–125 U/L
*Aspartate aminotransferase (AST, GOT at 30°C)	8–20 U/L	8–20 U/L
Bilirubin, serum (adult) Total // Direct	0.1–1.0 mg/dL // 0.0–0.3 mg/dL	2–17 μmol/L // 0–5 μmol/L
*Calcium, serum (Total)	8.4–10.2 mg/dL	2.1–2.8 mmol/L
*Cholesterol, serum (Total)	< 200 mg/dL	< 5.2 mmol/L
*Creatinine, serum (Total)	0.6–1.2 mg/dL	53–106 μmol/L
Electrolytes, serum		
Sodium	136–145 mEq/L	136–145 mmol/L
Chloride	95–105 mEq/L	95–105 mmol/L
* Potassium	3.5–5.0 mEq/L	3.5–5.0 mmol/L
Bicarbonate	22–28 mEq/L	22–28 mmol/L
Magnesium	1.5 mEq/L	0.75–1.0 mmol/L
Gases, arterial blood (room air)		
P_{O_2}	75–105 mm Hg	10.0–14.0 kPa
P_{CO_2}	33–44 mm Hg	4.4–5.9 kPa
pH	7.35–7.45	$[H^+]$ 36–44 nmol/L
*Glucose, serum	Fasting: 70–110 mg/dL 2-h postprandial: < 120 mg/dL	3.8–6.1 mmol/L < 6.6 mmol/L
Growth hormone – arginine stimulation	Fasting: < 5 ng/mL provocative stimuli: > 7 ng/mL	< 5 μg/L > 7 μg/L
Osmolality, serum	275–295 mOsm/kg	275–295 mOsm/kg
*Phosphatase (alkaline), serum (p-NPP at 30°C)	20–70 U/L	20–70 U/L
*Phosphorus (inorganic), serum	3.0–4.5 mg/dL	1.0–1.5 mmol/L
Prolactin, serum (hPRL)	< 20 ng/mL	< 20 μg/L
*Proteins, serum		
Total (recumbent)	6.0–7.8 g/dL	60–78 g/L
Albumin	3.5–5.5 g/dL	35–55 g/L
Globulins	2.3–3.5 g/dL	23–35 g/L
*Urea nitrogen, serum (BUN)	7–18 mg/dL	1.2–3.0 mmol/L
*Uric acid, serum	3.0–8.2 mg/dL	0.18–0.48 mmol/L

(continues)

Cerebrospinal Fluid	Reference Range	SI Reference Intervals
Glucose	40–70 mg/dL	2.2–3.9 mmol/L
Hematologic		
Erythrocyte count	Male: 4.3–5.9 million/mm^3 Female: 3.5–5.5 million/mm^3	4.3–5.9 × 10^{12}/L 3.5–5.5 × 10^{12}/L
Erythrocyte sedimentation rate (Westergen)	Male: 0–15 mm/h Female: 0–20 mm/h	0–15 mm/h 0–20 mm/h
Hematocrit	Male: 41–53% Female: 36–46%	0.41–0.53 0.36–0.46
Hemoglobin, blood	Male: 13.5–17.5 g/dL Female: 12.0–16.0 g/dL	2.09–2.71 mmol/L 1.86–2.48 mmol/L
Hemoglobin, plasma	1–4 mg/dL	0.16–0.62 μmol/L
Leukocyte count and differential		
Leukocyte count	4500–11,000/mm^3	4.5–11.0 × 10^9/L
Segmented neutrophils	54–62%	0.54–0.62
Band forms	3–5%	0.03–0.05
Eosinophils	1–3%	0.01–0.03
Basophils	0–0.75%	0–0.0075
Lymphocytes	25–33%	0.25–0.33
Monocytes	3–7%	0.03–0.07
Mean corpuscular hemoglobin	25.4–34.6 pg/cell	0.39–0.54 fmol/cell
Mean corpuscular volume	80–100 μm^3	80–100 fL
Partial thromboplastin time (activated)	25–40 seconds	25–40 seconds
Platelet count	150,000–400,000/mm^3	150–400 × 10^9/L
Prothrombin time	11–15 seconds	11–15 seconds
Reticulocyte count	0.5–1.5% of red cells	0.005–0.015
Sweat		
Chloride	0–35 mmol/L	0–35 mmol/L
Urine		
Proteins, total	< 150 mg/24 h	< 0.15 g/24 h

First Aid Checklist for the USMLE Step 1

This is an example of how you might use the information in Section I to prepare for the USMLE Step 1. Refer to corresponding topics in Section I for more details.

Years Prior

- ☐ Select top-rated review resources as study guides for first-year medical school courses.
- ☐ Ask for advice from those who have recently taken the USMLE Step 1.

Months Prior

- ☐ Review computer test format and registration information.
- ☐ Register six months in advance. Carefully verify name and address printed on scheduling permit. Call Prometric or go online for test date ASAP.
- ☐ Define goals for the USMLE Step 1 (eg, comfortably pass, beat the mean, ace the test).
- ☐ Set up a realistic timeline for study. Cover less crammable subjects first. Review subject-by-subject emphasis and clinical vignette format.
- ☐ Simulate the USMLE Step 1 to pinpoint strengths and weaknesses in knowledge and test-taking skills.
- ☐ Evaluate and choose study methods and materials (eg, review books, question banks).

Weeks Prior

- ☐ Simulate the USMLE Step 1 again. Assess how close you are to your goal.
- ☐ Pinpoint remaining weaknesses. Stay healthy (exercise, sleep).
- ☐ Verify information on admission ticket (eg, location, date).

One Week Prior

- ☐ Remember comfort measures (loose clothing, earplugs, etc).
- ☐ Work out test site logistics such as location, transportation, parking, and lunch.
- ☐ Call Prometric and confirm your exam appointment.

One Day Prior

- ☐ Relax.
- ☐ Lightly review short-term material if necessary. Skim high-yield facts.
- ☐ Get a good night's sleep.
- ☐ Make sure the name printed on your photo ID appears EXACTLY the same as the name printed on your scheduling permit.

Day of Exam

- ☐ Relax. Eat breakfast. Minimize bathroom breaks during the exam by avoiding excessive morning caffeine.
- ☐ Analyze and make adjustments in test-taking technique. You are allowed to review notes/study material during breaks on exam day.

After the Exam

- ☐ Celebrate, regardless.
- ☐ Send feedback to us on our website at **www.firstaidteam.com.**

SECTION I

Guide to Efficient Exam Preparation

"A mind of moderate capacity which closely pursues one study must infallibly arrive at great proficiency in that study."

—Mary Shelley, *Frankenstein*

"Finally, from so little sleeping and so much reading, his brain dried up and he went completely out of his mind."

—Miguel de Cervantes Saavedra, *Don Quixote*

"Sometimes the questions are complicated and the answers are simple."

—Dr. Seuss

"He who knows all the answers has not been asked all the questions."

—Confucius

▶ INTRODUCTION

Relax.

This section is intended to make your exam preparation easier, not harder. Our goal is to reduce your level of anxiety and help you make the most of your efforts by helping you understand more about the United States Medical Licensing Examination, Step 1 (USMLE Step 1). As a medical student, you are no doubt familiar with taking standardized examinations and quickly absorbing large amounts of material. When you first confront the USMLE Step 1, however, you may find it all too easy to become sidetracked from your goal of studying with maximal effectiveness. Common mistakes that students make when studying for Step 1 include the following:

- Starting to study (including *First Aid*) too late
- Starting to study intensely too early and burning out
- Starting to prepare for boards before creating a knowledge foundation
- Using inefficient or inappropriate study methods
- Buying the wrong resources or buying more resources than you can ever use
- Buying only one publisher's review series for all subjects
- Not using practice examinations to maximum benefit
- Not understanding how scoring is performed or what the score means
- Not using review books along with your classes
- Not analyzing and improving your test-taking strategies
- Getting bogged down by reviewing difficult topics excessively
- Studying material that is rarely tested on the USMLE Step 1
- Failing to master certain high-yield subjects owing to overconfidence
- Using *First Aid* as your sole study resource
- Trying to prepare for it all alone

In this section, we offer advice to help you avoid these pitfalls and be more productive in your studies.

> ▶ *The test at a glance:*
> - *8-hour exam*
> - *Total of 308 multiple choice items*
> - *7 test blocks (60 min/block)*
> - *44 test items per block*
> - *45 minutes of break time, plus another 15 if you skip the tutorial*

▶ USMLE STEP 1—THE BASICS

The USMLE Step 1 is the first of three examinations that you must pass in order to become a licensed physician in the United States. The USMLE is a joint endeavor of the National Board of Medical Examiners (NBME) and the Federation of State Medical Boards (FSMB). The USMLE serves as the single examination system for US medical students and international medical graduates (IMGs) seeking medical licensure in the United States.

The Step 1 exam includes test items drawn from the following content areas[1]:

DISCIPLINE

Behavioral Sciences
Biochemistry
Genetics
Gross Anatomy & Embryology
Histology & Cell Biology
Microbiology & Immunology
Nutrition
Pathology
Pharmacology
Physiology

ORGAN SYSTEM

Behavioral Health & Nervous Systems/Special Senses
Biostatistics & Epidemiology/Population Health
Blood & Lymphoreticular System
Cardiovascular System
Endocrine System
Gastrointestinal System
General Principles of Foundational Science
Immune System
Multisystem Processes & Disorders
Musculoskeletal, Skin, & Subcutaneous Tissue
Renal/Urinary System
Reproductive System
Respiratory System

In 2015, a new, detailed, 31-page content outline was released. However, it is too early to say how useful the information will be in determining high-yield topics.

How Is the Computer-Based Test (CBT) Structured?

The CBT Step 1 exam consists of one "optional" tutorial/simulation block and seven "real" question blocks of 44 questions each for a total of 308 questions, timed at 60 minutes per block. A short 11-question survey follows the last question block. The computer begins the survey with a prompt to proceed to the next block of questions.

Once an examinee finishes a particular question block on the CBT, he or she must click on a screen icon to continue to the next block. Examinees **cannot** go back and change their answers to questions from any previously completed block. However, changing answers is allowed **within** a block of questions as long as the block has not been ended and if time permits—**unless** the questions are part of a sequential item test set (see p. 4).

What Is the CBT Like?

Given the unique environment of the CBT, it's important that you become familiar ahead of time with what your test-day conditions will be like. In fact, you can easily add up to 15 minutes to your break time! This is because the 15-minute tutorial offered on exam day may be skipped if you are already familiar with the exam procedures and the testing interface. The 15 minutes is then added to your allotted break time of 45 minutes for a total of 1 hour of potential break time. You can download the tutorial from the USMLE website and do it before test day. This tutorial interface is very similar to the one you will use in the exam; learn it now and you can skip taking it during the exam, giving you up to 15 extra minutes of break time. You can also gain experience with the CBT format by taking the 132 practice questions available online or by signing up for a practice session at a test center.

▸ *If you know the format, you can skip the tutorial and add up to 15 minutes to your break time!*

For security reasons, examinees are not allowed to bring any personal electronic equipment into the testing area. This includes both digital and analog watches, iPods, tablets, calculators, cell phones, and electronic paging devices. Examinees are also prohibited from carrying in their books, notes, pens/pencils, and scratch paper. Food and beverages are also prohibited in the testing area. The testing centers are monitored by audio and video surveillance equipment. However, most testing centers allot each examinee a small locker outside the testing area in which he or she can store snacks, beverages, and personal items.

The typical question screen in the CBT consists of a question followed by a number of choices on which an examinee can click, together with several navigational buttons on the top of the screen. There is a countdown timer on the lower left corner of the screen as well. There is also a button that allows the examinee to mark a question for review. If a given question happens to be longer than the screen (which occurs very rarely), a scroll bar will appear on the right, allowing the examinee to see the rest of the question. Regardless of whether the examinee clicks on an answer choice or leaves it blank, he or she must click the "Next" button to advance to the next question.

▸ *Keyboard shortcuts:*
- *A, B, etc—letter choices*
- *Enter or spacebar—move to next question*
- *Esc—exit pop-up Lab and Exhibit windows*
- *Alt-T—countdown timers for current session and overall test*

The USMLE features a small number of media clips in the form of audio and/or video. There may even be a question with a multimedia heart sound simulation. In these questions, a digital image of a torso appears on the screen, and the examinee directs a digital stethoscope to various auscultation points to listen for heart and breath sounds. The USMLE orientation materials include several practice questions in these formats. During the exam tutorial, examinees are given an opportunity to ensure that both the audio headphones and the volume are functioning properly. If you are already familiar with the tutorial and planning on skipping it, first skip ahead to the section where you can test your headphones. After you are sure the headphones are working properly, proceed to the exam.

▸ *Heart sounds are tested via media questions. Make sure you know how different heart diseases sound on auscultation.*

▸ *Be sure to test your headphones during the tutorial.*

The USMLE also has a sequential item test format. These questions are grouped together in the list of questions on the left side of the screen and must be completed in order. After an examinee answers the first question, he or she will be given the option to proceed to the next item but will be warned that the answer to the first question will be locked. **After proceeding, examinees will not be able to change the answer selected for that question.**

The question stem and the answer chosen will be available to the examinee as he or she answers the next question(s) in the sequence.

> ▶ *Illustrations on the test include:*
> - *Gross specimen photos*
> - *Histology slides*
> - *Medical imaging (eg, x-ray, CT, MRI)*
> - *Electron micrographs*
> - *Line drawings*

The examinee can call up a window displaying normal laboratory values. In order to do so, he or she must click the "Lab" icon on the top part of the screen. Afterward, the examinee will have the option to choose between "Blood," "Cerebrospinal," "Hematologic," or "Sweat and Urine." The normal-values screen may obscure the question if it is expanded. The examinee may have to scroll down to search for the needed lab values. You might want to memorize some common lab values so you spend less time on questions that require you to analyze these.

> ▶ *Familiarize yourself with the commonly tested lab values.*

The CBT interface provides a running list of questions on the left part of the screen at all times. The software also permits examinees to highlight or cross out information by using their mouse. Finally, there is a "Notes" icon on the top part of the screen that allows students to write notes to themselves for review at a later time. Being familiar with these features can save time and may help you better organize the information you need to answer a question.

> ▶ *Ctrl-Alt-Delete are the keys of death during the exam. Don't touch them at the same time!*

For those who feel they might benefit, the USMLE offers an opportunity to take a simulated test, or "CBT Practice Session" at a Prometric center. Students are eligible to register for this three-and-one-half-hour practice session after they have received their scheduling permit.

The same USMLE Step 1 sample test items (150 questions) available on the USMLE website, www.usmle.org, are used at these sessions. **No new items will be presented.** The session is divided into a short tutorial and three 1-hour blocks of 44 test items each at a cost of $75, if your testing region is in the United States or Canada. Students receive a printed percent-correct score after completing the session. **No explanations of questions are provided.**

> ▶ *You can take a shortened CBT practice test at a Prometric center.*

You may register for a practice session online at www.usmle.org. A separate scheduling permit is issued for the practice session. Students should allow two weeks for receipt of this permit.

How Do I Register to Take the Exam?

Prometric test centers offer Step 1 on a year-round basis, except for the first two weeks in January and major holidays. The exam is given every day except Sunday at most centers. Some schools administer the exam on their own campuses. Check with the test center you want to use before making your exam plans.

> ▶ *The Prometric Web site will display a calendar with open test dates.*

US students can apply to take Step 1 at the NBME website. This application allows you to select one of 12 overlapping three-month blocks in which to be tested (eg, April–May–June, June–July–August). Choose your three-month eligibility period wisely. If you need to reschedule outside your initial three-month period, you can request a one-time extension of eligibility for the next contiguous three-month period, and pay a rescheduling fee. The application also includes a photo ID form that must be certified by an official at your medical school to verify your enrollment. After the NBME processes your application, it will send you a scheduling permit.

▶ *The confirmation emails that Prometric and NBME send are not the same as the scheduling permit.*

The scheduling permit you receive from the NBME will contain your USMLE identification number, the eligibility period in which you may take the exam, and two additional numbers. The first of these is known as your "scheduling number." You must have this number in order to make your exam appointment with Prometric. The second number is known as the "candidate identification number," or CIN. Examinees must enter their CINs at the Prometric workstation in order to access their exams. However, you will not be allowed to bring your permit into the exam and will be asked to copy your CIN onto your scratch paper. Prometric has no access to the codes. **Do not lose your permit!** You will not be allowed to take the exam unless you present this permit along with an unexpired, government-issued photo ID that includes your signature (such as a driver's license or passport). Make sure the name on your photo ID exactly matches the name that appears on your scheduling permit.

▶ *Test scheduling is done on a "first-come, first-served" basis. It's important to call and schedule an exam date as soon as you receive your scheduling permit.*

Once you receive your scheduling permit, you may access the Prometric website or call Prometric's toll-free number to arrange a time to take the exam. You may contact Prometric two weeks before the test date if you want to confirm identification requirements. Although requests for taking the exam may be completed more than six months before the test date, examinees will not receive their scheduling permits earlier than six months before the eligibility period. The eligibility period is the three-month period you have chosen to take the exam. Most medical students choose the April–June or June–August period. Because exams are scheduled on a "first-come, first-served" basis, it is recommended that you contact Prometric as soon as you receive your permit. After you've scheduled your exam, it's a good idea to confirm your exam appointment with Prometric at least one week before your test date. Prometric will provide appointment confirmation on a print-out and by email. Be sure to read the *2015 USMLE Bulletin of Information* for further details.

What If I Need to Reschedule the Exam?

You can change your test date and/or center by contacting Prometric at 1-800-MED-EXAM (1-800-633-3926) or www.prometric.com. Make sure to have your CIN when rescheduling. If you are rescheduling by phone, you must speak with a Prometric representative; leaving a voice-mail message will not suffice. To avoid a rescheduling fee, you will need to request a change at least 31 calendar days before your appointment. Please note that your rescheduled test date must fall within your assigned three-month eligibility period.

When Should I Register for the Exam?

▶ *Register six months in advance for seating and scheduling preference.*

You should plan to register as far in advance as possible ahead of your desired test date (eg, six months), but, depending on your particular test center, new dates and times may open closer to the date. Scheduling early will guarantee that you will get either your test center of choice or one within a 50-mile radius of your first choice. For most US medical students, the desired testing window is in June, since most medical school curricula for the second year end in May or June. Thus, US medical students should plan to register before January in anticipation of a June test date. The timing of the exam is more flexible for IMGs, as it is related only to when they finish exam preparation. Talk with upperclassmen who have already taken the test so you have real-life experience from students who went through a similar curriculum, then formulate your own strategy.

Where Can I Take the Exam?

Your testing location is arranged with Prometric when you call for your test date (after you receive your scheduling permit). For a list of Prometric locations nearest you, visit www.prometric.com.

How Long Will I Have to Wait Before I Get My Scores?

The USMLE reports scores in three to four weeks, unless there are delays in score processing. Examinees will be notified via email when their scores are available. By following the online instructions, examinees will be able to view, download, and print their score report. Additional information about score timetables and accessibility is available on the official USMLE website.

What About Time?

▶ *Gain extra break time by skipping the tutorial or finishing a block early.*

Time is of special interest on the CBT exam. Here's a breakdown of the exam schedule:

15 minutes	Tutorial (skip if familiar with test format and features)
7 hours	Seven 60-minute question blocks
45 minutes	Break time (includes time for lunch)

The computer will keep track of how much time has elapsed on the exam. However, the computer will show you only how much time you have remaining in a given block. Therefore, it is up to you to determine if you are pacing yourself properly (at a rate of approximately one question per 78 seconds).

The computer will not warn you if you are spending more than your allotted time for a break. You should therefore budget your time so that you can take a short break when you need one and have time to eat. You must be especially careful not to spend too much time in between blocks (you should keep track of how much time elapses from the time you finish a block of questions to the time you start the next block). After you finish one question block, you'll need to click to proceed to the next block of questions. If you do not click within 30 seconds, you will automatically be entered into a break period.

Forty-five minutes is the minimum break time for the day, but you are not required to use all of it, nor are you required to use any of it. You can gain extra break time (but not time for the question blocks) by skipping the tutorial or by finishing a block ahead of the allotted time. Any time remaining on the clock when you finish a block gets added to your remaining break time. Once a new question block has been started, you may not take a break until you have reached the end of that block. If you do so, this will be recorded as an "unauthorized break" and will be reported on your final score report.

▸ *Be careful to watch the clock on your break time.*

Finally, be aware that it may take a few minutes of your break time to "check out" of the secure resting room and then "check in" again to resume testing, so plan accordingly. The "check-in" process may include fingerprints, pocket checks, and metal detector scanning. Some students recommend pocketless clothing on exam day to streamline the process.

If I Freak Out and Leave, What Happens to My Score?

Your scheduling permit shows a CIN that you will need to enter to start your exam. Entering the CIN is the same as breaking the seal on a test book, and you are considered to have started the exam when you do so. However, no score will be reported if you do not complete the exam. In fact, if you leave at any time from the start of the test to the last block, no score will be reported. The fact that you started but did not complete the exam, however, will appear on your USMLE score transcript. Even though a score is not posted for incomplete tests, examinees may still get an option to request that their scores be calculated and reported if they desire; unanswered questions will be scored as incorrect.

The exam ends when all question blocks have been completed or when their time has expired. As you leave the testing center, you will receive a printed test-completion notice to document your completion of the exam. To receive an official score, you must finish the entire exam.

What Types of Questions Are Asked?

▸ *Nearly three fourths of Step 1 questions begin with a description of a patient.*

One-best-answer multiple choice items (either singly or as part of a sequential item set) are the only question type on the exam. Most questions consist of a clinical scenario or a direct question followed by a list of five or more options. You are required to select the single best answer among the options given. There are no "except," "not," or matching questions on the exam. A number of options may be partially correct, in which case you must select the option that best answers the question or completes the statement. Additionally, keep in mind that experimental questions may appear on the exam, which do not affect your score.

How Is the Test Scored?

Each Step 1 examinee receives an electronic score report that includes the examinee's pass/fail status, a three-digit test score, and a graphic depiction of the examinee's performance by discipline and organ system or subject area. The actual organ system profiles reported may depend on the statistical characteristics of a given administration of the examination.

The USMLE score report is divided into two sections: performance by discipline and performance by organ system. Each of the 308 questions (minus experimental questions) is tagged according to any or all relevant content areas. Your performance in each discipline and each organ system is represented by a line of X's, where the width of the line is related to the confidence interval for your performance, which is often a direct consequence of the total number of questions for each discipline/system. If any lines have an asterisk (*) at the far right, this means your performance was exemplary in that area—not necessarily representing a perfect score, but often close to it.

The NBME provides a three-digit test score based on the total number of items answered correctly on the examination (see Figure 1). Your three-digit score will be qualified by the mean and standard deviation of US and Canadian medical school first-time examinees. The translation from the lines of X's and number of asterisks you receive on your report to the three-digit score is unclear, but higher three-digit scores are associated with more asterisks.

Since some questions may be experimental and are not counted, it is possible to get different scores for the same number of correct answers. The most recent mean score was 230 with a standard deviation of 20.

▸ *The mean Step 1 score for US medical students continues to rise, from 200 in 1991 to 230 in 2015.*

A score of 192 or higher is required to pass Step 1. The NBME does not report the minimum number of correct responses needed to pass, but estimates that it is roughly 60–70%. The NBME may adjust the minimum passing score in the future, so please check the USMLE website or www.firstaidteam.com for updates.

According to the USMLE, medical schools receive a listing of total scores and pass/fail results plus group summaries by discipline and organ system. Students can withhold their scores from their medical school if they wish. Official USMLE transcripts, which can be sent on request to residency programs, include only total scores, not performance profiles.

FIGURE 1. Scoring Scale for the USMLE Step 1.

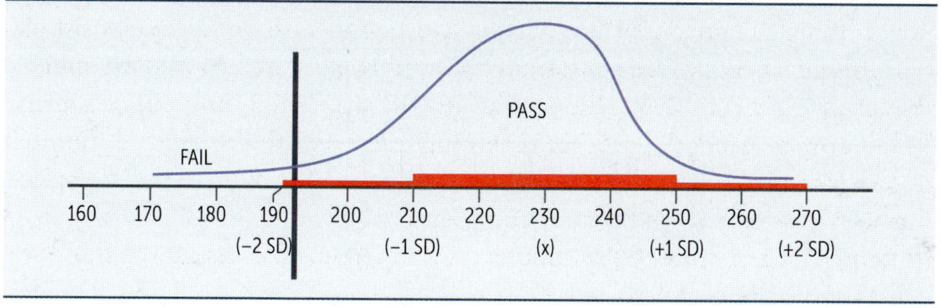

Consult the USMLE website or your medical school for the most current and accurate information regarding the examination.

What Does My Score Mean?

The most important point with the Step 1 score is passing versus failing. Passing essentially means, "Hey, you're on your way to becoming a fully licensed doc." As Table 1 shows, the majority of students pass the exam, so remember, we told you to relax.

Beyond that, the main point of having a quantitative score is to give you a sense of how well you've done on the exam and to help schools and residencies rank their students and applicants, respectively.

Official NBME/USMLE Resources

The NBME offers a Comprehensive Basic Science Examination (CBSE) for practice that is a shorter version of the Step 1. The CBSE contains four blocks of 50 questions each and covers material that is typically learned during the basic science years. Scores range from 45 to 95 and correlate with a Step 1 equivalent (see Table 2). The standard error of measurement is approximately 3 points, meaning a score of 80 would estimate the student's proficiency is somewhere between 77 and 83. In other words, the actual Step 1 score could be predicted to be between 218 and 232. Of course, these values do not correlate exactly, and they do not reflect different test preparation methods. Many schools use this test to gauge whether a student is expected to pass Step 1. If this test is offered by your school, it is usually conducted at the end of regular didactic time before any dedicated Step 1 preparation. If you do not encounter the CBSE before your dedicated study time, you need not worry about taking it. Use the information to help set realistic goals and timetables for your success.

▶ *Practice questions may be easier than the actual exam.*

TABLE 1. Passing Rates for the 2013–2014 USMLE Step 1.[2]

	2013		2014	
	No. Tested	% Passing	No. Tested	% Passing
Allopathic 1st takers	19,108	97%	19,582	96%
Repeaters	915	72%	812	68%
Allopathic total	20,023	95%	20,394	95%
Osteopathic 1st takers	2,680	94%	2,810	93%
Repeaters	46	74%	36	69%
Osteopathic total	2,726	94%	2,846	93%
Total US/Canadian	**22,749**	**95%**	**23,240**	**95%**
IMG 1st takers	14,649	79%	15,149	78%
Repeaters	3,772	44%	2,889	38%
IMG total	18,421	72%	18,038	72%
Total Step 1 examinees	**41,170**	**85%**	**41,278**	**85%**

The NBME also offers six forms of Comprehensive Basic Science Self-Assessment (CBSSA). Students who prepared for the exam using this web-based tool reported that they found the format and content highly indicative of questions tested on the actual exam. In addition, the CBSSA is a fair predictor of USMLE performance (see Table 3). The test interface, however, does not match the actual USMLE test interface, so practicing with these forms alone is not advised.

The CBSSA exists in two formats: standard-paced and self-paced, both of which consist of four sections of 50 questions each (for a total of 200 multiple choice items). The standard-paced format allows the user up to 65 minutes to complete each section, reflecting time limits similar to the actual exam. By contrast, the self-paced format places a 4:20 time limit on answering all multiple choice questions. Every few years, a new form is released and an older one is retired, reflecting changes in exam content.

Keep in mind that this bank of questions is available only on the web. The NBME requires that users log on, register, and start the test within 30 days of registration. Once the assessment has begun, users are required to complete the sections within 20 days. Following completion of the questions, the CBSSA provides a performance profile indicating the user's relative strengths and weaknesses, much like the report profile for the USMLE Step 1 exam. The profile is scaled with an average score of 500 and a standard deviation of 100. Please note that the CBSSAs do not list the correct answers to the questions at the end of the session. However, forms can be purchased with an extended feedback option; these tests show you which questions you answered incorrectly, but do not show you the correct answer or explain why your choice was wrong. Feedback from the self-assessment takes the form of a performance profile and nothing more. The NBME charges $50 for assessments without feedback and $60 for assessments with expanded feedback. The fees are payable by credit card or money order. For more information regarding the CBSE and the CBSSA, visit the NBME's website at www.nbme.org.

The NBME scoring system is weighted for each assessment exam. While some exams seem more difficult than others, the score reported takes into account these inter-test differences when predicting Step 1 performance. Also, while many students report seeing Step 1 questions "word-for-word" out of the assessments, the NBME makes special note that no live USMLE questions are shown on any NBME assessment.

Lastly, the International Foundations of Medicine (IFOM) offers a Basic Science Examination (BSE) practice exam at participating Prometric test centers for $200. Students may also take the self-assessment test online for $35 through the NBME's website. The IFOM BSE is intended to determine an examinee's relative areas of strength and weakness in general areas of basic science—not to predict performance on the USMLE Step 1 exam—and the content covered by the two examinations is somewhat different. However, because there is substantial overlap in content coverage and many IFOM items were previously used on the USMLE Step 1, it is possible to roughly

TABLE 2. CBSE to USMLE Score Prediction.

CBSE Score	Step 1 Equivalent
≥ 94	≥ 260
92	255
90	250
88	245
86	240
84	235
82	230
80	225
78	220
76	215
74	210
72	205
70	200
68	195
66	190
64	185
62	180
60	175
58	170
56	165
54	160
52	155
50	150
48	145
46	140
≤ 44	≤ 135

project IFOM performance onto the USMLE Step 1 score scale. More information is available at http://www.nbme.org/ifom/.

TABLE 3. CBSSA to USMLE Score Prediction.

CBSSA Score	Approximate USMLE Step 1 Score
150	153
200	164
250	175
300	185
350	196
400	207
450	217
500	228
550	239
600	249
650	260
700	271
750	281
800	292

▶ DEFINING YOUR GOAL

It is useful to define your own personal performance goal when approaching the USMLE Step 1. Your style and intensity of preparation can then be matched to your goal. Furthermore, your goal may depend on your school's requirements, your specialty choice, your grades to date, and your personal assessment of the test's importance. Do your best to define your goals early so that you can prepare accordingly.

Certain highly competitive residency programs, such as those in plastic surgery and orthopedic surgery, have acknowledged their use of Step 1 scores in the selection process. In such residency programs, greater emphasis may be placed on attaining a high score, so students who seek to enter these programs may wish to consider aiming for a very high score on the Step 1 exam (see Figure 2). At the same time, your Step 1 score is only one of a number of factors that are assessed when you apply for residency. In fact, many residency programs value other criteria such as letters of recommendation, third-year clerkship grades, honors, and research experience more than a high score on Step 1. Fourth-year medical students who have recently completed the residency application process can be a valuable resource in this regard.

▶ *Fourth-year medical students have the best feel for how Step 1 scores factor into the residency application process.*

▶ *Some competitive residency programs place more weight on Step 1 scores when choosing candidates to interview.*

▶ EXCELLING IN THE PRECLINICAL YEARS

Many students feel overwhelmed during the first few weeks of medical school and struggle to find a workable system. Strategies that worked during your undergraduate years may or may not work as you prepare for the USMLE

FIGURE 2. Median USMLE Step 1 Score by Specialty for Matched US Seniors.[a]

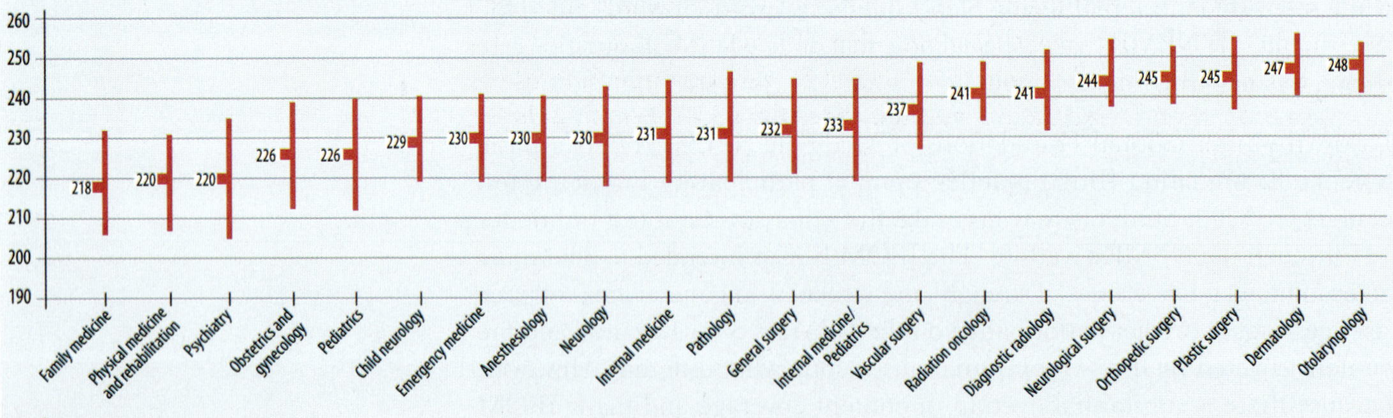

[a] Vertical lines show interquartile range.

Step 1. Below are three study methods to use during the preclinical years and their effectiveness for Step 1 preparation. Regardless of your choice, the foundation of knowledge you build during your basic science years is the most important resource for success on the USMLE Step 1.

Highlight, Read, and Reread

The most passive of the three methods, this generally consists of sitting through lectures and highlighting relevant material (sometimes in an assortment of colors). Notes are jotted in the margins, but the general bulk of information is in the same order presented by the various lecturers. Students then go home and reread the notes, focusing on the highlights. It is difficult to test integration of concepts. These notes (usually in the thousands of pages) are almost useless for Step 1 preparation.

Flash cards

There is no shortage of flash card applications, from make-your-own cards to purchasable premade decks. Self-made flash cards, if done correctly, offer the ability to objectively test necessary facts. Written in an open-ended format and coupled with spaced repetition, they train both recognition and recall. Apps exist for various smartphones and tablets, so the flash cards are always accessible. However, the ease of quickly creating digital cards and sharing can lead to flash card overload (it is unsustainable to make 50 flash cards per lecture!). Even at a modest pace, the thousands upon thousands of cards are too many for Step 1 preparation. Unless you have specified high-yield cards (and checked the content with high-yield resources), stick to premade cards by reputable sources that curate the vast amount of knowledge for you.

▸ *Watch out for flash card overload!*

Tables and Summaries

This is the most active (and time intensive) form of learning. It consists of integrating the pertinent information from paragraphs on each subject into tables that cut across topics within the same category. The key is to synthesize the sequentially presented material. Sensitive and specific findings should be highlighted. While many review sources offer this material in various styles and formats, your own class notes may in fact be concise enough to use as an adjunct for Step 1 preparation, and they have the added benefit of being organized to your liking.

▶ TIMELINE FOR STUDY

Before Starting

Your preparation for the USMLE Step 1 should begin when you enter medical school. Organize and commit to studying from the beginning so that when the time comes to prepare for the USMLE, you will be ready with a strong foundation.

Make a Schedule

▶ *Customize your schedule. Tackle your weakest section first.*

After you have defined your goals, map out a study schedule that is consistent with your objectives, your vacation time, the difficulty of your ongoing coursework, and your family and social commitments (see Figure 3). Determine whether you want to spread out your study time or concentrate it into 14-hour study days in the final weeks. Then factor in your own history in preparing for standardized examinations (eg, SAT, MCAT). Talk to students at your school who have recently taken Step 1. Ask them for their study schedules, especially those who have study habits and goals similar to yours.

Typically, US medical schools allot between four and eight weeks for dedicated Step 1 preparation. The time you dedicate to exam preparation will depend on your target score as well as your success in preparing yourself during the first two years of medical school. Some students reserve about a week at the end of their study period for final review; others save just a few days. When you have scheduled your exam date, do your best to adhere to it. Studies show that a later testing date does not translate into a higher score, so avoid pushing back your test date without good reason.[3]

▶ *"Crammable" subjects should be covered later and less crammable subjects earlier.*

Make your schedule realistic, and set achievable goals. Many students make the mistake of studying at a level of detail that requires too much time for a comprehensive review—reading *Gray's Anatomy* in a couple of days is not a realistic goal! Have one catch-up day per week of studying. No matter how well you stick to your schedule, unexpected events happen. But don't let yourself procrastinate because you have catch-up days; stick to your schedule as closely as possible and revise it regularly on the basis of your actual progress.

FIGURE 3. Typical Timeline for the USMLE Step 1.

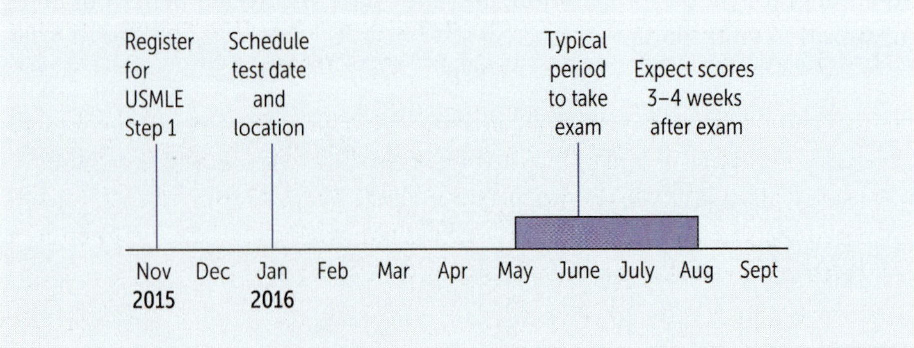

Be careful not to lose focus. Beware of feelings of inadequacy when comparing study schedules and progress with your peers. **Avoid others who stress you out.** Focus on a few top-rated resources that suit your learning style—not on some obscure books your friends may pass down to you. Accept the fact that you cannot learn it all.

You will need time for uninterrupted and focused study. Plan your personal affairs to minimize crisis situations near the date of the test. Allot an adequate number of breaks in your study schedule to avoid burnout. Maintain a healthy lifestyle with proper diet, exercise, and sleep.

▶ *Avoid burnout. Maintain proper diet, exercise, and sleep habits.*

Another important aspect of your preparation is your studying environment. **Study where you have always been comfortable studying.** Be sure to include everything you need close by (review books, notes, coffee, snacks, etc). If you're the kind of person who cannot study alone, form a study group with other students taking the exam. The main point here is to create a comfortable environment with minimal distractions.

Year(s) Prior

The knowledge you gained during your first two years of medical school and even during your undergraduate years should provide the groundwork on which to base your test preparation. Student scores on NBME subject tests (commonly known as "shelf exams") have been shown to be highly correlated with subsequent Step 1 scores.[4] Moreover, undergraduate science GPAs as well as MCAT scores are strong predictors of performance on the Step 1 exam.[5]

▶ *Buy review books early (first year) and use while studying for courses.*

We also recommend that you buy highly rated review books early in your first year of medical school and use them as you study throughout the two years. When Step 1 comes along, these books will be familiar and personalized to the way in which you learn. It is risky and intimidating to use unfamiliar review books in the final two or three weeks preceding the exam. Some students find it helpful to personalize and annotate *First Aid* throughout the curriculum.

Months Prior

Review test dates and the application procedure. Testing for the USMLE Step 1 is done on a year-round basis. If you have disabilities or special circumstances, contact the NBME as early as possible to discuss test accommodations (see the Section I Supplement at www.firstaidteam.com/bonus).

Use this time to finalize your ideal schedule. Consider upcoming breaks and whether you want to relax or study. Work backward from your test date to make sure you finish at least one question bank. Also add time to redo missed or flagged questions (which may be half the bank). This is the time to build a structured plan with enough flexibility for the realities of life.

▶ *Simulate the USMLE Step 1 under "real" conditions before beginning your studies.*

Begin doing blocks of questions from reputable question banks under "real" conditions. Don't use tutor mode until you're sure you can finish blocks in the allotted time. It is important to continue balancing success in your normal studies with the Step 1 test preparation process.

Weeks Prior (Dedicated Preparation)

- *In the final two weeks, focus on review, practice questions, and endurance. Stay confident!*

Your dedicated prep time may be one week or two months. You should have a working plan as you go into this period. Finish your school work strong, take a day off, and then get to work. Start by simulating a full-length USMLE Step 1 if you haven't yet done so. Consider doing one NBME CBSSA and the 150 free questions from the NBME website. Alternatively, you could choose 7 blocks of randomized questions from a commercial question bank. Make sure you get feedback on your strengths and weaknesses and adjust your studying accordingly. Many students study from review sources or comprehensive programs for part of the day, then do question blocks. Also, keep in mind that reviewing 46 questions can take upward of two hours. Feedback from CBSSA exams and question banks will help you focus on your weaknesses.

One Week Prior

- *One week before the test:*
  - *Sleep according to the same schedule you'll use on test day*
  - *Review the CBT tutorial one last time*
  - *Call Prometric to confirm test date and time*

Make sure you have your CIN (found on your scheduling permit) as well as other items necessary for the day of the examination, including a current driver's license or another form of photo ID with your signature (make sure the name on your **ID exactly** matches that on your scheduling permit). Confirm the Prometric testing center location and test time. Work out how you will get to the testing center and what parking and traffic problems you might encounter. Drive separately from other students taking the test on the same day, and exchange cell phone numbers in case of emergencies. If possible, visit the testing site to get a better idea of the testing conditions you will face. Determine what you will do for lunch. Make sure you have everything you need to ensure that you will be comfortable and alert at the test site. It may be beneficial to adjust your schedule to start waking up at the same time that you will on your test day. And of course, make sure to maintain a healthy lifestyle and get enough sleep.

One Day Prior

Try your best to relax and rest the night before the test. Double-check your admissions and test-taking materials as well as the comfort measures discussed earlier so that you will not have to deal with such details on the morning of the exam. At this point it will be more effective to review short-term memory material that you're already familiar with than to try to learn new material. The Rapid Review section at the end of this book is high yield for last-minute studying. Remember that regardless of how hard you have studied, you cannot know everything. There will be things on the exam that you have never even seen before, so do not panic. Do not underestimate your abilities.

Many students report difficulty sleeping the night prior to the exam. This is often exacerbated by going to bed much earlier than usual. Do whatever it takes to ensure a good night's sleep (eg, massage, exercise, warm milk, no back-lit screens at night). Do not change your daily routine prior to the exam. Exam day is not the day for a caffeine-withdrawal headache.

Morning of the Exam

On the morning of the Step 1 exam, wake up at your regular time and eat a normal breakfast. If you think it will help you, have a close friend or family member check to make sure you get out of bed. Make sure you have your scheduling permit admission ticket, test-taking materials, and comfort measures as discussed earlier. Wear loose, comfortable clothing. Plan for a variable temperature in the testing center. Arrive at the test site 30 minutes before the time designated on the admission ticket; however, do not come too early, as doing so may intensify your anxiety. When you arrive at the test site, the proctor should give you a USMLE information sheet that will explain critical factors such as the proper use of break time. Seating may be assigned, but ask to be reseated if necessary; you need to be seated in an area that will allow you to remain comfortable and to concentrate. Get to know your testing station, especially if you have never been in a Prometric testing center before. Listen to your proctors regarding any changes in instructions or testing procedures that may apply to your test site.

> ▶ *No notes, books, calculators, pagers, cell phones, recording devices, or watches of any kind are allowed in the testing area, but they are allowed in lockers.*

> ▶ *Arrive at the testing center 30 minutes before your scheduled exam time. If you arrive more than half an hour late, you will not be allowed to take the test.*

Finally, remember that it is natural (and even beneficial) to be a little nervous. Focus on being mentally clear and alert. Avoid panic. When you are asked to begin the exam, take a deep breath, focus on the screen, and then begin. Keep an eye on the timer. Take advantage of breaks between blocks to stretch, maybe do some jumping jacks, and relax for a moment with deep breathing or stretching.

After the Test

After you have completed the exam, be sure to have fun and relax regardless of how you may feel. Taking the test is an achievement in itself. Remember, you are much more likely to have passed than not. Enjoy the free time you have before your clerkships. Expect to experience some "reentry" phenomena as you try to regain a real life. Once you have recovered sufficiently from the test (or from partying), we invite you to send us your feedback, corrections, and suggestions for entries, facts, mnemonics, strategies, resource ratings, and the like (see p. xvii, How to Contribute). Sharing your experience will benefit fellow medical students and IMGs.

▶ STUDY MATERIALS

Quality Considerations

Although an ever-increasing number of review books and software are now available on the market, the quality of such material is highly variable. Some common problems are as follows:

- Certain review books are too detailed to allow for review in a reasonable amount of time or cover subtopics that are not emphasized on the exam.
- Many sample question books were originally written years ago and have not been adequately updated to reflect recent trends.
- Some question banks test to a level of detail that you will not find on the exam.

> ▶ *If a given review book is not working for you, stop using it no matter how highly rated it may be or how much it costs.*

Review Books

In selecting review books, be sure to weigh different opinions against each other, read the reviews and ratings in Section IV of this guide, examine the books closely in the bookstore, and choose carefully. You are investing not only money but also your limited study time. Do not worry about finding the "perfect" book, as many subjects simply do not have one, and different students prefer different formats. Supplement your chosen books with personal notes from other sources, including what you learn from question banks.

> ▶ *Charts and diagrams may be the best approach for physiology and biochemistry, whereas tables and outlines may be preferable for microbiology.*

There are two types of review books: those that are stand-alone titles and those that are part of a series. Books in a series generally have the same style, and you must decide if that style works for you. However, a given style is not optimal for every subject.

You should also find out which books are up to date. Some recent editions reflect major improvements, whereas others contain only cursory changes. Take into consideration how a book reflects the format of the USMLE Step 1.

Practice Tests

> ▶ *Most practice exams are shorter and less clinical than the real thing.*

Taking practice tests provides valuable information about potential strengths and weaknesses in your fund of knowledge and test-taking skills. Some students use practice examinations simply as a means of breaking up the monotony of studying and adding variety to their study schedule, whereas other students rely almost solely on practice. You should also subscribe to one or more high-quality question banks. In addition, students report that many current practice-exam books have questions that are, on average, shorter and less clinically oriented than those on the current USMLE Step 1.

Additionally, some students preparing for the Step 1 exam have started to incorporate case-based books intended primarily for clinical students on the wards or studying for the Step 2 CK exam. *First Aid Cases for the USMLE Step 1* aims to directly address this need.

After taking a practice test, spend time on each question and each answer choice whether you were right or wrong. There are important teaching points in each explanation. Knowing why a wrong answer choice is incorrect is just as important as knowing why the right answer is correct. Do not panic if your practice scores are low as many questions try to trick or distract you to highlight a certain point. Use the questions you missed or were unsure about to develop focused plans during your scheduled catch-up time.

▶ *Use practice tests to identify concepts and areas of weakness, not just facts that you missed.*

Textbooks and Course Syllabi

Limit your use of textbooks and course syllabi for Step 1 review. Many textbooks are too detailed for high-yield review and include material that is generally not tested on the USMLE Step 1 (eg, drug dosages, complex chemical structures). Syllabi, although familiar, are inconsistent across medical schools and frequently reflect the emphasis of individual faculty, which often does not correspond to that of the USMLE Step 1. Syllabi also tend to be less organized than top-rated books and generally contain fewer diagrams and study questions.

▶ TEST-TAKING STRATEGIES

Your test performance will be influenced by both your knowledge and your test-taking skills. You can strengthen your performance by considering each of these factors. Test-taking skills and strategies should be developed and perfected well in advance of the test date so that you can concentrate on the test itself. We suggest that you try the following strategies to see if they might work for you.

▶ *Practice! Develop your test-taking skills and strategies well before the test date.*

Pacing

You have seven hours to complete 308 questions. Note that each one-hour block contains 44 questions. This works out to about 82 seconds per question. If you find yourself spending too much time on a question, mark the question, make an educated guess, and move on. If time permits, come back to the question later. Remember that some questions may be experimental and do not count for points (and reassure yourself that these experimental questions are the ones that are stumping you). In the past, pacing errors have been detrimental to the performance of even highly prepared examinees. The bottom line is to keep one eye on the clock at all times!

▶ *Time management is an important skill for exam success.*

Dealing with Each Question

There are several established techniques for efficiently approaching multiple choice questions; find what works for you. One technique begins with identifying each question as easy, workable, or impossible. Your goal should be to answer all easy questions, resolve all workable questions in a reasonable amount of time, and make quick and intelligent guesses on all impossible questions. Most students read the stem, think of the answer, and turn immediately to the choices. A second technique is to first skim the answer choices to get a context, then read the last sentence of the question (the lead-in), and then read through the passage quickly, extracting only information relevant to answering the question. Try a variety of techniques on practice exams and see what works best for you. If you get overwhelmed, remember that a 30-second time out to refocus may get you back on track.

Guessing

There is **no penalty** for wrong answers. Thus, **no test block should be left with unanswered questions.** A hunch is probably better than a random guess. If you have to guess, we suggest selecting an answer you recognize over one with which you are totally unfamiliar.

Changing Your Answer

> ▶ *Go with your first hunch, unless you are certain that you are a good second-guesser.*

The conventional wisdom is not to change answers that you have already marked unless there is a convincing and logical reason to do so—in other words, go with your "first hunch." Many question banks tell you how many questions you changed from right to wrong, wrong to wrong, and wrong to right. Use this feedback to judge how good a second-guesser you are. If you have extra time, reread the question stem and make sure you didn't misinterpret the question.

▶ CLINICAL VIGNETTE STRATEGIES

> ▶ *Be prepared to read fast and think on your feet!*

In recent years, the USMLE Step 1 has become increasingly clinically oriented. This change mirrors the trend in medical education toward introducing students to clinical problem solving during the basic science years. The increasing clinical emphasis on Step 1 may be challenging to those students who attend schools with a more traditional curriculum.

What Is a Clinical Vignette?

> ▶ *Practice questions that include case histories or descriptive vignettes are critical for Step 1 preparation.*

A clinical vignette is a short (usually paragraph-long) description of a patient, including demographics, presenting symptoms, signs, and other information concerning the patient. Sometimes this paragraph is followed by a brief listing of important physical findings and/or laboratory results. The task of assimilating all this information and answering the associated question in the span of one minute can be intimidating. So be prepared to read quickly and think on your feet. Remember that the question is often indirectly asking something you already know.

Strategy

Remember that Step 1 vignettes usually describe diseases or disorders in their most classic presentation. So look for cardinal signs (eg, malar rash for SLE or nuchal rigidity for meningitis) in the narrative history. Be aware that the question will contain classic signs and symptoms instead of buzzwords. Sometimes the data from labs and the physical exam will help you confirm or reject possible diagnoses, thereby helping you rule answer choices in or out. In some cases, they will be a dead giveaway for the diagnosis.

▸ *Step 1 vignettes usually describe diseases or disorders in their most classic presentation.*

Making a diagnosis from the history and data is often not the final answer. Not infrequently, the diagnosis is divulged at the end of the vignette, after you have just struggled through the narrative to come up with a diagnosis of your own. The question might then ask about a related aspect of the diagnosed disease. Consider skimming the answer choices and lead-in before diving into a long stem. However, be careful with skimming the answer choices; going too fast may warp your perception of what the vignette is asking.

▸ IF YOU THINK YOU FAILED

After the test, many examinees feel that they have failed, and most are at the very least unsure of their pass/fail status. There are several sensible steps you can take to plan for the future in the event that you do not achieve a passing score. First, save and organize all your study materials, including review books, practice tests, and notes. Familiarize yourself with the reapplication procedures for Step 1, including application deadlines and upcoming test dates.

Make sure you know both your school's and the NBME's policies regarding retakes. The NBME allows a maximum of six attempts to pass each Step examination.[6] You may take Step 1 no more than three times within a 12-month period. Your fourth and subsequent attempts must be at least 12 months after your first attempt at that exam and at least six months after your most recent attempt at that exam.

▸ *If you pass Step 1 (score of 192 or above), you are not allowed to retake the exam.*

The performance profiles on the back of the USMLE Step 1 score report provide valuable feedback concerning your relative strengths and weaknesses. Study these profiles closely. Set up a study timeline to strengthen gaps in your knowledge as well as to maintain and improve what you already know. Do not neglect high-yield subjects. It is normal to feel somewhat anxious about retaking the test, but if anxiety becomes a problem, seek appropriate counseling.

▶ IF YOU FAILED

Even if you came out of the exam room feeling that you failed, seeing that failing grade can be traumatic, and it is natural to feel upset. Different people react in different ways: For some it is a stimulus to buckle down and study harder; for others it may "take the wind out of their sails" for a few days; and it may even lead to a reassessment of individual goals and abilities. In some instances, however, failure may trigger weeks or months of sadness, feelings of hopelessness, social withdrawal, and inability to concentrate—in other words, true clinical depression. If you think you are depressed, please seek help.

▶ TESTING AGENCIES

- **National Board of Medical Examiners (NBME) / USMLE Secretariat**
  Department of Licensing Examination Services
  3750 Market Street
  Philadelphia, PA 19104-3102
  (215) 590-9500 (operator) or
  (215) 590-9700 (automated information line)
  Fax: (215) 590-9457
  Email: webmail@nbme.org
  www.nbme.org

- **Educational Commission for Foreign Medical Graduates (ECFMG)**
  3624 Market Street
  Philadelphia, PA 19104-2685
  (215) 386-5900
  Fax: (215) 386-9196
  Email: info@ecfmg.org
  www.ecfmg.org

▶ REFERENCES

1. United States Medical Licensing Examination. Available at: http://www.usmle.org/bulletin/exam-content. Accessed October 20, 2015.
2. United States Medical Licensing Examination. 2014 Performance Data. Available at: http://www.usmle.org/performance-data/default.aspx#2014_step-1. Accessed October 20, 2015.
3. Pohl, Charles A., Robeson, Mary R., Hojat, Mohammadreza, and Veloski, J. Jon, "Sooner or Later? USMLE Step 1 Performance and Test Administration Date at the End of the Second Year," *Academic Medicine*, 2002, Vol. 77, No. 10, pp. S17–S19.
4. Holtman, Matthew C., Swanson, David B., Ripkey, Douglas R., and Case, Susan M., "Using Basic Science Subject Tests to Identify Students at Risk for Failing Step 1," *Academic Medicine*, 2001, Vol. 76, No. 10, pp. S48–S51.

5. Basco, William T., Jr., Way, David P., Gilbert, Gregory E., and Hudson, Andy, "Undergraduate Institutional MCAT Scores as Predictors of USMLE Step 1 Performance," *Academic Medicine*, 2002, Vol. 77, No. 10, pp. S13–S16.
6. United States Medical Licensing Examination. 2014 USMLE Bulletin of Information. http://www.usmle.org/pdfs/bulletin/2014bulletin.pdf. Accessed September 26, 2014.

▶ NOTES

SECTION I SUPPLEMENT

Special Situations

Please visit **www.usmle-rx.com/bonus/** to view this section.

NOTES

SECTION II

High-Yield General Principles

"There comes a time when for every addition of knowledge you forget something that you knew before. It is of the highest importance, therefore, not to have useless facts elbowing out the useful ones."

—Sir Arthur Conan Doyle, A *Study in Scarlet*

"Never regard study as a duty, but as the enviable opportunity to learn."

—Albert Einstein

"Live as if you were to die tomorrow. Learn as if you were to live forever."

—Gandhi

▶ HOW TO USE THE DATABASE

The 2016 edition of *First Aid for the USMLE Step 1* contains a revised and expanded database of basic science material that students, student authors, and faculty authors have identified as high yield for board review. The information is presented in a partially organ-based format. Hence, Section II is devoted to the foundational principles of behavioral science, biochemistry, microbiology, immunology, basic pathology, and basic pharmacology. Section III focuses on organ systems, with subsections covering the embryology, anatomy and histology, physiology, clinical pathology, and clinical pharmacology relevant to each. Each subsection is then divided into smaller topic areas containing related facts. Individual facts are generally presented in a three-column format, with the **Title** of the fact in the first column, the **Description** of the fact in the second column, and the **Mnemonic** or **Special Note** in the third column. Some facts do not have a mnemonic and are presented in a two-column format. Others are presented in list or tabular form in order to emphasize key associations.

The database structure used in Sections II and III is useful for reviewing material already learned. These sections are **not** ideal for learning complex or highly conceptual material for the first time.

The database of high-yield facts is not comprehensive. Use it to complement your core study material and not as your primary study source. The facts and notes have been condensed and edited to emphasize the essential material, and as a result, each entry is "incomplete" and arguably "over-simplified." Often, the more you research a topic, the more complex it becomes, with certain topics resisting simplification. Work with the material, add your own notes and mnemonics, and recognize that not all memory techniques work for all students.

We update the database of high-yield facts annually to keep current with new trends in boards emphasis, including clinical relevance. However, we must note that inevitably many other high-yield topics are not yet included in our database.

We actively encourage medical students and faculty to submit high-yield topics, well-written entries, diagrams, clinical images, and useful mnemonics so that we may enhance the database for future students. We also solicit recommendations of alternate tools for study that may be useful in preparing for the examination, such as charts, flash cards, apps, and online resources (see How to Contribute, p. xvii).

Image Acknowledgments

All images and diagrams marked with Rx are © USMLE-Rx.com (MedIQ Learning, LLC) and reproduced here by special permission. All images marked with RU are © Dr. Richard P. Usatine, author of *The Color Atlas of Family Medicine*, *The Color Atlas of Internal Medicine*, and *The Color Atlas of Pediatrics*, and are reproduced here by special permission (www.usatinemedia.com). Images and diagrams marked with * are adapted or reproduced with permission of other sources as listed on page 667. Images and diagrams with no acknowledgment are part of this book.

Disclaimer

The entries in this section reflect student opinions of what is high yield. Because of the diverse sources of material, no attempt has been made to trace or reference the origins of entries individually. We have regarded mnemonics as essentially in the public domain. Errata will gladly be corrected if brought to the attention of the authors, either through our online errata submission form at www.firstaidteam.com or directly by email to firstaidteam@yahoo.com.

NOTES

HIGH-YIELD PRINCIPLES IN

Behavioral Science

"It is a mathematical fact that fifty percent of all doctors graduate in the bottom half of their class."

—Author Unknown

"It's psychosomatic. You need a lobotomy. I'll get a saw."

—Calvin, "Calvin & Hobbes"

"There are two kinds of statistics: the kind you look up and the kind you make up."

—Rex Stout

"On a long enough time line, the survival rate for everyone drops to zero."

—Chuck Palahniuk

A heterogeneous mix of epidemiology, biostatistics, ethics, psychology, public health, and more falls under the heading of behavioral science. The exam has recently added an emphasis on patient safety and quality improvement topics. Many medical students do not diligently study this discipline because the material is felt to be easy or a matter of common sense. In our opinion, this is a missed opportunity.

Behavioral science questions may seem less concrete than questions from other disciplines, as they require an awareness of the psychosocial aspects of medicine. For example, if a patient does or says something, what should you do or say in response? These so-called quote questions now constitute much of the behavioral science section. Medical ethics and medical law are also appearing with increasing frequency. In addition, the key aspects of the doctor-patient relationship (eg, communication skills, open-ended questions, facilitation, silence) are high yield, as are biostatistics and epidemiology, which are the foundations of evidence-based medicine. Make sure you can apply biostatistical concepts such as sensitivity, specificity, and predictive values in a problem-solving format.

▶ BEHAVIORAL SCIENCE—EPIDEMIOLOGY/BIOSTATISTICS

Observational studies

STUDY TYPE	DESIGN	MEASURES/EXAMPLE
Cross-sectional study	Collects data from a group of people to assess frequency of disease (and related risk factors) at a particular point in time. Asks, "What is happening?"	Disease prevalence. Can show risk factor association with disease, but does not establish causality.
Case-control study	Compares a group of people with disease to a group without disease. Looks for prior exposure or risk factor. Asks, "What happened?"	Odds ratio (OR). "Patients with COPD had higher odds of a history of smoking than those without COPD."
Cohort study	Compares a group with a given exposure or risk factor to a group without such exposure. Looks to see if exposure affects the likelihood of disease. Can be prospective (asks, "Who will develop disease?") or historical (asks, "Who developed the disease [exposed vs nonexposed]?").	Relative risk (RR). "Smokers had a higher risk of developing COPD than nonsmokers."
Twin concordance study	Compares the frequency with which both monozygotic twins or both dizygotic twins develop the same disease.	Measures heritability and influence of environmental factors ("nature vs nurture").
Adoption study	Compares siblings raised by biological vs adoptive parents.	Measures heritability and influence of environmental factors.

Clinical trial

Experimental study involving humans. Compares therapeutic benefits of 2 or more treatments, or of treatment and placebo. Study quality improves when study is randomized, controlled, and double-blinded (ie, neither patient nor doctor knows whether the patient is in the treatment or control group). Triple-blind refers to the additional blinding of the researchers analyzing the data.

DRUG TRIALS	TYPICAL STUDY SAMPLE	PURPOSE
Phase I	Small number of healthy volunteers.	"Is it safe?" Assesses safety, toxicity, pharmacokinetics, and pharmacodynamics.
Phase II	Small number of patients with disease of interest.	"Does it work?" Assesses treatment efficacy, optimal dosing, and adverse effects.
Phase III	Large number of patients randomly assigned either to the treatment under investigation or to the best available treatment (or placebo).	"Is it as good or better?" Compares the new treatment to the current standard of care.
Phase IV	Postmarketing surveillance of patients after treatment is approved.	"Can it stay?" Detects rare or long-term adverse effects. Can result in treatment being withdrawn from market.

Evaluation of diagnostic tests

Uses 2 × 2 table comparing test results with the actual presence of disease. TP = true positive; FP = false positive; TN = true negative; FN = false negative.

Sensitivity and specificity are fixed properties of a test. PPV and NPV vary depending on disease prevalence.

	Disease ⊕	Disease ⊖	
Test ⊕	TP	FP	PPV = TP/(TP + FP)
Test ⊖	FN	TN	NPV = TN/(TN + FN)
	Sensitivity = TP/(TP + FN)	Specificity = TN/(TN + FP)	

Sensitivity (true-positive rate)	Proportion of all people with disease who test positive, or the probability that when the disease is present, the test is positive. Value approaching 100% is desirable for **ruling out** disease and indicates a **low false-negative rate**. High sensitivity test used for screening in diseases with low prevalence.	= TP / (TP + FN) = 1 – false-negative rate SN-N-OUT = highly SeNsitive test, when Negative, rules OUT disease If sensitivity is 100%, TP / (TP + FN) = 1, FN = 0, and all negatives must be TNs
Specificity (true-negative rate)	Proportion of all people without disease who test negative, or the probability that when the disease is absent, the test is negative. Value approaching 100% is desirable for **ruling in** disease and indicates a **low false-positive rate**. High specificity test used for confirmation after a positive screening test.	= TN / (TN + FP) = 1 – false-positive rate SP-P-IN = highly SPecific test, when Positive, rules IN disease If specificity is 100%, TN / (TN + FP) = 1, FP = 0, and all positives must be TPs
Positive predictive value	Proportion of positive test results that are true positive. Probability that a person who has a positive test result actually has the disease.	PPV = TP / (TP + FP) PPV varies directly with pretest probability (baseline risk, such as prevalence of disease): high pretest probability → high PPV
Negative predictive value	Proportion of negative test results that are true negative. Probability that a person with a negative test result actually does not have the disease.	NPV = TN / (TN + FN) NPV varies inversely with prevalence or pretest probability: high pretest probability → low NPV

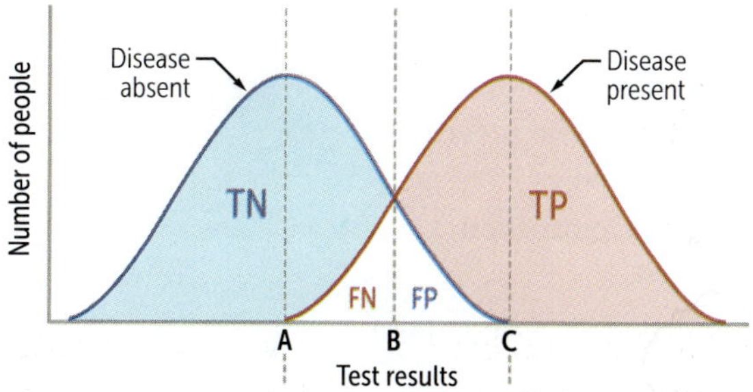

POSSIBLE CUTOFF VALUES
A = 100% sensitivity cutoff value
B = practical compromise between specificity and sensitivity
C = 100% specificity cutoff value

Lowering the cutoff point: **B** → **A** (↑ FP ↓ FN)	↑ Sensitivity ↑ NPV ↓ Specificity ↓ PPV
Raising the cutoff point: **B** → **C** (↑ FN ↓ FP)	↑ Specificity ↑ PPV ↓ Sensitivity ↓ NPV

Incidence vs prevalence

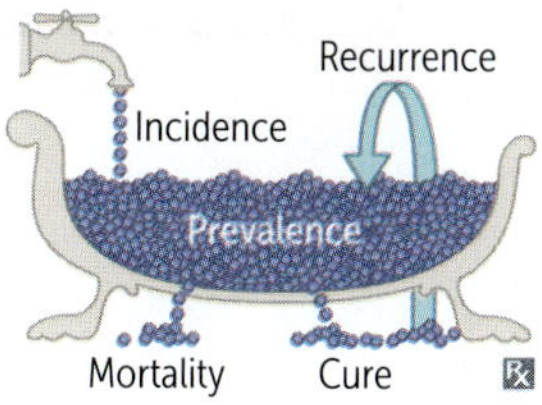

$$\text{Incidence rate} = \frac{\text{\# of new cases}}{\text{\# of people at risk}}$$ (during a specified time period)

Incidence looks at new cases (incidents).

$$\text{Prevalence} = \frac{\text{\# of existing cases}}{\text{Total \# of people in a population}}$$ (at a point in time)

Prevalence looks at all current cases.

Prevalence ≈ incidence for short duration disease (eg, common cold).

Prevalence > incidence for chronic diseases, due to large # of existing cases (eg, diabetes).

Prevalence ≈ pretest probability.

Quantifying risk

Definitions and formulas are based on the classic 2 × 2 or contingency table.

Risk factor or intervention	Disease ⊕	Disease ⊖
⊕	a	b
⊖	c	d

Odds ratio	Typically used in case-control studies. Odds that the group with the disease (cases) was exposed to a risk factor (a/c) divided by the odds that the group without the disease (controls) was exposed (b/d).	$OR = \frac{a/c}{b/d} = \frac{ad}{bc}$
Relative risk	Typically used in cohort studies. Risk of developing disease in the exposed group divided by risk in the unexposed group (eg, if 21% of smokers develop lung cancer vs 1% of nonsmokers, RR = 21/1 = 21). If prevalence is low, OR ≈ RR.	$RR = \frac{a/(a+b)}{c/(c+d)}$
Attributable risk	The difference in risk between exposed and unexposed groups, or the proportion of disease occurrences that are attributable to the exposure (eg, if risk of lung cancer in smokers is 21% and risk in nonsmokers is 1%, then 20% of the lung cancer risk in smokers is attributable to smoking).	$AR = \frac{a}{a+b} - \frac{c}{c+d}$
Relative risk reduction	The proportion of risk reduction attributable to the intervention as compared to a control (eg, if 2% of patients who receive a flu shot develop the flu, while 8% of unvaccinated patients develop the flu, then RR = 2/8 = 0.25, and RRR = 0.75).	$RRR = 1 - RR$
Absolute risk reduction	The difference in risk (not the proportion) attributable to the intervention as compared to a control (eg, if 8% of people who receive a placebo vaccine develop the flu vs 2% of people who receive a flu vaccine, then ARR = 8% – 2% = 6% = .06).	$ARR = \frac{c}{c+d} - \frac{a}{a+b}$
Number needed to treat	Number of patients who need to be treated for 1 patient to benefit.	$NNT = 1/ARR$
Number needed to harm	Number of patients who need to be exposed to a risk factor for 1 patient to be harmed.	$NNH = 1/AR$

Precision vs accuracy

Precision	The consistency and reproducibility of a test (reliability). The absence of random variation in a test.	Random error ↓ precision in a test. ↑ precision → ↓ standard deviation. ↑ precision → ↑ statistical power ($1 - \beta$).
Accuracy	The trueness of test measurements (validity). The absence of systematic error or bias in a test.	Systematic error ↓ accuracy in a test.

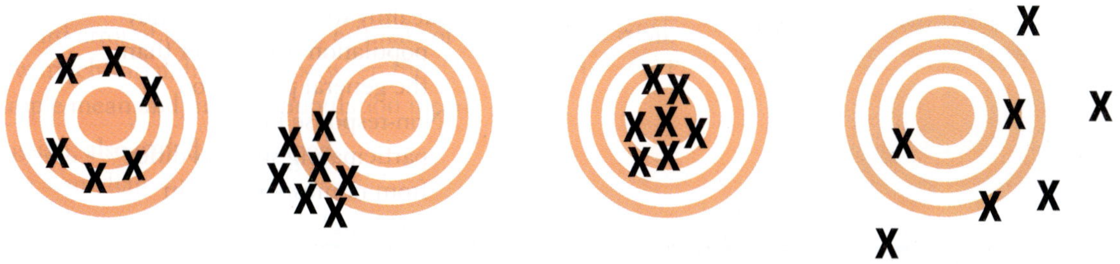

Accurate, not precise — Precise, not accurate — Accurate and precise — Not accurate, not precise

Outcomes of statistical hypothesis testing

Correct result	Stating that there is an effect or difference when one exists (null hypothesis rejected in favor of alternative hypothesis). Stating that there is not an effect or difference when none exists (null hypothesis not rejected).	
Incorrect result		
Type I error (α)	Stating that there is an effect or difference when none exists (null hypothesis incorrectly rejected in favor of alternative hypothesis). α is the probability of making a type I error. p is judged against a preset α level of significance (usually 0.05). If $p < 0.05$, then there is less than a 5% chance that the data will show something that is not really there.	Also known as false-positive error. α = you "**a**bserved" a difference that did not exist. You can never "prove" the alternate hypothesis, but you can reject the null hypothesis as being very unlikely.
Type II error (β)	Stating that there is not an effect or difference when one exists (null hypothesis is not rejected when it is in fact false). β is the probability of making a type II error. β is related to statistical power $(1 - \beta)$, which is the probability of rejecting the null hypothesis when it is false. ↑ power and ↓ β by: ▪ ↑ sample size ▪ ↑ expected effect size ▪ ↑ precision of measurement	Also known as false-negative error. β = you were **bl**inded by the truth. If you ↑ sample size, you ↑ power. There is **power in numbers**.

Confidence interval	Range of values within which the true mean of the population is expected to fall, with a specified probability. CI = mean ± Z(SEM). The 95% CI (corresponding to $p = .05$) is often used. For the 95% CI, Z = 1.96. For the 99% CI, Z = 2.58.	If the 95% CI for a mean difference between 2 variables includes 0, then there is no significant difference and H_0 is not rejected. If the 95% CI for odds ratio or relative risk includes 1, H_0 is not rejected. If the CIs between 2 groups do not overlap → statistically significant difference exists. If the CIs between 2 groups overlap → usually no significant difference exists.

Common statistical tests

t-test	Checks differences between **means** of **2** groups.	Tea is **meant** for **2**. Example: comparing the mean blood pressure between men and women.
ANOVA	Checks differences between means of **3** or more groups.	**3** words: **AN**alysis **Of** **VA**riance. Example: comparing the mean blood pressure between members of 3 different ethnic groups.
Chi-square (χ^2)	Checks differences between 2 or more percentages or proportions of **categorical** outcomes (not mean values).	Pronounce **Chi-tegorical**. Example: comparing the percentage of members of 3 different ethnic groups who have essential hypertension.

Pearson correlation coefficient (*r*)

r is always between −1 and +1. The closer the absolute value of *r* is to 1, the stronger the linear correlation between the 2 variables.
Positive *r* value → positive correlation (as one variable ↑, the other variable ↑).
Negative *r* value → negative correlation (as one variable ↑, the other variable ↓).
Coefficient of determination = r^2 (value that is usually reported).

▶ BEHAVIORAL SCIENCE—ETHICS

Core ethical principles

Autonomy	Obligation to respect patients as individuals (truth-telling, confidentiality), to create conditions necessary for autonomous choice (informed consent), and to honor their preference in accepting or not accepting medical care.
Beneficence	Physicians have a special ethical (fiduciary) duty to act in the patient's best interest. May conflict with autonomy (an informed patient has the right to decide) or what is best for society (eg, mandatory TB treatment). Traditionally, patient interest supersedes.
Nonmaleficence	"Do no harm." Must be balanced against beneficence; if the benefits outweigh the risks, a patient may make an informed decision to proceed (most surgeries and medications fall into this category).
Justice	To treat persons fairly and equitably. This does not always imply equally (eg, triage).

Informed consent	A process (not just a document/signature) that requires: ▪ Disclosure: discussion of pertinent information ▪ Understanding: ability to comprehend ▪ Capacity: ability to reason and make one's own decisions (distinct from competence, a legal determination) ▪ Voluntariness: freedom from coercion and manipulation Patients must have an intelligent understanding of their diagnosis and the risks/benefits of proposed treatment and alternative options, including no treatment. Patient must be informed that he or she can revoke written consent at any time, even orally.	Exceptions to informed consent: ▪ Patient lacks decision-making capacity or is legally incompetent ▪ Implied consent in an emergency ▪ Therapeutic privilege—withholding information when disclosure would severely harm the patient or undermine informed decision-making capacity ▪ Waiver—patient explicitly waives the right of informed consent
Consent for minors	A minor is generally any person < 18 years old. Parental consent laws in relation to health care vary by state. In general, parental consent should be obtained unless emergent treatment is required (eg, blood transfusion) even if it opposes parental religious/cultural beliefs, or if a minor is legally emancipated (eg, is married, is self supporting, or is in the military).	Situations in which parental consent is usually not required: ▪ **Sex** (contraception, STIs, pregnancy) ▪ **Drugs** (substance abuse) ▪ **Rock and roll** (emergency/trauma) Physicians should always encourage healthy minor-guardian communication.
Decision-making capacity	Physician must determine whether the patient is psychologically and legally capable of making a particular health care decision. Components: ▪ Patient is ≥ 18 years old or otherwise legally emancipated ▪ Patient makes and communicates a choice ▪ Patient is informed (knows and understands) ▪ Decision remains stable over time ▪ Decision is consistent with patient's values and goals, not clouded by a mood disorder ▪ Decision is not a result of altered mental status (eg, delirium, psychosis, intoxication)	

Advance directives	Instructions given by a patient in anticipation of the need for a medical decision. Details vary per state law.
Oral advance directive	Incapacitated patient's prior oral statements commonly used as guide. Problems arise from variance in interpretation. If patient was informed, directive was specific, patient made a choice, and decision was repeated over time to multiple people, then the oral directive is more valid.
Living will (written advance directive)	Describes treatments the patient wishes to receive or not receive if he/she loses decision-making capacity. Usually, patient directs physician to withhold or withdraw life-sustaining treatment if he/she develops a terminal disease or enters a persistent vegetative state.
Medical power of attorney	Patient designates an agent to make medical decisions in the event that he/she loses decision-making capacity. Patient may also specify decisions in clinical situations. Can be revoked by patient if decision-making capacity is intact. More flexible than a living will.

Surrogate decision-maker	If a patient loses decision-making capacity and has not prepared an advance directive, individuals (surrogates) who know the patient must determine what the patient would have done. Priority of surrogates: spouse > adult children > parents > adult siblings > other relatives.

Confidentiality

Confidentiality respects patient privacy and autonomy. If patient is not present or is incapacitated, disclosing information to family and friends should be guided by professional judgment of patient's best interest. The patient may voluntarily waive the right to confidentiality (eg, insurance company request).

General principles for exceptions to confidentiality:

- Potential physical harm to others is serious and imminent
- Likelihood of harm to self is great
- No alternative means exists to warn or to protect those at risk
- Physicians can take steps to prevent harm

Examples of exceptions to patient confidentiality (many are state-specific) include:

- Reportable diseases (eg, STIs, TB, hepatitis, food poisoning)—physicians may have a duty to warn public officials, who will then notify people at risk
- The Tarasoff decision—California Supreme Court decision requiring physician to directly inform and protect potential victim from harm
- Child and/or elder abuse
- Impaired automobile drivers (eg, epileptics)
- Suicidal/homicidal patients

Ethical situations

SITUATION	APPROPRIATE RESPONSE
Patient is not adherent.	Attempt to identify the reason for nonadherence and determine his/her willingness to change; do not coerce the patient into adhering or refer him/her to another physician.
Patient desires an unnecessary procedure.	Attempt to understand why the patient wants the procedure and address underlying concerns. Do not refuse to see the patient or refer him/her to another physician. Avoid performing unnecessary procedures.
Patient has difficulty taking medications.	Provide written instructions; attempt to simplify treatment regimens; use teach-back method (ask patient to repeat regimen back to physician) to ensure comprehension.
Family members ask for information about patient's prognosis.	Avoid discussing issues with relatives without the patient's permission.
A patient's family member asks you not to disclose the results of a test if the prognosis is poor because the patient will be "unable to handle it."	Attempt to identify why the family member believes such information would be detrimental to the patient's condition. Explain that as long as the patient has decision-making capacity and does not indicate otherwise, communication of information concerning his/her care will not be withheld.
A 17-year-old girl is pregnant and requests an abortion.	Many states require parental notification or consent for minors for an abortion. Unless there are specific medical risks associated with pregnancy, a physician should not sway the patient's decision for an elective abortion (regardless of maternal age or fetal condition).
A 15-year-old girl is pregnant and wants to keep the child. Her parents want you to tell her to give the child up for adoption.	The patient retains the right to make decisions regarding her child, even if her parents disagree. Provide information to the teenager about the practical issues of caring for a baby. Discuss the options, if requested. Encourage discussion between the teenager and her parents to reach the best decision.
A terminally ill patient requests physician assistance in ending his/her own life.	In the overwhelming majority of states, refuse involvement in any form of physician-assisted suicide. Physicians may, however, prescribe medically appropriate analgesics that coincidentally shorten the patient's life.
Patient is suicidal.	Assess the seriousness of the threat. If it is serious, suggest that the patient remain in the hospital voluntarily; patient can be hospitalized involuntarily if he/she refuses.
Patient states that he/she finds you attractive.	Ask direct, closed-ended questions and use a chaperone if necessary. Romantic relationships with patients are never appropriate.
A woman who had a mastectomy says she now feels "ugly."	Find out why the patient feels this way. Do not offer falsely reassuring statements (eg, "You still look good").
Patient is angry about the long time he/she spent in the waiting room.	Acknowledge the patient's anger, but do not take a patient's anger personally. Apologize for any inconvenience. Stay away from efforts to explain the delay.
Patient is upset with the way he/she was treated by another doctor.	Suggest that the patient speak directly to that physician regarding his/her concerns. If the problem is with a member of the office staff, tell the patient you will speak to that person.
An invasive test is performed on the wrong patient.	Regardless of the outcome, a physician is ethically obligated to inform a patient that a mistake has been made.
A patient requires a treatment not covered by his/her insurance.	Never limit or deny care because of the expense in time or money. Discuss all treatment options with patients, even if some are not covered by their insurance companies.
A 7-year-old boy loses a sister to cancer and now feels responsible.	At ages 5–7, children begin to understand that death is permanent, that all life functions end completely at death, and that everything that is alive eventually dies. Provide a direct, concrete description of his sister's death. Avoid clichés and euphemisms. Reassure that the boy is not responsible. Identify and normalize fears and feelings. Encourage play and healthy coping behaviors (eg, remembering her in his own way).

▶ BEHAVIORAL SCIENCE—DEVELOPMENT AND AGING

Early developmental milestones

Milestone dates are ranges that have been approximated and vary by source. Children not meeting milestones may need assessment for potential developmental delay.

AGE	MOTOR	SOCIAL	VERBAL/COGNITIVE
Infant	**Parents**	**Start**	**Observing,**
0–12 mo	Primitive reflexes disappear—Moro (by 3 mo), rooting (by 4 mo), palmar (by 6 mo), Babinski (by 12 mo) Posture—lifts head up prone (by 1 mo), rolls and sits (by 6 mo), crawls (by 8 mo), stands (by 10 mo), walks (by 12–18 mo) Picks—passes toys hand to hand (by 6 mo), Pincer grasp (by 10 mo) Points to objects (by 12 mo)	Social smile (by 2 mo) Stranger anxiety (by 6 mo) Separation anxiety (by 9 mo)	Orients—first to voice (by 4 mo), then to name and gestures (by 9 mo) Object permanence (by 9 mo) Oratory—says "mama" and "dada" (by 10 mo)
Toddler	**Child**	**Rearing**	**Working,**
12–36 mo	Cruises, takes first steps (by 12 mo) Climbs stairs (by 18 mo) Cubes stacked—number = age (yr) × 3 Cultured—feeds self with fork and spoon (by 20 mo) Kicks ball (by 24 mo)	Recreation—parallel play (by 24–36 mo) Rapprochement—moves away from and returns to mother (by 24 mo) Realization—core gender identity formed (by 36 mo)	Words—200 words by age 2 (2 zeros), 2-word sentences
Preschool	**Don't**	**Forget, they're still**	**Learning!**
3–5 yr	Drive—tricycle (3 wheels at 3 yr) Drawings—copies line or circle, stick figure (by 4 yr) Dexterity—hops on one foot (by 4 yr), uses buttons or zippers, grooms self (by 5 yr)	Freedom—comfortably spends part of day away from mother (by 3 yr) Friends—cooperative play, has imaginary friends (by 4 yr)	Language—1000 words by age 3 (3 zeros), uses complete sentences and prepositions (by 4 yr) Legends—can tell detailed stories (by 4 yr)

Changes in the elderly

Sexual changes:
- Men—slower erection/ejaculation, longer refractory period
- Women—vaginal shortening, thinning, and dryness

Sleep patterns: ↓ REM and slow-wave sleep; ↑ sleep onset latency and ↑ early awakenings
↑ suicide rate
↓ vision, hearing, immune response, bladder control
↓ renal, pulmonary, GI function
↓ muscle mass, ↑ fat

Libido is stable in men but decreases in women after menopause.
Intelligence does not decrease.

Presbycusis—sensorineural hearing loss (often of higher frequencies) due to destruction of hair cells at the cochlear base (preserved low-frequency hearing at apex).

▸ BEHAVIORAL SCIENCE—PUBLIC HEALTH

Disease prevention

Primary	Prevent disease before it occurs (eg, HPV vaccination)	
Secondary	Screen early for and manage existing but asymptomatic disease (eg, Pap smear for cervical cancer)	
Tertiary	Treatment to reduce complications from disease that is ongoing or has long-term effects (eg, chemotherapy)	**Quaternary**—identifying patients at risk of unnecessary treatment, protecting from the harm of new interventions

Medicare and Medicaid

Medicare and Medicaid—federal programs that originated from amendments to the Social Security Act.
Medicare is available to patients ≥ 65 years old, < 65 with certain disabilities, and those with end-stage renal disease.
Medicaid is joint federal and state health assistance for people with very low income.

MedicarE is for Elderly.
MedicaiD is for Destitute.

The 4 parts of Medicare:
- Part A: Hospital insurance
- Part B: Basic medical bills (eg, doctor's fees, diagnostic testing)
- Part C: (Parts A+B) delivered by approved private companies
- Part D: Prescription drugs

Common causes of death (US) by age

	< 1 YR	1–14 YR	15–34 YR	35–44 YR	45–64 YR	65+ YR
#1	Congenital malformations	Unintentional injury	Unintentional injury	Unintentional injury	Cancer	Heart disease
#2	Preterm birth	Cancer	Suicide	Cancer	Heart disease	Cancer
#3	SIDS	Congenital malformations	Homicide	Heart disease	Unintentional injury	Chronic respiratory disease

Hospitalized conditions with frequent readmissions

	MEDICARE	MEDICAID	PRIVATE INSURANCE	UNINSURED
#1	Congestive HF	Mood disorders	Maintenance of chemotherapy or radiotherapy	Mood disorders
#2	Septicemia	Schizophrenia/ psychotic disorders	Mood disorders	Alcohol-related disorders
#3	Pneumonia	Diabetes mellitus with complications	Complications of surgical procedures or medical care	Diabetes mellitus with complications

Readmission for any reason within 30 days of original admission.

Safety culture

Organizational environment in which everyone can freely bring up safety concerns without fear of censure. Facilitates error identification.

Event reporting systems collect data on errors for internal and external monitoring.

Human factors design

Forcing functions (those that prevent undesirable actions [eg, connecting feeding syringe to IV tubing]) are the most effective.
Standardization improves process reliability (eg, clinical pathways, guidelines, checklists).
Simplification reduces wasteful activities (eg, consolidating electronic medical records [EMRs]).

Deficient designs hinder workflow and lead to staff workarounds that bypass safety features (eg, patient ID barcodes affixed to computers due to unreadable wristbands).

PDSA cycle

Process improvement model to test changes in real clinical setting. Impact on patients:
- Plan—define problem and solution
- Do—test new process
- Study—measure and analyze data
- Act—integrate new process into regular workflow

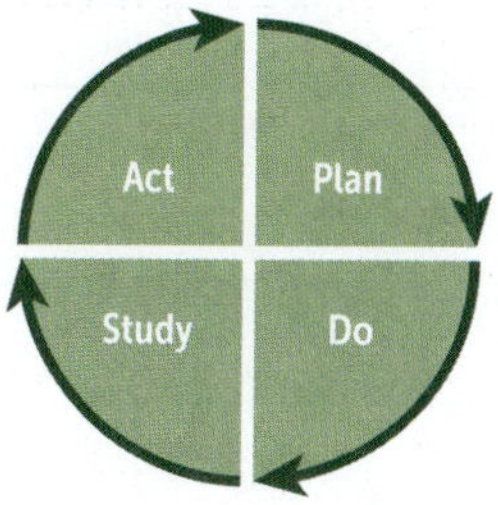

Quality measurements Plotted on run and control charts.

	MEASURE	EXAMPLE
Outcome	Impact on patients	Average HbA_{1c} of patients with diabetes
Process	Performance of system as planned	Ratio of patients whose HbA_{1c} was measured in the past 6 months
Balancing	Impact on other systems/outcomes	Incidence of hypoglycemia among those patients

Swiss cheese model In complex organizations, flaws in multiple processes and systems may align to cause patient harm. Focuses on systems and conditions rather than an individual's error.

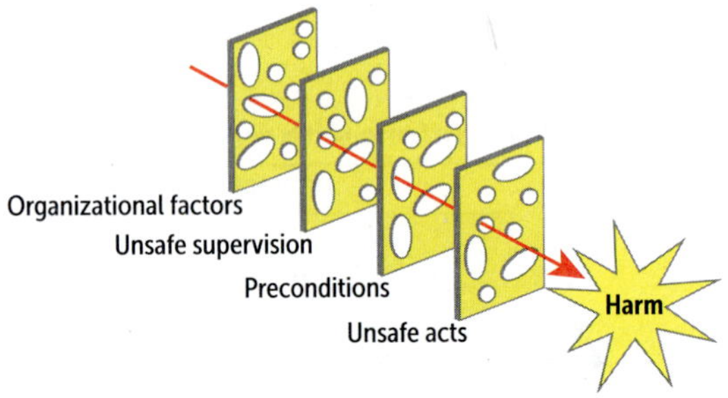

Types of medical errors	May involve patient identification, diagnosis, monitoring, nosocomial infection, medications, procedures, devices, documentation, handoffs. Errors causing harmful outcomes must be disclosed to patients.	
Active error	Occurs at level of frontline operator (eg, wrong IV pump dose programmed).	Immediate impact.
Latent error	Occurs in processes indirect from operator but impacts patient care (eg, different types of IV pumps used within same hospital).	Accident waiting to happen.

Medical error analysis		
Root cause analysis	Uses records and participant interviews to identify all the underlying problems that led to an error. Categories of causes include process, people (providers or patients), environment, equipment, materials, management.	**R**etrospective approach applied after failure event to prevent recurrence. Plotted on fishbone (Ishikawa, cause-and-effect) diagram. Fix causes with corrective action plan.
Failure mode and effects analysis	Uses inductive reasoning to identify all the ways a process might fail and prioritize these by their probability of occurrence and impact on patients.	**F**orward-looking approach applied before process implementation to prevent failure occurrence.

HIGH-YIELD PRINCIPLES IN

Biochemistry

"Biochemistry is the study of carbon compounds that crawl."

—Mike Adams

"We think we have found the basic mechanism by which life comes from life."

—Francis H. C. Crick

This high-yield material includes molecular biology, genetics, cell biology, and principles of metabolism (especially vitamins, cofactors, minerals, and single-enzyme-deficiency diseases). When studying metabolic pathways, emphasize important regulatory steps and enzyme deficiencies that result in disease, as well as reactions targeted by pharmacologic interventions. For example, understanding the defect in Lesch-Nyhan syndrome and its clinical consequences is higher yield than memorizing every intermediate in the purine salvage pathway. Do not spend time on hard-core organic chemistry, mechanisms, or physical chemistry. Detailed chemical structures are infrequently tested; however, many structures have been included here to help students learn reactions and the important enzymes involved. Familiarity with the biochemical techniques that have medical relevance—such as ELISA, immunoelectrophoresis, Southern blotting, and PCR—is useful. Review the related biochemistry when studying pharmacology or genetic diseases as a way to reinforce and integrate the material.

▶ BIOCHEMISTRY—MOLECULAR

Chromatin structure

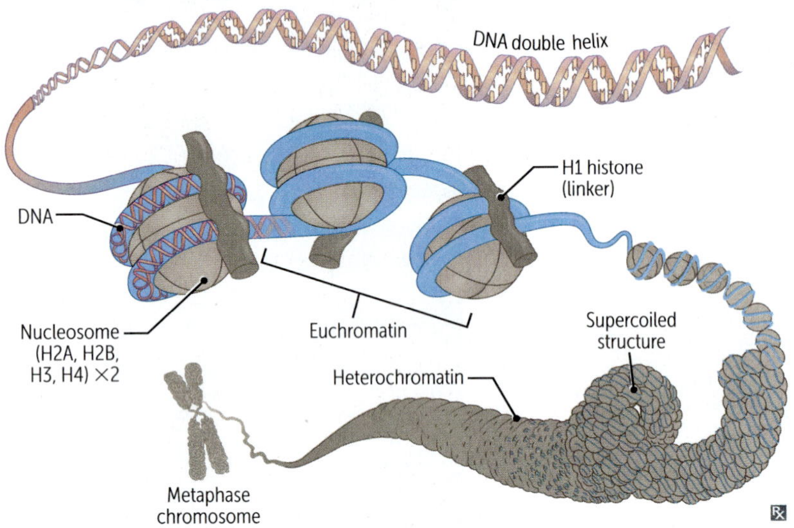

DNA exists in the condensed, chromatin form in order to fit into the nucleus. Negatively charged DNA loops twice around positively charged histone octamer to form nucleosome "**beads on a string**." Histones are rich in the amino acids lysine and arginine. H1 binds to the nucleosome and to "linker DNA," thereby stabilizing the chromatin fiber.

In mitosis, DNA condenses to form chromosomes. DNA and histone synthesis occur during S phase.

Heterochromatin	Condensed, appears darker on EM. Transcriptionally inactive, sterically inaccessible.	**H**etero**C**hromatin = **H**ighly **C**ondensed. Barr bodies (inactive X chromosomes) are heterochromatin.
Euchromatin	Less condensed, appears lighter on EM. Transcriptionally active, sterically accessible.	*Eu* = true, "truly transcribed."
DNA methylation	Template strand cytosine and adenine are methylated in DNA replication, which allows mismatch repair enzymes to distinguish between old and new strands in prokaryotes.	
	DNA methylation at CpG islands represses transcription.	CpG **M**ethylation **M**akes DNA **M**ute.
Histone methylation	Usually reversibly represses DNA transcription, but can activate it in some cases depending on methylation location.	Histone **M**ethylation **M**ostly **M**akes DNA **M**ute.
Histone acetylation	Relaxes DNA coiling, allowing for transcription.	Histone **A**cetylation makes DNA **A**ctive.

Nucleotides

NucleoSide = base + (deoxy)ribose (Sugar).
NucleoTide = base + (deoxy)ribose + phosphaTe; linked by 3′-5′ phosphodiester bond.
PURines (A,G)—2 rings.
PYrimidines (C,U,T)—1 ring.

PURe As Gold.
CUT the PY (pie).
Thymine has a methyl.

Deamination of cytosine makes uracil.
Uracil found in RNA; thymine in DNA.

G-C bond (3 H bonds) stronger than A-T bond (2 H bonds). ↑ G-C content → ↑ melting temperature of DNA.

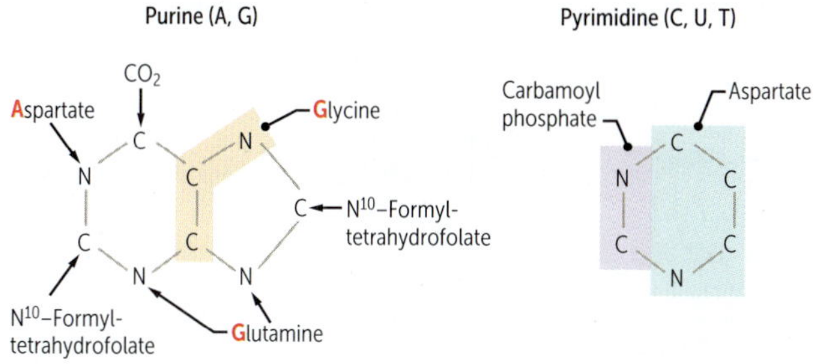

GAG—Amino acids necessary for purine synthesis:
Glycine
Aspartate
Glutamine

De novo pyrimidine and purine synthesis

Various immunosuppressive, antineoplastic, and antibiotic drugs function by interfering with nucleotide synthesis:

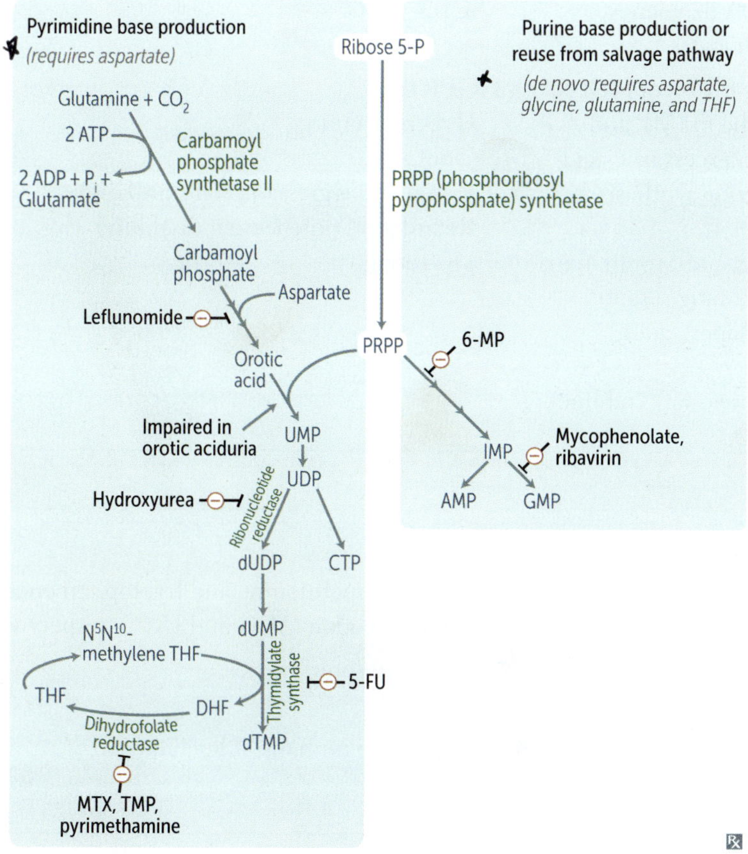

Disrupt pyrimidine synthesis:

- Leflunomide: inhibits dihydroorotate dehydrogenase
- Methotrexate (MTX), trimethoprim (TMP), and pyrimethamine: inhibit dihydrofolate reductase (↓ deoxythymidine monophosphate [dTMP]) in humans, bacteria, and protozoa, respectively
- 5-fluorouracil (5-FU): forms 5-F-dUMP, which inhibits thymidylate synthase (↓ dTMP)

Disrupt purine synthesis:

- 6-mercaptopurine (6-MP) and its prodrug azathioprine: inhibit de novo purine synthesis
- Mycophenolate and ribavirin: inhibit inosine monophosphate dehydrogenase

Disrupts purine and pyrimidine synthesis:

- Hydroxyurea: inhibits ribonucleotide reductase

Purine salvage deficiencies

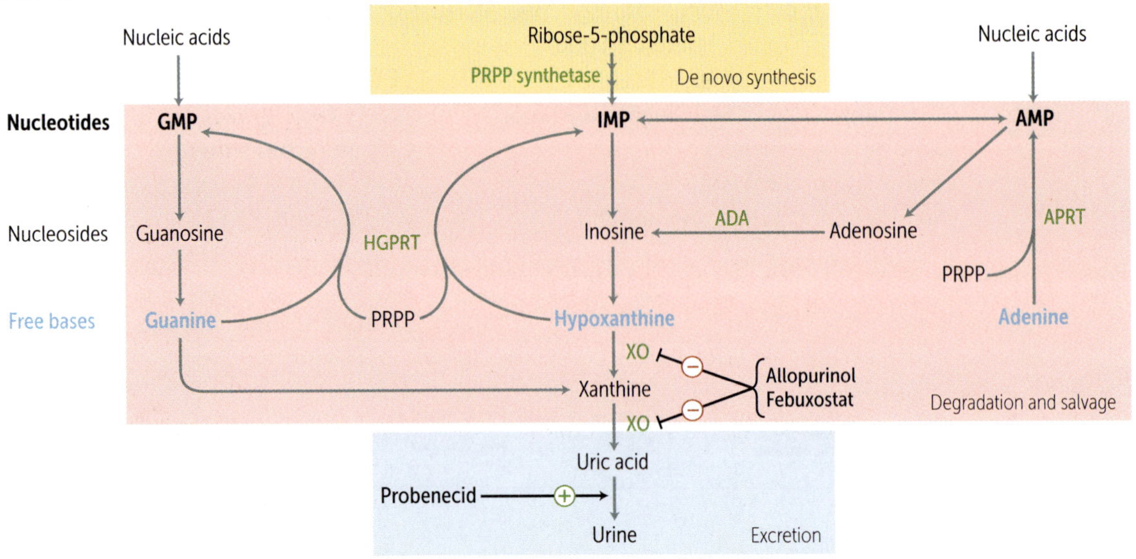

ADA, adenosine deaminase; APRT, adenine phosphoribosyltransferase;
HGPRT, hypoxanthine guanine phosphoribosyltransferase; XO, xanthine oxidase.

Adenosine deaminase deficiency	ADA is required for degradation of adenosine and deoxyadenosine. In ADA deficiency, ↑ dATP → toxicity in lymphocytes.	One of the major causes of autosomal recessive SCID.
Lesch-Nyhan syndrome	Defective purine salvage due to absent **HGPRT**, which converts hypoxanthine to IMP and guanine to GMP. Results in excess uric acid production and de novo purine synthesis. X-linked recessive. Findings: intellectual disability, self-mutilation, aggression, hyperuricemia (orange "sand" [sodium urate crystals] in diaper), gout, dystonia. Treatment: allopurinol or febuxostat (2nd line).	**HGPRT**: **H**yperuricemia **G**out **P**issed off (aggression, self-mutilation) **R**etardation (intellectual disability) Dys**T**onia

Genetic code features

Unambiguous	Each codon specifies only 1 amino acid.	
Degenerate/ redundant	Most amino acids are coded by multiple codons.	Exceptions: methionine and tryptophan encoded by only 1 codon (AUG and UGG, respectively).
Commaless, nonoverlapping	Read from a fixed starting point as a continuous sequence of bases.	Exceptions: some viruses.
Universal	Genetic code is conserved throughout evolution.	Exception in humans: mitochondria.

DNA replication	Eukaryotic DNA replication is more complex than the prokaryotic process but uses many enzymes analogous to those listed below. In both prokaryotes and eukaryotes, DNA replication is semiconservative and involves both continuous and discontinuous (Okazaki fragment) synthesis.	
[A] Origin of replication	Particular consensus sequence of base pairs in genome where DNA replication begins. May be single (prokaryotes) or multiple (eukaryotes).	AT-rich sequences are found in promoters and origins of replication.
[B] Replication fork	Y-shaped region along DNA template where leading and lagging strands are synthesized.	
[C] Helicase	Unwinds DNA template at replication fork.	
[D] Single-stranded binding proteins	Prevent strands from reannealing.	
[E] DNA topoisomerases	Create a single- or double-stranded break in the helix to add or remove supercoils.	Topoisomerase inhibitors: fluoroquinolones—prokaryotic topoisomerase II [DNA gyrase] and topoisomerase IV; e**topo**side/ten**ipo**side—eukaryotic **topo**isomerase II.
[F] Primase	Makes an RNA primer on which DNA polymerase III can initiate replication.	
[G] DNA polymerase III	Prokaryotic only. Elongates leading strand by adding deoxynucleotides to the 3′ end. Elongates lagging strand until it reaches primer of preceding fragment. 3′ → 5′ exonuclease activity "proofreads" each added nucleotide.	DNA polymerase III has 5′ → 3′ synthesis and proofreads with 3′ → 5′ exonuclease.
[H] DNA polymerase I	Prokaryotic only. Degrades RNA primer; replaces it with DNA.	Has same functions as DNA polymerase III but also excises RNA primer with 5′ → 3′ exonuclease.
[I] DNA ligase	Catalyzes the formation of a phosphodiester bond within a strand of double-stranded DNA (ie, joins Okazaki fragments).	
Telomerase	An RNA-dependent DNA polymerase that adds DNA to 3′ ends of chromosomes to avoid loss of genetic material with every duplication. Eukaryotes only.	Often dysregulated in cancer cells, allowing unlimited replication.

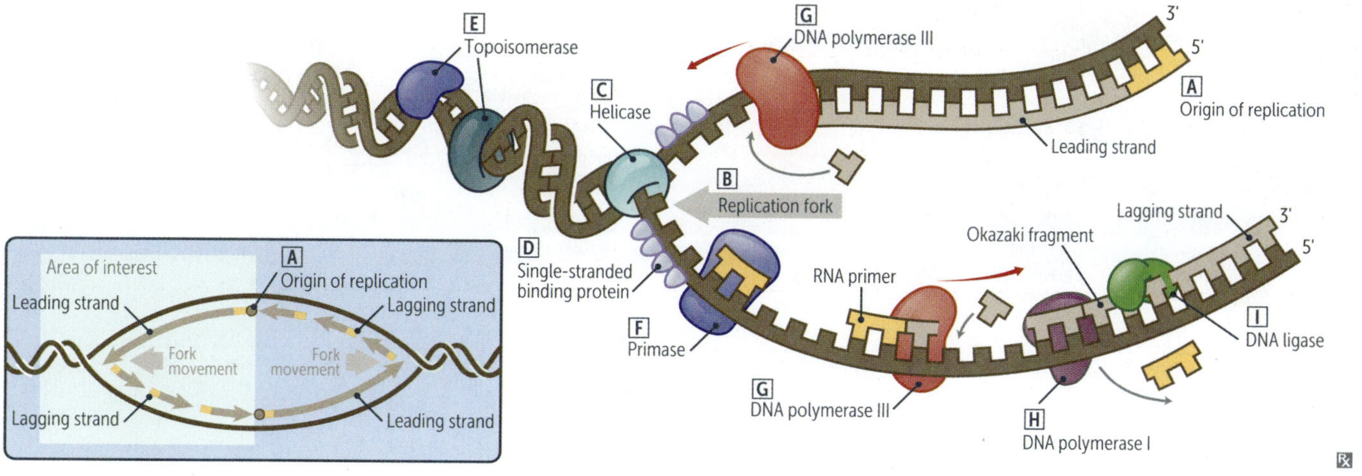

Mutations in DNA	Severity of damage: silent << missense < nonsense < frameshift. For point (silent, missense, and nonsense) mutations: ▪ Transition—purine to purine (eg, A to G) or pyrimidine to pyrimidine (eg, C to T). ▪ Transversion—purine to pyrimidine (eg, A to T) or pyrimidine to purine (eg, C to G).	
Silent	Nucleotide substitution but codes for same (synonymous) amino acid; often base change in 3rd position of codon (tRNA wobble).	
Missense	Nucleotide substitution resulting in changed amino acid (called conservative if new amino acid is similar in chemical structure).	Sickle cell disease (substitution of glutamic acid with valine).
Nonsense	Nucleotide substitution resulting in early **stop** codon. Usually results in nonfunctional protein.	**Stop** the **nonsense**!
Frameshift	Deletion or insertion of a number of nucleotides not divisible by 3, resulting in misreading of all nucleotides downstream. Protein may be shorter or longer, and its function may be disrupted or altered.	Duchenne muscular dystrophy, Tay-Sachs disease.
Splice site	Mutation at a splice site → retained intron in the mRNA → protein with impaired or altered function.	Rare cause of cancers, dementia, epilepsy, some types of β-thalassemia.

Lac operon

Classic example of a genetic response to an environmental change. Glucose is the preferred metabolic substrate in *E coli*, but when glucose is absent and lactose is available, the *lac* operon is activated to switch to lactose metabolism. Mechanism of shift:

- Low glucose → ↑ adenylate cyclase (adenylyl cyclase) activity → ↑ generation of cAMP from ATP → activation of catabolite activator protein (CAP) → ↑ transcription.
- High lactose → unbinds repressor protein from repressor/operator site → ↑ transcription.

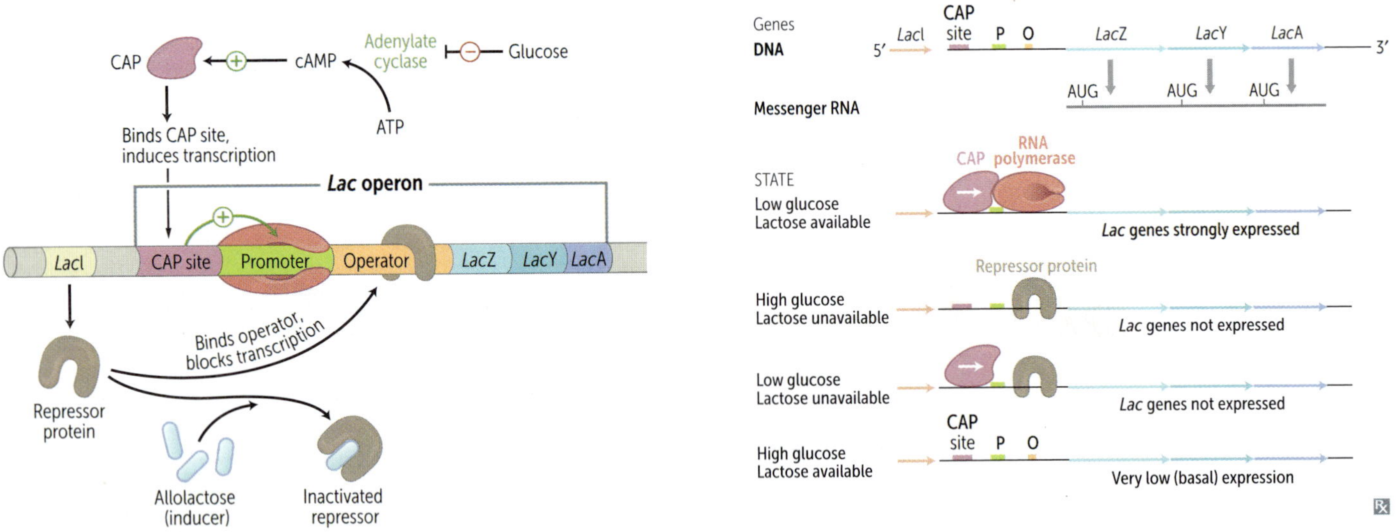

DNA repair

Single strand		
Nucleotide excision repair	Specific endonucleases release the oligonucleotides containing damaged bases; DNA polymerase and ligase fill and reseal the gap, respectively. Repairs bulky helix-distorting lesions. Occurs in G_1 phase of cell cycle.	Defective in xeroderma pigmentosum, which prevents repair of pyrimidine dimers because of ultraviolet light exposure.
Base excision repair	Base-specific glycosylase removes altered base and creates AP site (apurinic/apyrimidinic). One or more nucleotides are removed by AP-endonuclease, which cleaves the 5′ end. Lyase cleaves the 3′ end. DNA polymerase-β fills the gap and DNA ligase seals it. Occurs throughout cell cycle.	Important in repair of spontaneous/toxic deamination.
Mismatch repair	Newly synthesized strand is recognized, mismatched nucleotides are removed, and the gap is filled and resealed. Occurs predominantly in G_2 phase of cell cycle.	Defective in Lynch syndrome (hereditary nonpolyposis colorectal cancer [HNPCC]).
Double strand		
Nonhomologous end joining	Brings together 2 ends of DNA fragments to repair double-stranded breaks. No requirement for homology. Some DNA may be lost.	Mutated in ataxia telangiectasia; Fanconi anemia.

DNA/RNA/protein synthesis direction	DNA and RNA are both synthesized 5′ → 3′. The 5′ end of the incoming nucleotide bears the triphosphate (energy source for bond). Protein synthesis is N-terminus to C-terminus.	mRNA is read 5′ to 3′. The triphosphate bond is the target of the 3′ hydroxyl attack. Drugs blocking DNA replication often have modified 3′ OH, preventing addition of the next nucleotide ("chain termination").

Start and stop codons

mRNA start codons	AUG (or rarely GUG).	AUG inAUGurates protein synthesis.
Eukaryotes	Codes for methionine, which may be removed before translation is completed.	
Prokaryotes	Codes for N-formylmethionine (fMet).	fMet stimulates neutrophil chemotaxis.
mRNA stop codons	UGA, UAA, UAG.	UGA = U Go Away. UAA = U Are Away. UAG = U Are Gone.

Functional organization of a eukaryotic gene

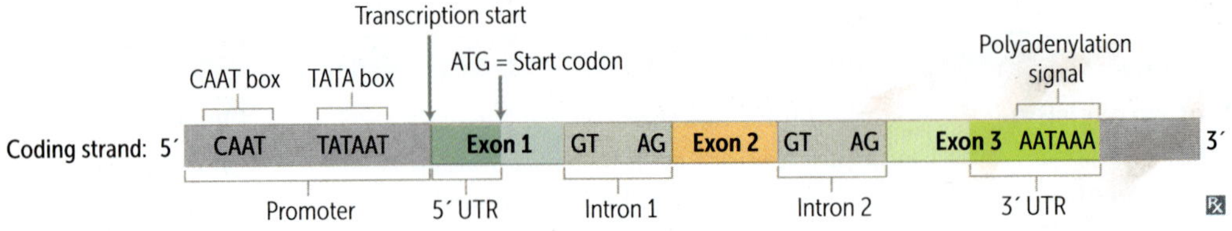

Regulation of gene expression

Promoter	Site where RNA polymerase II and multiple other transcription factors bind to DNA upstream from gene locus (AT-rich upstream sequence with TATA and CAAT boxes).	Promoter mutation commonly results in dramatic ↓ in level of gene transcription.
Enhancer	Stretch of DNA that alters gene expression by binding transcription factors.	Enhancers and silencers may be located close to, far from, or even within (in an intron) the gene whose expression it regulates.
Silencer	Site where negative regulators (repressors) bind.	

RNA polymerases

Eukaryotes	RNA polymerase I makes **r**RNA (most numerous RNA, **r**ampant). RNA polymerase II makes **m**RNA (largest RNA, **m**assive). RNA polymerase III makes 5S rRNA, **t**RNA (smallest RNA, **t**iny). No proofreading function, but can initiate chains. RNA polymerase II opens DNA at promoter site.	I, II, and III are numbered in the same order that their products are used in protein synthesis: large ribosomal RNA, mRNA, then small RNAs. α-amanitin, found in *Amanita phalloides* (death cap mushrooms), inhibits RNA polymerase II. Causes severe hepatotoxicity if ingested. Rifampin inhibits RNA polymerase in prokaryotes. Actinomycin D inhibits RNA polymerase in both prokaryotes and eukaryotes.
Prokaryotes	1 RNA polymerase (multisubunit complex) makes all 3 kinds of RNA.	

RNA processing (eukaryotes)

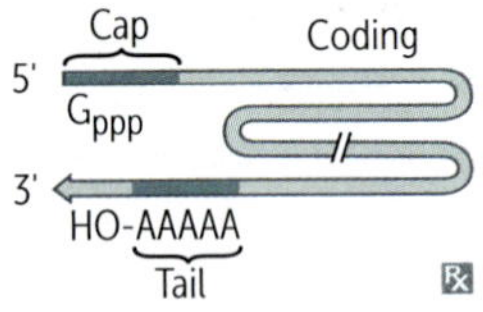

Initial transcript is called heterogeneous nuclear RNA (hnRNA). hnRNA is then modified and becomes mRNA.

The following processes occur in the nucleus following transcription:

- Capping of 5′ end (addition of 7-methylguanosine cap)
- Polyadenylation of 3′ end (≈ 200 A's)
- Splicing out of introns

Capped, tailed, and spliced transcript is called mRNA.

mRNA is transported out of the nucleus into the cytosol, where it is translated.

mRNA quality control occurs at cytoplasmic processing bodies (P-bodies), which contain exonucleases, decapping enzymes, and microRNAs; mRNAs may be stored in P-bodies for future translation.

Poly-A polymerase does not require a template.

AAUAAA = polyadenylation signal.

Splicing of pre-mRNA

❶ Primary transcript combines with small nuclear ribonucleoproteins (snRNPs) and other proteins to form spliceosome.

❷ Lariat-shaped (looped) intermediate is generated.

❸ Lariat is released to precisely remove intron and join 2 exons.

Antibodies to spliceosomal snRNPs (anti-Smith antibodies) are highly specific for SLE. Anti-U1 RNP antibodies are highly associated with mixed connective tissue disease (MCTD).

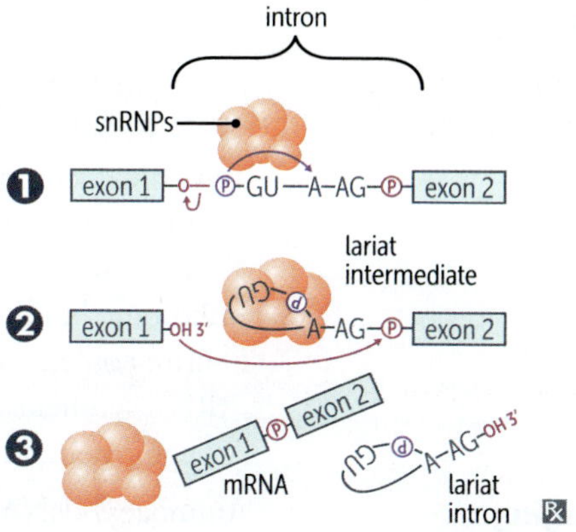

Introns vs exons

Exons contain the actual genetic information coding for protein.

Introns are intervening noncoding segments of DNA.

Different exons are frequently combined by alternative splicing to produce a larger number of unique proteins.

Introns are intervening sequences and stay in the nucleus, whereas exons exit and are expressed.

Abnormal splicing variants are implicated in oncogenesis and many genetic disorders (eg, β-thalassemia).

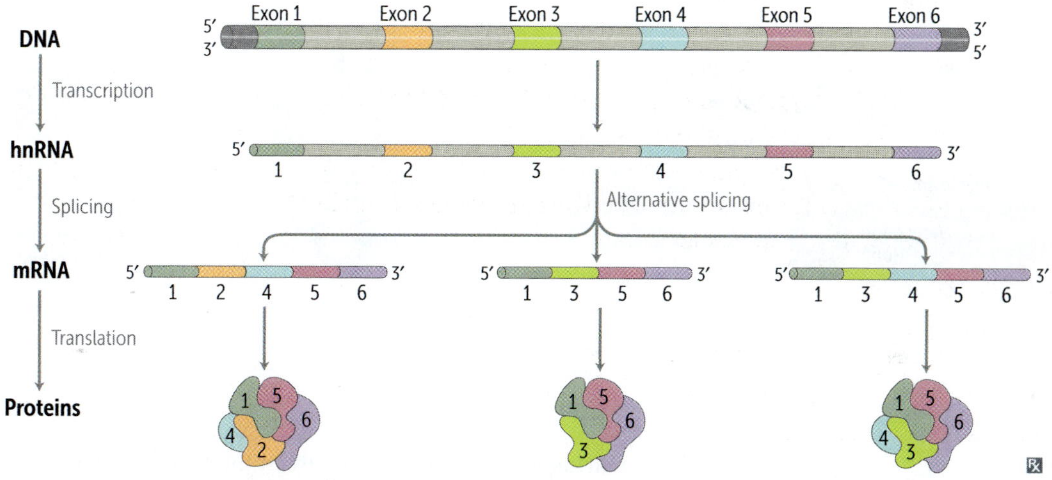

microRNAs

Small, noncoding RNA molecules that posttranscriptionally regulate protein expression. Introns can contain microRNA (miRNA) genes. They can have multiple mRNA targets, typically related to complementary base pairing. miRNA → degradation or inactivation of target mRNA → ↓ translation into protein. Abnormal expression of miRNAs contributes to certain malignancies (eg, by silencing an mRNA from a tumor suppressor gene).

tRNA

Structure

75–90 nucleotides, 2° structure, cloverleaf form, anticodon end is opposite 3′ aminoacyl end. All tRNAs, both eukaryotic and prokaryotic, have CCA at 3′ end along with a high percentage of chemically modified bases. The amino acid is covalently bound to the 3′ end of the tRNA. CCA Can Carry Amino acids.

T-arm: contains the TΨC (ribothymidine, pseudouridine, cytidine) sequence necessary for tRNA-ribosome binding.

D-arm: contains dihydrouridine residues necessary for tRNA recognition by the correct aminoacyl-tRNA synthetase.

Acceptor stem: the 5′-CCA-3′ is the amino acid acceptor site.

Charging

Aminoacyl-tRNA synthetase (1 per amino acid; "matchmaker"; uses ATP) scrutinizes amino acid before and after it binds to tRNA. If incorrect, bond is hydrolyzed. The amino acid-tRNA bond has energy for formation of peptide bond. A mischarged tRNA reads usual codon but inserts wrong amino acid.

Aminoacyl-tRNA synthetase and binding of charged tRNA to the codon are responsible for accuracy of amino acid selection.

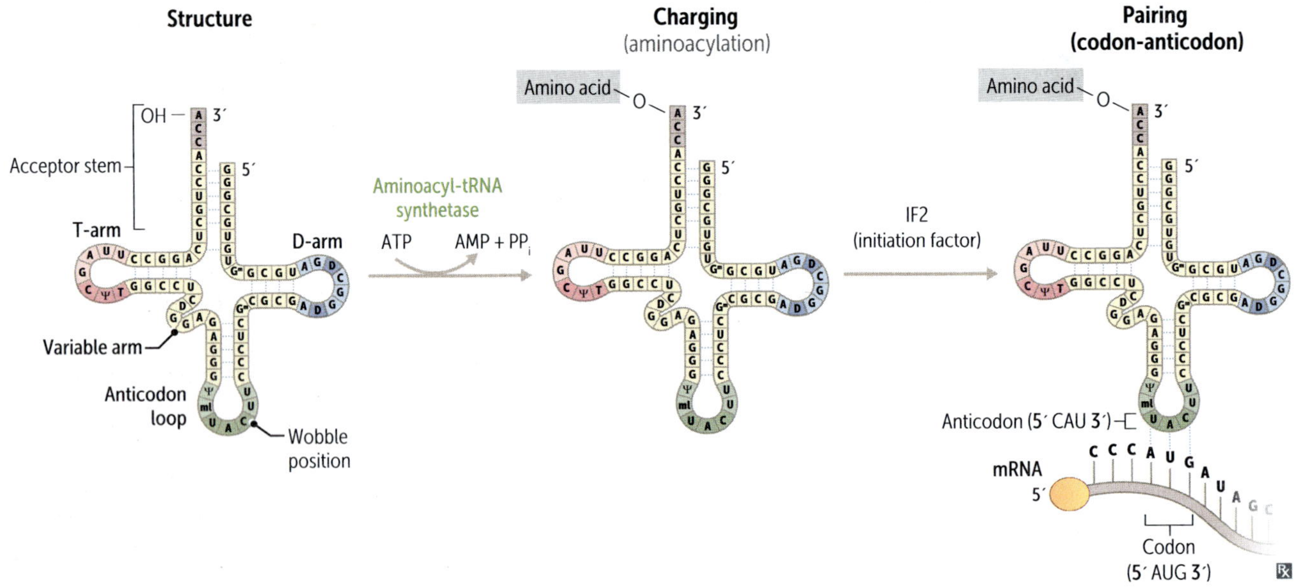

Wobble

Accurate base pairing is usually required only in the first 2 nucleotide positions of an mRNA codon, so codons differing in the 3rd "wobble" position may code for the same tRNA/amino acid (as a result of degeneracy of genetic code).

Protein synthesis

Initiation	Initiated by GTP hydrolysis; initiation factors (eukaryotic IFs) help assemble the 40S ribosomal subunit with the initiator tRNA and are released when the mRNA and the ribosomal 60S subunit assemble with the complex.	Eukaryotes: 40S + 60S → 80S (Even). PrOkaryotes: 30S + 50S → 70S (Odd). ATP—tRNA Activation (charging). GTP—tRNA Gripping and Going places (translocation).
Elongation	1. Aminoacyl-tRNA binds to A site (except for initiator methionine) 2. rRNA ("ribozyme") catalyzes peptide bond formation, transfers growing polypeptide to amino acid in A site 3. Ribosome advances 3 nucleotides toward 3′ end of mRNA, moving peptidyl tRNA to P site (translocation)	Think of "going APE": A site = incoming Aminoacyl-tRNA. P site = accommodates growing Peptide. E site = holds Empty tRNA as it Exits.
Termination	Stop codon is recognized by release factor, and completed polypeptide is released from ribosome.	

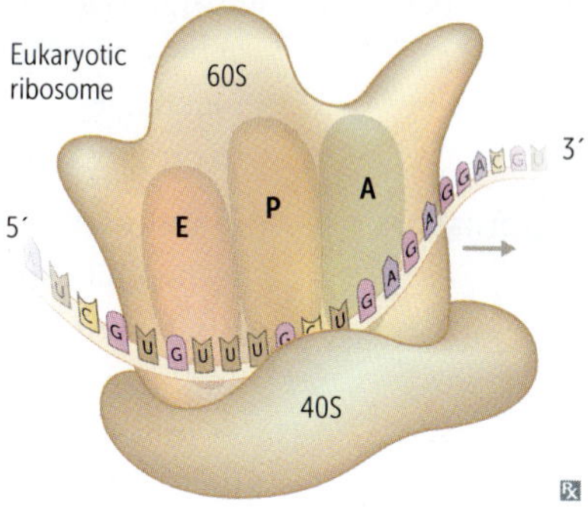

Posttranslational modifications

Trimming	Removal of N- or C-terminal propeptides from zymogen to generate mature protein (eg, trypsinogen to trypsin).
Covalent alterations	Phosphorylation, glycosylation, hydroxylation, methylation, acetylation, and ubiquitination.

Chaperone protein	Intracellular protein involved in facilitating and/or maintaining protein folding. For example, in yeast, heat shock proteins (eg, Hsp60) are expressed at high temperatures to prevent protein denaturing/misfolding.

▶ BIOCHEMISTRY—CELLULAR

Cell cycle phases — Checkpoints control transitions between phases of cell cycle. This process is regulated by cyclins, cyclin-dependent kinases (CDKs), and tumor suppressors. M phase (shortest phase of cell cycle) includes mitosis (prophase, prometaphase, metaphase, anaphase, telophase) and cytokinesis (cytoplasm splits in two). G_1 and G_0 are of variable duration.

REGULATION OF CELL CYCLE

CDKs	Constitutive and inactive.
Cyclins	Regulatory proteins that control cell cycle events; phase specific; activate CDKs.
Cyclin-CDK complexes	Phosphorylate other proteins to coordinate cell cycle progression; must be activated and inactivated at appropriate times for cell cycle to progress.
Tumor suppressors	p53 induces p21, which inhibits CDKs → hypophosphorylation (activation) of Rb. Hypophosphorylated Rb binds to and inactivates transcription factor E2F → inhibition of G_1-S progression. Mutations in these genes result in unrestrained cell division (eg, Li-Fraumeni syndrome).

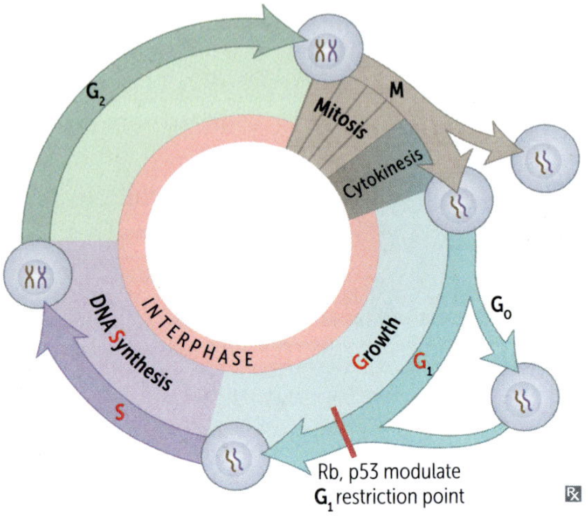

CELL TYPES

Permanent	Remain in G_0, regenerate from stem cells.	Neurons, skeletal and cardiac muscle, RBCs.
Stable (quiescent)	Enter G_1 from G_0 when stimulated.	Hepatocytes, lymphocytes.
Labile	Never go to G_0, divide rapidly with a short G_1. Most affected by chemotherapy.	Bone marrow, gut epithelium, skin, hair follicles, germ cells.

Rough endoplasmic reticulum	Site of synthesis of secretory (exported) proteins and of N-linked oligosaccharide addition to many proteins. Nissl bodies (RER in neurons)—synthesize peptide neurotransmitters for secretion. Free ribosomes—unattached to any membrane; site of synthesis of cytosolic and organellar proteins.	Mucus-secreting goblet cells of the small intestine and antibody-secreting plasma cells are rich in RER.
Smooth endoplasmic reticulum	Site of steroid synthesis and detoxification of drugs and poisons. Lacks surface ribosomes.	Liver hepatocytes and steroid hormone–producing cells of the adrenal cortex and gonads are rich in SER.

Cell trafficking

Golgi is the distribution center for proteins and lipids from the ER to the vesicles and plasma membrane. Modifies N-oligosaccharides on asparagine. Adds O-oligosaccharides on serine and threonine. Adds mannose-6-phosphate to proteins for trafficking to lysosomes.

Endosomes are sorting centers for material from outside the cell or from the Golgi, sending it to lysosomes for destruction or back to the membrane/Golgi for further use.

I-cell disease (inclusion cell disease/mucolipidosis type II)—inherited lysosomal storage disorder; defect in N-acetylglucosaminyl-1-phosphotransferase → failure of the Golgi to phosphorylate mannose residues (ie, ↓ mannose-6-phosphate) on glycoproteins → proteins are secreted extracellularly rather than delivered to lysosomes. Results in coarse facial features, clouded corneas, restricted joint movement, and high plasma levels of lysosomal enzymes. Often fatal in childhood.

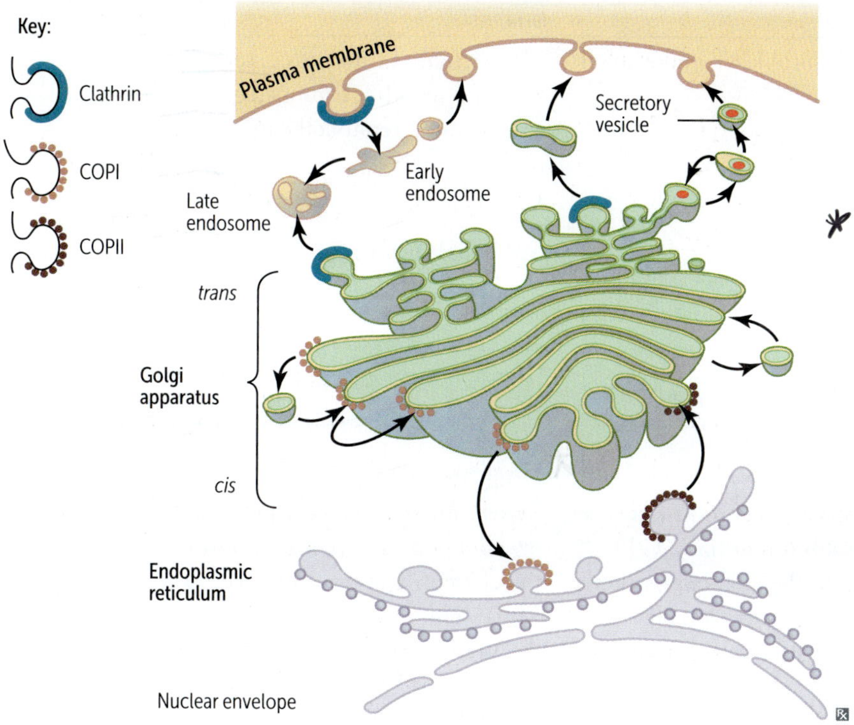

Signal recognition particle (SRP)

Abundant, cytosolic ribonucleoprotein that traffics proteins from the ribosome to the RER. Absent or dysfunctional SRP → proteins accumulate in the cytosol.

Vesicular trafficking proteins

COPI: Golgi → Golgi (retrograde); *cis*-Golgi → ER.

COPII: ER → *cis*-Golgi (anterograde).

Clathrin: *trans*-Golgi → lysosomes; plasma membrane → endosomes (receptor-mediated endocytosis [eg, LDL receptor activity]).

Peroxisome

Membrane-enclosed organelle involved in catabolism of very-long-chain fatty acids (through β-oxidation), branched-chain fatty acids, amino acids, and ethanol.

Proteasome

Barrel-shaped protein complex that degrades damaged or ubiquitin-tagged proteins. Defects in the ubiquitin-proteasome system have been implicated in some cases of Parkinson disease.

Cytoskeletal elements A network of protein fibers within the cytoplasm that supports cell structure, cell and organelle movement, and cell division.

TYPE OF FILAMENT	PREDOMINANT FUNCTION	EXAMPLES
Microfilaments	Muscle contraction, cytokinesis	Actin, microvilli.
Intermediate filaments	Maintain cell structure	Vimentin, desmin, cytokeratin, lamins, glial fibrillary acid proteins (GFAP), neurofilaments.
Microtubules	Movement, cell division	Cilia, flagella, mitotic spindle, axonal trafficking, centrioles.

Immunohistochemical stains for intermediate filaments

STAIN	CELL TYPE	IDENTIFIES
Vimentin	Mesenchymal tissue (eg, fibroblasts, endothelial cells, macrophages)	Mesenchymal tumors (eg, sarcoma), but also many other tumors (eg, endometrial carcinoma, renal cell carcinoma, and meningiomas)
DesMin	Muscle	Muscle tumors (eg, rhabdomyosarcoma)
Cytokeratin	Epithelial cells	Epithelial tumors (eg, squamous cell carcinoma)
GFAP	NeuroGlia (eg, astrocytes, Schwann cells, oligodendroglia)	Astrocytoma, glioblastoma
Neurofilaments	Neurons	Neuronal tumors (eg, neuroblastoma)

Microtubule

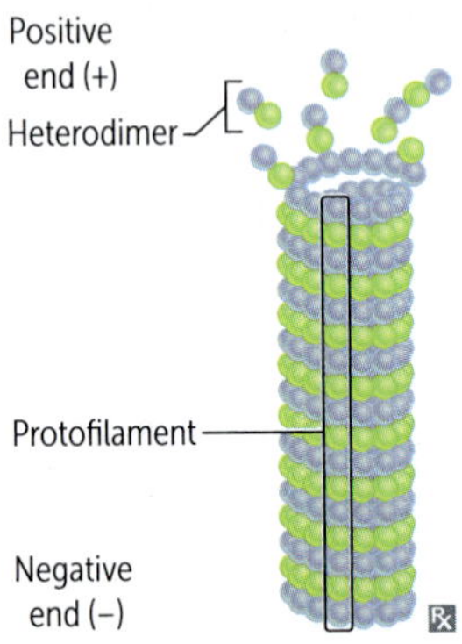

Cylindrical outer structure composed of a helical array of polymerized heterodimers of α- and β-tubulin. Each dimer has 2 GTP bound. Incorporated into flagella, cilia, mitotic spindles. Grows slowly, collapses quickly. Also involved in slow axoplasmic transport in neurons.

Molecular motor proteins—transport cellular cargo toward opposite ends of microtubule tracks.

- Dynein—retrograde to microtubule (+ → −).
- Kinesin—anterograde to microtubule (− → +).

Drugs that act on microtubules (Microtubules Get Constructed Very Poorly):

- Mebendazole (antihelminthic)
- Griseofulvin (antifungal)
- Colchicine (antigout)
- Vincristine/Vinblastine (anticancer)
- Paclitaxel (anticancer)

Cilia structure

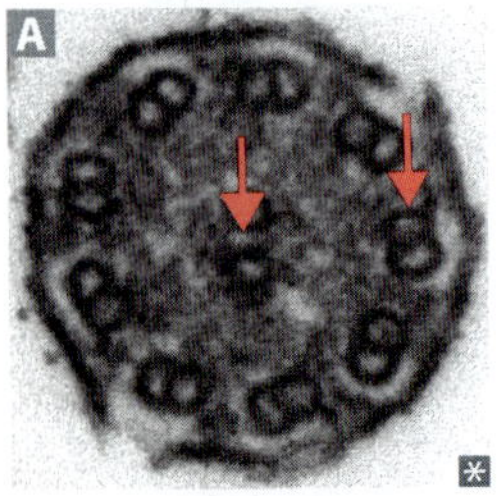

9 + 2 arrangement of microtubule doublets (arrows in A). The base of a cilium below the cell membrane, called the basal body, consists of 9 microtubule triplets with no central microtubules.

Axonemal dynein—ATPase that links peripheral 9 doublets and causes bending of cilium by differential sliding of doublets.

Kartagener syndrome (1° ciliary dyskinesia)—immotile cilia due to a dynein arm defect. Results in male and female infertility due to immotile sperm and dysfunctional fallopian tube cilia, respectively; ↑ risk of ectopic pregnancy. Can cause bronchiectasis, recurrent sinusitis, and situs inversus (eg, dextrocardia on CXR).

Plasma membrane composition

Asymmetric lipid bilayer.
Contains cholesterol, phospholipids, sphingolipids, glycolipids, and proteins. Fungal membranes contain ergosterol.

Sodium-potassium pump

Na^+-K^+ ATPase is located in the plasma membrane with ATP site on cytosolic side. For each ATP consumed, $3Na^+$ go out of the cell (pump phosphorylated) and $2K^+$ come into the cell (pump dephosphorylated).

Ouabain inhibits by binding to K^+ site.
Cardiac glycosides (digoxin and digitoxin) directly inhibit the Na^+-K^+ ATPase, which leads to indirect inhibition of Na^+/Ca^{2+} exchange → ↑ $[Ca^{2+}]_i$ → ↑ cardiac contractility.

- Na powers by going into cell to kick Ca out

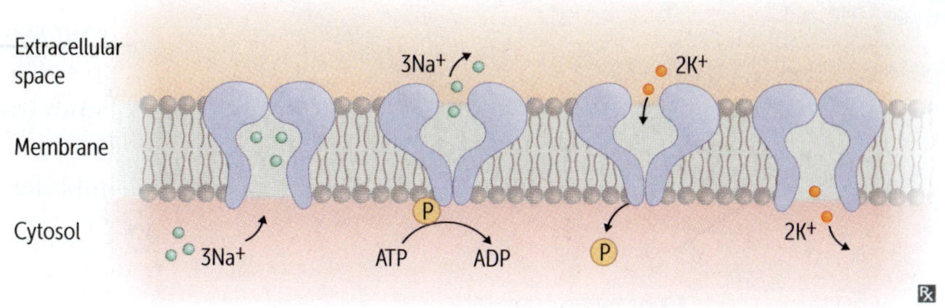

Collagen	Most abundant protein in the human body. Extensively modified by posttranslational modification. Organizes and strengthens extracellular matrix. → no wrinkles	Be (So Totally) Cool, Read Books.
Type I	Most common (90%)—Bone (made by osteoblasts), Skin, Tendon, dentin, fascia, cornea, late wound repair.	Type I: bone. ↓ production in osteogenesis imperfecta type I.
Type II	Cartilage (including hyaline), vitreous body, nucleus pulposus.	Type II: cartwolage.
Type III	Reticulin—skin, blood vessels, uterus, fetal tissue, granulation tissue.	Type III: deficient in the uncommon, vascular type of Ehlers-Danlos syndrome (ThreE D).
Type IV	Basement membrane, basal lamina, lens.	Type IV: under the floor (basement membrane). Defective in Alport syndrome; targeted by autoantibodies in Goodpasture syndrome.

Collagen synthesis and structure

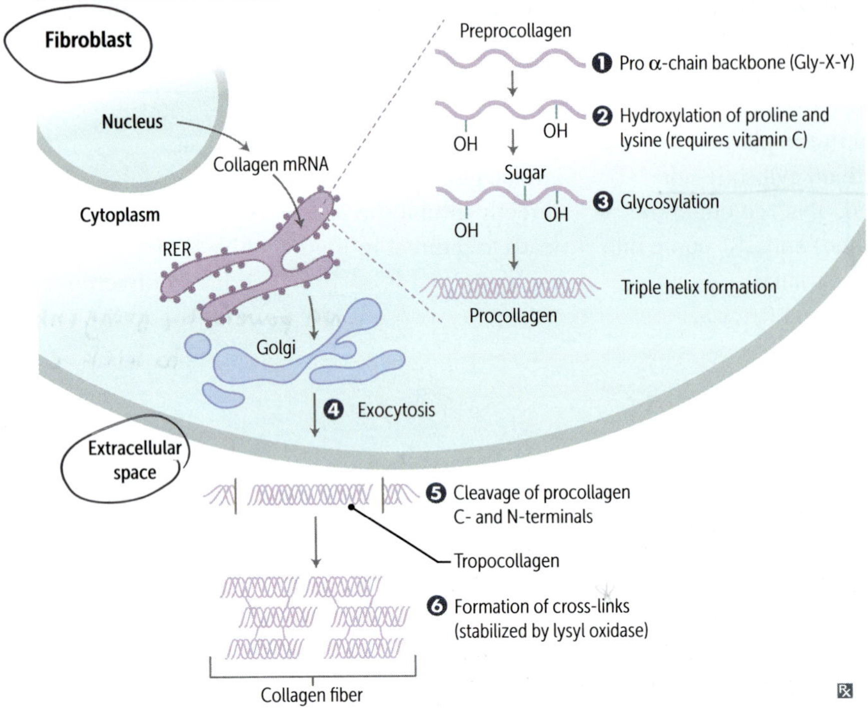

❶ Synthesis—translation of collagen α chains (preprocollagen)—usually Gly-X-Y (X and Y are proline or lysine). Glycine content best reflects collagen synthesis (collagen is ⅓ glycine). * wow

❷ Hydroxylation—hydroxylation of specific proline and lysine residues. Requires vitamin C; deficiency → scurvy. *

❸ Glycosylation—glycosylation of pro-α-chain hydroxylysine residues and formation of procollagen via hydrogen and disulfide bonds (triple helix of 3 collagen α chains). Problems forming triple helix → osteogenesis imperfecta.

❹ Exocytosis—exocytosis of procollagen into extracellular space.

❺ Proteolytic processing—cleavage of disulfide-rich terminal regions of procollagen → insoluble tropocollagen.

❻ Cross-linking—reinforcement of many staggered tropocollagen molecules by covalent lysine-hydroxylysine cross-linkage (by copper-containing lysyl oxidase) to make collagen fibrils. Problems with cross-linking → Ehlers-Danlos syndrome, Menkes disease.

Osteogenesis imperfecta

Genetic bone disorder (brittle bone disease) caused by a variety of gene defects (most commonly *COL1A1* and *COL1A2*).

Most common form is autosomal dominant with ↓ production of otherwise normal type I collagen. Manifestations can include:

- Multiple fractures with minimal trauma A B; may occur during the birth process
- Blue sclerae C due to the translucent connective tissue over choroidal veins
- Hearing loss (abnormal ossicles)
- Some forms have tooth abnormalities, including opalescent teeth that wear easily due to lack of dentin (dentinogenesis imperfecta)

May be confused with child abuse.

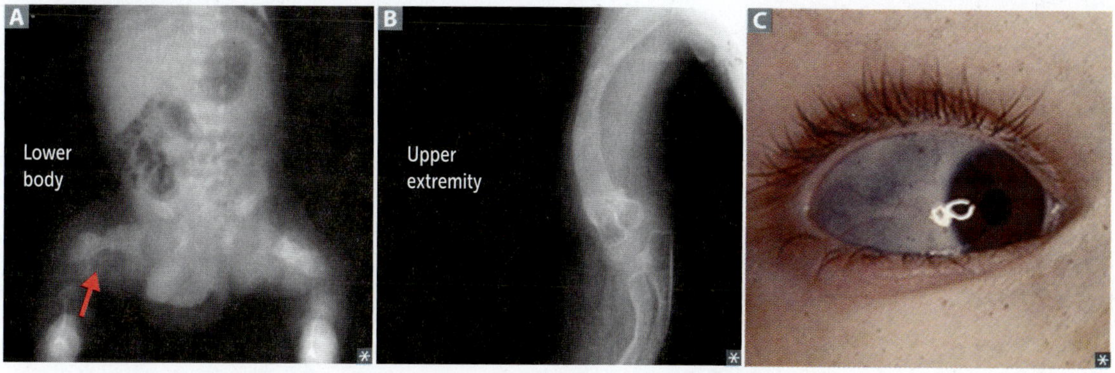

Ehlers-Danlos syndrome

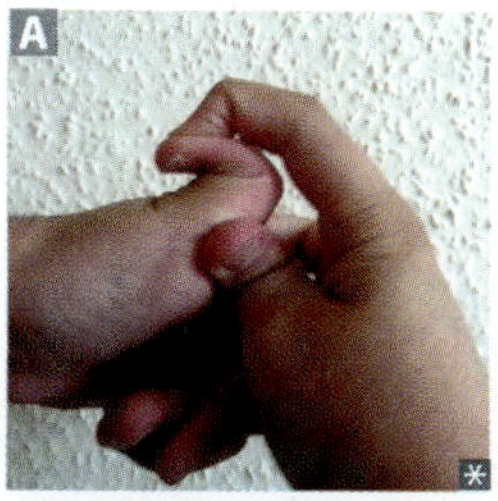

Faulty collagen synthesis causing hyperextensible skin, tendency to bleed (easy bruising), and hypermobile joints A.

Multiple types. Inheritance and severity vary. Can be autosomal dominant or recessive. May be associated with joint dislocation, berry and aortic aneurysms, organ rupture.

Hyperext skin, joints, bleeds

Hypermobility type (joint instability): most common type.

Classical type (joint and skin symptoms): caused by a mutation in type V collagen.

Vascular type (vascular and organ rupture): deficient type III collagen.

Menkes disease

X-linked recessive connective tissue disease caused by impaired copper absorption and transport due to defective Menkes protein (ATP7A). Leads to ↓ activity of lysyl oxidase (copper is a necessary cofactor). Results in brittle, "kinky" hair, growth retardation, and hypotonia.

Elastin

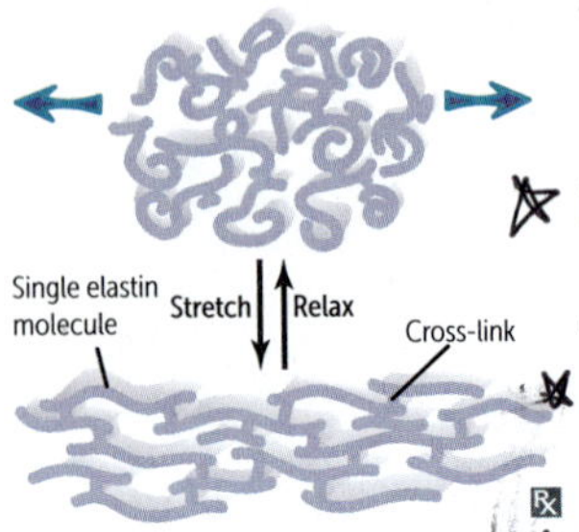

Stretchy protein within skin, lungs, large arteries, elastic ligaments, vocal cords, ligamenta flava (connect vertebrae → relaxed and stretched conformations).

Rich in nonhydroxylated proline, glycine, and lysine residues.

Tropoelastin with fibrillin scaffolding.

Cross-linking takes place extracellularly and gives elastin its elastic properties.

Broken down by elastase, which is normally inhibited by α_1-antitrypsin.

Marfan syndrome—caused by a defect in fibrillin, a glycoprotein that forms a sheath around elastin.

Emphysema—can be caused by α_1-antitrypsin deficiency, resulting in excess elastase activity.

Wrinkles of aging are due to ↓ collagen and elastin production.

▸ BIOCHEMISTRY—LABORATORY TECHNIQUES

Polymerase chain reaction

Molecular biology laboratory procedure used to amplify a desired fragment of DNA. Useful as a diagnostic tool (eg, neonatal HIV, herpes encephalitis).

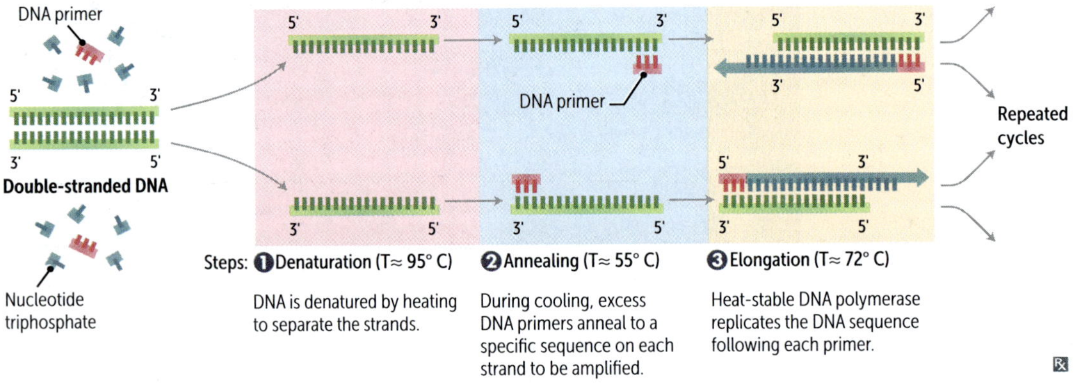

- gel elechoph = sep by charge & size

Blotting procedures

Southern blot	1. **DNA** sample is enzymatically cleaved into smaller pieces, which are separated on a gel by electrophoresis, and then transferred to a filter. (more stable) 2. Filter is exposed to radiolabeled DNA probe that recognizes and anneals to its complementary strand. → the gene A of our interest 3. Resulting double-stranded, labeled piece of DNA is visualized when filter is exposed to film. → XRAY. Pop up on the film	SNoW DRoP: Southern = DNA Northern = RNA Western = Protein - want to see if gene A is in that cup of DNA. cleave the cup of dna ①
Northern blot	Similar to Southern blot, except that an **RNA** sample is electrophoresed. Useful for studying mRNA levels, which are reflective of gene expression.	
Western blot	Sample protein is separated via gel electrophoresis and transferred to a membrane. Labeled antibody is used to bind to relevant **protein**. Confirmatory test for HIV after ⊕ ELISA.	Protein gel electrophor sep. Antibody binds.
Southwestern blot	Identifies **DNA-binding proteins** (eg, transcription factors) using labeled oligonucleotide probes.	

Flow cytometry

Laboratory technique to assess size, granularity, and protein expression (immunophenotype) of individual cells in a sample.

Commonly used in workup of hematologic abnormalities (eg, paroxysmal nocturnal hemoglobinuria, fetal RBCs in mother's blood) and immunodeficiencies (eg, CD4 cell count in HIV).

Cells are tagged with antibodies specific to surface or intracellular proteins. Antibodies are then tagged with a unique fluorescent dye. Sample is analyzed one cell at a time by focusing a laser on the cell and measuring light scatter and intensity of fluorescence.

Data are plotted either as histogram (one measure) or scatter plot (any two measures, as shown). In illustration:

- Cells in left lower quadrant ⊖ for both CD8 and CD3.
- Cells in right lower quadrant ⊕ for CD8. (Right lower quadrant is empty because all CD8-expressing cells also express CD3.)
- Cells in left upper quadrant ⊕ for CD3.
- Cells in right upper quadrant ⊕ for CD8 and CD3 (red + blue → purple).

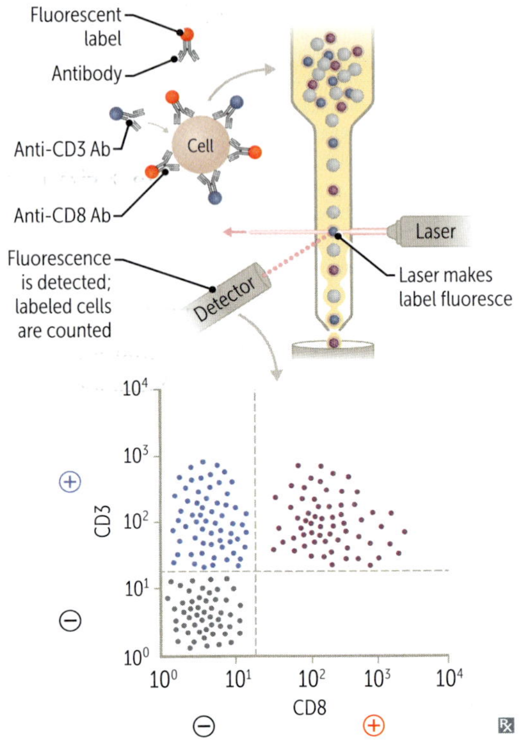

Microarrays

Thousands of nucleic acid sequences are arranged in grids on glass or silicon. DNA or RNA probes are hybridized to the chip, and a scanner detects the relative amounts of complementary binding.

Used to profile gene expression levels of thousands of genes simultaneously to study certain diseases and treatments. Able to detect single nucleotide polymorphisms (SNPs) and copy number variations (CNVs) for a variety of applications including genotyping, clinical genetic testing, forensic analysis, cancer mutations, and genetic linkage analysis.

Enzyme-linked immunosorbent assay	Immunologic test used to detect the presence of either a specific antigen (eg, HBsAg) or antibody (eg, anti-HBs) in a patient's blood sample. Detection involves the use of an antibody linked to an enzyme. Added substrate reacts with enzyme, producing a detectable signal (eg, color change). Major ELISA variations include direct, sandwich, and competitive. Can have high sensitivity and specificity.
Karyotyping	A process in which metaphase chromosomes are stained, ordered, and numbered according to morphology, size, arm-length ratio, and banding pattern. Can be performed on a sample of blood, bone marrow, amniotic fluid, or placental tissue. Used to diagnose chromosomal imbalances (eg, autosomal trisomies, sex chromosome disorders).
Fluorescence in situ hybridization	Fluorescent DNA or RNA probe binds to specific gene site of interest on chromosomes. Used for specific localization of genes and direct visualization of chromosomal anomalies at the molecular level. ▪ Microdeletion—no fluorescence on a chromosome compared to fluorescence at the same locus on the second copy of that chromosome ▪ Translocation—fluorescence outside the original chromosome ▪ Duplication—extra site of fluorescence on one chromosome relative to its homologous chromosome
Cloning methods	Cloning is the production of a recombinant DNA molecule that is self-perpetuating. Steps: 1. Isolate eukaryotic mRNA (post-RNA processing steps) of interest. 2. Expose mRNA to reverse transcriptase to produce cDNA (lacks introns). 3. Insert cDNA fragments into bacterial plasmids containing antibiotic resistance genes. 4. Transform recombinant plasmid into bacteria. 5. Surviving bacteria on antibiotic medium produce cloned DNA (copies of cDNA).

Gene expression modifications	Transgenic strategies in mice involve: ▪ Random insertion of gene into mouse genome ▪ Targeted insertion or deletion of gene through homologous recombination with mouse gene	Knock-**out** = removing a gene, taking it **out**. Knock-**in** = **in**serting a gene.
Cre-lox system	Can inducibly manipulate genes at specific developmental points (eg, to study a gene whose deletion causes embryonic death).	
RNA interference	dsRNA is synthesized that is complementary to the mRNA sequence of interest. When transfected into human cells, dsRNA separates and promotes degradation of target mRNA, "knocking down" gene expression.	

▸ BIOCHEMISTRY—GENETICS

Genetic terms

TERM	DEFINITION	EXAMPLE
Codominance	Both alleles contribute to the phenotype of the heterozygote.	Blood groups A, B, AB; α_1-antitrypsin deficiency.
Variable expressivity	Phenotype varies among individuals with same genotype.	2 patients with neurofibromatosis type 1 (NF1) may have varying disease severity.
Incomplete penetrance	Not all individuals with a mutant genotype show the mutant phenotype.	*BRCA1* gene mutations do not always result in breast or ovarian cancer.
Pleiotropy	One gene contributes to multiple phenotypic effects.	Untreated phenylketonuria (PKU) manifests with light skin, intellectual disability, and musty body odor.
Anticipation	Increased severity or earlier onset of disease in succeeding generations.	Trinucleotide repeat diseases (eg, Huntington disease).
Loss of heterozygosity	If a patient inherits or develops a mutation in a tumor suppressor gene, the complementary allele must be deleted/mutated before cancer develops. This is not true of oncogenes.	Retinoblastoma and the "two-hit hypothesis," Lynch syndrome (HNPCC), Li-Fraumeni syndrome.
Dominant negative mutation	Exerts a dominant effect. A heterozygote produces a nonfunctional altered protein that also prevents the normal gene product from functioning.	Mutation of a transcription factor in its allosteric site. Nonfunctioning mutant can still bind DNA, preventing wild-type transcription factor from binding.
Linkage disequilibrium	Tendency for certain alleles at 2 linked loci to occur together more or less often than expected by chance. Measured in a population, not in a family, and often varies in different populations.	

Genetic terms *(continued)*

TERM	DEFINITION	EXAMPLE
Mosaicism	Presence of genetically distinct cell lines in the same individual. Somatic mosaicism—mutation arises from mitotic errors after fertilization and propagates through multiple tissues or organs. Gonadal mosaicism—mutation only in egg or sperm cells.	**McCune-Albright syndrome**—due to mutation affecting G-protein signaling. Presents with unilateral café-au-lait spots, polyostotic fibrous dysplasia, precocious puberty, multiple endocrine abnormalities. Lethal if mutation occurs before fertilization (affecting all cells), but survivable in patients with mosaicism.
Locus heterogeneity	Mutations at different loci can produce a similar phenotype.	Albinism.
Allelic heterogeneity	Different mutations in the same locus produce the same phenotype.	β-thalassemia.
Heteroplasmy	Presence of both normal and mutated mtDNA, resulting in variable expression in mitochondrially inherited disease.	
Uniparental disomy	Offspring receives 2 copies of a chromosome from 1 parent and no copies from the other parent. Heterodisomy (heterozygous) indicates a meiosis I error. Isodisomy (homozygous) indicates a meiosis II error or postzygotic chromosomal duplication of one of a pair of chromosomes, and loss of the other of the original pair.	Uniparental is eUploid (correct number of chromosomes), not aneuploid. Most occurrences of UPD → normal phenotype. Consider UPD in an individual manifesting a recessive disorder when only one parent is a carrier.

Hardy-Weinberg population genetics

	pA	*qa*
pA	*AA* $p \times p = p^2$	*Aa* $p \times q$
qa	*Aa* $p \times q$	*aa* $q \times q = q^2$

If a population is in Hardy-Weinberg equilibrium and if p and q are the frequencies of separate alleles, then: $p^2 + 2pq + q^2 = 1$ and $p + q = 1$, which implies that:

p^2 = frequency of homozygosity for allele p

q^2 = frequency of homozygosity for allele q

$2pq$ = frequency of heterozygosity (carrier frequency, if an autosomal recessive disease).

The frequency of an X-linked recessive disease in males = q and in females = q^2.

Hardy-Weinberg law assumptions include:

- No mutation occurring at the locus
- Natural selection is not occurring
- Completely random mating
- No net migration

Imprinting	At some loci, only one allele is active; the other is inactive (imprinted/inactivated by methylation). With one allele inactivated, deletion of the active allele → disease.	Both Prader-Willi and Angelman syndromes are due to mutation or deletion of genes on chromosome 15.
Prader-Willi syndrome	Maternal imprinting: gene from mom is normally silent and Paternal gene is deleted/mutated. Results in hyperphagia, obesity, intellectual disability, hypogonadism, and hypotonia.	25% of cases due to maternal uniparental disomy (two maternally imprinted genes are received; no paternal gene received).
AngelMan syndrome	Paternal imprinting: gene from dad is normally silent and Maternal gene is deleted/mutated. Results in inappropriate laughter ("happy puppet"), seizures, ataxia, and severe intellectual disability.	5% of cases due to paternal uniparental disomy (two paternally imprinted genes are received; no maternal gene received).

Modes of inheritance

Autosomal dominant 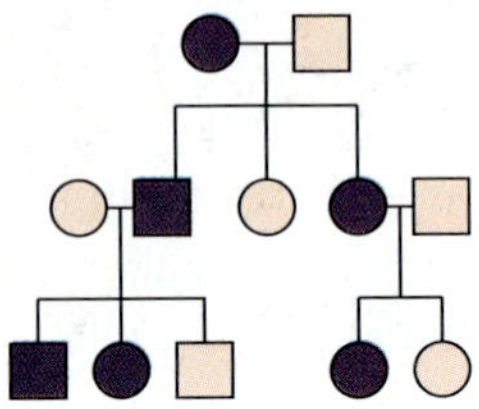	Often due to defects in structural genes. Many generations, both male and female, affected.	Often pleiotropic (multiple apparently unrelated effects) and variably expressive (different between individuals). Family history crucial to diagnosis. With one affected (heterozygous) parent, on average, ½ of children affected.
Autosomal recessive 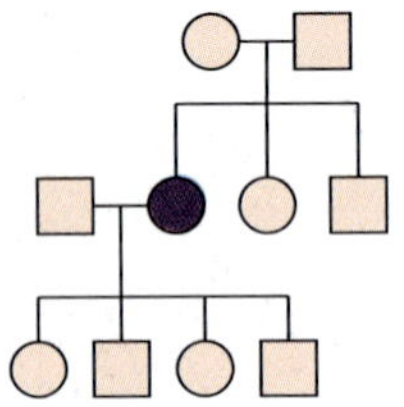	Often due to enzyme deficiencies. Usually seen in only 1 generation.	Commonly more severe than dominant disorders; patients often present in childhood. ↑ risk in consanguineous families. With 2 carrier (heterozygous) parents, on average: ¼ of children will be affected (homozygous), ½ of children will be carriers, and ¼ of children will be neither affected nor carriers.
X-linked recessive 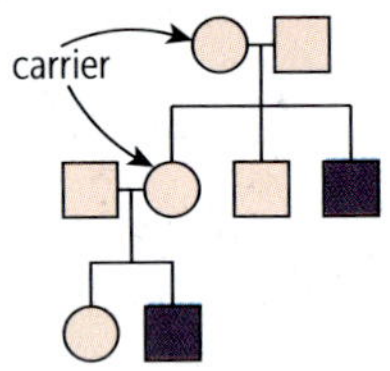	Sons of heterozygous mothers have a 50% chance of being affected. No male-to-male transmission. Skips generations.	Commonly more severe in males. Females usually must be homozygous to be affected.
X-linked dominant 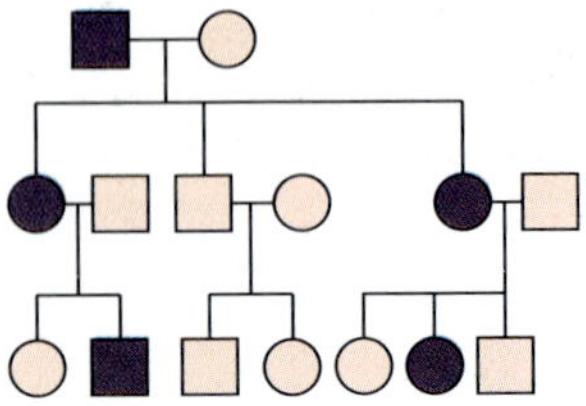	Transmitted through both parents. Mothers transmit to 50% of daughters and sons; fathers transmit to all daughters but no sons.	**Hypophosphatemic rickets**—formerly known as vitamin D–resistant rickets. Inherited disorder resulting in ↑ phosphate wasting at proximal tubule. Results in rickets-like presentation. Other examples: Rett syndrome, fragile X syndrome, Alport syndrome.
Mitochondrial inheritance 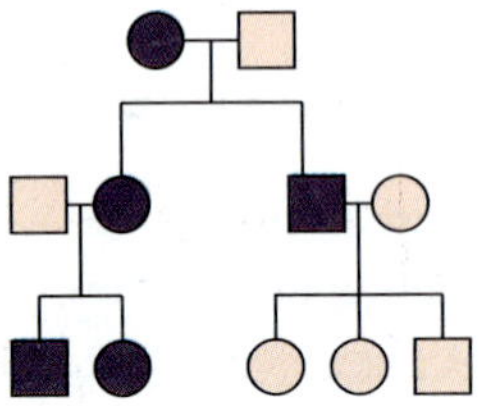	Transmitted only through the mother. All offspring of affected females may show signs of disease.	Variable expression in a population or even within a family due to heteroplasmy. **Mitochondrial myopathies**—rare disorders; often present with myopathy, lactic acidosis, and CNS disease, eg, MELAS syndrome (mitochondrial encephalopathy, lactic acidosis, and stroke-like episodes). 2° to failure in oxidative phosphorylation. Muscle biopsy often shows "ragged red fibers."

□ = unaffected male; ■ = affected male; ○ = unaffected female; ● = affected female.

Melas - every organ
has mitoch
so Sx widespread
↳ DM, Deaf
HARD to Dx

Autosomal dominant diseases

Achondroplasia	Mutation of fibroblast growth factor receptor 3 (*FGFR3*) inhibits chondrocyte proliferation. Most common cause of dwarfism; limb length affected more than head or torso size. Full penetrance.
Autosomal dominant polycystic kidney disease	Bilateral, massive enlargement of kidneys due to multiple large cysts. 85% of cases are due to mutation in *PKD1* (chromosome 16; 16 letters in "polycystic kidney"); remainder due to mutation in *PKD2* (chromosome 4).
Familial adenomatous polyposis	Colon becomes covered with adenomatous polyps after puberty. Progresses to colon cancer unless colon is resected. Mutations on chromosome 5q (*APC* gene); 5 letters in "polyp."
Familial hypercholesterolemia	Elevated LDL due to defective or absent LDL receptor. Leads to severe atherosclerotic disease early in life, corneal arcus, tendon xanthomas (classically in the Achilles tendon).
Hereditary hemorrhagic telangiectasia	Inherited disorder of blood vessels. Findings: branching skin lesions (telangiectasias), recurrent epistaxis, skin discolorations, arteriovenous malformations (AVMs), GI bleeding, hematuria. Also known as Osler-Weber-Rendu syndrome.
Hereditary spherocytosis	Spheroid erythrocytes due to spectrin or ankyrin defect; hemolytic anemia; ↑ MCHC, ↑ RDW. Treatment: splenectomy.
Huntington disease	Findings: depression, progressive dementia, choreiform movements, and caudate atrophy. ↑ dopamine, ↓ GABA, ↓ ACh in the brain. Gene on chromosome 4; trinucleotide repeat disorder: $(CAG)_n$. Demonstrates anticipation: ↑ repeats → ↓ age of onset. "Hunting 4 CAGs."
Li-Fraumeni syndrome	Abnormalities in *TP53* → multiple malignancies at an early age. Also known as SBLA cancer syndrome (sarcoma, breast, leukemia, adrenal gland).
Marfan syndrome	*FBN1* gene mutation on chromosome 15 → defective fibrillin (scaffold for elastin) → connective tissue disorder affecting skeleton, heart, and eyes. Findings: tall with long extremities, pectus excavatum, hypermobile joints, and long, tapering fingers and toes (arachnodactyly); cystic medial necrosis of aorta → aortic incompetence and dissecting aortic aneurysms; floppy mitral valve. Subluxation of lenses, typically upward and temporally.
Multiple endocrine neoplasias (MEN)	Several distinct syndromes (1, 2A, 2B) characterized by familial tumors of endocrine glands, including those of the pancreas, parathyroid, pituitary, thyroid, and adrenal medulla. MEN 1 is associated with *MEN1* gene, MEN 2A and 2B are associated with *RET* gene.
Neurofibromatosis type 1 (von Recklinghausen disease)	Neurocutaneous disorder characterized by café-au-lait spots, cutaneous neurofibromas, optic gliomas, pheochromocytomas, Lisch nodules (pigmented iris hamartomas). 100% penetrance, variable expression. Caused by mutations in the *NF1* gene on chromosome 17; 17 letters in "von Recklinghausen."
Neurofibromatosis type 2	Findings: bilateral acoustic schwannomas, juvenile cataracts, meningiomas, and ependymomas. *NF2* gene on chromosome 22; type 2 = 22.
Tuberous sclerosis	Neurocutaneous disorder with multi-organ system involvement, characterized by numerous benign hamartomas. Variable expression.
von Hippel-Lindau disease	Disorder characterized by development of numerous tumors, both benign and malignant. Associated with deletion of *VHL* gene (tumor suppressor) on chromosome 3 (3p). Von Hippel-Lindau = 3 words for chromosome 3.

VHL
- Hemangioblastomas - 60-80%.
  - cerebrallum
  - Spinal cord, brainstem
- kidney cancer
  - 40%, Most common cause of death.
- Eye = 60% hemangiob.

Autosomal recessive diseases

Albinism, autosomal recessive polycystic kidney disease (ARPKD), cystic fibrosis, glycogen storage diseases, hemochromatosis, Kartagener syndrome, mucopolysaccharidoses (except Hunter syndrome), phenylketonuria, sickle cell anemia, sphingolipidoses (except Fabry disease), thalassemias, Wilson disease.

Cystic fibrosis

GENETICS	Autosomal recessive; defect in *CFTR* gene on chromosome 7; commonly a deletion of Phe508. Most common lethal genetic disease in Caucasian population.
PATHOPHYSIOLOGY	*CFTR* encodes an ATP-gated Cl^- channel that secretes Cl^- in lungs and GI tract, and reabsorbs Cl^- in sweat glands. Most common mutation → misfolded protein → protein retained in RER and not transported to cell membrane, causing ↓ Cl^- (and H_2O) secretion; ↑ intracellular Cl^- results in compensatory ↑ Na^+ reabsorption via epithelial Na^+ channels → ↑ H_2O reabsorption → abnormally thick mucus secreted into lungs and GI tract. ↑ Na^+ reabsorption also causes more negative transepithelial potential difference.
DIAGNOSIS	↑ Cl^- concentration (> 60 mEq/L) in sweat is diagnostic. Can present with contraction alkalosis and hypokalemia (ECF effects analogous to a patient taking a loop diuretic) because of ECF H_2O/Na^+ losses and concomitant renal K^+/H^+ wasting. ↑ immunoreactive trypsinogen (newborn screening).
COMPLICATIONS	Recurrent pulmonary infections (eg, *S aureus* [early infancy], *P aeruginosa* [adolescence]), chronic bronchitis and bronchiectasis → reticulonodular pattern on CXR. Pancreatic insufficiency, malabsorption with steatorrhea, fat-soluble vitamin deficiencies (A, D, E, K), biliary cirrhosis, liver disease. Meconium ileus in newborns. Infertility in men (absence of vas deferens, spermatogenesis may be unaffected) and subfertility in women (amenorrhea, abnormally thick cervical mucus). Nasal polyps, clubbing of nails.
TREATMENT	Multifactorial: chest physiotherapy, albuterol, aerosolized dornase alfa (DNAse), and hypertonic saline facilitate mucus clearance. Azithromycin used as anti-inflammatory agent. Pancreatic enzymes for insufficiency.

X-linked recessive disorders

Ornithine transcarbamylase deficiency, Fabry disease, Wiskott-Aldrich syndrome, Ocular albinism, G6PD deficiency, Hunter syndrome, Bruton agammaglobulinemia, Hemophilia A and B, Lesch-Nyhan syndrome, Duchenne (and Becker) muscular dystrophy.

Female carriers can be variably affected depending on the percentage inactivation of the X chromosome carrying the mutant vs normal gene.

Oblivious Female Will Often Give Her Boys Her x-Linked Disorders

Muscular dystrophies

Duchenne 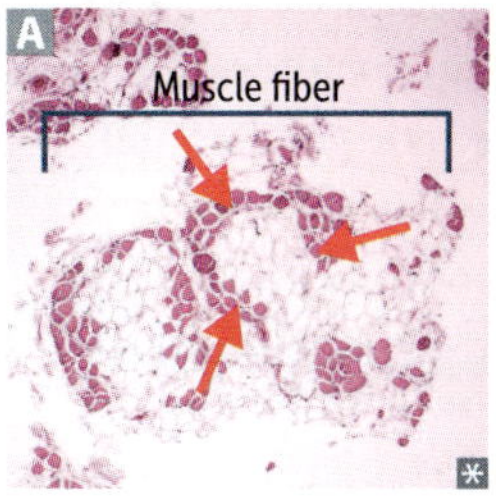	X-linked disorder typically due to **frameshift** or nonsense mutations → truncated dystrophin protein → inhibited muscle regeneration. Weakness begins in pelvic girdle muscles and progresses superiorly. Pseudohypertrophy of calf muscles due to fibrofatty replacement of muscle A. Gower maneuver—patients use upper extremities to help them stand up. Waddling gait. Onset before 5 years of age. Dilated cardiomyopathy is common cause of death.	Duchenne = deleted dystrophin. Dystrophin gene (*DMD*) is the largest protein-coding human gene → ↑ chance of spontaneous mutation. Dystrophin helps anchor muscle fibers, primarily in skeletal and cardiac muscle. It connects the intracellular cytoskeleton (actin) to the transmembrane proteins α- and β-dystroglycan, which are connected to the extracellular matrix (ECM). Loss of dystrophin results in myonecrosis. ↑ CK and aldolase are seen; Western blot and muscle biopsy confirm diagnosis.
Becker	X-linked disorder typically due to **non-frameshift** insertions in dystrophin gene (partially functional instead of truncated). Less severe than Duchenne. Onset in adolescence or early adulthood. (later)	Deletions can cause both Duchenne and Becker.
Myotonic type 1	Autosomal dominant. CTG trinucleotide repeat expansion in the *DMPK* gene → abnormal expression of myotonin protein kinase → myotonia, muscle wasting, cataracts, testicular atrophy, frontal balding, arrhythmia.	My Tonia, My Testicles (testicular atrophy), My Toupee (frontal balding), My Ticker (arrhythmia).

Fragile X syndrome	X-linked dominant inheritance. Trinucleotide repeat in *FMR1* gene → methylation → ↓ expression. The 2nd most common cause of genetic intellectual disability (after Down syndrome). Findings: post-pubertal macroorchidism (enlarged testes), long face with a large jaw, large everted ears, autism, mitral valve prolapse.	Trinucleotide repeat disorder $(CGG)_n$. Fragile X = eXtra large testes, jaw, ears.
Trinucleotide repeat expansion diseases	Huntington disease, myotonic dystrophy, Friedreich ataxia, fragile X syndrome. Fragile X syndrome = $(CGG)_n$. Friedreich ataxia = $(GAA)_n$. Huntington disease = $(CAG)_n$. Myotonic dystrophy = $(CTG)_n$.	Try (trinucleotide) hunting for my fried eggs (X). X-Girlfriend's First Aid Helped Ace My Test. May show genetic anticipation (disease severity ↑ and age of onset ↓ in successive generations).

Autosomal trisomies

Down syndrome (trisomy 21)	Findings: intellectual disability, flat facies, prominent epicanthal folds, single palmar crease, gap between 1st 2 toes, duodenal atresia, Hirschsprung disease, congenital heart disease (eg, atrioventricular septal defect), Brushfield spots. Associated with early-onset Alzheimer disease (chromosome 21 codes for amyloid precursor protein) and ↑ risk of ALL and AML. 95% of cases due to meiotic nondisjunction (↑ with advanced maternal age; from 1:1500 in women < 20 to 1:25 in women > 45 years old). 4% of cases due to unbalanced Robertsonian translocation, most typically between chromosomes 14 and 21. 1% of cases due to mosaicism (no maternal association; post-fertilization mitotic error).	Incidence 1:700. Drinking age (21). Most common viable chromosomal disorder and most common cause of genetic intellectual disability. First-trimester ultrasound commonly shows ↑ nuchal translucency and hypoplastic nasal bone; ↓ serum PAPP-A, ↑ free β-hCG. Second-trimester quad screen shows ↓ α-fetoprotein, ↑ β-hCG, ↓ estriol, ↑ inhibin A.
Edwards syndrome (trisomy 18)	Findings: severe intellectual disability, rocker-bottom feet, micrognathia (small jaw), low-set Ears, clenched hands with overlapping fingers, prominent occiput, congenital heart disease. Death usually occurs within 1 year of birth.	Incidence 1:8000. Election age (18). 2nd most common trisomy resulting in live birth (most common is Down syndrome). PAPP-A and free β-hCG are ↓ in first trimester. Quad screen shows ↓ α-fetoprotein, ↓ β-hCG, ↓ estriol, ↓ or normal inhibin A.
Patau syndrome (trisomy 13)	Findings: severe intellectual disability, rocker-bottom feet, microphthalmia, microcephaly, cleft liP/Palate, holoProsencephaly, Polydactyly, congenital heart disease, cutis aplasia. Death usually occurs within 1 year of birth.	Incidence 1:15,000. Puberty (13). First-trimester pregnancy screen shows ↓ free β-hCG, ↓ PAPP-A.

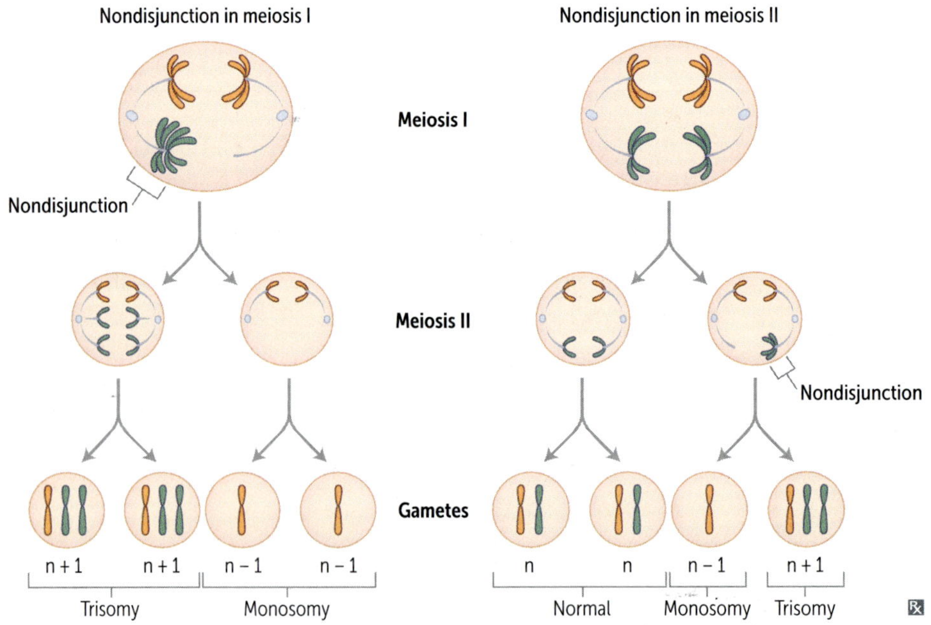

Genetic disorders by chromosome

CHROMOSOME	SELECTED EXAMPLES
3	von Hippel-Lindau disease, renal cell carcinoma
4	ADPKD (*PKD2*), achondroplasia, Huntington disease
5	Cri-du-chat syndrome, familial adenomatous polyposis
6	Hemochromatosis (*HFE*)
7	Williams syndrome, cystic fibrosis
9	Friedreich ataxia
11	Wilms tumor, β-globin gene defects (eg, sickle cell disease, β-thalassemia)
13	Patau syndrome, Wilson disease, retinoblastoma (*RB1*), *BRCA2*
15	Prader-Willi syndrome, Angelman syndrome, Marfan syndrome
16	ADPKD (*PKD1*), α-globin gene defects (eg, α-thalassemia)
17	Neurofibromatosis type 1, *BRCA1*
18	Edwards syndrome
21	Down syndrome
22	Neurofibromatosis type 2, DiGeorge syndrome (22q11)
X	Fragile X syndrome, X-linked agammaglobulinemia, Klinefelter syndrome (XXY)

Robertsonian translocation

Chromosomal translocation that commonly involves chromosome pairs 13, 14, 15, 21, and 22. One of the most common types of translocation. Occurs when the long arms of 2 acrocentric chromosomes (chromosomes with centromeres near their ends) fuse at the centromere and the 2 short arms are lost. Balanced translocations normally do not cause any abnormal phenotype. Unbalanced translocations can result in miscarriage, stillbirth, and chromosomal imbalance (eg, Down syndrome, Patau syndrome).

Cri-du-chat syndrome

Congenital microdeletion of short arm of chromosome 5 (46,XX or XY, 5p−).
Findings: microcephaly, moderate to severe intellectual disability, high-pitched crying/**mewing**, epicanthal folds, cardiac abnormalities (VSD).

Cri du chat = cry of the **cat**.

Williams syndrome

Congenital microdeletion of long arm of chromosome 7 (deleted region includes elastin gene).
Findings: distinctive "elfin" facies, intellectual disability, hypercalcemia (↑ sensitivity to vitamin D), well-developed verbal skills, extreme friendliness with strangers, cardiovascular problems.

22q11 deletion syndromes	Microdeletion at chromosome 22q11 → variable presentations including Cleft palate, Abnormal facies, Thymic aplasia → T-cell deficiency, Cardiac defects, and Hypocalcemia 2° to parathyroid aplasia. DiGeorge syndrome—thymic, parathyroid, and cardiac defects. Velocardiofacial syndrome—palate, facial, and cardiac defects.	CATCH-22. Due to aberrant development of 3rd and 4th branchial pouches.

▶ BIOCHEMISTRY—NUTRITION

Vitamins: fat soluble	A, D, E, K. Absorption dependent on gut and pancreas. Toxicity more common than for water-soluble vitamins because fat-soluble vitamins accumulate in fat.	Malabsorption syndromes with steatorrhea, such as cystic fibrosis and sprue, or mineral oil intake can cause fat-soluble vitamin deficiencies.
Vitamins: water soluble	B_1 (thiamine: TPP) B_2 (riboflavin: FAD, FMN) B_3 (niacin: NAD^+) B_5 (pantothenic acid: CoA) B_6 (pyridoxine: PLP) B_7 (biotin) B_9 (folate) B_{12} (cobalamin) C (ascorbic acid)	All wash out easily from body except B_{12} and B_9 (folate). B_{12} stored in liver for ~ 3–4 years. B_9 stored in liver for ~ 3–4 months. B-complex deficiencies often result in dermatitis, glossitis, and diarrhea. Can be coenzymes (eg, ascorbic acid) or precursors to organic cofactors (eg, FAD, NAD^+).

Vitamin A (retinol)

FUNCTION	Antioxidant; constituent of visual pigments (**retinal**); essential for normal differentiation of epithelial cells into specialized tissue (pancreatic cells, mucus-secreting cells); prevents squamous metaplasia. Used to treat measles and AML subtype M3.	**Retin**ol is vitamin **A**, so think **retin-A** (used topically for wrinkles and **A**cne). Found in liver and leafy vegetables. Use oral isotretinoin to treat severe cystic acne. Use *all*-trans retinoic acid to treat acute promyelocytic leukemia.
DEFICIENCY	Night blindness (nyctalopia); dry, scaly skin (xerosis cutis); corneal degeneration (keratomalacia); Bitot spots on conjunctiva; immunosuppression.	Bitot = build up of desquamated keratin epith cells -on lateral part of eye - From long term xerosis (dryness) of bulbar conjunctiva.
EXCESS	Acute toxicity—nausea, vomiting, vertigo, and blurred vision. Chronic toxicity—alopecia, dry skin (eg, scaliness), hepatic toxicity and enlargement, arthralgias, and pseudotumor cerebri. Teratogenic (cleft palate, cardiac abnormalities), therefore a ⊖ pregnancy test and two forms of contraception are required before isotretinoin (vitamin A derivative) is prescribed.	**Isotret**inoin **is terat**ogenic.

Vitamin B_1 (thiamine)

FUNCTION	In thiamine pyrophosphate (TPP), a cofactor for several dehydrogenase enzyme reactions: ▪ Pyruvate dehydrogenase (links glycolysis to TCA cycle) → That's why in alc. O.D u need Thiam w/ gluc infusion ▪ α-ketoglutarate dehydrogenase (TCA cycle) ▪ Transketolase (HMP shunt) ▪ Branched-chain ketoacid dehydrogenase	Think **ATP**: **α**-ketoglutarate dehydrogenase, **T**ransketolase, and **P**yruvate dehydrogenase. Spell beriberi as **B**er**1B**er**1** to remember vitamin B_1. Wernicke-Korsakoff syndrome—confusion, ophthalmoplegia, ataxia (classic triad) + confabulation, personality change, memory loss (permanent). Damage to medial dorsal nucleus of thalamus, mammillary bodies. MDN
DEFICIENCY	Impaired glucose breakdown → ATP depletion worsened by glucose infusion; highly aerobic tissues (eg, brain, heart) are affected first. Wernicke-Korsakoff syndrome and beriberi. Seen in malnutrition and alcoholism (2° to malnutrition and malabsorption). Diagnosis made by ↑ in RBC transketolase activity following vitamin B_1 administration.	Dry beriberi—polyneuritis, symmetrical muscle wasting. Wet beriberi—high-output cardiac failure (dilated cardiomyopathy), edema. BeriBeri = inflam of nerves + HF from ↓ B_1

Wernicke
- possibly reversible.
- triad as above
- untreated goes to korsakoff (a severe antergrade amnesia w/ confab → Dr. Coppolas ex)
- I think Korsakoff is calmer

Vit A – imp for vision
D – imp for bone dev.

*BOTH imp in immune regul. (paracrine & autocrine)

Vitamin B_2 (riboflavin)

FUNCTION	Component of flavins FAD and FMN, used as cofactors in redox reactions, eg, the succinate dehydrogenase reaction in the TCA cycle.	FAD and FMN are derived from riboFlavin ($B_2 \approx 2$ ATP).
DEFICIENCY	Cheilosis (inflammation of lips, scaling and fissures at the corners of the mouth), Corneal vascularization.	The 2 C's of B_2.

lips (flavor)

Vitamin B_3 (niacin)

FUNCTION	Constituent of NAD^+, $NADP^+$ (used in redox reactions). Derived from tryptophan. Synthesis requires vitamins B_2 and B_6. Used to treat dyslipidemia; lowers levels of VLDL and raises levels of HDL.	NAD derived from Niacin ($B_3 \approx 3$ ATP).
DEFICIENCY 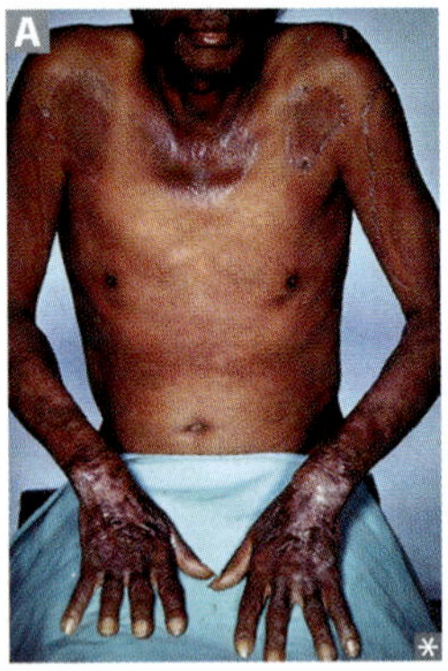	Glossitis. Severe deficiency leads to pellagra, which can be caused by Hartnup disease, malignant carcinoid syndrome (↑ tryptophan metabolism), and isoniazid (↓ vitamin B_6). Symptoms of pellagra: Diarrhea, Dementia (also hallucinations), Dermatitis (C3/C4 dermatome circumferential "broad collar" rash [Casal necklace], hyperpigmentation of sun-exposed limbs A).	The 3 D's of B_3. **Hartnup disease**—autosomal recessive. Deficiency of neutral amino acid (eg, tryptophan) transporters in proximal renal tubular cells and on enterocytes → neutral aminoaciduria and ↓ absorption from the gut → ↓ tryptophan for conversion to niacin → pellagra-like symptoms. Treat with high-protein diet and nicotinic acid.
EXCESS	Facial flushing (induced by prostaglandin, not histamine; can avoid by taking aspirin with niacin), hyperglycemia, hyperuricemia.	

Vitamin B_5 (pantothenic acid)

FUNCTION	Essential component of coenzyme A (CoA, a cofactor for acyl transfers) and fatty acid synthase.	B_5 is "pento"thenic acid.
DEFICIENCY	Dermatitis, enteritis, alopecia, adrenal insufficiency.	

Vitamin B_6 (pyridoxine)

FUNCTION - obvi. very imp. for brain (neurotrans)	Converted to pyridoxal phosphate (PLP), a cofactor used in transamination (eg, ALT and AST), decarboxylation reactions, glycogen phosphorylase. Synthesis of cystathionine, heme, niacin, histamine, and neurotransmitters including serotonin, epinephrine, norepinephrine (NE), dopamine, and GABA.
DEFICIENCY	Convulsions, hyperirritability, peripheral neuropathy (deficiency inducible by isoniazid and oral contraceptives), sideroblastic anemias due to impaired hemoglobin synthesis and iron excess.

Body said "wait our heme is low lets ↑ all the nutrients it needs to make more. All ↑ but B6 = ↑ Fe

Vitamin B_7 (biotin)

FUNCTION	Cofactor for carboxylation enzymes (which add a 1-carbon group): ▪ Pyruvate carboxylase: pyruvate (3C) → oxaloacetate (4C) ▪ Acetyl-CoA carboxylase: acetyl-CoA (2C) → malonyl-CoA (3C) ▪ Propionyl-CoA carboxylase: propionyl-CoA (3C) → methylmalonyl-CoA (4C)	"**Avid**in in egg whites **avid**ly binds biotin."
DEFICIENCY	Relatively rare. Dermatitis, alopecia, enteritis. Caused by antibiotic use or excessive ingestion of raw egg whites.	

Vitamin B_9 (folate)

FUNCTION	Converted to tetrahydrofolic acid (THF), a coenzyme for 1-carbon transfer/methylation reactions. Important for the synthesis of nitrogenous bases in DNA and RNA.	Found in leafy green vegetables. Absorbed in jejunum. **Fol**ate from **fol**iage. Small reserve pool stored primarily in the liver.
DEFICIENCY	Macrocytic, megaloblastic anemia; 75 ✱hypersegmented polymorphonuclear cells (PMNs); glossitis; no neurologic symptoms (as opposed to vitamin B_{12} deficiency). Labs: ↑ homocysteine, normal methylmalonic acid levels. Most common vitamin deficiency in the United States. Seen in alcoholism and pregnancy.	Deficiency can be caused by several drugs (eg, phenytoin, sulfonamides, methotrexate). Supplemental maternal folic acid in early pregnancy ↓ risk of neural tube defects.

Dehydrogenase rxns → B1 thiamine
Decarboxylat → Vit B6 pyridoxine
Carboxylation → B7 biotin
Redox = B2 riboflavin (FAD, FMN)
B3 niacin (NAD, NADP+)

Vitamin B_{12} (cobalamin)

FUNCTION	Cofactor for methionine synthase (transfers CH_3 groups as methylcobalamin) and methylmalonyl-CoA mutase.	Found in animal products. Synthesized only by microorganisms. Very large reserve pool (several years) stored primarily in the liver. Deficiency caused by malabsorption (eg, sprue, enteritis, *Diphyllobothrium latum*), lack of intrinsic factor (pernicious anemia, gastric bypass surgery), absence of terminal ileum (surgical resection, eg, for Crohn disease), or insufficient intake (eg, veganism). Anti-intrinsic factor antibodies diagnostic for pernicious anemia.
DEFICIENCY	Macrocytic, megaloblastic anemia; hypersegmented PMNs; paresthesias and subacute combined degeneration (degeneration of dorsal columns, lateral corticospinal tracts, and spinocerebellar tracts) due to abnormal myelin. Associated with ↑ serum homocysteine and methylmalonic acid levels. Prolonged deficiency → irreversible nerve damage.	

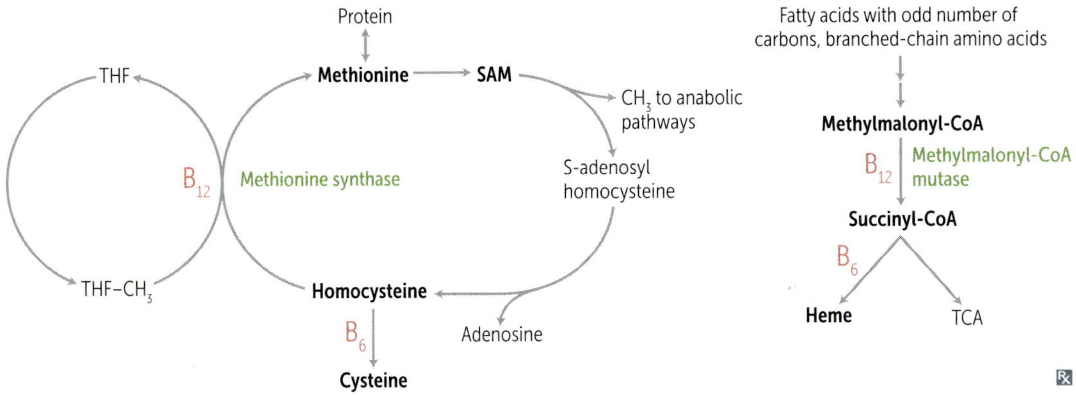

Vitamin C (ascorbic acid)

FUNCTION	Antioxidant; also facilitates iron absorption by reducing it to Fe^{2+} state. Necessary for hydroxylation of proline and lysine in collagen synthesis. Necessary for dopamine β-hydroxylase, which converts dopamine to NE.	Found in fruits and vegetables. Pronounce "**absorb**ic" acid. Ancillary treatment for methemoglobinemia by reducing Fe^{3+} to Fe^{2+}.
DEFICIENCY	Scurvy—swollen gums, bruising, petechiae, hemarthrosis, anemia, poor wound healing, perifollicular and subperiosteal hemorrhages, "corkscrew" hair. Weakened immune response.	Vitamin **C** deficiency causes s**C**urvy due to a **C**ollagen synthesis defect.
EXCESS	Nausea, vomiting, diarrhea, fatigue, calcium oxalate nephrolithiasis. Can ↑ risk of iron toxicity in predisposed individuals (eg, those with transfusions, hereditary hemochromatosis).	

Vitamin D

D_2 = ergocalciferol—ingested from plants.
D_3 = cholecalciferol—consumed in milk, formed in sun-exposed skin (stratum basale).
25-OH D_3 = storage form.
1,25-$(OH)_2$ D_3 (calcitriol) = active form.

FUNCTION	↑ intestinal absorption of calcium and phosphate, ↑ bone mineralization at low levels, ↑ bone resorption at higher levels.
DEFICIENCY	Rickets A in children (bone pain and deformity), osteomalacia in adults (bone pain and muscle weakness), hypocalcemic tetany. Breastfed infants should receive oral vitamin D. Deficiency is exacerbated by low sun exposure, pigmented skin, prematurity.
EXCESS	Hypercalcemia, hypercalciuria, loss of appetite, stupor. Seen in granulomatous disease (↑ activation of vitamin D by epithelioid macrophages).

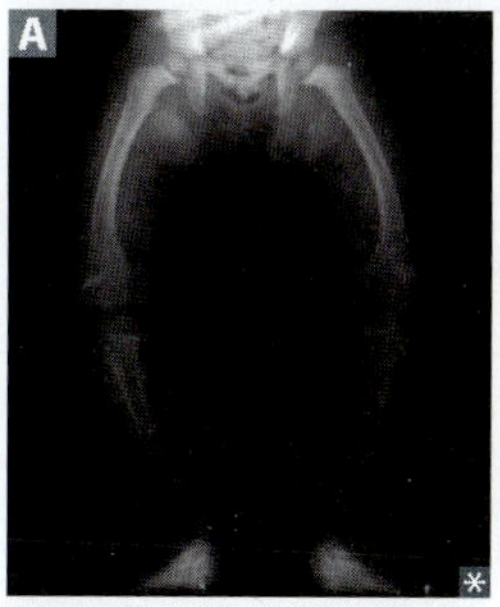

Vitamin E (tocopherol/tocotrienol)

FUNCTION	Antioxidant (protects RBCs and membranes from free radical damage).	Can enhance anticoagulant effects of warfarin.
DEFICIENCY	Hemolytic anemia, acanthocytosis, muscle weakness, posterior column and spinocerebellar tract demyelination.	Neurologic presentation may appear similar to vitamin B_{12} deficiency, but without megaloblastic anemia, hypersegmented neutrophils, or ↑ serum methylmalonic acid levels.

Vitamin K (phytomenadione, phylloquinone, phytonadione)

FUNCTION	Cofactor for the γ-carboxylation of glutamic acid residues on various proteins required for blood clotting. Synthesized by intestinal flora.	**K** is for **K**oagulation. Necessary for the maturation of clotting factors II, VII, IX, X, and proteins C and S. Warfarin—vitamin K antagonist.
DEFICIENCY	Neonatal hemorrhage with ↑ PT and ↑ aPTT but normal bleeding time (neonates have sterile intestines and are unable to synthesize vitamin K). Can also occur after prolonged use of broad-spectrum antibiotics.	Not in breast milk; neonates are given vitamin K injection at birth to prevent hemorrhagic disease of the newborn.

Zinc

FUNCTION	Mineral essential for the activity of 100+ enzymes. Important in the formation of zinc fingers (transcription factor motif).
DEFICIENCY 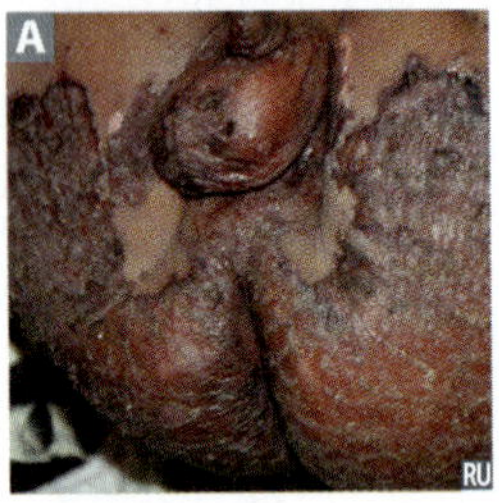	Delayed wound healing, hypogonadism, ↓ adult hair (axillary, facial, pubic), dysgeusia, anosmia, acrodermatitis enteropathica A. May predispose to alcoholic cirrhosis.

Malnutrition

Kwashiorkor 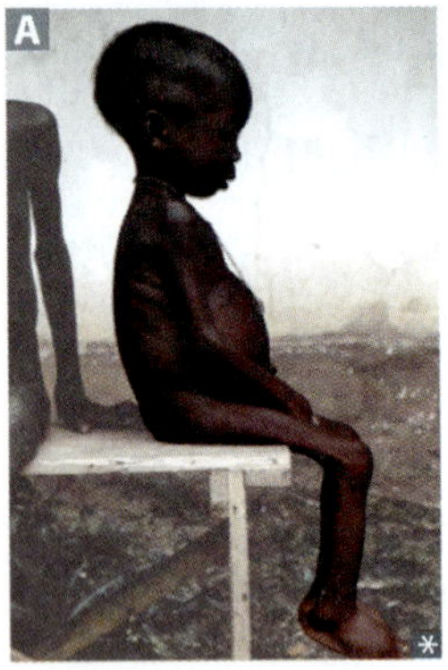	Protein malnutrition resulting in skin lesions, edema due to ↓ plasma oncotic pressure, liver malfunction (fatty change due to ↓ apolipoprotein synthesis). Clinical picture is small child with swollen abdomen A.	Kwashiorkor results from a protein-deficient MEAL: Malnutrition Edema Anemia Liver (fatty)
Marasmus	Total calorie malnutrition resulting in emaciation (tissue and muscle wasting, loss of subcutaneous fat); +/– edema.	Marasmus results in Muscle wasting.

Ethanol metabolism

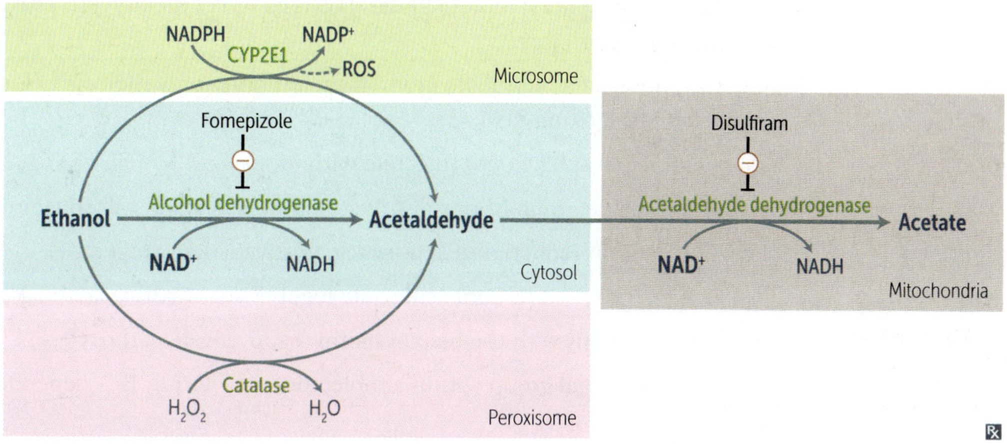

Fomepizole—inhibits alcohol dehydrogenase and is an antidote for methanol or ethylene glycol poisoning.

Disulfiram—inhibits acetaldehyde dehydrogenase (acetaldehyde accumulates, contributing to hangover symptoms).

NAD^+ is the limiting reagent.

Alcohol dehydrogenase operates via zero-order kinetics.

Ethanol metabolism ↑ $NADH/NAD^+$ ratio in liver, causing:

- Pyruvate → lactate (lactic acidosis).
- Oxaloacetate → malate (prevents gluconeogenesis → fasting hypoglycemia)
- Dihydroxyacetone phosphate → glycerol-3-phosphate (combines with fatty acids to make triglycerides → hepatosteatosis)

End result is clinical picture seen in chronic alcoholism.

Additionally, ↑ $NADH/NAD^+$ ratio disfavors TCA production of NADH → ↑ utilization of acetyl-CoA for ketogenesis (→ ketoacidosis) and lipogenesis (→ hepatosteatosis).

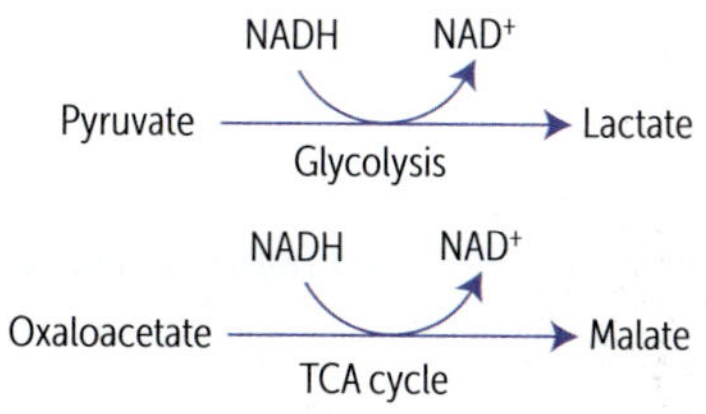

▶ BIOCHEMISTRY—METABOLISM

Metabolism sites

Mitochondria	Fatty acid oxidation (β-oxidation), acetyl-CoA production, TCA cycle, oxidative phosphorylation, ketogenesis.
Cytoplasm	Glycolysis, HMP shunt, and synthesis of steroids (SER), proteins (ribosomes, RER), fatty acids, cholesterol, and nucleotides.
Both	Heme synthesis, Urea cycle, Gluconeogenesis. HUGs take two (ie, both).

Enzyme terminology	An enzyme's name often describes its function. For example, glucokinase is an enzyme that catalyzes the phosphorylation of glucose using a molecule of ATP. The following are commonly used enzyme descriptors.
Kinase	Catalyzes transfer of a phosphate group from a high-energy molecule (usually ATP) to a substrate (eg, phosphofructokinase).
Phosphorylase	Adds inorganic phosphate onto substrate without using ATP (eg, glycogen phosphorylase).
Phosphatase	Removes phosphate group from substrate (eg, fructose-1,6-bisphosphatase).
Dehydrogenase	Catalyzes oxidation-reduction reactions (eg, pyruvate dehydrogenase).
Hydroxylase	Adds hydroxyl group (–OH) onto substrate (eg, tyrosine hydroxylase).
Carboxylase	Transfers CO_2 groups with the help of biotin (eg, pyruvate carboxylase).
Mutase	Relocates a functional group within a molecule (eg, vitamin B_{12}–dependent methylmalonyl-CoA mutase).

Rate-determining enzymes of metabolic processes

PROCESS	ENZYME	REGULATORS
Glycolysis	Phosphofructokinase-1 (PFK-1)	AMP ⊕, fructose-2,6-bisphosphate ⊕ ATP ⊖, citrate ⊖
Gluconeogenesis	Fructose-1,6-bisphosphatase	AMP ⊖, fructose-2,6-bisphosphate ⊖
TCA cycle	Isocitrate dehydrogenase	ADP ⊕ ATP ⊖, NADH ⊖
Glycogenesis	Glycogen synthase	Glucose-6-phosphate ⊕, insulin ⊕, cortisol ⊕ Epinephrine ⊖, glucagon ⊖
Glycogenolysis	Glycogen phosphorylase	Epinephrine ⊕, glucagon ⊕, AMP ⊕ Glucose-6-phosphate ⊖, insulin ⊖, ATP ⊖
HMP shunt	Glucose-6-phosphate dehydrogenase (G6PD)	$NADP^+$ ⊕ NADPH ⊖
De novo pyrimidine synthesis	Carbamoyl phosphate synthetase II	ATP ⊕, PRPP ⊕ UTP ⊖
De novo purine synthesis	Glutamine-phosphoribosylpyrophosphate (PRPP) amidotransferase	AMP ⊖, inosine monophosphate (IMP) ⊖, GMP ⊖
Urea cycle	Carbamoyl phosphate synthetase I	N-acetylglutamate ⊕
Fatty acid synthesis	Acetyl-CoA carboxylase (ACC)	Insulin ⊕, citrate ⊕ Glucagon ⊖, palmitoyl-CoA ⊖
Fatty acid oxidation	Carnitine acyltransferase I	Malonyl-CoA ⊖
Ketogenesis	HMG-CoA synthase	
Cholesterol synthesis	HMG-CoA reductase	Insulin ⊕, thyroxine ⊕ Glucagon ⊖, cholesterol ⊖

Summary of pathways

1. Galactokinase *(mild galactosemia)*
2. Galactose-1-phosphate uridyltransferase *(severe galactosemia)*
3. Hexokinase/glucokinase
4. Glucose-6-phosphatase *(von Gierke disease)*
5. Glucose-6-phosphate dehydrogenase
6. Transketolase
7. Phosphofructokinase-1
8. Fructose-1,6-bisphosphatase
9. Fructokinase *(essential fructosuria)*
10. Aldolase B *(fructose intolerance)*
11. Aldolase B *(liver)*, A *(muscle)*
12. Pyruvate kinase
13. Pyruvate dehydrogenase
14. HMG-CoA reductase
15. Pyruvate carboxylase
16. PEP carboxykinase
17. Citrate synthase
18. Isocitrate dehydrogenase
19. α-ketoglutarate dehydrogenase
20. Ornithine transcarbamylase
21. Propionyl-CoA carboxylase

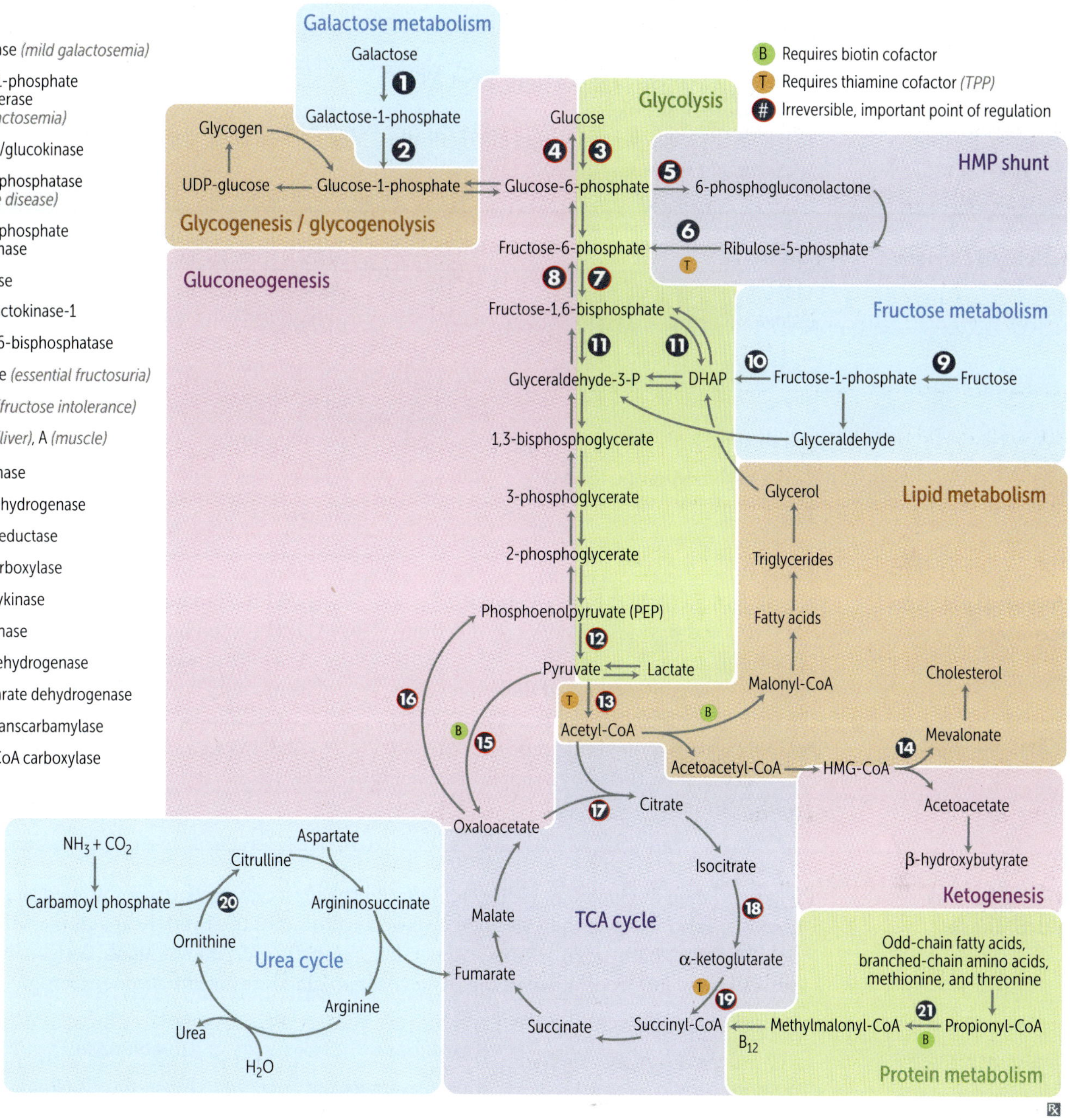

- notice how ↑ your diet gluc ↑ Triglyc & cholest. via acetyl CoA.

ATP production

Aerobic metabolism of glucose produces 32 net ATP via malate-aspartate shuttle (heart and liver), 30 net ATP via glycerol-3-phosphate shuttle (muscle).
Anaerobic glycolysis produces only 2 net ATP per glucose molecule.
ATP hydrolysis can be coupled to energetically unfavorable reactions.

Arsenic causes glycolysis to produce zero net ATP.

Activated carriers

CARRIER MOLECULE	CARRIED IN ACTIVATED FORM
ATP	Phosphoryl groups
NADH, NADPH, $FADH_2$	Electrons
CoA, lipoamide	Acyl groups
Biotin	CO_2
Tetrahydrofolates	1-carbon units
S-adenosylmethionine (SAM)	CH_3 groups
TPP	Aldehydes

Universal electron acceptors

Nicotinamides (NAD^+ from vitamin B_3, $NADP^+$) and flavin nucleotides (FAD^+ from vitamin B_2).
NAD^+ is generally used in **catabolic** processes to carry reducing equivalents away as NADH.
NADPH is used in **anabolic** processes (steroid and fatty acid synthesis) as a supply of reducing equivalents.

NADPH is a product of the HMP shunt.
NADPH is used in:
- Anabolic processes
- Respiratory burst
- Cytochrome P-450 system
- Glutathione reductase

Hexokinase vs glucokinase

Phosphorylation of glucose to yield glucose-6-phosphate serves as the 1st committed step of glycolysis (also serves as the 1st step of glycogen synthesis in the liver). Reaction is catalyzed by either hexokinase or glucokinase, depending on the tissue. At low glucose concentrations, hexokinase sequesters glucose in the tissue. At high glucose concentrations, excess glucose is stored in the liver.

	Hexokinase	Glucokinase
Location	Most tissues, except liver and pancreatic β cells	Liver, β cells of pancreas
K_m	Lower (↑ affinity)	Higher (↓ affinity)
V_{max}	Lower (↓ capacity)	Higher (↑ capacity)
Induced by insulin	No	Yes
Feedback-inhibited by glucose-6-phosphate	Yes	No
Gene mutation associated with maturity-onset diabetes of the young (MODY)	No	Yes

Glycolysis regulation, key enzymes

Net glycolysis (cytoplasm):
Glucose + 2 P_i + 2 ADP + 2 NAD^+ → 2 pyruvate + 2 ATP + 2 NADH + 2 H^+ + 2 H_2O.

Equation not balanced chemically, and exact balanced equation depends on ionization state of reactants and products.

REQUIRE ATP

Glucose —(Hexokinase/glucokinase[a])→ Glucose-6-P

Glucose-6-P ⊖ hexokinase.
Fructose-6-P ⊖ glucokinase.

Fructose-6-P —(Phosphofructokinase-1 (rate-limiting step))→ Fructose-1,6-BP

AMP ⊕, fructose-2,6-bisphosphate ⊕.
ATP ⊖, citrate ⊖.

[a]Glucokinase in liver and β cells of pancreas; hexokinase in all other tissues.

PRODUCE ATP

1,3-BPG ⇄(Phosphoglycerate kinase) 3-PG

Phosphoenolpyruvate —(Pyruvate kinase)→ Pyruvate

Fructose-1,6-bisphosphate ⊕.
ATP ⊖, alanine ⊖.

Regulation by fructose-2,6-bisphosphate

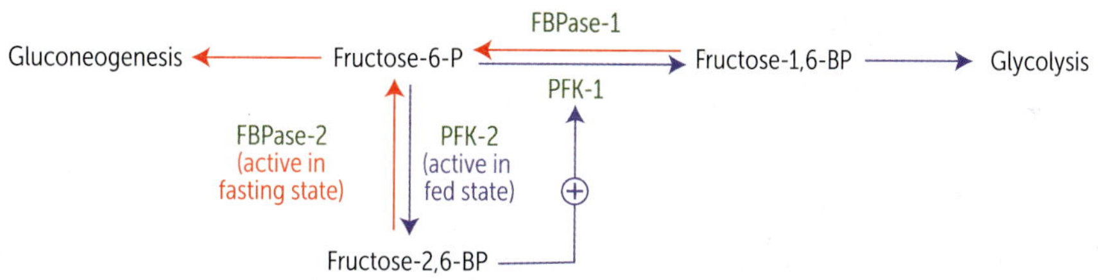

FBPase-2 (fructose bisphosphatase-2) and PFK-2 (phosphofructokinase-2) are the same bifunctional enzyme whose function is reversed by phosphorylation by protein kinase A.

Fasting state: ↑ glucagon → ↑ cAMP → ↑ protein kinase A → ↑ FBPase-2, ↓ PFK-2, less glycolysis, more gluconeogenesis.

Fed state: ↑ insulin → ↓ cAMP → ↓ protein kinase A → ↓ FBPase-2, ↑ PFK-2, more glycolysis, less gluconeogenesis.

Pyruvate dehydrogenase complex

Mitochondrial enzyme complex linking glycolysis and TCA cycle. Differentially regulated in fed/fasting states (active in fed state).

Reaction: pyruvate + NAD^+ + CoA → acetyl-CoA + CO_2 + NADH.

The complex contains 3 enzymes that require 5 cofactors:

1. **T**hiamine pyrophosphate (B_1)
2. **L**ipoic acid
3. **C**oA (B_5, pantothenic acid)
4. **F**AD (B_2, riboflavin)
5. **N**AD (B_3, niacin)

Activated by:
- ↑ NAD^+/NADH ratio
- ↑ ADP
- ↑ Ca^{2+}

The complex is similar to the α-ketoglutarate dehydrogenase complex (same cofactors, similar substrate and action), which converts α-ketoglutarate → succinyl-CoA (TCA cycle).

TLC For **N**ancy.

Arsenic inhibits lipoic acid. Findings: vomiting, rice-water stools, garlic breath.

Pyruvate dehydrogenase complex deficiency	Causes a buildup of pyruvate that gets shunted to lactate (via LDH) and alanine (via ALT). X-linked.	
FINDINGS	Neurologic defects, lactic acidosis, ↑ serum alanine starting in infancy.	
TREATMENT	↑ intake of ketogenic nutrients (eg, high fat content or ↑ lysine and leucine).	Lysine and Leucine—the onLy pureLy ketogenic amino acids.

Pyruvate metabolism

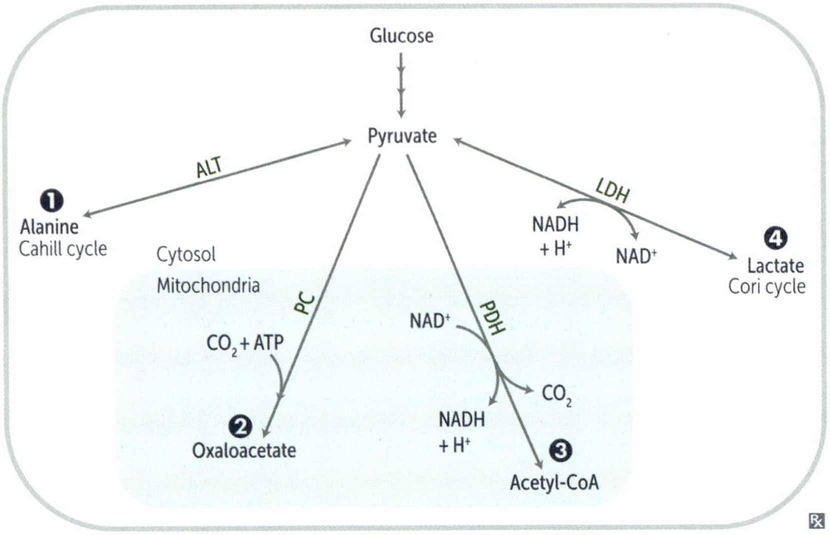

Functions of different pyruvate metabolic pathways (and their associated cofactors):

1. Alanine aminotransferase (B_6): alanine carries amino groups to the liver from muscle
2. Pyruvate carboxylase (biotin): oxaloacetate can replenish TCA cycle or be used in gluconeogenesis
3. Pyruvate dehydrogenase (B_1, B_2, B_3, B_5, lipoic acid): transition from glycolysis to the TCA cycle
4. Lactic acid dehydrogenase (B_3): end of anaerobic glycolysis (major pathway in RBCs, WBCs, kidney medulla, lens, testes, and cornea)

TCA cycle (Krebs cycle)

Pyruvate → acetyl-CoA produces 1 NADH, 1 CO_2.

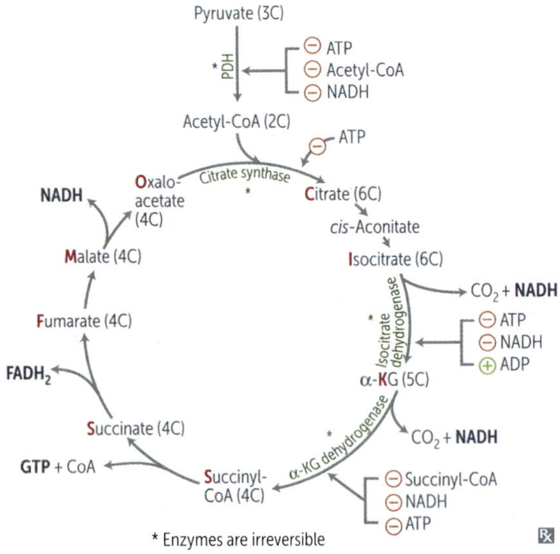

The TCA cycle produces 3 NADH, 1 $FADH_2$, 2 CO_2, 1 GTP per acetyl-CoA = 10 ATP/acetyl-CoA (2× everything per glucose). TCA cycle reactions occur in the mitochondria.

α-ketoglutarate dehydrogenase complex requires the same cofactors as the pyruvate dehydrogenase complex (B_1, B_2, B_3, B_5, lipoic acid).

Citrate Is Krebs' Starting Substrate For Making Oxaloacetate.

Electron transport chain and oxidative phosphorylation

NADH electrons from glycolysis enter mitochondria via the malate-aspartate or glycerol-3-phosphate shuttle. $FADH_2$ electrons are transferred to complex II (at a lower energy level than NADH). The passage of electrons results in the formation of a proton gradient that, coupled to oxidative phosphorylation, drives the production of ATP.

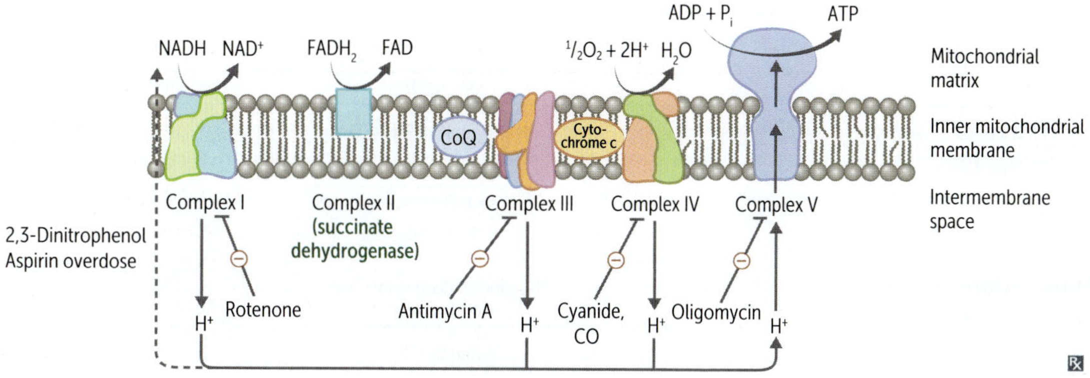

ATP PRODUCED VIA ATP SYNTHASE		
	1 NADH → 2.5 ATP; 1 $FADH_2$ → 1.5 ATP.	
OXIDATIVE PHOSPHORYLATION POISONS		
Electron transport inhibitors	Directly inhibit electron transport, causing a ↓ proton gradient and block of ATP synthesis.	RotenONE: complex ONE inhibitor. "An-3-mycin" (antimycin) A: complex 3 inhibitor. CO/CN: complex 4 inhibitors (4 letters).
ATP synthase inhibitors	Directly inhibit mitochondrial ATP synthase, causing an ↑ proton gradient. No ATP is produced because electron transport stops.	Oligomycin.
Uncoupling agents	↑ permeability of membrane, causing a ↓ proton gradient and ↑ O_2 consumption. ATP synthesis stops, but electron transport continues. Produces heat.	2,4-Dinitrophenol (used illicitly for weight loss), aspirin (fevers often occur after aspirin overdose), thermogenin in brown fat.

Gluconeogenesis, irreversible enzymes		Pathway Produces Fresh Glucose.
Pyruvate carboxylase	In mitochondria. Pyruvate → oxaloacetate.	Requires biotin, ATP. Activated by acetyl-CoA.
Phosphoenolpyruvate carboxykinase	In cytosol. Oxaloacetate → phosphoenolpyruvate.	Requires GTP.
Fructose-1,6-bisphosphatase	In cytosol. Fructose-1,6-bisphosphate → fructose-6-phosphate.	Citrate ⊕, fructose 2,6-bisphosphate ⊖.
Glucose-6-phosphatase	In ER. Glucose-6-phosphate → glucose.	

Occurs primarily in liver; serves to maintain euglycemia during fasting. Enzymes also found in kidney, intestinal epithelium. Deficiency of the key gluconeogenic enzymes causes hypoglycemia. (Muscle cannot participate in gluconeogenesis because it lacks glucose-6-phosphatase).

Odd-chain fatty acids yield 1 propionyl-CoA during metabolism, which can enter the TCA cycle (as succinyl-CoA), undergo gluconeogenesis, and serve as a glucose source. Even-chain fatty acids cannot produce new glucose, since they yield only acetyl-CoA equivalents.

HMP shunt (pentose phosphate pathway)

Provides a source of NADPH from abundantly available glucose-6-P (NADPH is required for reductive reactions, eg, glutathione reduction inside RBCs, fatty acid and cholesterol biosynthesis). Additionally, this pathway yields ribose for nucleotide synthesis and glycolytic intermediates. 2 distinct phases (oxidative and nonoxidative), both of which occur in the cytoplasm. No ATP is used or produced.

Sites: lactating mammary glands, liver, adrenal cortex (sites of fatty acid or steroid synthesis), RBCs.

REACTIONS	KEY ENZYMES	PRODUCTS
Oxidative (irreversible)	Glucose-6-P_i → (NADP⁺ → NADPH; NADPH ⊖) **Glucose-6-P dehydrogenase** — Rate-limiting step	CO_2 2 NADPH Ribulose-5-P_i
Nonoxidative (reversible)	Ribulose-5-P_i ⟷ **Phosphopentose isomerase, transketolases** — Requires B_1	Ribose-5-P_i Glyceraldehyde-3-phosphate Fructose-6-P

Glucose-6-phosphate dehydrogenase deficiency

NADPH is necessary to keep glutathione reduced, which in turn detoxifies free radicals and peroxides. ↓ NADPH in RBCs leads to hemolytic anemia due to poor RBC defense against oxidizing agents (eg, fava beans, sulfonamides, primaquine, antituberculosis drugs). Infection (most common cause) can also precipitate hemolysis; inflammatory response produces free radicals that diffuse into RBCs, causing oxidative damage.

X-linked recessive disorder; most common human enzyme deficiency; more prevalent among African Americans. ↑ malarial resistance.

Heinz bodies—denatured **He**moglobin precipitates within RBCs due to oxidative stress.

Bite cells—result from the phagocytic removal of **Heinz** bodies by splenic macrophages. Think, "**Bite** into some **Heinz** ketchup."

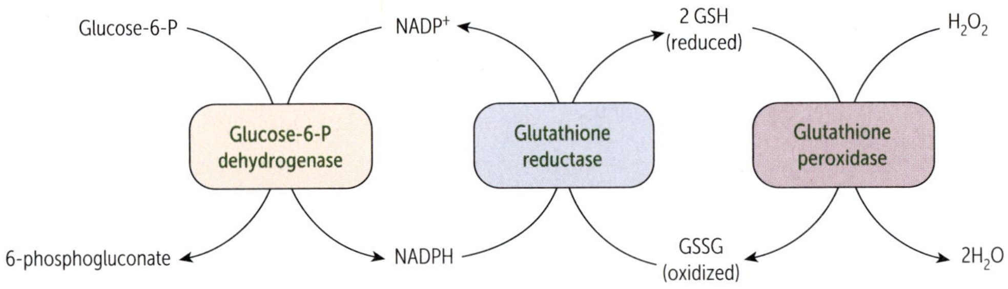

Disorders of fructose metabolism

Essential fructosuria	Involves a defect in **fructokinase**. Autosomal recessive. A benign, asymptomatic condition, since fructose is not trapped in cells. Symptoms: fructose appears in blood and urine. Disorders of fructose metabolism cause milder symptoms than analogous disorders of galactose metabolism.
Fructose intolerance	Hereditary deficiency of **aldolase B**. Autosomal recessive. Fructose-1-phosphate accumulates, causing a ↓ in available phosphate, which results in inhibition of glycogenolysis and gluconeogenesis. Symptoms present following consumption of fruit, juice, or honey. Urine dipstick will be ⊖ (tests for glucose only); reducing sugar can be detected in the urine (nonspecific test for inborn errors of carbohydrate metabolism). Symptoms: hypoglycemia, jaundice, cirrhosis, vomiting. Treatment: ↓ intake of both fructose and sucrose (glucose + fructose).

Fructose metabolism (liver)

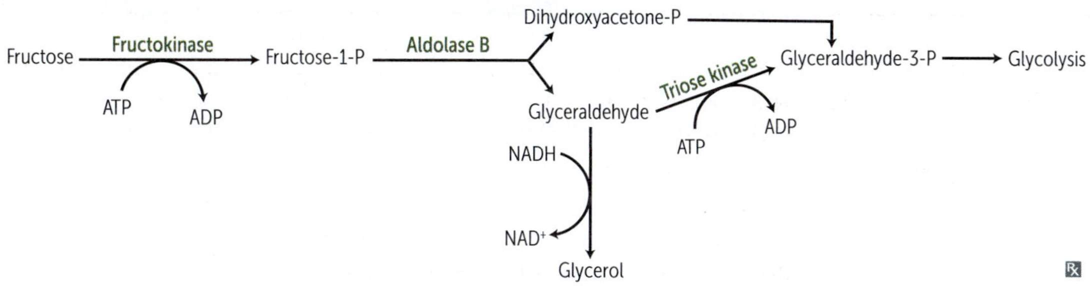

Disorders of galactose metabolism

Galactokinase deficiency	Hereditary deficiency of **galactokinase**. Galactitol accumulates if galactose is present in diet. Relatively mild condition. Autosomal recessive. Symptoms develop when infant begins feeding (lactose present in breast milk and routine formula). Symptoms: galactose appears in blood (galactosemia) and urine (galactosuria); infantile cataracts. May present as failure to track objects or to develop a social smile.
Classic galactosemia	Absence of **galactose-1-phosphate uridyltransferase**. Autosomal recessive. Damage is caused by accumulation of toxic substances (including galactitol, which accumulates in the lens of the eye). Symptoms: failure to thrive, jaundice, hepatomegaly, infantile cataracts, intellectual disability. Can lead to *E coli* sepsis in neonates. Treatment: exclude galactose and lactose (galactose + glucose) from diet.

Galactose metabolism

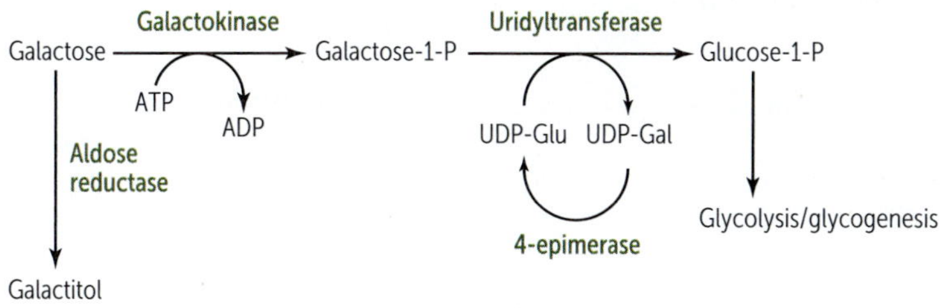

Fructose is to **A**ldolase **B** as **G**alactose is to **U**ridyl**T**ransferase (**FAB GUT**).

The more serious defects lead to PO_4^{3-} depletion.

Sorbitol

An alternative method of trapping glucose in the cell is to convert it to its alcohol counterpart, called sorbitol, via aldose reductase. Some tissues then convert sorbitol to fructose using sorbitol dehydrogenase; tissues with an insufficient amount/activity of this enzyme are at risk for intracellular sorbitol accumulation, causing osmotic damage (eg, cataracts, retinopathy, and peripheral neuropathy seen with chronic hyperglycemia in diabetes).

High blood levels of galactose also result in conversion to the osmotically active galactitol via aldose reductase.

Liver, ovaries, and seminal vesicles have both enzymes.

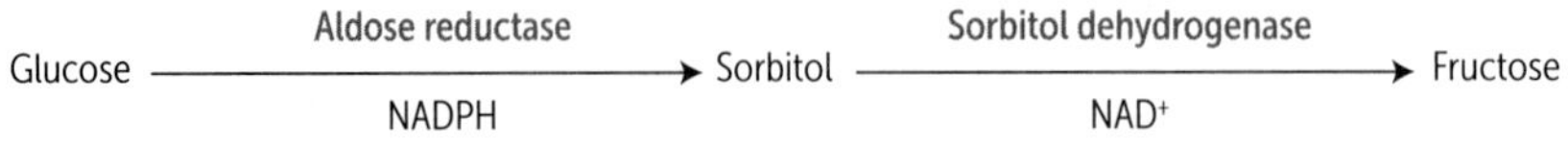

Schwann cells, retina, and kidneys have only aldose reductase. Lens has primarily aldose reductase.

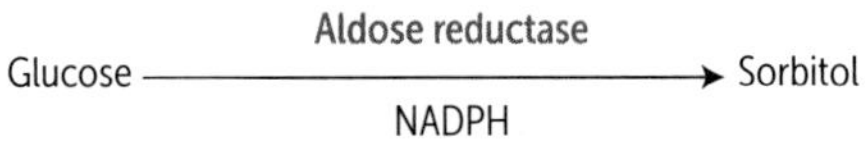

Lactase deficiency	Insufficient lactase enzyme → dietary lactose intolerance. Lactase functions on the brush border to digest lactose (in human and cow milk) into glucose and galactose. Primary: age-dependent decline after childhood (absence of lactase-persistent allele), common in people of Asian, African, or Native American descent. Secondary: loss of brush border due to gastroenteritis (eg, rotavirus), autoimmune disease, etc. Congenital lactase deficiency: rare, due to defective gene. Stool demonstrates ↓ pH and breath shows ↑ hydrogen content with lactose hydrogen breath test. Intestinal biopsy reveals normal mucosa in patients with hereditary lactose intolerance.
FINDINGS	Bloating, cramps, flatulence, osmotic diarrhea.
TREATMENT	Avoid dairy products or add lactase pills to diet; lactose-free milk.

Amino acids	Only L-amino acids are found in proteins.	
Essential	Glucogenic: methionine (Met), valine (Val), histidine (His). Glucogenic/ketogenic: isoleucine (Ile), phenylalanine (Phe), threonine (Thr), tryptophan (Trp). Ketogenic: leucine (Leu), lysine (Lys).	All essential amino acids need to be supplied in the diet.
Acidic	Aspartic acid (Asp) and glutamic acid (Glu). Negatively charged at body pH.	
Basic	Arginine (Arg), lysine (Lys), histidine (His). Arg is most basic. His has no charge at body pH.	Arg and His are required during periods of growth. Arg and Lys are ↑ in histones, which bind negatively charged DNA.

Urea cycle

Amino acid catabolism results in the formation of common metabolites (eg, pyruvate, acetyl-CoA), which serve as metabolic fuels. Excess nitrogen (NH_3) generated by this process is converted to urea and excreted by the kidneys.

Ordinarily, Careless Crappers Are Also Frivolous About Urination.

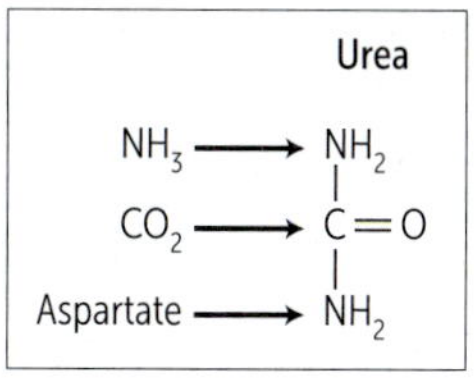

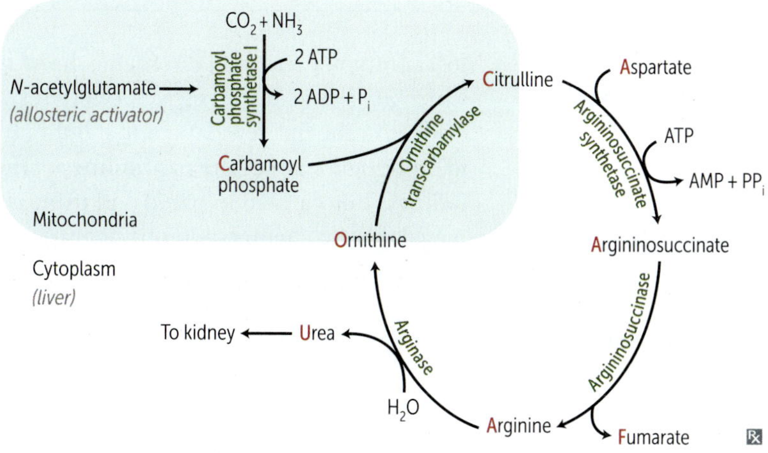

Transport of ammonia by alanine and glutamate

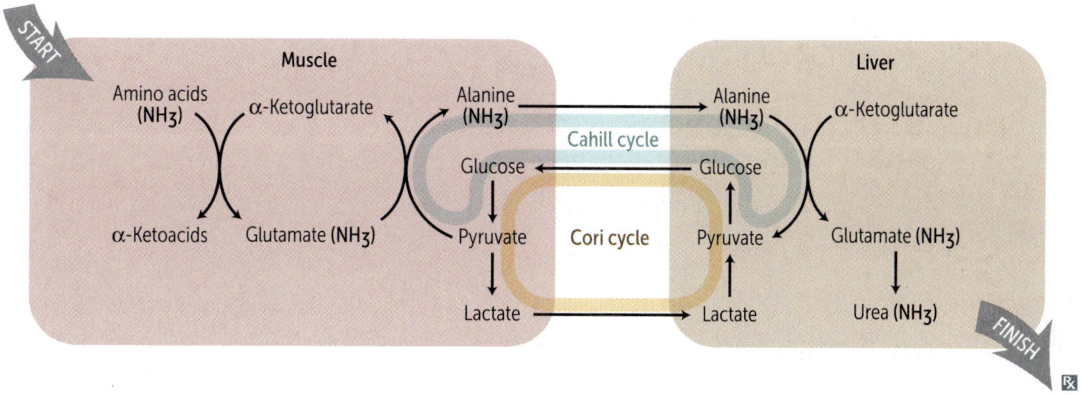

Hyperammonemia

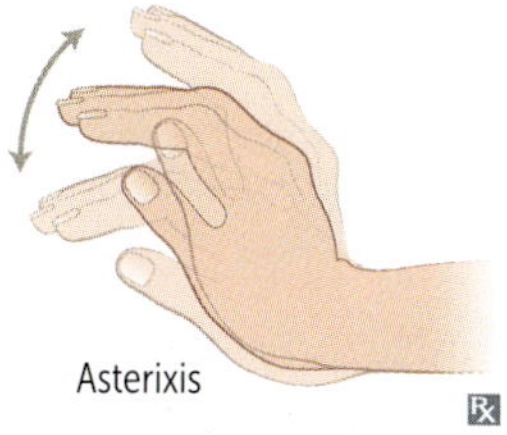

Can be acquired (eg, liver disease) or hereditary (eg, urea cycle enzyme deficiencies).

Results in excess NH_3, which depletes α-ketoglutarate, leading to inhibition of TCA cycle.

Treatment: limit protein in diet.

May be given to ↓ ammonia levels:

- Lactulose to acidify the GI tract and trap NH_4^+ for excretion.
- Rifaximin to ↓ colonic ammoniagenic bacteria.
- Benzoate, phenylacetate, or phenylbutyrate to bind to NH_4^+ and lead to excretion.

Ammonia accumulation—tremor (asterixis), slurring of speech, somnolence, vomiting, cerebral edema, blurring of vision.

N-acetylglutamate synthase deficiency

Required cofactor for carbamoyl phosphate synthetase I. Absence of N-acetylglutamate → hyperammonemia.

Presents in neonates as poorly regulated respiration and body temperature, poor feeding, developmental delay, intellectual disability (identical to presentation of carbamoyl phosphate synthetase I deficiency).

Ornithine transcarbamylase deficiency

Most common urea cycle disorder. X-linked recessive (vs other urea cycle enzyme deficiencies, which are autosomal recessive). Interferes with the body's ability to eliminate ammonia. Often evident in the first few days of life, but may present later. Excess carbamoyl phosphate is converted to orotic acid (part of the pyrimidine synthesis pathway).

Findings: ↑ orotic acid in blood and urine, ↓ BUN, symptoms of hyperammonemia. No megaloblastic anemia (vs orotic aciduria).

Amino acid derivatives

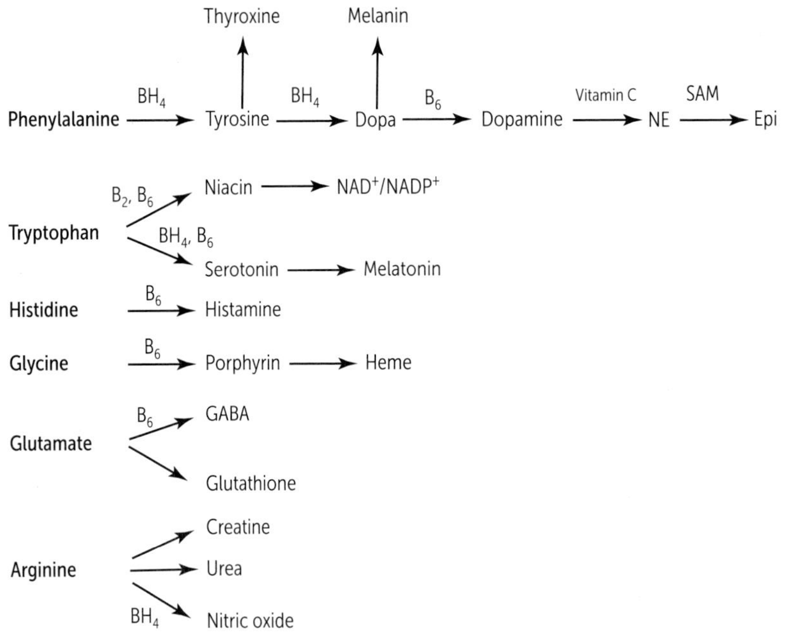

Catecholamine synthesis/tyrosine catabolism

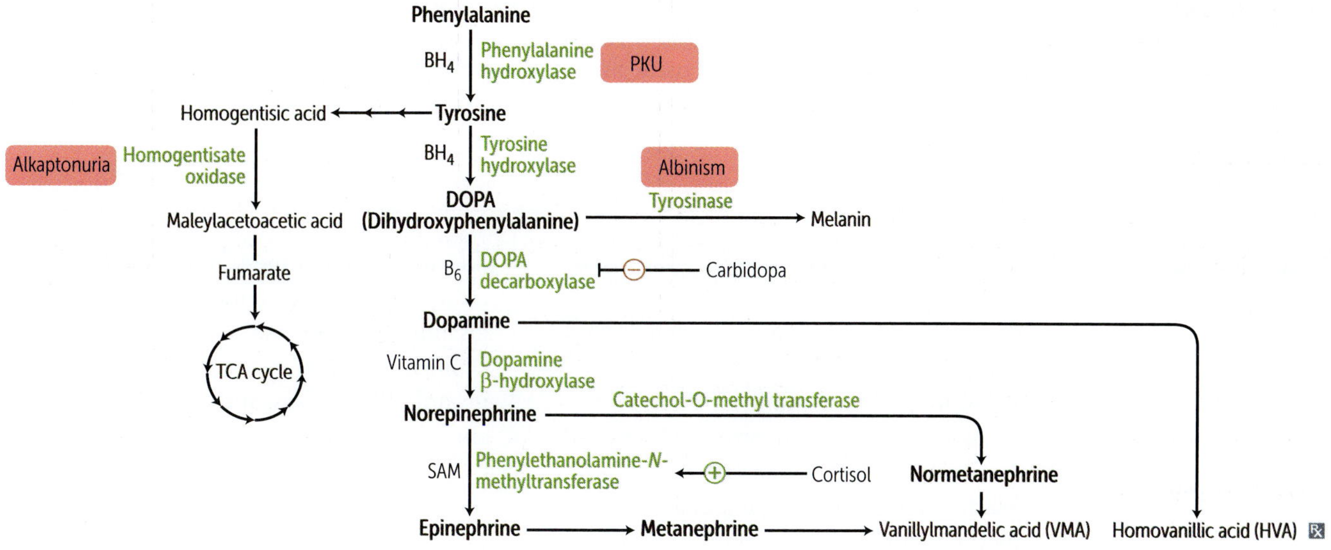

Phenylketonuria

Due to ↓ phenylalanine hydroxylase or ↓ tetrahydrobiopterin cofactor (malignant PKU). Tyrosine becomes essential. ↑ phenylalanine → excess phenylketones in urine.

Findings: intellectual disability, growth retardation, seizures, fair skin, eczema, musty body odor.

Treatment: ↓ phenylalanine and ↑ tyrosine in diet, tetrahydrobiopterin supplementation.

Maternal PKU—lack of proper dietary therapy during pregnancy. Findings in infant: microcephaly, intellectual disability, growth retardation, congenital heart defects.

Autosomal recessive. Incidence ≈ 1:10,000.

Screening occurs 2–3 days after birth (normal at birth because of maternal enzyme during fetal life).

Phenylketones—phenylacetate, phenyllactate, and phenylpyruvate.

Disorder of **aromatic** amino acid metabolism → musty body **odor**.

PKU patients must avoid the artificial sweetener aspartame, which contains phenylalanine.

Maple syrup urine disease

Blocked degradation of **branched** amino acids (**I**soleucine, **L**eucine, **V**aline) due to ↓ branched-chain α-ketoacid dehydrogenase (B_1). Causes ↑ α-ketoacids in the blood, especially those of leucine.

Causes severe CNS defects, intellectual disability, and death.

Treatment: restriction of isoleucine, leucine, valine in diet, and thiamine supplementation.

Autosomal recessive.

Presentation: vomiting, poor feeding, urine smells like maple syrup/burnt sugar.

I Love **V**ermont **maple syrup** from maple trees (with **B_1ranches**).

Alkaptonuria

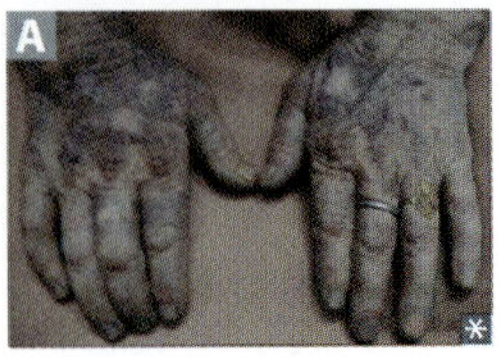

Congenital deficiency of homogentisate oxidase in the degradative pathway of tyrosine to fumarate → pigment-forming homogentisic acid accumulates in tissue A. Autosomal recessive. Usually benign.

Findings: bluish-black connective tissue and sclerae (ochronosis); urine turns black on prolonged exposure to air. May have debilitating arthralgias (homogentisic acid toxic to cartilage).

Homocystinuria

Types (all autosomal recessive):

- Cystathionine synthase deficiency (treatment: ↓ methionine, ↑ cysteine, ↑ B_{12} and folate in diet)
- ↓ affinity of cystathionine synthase for pyridoxal phosphate (treatment: ↑↑ B_6 and ↑ cysteine in diet)
- Methionine synthase (homocysteine methyltransferase) deficiency (treatment: ↑ methionine in diet)

All forms result in excess homocysteine.

Findings: ↑↑ homocysteine in urine, intellectual disability, osteoporosis, marfanoid habitus, kyphosis, lens subluxation (downward and inward), thrombosis, and atherosclerosis (stroke and MI).

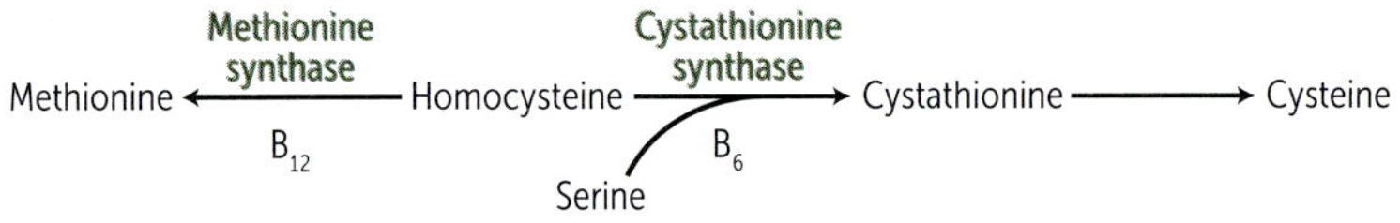

Cystinuria

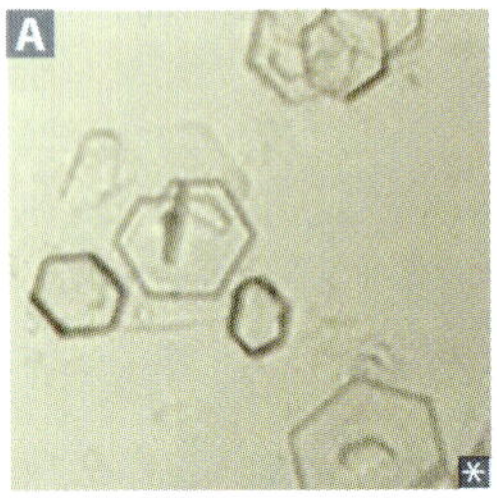

Hereditary defect of renal PCT and intestinal amino acid transporter that prevents reabsorption of **C**ystine, **O**rnithine, **L**ysine, and **A**rginine (**COLA**).

Excess cystine in the urine can lead to recurrent precipitation of hexagonal cystine stones A.

Treatment: urinary alkalinization (eg, potassium citrate, acetazolamide) and chelating agents (eg, penicillamine) ↑ solubility of cystine stones; good hydration.

Autosomal recessive. Common (1:7000).

Urinary cyanide-nitroprusside test is diagnostic.

Cystine is made of 2 cysteines connected by a disulfide bond.

Glycogen regulation by insulin and glucagon/epinephrine

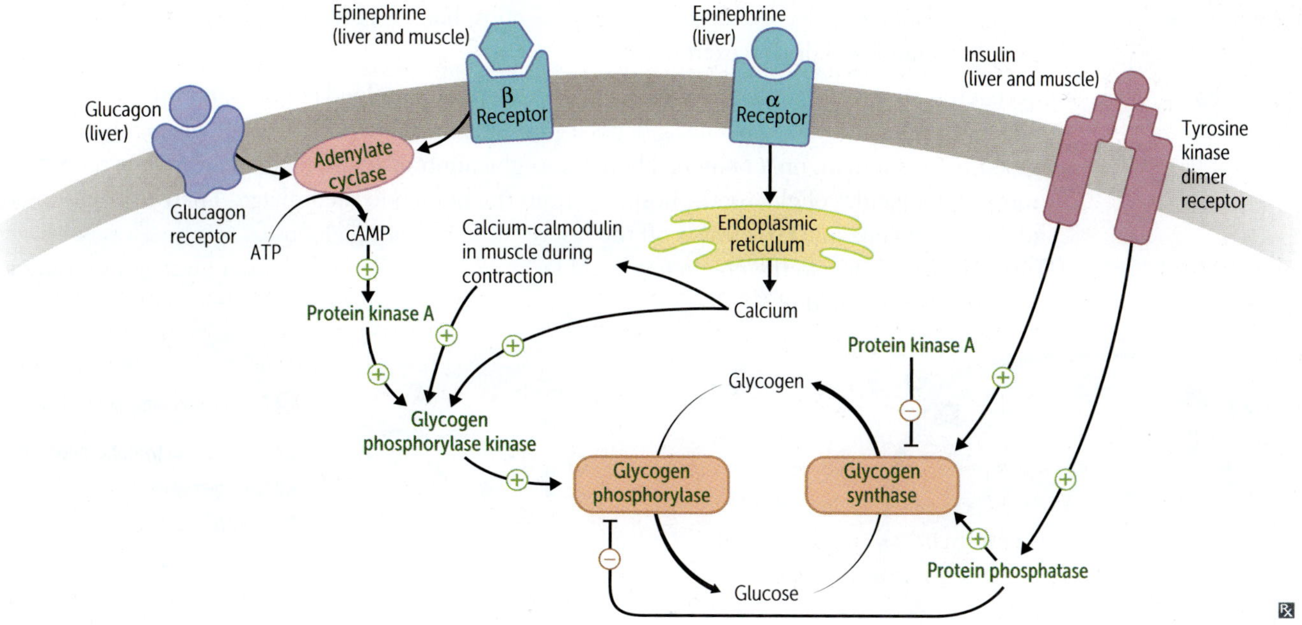

Glycogen	Branches have α-(1,6) bonds; linkages have α-(1,4) bonds.
Skeletal muscle	Glycogen undergoes glycogenolysis → glucose-1-phosphate → glucose-6-phosphate, which is rapidly metabolized during exercise.
Hepatocytes	Glycogen is stored and undergoes glycogenolysis to maintain blood sugar at appropriate levels. Glycogen phosphorylase liberates glucose-1-phosphate residues off branched glycogen until 4 glucose units remain on a branch. Then 4-α-D-glucanotransferase (debranching enzyme ❺) moves 3 molecules of glucose-1-phosphate from the branch to the linkage. Then α-1,6 glucosidase (debranching enzyme ❻) cleaves off the last residue, liberating glucose. "Limit dextrin" refers to the one to four residues remaining on a branch after glycogen phosphorylase has already shortened it.

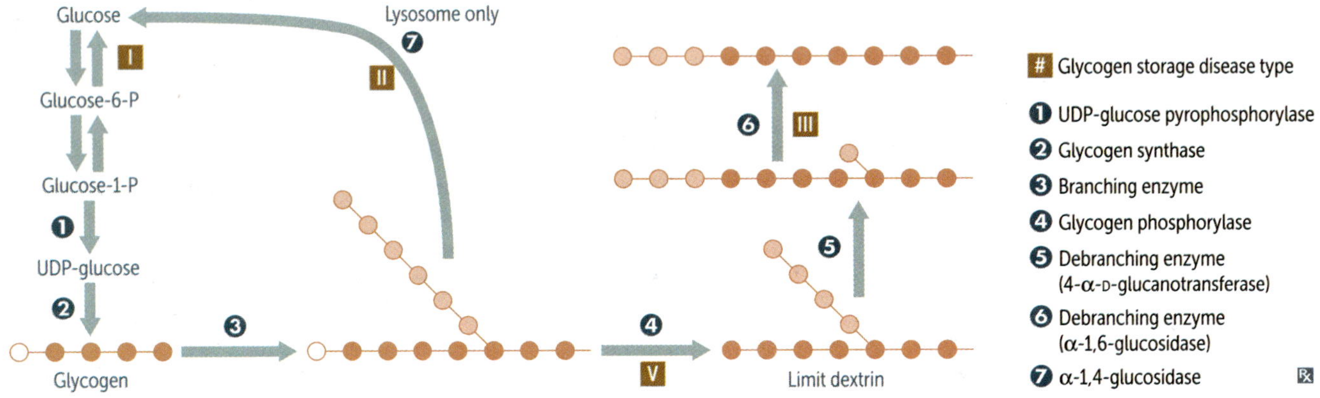

Note: A small amount of glycogen is degraded in lysosomes by α-1,4-glucosidase (acid maltase).

Glycogen storage diseases

12 types, all resulting in abnormal glycogen metabolism and an accumulation of glycogen within cells. Periodic acid–Schiff stain identifies glycogen and is useful in identifying these diseases.

Very Poor Carbohydrate Metabolism.
Types I, II, III, and V are autosomal recessive.

DISEASE	FINDINGS	DEFICIENT ENZYME	COMMENTS
Von Gierke disease (type I)	Severe fasting hypoglycemia, ↑↑ Glycogen in liver, ↑ blood lactate, ↑ triglycerides, ↑ uric acid (Gout), and hepatomegaly.	Glucose-6-phosphatase	Treatment: frequent oral glucose/cornstarch; avoidance of fructose and galactose Impaired gluconeogenesis and glycogenolysis
Pompe disease (type II)	Cardiomegaly, hypertrophic cardiomyopathy, exercise intolerance, and systemic finds leading to early death.	Lysosomal α-1,4-glucosidase with α-1,6-glucosidase activity (acid maltase)	Pompe trashes the Pump (heart, liver, and muscle)
Cori disease (type III)	Milder form of von Gierke (type I) with normal blood lactate levels. Accumulation of limit dextrin–like structures in cytosol.	Debranching enzyme (α-1,6-glucosidase)	Gluconeogenesis is intact
McArdle disease (type V)	↑ glycogen in muscle, but muscle cannot break it down → painful Muscle cramps, Myoglobinuria (red urine) with strenuous exercise, and arrhythmia from electrolyte abnormalities. Second-wind phenomenon noted during exercise due to ↑ muscular blood flow.	Skeletal muscle glycogen phosphorylase (Myophosphorylase)	Blood glucose levels typically unaffected McArdle = Muscle

Lysosomal storage diseases

Each is caused by a deficiency in one of the many lysosomal enzymes. Results in an accumulation of abnormal metabolic products.

DISEASE	FINDINGS	DEFICIENT ENZYME	ACCUMULATED SUBSTRATE	INHERITANCE
Sphingolipidoses				
Fabry disease 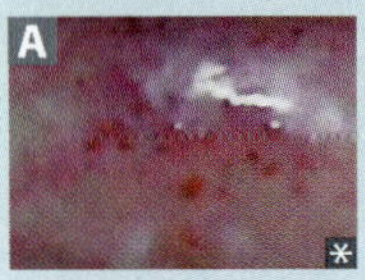	Early: Triad of episodic peripheral neuropathy, angiokeratomas A, hypohidrosis. Late: progressive renal failure, cardiovascular disease.	❷ α-galactosidase A	Ceramide trihexoside	XR
Gaucher disease 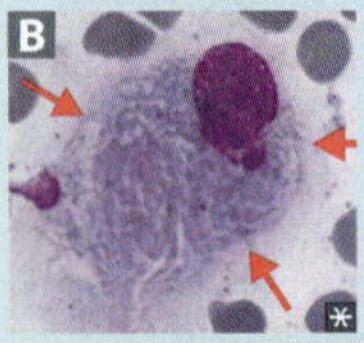	Most common. Hepatosplenomegaly, pancytopenia, osteoporosis, aseptic necrosis of femur, bone crises, Gaucher cells B (lipid-laden macrophages resembling crumpled tissue paper).	❺ Glucocerebrosidase (β-glucosidase); treat with recombinant glucocerebrosidase	Glucocerebroside	AR
Niemann-Pick disease 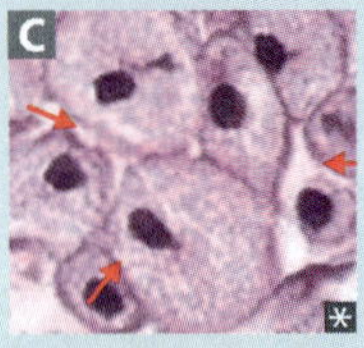	Progressive neurodegeneration, hepatosplenomegaly, foam cells (lipid-laden macrophages) C, "cherry-red" spot on macula D.	❻ Sphingomyelinase	Sphingomyelin	AR
Tay-Sachs disease 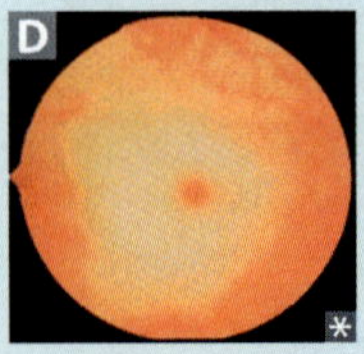	Progressive neurodegeneration, developmental delay, "cherry-red" spot on macula D, lysosomes with onion skin, no hepatosplenomegaly (vs Niemann-Pick).	❶ Hexosaminidase A	GM_2 ganglioside	AR
Krabbe disease	Peripheral neuropathy, developmental delay, optic atrophy, globoid cells.	❹ Galactocerebrosidase	Galactocerebroside, psychosine	AR
Metachromatic leukodystrophy	Central and peripheral demyelination with ataxia, dementia.	❸ Arylsulfatase A	Cerebroside sulfate	AR
Mucopolysaccharidoses				
Hurler syndrome	Developmental delay, gargoylism, airway obstruction, corneal clouding, hepatosplenomegaly.	α-L-iduronidase	Heparan sulfate, dermatan sulfate	AR
Hunter syndrome	Mild Hurler + aggressive behavior, no corneal clouding.	Iduronate sulfatase	Heparan sulfate, dermatan sulfate	XR

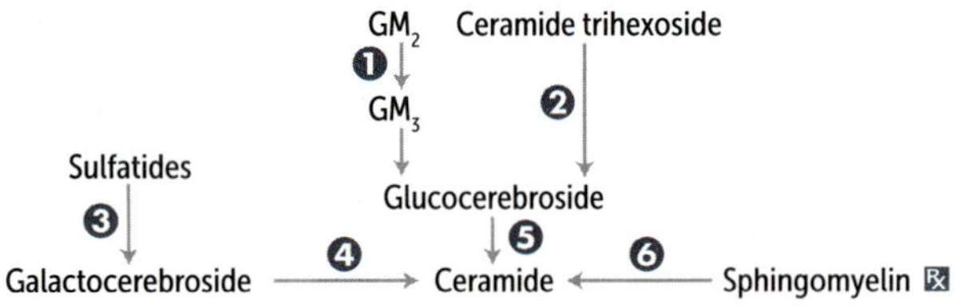

No man picks (**Niemann-Pick**) his nose with his **sphinger** (**sphingo**myelinase).

Tay-Sa**X** lacks he**X**osaminidase.

Hunters see clearly (no corneal clouding) and aggressively aim for the **X** (**X**-linked recessive).

↑ incidence of Tay-Sachs, Niemann-Pick, and some forms of Gaucher disease in Ashkenazi Jews.

Fatty acid metabolism

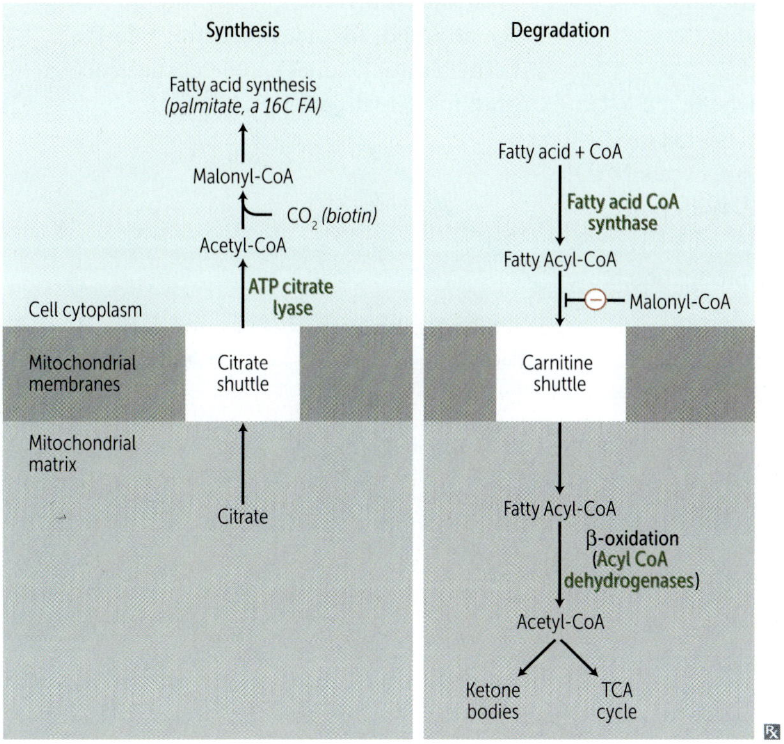

Fatty acid synthesis requires transport of citrate from mitochondria to cytosol. Predominantly occurs in liver, lactating mammary glands, and adipose tissue.

Long-chain fatty acid (LCFA) degradation requires carnitine-dependent transport into the mitochondrial matrix.

"**SY**trate" = **SY**nthesis.
CARnitine = **CAR**nage of fatty acids.

Systemic 1° carnitine deficiency—inherited defect in transport of LCFAs into the mitochondria → toxic accumulation. Causes weakness, hypotonia, and hypoketotic hypoglycemia.

Medium-chain acyl-CoA dehydrogenase deficiency

Autosomal recessive disorder of fatty acid oxidation. ↓ ability to break down fatty acids into acetyl-CoA → accumulation of 8- to 10-carbon fatty acyl carnitines in the blood and hypoketotic hypoglycemia. May present in infancy or early childhood with vomiting, lethargy, seizures, coma, and liver dysfunction.

Minor illness can lead to sudden death. Treat by avoiding fasting.

Ketone bodies

In the liver, fatty acids and amino acids are metabolized to acetoacetate and β-hydroxybutyrate (to be used in muscle and brain).

In prolonged starvation and diabetic ketoacidosis, oxaloacetate is depleted for gluconeogenesis. In alcoholism, excess NADH shunts oxaloacetate to malate. Both processes cause a buildup of acetyl-CoA, which shunts glucose and FFA toward the production of ketone bodies.

Ketone bodies: acetone, acetoacetate, β-hydroxybutyrate.

Breath smells like acetone (fruity odor).

Urine test for ketones can detect acetoacetate, but not β-hydroxybutyrate.

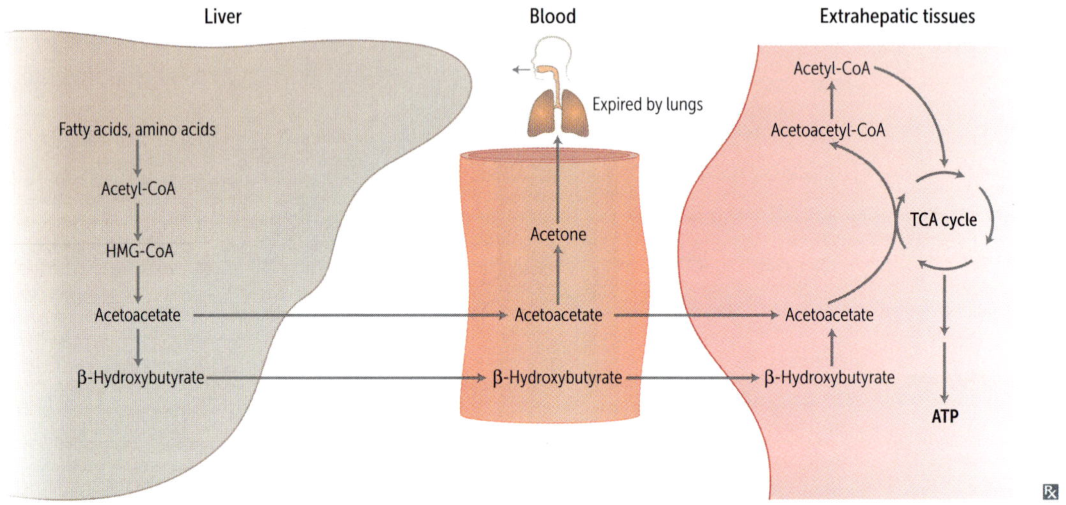

Metabolic fuel use

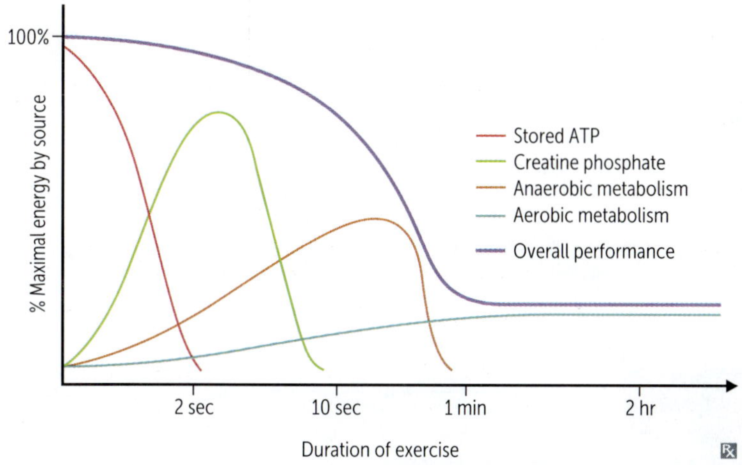

1 g protein or carbohydrate = 4 kcal.
1 g fat = 9 kcal.
1 g alcohol = 7 kcal.

Fasting and starvation

Priorities are to supply sufficient glucose to the brain and RBCs and to preserve protein.

Fed state (after a meal)	Glycolysis and aerobic respiration.	Insulin stimulates storage of lipids, proteins, and glycogen.
Fasting (between meals)	Hepatic glycogenolysis (major); hepatic gluconeogenesis, adipose release of FFA (minor).	Glucagon and epinephrine stimulate use of fuel reserves.
Starvation days 1–3	Blood glucose levels maintained by: ▪ Hepatic glycogenolysis ▪ Adipose release of FFA ▪ Muscle and liver, which shift fuel use from glucose to FFA ▪ Hepatic gluconeogenesis from peripheral tissue lactate and alanine, and from adipose tissue glycerol and propionyl-CoA (from odd-chain FFA—the only triacylglycerol components that contribute to gluconeogenesis)	Glycogen reserves depleted after day 1. RBCs lack mitochondria and therefore cannot use ketones.
Starvation after day 3	Adipose stores (ketone bodies become the main source of energy for the brain). After these are depleted, vital protein degradation accelerates, leading to organ failure and death. Amount of excess stores determines survival time.	

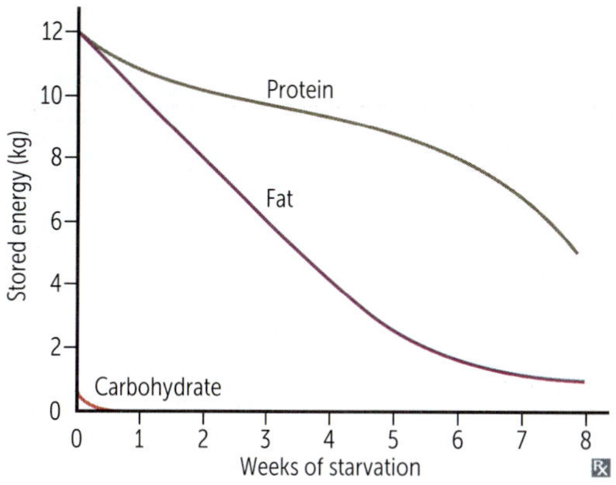

Cholesterol synthesis

Cholesterol needed to maintain cell membrane integrity and to synthesize bile acid, steroids, and vitamin D.

Rate-limiting step catalyzed by HMG-CoA reductase (induced by insulin), which converts HMG-CoA to mevalonate. ⅔ of plasma cholesterol esterified by lecithin-cholesterol acyltransferase (LCAT).

Statins (eg, atorvastatin) competitively and reversibly inhibit HMG-CoA reductase.

Lipid transport, key enzymes

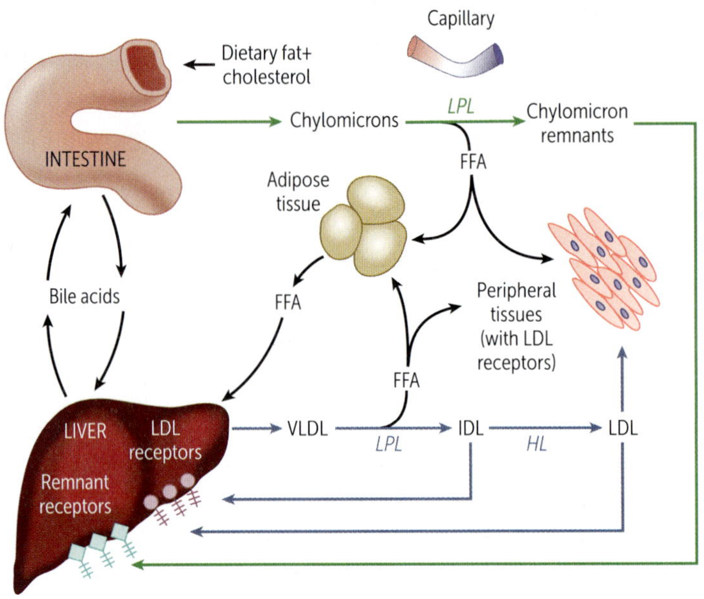

Pancreatic lipase—degradation of dietary triglycerides (TGs) in small intestine.
Lipoprotein lipase (LPL)—degradation of TGs circulating in chylomicrons and VLDLs. Found on vascular endothelial surface.
Hepatic TG lipase (HL)—degradation of TGs remaining in IDL.
Hormone-sensitive lipase—degradation of TGs stored in adipocytes.

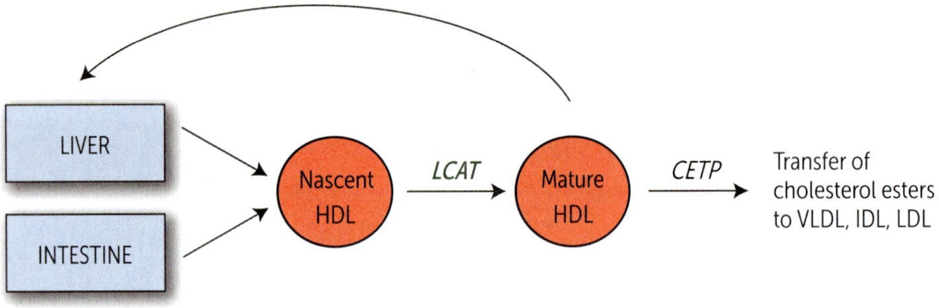

LCAT—catalyzes esterification of cholesterol.
Cholesterol ester transfer protein (CETP)—mediates transfer of cholesterol esters to other lipoprotein particles.

Major apolipoproteins

Apolipoprotein	Function	Chylomicron	Chylomicron remnant	VLDL	IDL	LDL	HDL
E	Mediates remnant uptake	✓	✓	✓	✓		✓
A-I	Activates LCAT	✓					✓
C-II	Lipoprotein lipase cofactor	✓		✓			✓
B-48	Mediates chylomicron secretion	✓	✓				
B-100	Binds LDL receptor			✓	✓	✓	

Lipoprotein functions	Lipoproteins are composed of varying proportions of cholesterol, TGs, and phospholipids. LDL and HDL carry the most cholesterol.	
	LDL transports cholesterol from liver to tissues.	LDL is Lousy.
	HDL transports cholesterol from periphery to liver.	HDL is Healthy.
Chylomicron	Delivers dietary TGs to peripheral tissue. Delivers cholesterol to liver in the form of chylomicron remnants, which are mostly depleted of their TGs. Secreted by intestinal epithelial cells.	
VLDL	Delivers hepatic TGs to peripheral tissue. Secreted by liver.	
IDL	Formed in the degradation of VLDL. Delivers TGs and cholesterol to liver.	
LDL	Delivers hepatic cholesterol to peripheral tissues. Formed by hepatic lipase modification of IDL in the liver and peripheral tissue. Taken up by target cells via receptor-mediated endocytosis.	
HDL	Mediates reverse cholesterol transport from periphery to liver. Acts as a repository for apolipoproteins C and E (which are needed for chylomicron and VLDL metabolism). Secreted from both liver and intestine. Alcohol ↑ synthesis.	

Familial dyslipidemias

TYPE	INHERITANCE	PATHOGENESIS	↑ BLOOD LEVEL	CLINICAL
I—Hyper-chylomicronemia	AR	Lipoprotein lipase or apolipoprotein C-II deficiency	Chylomicrons, TG, cholesterol	Pancreatitis, hepatosplenomegaly, and eruptive/pruritic xanthomas (no ↑ risk for atherosclerosis). Creamy layer in supernatant.
IIa—Familial hyper-cholesterolemia	AD	Absent or defective LDL receptors	LDL, cholesterol	Heterozygotes (1:500) have cholesterol ≈ 300mg/dL; homozygotes (very rare) have cholesterol ≈ 700+ mg/dL. Accelerated atherosclerosis (may have MI before age 20), tendon (Achilles) xanthomas, and corneal arcus.
IV—Hyper-triglyceridemia	AD	Hepatic overproduction of VLDL	VLDL, TG	Hypertriglyceridemia (> 1000 mg/dL) can cause acute pancreatitis.

NOTES

HIGH-YIELD PRINCIPLES IN

Microbiology

"Support bacteria. They're the only culture some people have."

—Steven Wright

"What lies behind us and what lies ahead of us are tiny matters compared to what lies within us."

—Henry S. Haskins

"Infectious disease is merely a disagreeable instance of a widely prevalent tendency of all living creatures to save themselves the bother of building, by their own efforts, the things they require."

—Hans Zinsser

This high-yield material covers the basic concepts of microbiology. The emphasis in previous examinations has been approximately 40% bacteriology (20% basic, 20% quasi-clinical), 25% immunology, 25% virology (10% basic, 15% quasi-clinical), 5% parasitology, and 5% mycology.

Microbiology questions on the Step 1 exam often require two (or more) steps: Given a certain clinical presentation, you will first need to identify the most likely causative organism, and you will then need to provide an answer regarding some feature of that organism. For example, a description of a child with fever and a petechial rash will be followed by a question that reads, "From what site does the responsible organism usually enter the blood?"

This section therefore presents organisms in two major ways: in individual microbial "profiles" and in the context of the systems they infect and the clinical presentations they produce. You should become familiar with both formats. When reviewing the systems approach, remind yourself of the features of each microbe by returning to the individual profiles. Also be sure to memorize the laboratory characteristics that allow you to identify microbes.

▸ MICROBIOLOGY—BASIC BACTERIOLOGY

Bacterial structures

STRUCTURE	CHEMICAL COMPOSITION	FUNCTION
Appendages		
Flagellum	Proteins.	Motility.
Pilus/fimbria	Glycoprotein.	Mediate adherence of bacteria to cell surface; sex pilus forms during conjugation.
Specialized structures		
Spore	Keratin-like coat; dipicolinic acid; peptidoglycan, DNA.	Gram ⊕ only. Survival: resist dehydration, heat, chemicals.
Cell envelope		
Capsule	Organized, discrete polysaccharide layer (except poly-D glutamate on *B anthracis*).	Protects against phagocytosis.
Glycocalyx	Loose network of polysaccharides.	Mediates adherence to surfaces, especially foreign surfaces (eg, indwelling catheters).
Outer membrane	Outer leaflet: contains endotoxin (LPS/LOS). Embedded proteins: porins and other outer membrane proteins (OMPs) Inner leaflet: phospholipids.	Gram ⊖ only. Endotoxin: lipid A induces TNF and IL-1; O polysaccharide component antigenic. Most OMPs are antigenic. Porins: transport across outer membrane.
Periplasm	Space between cytoplasmic membrane and outer membrane in gram ⊖ bacteria. (Peptidoglycan in middle.)	Gram ⊖ only. Accumulates components exiting gram ⊖ cells, including hydrolytic enzymes (eg, β-lactamases).
Cell wall	Peptidoglycan is a sugar backbone with peptide side chains cross-linked by transpeptidase.	Net-like structure gives rigid support, protects against osmotic pressure damage.
Cytoplasmic membrane	Phospholipid bilayer sac with embedded proteins (eg, penicillin-binding proteins [PBPs]) and other enzymes. Lipoteichoic acids (gram ⊕ only) extend from membrane to exterior.	Site of oxidative and transport enzymes; PBPs involved in cell wall synthesis. Lipoteichoic acids induce TNF and IL-1.

Cell walls

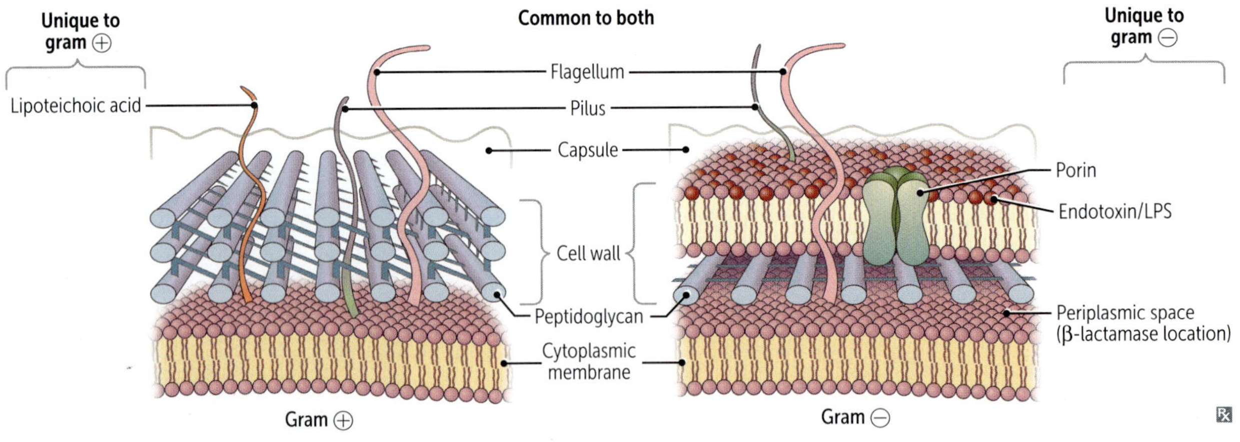

Bacterial taxonomy

MORPHOLOGY	Gram ⊕ examples	Gram ⊖ examples
Spherical (coccus)	*Staphylococcus* (clusters) *Streptococcus* (chains or pairs)	*Moraxella catarrhalis* *Neisseria*
Rod (bacillus)	*Bacillus* *Clostridium* *Corynebacterium* *Gardnerella* (gram variable) *Lactobacillus* *Listeria* *Mycobacterium* (acid fast) *Propionibacterium*	Enterics: ▪ *Bacteroides* ▪ *Campylobacter* ▪ *E coli* ▪ *Enterobacter* ▪ *Helicobacter* ▪ *Klebsiella* ▪ *Proteus* ▪ *Pseudomonas* ▪ *Salmonella* ▪ *Serratia* ▪ *Shigella* ▪ *Vibrio* ▪ *Yersinia* Respiratory: ▪ *Bordetella* ▪ *Burkholderia cepacia* ▪ *Haemophilus* (pleomorphic) ▪ *Legionella* (silver stain) Zoonotic: ▪ *Bartonella* ▪ *Brucella* ▪ *Francisella* ▪ *Pasteurella*
Branching filamentous	*Actinomyces* *Nocardia* (weakly acid fast)	
Pleomorphic		Chlamydiae (Giemsa) Rickettsiae (Giemsa)
Spiral		Spirochetes: ▪ *Borrelia* (Giemsa) ▪ *Leptospira* ▪ *Treponema*
No cell wall	*Mycoplasma*, *Ureaplasma* (contain sterols, which do not Gram stain)	

Stains

Gram stain	First-line lab test in bacterial identification. Bacteria with thick peptidoglycan layer retain crystal violet dye (gram ⊕); bacteria with thin peptidoglycan layer turn red or pink (gram ⊖) with counterstain.	
	The bugs below do not Gram stain well.	**T**hese **M**icrobes **M**ay **L**ack **R**eal **C**olor
	Treponema, *Leptospira*	Too thin to be visualized.
	Mycobacteria	Cell wall has high lipid content.
	***M**ycoplasma*, *Ureaplasma*	No cell wall.
	***L**egionella*, ***R**ickettsia*, ***C**hlamydia*, *Bartonella*, *Ehrlichia*, *Anaplasma*	Primarily intracellular; also, *Chlamydia* lack classic peptidoglycan because of ↓ muramic acid.
Giemsa stain	***C**hlamydia*, ***B**orrelia*, ***R**ickettsia*, **T**rypanosomes A, ***P**lasmodium*	**C**ertain **B**ugs **R**eally **T**ry my **P**atience.
Periodic acid–Schiff stain	Stains **glycogen**, mucopolysaccharides; used to diagnose Whipple disease (*Tropheryma whipplei* B)	**PaS**s the **sugar**.
Ziehl-Neelsen stain (carbol fuchsin)	Acid-fast bacteria, eg, *Mycobacteria* C (stains mycolic acid in cell wall), *Nocardia*; protozoa, eg, *Cryptosporidium* oocysts	Alternative is auramine-rhodamine stain for screening (inexpensive, more sensitive but less specific).
India ink stain	*Cryptococcus neoformans* D; mucicarmine can also be used to stain thick polysaccharide capsule red	
Silver stain	Fungi (eg, *Coccidioides* E, *Pneumocystis jirovecii*), *Legionella*, *Helicobacter pylori*	
Fluorescent antibody stain	Used to identify many bacteria and viruses.	Example is FTA-ABS for confirming syphilis.

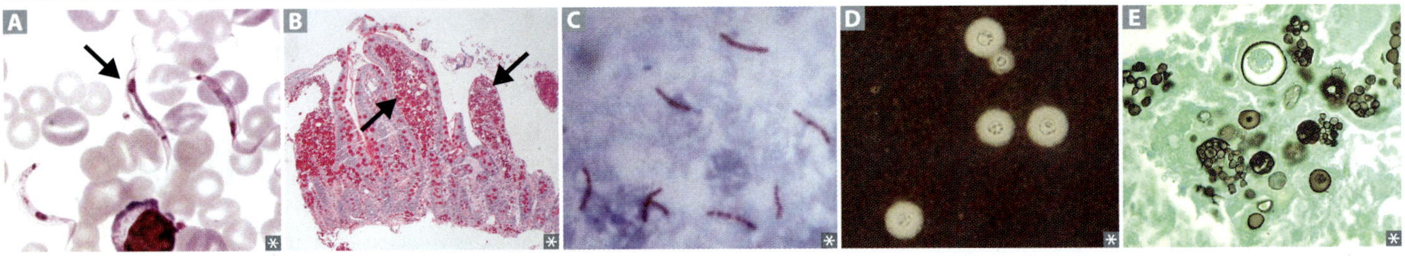

Properties of growth media

Properties of growth media	The same type of media can possess both (or neither) of these properties.
Selective media	Favors the growth of particular organism while preventing growth of other organisms, eg, Thayer-Martin agar contains antibiotics that allow the selective growth of *Neisseria* by inhibiting the growth of other sensitive organisms.
Indicator (differential) media	Yields a color change in response to the metabolism of certain organisms, eg, MacConkey agar contains a pH indicator; a lactose fermenter like *E coli* will convert lactose to acidic metabolites → color change.

Giemsa stain = used to stain periph blood smear & BM smear
The eiosin Y turns cytop orange/pink
methylene blue / azure B stains nucleus blue/purple

Special culture requirements

BUG	MEDIA USED FOR ISOLATION	MEDIA CONTENTS/OTHER
H influenzae	Chocolate agar	Factors V (NAD^+) and X (hematin)
N gonorrhoeae, *N meningitidis*	Thayer-Martin agar	Selectively favors growth of *Neisseria* by inhibiting growth of gram ⊕ organisms with **V**ancomycin, gram ⊖ organisms except *Neisseria* with **T**rimethoprim and **C**olistin, and fungi with **N**ystatin **V**ery **T**ypically **C**ultures ***N**eisseria*
B pertussis	Bordet-Gengou agar (**Bordet** for ***Bordet**ella*) Regan-Lowe medium	Potato Charcoal, blood, and antibiotic
C diphtheriae	Tellurite agar, Löffler medium	
M tuberculosis	Löwenstein-Jensen agar	
M pneumoniae	Eaton agar	Requires cholesterol
Lactose-fermenting enterics	MacConkey agar	Fermentation produces acid, causing colonies to turn pink
E coli	Eosin–methylene blue (EMB) agar	Colonies with green metallic sheen
Legionella	Charcoal yeast extract agar buffered with cysteine and iron	
Fungi	**Sab**ouraud agar	"**Sab**'s a **fun guy**!"

Aerobes

Use an O_2-dependent system to generate ATP. Examples include ***N**ocardia*, ***P**seudomonas aeruginosa*, and *Myco**B**acterium tuberculosis*.
Reactivation of *M tuberculosis* (eg, after immunocompromise or TNF-α inhibitor use) has a predilection for the apices of the lung.

Nagging **P**ests **M**ust **B**reathe.

Anaerobes

Examples include ***C**lostridium*, ***B**acteroides*, ***F**usobacterium*, and ***A**ctinomyces*. They lack catalase and/or superoxide dismutase and are thus susceptible to oxidative damage. Generally foul smelling (short-chain fatty acids), are difficult to culture, and produce gas in tissue (CO_2 and H_2).

Anaerobes **C**an't **B**reathe **F**resh **A**ir.
Anaerobes are normal flora in GI tract, typically pathogenic elsewhere. Amin**O_2**glycosides are ineffective against anaerobes because these antibiotics require **O_2** to enter into bacterial cell.

catalase = $2H_2O_2 \longrightarrow 2H_2O + O_2$

$2O_2^- \xrightarrow{SOD} O_2 + H_2O_2$

Intracellular bugs

Obligate intracellular	*Rickettsia*, *CHlamydia*, *COxiella*. Rely on host ATP.	Stay inside (cells) when it is Really CHilly and COld.
Facultative intracellular	*Salmonella*, *Neisseria*, *Brucella*, *Mycobacterium*, *Listeria*, *Francisella*, *Legionella*, *Yersinia pestis*.	Some Nasty Bugs May Live FacultativeLY.

Encapsulated bacteria

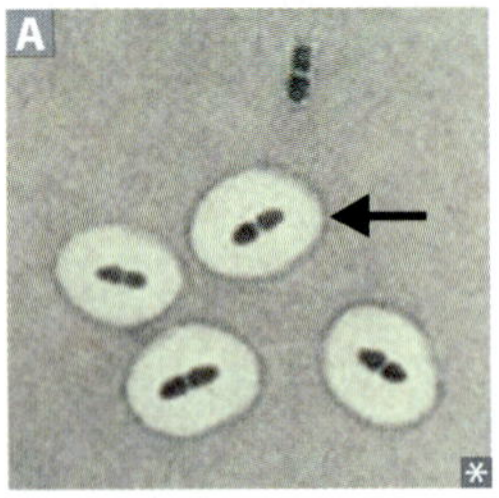

Examples are *Pseudomonas aeruginosa*, *Streptococcus pneumoniae* A, *Haemophilus Influenzae* type B, *Neisseria meningitidis*, *Escherichia coli*, *Salmonella*, *Klebsiella pneumoniae*, and group B Strep. Their capsules serve as an antiphagocytic virulence factor.

Capsular polysaccharide + protein conjugate serves as an antigen in vaccines.

Please SHINE my SKiS.

Are opsonized, and then cleared by spleen. Asplenics have ↓ opsonizing ability and thus ↑ risk for severe infections. Give *S pneumoniae*, *H influenzae*, *N meningitidis* vaccines.

Encapsulated bacteria vaccines

Some vaccines containing polysaccharide capsule antigens are conjugated to a carrier protein, enhancing immunogenicity by promoting T-cell activation and subsequent class switching. A polysaccharide antigen alone cannot be presented to T cells.

Pneumococcal vaccine: PCV (pneumococcal conjugate vaccine, ie, Prevnar); PPSV (pneumococcal polysaccharide vaccine with no conjugated protein, ie, Pneumovax)

H influenzae type B (conjugate vaccine)

Meningococcal vaccine (conjugate vaccine)

Urease-positive organisms

Proteus, *Cryptococcus*, *H pylori*, *Ureaplasma*, *Nocardia*, *Klebsiella*, *S epidermidis*, *S saprophyticus*. Potentiate struvite (ammonium magnesium phosphate) stones. Urease hydrolyzes urea to release ammonia and CO_2 → ↑ pH.

Pee CHUNKSS.

Catalase-positive organisms

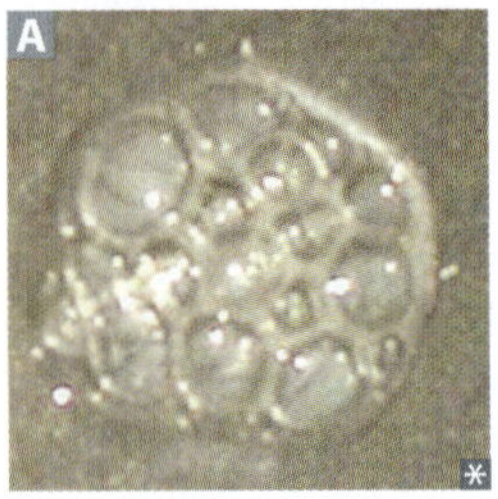

Catalase degrades H_2O_2 into H_2O and bubbles of O_2 A before it can be converted to microbicidal products by the enzyme myeloperoxidase. People with chronic granulomatous disease (NADPH oxidase deficiency) have recurrent infections with certain catalase ⊕ organisms.

Examples: *Nocardia*, *Pseudomonas*, *Listeria*, *Aspergillus*, *Candida*, *E coli*, Staphylococci, *Serratia*, *B cepacia*, *H pylori*.

Cats Need PLACESS to Belch their Hairballs.

Pigment-producing bacteria	*Actinomyces israelii*—yellow "sulfur" granules, which are composed of filaments of bacteria.	Israel has yellow sand.
	S aureus—yellow pigment.	*Aureus* (Latin) = gold.
	P aeruginosa—blue-green pigment.	Aerugula is green.
	Serratia marcescens—red pigment.	*Serratia marcescens*—think red maraschino cherries.

In vivo biofilm-producing bacteria	*S epidermidis*	Catheter and prosthetic device infections
	Viridans streptococci (*S mutans*, *S sanguinis*)	Dental plaques, infective endocarditis
	P aeruginosa	Respiratory tree colonization in cystic fibrosis patients, contact lens–associated keratitis
	Nontypeable (unencapsulated) *H influenza*	Otitis media

Bacterial virulence factors	These promote evasion of host immune response.
Protein A	Binds Fc region of IgG. Prevents opsonization and phagocytosis. Expressed by *S aureus*.
IgA protease	Enzyme that cleaves IgA. Secreted by *S pneumoniae*, *H influenzae* type B, and *Neisseria* (SHiN) in order to colonize respiratory mucosa.
M protein	Helps prevent phagocytosis. Expressed by group A streptococci. Shares similar epitopes to human cellular proteins (molecular mimicry); possibly underlies the autoimmune response seen in acute rheumatic fever.

Type III secretion system	Also known as "injectisome." Needle-like protein appendage facilitating direct delivery of toxins from certain gram ⊖ bacteria (eg, *Pseudomonas*, *Salmonella*, *Shigella*, *E coli*) to eukaryotic host cell.

Bacterial genetics

Transformation	Ability to take up naked DNA (ie, from cell lysis) from environment (also known as "competence"). A feature of many bacteria, especially **S** *pneumoniae*, **H** *influenzae* type B, and **N***eisseria* (**SHiN**). Any DNA can be used. Adding deoxyribonuclease to environment will degrade naked DNA in medium → no transformation seen.
Conjugation	
$F^+ \times F^-$	F^+ plasmid contains genes required for sex pilus and conjugation. Bacteria without this plasmid are termed F^-. Sex pilus on F^+ bacterium contacts F^- bacterium. A single strand of plasmid DNA is transferred across the conjugal bridge ("mating bridge"). No transfer of chromosomal DNA.
Hfr $\times F^-$	F^+ plasmid can become incorporated into bacterial chromosomal DNA, termed high-frequency recombination (Hfr) cell. Replication of incorporated plasmid DNA may include some flanking chromosomal DNA. Transfer of plasmid and chromosomal genes.
Transposition	Segment of DNA (eg, transposon) that can "jump" (excision and reintegration) from one location to another, can transfer genes from plasmid to chromosome and vice versa. When excision occurs, may include some flanking chromosomal DNA, which can be incorporated into a plasmid and transferred to another bacterium (eg, *van*A gene from vancomycin-resistant *Enterococcus* to *S aureus*).
Transduction	
Generalized	A "packaging" event. Lytic phage infects bacterium, leading to cleavage of bacterial DNA. Parts of bacterial chromosomal DNA may become packaged in phage capsid. Phage infects another bacterium, transferring these genes.
Specialized	An "excision" event. Lysogenic phage infects bacterium; viral DNA incorporates into bacterial chromosome. When phage DNA is excised, flanking bacterial genes may be excised with it. DNA is packaged into phage capsid and can infect another bacterium. Genes for the following 5 bacterial toxins are encoded in a lysogenic phage (**ABCD'S**): ▪ Group **A** strep erythrogenic toxin ▪ **B**otulinum toxin ▪ **C**holera toxin ▪ **D**iphtheria toxin ▪ **S**higa toxin

Spore-forming bacteria

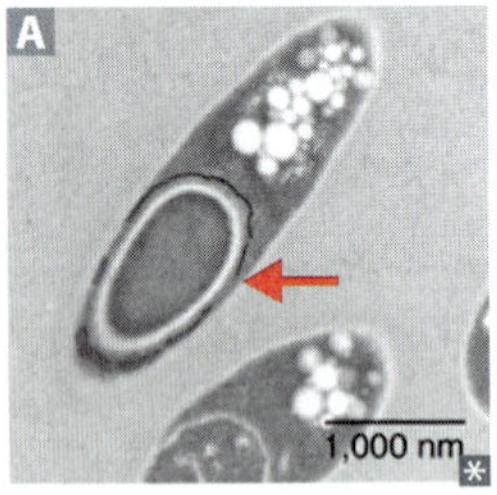

Some bacteria can form spores A at the end of the stationary phase when nutrients are limited.

Spores are highly resistant to heat and chemicals. Have dipicolinic acid in their core. Have no metabolic activity. Must autoclave to potentially kill spores (as is done to surgical equipment) by steaming at 121°C for 15 minutes.

Bacillus anthracis	Anthrax
Bacillus cereus	Food poisoning
Clostridium botulinum	Botulism
Clostridium difficile	Pseudomembranous colitis
Clostridium perfringens	Gas gangrene
Clostridium tetani	Tetanus

Main features of exotoxins and endotoxins

PROPERTY	Exotoxin	Endotoxin
SOURCE	Certain species of gram ⊕ and gram ⊖ bacteria	Outer cell membrane of most gram ⊖ bacteria
SECRETED FROM CELL	Yes	No
CHEMISTRY	Polypeptide	Lipid A component of LPS (structural part of bacteria; released when lysed)
LOCATION OF GENES	Plasmid or bacteriophage	Bacterial chromosome
ADVERSE EFFECTS	High (fatal dose on the order of 1 μg)	Low (fatal dose on the order of hundreds of micrograms)
CLINICAL EFFECTS	Various effects (see following pages)	Fever, shock (hypotension), DIC
MODE OF ACTION	Various modes (see following pages)	Induces TNF, IL-1, and IL-6
ANTIGENICITY	Induces high-titer antibodies called antitoxins	Poorly antigenic
VACCINES	Toxoids used as vaccines	No toxoids formed and no vaccine available
HEAT STABILITY	Destroyed rapidly at 60°C (except staphylococcal enterotoxin)	Stable at 100°C for 1 hr
TYPICAL DISEASES	Tetanus, botulism, diphtheria	Meningococcemia; sepsis by gram ⊖ rods

Bugs with exotoxins

BACTERIA	TOXIN	MECHANISM	MANIFESTATION
Inhibit protein synthesis			
Corynebacterium diphtheriae	Diphtheria toxin[a]	Inactivate elongation factor (EF-2)	Pharyngitis with pseudomembranes in throat and severe lymphadenopathy (bull neck)
Pseudomonas aeruginosa	Exotoxin A[a]		Host cell death
***Shigella* spp.**	Shiga toxin (ST)[a]	Inactivate 60S ribosome by removing adenine from rRNA	GI mucosal damage → dysentery; ST also enhances cytokine release, causing hemolytic-uremic syndrome (HUS)
Enterohemorrhagic *E coli* (EHEC)	Shiga-like toxin (SLT)[a]		SLT enhances cytokine release, causing HUS (prototypically in EHEC serotype O157:H7). Unlike *Shigella*, EHEC does not invade host cells
Increase fluid secretion			
Enterotoxigenic *E coli* (ETEC)	Heat-**labile** toxin (LT)[a]	Overactivates adenylate cyclase (↑ cAMP) → ↑ Cl^- secretion in gut and H_2O efflux	Watery diarrhea: "**labile** in the **A**ir (**A**denylate cyclase), **stable** on the **G**round (**G**uanylate cyclase)"
	Heat-**stable** toxin (ST)	Overactivates guanylate cyclase (↑ c**G**MP) → ↓ resorption of NaCl and H_2O in gut	
Bacillus anthracis	Edema toxin[a]	Mimics the adenylate cyclase enzyme (↑ cAMP)	Likely responsible for characteristic edematous borders of black eschar in cutaneous anthrax
Vibrio cholerae	Cholera toxin[a]	Overactivates adenylate cyclase (↑ cAMP) by permanently activating G_s → ↑ Cl^- secretion in gut and H_2O efflux	Voluminous "rice-water" diarrhea
Inhibit phagocytic ability			
Bordetella pertussis	Pertussis toxin[a]	Overactivates adenylate cyclase (↑ cAMP) by disabling G_i, impairing phagocytosis to permit survival of microbe	**Whooping cough**—child coughs on expiration and "whoops" on inspiration (toxin may not actually be a cause of cough; can cause "100-day cough" in adults)
Inhibit release of neurotransmitter			
Clostridium tetani	Tetanospasmin[a]	Both are proteases that cleave SNARE (soluble NSF attachment protein receptor), a set of proteins required for neurotransmitter release via vesicular fusion	Spastic paralysis, risus sardonicus, and "lockjaw"; toxin prevents release of **inhibitory** (GABA and glycine) neurotransmitters from Renshaw cells in spinal cord
Clostridium botulinum	Botulinum toxin[a]		Flaccid paralysis, floppy baby; toxin prevents release of **stimulatory** (ACh) signals at neuromuscular junctions → flaccid paralysis

[a]An AB toxin (aka, two-component toxin [or three for anthrax]) with **B** enabling **b**inding and triggering uptake (endocytosis) of the **a**ctive **A** component. The A components are usually ADP ribosyltransferases; others have enzymatic activities as listed in chart.

Bugs with exotoxins *(continued)*

BACTERIA	TOXIN	MECHANISM	MANIFESTATION
Lyse cell membranes			
Clostridium perfringens	Alpha toxin	Phospholipase (lecithinase) that degrades tissue and cell membranes	Degradation of phospholipids → myonecrosis ("gas gangrene") and hemolysis ("double zone" of hemolysis on blood agar)
Streptococcus pyogenes	Streptolysin O	Protein that degrades cell membrane	Lyses RBCs; contributes to β-hemolysis; host antibodies against toxin (ASO) used to diagnose rheumatic fever (do not confuse with immune complexes of poststreptococcal glomerulonephritis)
Superantigens causing shock			
Staphylococcus aureus	Toxic shock syndrome toxin (TSST-1)	Binds to MHC II and TCR outside of antigen binding site to cause overwhelming release of IL-1, IL-2, IFN-γ, and TNF-α → shock	Toxic shock syndrome: fever, rash, shock; other toxins cause scalded skin syndrome (exfoliative toxin) and food poisoning (enterotoxin)
Streptococcus pyogenes	Exotoxin A		Toxic shock syndrome: fever, rash, shock

Endotoxin

LPS found in outer membrane of gram ⊖ bacteria (both cocci and rods). Composed of O antigen + core polysaccharide + lipid A (the toxic component).

Released upon cell lysis or by living cells by blebs detaching from outer surface membrane (vs exotoxin, which is actively secreted).

Three main effects: macrophage activation (TLR4), complement activation, and tissue factor activation.

ENDOTOXINS:
- **E**dema
- **N**itric oxide
- **D**IC/**D**eath
- **O**uter membrane
- **T**NF-α
- **O**-antigen + core polysaccharide + lipid A
- e**X**tremely heat stable
- **I**L-1 and **I**L-6
- **N**eutrophil chemotaxis
- **S**hock

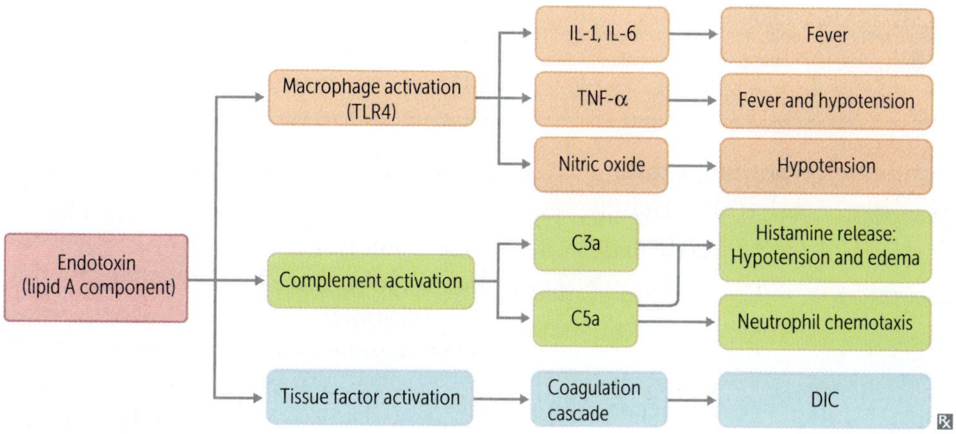

▸ MICROBIOLOGY—CLINICAL BACTERIOLOGY

Gram-positive lab algorithm

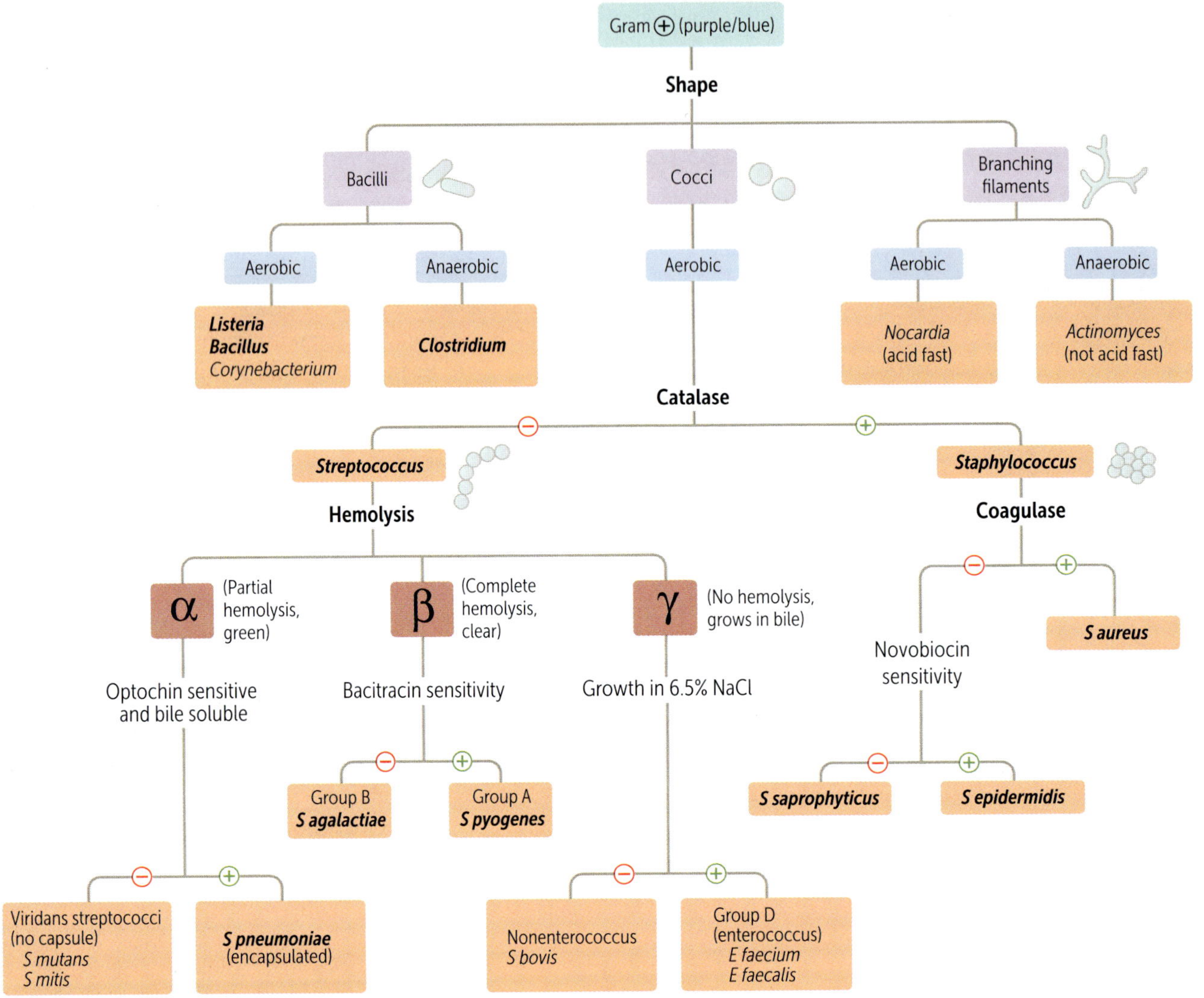

Important **tests** are in **bold**. Important ***pathogens*** are in ***bold italics***.
Note: Enterococcus is either α- or γ-hemolytic.

Gram-positive cocci antibiotic tests

Staphylococci	**NO**vobiocin—***S**aprophyticus* is **R**esistant; ***E**pidermidis* is **S**ensitive.	On the office's "**staph**" retreat, there was **NO StRES**s.
Streptococci	**O**ptochin—***V**iridans* is **R**esistant; ***P**neumoniae* is **S**ensitive.	**OVRPS** (overpass).
	Bacitracin—group **B** strep are **R**esistant; group **A** strep are **S**ensitive.	**B-BRAS**.

α-hemolytic bacteria

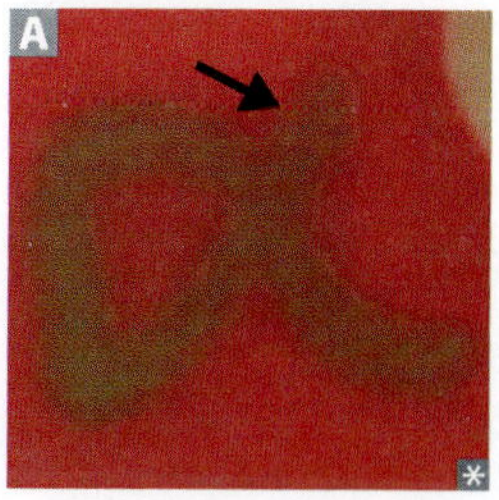

Gram ⊕ cocci. Partial reduction of hemoglobin causes greenish or brownish color without clearing around growth on blood agar A. Include the following organisms:

- *Streptococcus pneumoniae* (catalase ⊖ and optochin sensitive)
- Viridans streptococci (catalase ⊖ and optochin resistant)

β-hemolytic bacteria

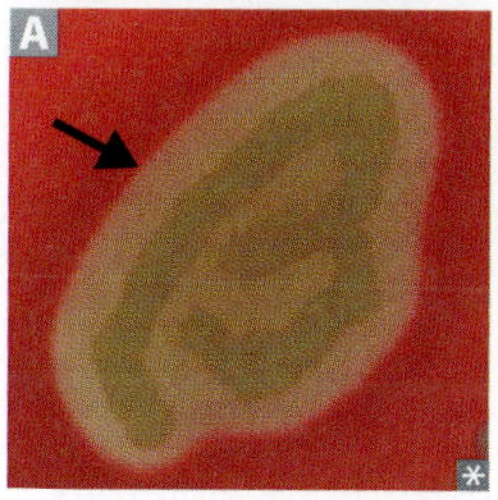

Gram ⊕ cocci. Complete lysis of RBCs → clear area surrounding colony on blood agar A. Include the following organisms:

- *Staphylococcus aureus* (catalase and coagulase ⊕)
- *Streptococcus pyogenes*—group A strep (catalase ⊖ and bacitracin sensitive)
- *Streptococcus agalactiae*—group B strep (catalase ⊖ and bacitracin resistant)

Staphylococcus aureus

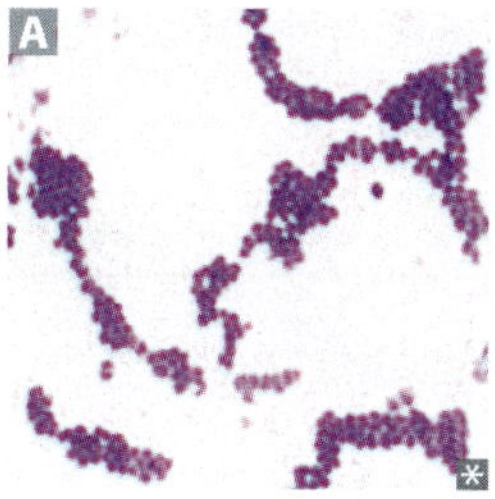

Gram ⊕, β-hemolytic, catalase ⊕, coagulase ⊕ cocci in clusters A. Protein A (virulence factor) binds Fc-IgG, inhibiting complement activation and phagocytosis. Commonly colonizes the nares.

Causes:

- Inflammatory disease—skin infections, organ abscesses, pneumonia (often after influenza virus infection), endocarditis, septic arthritis, and osteomyelitis.
- Toxin-mediated disease—toxic shock syndrome (TSST-1), scalded skin syndrome (exfoliative toxin), rapid-onset food poisoning (enterotoxins).
- MRSA (methicillin-resistant *S aureus*) infection—important cause of serious nosocomial and community-acquired infections; resistant to methicillin and nafcillin because of altered penicillin-binding protein.

TSST-1 is a superantigen that binds to MHC II and T-cell receptor, resulting in polyclonal T-cell activation.

Staphylococcal toxic shock syndrome (TSS) presents as fever, vomiting, rash, desquamation, shock, end-organ failure. TSS results in ↑ AST, ↑ ALT, ↑ bilirubin. Associated with prolonged use of vaginal tampons or nasal packing.

Compare with *Streptococcus pyogenes* TSS (a toxic shock–like syndrome associated with painful skin infection).

S aureus food poisoning due to ingestion of preformed toxin → short incubation period (2–6 hr) followed by nonbloody diarrhea and emesis. Enterotoxin is heat stable → not destroyed by cooking.

Staph make catalase because they have more "**staff**." Bad staph (*aureus*) make coagulase and toxins. Forms fibrin clot around self → abscess.

Staphylococcus epidermidis

Gram ⊕, catalase ⊕, coagulase ⊖, urease ⊕ cocci in clusters. Novobiocin sensitive.

Normal flora of skin; contaminates blood cultures.

Infects prosthetic devices (eg, hip implant, heart valve) and IV catheters by producing adherent biofilms.

Staphylococcus saprophyticus

Gram ⊕, catalase ⊕, coagulase ⊖, urease ⊕ cocci in clusters. Novobiocin resistant.
Normal flora of female genital tract and perineum.
Second most common cause of uncomplicated UTI in young women (most common cause is *E coli*).

Streptococcus pneumoniae

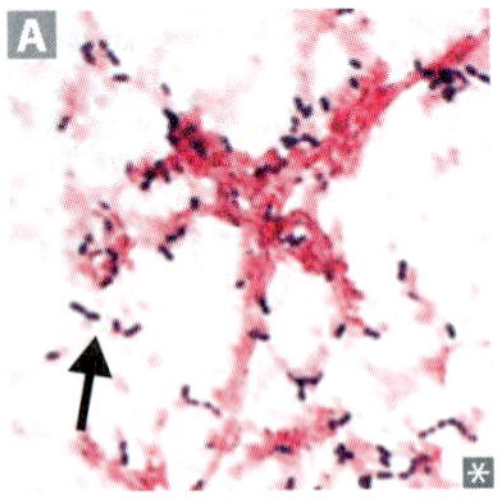

Gram ⊕, lancet-shaped diplococci A. Encapsulated. IgA protease. Optochin sensitive. Most common cause of:

- Meningitis
- Otitis media (in children)
- Pneumonia
- Sinusitis

Pneumococcus is associated with "rusty" sputum, sepsis in patients with sickle cell disease and splenectomy.
No virulence without capsule.

Viridans group streptococci

Gram ⊕, α-hemolytic cocci. They are normal flora of the oropharynx that cause dental caries (*Streptococcus mutans* and *S mitis*) and subacute bacterial endocarditis at damaged **heart** valves (*S sanguinis*). Resistant to optochin, differentiating them from *S pneumoniae*, which is α-hemolytic but is optochin sensitive.

Sanguinis = **blood**. Think, "there is lots of **blood** in the **heart**" (endocarditis). *S sanguinis* makes dextrans, which bind to fibrin-platelet aggregates on damaged heart valves.
Viridans group strep live in the mouth because they are not afraid **of-the-chin** (**op-to-chin** resistant).

Streptococcus pyogenes (group A streptococci)

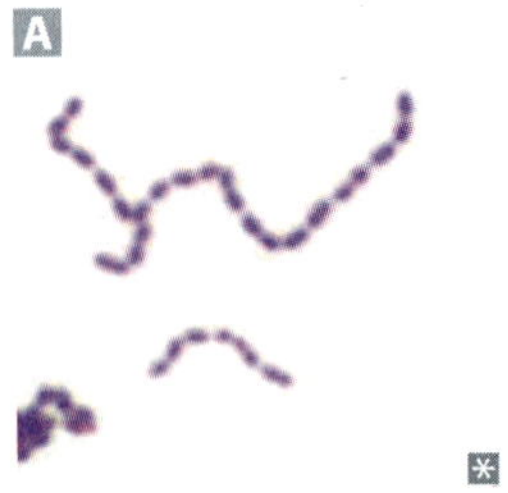

Gram ⊕ cocci. Group A strep A cause:

- Pyogenic—pharyngitis, cellulitis, impetigo, erysipelas
- Toxigenic—scarlet fever, toxic shock–like syndrome, necrotizing fasciitis
- Immunologic—rheumatic fever, glomerulonephritis

Bacitracin sensitive, β-hemolytic, pyrrolidonyl arylamidase (PYR) ⊕. Antibodies to M protein enhance host defenses against *S pyogenes* but can give rise to rheumatic fever.
ASO titer detects recent *S pyogenes* infection.

J♥NES (major criteria for acute rheumatic fever):
- **J**oints—polyarthritis
- **♥**—carditis
- **N**odules (subcutaneous)
- **E**rythema marginatum
- **S**ydenham chorea

Pharyngitis can result in rheumatic "**ph**ever" and glomerulone**ph**ritis.
Impetigo usually precedes glomerulonephritis.
Scarlet fever—blanching, sandpaper-like body rash, strawberry tongue, and circumoral pallor in the setting of group A streptococcal pharyngitis (erythrogenic toxin ⊕).

Streptococcus agalactiae **(group B streptococci)**	Gram ⊕ cocci, bacitracin resistant, β-hemolytic, colonizes vagina; causes pneumonia, meningitis, and sepsis, mainly in **babies**. Produces CAMP factor, which enlarges the area of hemolysis formed by *S aureus*. (Note: CAMP stands for the authors of the test, not cyclic AMP.) Hippurate test ⊕, PYR ⊖. Screen pregnant women at 35–37 weeks of gestation. Patients with ⊕ culture receive intrapartum penicillin prophylaxis.	Group **B** for **B**abies!
Streptococcus bovis	Gram ⊕ cocci, colonizes the gut. *S gallolyticus* (*S bovis* biotype 1) can cause bacteremia and subacute endocarditis and is associated with colon cancer.	**B**ovis in the **b**lood = **c**ancer in the **c**olon.
Enterococci	Gram ⊕ cocci. Enterococci (*E faecalis* and *E faecium*) are normal colonic flora that are penicillin G resistant and cause UTI, biliary tract infections, and subacute endocarditis (following GI/GU procedures). Catalase ⊖, PYR ⊕, variable hemolysis. VRE (vancomycin-resistant enterococci) are an important cause of nosocomial infection.	Enterococci, hardier than nonenterococcal group D, can grow in 6.5% NaCl and bile (lab test). *Entero* = intestine, *faecalis* = feces, *strepto* = twisted (chains), *coccus* = berry.
Bacillus anthracis	Gram ⊕, spore-forming rod that produces anthrax toxin. The only bacterium with a polypeptide capsule (contains D-glutamate).	
Cutaneous anthrax	Painless papule surrounded by vesicles → ulcer with black eschar (A) (painless, necrotic) → uncommonly progresses to bacteremia and death.	
Pulmonary anthrax	Inhalation of spores → flu-like symptoms that rapidly progress to fever, pulmonary hemorrhage, mediastinitis, and shock. Also known as woolsorter's disease	

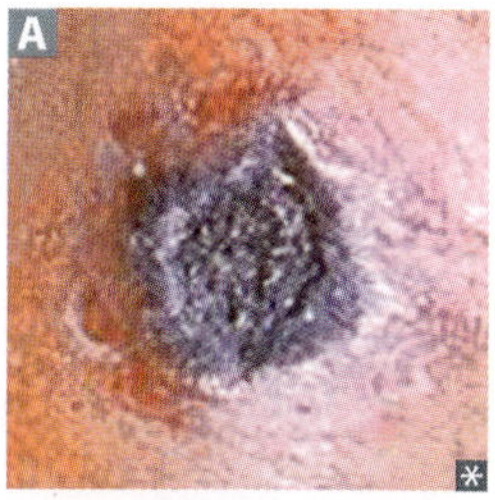

Bacillus cereus	Gram ⊕ rod. Causes food poisoning. Spores survive cooking rice. Keeping rice warm results in germination of spores and enterotoxin formation. Emetic type usually seen with rice and pasta. Nausea and vomiting within 1–5 hr. Caused by cereulide, a preformed toxin. Diarrheal type causes watery, nonbloody diarrhea and GI pain within 8–18 hr.	Reheated rice syndrome.
Clostridia (with exotoxins)	Gram ⊕, spore-forming, obligate anaerobic rods.	
C tetani	Produces tetano**spas**min, an exotoxin causing tetanus. Tetanus toxin (and botulinum toxin) are proteases that cleave SNARE proteins for neurotransmitters. Blocks release of inhibitory neurotransmitters, GABA and glycine, from Renshaw cells in spinal cord. Causes **spas**tic paralysis, trismus (lockjaw), risus sardonicus (raised eyebrows and open grin). Prevent with tetanus vaccine. Treat with antitoxin +/– vaccine booster, diazepam (for muscle spasms), and wound debridement.	**Tet**anus is **tet**anic paralysis.
C botulinum	Produces a heat-labile toxin that inhibits ACh release at the neuromuscular junction, causing botulism. In adults, disease is caused by ingestion of preformed toxin. In babies, ingestion of spores (eg, in honey) leads to disease (**floppy** baby syndrome). Treat with antitoxin.	***Bot**ulinum* is from bad **bot**tles of food, juice, and honey (causes a descending **flaccid** paralysis). Local botox injections used to treat focal dystonia, achalasia, and muscle spasms. Also used for cosmetic reduction of facial wrinkles.
C perfringens 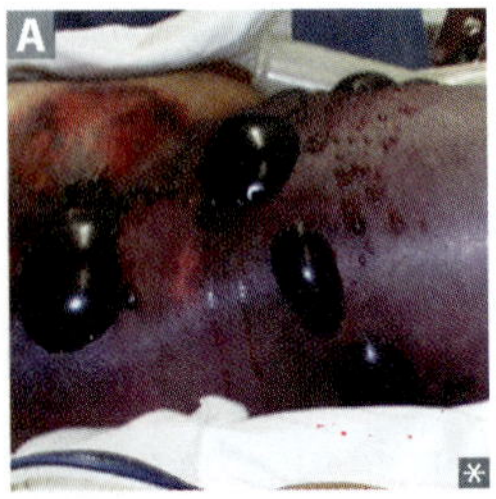	Produces α toxin (lecithinase, a phospholipase) that can cause myonecrosis (gas gangrene A) and hemolysis. Spores can survive in undercooked food; when ingested, bacteria release heat-labile enterotoxin → food poisoning.	***Perf**ringens* **perf**orates a gangrenous leg.
C difficile 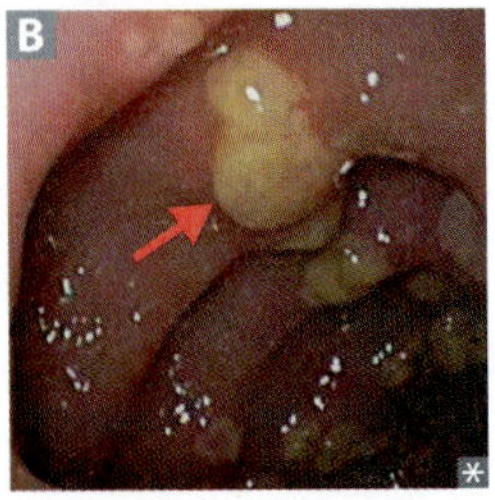	Produces 2 toxins. Toxin A, enterotoxin, binds to the brush border of the gut. Toxin B, cytotoxin, causes cytoskeletal disruption via actin depolymerization → diarrhea → pseudomembranous colitis B. Often 2° to antibiotic use, especially clindamycin or ampicillin; associated with PPI use. Diagnosed by detecting one or both toxins in stool by PCR.	***Di**fficile* causes **di**arrhea. Treatment: metronidazole or oral vancomycin. For recurrent cases, consider repeating prior regimen, fidaxomicin, or fecal microbiota transplant.

Corynebacterium diphtheriae

A
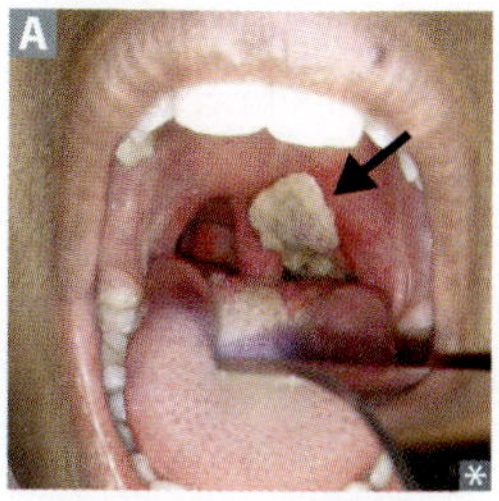

Gram ⊕ rod. Causes diphtheria via exotoxin encoded by β-prophage. Potent exotoxin inhibits protein synthesis via ADP-ribosylation of EF-2.

Symptoms include pseudomembranous pharyngitis (grayish-white membrane A) with lymphadenopathy, myocarditis, and arrhythmias.

Lab diagnosis based on gram ⊕ rods with metachromatic (blue and red) granules and ⊕ Elek test for toxin.

Toxoid vaccine prevents diphtheria.

Coryne = club shaped.

Black colonies on cystine-tellurite agar.

ABCDEFG:

- **A**DP-ribosylation
- **β**-prophage
- ***C****orynebacterium*
- ***D****iphtheriae*
- **E**longation **F**actor 2
- **G**ranules

Listeria monocytogenes

A
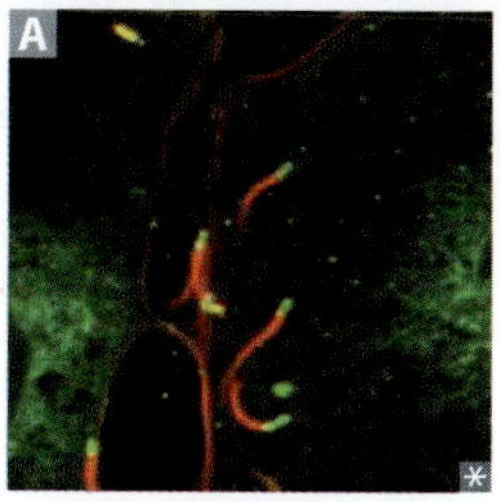

Gram ⊕, facultative intracellular rod; acquired by ingestion of unpasteurized dairy products and cold deli meats, via transplacental transmission, or by vaginal transmission during birth.

Forms "rocket tails" (red in A) via actin polymerization that allow intracellular movement and cell-to-cell spread across cell membranes, thereby avoiding antibody. Characteristic tumbling motility in broth.

* Can cause amnionitis, septicemia, and spontaneous abortion in pregnant women; granulomatosis infantiseptica; neonatal meningitis; meningitis in immunocompromised patients; mild, self-limited gastroenteritis in healthy individuals.

Treatment: ampicillin in infants, immunocompromised, and the elderly as empirical treatment of meningitis.

Nocardia vs *Actinomyces*

A
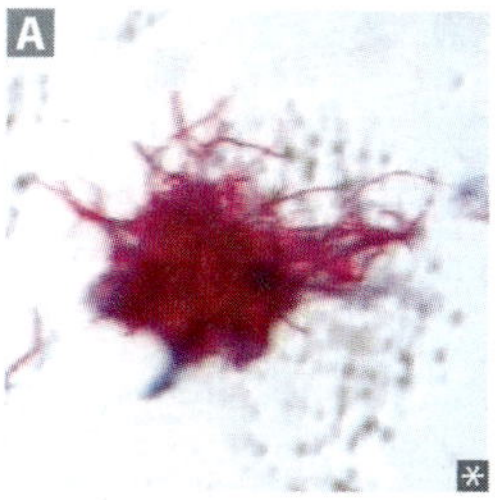

B
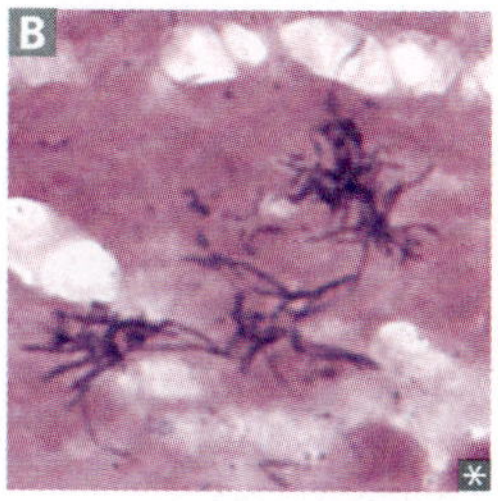

Both are gram ⊕ and form long, branching filaments resembling fungi.

Nocardia	*Actinomyces*
Aerobe	Anaerobe
Acid fast (weak) A	Not acid fast B
Found in soil	Normal oral, reproductive, and GI flora
* Causes pulmonary infections in immunocompromised (can mimic TB but with ⊖ PPD); cutaneous infections after trauma in immunocompetent	Causes oral/facial abscesses that drain through sinus tracts, forms yellow "sulfur granules;" can also cause PID with IUDs
Treat with sulfonamides (TMP-SMX)	Treat with penicillin

Treatment is a **SNAP**: **S**ulfonamides—***N****ocardia*; ***A****ctinomyces*—**P**enicillin

fastid - CO_2. (weeks)
molar tooth colonies

Actinomycetes group = Nocard, Actinomyces, M.TB, C-dipth, Streptomyces

Primary and secondary tuberculosis

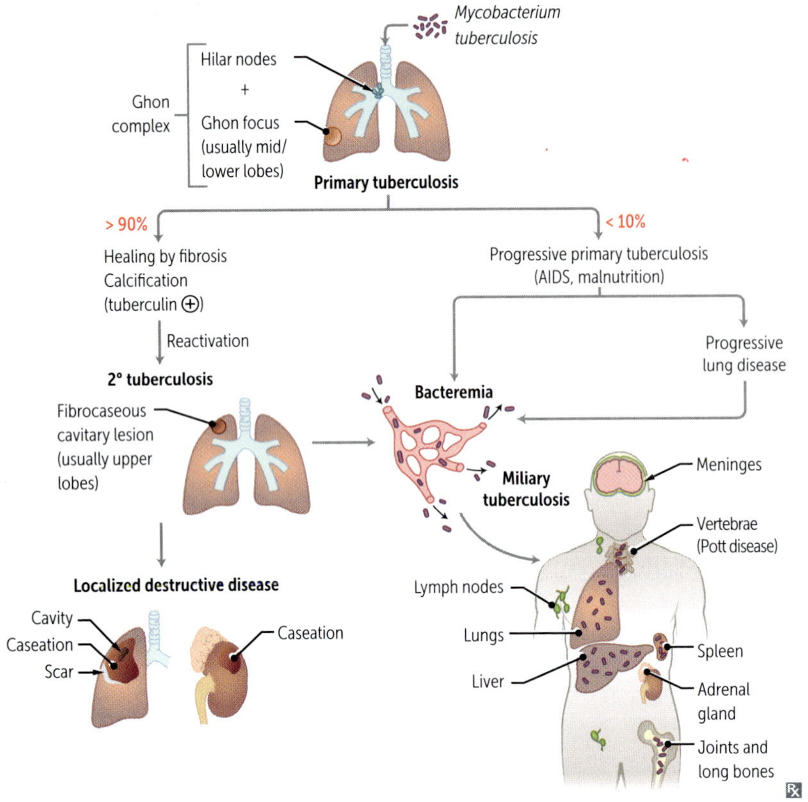

PPD ⊕ if current infection or past exposure.
PPD ⊖ if no infection and in sarcoidosis.
Interferon-γ release assay (IGRA) has fewer false positives from BCG vaccination.
Caseating granulomas **A** with central necrosis (upper left) and Langerhans giant cells (arrow) are characteristic of 2° tuberculosis.

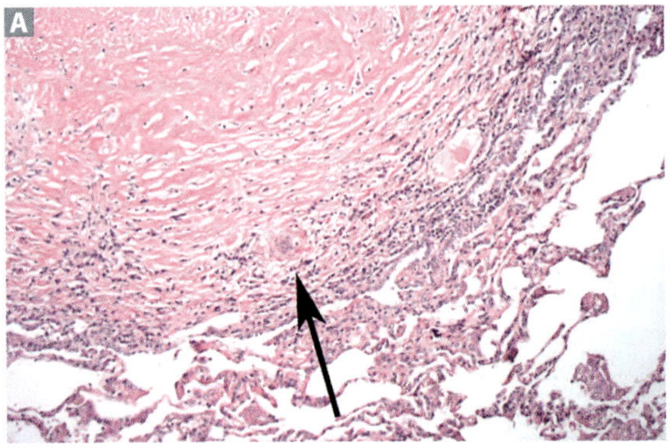

Mycobacteria

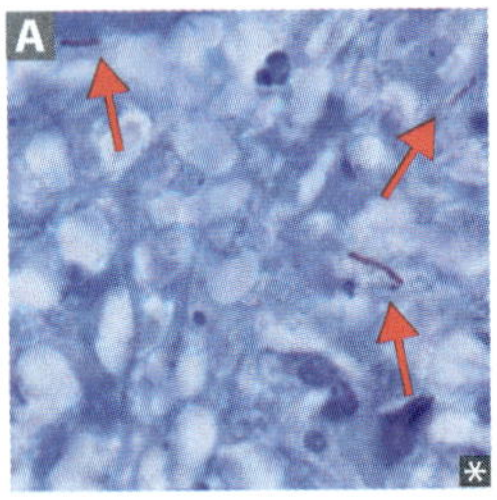

Mycobacterium tuberculosis (TB, often resistant to multiple drugs).
M avium–intracellulare (causes disseminated, non-TB disease in AIDS; often resistant to multiple drugs). Prophylaxis with azithromycin when CD4+ count < 50 cells/mm^3.
M scrofulaceum (cervical lymphadenitis in children).
M marinum (hand infection in aquarium handlers).
All mycobacteria are acid-fast organisms (pink rods; arrows in **A**).

TB symptoms include fever, night sweats, weight loss, cough (nonproductive or productive), hemoptysis.
Cord factor creates a "serpentine cord" appearance in virulent *M tuberculosis* strains; inhibits macrophage maturation and induces release of TNF-α. Sulfatides (surface glycolipids) inhibit phagolysosomal fusion.

Leprosy (Hansen disease)

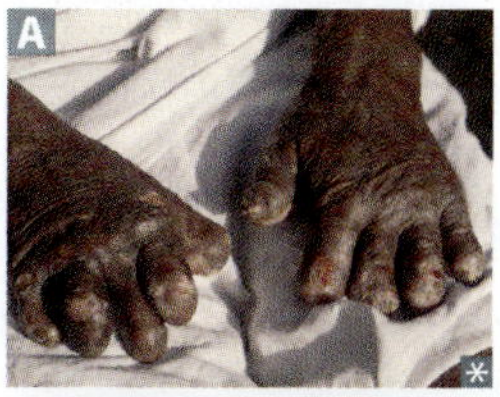

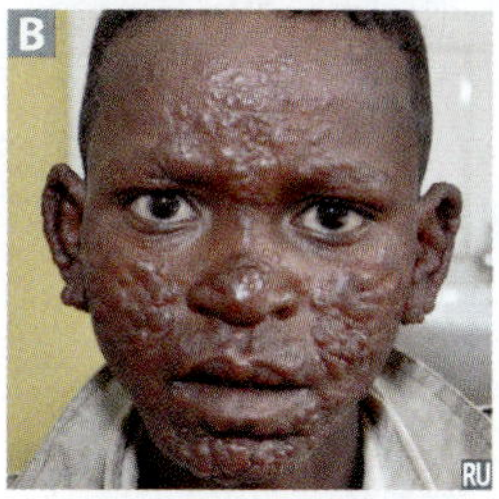

Caused by *Mycobacterium leprae*, an acid-fast bacillus that likes cool temperatures (infects skin and superficial nerves—"glove and stocking" loss of sensation A) and cannot be grown in vitro. Reservoir in United States: armadillos.

Hansen disease has 2 forms:

- Lepromatous—presents diffusely over the skin, with leonine (lion-like) facies B, and is communicable; characterized by low cell-mediated immunity with a humoral Th2 response. Lepromatous form can be lethal.
- Tuberculoid—limited to a few hypoesthetic, hairless skin plaques; characterized by high cell-mediated immunity with a largely Th1-type immune response.

Treatment: dapsone and rifampin for tuberculoid form; clofazimine is added for lepromatous form.

Gram-negative lab algorithm

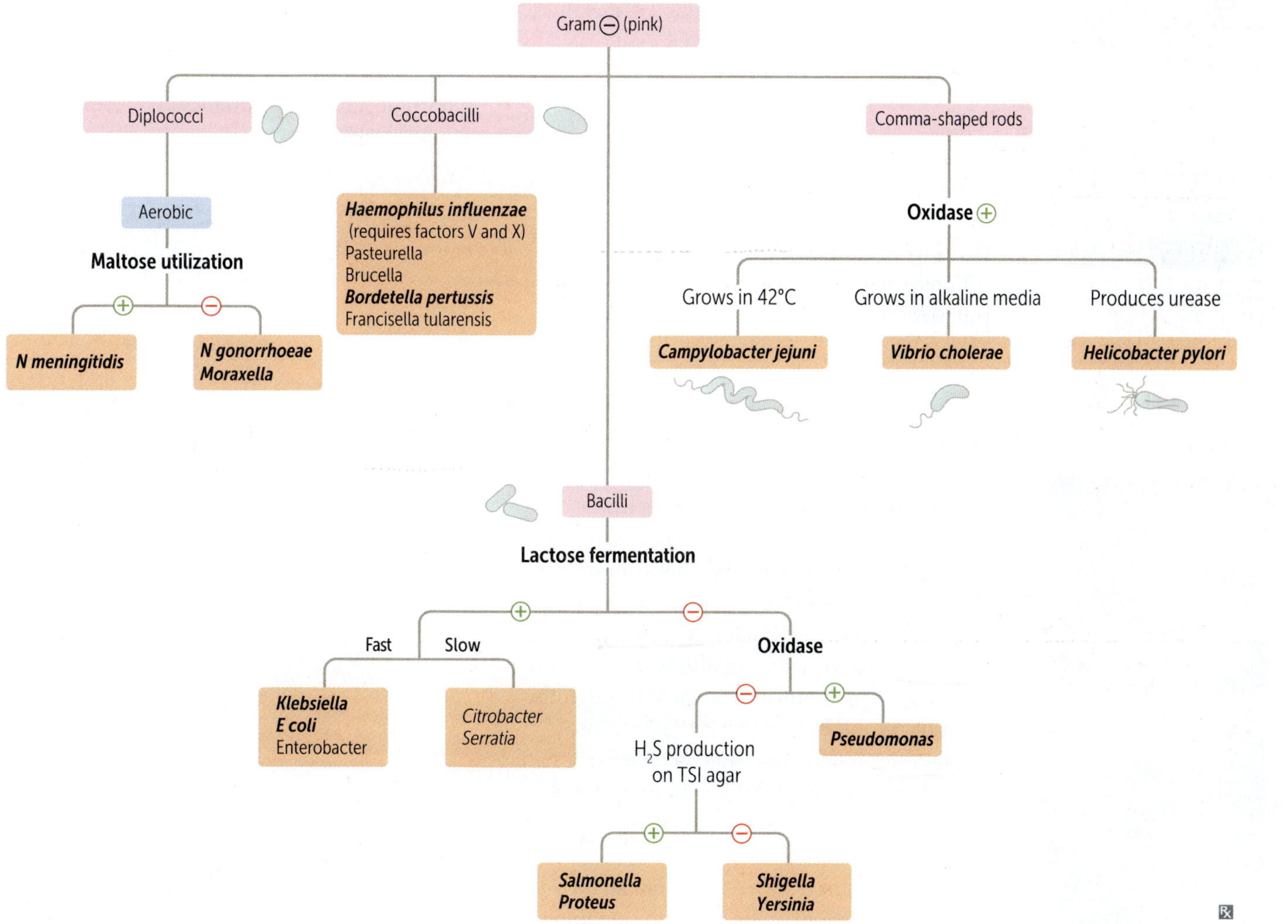

Important **tests** are in **bold.** Important ***pathogens*** are in ***bold italics.***

Lactose-fermenting enteric bacteria

Fermentation of **lactose** → pink colonies on MacCon**key** agar. Examples include ***K**lebsiella*, ***E** coli*, ***E**nterobacter*, and ***S**erratia* (weak fermenter). *E coli* produces β-galactosidase, which breaks down lactose into glucose and galactose.

Lactose is **key**.
Test with MacCon**KEE'S** agar.
EMB agar—lactose fermenters grow as purple/black colonies. *E coli* grows colonies with a green sheen.

Neisseria

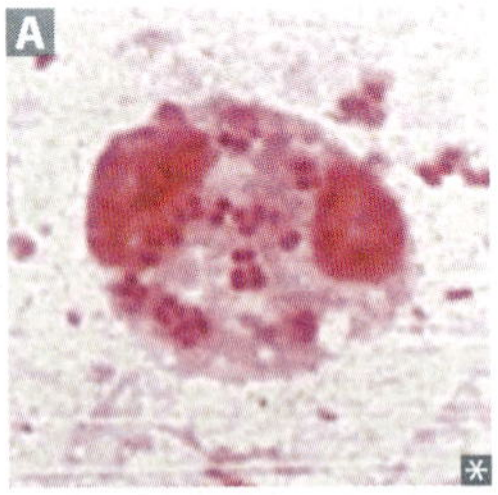

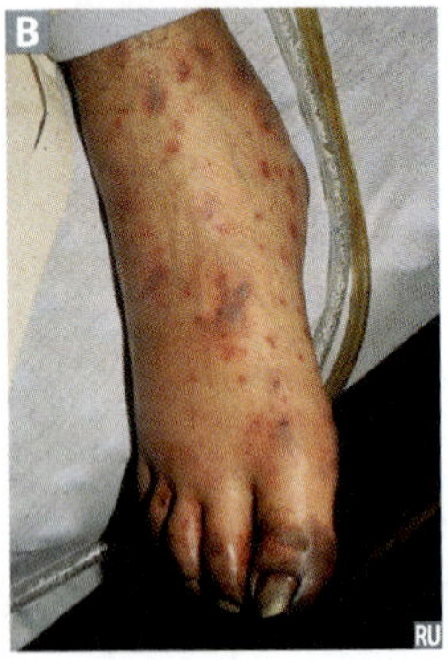

Gram ⊖ diplococci. Metabolize glucose and produce IgA proteases. *N gonorrhoeae* is often intracellular (within neutrophils) A.

Menin**G**ococci ferment **M**altose and **G**lucose.
Gonococci ferment **G**lucose.

Gonococci	Meningococci
No polysaccharide capsule	Polysaccharide capsule
No maltose metabolized	Maltose fermentation
No vaccine due to antigenic variation of pilus proteins	Vaccine (type B vaccine not widely available)
Sexually or perinatally transmitted	Transmitted via respiratory and oral secretions
Causes gonorrhea, septic arthritis, neonatal conjunctivitis, pelvic inflammatory disease (PID), and Fitz-Hugh–Curtis syndrome	Causes meningococcemia with petechial hemorrhages and gangrene of toes B, meningitis, Waterhouse-Friderichsen syndrome (adrenal insufficiency, fever, DIC, shock) syndrome
Condoms ↓ sexual transmission, erythromycin eye ointment prevents neonatal blindness	Rifampin, ciprofloxacin, or ceftriaxone prophylaxis in close contacts
Treatment: ceftriaxone + (azithromycin or doxycycline) for possible chlamydial coinfection	Treatment: ceftriaxone or penicillin G

Haemophilus influenzae

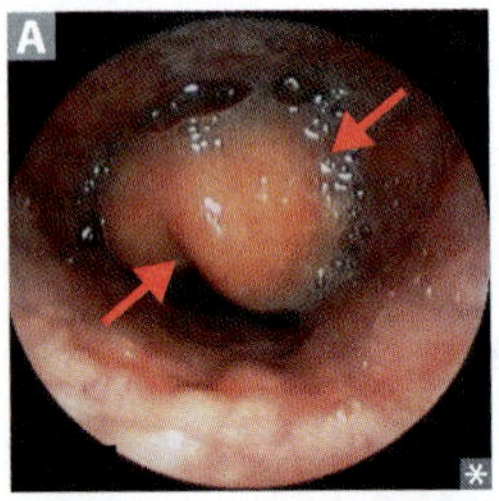

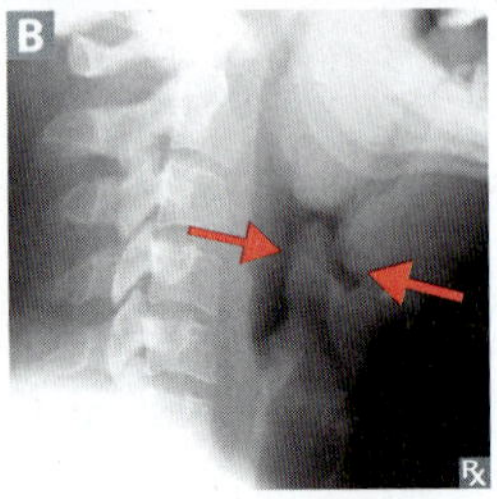

Small gram ⊖ (coccobacillary) rod. Aerosol transmission. Nontypeable (unencapsulated) strains are the most common cause of mucosal infections (otitis media, conjunctivitis, bronchitis) as well as invasive infections since the vaccine for capsular type b was introduced. Produces IgA protease. Culture on chocolate agar, which contains factors V (NAD^+) and X (hematin) for growth; can also be grown with *S aureus*, which provides factor V through the hemolysis of RBCs. *Ha**EMOP**hilus* causes **E**piglottitis (endoscopic appearance in A, can be "cherry red" in children; "thumbprint sign" on x-ray B), **M**eningitis, **O**titis media, and **P**neumonia.
Treatment: amoxicillin +/– clavulanate for mucosal infections; ceftriaxone for meningitis; rifampin prophylaxis for close contacts.

Vaccine contains type b capsular polysaccharide and PRP (polyribosylribitol phosphate) conjugated to diphtheria toxoid or other protein. Given between 2 and 18 months of age.
Does not cause the flu (influenza virus does).

Bordetella pertussis

Gram ⊖, aerobic coccobacillus. Virulence factors include pertussis toxin (disables G_i) and tracheal cytotoxin. Causes whooping cough. Prevented by Tdap, DTaP vaccines. May be mistaken as viral infection due to lymphocytic infiltrate resulting from immune response.

Legionella pneumophila

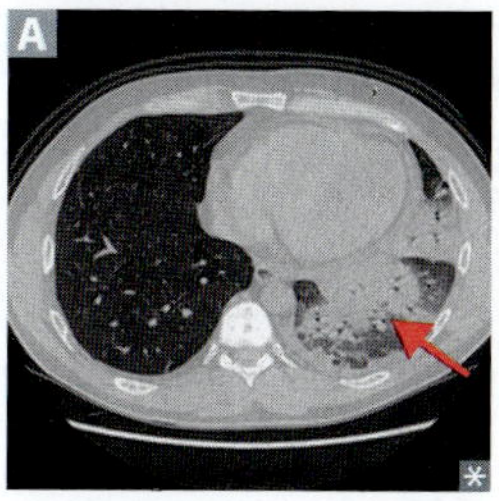

Gram ⊖ rod. Gram stains poorly—use **silver** stain. Grow on **charcoal** yeast extract medium with **iron** and **cysteine**. Detected by presence of antigen in urine. Labs may show hyponatremia. Aerosol transmission from environmental water source habitat (eg, air conditioning systems, hot water tanks). No person-to-person transmission.

Treatment: macrolide or quinolone.

Legionnaires' disease—severe pneumonia (often unilateral and lobar A), fever, GI and CNS symptoms. Common in smokers and in chronic lung disease.

Pontiac fever—mild flu-like syndrome.

Think of a French **legionnaire** (soldier) with his **silver** helmet, sitting around a campfire (**charcoal**) with his **iron** dagger—he is no **sissy** (cysteine).

Pseudomonas aeruginosa

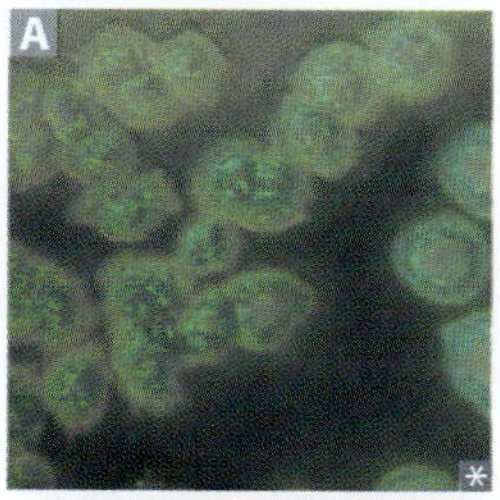

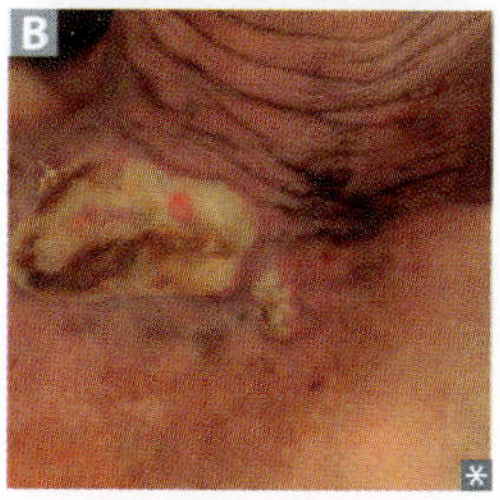

Aerobic, motile, gram ⊖ rod. Non-lactose fermenting, oxidase ⊕. Produces pyocyanin (blue-green pigment A); has a grape-like odor. Produces endotoxin (fever, shock), exotoxin A (inactivates EF-2), phospholipase C (degrades cell membranes), and pyocyanin (generates reactive oxygen species).

PSEUDOMONAS is associated with:
- **P**neumonia, pyocyanin
- **S**epsis
- **E**cthyma gangrenosum
- **U**TIs
- **D**iabetes, drug use
- **O**steomyelitis (eg, puncture wounds)
- **M**ucoid polysaccharide capsule
- **O**titis externa (swimmer's ear)
- **N**osocomial infections (catheters, equipment)
- exotoxin **A**
- **S**kin infections (hot tub folliculitis)

Treatments include "**CAMPFIRE**" drugs:
- **C**arbapenems
- **A**minoglycosides
- **M**onobactams
- **P**olymyxins (eg, polymyxin B, colistin)
- **F**luoroquinolones (eg, ciprofloxacin, levofloxacin)
- Th**IR**d- and fourth-generation cephalosporins (eg, ceftazidime, cefepime)
- **E**xtended-spectrum penicillins (eg, piperacillin, ticarcillin)

Aeruginosa—**aer**obic.

Mucoid polysaccharide capsule may contribute to chronic pneumonia in cystic fibrosis patients due to biofilm formation.

Can cause wound infection in burn victims.

Frequently found in water → hot tub folliculitis.

Ecthyma gangrenosum—rapidly progressive, necrotic cutaneous lesion B caused by *Pseudomonas* bacteremia. Typically seen in immunocompromised patients.

Inactiv EF2 = Pseudomonas Aerug. Coryne dipth

E coli

Gram ⊖ rod. *E coli* virulence factors: fimbriae—cystitis and pyelonephritis (P-pili); K capsule—pneumonia, neonatal meningitis; LPS endotoxin—septic shock.

STRAIN	TOXIN AND MECHANISM	PRESENTATION
EIEC	Microbe invades intestinal mucosa and causes necrosis and inflammation.	Invasive; dysentery. Clinical manifestations similar to *Shigella*.
ETEC	Produces heat-labile and heat-stable enteroToxins. No inflammation or invasion.	Travelers' diarrhea (watery).
EPEC	No toxin produced. Adheres to apical surface, flattens villi, prevents absorption.	Diarrhea, usually in children (Pediatrics).
EHEC	O157:H7 is most common serotype in US. Often transmitted via undercooked meat, raw leafy vegetables. Shiga-like toxin causes **hemolytic-uremic syndrome**: triad of anemia, thrombocytopenia, and acute renal failure due to microthrombi forming on damaged endothelium → mechanical hemolysis (with schistocytes on peripheral blood smear), platelet consumption, and ↓ renal blood flow.	Dysentery (toxin alone causes necrosis and inflammation). Does not ferment sorbitol (distinguishes EHEC from other *E coli*). Hemorrhagic, Hamburgers, Hemolytic-uremic syndrome.

Klebsiella

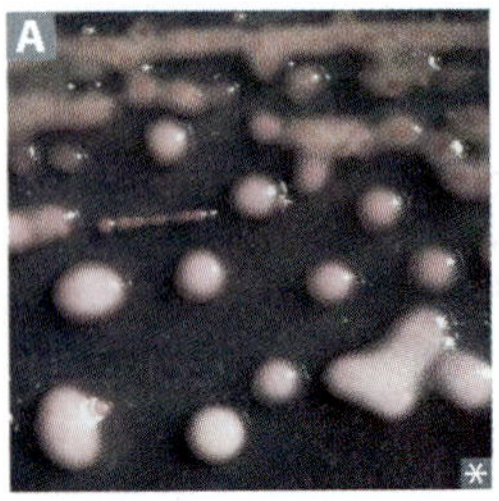

Gram ⊖ rod; intestinal flora that causes lobar pneumonia in alcoholics and diabetics when aspirated. Very mucoid colonies A caused by abundant polysaccharide capsules. Dark red "currant jelly" sputum (blood/mucus).
Also cause of nosocomial UTIs.

4 A's of *KlebsiellA*:
- Aspiration pneumonia
- Abscess in lungs and liver
- Alcoholics
- di-A-betics

Campylobacter jejuni

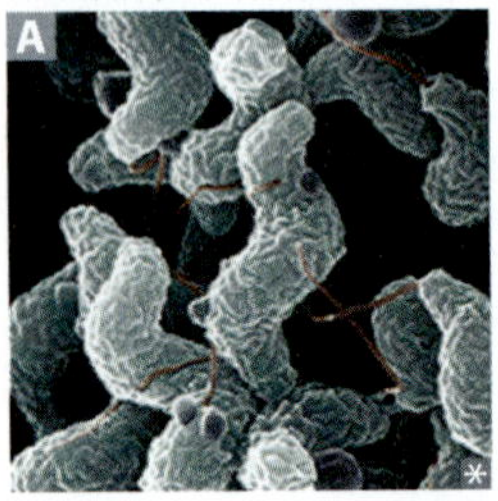

Gram ⊖, comma or S shaped (with polar flagella) A, oxidase ⊕, grows at 42°C ("*Campylobacter* likes the hot campfire"). Major cause of bloody diarrhea, especially in children. Fecal-oral transmission through person-to-person contact or via ingestion of undercooked contaminated poultry or meat, unpasteurized milk. Contact with infected animals (dogs, cats, pigs) is also a risk factor. Common antecedent to Guillain-Barré syndrome and reactive arthritis.

Salmonella vs _Shigella_

Both *Salmonella* and *Shigella* are gram ⊖ rods, non-lactose fermenters, oxidase ⊖, and can invade the GI tract via M cells of Peyer patches.

	Salmonella typhi	***Salmonella* spp. (except *S typhi*)**	***Shigella***
RESERVOIRS	Humans only	Humans and animals	Humans only
SPREAD	Can disseminate hematogenously	Can disseminate hematogenously	Cell to cell; no hematogenous spread
H_2S PRODUCTION	Yes	Yes	No
FLAGELLA	Yes (**salmon swim**)	Yes (**salmon swim**)	No
VIRULENCE FACTORS	Endotoxin; Vi capsule	Endotoxin	Endotoxin; Shiga toxin (enterotoxin)
INFECTIOUS DOSE (ID_{50})	High—large inoculum required because organism inactivated by gastric acids	High	Low—very small inoculum required; resistant to gastric acids
EFFECT OF ANTIBIOTICS ON FECAL EXCRETION	Prolongs duration	Prolongs duration	Shortens duration
IMMUNE RESPONSE	Primarily monocytes	PMNs in disseminated disease	Primarily PMN infiltration
GI MANIFESTATIONS	Constipation, followed by diarrhea	Diarrhea (possibly bloody)	Bloody diarrhea (bacillary dysentery)
VACCINE	Oral vaccine contains live attenuated *S typhi* IM vaccine contains Vi capsular polysaccharide	No vaccine	No vaccine
UNIQUE PROPERTIES	▪ Causes typhoid fever (rose spots on abdomen, constipation, abdominal pain, fever); treat with ceftriaxone or fluoroquinolone ▪ Carrier state with gallbladder colonization	▪ Poultry, eggs, pets, and turtles are common sources ▪ Antibiotics not indicated ▪ Gastroenteritis is usually caused by non-typhoidal *Salmonella*	▪ **Four F's**: **F**ingers, **F**lies, **F**ood, **F**eces ▪ In order of decreasing severity (less toxin produced): *S dysenteriae*, *S flexneri*, *S boydii*, *S sonnei* ▪ Invasion is the key to pathogenicity; organisms that produce little toxin can cause disease due to invasion

Vibrio cholerae

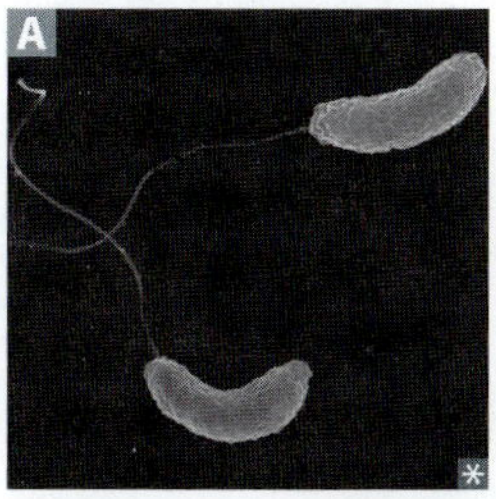

Gram ⊖, flagellated, comma shaped **A**, oxidase ⊕, grows in alkaline media. Endemic to developing countries. Produces profuse rice-water diarrhea via enterotoxin that permanently activates G_s, ↑ cAMP. Sensitive to stomach acid (acid labile); requires large inoculum (high ID_{50}) unless host has ↓ gastric acidity. Prompt oral rehydration is necessary.

Yersinia enterocolitica

Gram ⊖ rod. Usually transmitted from pet feces (eg, puppies), contaminated milk, or pork. Causes acute diarrhea or pseudoappendicitis (right lower abdominal pain due to mesenteric adenitis and/or terminal ileitis).

Helicobacter pylori

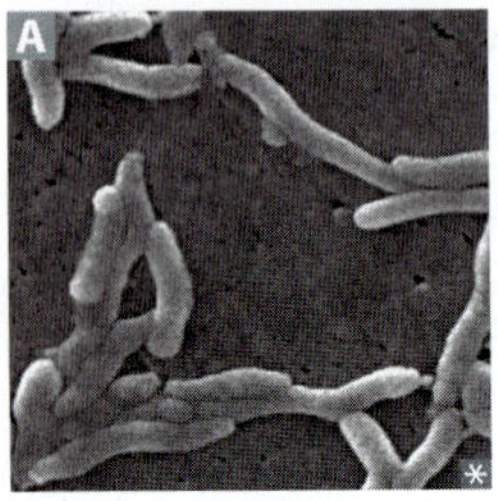

Curved, terminally flagellated, gram ⊖ rod A that is **triple** ⊕: catalase ⊕, oxidase ⊕, and urease ⊕ (can use urea breath test or fecal antigen test for diagnosis). Urease produces ammonia, creating an alkaline environment, which helps *H pylori* survive in acidic mucosa. Colonizes mainly antrum of stomach; causes gastritis and peptic ulcers (especially duodenal). Risk factor for peptic ulcer disease, gastric adenocarcinoma, and MALT lymphoma.

Most common initial treatment is **triple** therapy: **A**moxicillin (metronidazole if penicillin allergy) + **C**larithromycin + **P**roton pump inhibitor; **A**ntibiotics **C**ure ***P**ylori*.

Spirochetes

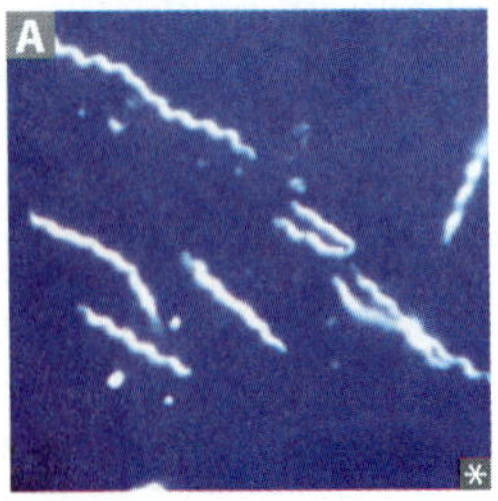

Spiral-shaped bacteria A with axial filaments. Includes ***B**orrelia* (big size), ***L**eptospira*, and ***T**reponema*. Only *Borrelia* can be visualized using aniline dyes (Wright or Giemsa stain) in light microscopy due to size. *Treponema* is visualized by dark-field microscopy or direct fluorescent antibody (DFA) microscopy.

BLT.
***B**orrelia* is **B**ig.

Leptospira interrogans

Spirochete found in water contaminated with animal urine, causes **leptospirosis**—flu-like symptoms, myalgias (classically of calves), jaundice, photophobia with conjunctival suffusion (erythema without exudate). Prevalent among surfers and in tropics (eg, Hawaii).

Weil disease (icterohemorrhagic leptospirosis)—severe form with jaundice and azotemia from liver and kidney dysfunction, fever, hemorrhage, and anemia.

Lyme disease

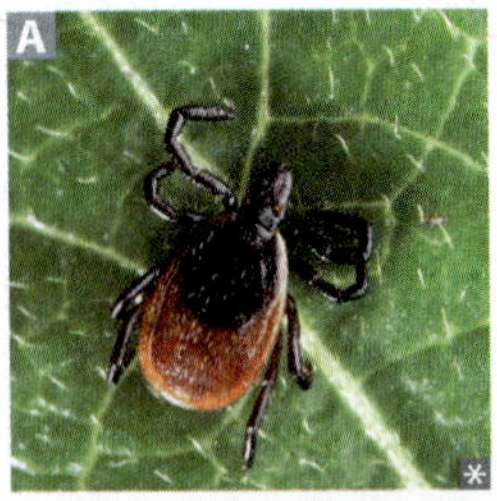

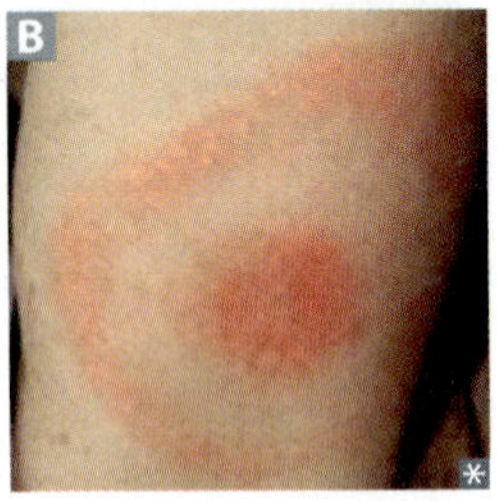

Caused by *Borrelia burgdorferi*, which is transmitted by the *Ixodes* deer tick A (also vector for *Anaplasma* spp. and protozoa *Babesia*). Natural reservoir is the mouse.

Mice are important to tick life cycle.

Common in northeastern United States.

Stage 1—early localized: erythema migrans B, flu-like symptoms.

Stage 2—early disseminated: secondary lesions, carditis, AV block, facial nerve (Bell) palsy, migratory myalgias/transient arthritis.

Stage 3—late disseminated: encephalopathies, chronic arthritis.

A Key **Lyme** pie to the **FACE**:
- **F**acial nerve palsy (typically bilateral)
- **A**rthritis
- **C**ardiac block
- **E**rythema migrans

Syphilis	Caused by spirochete *Treponema pallidum*.
Primary syphilis	Localized disease presenting with **painless** chancre A. If available, use dark-field microscopy to visualize treponemes in fluid from chancre B. VDRL ⊕ in ~ 80%.
Secondary syphilis	Disseminated disease with constitutional symptoms, maculopapular rash C (including palms D and soles), condylomata lata E (smooth, moist, painless, wart-like white lesions on genitals), lymphadenopathy, patchy hair loss; also confirmable with dark-field microscopy. Serologic testing: VDRL/RPR (nonspecific), confirm diagnosis with specific test (eg, FTA-ABS). **S**econdary syphilis = **S**ystemic. Latent syphilis (⊕ serology without symptoms) may follow.
Tertiary syphilis	Gummas F (chronic granulomas), aortitis (vasa vasorum destruction), neurosyphilis (tabes dorsalis, "general paresis"), Argyll Robertson pupil (constricts with accommodation but is not reactive to light; also called "prostitute's pupil" since it accommodates but does not react). Signs: broad-based ataxia, ⊕ Romberg, Charcot joint, stroke without hypertension. For neurosyphilis: test spinal fluid with VDRL, FTA-ABS, and PCR.
Congenital syphilis	Presents with facial abnormalities such as rhagades (linear scars at angle of mouth, black arrow in G), snuffles (nasal discharge, red arrow in G), saddle nose, notched (Hutchinson) teeth H, mulberry molars, and short maxilla; saber shins; CN VIII deafness. To prevent, treat mother early in pregnancy, as placental transmission typically occurs after first trimester.

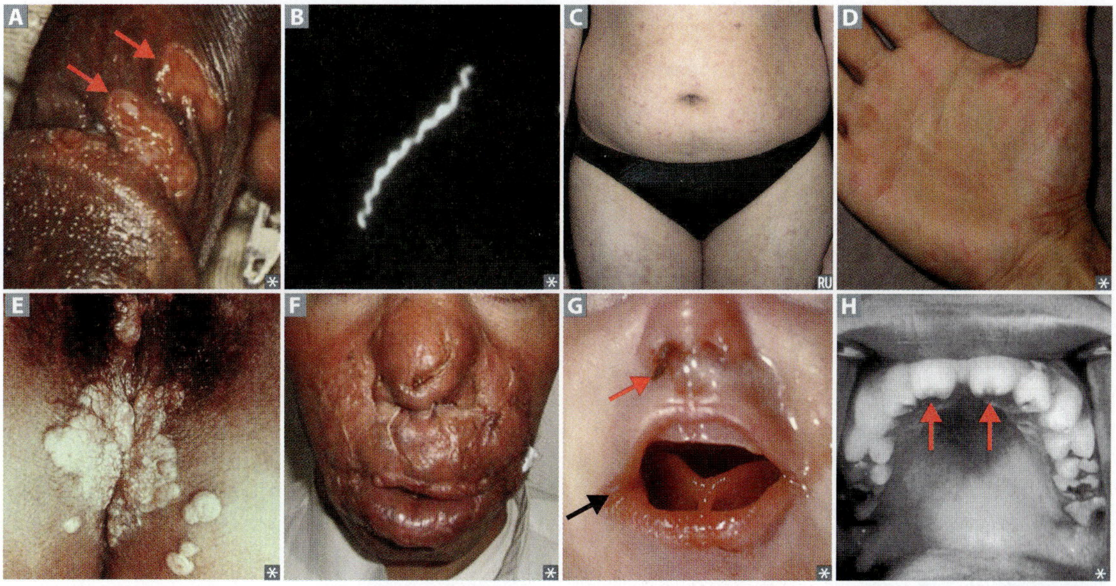

VDRL false positives	VDRL detects nonspecific antibody that reacts with beef cardiolipin. Inexpensive, widely available test for syphilis, quantitative, sensitive but not specific.	False-positive results on **VDRL** with: **V**iral infection (eg, EBV, hepatitis) **D**rugs **R**heumatic fever **L**upus and leprosy

Jarisch-Herxheimer reaction	Flu-like syndrome (fever, chills, headache, myalgia) after antibiotics are started; due to killed bacteria (usually spirochetes) releasing toxins.

Zoonotic bacteria

Zoonosis: infectious disease transmitted between animals and humans.

SPECIES	DISEASE	TRANSMISSION AND SOURCE
***Anaplasma* spp.**	Anaplasmosis	*Ixodes* ticks (live on deer and mice)
***Bartonella* spp.**	Cat scratch disease, bacillary angiomatosis	Cat scratch
Borrelia burgdorferi	Lyme disease	*Ixodes* ticks (live on deer and mice)
Borrelia recurrentis	Relapsing fever	Louse (recurrent due to variable surface antigens)
***Brucella* spp.**	Brucellosis/undulant fever	Unpasteurized dairy
Campylobacter	Bloody diarrhea	Feces from infected pets/animals; contaminated meats/foods/hands
Chlamydophila psittaci	Psittacosis	Parrots, other birds
Coxiella burnetii	Q fever	Aerosols of cattle/sheep amniotic fluid
Ehrlichia chaffeensis	Ehrlichiosis	*Amblyomma* (Lone Star tick)
Francisella tularensis	Tularemia	Ticks, rabbits, deer flies
***Leptospira* spp.**	Leptospirosis	Animal urine in water; recreational water use
Mycobacterium leprae	Leprosy	Humans with lepromatous leprosy; armadillo (rare)
Pasteurella multocida	Cellulitis, osteomyelitis	Animal bite, cats, dogs
Rickettsia prowazekii	Epidemic typhus	Human to human via human body louse
Rickettsia rickettsii	Rocky Mountain spotted fever	*Dermacentor* (dog tick)
Rickettsia typhi	Endemic typhus	Fleas
***Salmonella* spp. (except *S typhi*)**	Diarrhea (which may be bloody), vomiting, fever, abdominal cramps	Reptiles and poultry
Yersinia pestis	Plague	Fleas (rats and prairie dogs are reservoirs)

Gardnerella vaginalis

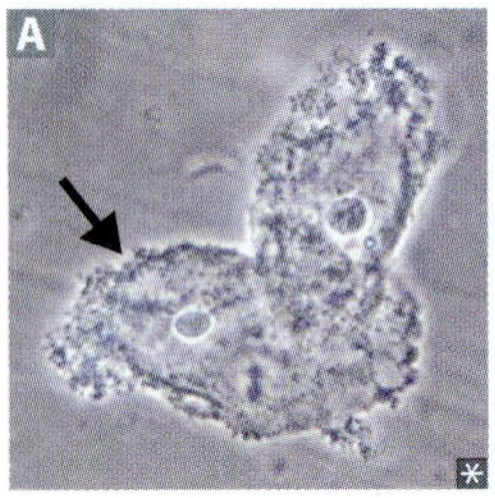

A pleomorphic, gram-variable rod involved in bacterial vaginosis. Presents as a gray vaginal discharge with a fishy smell; nonpainful (vs vaginitis). Associated with sexual activity, but not sexually transmitted. Bacterial vaginosis is also characterized by overgrowth of certain anaerobic bacteria in vagina. Clue cells (vaginal epithelial cells covered with *Gardnerella*) have stippled appearance along outer margin (arrow in A).

Treatment: metronidazole or clindamycin.

I don't have a clue why I smell fish in the vagina garden!

Amine whiff test—mixing discharge with 10% KOH enhances fishy odor.

Rickettsial diseases and vector-borne illnesses Treatment for all: doxycycline.

RASH COMMON		
Rocky Mountain spotted fever	*Rickettsia rickettsii*, vector is tick. Despite its name, disease occurs primarily in the South Atlantic states, especially North Carolina. Rash typically starts at wrists A and ankles and then spreads to trunk, palms, and soles.	Classic triad—headache, fever, rash (vasculitis). Palms and soles rash is seen in Coxsackievirus A infection (hand, foot, and mouth disease), Rocky Mountain spotted fever, and 2° Syphilis (you drive CARS using your palms and soles).
Typhus	Endemic (fleas)—*R typhi*. Epidemic (human body louse)—*R prowazekii*. Rash starts centrally and spreads out, sparing palms and soles.	*Rickettsii* on the wRists, Typhus on the Trunk.
RASH RARE		
Ehrlichiosis	*Ehrlichia*, vector is tick. Monocytes with morulae B (mulberry-like inclusions) in cytoplasm.	MEGA berry— Monocytes = Ehrlichiosis Granulocytes = Anaplasmosis
Anaplasmosis	*Anaplasma*, vector is tick. Granulocytes with morulae C in cytoplasm.	
Q fever	*Coxiella burnetii*, no arthropod vector. Spores inhaled as aerosols from cattle/sheep amniotic fluid. Presents as pneumonia. Most common cause of culture ⊖ endocarditis.	Q fever is Queer because it has no rash or vector and its causative organism can survive outside in its endospore form. Not in the *Rickettsia* genus, but closely related.

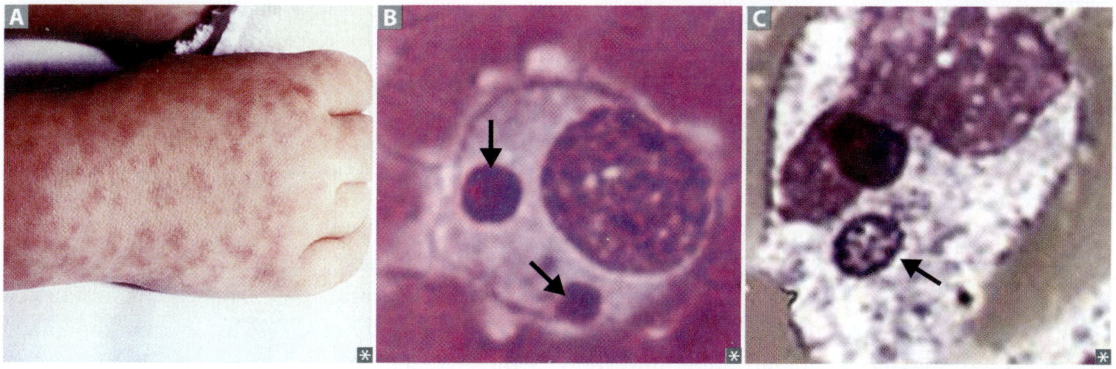

Chlamydiae

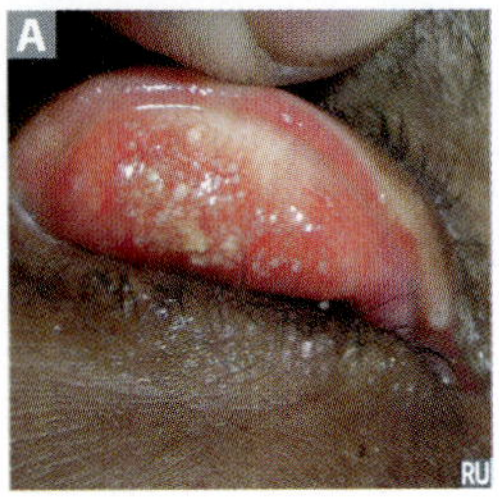

Chlamydiae cannot make their own ATP. They are obligate intracellular organisms that cause mucosal infections. 2 forms:

- **E**lementary body (small, dense) is "**E**nfectious" and **E**nters cell via **E**ndocytosis; transforms into reticulate body.
- **R**eticulate body **R**eplicates in cell by fission; **R**eorganizes into elementary bodies.

Chlamydia trachomatis causes reactive arthritis (Reiter syndrome), follicular conjunctivitis A, nongonococcal urethritis, and PID.

Chlamydophila pneumoniae and *Chlamydophila psittaci* cause atypical pneumonia; transmitted by aerosol.

Treatment: azithromycin (favored because one-time treatment) or doxycycline.

Chlamys = cloak (intracellular).

C *psittaci*—has an avian reservoir (**p**arrots), causes atypical **p**neumonia.

Lab diagnosis: cytoplasmic inclusions seen on Giemsa or fluorescent antibody–stained smear.

The chlamydial cell wall lacks classic peptidoglycan (due to reduced muramic acid), rendering β-lactam antibiotics less effective.

Chlamydia trachomatis serotypes

Types A, B, and C	Chronic infection, cause blindness due to follicular conjunctivitis in Africa.	**ABC** = **A**frica, **B**lindness, **C**hronic infection.
Types D–K	Urethritis/PID, ectopic pregnancy, neonatal pneumonia (staccato cough) with eosinophilia, neonatal conjunctivitis.	D–K = everything else. Neonatal disease can be acquired during passage through infected birth canal.
Types **L**1, **L**2, and **L**3	**L**ymphogranuloma venereum—small, painless ulcers on genitals → swollen, painful inguinal lymph nodes that ulcerate (buboes). Treat with doxycycline.	

Mycoplasma pneumoniae

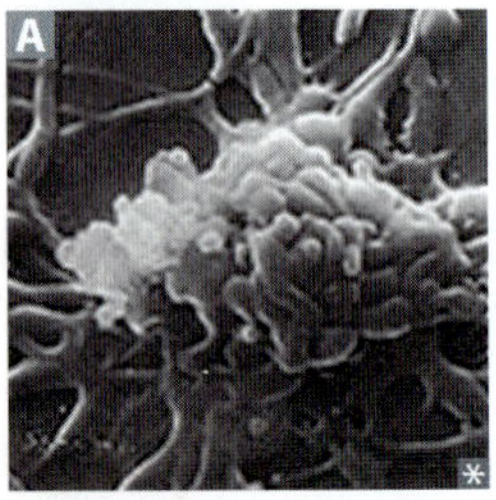

Classic cause of atypical "walking" pneumonia (insidious onset, headache, nonproductive cough, patchy or diffuse interstitial infiltrate). X-ray looks worse than patient. High titer of **cold** agglutinins (IgM), which can agglutinate or lyse RBCs. Grown on Eaton agar.

Treatment: macrolides, doxycycline, or fluoroquinolone (penicillin ineffective since *Mycoplasma* have no cell wall).

No cell wall. Not seen on Gram stain. Pleomorphic A.

Bacterial membrane contains sterols for stability.

Mycoplasmal pneumonia is more common in patients < 30 years old.

Frequent outbreaks in military recruits and prisons.

Mycoplasma gets **cold** without a **coat** (cell wall).

▸ MICROBIOLOGY—MYCOLOGY

Systemic mycoses

All of the following can cause pneumonia and can disseminate. All are caused by dimorphic fungi: **cold** (20°C) = **mold**; **heat** (37°C) = **yeast**. The only exception is coccidioidomycosis, which is a spherule (not yeast) in tissue. Treatment: fluconazole or itraconazole for **local** infection; amphotericin B for **systemic** infection. Systemic mycoses can form granulomas (like TB) but cannot be transmitted person-to-person (unlike TB). Asymp/mild URI (most), pneumo, dissemin granulom

DISEASE	ENDEMIC LOCATION AND PATHOLOGIC FEATURES	NOTES
Histoplasmosis 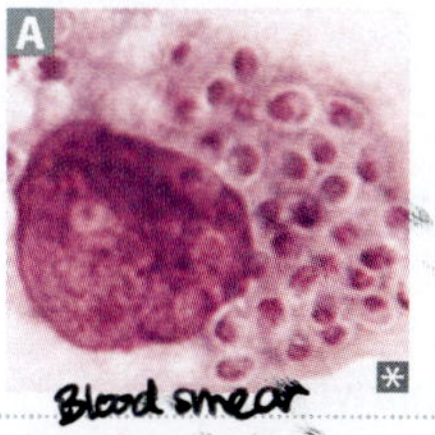 Blood smear	Mississippi and Ohio River valleys. Macrophage filled with *Histoplasma* (smaller than RBC) A. oval bud yeast in them Tear Drop microconidia	**H**isto **h**ides (within macrophages). Bird (eg, starlings) or bat droppings. - Fac intra - Reticuendo cells - make alkaline - bicarb, ammonia in phagolysos = inactive - Calcif granul in spleen/lung = prev. infect
Blastomycosis 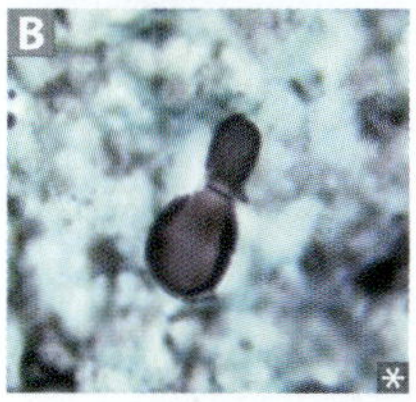	Eastern United States and Central America. Causes inflammatory lung disease and can disseminate to skin and bone. Forms granulomatous nodules. Broad-base budding (same size as RBC) B.	**B**lasto **b**uds **b**roadly. Healthy ppl Rapidly fatal. Must tx w/ itraconaz or ampho B
Coccidioidomycosis 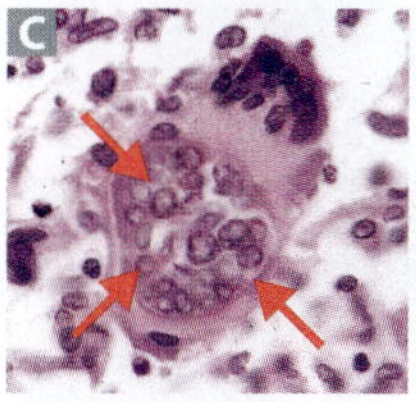	Southwestern United States, California. Causes pneumonia and meningitis; can disseminate to skin and bone. Case rate ↑ after earthquakes (spores in dust thrown into air → inhaled → spherules in lung). Spherule (much larger than RBC) filled with endospores C.	**C**occidio **c**rowds endospores. "(San Joaquin) Valley fever" "Desert bumps" = erythema nodosum "Desert rheumatism" = arthralgias
Paracoccidioidomycosis 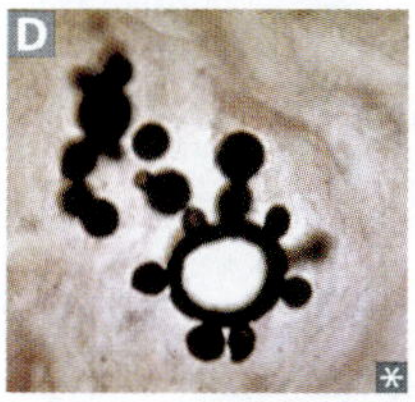	**Latin America.** Budding yeast with "**captain's wheel**" formation (much larger than RBC) D.	**Para**coccidio **parasails** with the **captain's wheel** all the way to **Latin America**.

Cutaneous mycoses

Tinea (dermatophytes)	Tinea is the clinical name given to dermatophyte (cutaneous fungal) infections. Dermatophytes include *Microsporum*, *Trichophyton*, and *Epidermophyton*. Branching septate hyphae visible on KOH preparation with blue fungal stain A.
Tinea capitis	Occurs on head, scalp. Associated with lymphadenopathy, alopecia, scaling B. T. tonsurans, M. canis
Tinea corporis	Occurs on torso. Characterized by erythematous scaling rings ("ringworm") and central clearing C. Can be acquired from contact with an infected cat or dog.
Tinea cruris	Occurs in inguinal area D. Often does not show the central clearing seen in tinea corporis. { all red
Tinea pedis	Three varieties: ▪ Interdigital E; most common ▪ Moccasin distribution F ▪ Vesicular type
Tinea unguium	Onychomycosis; occurs on nails.
Tinea (pityriasis) versicolor	Caused by *Malassezia* spp. (*Pityrosporum* spp.), a yeast-like fungus (not a dermatophyte despite being called tinea). Degradation of lipids produces acids that damage melanocytes and cause hypopigmented G and/or pink patches. Can occur any time of year, but more common in summer (hot, humid weather). "Spaghetti and meatballs" appearance on microscopy H. Treatment: selenium sulfide, topical and/or oral antifungal medications.

- the only human to human = Trich. tonsurans
Epid floccosum

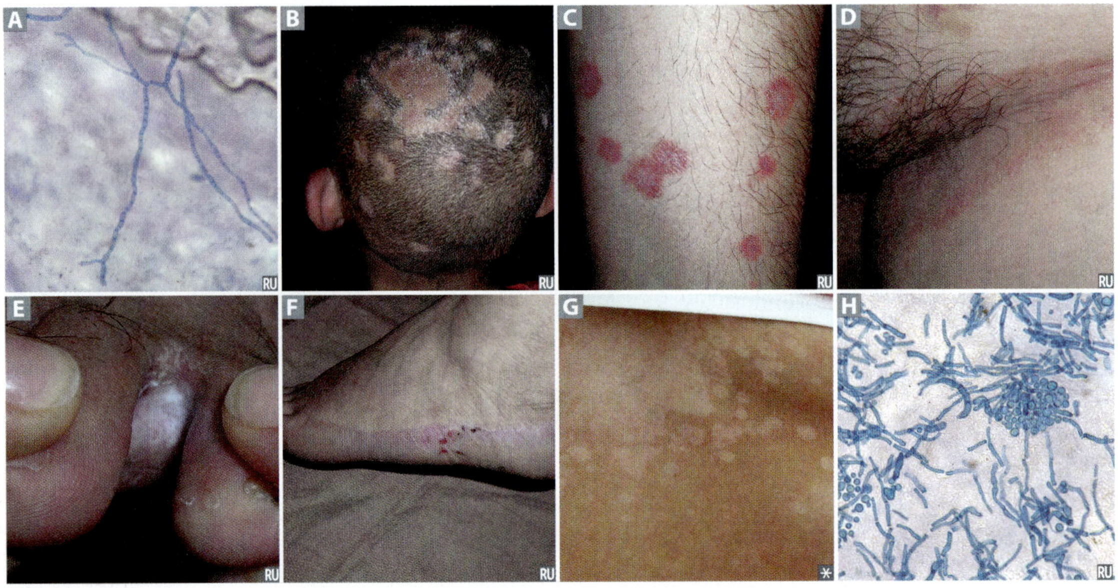

Trich = irreg, broad, branched septae
balloon like

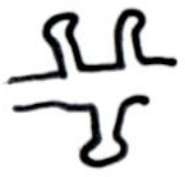

+ hair, skin, nail

Microsporum =

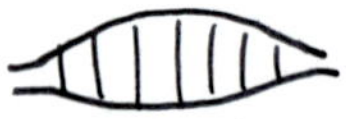

spindle shaped, thick walled, large + hair, skin

Epidermophyton =

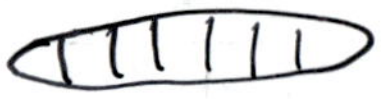

smooth, thin walled + skin, nail

Opportunistic fungal infections

Candida albicans	*alba* = white. Dimorphic; forms pseudohyphae and budding yeasts at 20°C **A**, germ tubes at 37°C **B**. Systemic or superficial fungal infection. Causes oral **C** and esophageal thrush in immunocompromised (neonates, steroids, diabetes, AIDS), vulvovaginitis (diabetes, use of antibiotics), diaper rash, endocarditis (IV drug users), disseminated candidiasis (to any organ), chronic mucocutaneous candidiasis. Treatment: topical azole for vaginal; nystatin, fluconazole, or caspofungin for oral/esophageal; fluconazole, caspofungin, or amphotericin B for systemic.
Aspergillus fumigatus	Septate hyphae that branch at 45° **A**cute **A**ngle **D**. Produces conidia in radiating chains at end of conidiophore **E**. Causes invasive aspergillosis, especially in immunocompromised and those with chronic granulomatous disease. Can cause aspergillomas in pre-existing lung cavities, especially after TB infection. Some species of *Aspergillus* produce **A**flatoxins, which are associated with hepatocellular carcinoma. Allergic bronchopulmonary aspergillosis (ABPA): hypersensitivity response associated with asthma and cystic fibrosis; may cause bronchiectasis and eosinophilia.
Cryptococcus neoformans	5–10 μm with narrow budding. Heavily encapsulated yeast. Not dimorphic. Found in soil, pigeon droppings. Acquired through inhalation with hematogenous dissemination to meninges. Culture on Sabouraud agar. Highlighted with India ink (clear halo **F**) and mucicarmine (red inner capsule **G**). Latex agglutination test detects polysaccharide capsular antigen and is more specific. Causes cryptococcosis, cryptococcal meningitis, cryptococcal encephalitis ("soap bubble" lesions in brain), primarily in immunocompromised.
***Mucor* and *Rhizopus* spp.**	Irregular, broad, nonseptate hyphae branching at wide angles **H**. Mucormycosis. Causes disease mostly in ketoacidotic diabetic and/or neutropenic patients (eg, leukemia). Fungi proliferate in blood vessel walls, penetrate cribriform plate, and enter brain. Rhinocerebral, frontal lobe abscess; cavernous sinus thrombosis. Headache, facial pain, black necrotic eschar on face; may have cranial nerve involvement. Treatment: surgical debridement, amphotericin B.

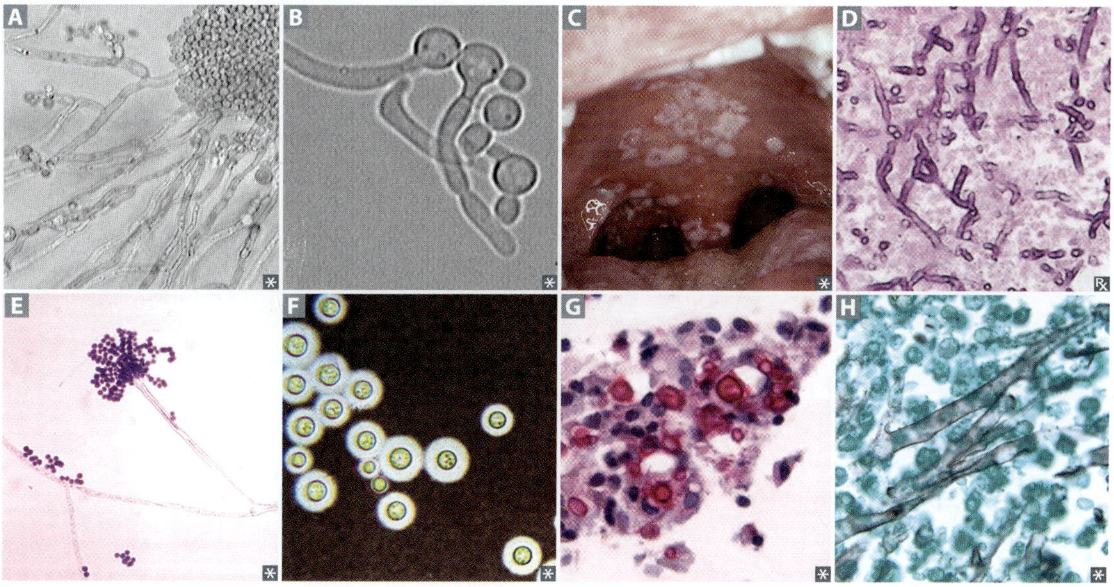

Pneumocystis jirovecii

Causes *Pneumocystis* pneumonia (PCP), a diffuse interstitial pneumonia A. Yeast-like fungus (originally classified as protozoan). Inhaled. Most infections are asymptomatic. Immunosuppression (eg, AIDS) predisposes to disease. Diffuse, bilateral ground-glass opacities on CXR/CT B. Diagnosed by lung biopsy or lavage. Disc-shaped yeast seen on methenamine silver stain of lung tissue C.

Treatment/prophylaxis: TMP-SMX, pentamidine, dapsone (prophylaxis only), atovaquone. Start prophylaxis when CD4+ count drops to < 200 cells/mm^3 in HIV patients.

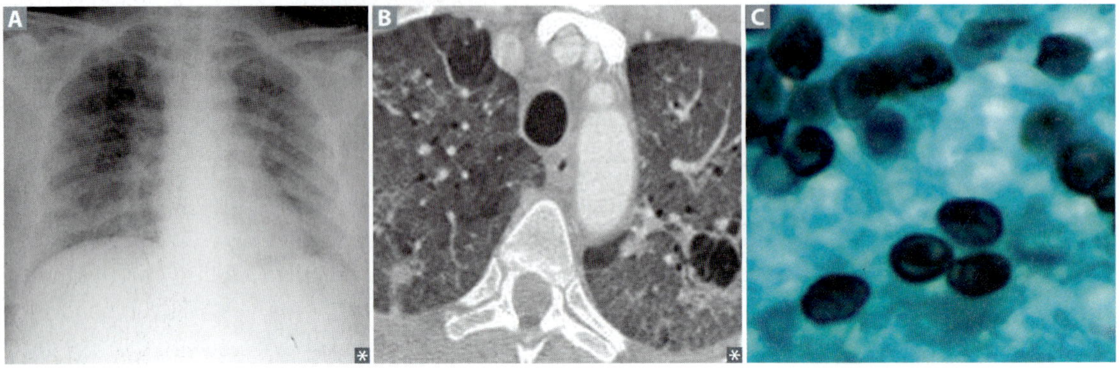

Sporothrix schenckii

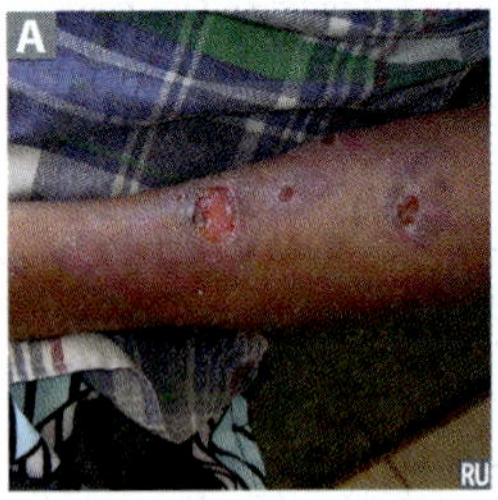

Sporotrichosis. Dimorphic, cigar-shaped budding yeast that grows in branching hyphae with **rose**ttes of conidia; lives on vegetation. When spores are traumatically introduced into the skin, typically by a thorn ("**rose** gardener's" disease), causes local pustule or ulcer A with nodules along draining lymphatics (ascending lymphangitis). Disseminated disease possible in immunocompromised host.

Treatment: itraconazole or **pot**assium iodide.

"Plant a **rose** in the **pot**."

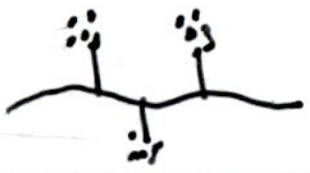

▶ MICROBIOLOGY—PARASITOLOGY

Protozoa—GI infections

ORGANISM	DISEASE	TRANSMISSION	DIAGNOSIS	TREATMENT
Giardia lamblia	**Giardiasis**—bloating, flatulence, foul-smelling, fatty diarrhea (often seen in campers/hikers)—think **fat**-rich **Ghirardelli** chocolates for **fatty** stools of ***Giardia***	Cysts in water	Multinucleated trophozoites A or cysts B in stool	Metronidazole
Entamoeba histolytica	**Amebiasis**—bloody diarrhea (dysentery), liver abscess ("anchovy paste" exudate), RUQ pain; histology shows flask-shaped ulcer	Cysts in water	Serology and/or trophozoites (with engulfed RBCs C in the cytoplasm) or cysts with up to 4 nuclei D in stool	Metronidazole; iodoquinol for asymptomatic cyst passers
Cryptosporidium	Severe diarrhea in AIDS Mild disease (watery diarrhea) in immunocompetent hosts	Oocysts in water	Oocysts on acid-fast stain E	Prevention (by filtering city water supplies); nitazoxanide in immunocompetent hosts

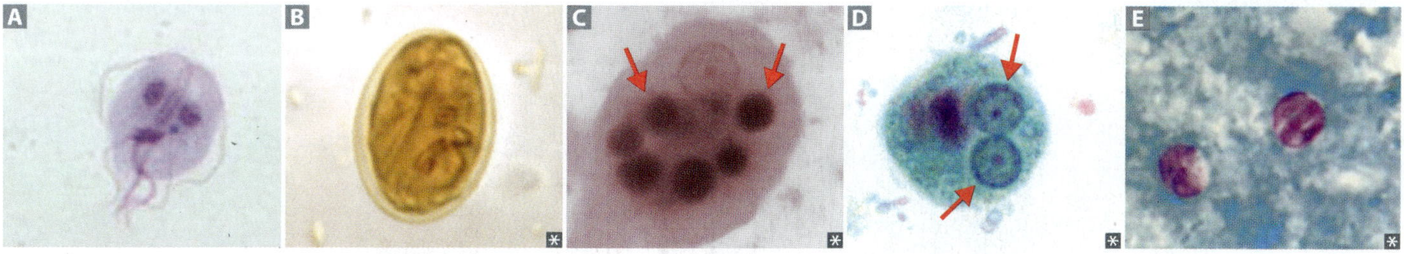

Protozoa—CNS infections

ORGANISM	DISEASE	TRANSMISSION	DIAGNOSIS	TREATMENT
Toxoplasma gondii	Congenital toxoplasmosis = classic triad of chorioretinitis, hydrocephalus, and intracranial calcifications; reactivation in AIDS → brain abscess seen as ring-enhancing lesions on MRI A	Cysts in meat (most common); oocysts in cat feces; crosses placenta (pregnant women should avoid cats)	Serology, biopsy (tachyzoite) B	Sulfadiazine + pyrimethamine
Naegleria fowleri	Rapidly fatal meningoencephalitis	Swimming in **freshwater** lakes (think **Nalgene** bottle filled with **fresh water** containing ***Naegleria***); enters via cribriform plate	Amoebas in spinal fluid C	Amphotericin B has been effective for a few survivors
Trypanosoma brucei	**African sleeping sickness**—enlarged lymph nodes, recurring fever (due to antigenic variation), somnolence, coma Two subspecies: *Trypanosoma brucei rhodesiense*, *Trypanosoma brucei gambiense*	Tsetse fly, a painful bite	Trypomastigote in blood smear D	**Sur**amin for blood-borne disease or **mela**rsoprol for CNS penetration ("it **sure** is nice to go to sleep"; **mela**tonin helps with sleep)

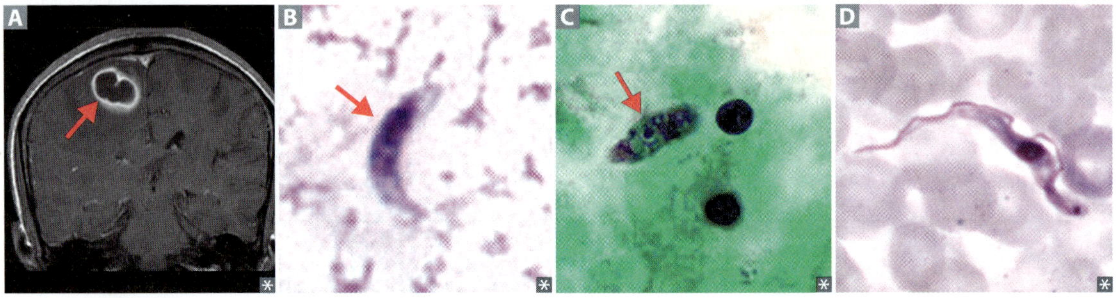

Protozoa—hematologic infections

ORGANISM	DISEASE	TRANSMISSION	DIAGNOSIS	TREATMENT
Plasmodium ***P vivax/ovale*** ***P falciparum*** ***P malariae*** 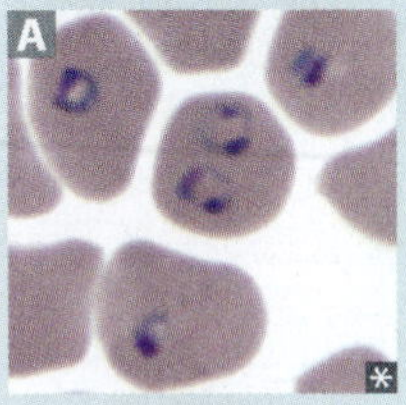 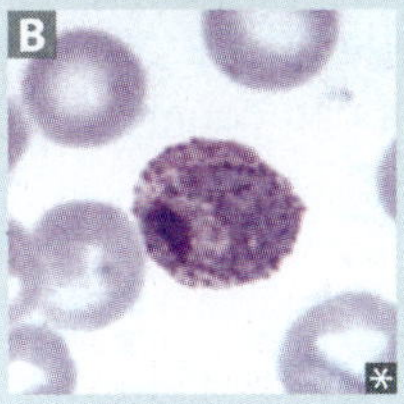	**Malaria**—fever, headache, anemia, splenomegaly *P vivax/ovale*—48-hr cycle (tertian; includes fever on first day and third day, thus fevers are actually 48 hr apart); dormant form (hypnozoite) in liver *P falciparum*—severe; irregular fever patterns; parasitized RBCs occlude capillaries in brain (cerebral malaria), kidneys, lungs *P malariae*—72-hr cycle (quartan)	*Anopheles* mosquito	Blood smear: trophozoite ring form within RBC A, schizont containing merozoites; red granules (Schüffner stippling) B throughout RBC cytoplasm seen with *P vivax/ovale* - looks like an eios.	Chloroquine (for sensitive species), which blocks *Plasmodium* heme polymerase; if resistant, use mefloquine or atovaquone/proguanil If life-threatening, use intravenous quinidine or artesunate (test for G6PD deficiency) For *P vivax/ovale*, add primaquine for hypnozoite (test for G6PD deficiency)
Babesia 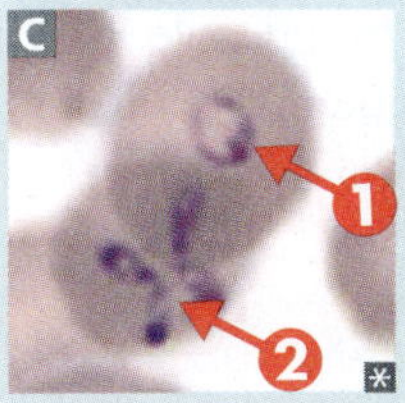	**Babesiosis**—fever and hemolytic anemia; predominantly in northeastern United States; ★ asplenia ↑ risk of severe disease	*Ixodes* tick (same as *Borrelia burgdorferi* of Lyme disease; may often coinfect humans)	Blood smear: ring form C1, "Maltese cross" C2; PCR	Atovaquone + azithromycin

- Infect RBC
- Summer flu, hemolyt anemia +/- HSM
- lysis releases merozoites
  - escapes "parasitophorous" vacuole

Protozoa—others

ORGANISM	DISEASE	TRANSMISSION	DIAGNOSIS	TREATMENT
Visceral infections				
Trypanosoma cruzi 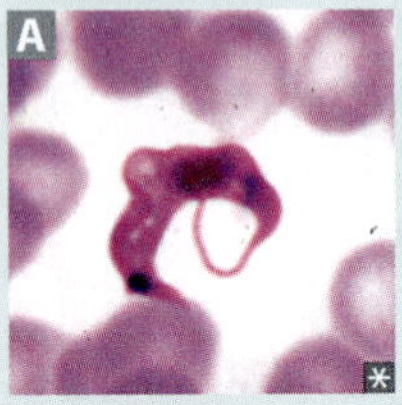	**Chagas disease**—dilated cardiomyopathy with apical atrophy, megacolon, megaesophagus; predominantly in South America Unilateral periorbital swelling (Romaña sign) characteristic of acute stage	Reduviid bug ("**kiss**ing bug") feces, deposited in a painless bite (much like a **kiss**)	Trypomastigote in blood smear A	**Benz**nidazole or ni**fur**timox; **Cruz**ing in my **Benz**, with a **fur** coat on
Leishmania donovani 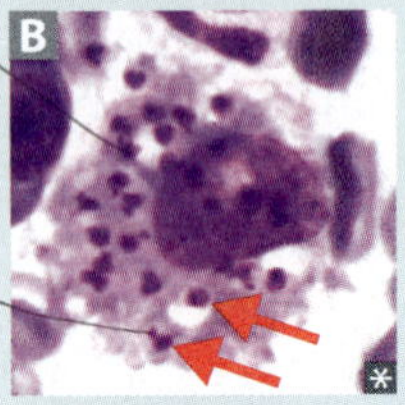	**Visceral leishmaniasis (kala-azar)**—spiking fevers, hepatosplenomegaly, pancytopenia (India) **Cutaneous leishmaniasis**—skin ulcers (Brazil, Afghan)	Sandfly painless	Macrophages containing amastigotes B Dx = BM / skin microscopy	Amphotericin B, sodium stibogluconate
Sexually transmitted infections				
Trichomonas vaginalis 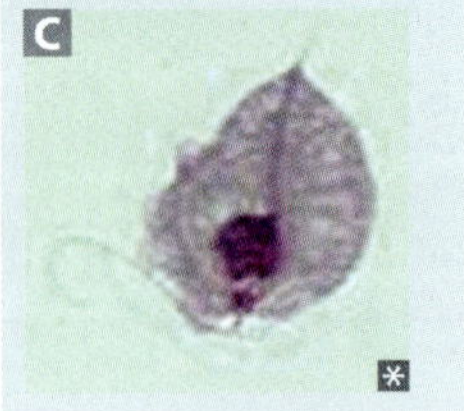	**Vaginitis**—foul-smelling, greenish discharge; itching and burning; do not confuse with *Gardnerella vaginalis*, a gram-variable bacterium associated with bacterial vaginosis	Sexual (cannot exist outside human because it cannot form cysts)	Trophozoites (motile) C on wet mount; "strawberry cervix"	Metronidazole for patient and partner (prophylaxis)

Nematode routes of infection

Ingested—*Enterobius*, *Ascaris*, *Toxocara*, *Trichinella* — You'll get sick if you **EATT** these!

Cutaneous—*Strongyloides*, *Ancylostoma*, *Necator* — These get into your feet from the **SAN**d.

Bites—*Loa loa*, *Onchocerca volvulus*, *Wuchereria bancrofti* — Lay **LOW** to avoid getting bitten.

Immune response to helminths

Eosinophils act by type I and type II hypersensitivity reactions in responding to helminths. Type I—neutralization of histamine and leukotrienes. Type II—eosinophils attach to surface of helminths via IgE and release cytotoxins (eg, major basic protein) contained in their granules.

Nematodes (roundworms)

ORGANISM	DISEASE	TRANSMISSION	TREATMENT
Intestinal			
***Enterobius vermicularis* (pinworm)**	Intestinal infection causing anal pruritus (diagnosed by seeing egg A via the tape test)	Fecal-oral	**Bend**azoles (because worms are **bend**y)
***Ascaris lumbricoides* (giant roundworm)**	Intestinal infection with possible obstruction at ileocecal valve	Fecal-oral; eggs visible in feces under microscope B	Bendazoles
***Strongyloides stercoralis* (threadworm)**	Intestinal infection causing vomiting, diarrhea, epigastric pain (may mimic peptic ulcer)	Larvae in soil penetrate the skin	Ivermectin or bendazoles
***Ancylostoma duodenale, Necator americanus* (hookworms)**	Intestinal infection causing anemia by sucking blood from intestinal wall. **Cutaneous larva migrans**—pruritic, serpiginous rash from walking barefoot on contaminated beach.	Larvae penetrate skin	Bendazoles or pyrantel pamoate
Trichinella spiralis	Intestinal infection; larvae enter bloodstream and encyst in striated muscle cells → inflammation of muscle. **Trichinosis**—fever, vomiting, nausea, periorbital edema, myalgia.	Fecal-oral; undercooked meat (especially pork)	Bendazoles
Tissue			
Toxocara canis	**Visceral larva migrans**—nematodes migrate to blood through intestinal wall causing inflammation and damage. Organs frequently affected include the heart (myocarditis), liver, and CNS (seizures, coma).	Fecal-oral	Bendazoles
Onchocerca volvulus	Skin changes, loss of elastic fibers, and river blindness (**black** flies, **black** skin nodules, "**black** sight"); allergic reaction to microfilaria possible.	Female blackfly	Ivermectin (**iver**mectin for **river** blindness)
Loa loa	Swelling in skin, worm in conjunctiva	Deer fly, horse fly, mango fly	Diethylcarbamazine
Wuchereria bancrofti	**Elephantiasis**—worms invade lymph nodes and cause inflammation, which can block lymphatic vessels C, takes 9 mo–1 yr after bite to become symptomatic.	Female mosquito	Diethylcarbamazine

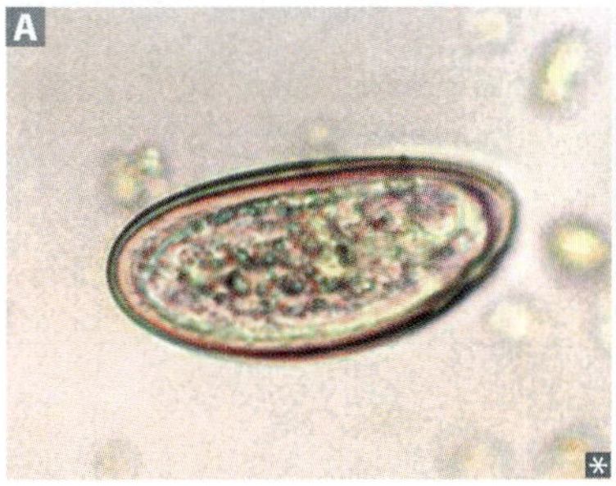
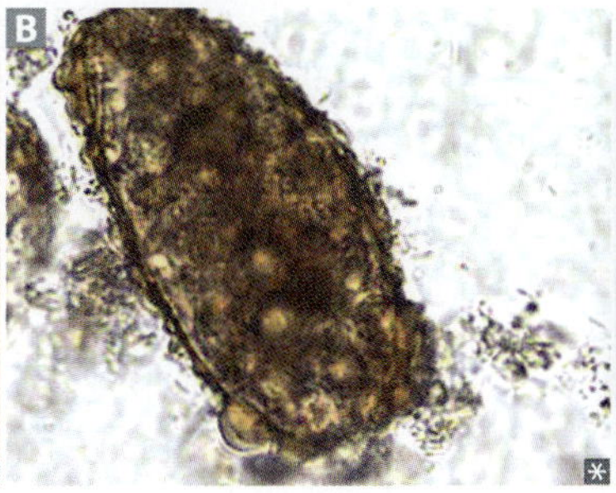
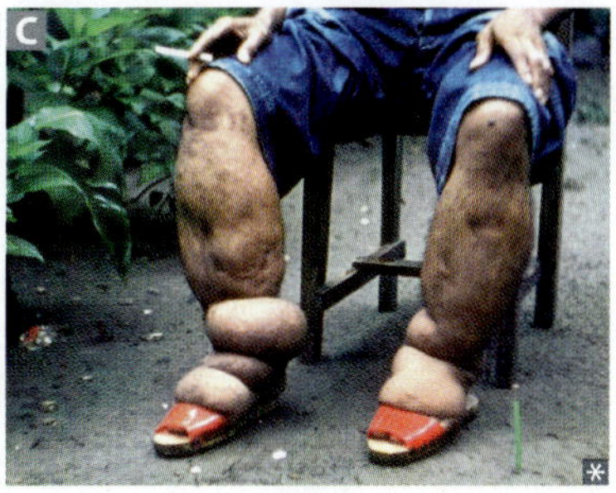

Cestodes (tapeworms)

ORGANISM	DISEASE	TRANSMISSION	TREATMENT
Taenia solium **A**	Intestinal tapeworm	Ingestion of larvae encysted in undercooked pork	Praziquantel
	Cysticercosis, neurocysticercosis **B**	Ingestion of eggs contaminated with human feces	Praziquantel; albendazole for neurocysticercosis
Diphyllobothrium latum	Vitamin B_{12} deficiency (tapeworm competes for B_{12} in intestine) → megaloblastic anemia	Ingestion of larvae from raw freshwater fish	Praziquantel
Echinococcus granulosus **C**	Hydatid cysts **D** in liver **E**, causing anaphylaxis if antigens released (hydatid cyst injected with ethanol or hypertonic saline to kill daughter cysts before removal)	Ingestion of eggs from dog feces Sheep are an intermediate host	Albendazole

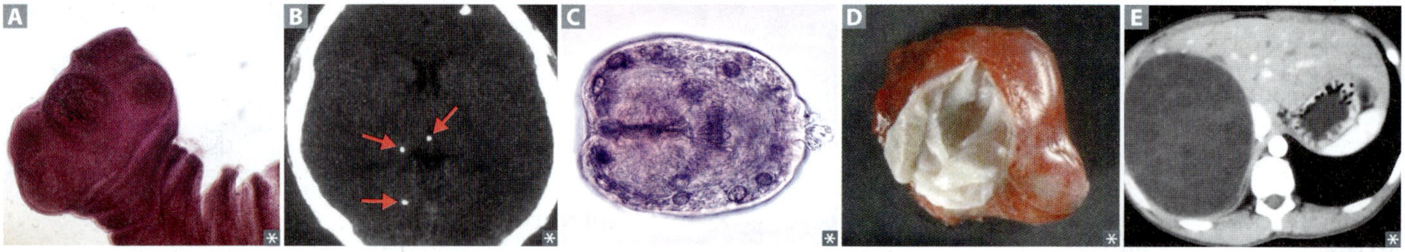

Trematodes (flukes)

ORGANISM	DISEASE	TRANSMISSION	TREATMENT
Schistosoma A 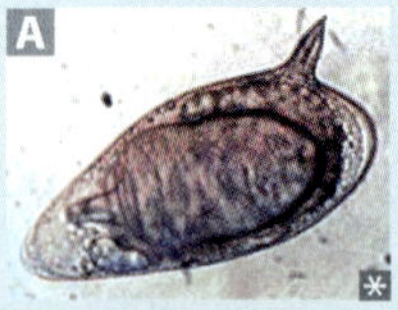 B 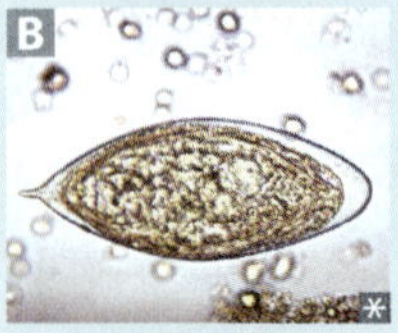	Liver and spleen enlargement (*S mansoni*, egg with lateral spine **A**), fibrosis, and inflammation Chronic infection with *S haematobium* (egg with terminal spine **B**) can lead to squamous cell carcinoma of the bladder (painless hematuria) and pulmonary hypertension	Snails are host; cercariae penetrate skin of humans	Praziquantel
Clonorchis sinensis	Biliary tract inflammation → pigmented gallstones Associated with cholangiocarcinoma	Undercooked fish	Praziquantel

Parasite hints

ASSOCIATIONS	ORGANISM
Biliary tract disease, cholangiocarcinoma	*Clonorchis sinensis*
Brain cysts, seizures	*Taenia solium* (neurocysticercosis)
Hematuria, squamous cell bladder cancer	*Schistosoma haematobium*
Liver (hydatid) cysts	*Echinococcus granulosus*
Microcytic anemia	*Ancylostoma*, *Necator*
Myalgias, periorbital edema	*Trichinella spiralis*
Perianal pruritus	*Enterobius*
Portal hypertension	*Schistosoma mansoni*, *Schistosoma japonicum*
Vitamin B_{12} deficiency	*Diphyllobothrium latum*

Ectoparasites

Scabies (*Sarcoptes scabiei*)

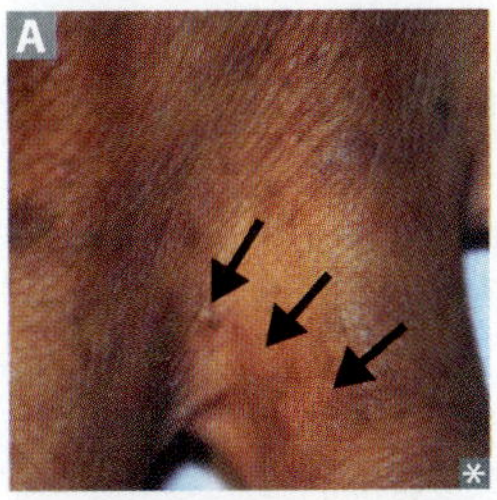

Mites that burrow into the stratum corneum and cause pruritis. Causes serpiginous burrows (lines) in webspace of hands and feet A.

Common in children, crowded populations (jails, nursing homes); transmission through fomites.

Treatment: permethrin cream, washing/drying all clothing/bedding, treat close contacts.

Lice (*Pediculus humanus*/ *Phthirus pubis*)

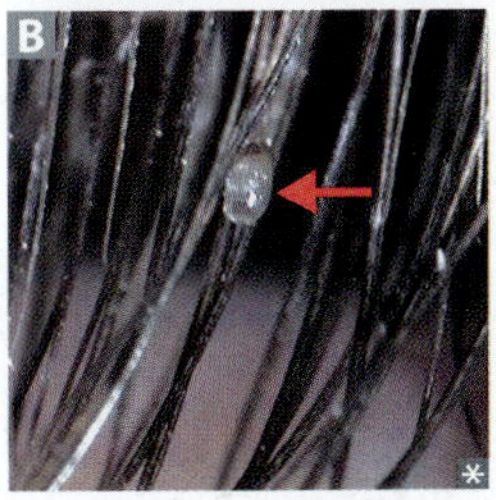

Blood-sucking insects that prefer to live on clothing. Cause intense pruritis, pink macules and papules commonly in intertriginous regions.

Can transmit *Rickettsia prowazekii* (typhus), *Borrelia recurrentis* (relapsing fever), *Bartonella quintana* (trench fever).

Treatment includes pyrethroids, malathion, or ivermectin lotion, and nit B combing. Children with head lice can be treated at home without interrupting school.

▶ MICROBIOLOGY—VIROLOGY

Viral structure—general features

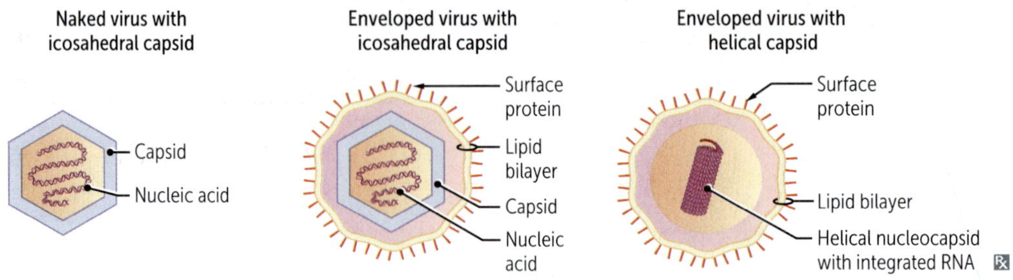

Viral genetics

Recombination	Exchange of genes between 2 chromosomes by crossing over within regions of significant base sequence homology.
Reassortment	When viruses with segmented genomes (eg, influenza virus) exchange genetic material. For example, the 2009 novel H1N1 influenza A pandemic emerged via complex viral reassortment of genes from human, swine, and avian viruses. Has potential to cause antigenic shift.
Complementation	When 1 of 2 viruses that infect the cell has a mutation that results in a nonfunctional protein, the nonmutated virus "complements" the mutated one by making a functional protein that serves both viruses. For example, hepatitis D virus requires the presence of replicating hepatitis B virus to supply HBsAg, the envelope protein for HDV.
Phenotypic mixing	Occurs with simultaneous infection of a cell with 2 viruses. Genome of virus A can be partially or completely coated (forming pseudovirion) with the surface proteins of virus B. Type B protein coat determines the tropism (infectivity) of the hybrid virus. However, the progeny from this infection have a type A coat that is encoded by its type A genetic material.

Viral vaccines

Live attenuated vaccines	Induce humoral and cell-mediated immunity but have reverted to virulence on rare occasions. **Live** attenuated: **small**pox, **yellow** fever, **rota**virus, **chicken**pox (VZV), **Sabin** polio virus, **MMR**, **In**fluenza (**in**tranasal).	No booster needed for live attenuated vaccines. Dangerous to give live vaccines to immunocompromised patients. Close contacts may be vaccinated with live vaccines (except live polio or influenza). "**Live**! One night only! See **small yellow rotat**ing **chickens** get vaccinated with **Sabin** and **MMR**! **I**t's **in**credible!" MMR = measles, mumps, rubella; live attenuated vaccine that can be given to HIV ⊕ patients who do not show signs of immunodeficiency.
Killed	**R**abies, **I**nfluenza (injected), Salk **P**olio, and H**A**V vaccines. Killed/inactivated vaccines induce only humoral immunity but are stable.	Sal**K** = **K**illed. **RIP A**lways.
Subunit	HBV (antigen = HBsAg), HPV (types 6, 11, 16, and 18).	

DNA viral genomes	All DNA viruses except the Parvoviridae are dsDNA. All are linear except papilloma-, polyoma-, and hepadnaviruses (circular).	All are dsDNA (like our cells), except "**part-of-a-virus**" (**parvovirus**) is ssDNA. *Parvus* = small.
RNA viral genomes	All RNA viruses except Reoviridae are ssRNA. ⊕ stranded RNA viruses: I went to a **retro** (**retro**virus) **toga** (**toga**virus) party, where I drank **flav**ored (**flav**ivirus) **Corona** (**corona**virus) and ate **hippie** (**hepe**virus) **Cali**fornia (**cali**civirus) **pic**kles (**pic**ornavirus).	All are ssRNA (like our mRNA), except "**repeato**-virus" (**reo**virus) is dsRNA.

Naked viral genome infectivity

Purified nucleic acids of most dsDNA (except poxviruses and HBV) and ⊕ strand ssRNA (≈ mRNA) viruses are infectious. Naked nucleic acids of ⊖ strand ssRNA and dsRNA viruses are not infectious. They require polymerases contained in the complete virion.

Viral replication

DNA viruses	All replicate in the nucleus (except poxvirus).
RNA viruses	All replicate in the cytoplasm (except influenza virus and retroviruses).

Viral envelopes	**Naked** (nonenveloped) viruses include **P**apillomavirus, **A**denovirus, **P**arvovirus, **P**olyomavirus, **C**alicivirus, **P**icornavirus, **R**eovirus, and **Hep**evirus. Generally, enveloped viruses acquire their envelopes from plasma membrane when they exit from cell. Exceptions include herpesviruses, which acquire envelopes from nuclear membrane.	Give **PAPP** smears and **CPR** to a **naked hip**pie (**hep**evirus). DNA = **PAPP**; RNA = **CPR** and **hep**evirus.

DNA virus characteristics

Some general rules—all DNA viruses:

GENERAL RULE	COMMENTS
Are **HHAPPPP**y viruses	**H**epadna, **H**erpes, **A**deno, **P**ox, **P**arvo, **P**apilloma, **P**olyoma.
Are double stranded	Except parvo (single stranded).
Have linear genomes	Except papilloma and polyoma (circular, supercoiled) and hepadna (circular, incomplete).
Are icosahedral	Except pox (complex).
Replicate in the nucleus	Except pox (carries own DNA-dependent RNA polymerase).

DNA viruses

VIRAL FAMILY	ENVELOPE	DNA STRUCTURE	MEDICAL IMPORTANCE
Herpesviruses	Yes	DS and linear	See Herpesviruses entry
Poxvirus	Yes	DS and linear (largest DNA virus)	Smallpox eradicated world wide by use of the live-attenuated vaccine Cowpox ("milkmaid blisters") **Molluscum contagiosum**—flesh-colored papule with central umbilication
Hepadnavirus	Yes	Partially DS and circular	HBV: ▪ Acute or chronic hepatitis ▪ Not a retrovirus but has reverse transcriptase
Adenovirus A 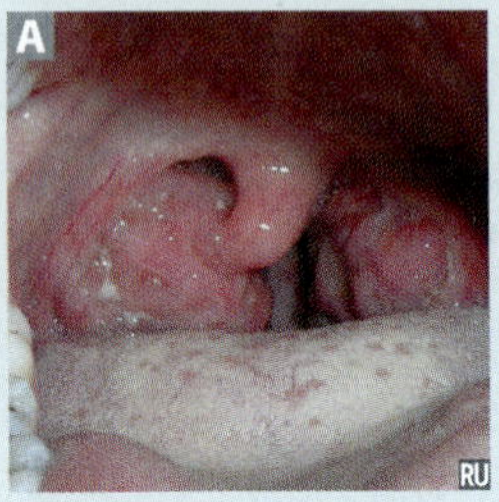	No	DS and linear	Febrile pharyngitis A—sore throat Acute hemorrhagic cystitis Pneumonia Conjunctivitis—"pink eye"
Papillomavirus	No	DS and circular	HPV–warts (serotypes 1, 2, 6, 11), CIN, cervical cancer (most commonly 16, 18)
Polyomavirus	No	DS and circular	JC virus—progressive multifocal leukoencephalopathy (PML) in HIV BK virus—transplant patients, commonly targets kidney **JC**: **J**unky **C**erebrum; **BK**: **B**ad **K**idney
Parvovirus	No	SS and linear (smallest DNA virus)	B19 virus—aplastic crises in sickle cell disease, "slapped cheeks" rash in children (erythema infectiosum, or fifth disease) RBC destruction in fetus leads to hydrops fetalis and death, in adults leads to pure RBC aplasia and rheumatoid arthritis–like symptoms

Herpesviruses

Enveloped, DS and linear viruses

VIRUS	ROUTE OF TRANSMISSION	CLINICAL SIGNIFICANCE	NOTES
Herpes simplex virus-1	Respiratory secretions, saliva	Gingivostomatitis, keratoconjunctivitis A, herpes labialis B, herpetic whitlow on finger, temporal lobe encephalitis.	Most common cause of sporadic encephalitis, can present as altered mental status, seizures, and/or aphasia.
Herpes simplex virus-2	Sexual contact, perinatal	Herpes genitalis C, neonatal herpes.	Latent in sacral ganglia. Viral meningitis more common with HSV-2 than with HSV-1.
Varicella-Zoster virus (HHV-3)	Respiratory secretions	Varicella-zoster (chickenpox D, shingles E), encephalitis, pneumonia. Most common complication of shingles is post-herpetic neuralgia.	Latent in dorsal root or trigeminal ganglia. —random
Epstein-Barr virus (HHV-4)	Respiratory secretions, saliva; aka "kissing disease," (common in teens, young adults)	Mononucleosis—fever, hepatosplenomegaly, pharyngitis, and lymphadenopathy (especially posterior cervical nodes F). Avoid contact sports until resolution due to risk of splenic rupture. Associated with lymphomas (eg, endemic Burkitt lymphoma), nasopharyngeal carcinoma.	Infects B cells through CD21. Atypical lymphocytes on peripheral blood smear G—not infected B cells but reactive cytotoxic T cells. ⊕ Monospot test—heterophile antibodies detected by agglutination of sheep or horse RBCs.
Cytomegalovirus (HHV-5)	Congenital transfusion, sexual contact, saliva, urine, transplant	Mononucleosis (⊖ Monospot) in (milder) immunocompetent patients; infection in immunocompromised patients, especially pneumonia in transplant patients; AIDS **retinitis** ("**sight**omegalovirus"): hemorrhage, cotton-wool exudates, vision loss. Congenital CMV — petech rash, microceph, jaundice	Infected cells have characteristic "owl eye" inclusions H. Latent in mononuclear cells.
Human herpesviruses 6 and 7	Saliva	Roseola infantum (exanthem subitum): high fevers for several days that can cause seizures, followed by diffuse macular rash I. HHV-7—less common cause of roseola.	
Human herpesvirus 8	Sexual contact	Kaposi sarcoma (neoplasm of endothelial cells). Seen in HIV/AIDS and transplant patients. Dark/violaceous plaques or nodules J representing vascular proliferations.	Can also affect GI and lungs.

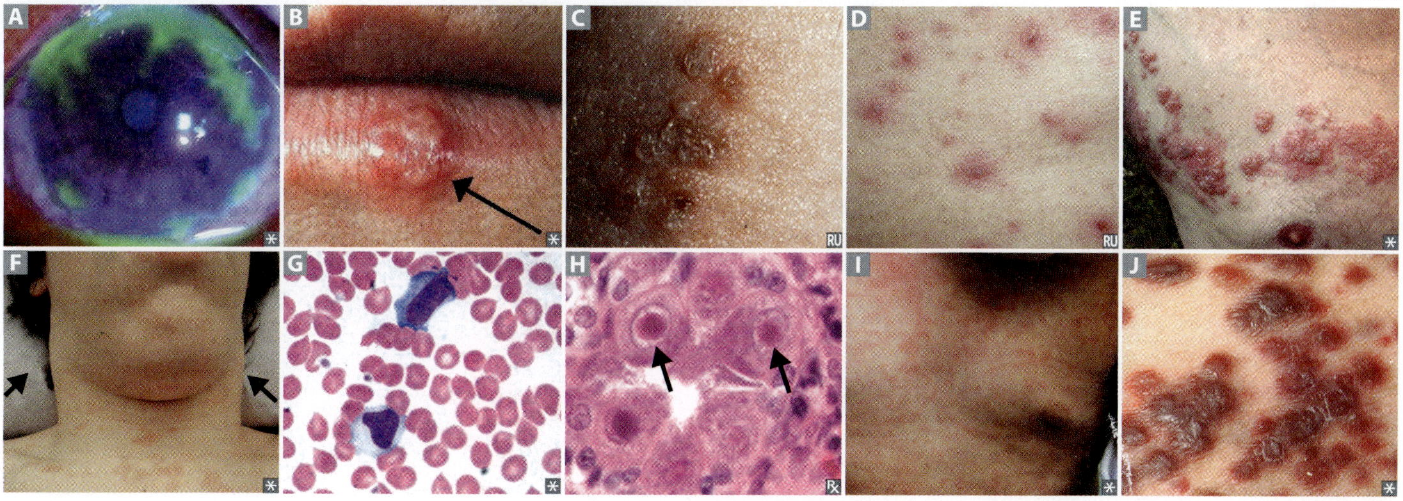

HSV identification

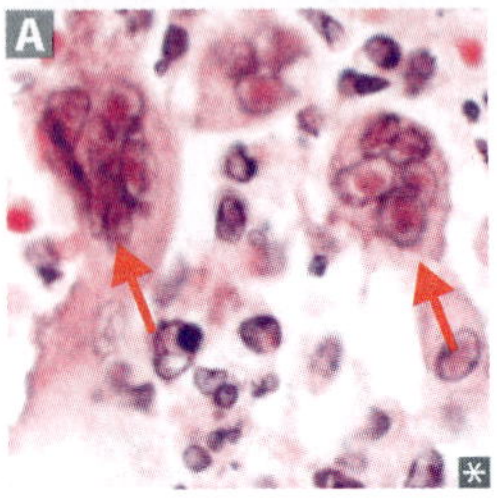

Viral culture for skin/genitalia.
CSF PCR for herpes encephalitis.
Tzanck test—a smear of an opened skin vesicle to detect multinucleated giant cells A commonly seen in HSV-1, HSV-2, and VZV infection.
Intranuclear inclusions also seen with HSV-1, HSV-2, VZV.
Tzanck heavens I do not have herpes.

Receptors used by viruses

VIRUS	RECEPTORS
CMV	Integrins (heparan sulfate)
EBV	CD21
HIV	CD4, CXCR4, CCR5
Rabies	Nicotinic AChR
Rhinovirus	ICAM-1

RNA viruses

VIRAL FAMILY	ENVELOPE	RNA STRUCTURE	CAPSID SYMMETRY	MEDICAL IMPORTANCE
Reoviruses	No	DS linear 10–12 segments	Icosahedral (double)	Coltivirus[a]—Colorado tick fever Rotavirus—#1 cause of fatal diarrhea in children
Picornaviruses	No	SS ⊕ linear	Icosahedral	**P**oliovirus—polio-Salk/Sabin vaccines—IPV/OPV **E**chovirus—aseptic meningitis **R**hinovirus—“common cold” **C**oxsackievirus—aseptic meningitis; herpangina (mouth blisters, fever); hand, foot, and mouth disease; myocarditis; pericarditis **H**AV—acute viral hepatitis **PERCH**
Hepevirus	No	SS ⊕ linear	Icosahedral	HEV
Caliciviruses	No	SS ⊕ linear	Icosahedral	Norovirus—viral gastroenteritis
Flaviviruses	Yes	SS ⊕ linear	Icosahedral	HCV Yellow fever[a] Dengue[a] St. Louis encephalitis[a] West Nile virus[a]
Togaviruses	Yes	SS ⊕ linear	Icosahedral	Rubella Eastern equine encephalitis[a] Western equine encephalitis[a]
Retroviruses	Yes	SS ⊕ linear 2 copies	Icosahedral (HTLV), complex and conical (HIV)	Have reverse transcriptase HTLV—T-cell leukemia HIV—AIDS
Coronaviruses	Yes	SS ⊕ linear	Helical	“Common cold,” SARS, MERS
Orthomyxoviruses	Yes	SS ⊖ linear 8 segments	Helical	Influenza virus
Paramyxoviruses	Yes	SS ⊖ linear Nonsegmented	Helical	**P**a**R**a**M**yxovirus: **P**arainfluenza—croup **R**SV—bronchiolitis in babies; **R**x—ribavirin **M**easles, **M**umps
Rhabdoviruses	Yes	SS ⊖ linear	Helical	Rabies
Filoviruses	Yes	SS ⊖ linear	Helical	Ebola/Marburg hemorrhagic fever—often fatal!
Arenaviruses	Yes	SS ⊕ or ⊖ circular 2 segments	Helical	LCMV—lymphocytic choriomeningitis virus Lassa fever encephalitis—spread by rodents
Bunyaviruses	Yes	SS ⊖ circular 3 segments	Helical	California encephalitis[a] Sandfly/Rift Valley fevers[a] Crimean-Congo hemorrhagic fever[a] Hantavirus—hemorrhagic fever, pneumonia
Delta virus	Yes	SS ⊖ circular	Uncertain	HDV is a “defective” virus that requires the presence of HBV to replicate

SS, single-stranded; DS, double-stranded; ⊕, positive sense; ⊖, negative sense; [a]= **arbo**virus, **ar**thropod **bo**rne (mosquitoes, ticks).

Negative-stranded viruses	Must transcribe ⊖ strand to ⊕. Virion brings its own RNA-dependent RNA polymerase. They include **A**renaviruses, **B**unyaviruses, **P**aramyxoviruses, **O**rthomyxoviruses, **F**iloviruses, and **R**habdoviruses.	**A**lways **B**ring **P**olymerase **O**r **F**ail **R**eplication.
Segmented viruses	All are RNA viruses. They include **B**unyaviruses, **O**rthomyxoviruses (influenza viruses), **A**renaviruses, and **R**eoviruses.	**BOAR**.
Picornavirus	Includes **P**oliovirus, **E**chovirus, **R**hinovirus, **C**oxsackievirus, and **H**AV. RNA is translated into 1 large polypeptide that is cleaved by proteases into functional viral proteins. Can cause aseptic (viral) meningitis (except rhinovirus and HAV). All are enteroviruses (fecal-oral spread) except rhinovirus.	Pico**RNA**virus = small **RNA** virus. **PERCH** on a "**peak**" (**pico**).
Rhinovirus	A picornavirus. Nonenveloped RNA virus. Cause of common cold; > 100 serologic types. Acid labile—destroyed by stomach acid; therefore, does not infect the GI tract (unlike the other picornaviruses).	**Rhino** has a runny **nose**.
Yellow fever virus 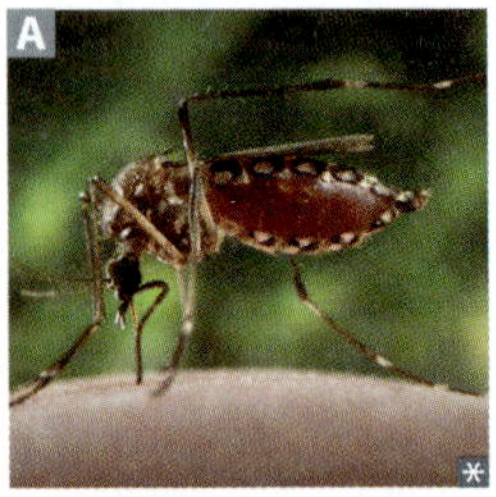	A flavivirus (also an arbovirus) transmitted by *Aedes* mosquitoes A. Virus has a monkey or human reservoir. Symptoms: high fever, black vomitus, and jaundice. May see Councilman bodies (eosinophilic apoptotic globules) on liver biopsy.	*Flavi* = yellow, jaundice.
Rotavirus 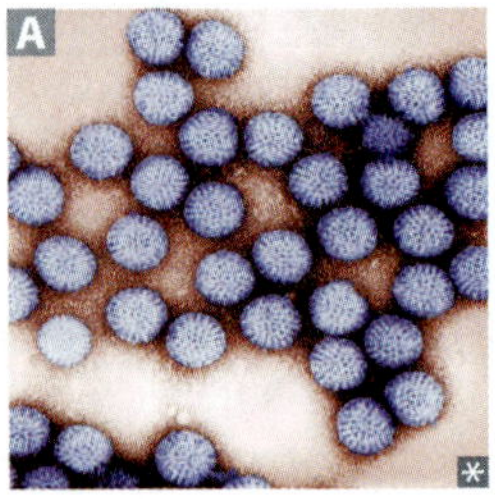	Rotavirus A, the most important global cause of infantile gastroenteritis, is a segmented dsRNA virus (a reovirus). Major cause of acute diarrhea in the United States during winter, especially in day care centers, kindergartens. Villous destruction with atrophy leads to ↓ absorption of Na^+ and loss of K^+.	**ROTA**virus = **R**ight **O**ut **T**he **A**nus. CDC recommends routine vaccination of all infants.

Influenza viruses

Orthomyxoviruses. Enveloped, ⊖ ssRNA viruses with 8-segment genome. Contain hemagglutinin (promotes viral entry) and neuraminidase (promotes progeny virion release) antigens. Patients at risk for fatal bacterial superinfection, most commonly *S aureus*, *S pneumoniae*, and *H influenzae*.

Reformulated vaccine ("the flu shot") contains viral strains most likely to appear during the flu season, due to the virus' rapid genetic change.
Killed viral vaccine is most frequently used.
Live attenuated vaccine contains temperature-sensitive mutant that replicates in the nose but not in the lung; administered intranasally.

Genetic shift/ antigenic shift

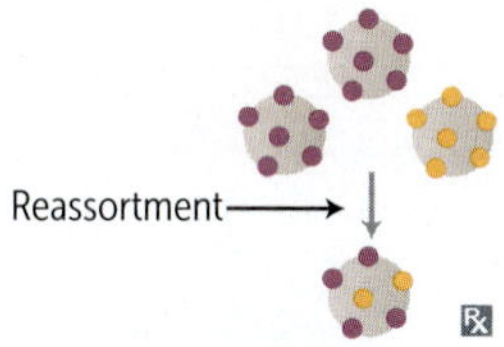

Causes pandemics. Reassortment of viral genome segments, such as when segments of human flu A virus reassort with swine flu A virus.

Sudden shift is more deadly than gradual drift.

Genetic drift/ antigenic drift

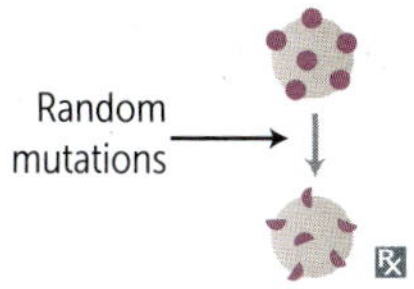

Causes epidemics. Minor (antigenic drift) changes based on random mutation in hemagglutinin or neuraminidase genes.

Rubella virus

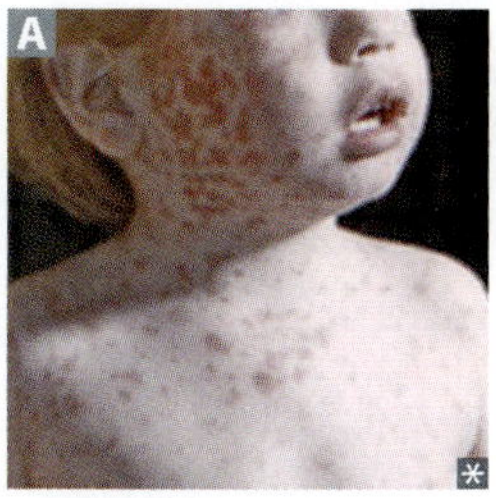

A togavirus. Causes rubella, once known as German (3-day) measles. Fever, postauricular and other lymphadenopathy, arthralgias, and fine, confluent rash that starts on face and spreads centrifugally to involve trunk and extremities **A**. Causes mild disease in children but serious congenital disease (a ToRCHeS infection). Congenital rubella findings include "blueberry muffin" appearance due to dermal extramedullary hematopoiesis.

Paramyxoviruses

Paramyxoviruses cause disease in children. They include those that cause parainfluenza (croup: seal-like barking cough), mumps, and measles as well as RSV, which causes respiratory tract infection (bronchiolitis, pneumonia) in infants. All contain surface F (fusion) protein, which causes respiratory epithelial cells to fuse and form multinucleated cells. Palivizumab (monoclonal antibody against F protein) prevents pneumonia caused by RSV infection in premature infants.

Croup (acute laryngotracheobronchitis)

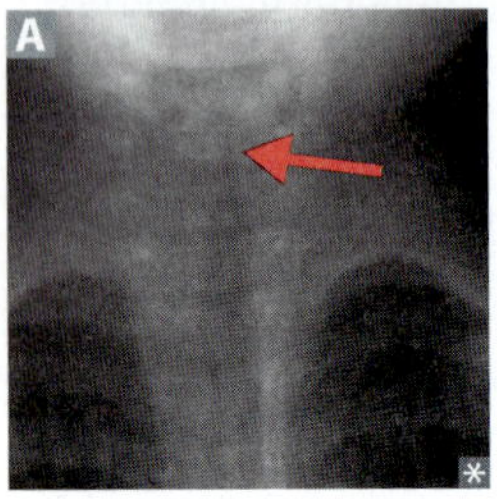

Caused by parainfluenza viruses (paramyxovirus). Results in a "seal-like" barking cough and inspiratory stridor. Narrowing of upper trachea and subglottis leads to characteristic steeple sign on x-ray A. Severe croup can result in pulsus paradoxus 2° to upper airway obstruction.

Measles (rubeola) virus

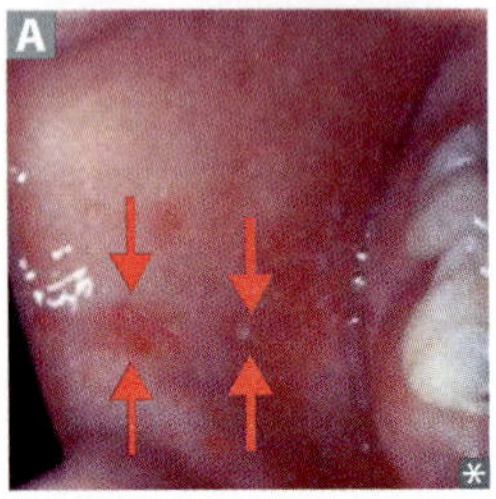

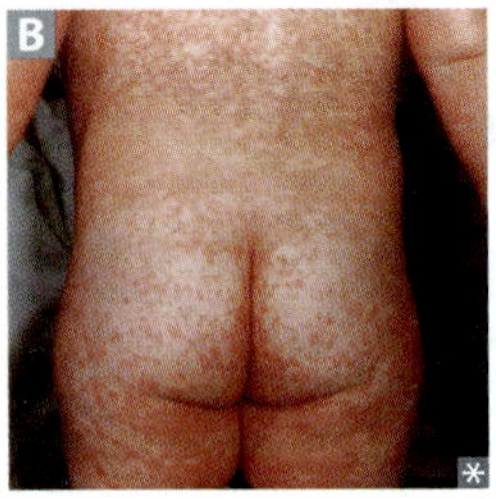

A paramyxovirus that causes measles. Usual presentation involves prodromal fever with cough, coryza, and conjunctivitis, then eventually Koplik spots (bright red spots with blue-white center on buccal mucosa A), followed 1–2 days later by a maculopapular rash B that starts at the head/neck and spreads downward. Lymphadenitis with Warthin-Finkeldey giant cells (fused lymphocytes) in a background of paracortical hyperplasia. SSPE (subacute sclerosing panencephalitis, occurring years later), encephalitis (1:2000), and giant cell pneumonia (rarely, in immunosuppressed) are possible sequelae.

3 C's of measles:
- Cough
- Coryza
- Conjunctivitis

Vitamin A supplementation can reduce morbidity and mortality from measles, particularly in malnourished children.

Mumps virus

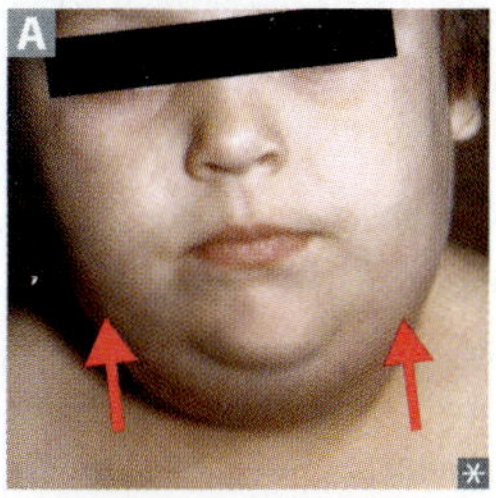

A paramyxovirus that causes mumps, uncommon due to effectiveness of MMR vaccine.

Symptoms: **P**arotitis A, **O**rchitis (inflammation of testes), aseptic **M**eningitis, and **P**ancreatitis. Can cause sterility (especially after puberty).

Mumps makes your parotid glands and testes as big as **POM-P**oms.

Rabies virus

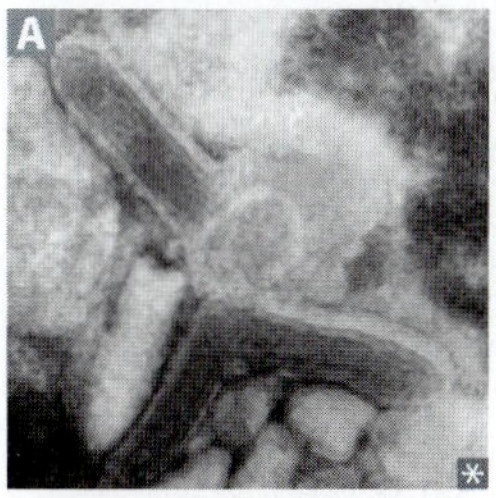

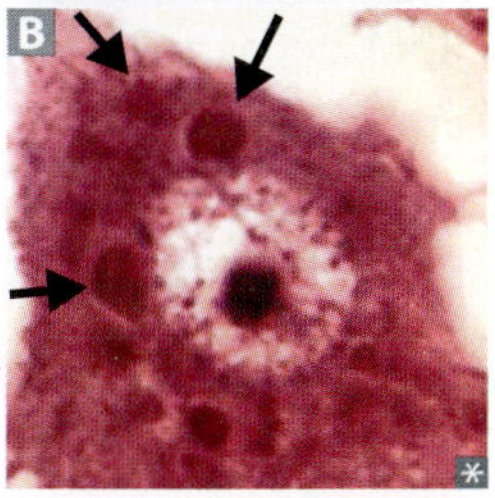

Bullet-shaped virus A. Negri bodies (cytoplasmic inclusions B) commonly found in Purkinje cells of cerebellum and in hippocampal neurons. Rabies has long incubation period (weeks to months) before symptom onset. Postexposure prophylaxis is wound cleaning plus immunization with killed vaccine and rabies immunoglobulin. Example of passive-active immunity.

I never Knew!

Travels to the CNS by migrating in a retrograde fashion up nerve axons after binding to ACh receptors.

Progression of disease: fever, malaise → agitation, photophobia, hydrophobia, hypersalivation → paralysis, coma → death.

Infection more commonly from bat, raccoon, and skunk bites than from dog bites in the United States; aerosol transmission (eg, bat caves) also possible.

Ebola virus

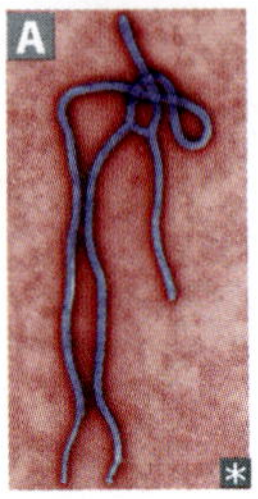

A filovirus **A** that targets endothelial cells, phagocytes, hepatocytes. Following an incubation period of up to 21 days, presents with abrupt onset of flu-like symptoms, diarrhea/vomiting, high fever, myalgia. Can progress to DIC, diffuse hemorrhage, shock. Diagnosed with RT-PCR within 48 hr of symptom onset. High mortality rate.

Transmission requires direct contact with bodily fluids, fomites (including dead bodies), infected bats or primates (apes/monkeys); high incidence of nosocomial infection.

Supportive care, no definitive treatment. Strict isolation of infected individuals and barrier practices for health care workers are key to preventing transmission.

Hepatitis viruses

Signs and symptoms of all hepatitis viruses: episodes of fever, jaundice, ↑ ALT and AST. Naked viruses (HAV and HEV) lack an envelope and are not destroyed by the gut: the **vowels** hit your **bowels**.

HBV DNA polymerase has DNA- and RNA-dependent activities. Upon entry into nucleus, the polymerase completes the partial dsDNA. Host RNA polymerase transcribes mRNA from viral DNA to make viral proteins. The DNA polymerase then reverse transcribes viral RNA to DNA, which is the genome of the progeny virus.

HCV lacks 3′-5′ exonuclease activity → variation in antigenic structures of HCV envelope proteins. Host antibody production lags behind production of new mutant strains of HCV.

Virus	HAV	HBV	HCV	HDV	HEV
FAMILY	RNA picornavirus	DNA hepadnavirus	RNA flavivirus	RNA deltavirus	RNA hepevirus
TRANSMISSION	Fecal-oral (shellfish, travelers, day care)	Parenteral (Blood), sexual (Baby-making), perinatal (Birthing)	Primarily blood (IVDU, post-transfusion)	Parenteral, sexual, perinatal	Fecal-oral, especially waterborne
INCUBATION	Short (weeks)	Long (months)	Long	Superinfection (HDV after HBV) = short Coinfection (HDV with HBV) = long	Short
CLINICAL COURSE	Asymptomatic (usually), Acute	★ Initially like serum sickness (fever, arthralgias, rash); may progress to carcinoma	May progress to Cirrhosis or Carcinoma	Similar to HBV	★ Fulminant hepatitis in Expectant (pregnant) women
PROGNOSIS	Good	★ Most adults have full resolution, minority have chronic infection	Majority develop stable, Chronic hepatitis C	Superinfection → worse prognosis	High mortality in pregnant women
HCC RISK	No	Yes	Yes	Yes	No
LIVER BIOPSY	Hepatocyte swelling, monocyte infiltration, Councilman bodies	Granular eosinophilic "ground glass" appearance; cytotoxic T cells mediate damage	Lymphoid aggregates with focal areas of macrovesicular steatosis	Similar to HBV	Patchy necrosis
NOTES	No carrier state ("Alone")	Carrier state common	Carrier state common	Defective virus, Depends on HBV	Enteric, Epidemic, no carrier state

councilman body = a dying hepatocyte shrinks to form an eosinoph. body.

Hepatitis serologic markers

Anti-HAV (IgM)	IgM antibody to HAV; best test to detect acute hepatitis A.
Anti-HAV (IgG)	IgG antibody indicates prior HAV infection and/or prior vaccination; protects against reinfection.
HBsAg	Antigen found on surface of HBV; indicates hepatitis B infection.
Anti-HBs	Antibody to HBsAg; indicates immunity to hepatitis B.
HBcAg	Antigen associated with core of HBV.
Anti-HBc	Antibody to HBcAg; IgM = acute/recent infection; IgG = prior exposure or chronic infection. IgM anti-HBc may be the sole ⊕ marker of infection during window period.
HBeAg	Secreted by infected hepatocyte into circulation. Not part of mature HBV virion. Indicates active viral replication and therefore high transmissibility.
Anti-HBe	Antibody to HBeAg; indicates low transmissibility.

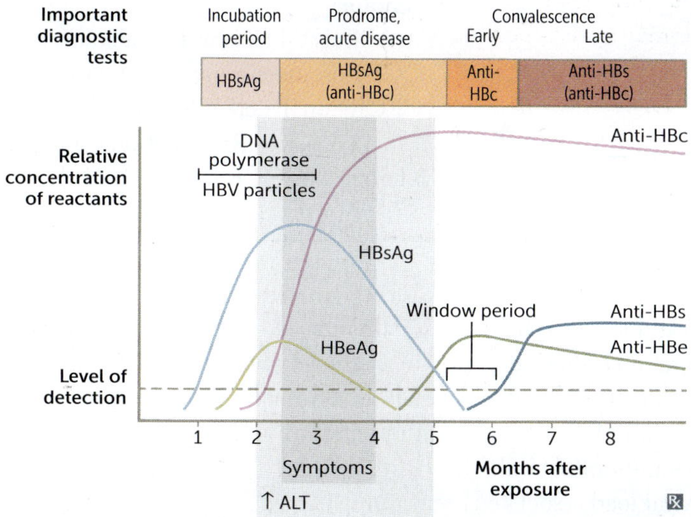

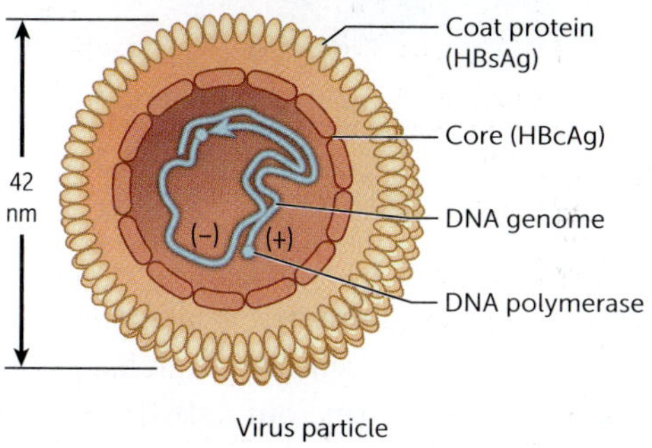

	HBsAg	Anti-HBs	HBeAg	Anti-HBe	Anti-HBc
Acute HBV	✓		✓		IgM
Window				✓	IgM
Chronic HBV (high infectivity)	✓		✓		IgG
Chronic HBV (low infectivity)	✓			✓	IgG
Recovery		✓		✓	IgG
Immunized		✓			

HIV

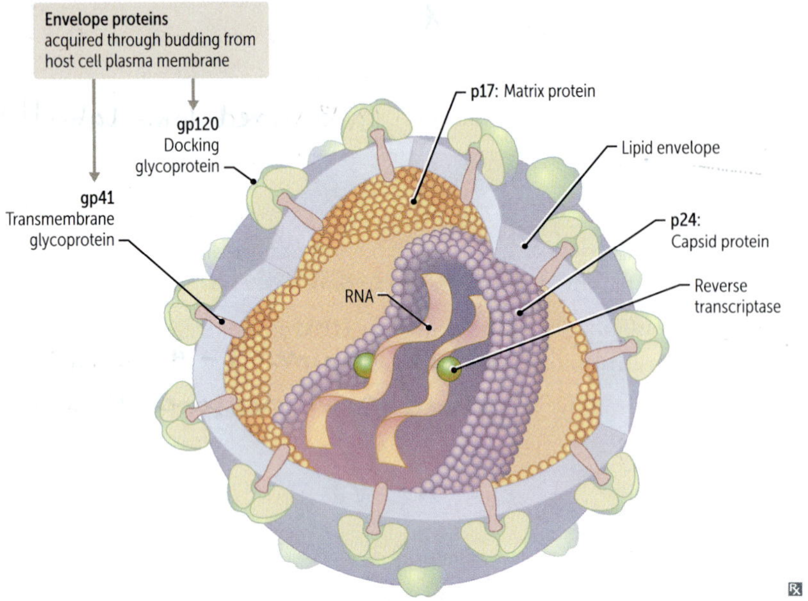

Diploid genome (2 molecules of RNA).

The 3 structural genes (protein coded for):

- *env* (gp120 and gp41):
  - Formed from cleavage of gp160 to form envelope glycoproteins.
  - gp120—attachment to host CD4+ T cell.
  - gp41—fusion and entry.
- *gag* (p24 and p17—capsid and matrix proteins, respectively.
- *pol*—reverse transcriptase, aspartate protease, integrase.

Reverse transcriptase synthesizes dsDNA from genomic RNA; dsDNA integrates into host genome.

Virus binds CD4 as well as a coreceptor, either CCR5 on macrophages (early infection) or CXCR4 on T cells (late infection).

Homozygous CCR5 mutation = immunity.

Heterozygous CCR5 mutation = slower course.

HIV diagnosis

Presumptive diagnosis made with ELISA (sensitive, high false ⊕ rate and low threshold, **rule out** test); ⊕ results are then confirmed with Western blot assay (specific, low false ⊕ rate and high threshold, rule in test).

Viral load tests determine the amount of viral RNA in the plasma. High viral load associated with poor prognosis. Also use viral load to monitor effect of drug therapy.

AIDS diagnosis ≤ 200 CD4+ cells/mm^3 (normal: 500–1500 cells/mm^3). HIV⊕ with AIDS-defining condition (eg, *Pneumocystis* pneumonia) or CD4+ percentage < 14%.

ELISA/Western blot tests look for antibodies to viral proteins; these tests often are falsely ⊖ in the first 1–2 months of HIV infection and falsely ⊕ initially in babies born to infected mothers (anti-gp120 crosses placenta).

Time course of untreated HIV infection

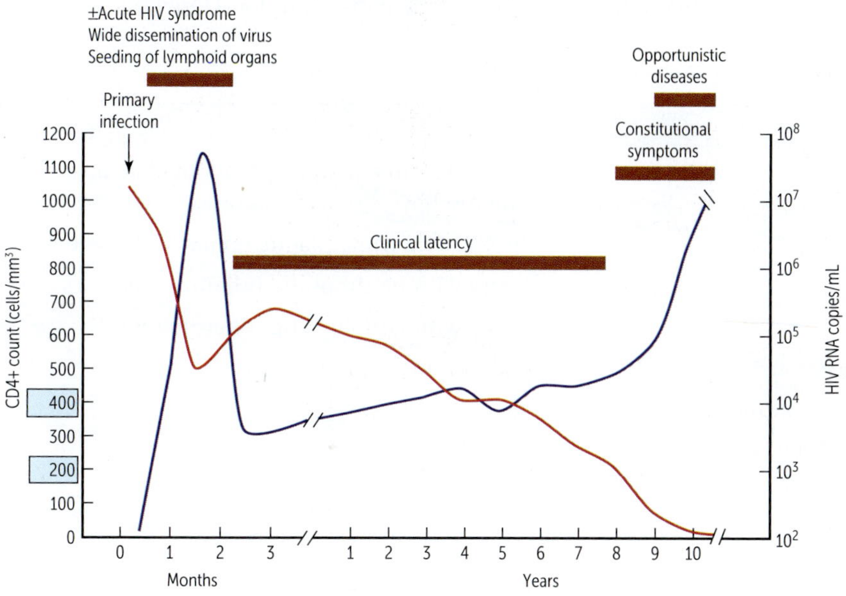

Red line = CD4+ T cell count (cells/mm^3); blue line = HIV RNA copies/mL plasma.

Blue boxes on vertical CD4+ count axis indicate moderate immunocompromise (< 400 CD4+ cells/mm^3) and when AIDS-defining illnesses emerge (< 200 CD4+ cells/mm^3).

Most patients who do not receive treatment eventually die of complications of HIV infection.

Four stages of untreated infection:
1. Flu-like (acute)
2. Feeling fine (latent)
3. Falling count
4. Final crisis

During latent phase, virus replicates in lymph nodes.

Common diseases of HIV-positive adults

As CD4+ cell count ↓, risks of reactivation of past infections (eg, TB, HSV, shingles), dissemination of bacterial infections and fungal infections (eg, coccidioidomycosis), and non-Hodgkin lymphomas ↑.

PATHOGEN	PRESENTATION	FINDINGS
CD4+ cell count < 500/mm^3		
Candida albicans	Oral thrush	Scrapable white plaque, pseudohyphae on microscopy
EBV	Oral hairy leukoplakia	Unscrapable white plaque on lateral tongue
Bartonella henselae	Bacillary angiomatosis	Biopsy with neutrophilic inflammation
HHV-8	Kaposi sarcoma	Biopsy with lymphocytic inflammation
Cryptosporidium spp.	Chronic, watery diarrhea	Acid-fast oocysts in stool
HPV	Squamous cell carcinoma, commonly of anus (men who have sex with men) or cervix (women)	
CD4+ cell count < 200/mm^3		
HIV	Dementia	
JC virus (reactivation)	Progressive multifocal leukoencephalopathy	Nonenhancing areas of demyelination on MRI
Pneumocystis jirovecii	*Pneumocystis* pneumonia	"Ground-glass" opacities on CXR
CD4+ cell count < 100/mm^3		
Aspergillus fumigatus	Hemoptysis, pleuritic pain	Cavitation or infiltrates on chest imaging
Cryptococcus neoformans	Meningitis	Encapsulated yeast on India ink stain or capsular antigen ⊕
Candida albicans	Esophagitis	White plaques on endoscopy; yeast and pseudohyphae on biopsy
CMV	Retinitis, esophagitis, colitis, pneumonitis, encephalitis	Linear ulcers on endoscopy, cotton-wool spots on fundoscopy Biopsy reveals cells with intranuclear (owl eye) inclusion bodies
EBV	B-cell lymphoma (eg, non-Hodgkin lymphoma, CNS lymphoma)	CNS lymphoma—ring enhancing, may be solitary (vs *Toxoplasma*)
Histoplasma capsulatum	Fever, weight loss, fatigue, cough, dyspnea, nausea, vomiting, diarrhea	Oval yeast cells within macrophages
Mycobacterium avium–intracellulare, *Mycobacterium avium* complex	Nonspecific systemic symptoms (fever, night sweats, weight loss) or focal lymphadenitis	
Toxoplasma gondii	Brain abscesses	Multiple ring-enhancing lesions on MRI

Prions

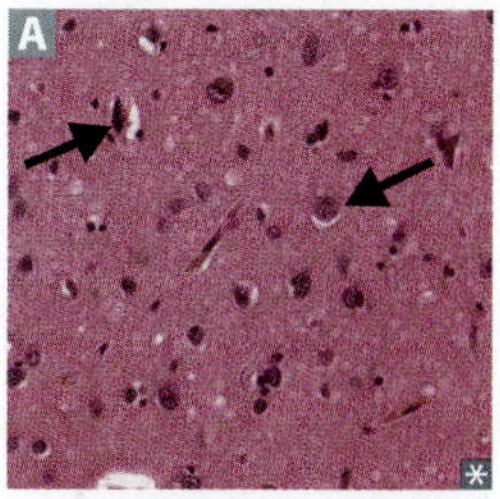

Prion diseases are caused by the conversion of a normal (predominantly α-helical) protein termed prion protein (PrP^c) to a β-pleated form (PrP^{sc}), which is transmissible via CNS-related tissue (iatrogenic CJD) or food contaminated by BSE-infected animal products (variant CJD). PrP^{sc} resists protease degradation and facilitates the conversion of still more PrP^c to PrP^{sc}. Resistant to standard sterilizing procedures, including standard autoclaving. Accumulation of PrP^{sc} results in spongiform encephalopathy A and dementia, ataxia, and death.

Creutzfeldt-Jakob disease—rapidly progressive dementia, typically sporadic (some familial forms).
Bovine spongiform encephalopathy (BSE)—also known as "mad cow disease."
Kuru—acquired prion disease noted in tribal populations practicing human cannibalism.

▶ MICROBIOLOGY—SYSTEMS

Normal flora: dominant

LOCATION	MICROORGANISM
Skin	*S epidermidis*
Nose	*S epidermidis*; colonized by *S aureus*
Oropharynx	Viridans group streptococci
Dental plaque	*S mutans*
Colon	*B fragilis* > *E coli*
Vagina	*Lactobacillus*, colonized by *E coli* and group B strep

Neonates delivered by C-section have no flora but are rapidly colonized after birth.

Bugs causing food poisoning

S aureus and *B cereus* food poisoning starts quickly and ends quickly.

MICROORGANISM	SOURCE OF INFECTION
B cereus	Reheated rice. "Food poisoning from reheated rice? **Be serious**!" (***B cereus***)
C botulinum	Improperly canned foods (toxins), raw honey (spores)
C perfringens	Reheated meat
E coli O157:H7	Undercooked meat
Salmonella	Poultry, meat, and eggs
S aureus	Meats, mayonnaise, custard; preformed toxin
V parahaemolyticus and *V vulnificus*[a]	Contaminated seafood

[a] *V vulnificus* can also cause wound infections from contact with contaminated water or shellfish.

Bugs causing diarrhea

Bloody diarrhea	
Campylobacter	Comma- or S-shaped organisms; growth at 42°C
E histolytica	Protozoan; amebic dysentery; liver abscess
Enterohemorrhagic *E coli*	O157:H7; can cause HUS; makes Shiga-like toxin
Enteroinvasive *E coli*	Invades colonic mucosa
Salmonella	Lactose ⊖; flagellar motility; has animal reservoir, especially poultry and eggs
Shigella	Lactose ⊖; very low ID_{50}; produces Shiga toxin (human reservoir only); bacillary dysentery
Y enterocolitica	Day care outbreaks, pseudoappendicitis
Watery diarrhea	
C difficile	Pseudomembranous colitis; caused by antibiotics; occasionally bloody diarrhea
C perfringens	Also causes gas gangrene
Enterotoxigenic *E coli*	Travelers' diarrhea; produces heat-labile (LT) and heat-stable (ST) toxins
Protozoa	*Giardia*, *Cryptosporidium*
V cholerae	Comma-shaped organisms; rice-water diarrhea; often from infected seafood
Viruses	Rotavirus, norovirus, adenovirus

Common causes of pneumonia

NEONATES (< 4 WK)	CHILDREN (4 WK–18 YR)	ADULTS (18–40 YR)	ADULTS (40–65 YR)	ELDERLY
Group B streptococci *E coli*	Viruses (**R**SV) ***M**ycoplasma* ***C** trachomatis* (infants–3 yr) ***C** pneumoniae* (school-aged children) ***S** pneumoniae* **R**unts **M**ay **C**ough **C**hunky **S**putum	*Mycoplasma* *C pneumoniae* *S pneumoniae* Viruses (eg, influenza)	*S pneumoniae* *H influenzae* Anaerobes Viruses *Mycoplasma*	*S pneumoniae* Influenza virus Anaerobes *H influenzae* Gram ⊖ rods

Special groups	
Alcoholic	*Klebsiella*, anaerobes (eg, *Peptostreptococcus*, *Fusobacterium*, *Prevotella*, *Bacteroides*)
IV drug users	*S pneumoniae*, *S aureus*
Aspiration	Anaerobes
Atypical	*Mycoplasma*, *Legionella*, *Chlamydia*
Cystic fibrosis	*Pseudomonas*, *S aureus*, *S pneumoniae*, *Burkholderia cepacia*
Immunocompromised	*S aureus*, enteric gram ⊖ rods, fungi, viruses, *P jirovecii* (with HIV)
Nosocomial (hospital acquired)	*S aureus*, *Pseudomonas*, other enteric gram ⊖ rods
Postviral	*S pneumoniae*, *S aureus*, *H influenzae*

Common causes of meningitis

NEWBORN (0–6 MO)	CHILDREN (6 MO–6 YR)	6–60 YR	60 YR +
Group B streptococci	*S pneumoniae*	*S pneumoniae*	*S pneumoniae*
E coli	*N meningitidis*	*N meningitidis* (#1 in teens)	Gram ⊖ rods
Listeria	*H influenzae* type B	Enteroviruses	*Listeria*
	Enteroviruses	HSV	

Give ceftriaxone and vancomycin empirically (add ampicillin if *Listeria* is suspected).
Viral causes of meningitis: enteroviruses (especially coxsackievirus), HSV-2 (HSV-1 = encephalitis), HIV, West Nile virus (also causes encephalitis), VZV.
In HIV: *Cryptococcus* spp.
Note: Incidence of *H influenzae* meningitis has ↓ greatly with introduction of the conjugate *H influenzae* vaccine in last 10–15 years. Today, cases are usually seen in unimmunized children.

CSF findings in meningitis

	OPENING PRESSURE	CELL TYPE	PROTEIN	SUGAR
Bacterial	↑	↑ PMNs	↑	↓
Fungal/TB	↑	↑ lymphocytes	↑	↓
Viral	Normal/↑	↑ lymphocytes	Normal/↑	Normal

Infections causing brain abscess

Most commonly viridans streptococci and *Staphylococcus aureus*. If dental infection or extraction precedes abscess, oral anaerobes commonly involved.
Multiple abscesses are usually from bacteremia; single lesions from contiguous sites: otitis media and mastoiditis → temporal lobe and cerebellum; sinusitis or dental infection → frontal lobe.
Toxoplasma reactivation in AIDS.

Osteomyelitis

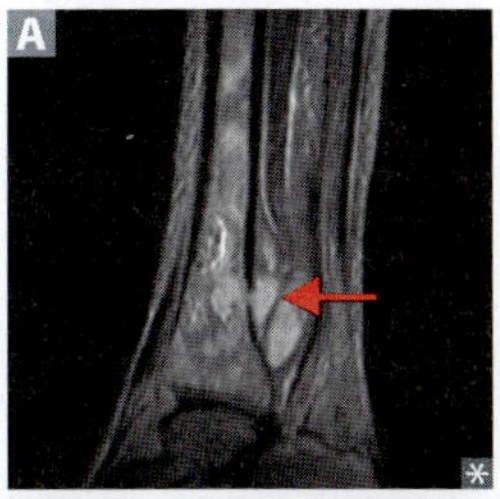

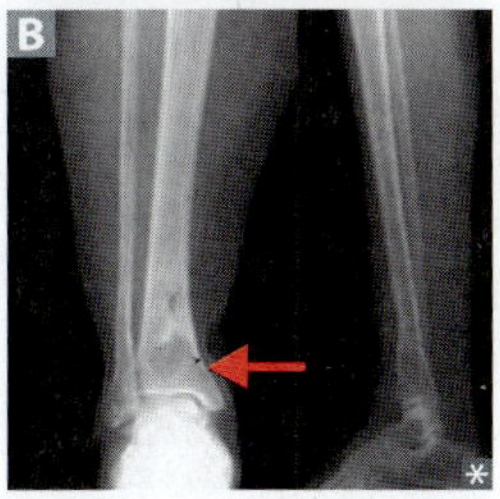

RISK FACTOR	ASSOCIATED INFECTION
Assume if no other information is available	*S aureus* (most common overall)
Sexually active	*Neisseria gonorrhoeae* (rare), septic arthritis more common
Sickle cell disease	*Salmonella* and *S aureus*
Prosthetic joint replacement	*S aureus* and *S epidermidis*
Vertebral involvement	*S aureus*, *Mycobacterium tuberculosis* (Pott disease)
Cat and dog bites	*Pasteurella multocida*
IV drug abuse	*Pseudomonas*, *Candida*, *S aureus* are most common

Elevated C-reactive protein (CRP) and erythrocyte sedimentation rate common but nonspecific.
MRI is best for detecting acute infection and detailing anatomic involvement A. Radiographs are insensitive early but can be useful in chronic osteomyelitis B.

Urinary tract infections

Cystitis presents with dysuria, frequency, urgency, suprapubic pain, and WBCs (but not WBC casts) in urine. Primarily caused by ascension of microbes from urethra to bladder. Males—infants with congenital defects, vesicoureteral reflux. Elderly—enlarged prostate. Ascension to kidney results in pyelonephritis, which presents with fever, chills, flank pain, costovertebral angle tenderness, hematuria, and WBC casts.

Ten times more common in women (shorter urethras colonized by fecal flora). Other predisposing factors: obstruction, kidney surgery, catheterization, GU malformation, diabetes, pregnancy.

UTI bugs

SPECIES	FEATURES	COMMENTS
Escherichia coli	Leading cause of UTI. Colonies show green metallic sheen on EMB agar.	Diagnostic markers: ⊕ Leukocyte esterase = evidence of WBC activity. ⊕ Nitrite test = reduction of urinary nitrates by bacterial species (eg, *E coli*). ⊕ Urease test = urease-producing bugs (eg, *Proteus*, *Klebsiella*).
Staphylococcus saprophyticus	2nd leading cause of UTI in sexually active women.	
Klebsiella pneumoniae	3rd leading cause of UTI. Large mucoid capsule and viscous colonies.	
Serratia marcescens	Some strains produce a red pigment; often nosocomial and drug resistant.	
Enterococcus	Often nosocomial and drug resistant.	
Proteus mirabilis	Motility causes "swarming" on agar; produces urease; associated with struvite stones.	
Pseudomonas aeruginosa	Blue-green pigment and fruity odor; usually nosocomial and drug resistant.	

Common vaginal infections

	Bacterial vaginosis	*Trichomonas* vaginitis	*Candida* vulvovaginitis
SIGNS AND SYMPTOMS	No inflammation Thin, white discharge A with fishy odor	Inflammation ("strawberry cervix") Frothy, yellow-green, foul-smelling discharge	Inflammation Thick, white, "cottage cheese" discharge C
LAB FINDINGS	Clue cells pH > 4.5	Motile trichomonads B pH > 4.5	Pseudohyphae pH normal (4.0–4.5)
TREATMENT	Metronidazole	Metronidazole Treat sexual partner(s)	-azoles

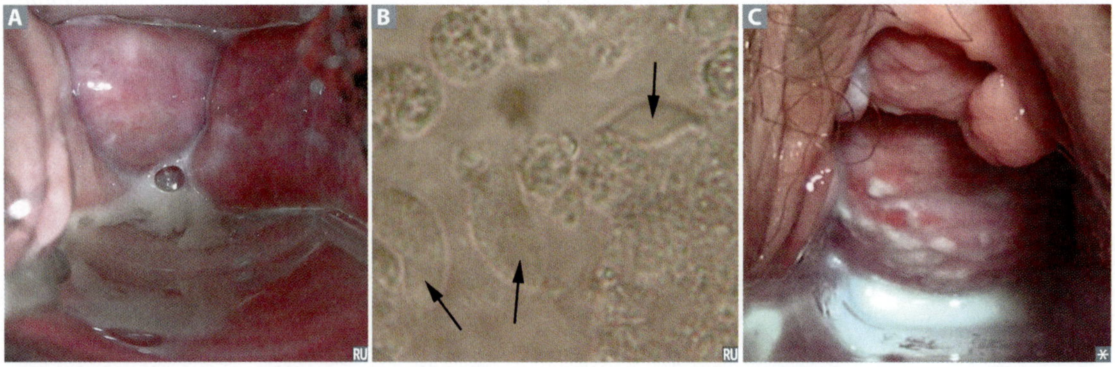

ToRCHeS infections

Microbes that may pass from mother to fetus. Transmission is transplacental in most cases, or via delivery (especially HSV-2). Nonspecific signs common to many **ToRCHeS** infections include hepatosplenomegaly, jaundice, thrombocytopenia, and growth retardation.

Other important infectious agents include *Streptococcus agalactiae* (group B streptococci), *E coli*, and *Listeria monocytogenes*—all causes of meningitis in neonates. Parvovirus B19 causes hydrops fetalis.

AGENT	MODES OF MATERNAL TRANSMISSION	MATERNAL MANIFESTATIONS	NEONATAL MANIFESTIONS
***To**xoplasma gondii* 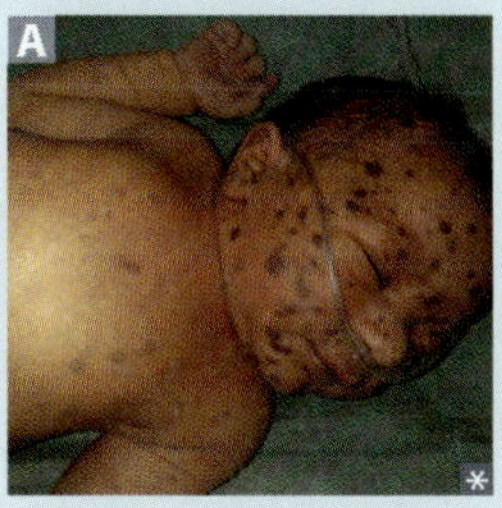	Cat feces or ingestion of undercooked meat	Usually asymptomatic; lymphadenopathy (rarely)	Classic triad: chorioretinitis, hydrocephalus, and intracranial calcifications, +/– "blueberry muffin" rash A.
Rubella	Respiratory droplets	Rash, lymphadenopathy, polyarthritis, polyarthralgia	Classic triad: abnormalities of eye (cataract) and ear (deafness) and congenital heart disease (PDA); ± "blueberry muffin" rash. "**I** (eye) ♥ **ruby** (**rub**ella) **ear**rings."
Cytomegalovirus 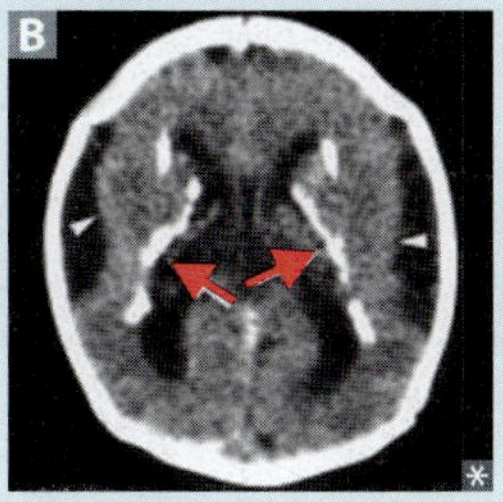	Sexual contact, organ transplants	Usually asymptomatic; mononucleosis-like illness	Hearing loss, seizures, petechial rash, "blueberry muffin" rash, periventricular calcifications B
HIV	Sexual contact, needlestick	Variable presentation depending on CD4+ cell count	Recurrent infections, chronic diarrhea
Herpes simplex virus-2	Skin or mucous membrane contact	Usually asymptomatic; herpetic (vesicular) lesions	Encephalitis, herpetic (vesicular) lesions
Syphilis	Sexual contact	Chancre (1°) and disseminated rash (2°) are the two stages likely to result in fetal infection	Often results in stillbirth, hydrops fetalis; if child survives, presents with facial abnormalities (eg, notched teeth, saddle nose, short maxilla), saber shins, CN VIII deafness

Red rashes of childhood

AGENT	ASSOCIATED SYNDROME/DISEASE	CLINICAL PRESENTATION
Coxsackievirus type A	Hand-foot-mouth disease	Oval-shaped vesicles on palms and soles A; vesicles and ulcers in oral mucosa
Human herpesvirus 6	Roseola (exanthem subitum)	Asymptomatic rose-colored macules appear on body after several days of high fever; can present with febrile seizures; usually affects infants
Measles virus	Measles (rubeola)	Beginning at head and moving down; rash is preceded by cough, coryza, conjunctivitis, and blue-white (Koplik) spots on buccal mucosa
Parvovirus B19	Erythema infectiosum (fifth disease)	"Slapped cheek" rash on face B (can cause hydrops fetalis in pregnant women)
Rubella virus	Rubella (German measles)	Pink coalescing macules begin at head and move down → fine desquamating truncal rash; postauricular lymphadenopathy
Streptococcus pyogenes	Scarlet fever	Erythematous, sandpaper-like rash C with fever and sore throat
Varicella-Zoster virus	Chickenpox	Vesicular rash begins on trunk; spreads to face and extremities with lesions of different stages

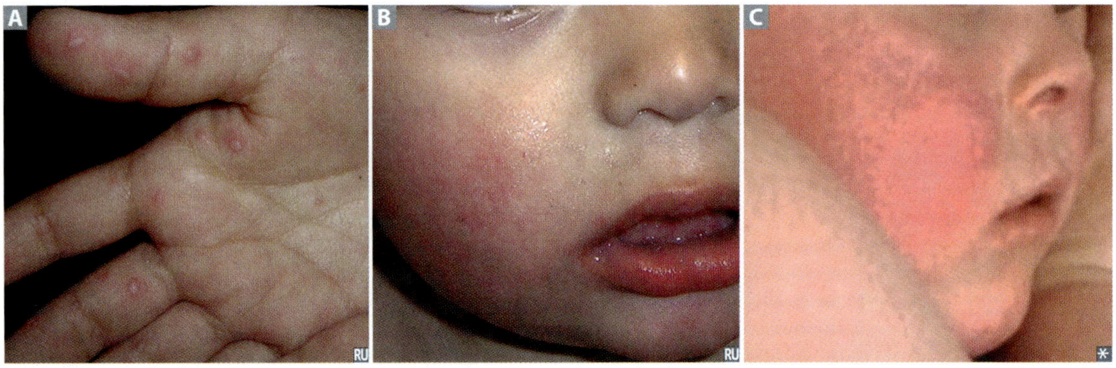

Sexually transmitted infections

DISEASE	CLINICAL FEATURES	ORGANISM
AIDS	Opportunistic infections, Kaposi sarcoma, lymphoma	HIV
Chancroid	Painful genital ulcer with exudate, inguinal adenopathy	*Haemophilus* ***ducreyi*** (it's so painful, you "**do cry**")
Chlamydia	Urethritis, cervicitis, epididymitis, conjunctivitis, reactive arthritis, PID	*Chlamydia trachomatis* (D–K)
Condylomata acuminata	Genital warts, koilocytes	HPV-6 and -11
Genital herpes	Painful penile, vulvar, or cervical vesicles and ulcers; can cause systemic symptoms such as fever, headache, myalgia	HSV-2, less commonly HSV-1
Gonorrhea	Urethritis, cervicitis, PID, prostatitis, epididymitis, arthritis, creamy purulent discharge	*Neisseria gonorrhoeae*
Hepatitis B	Jaundice	HBV
Lymphogranuloma venereum	Infection of lymphatics; painless genital ulcers, painful lymphadenopathy (ie, buboes)	*C trachomatis* (L1–L3)
Primary syphilis	Painless chancre	*Treponema pallidum*
Secondary syphilis	Fever, lymphadenopathy, skin rashes, condylomata lata	
Tertiary syphilis	Gummas, tabes dorsalis, general paresis, aortitis, Argyll Robertson pupil	
Trichomoniasis	Vaginitis, strawberry cervix, motile in wet prep	*Trichomonas vaginalis*

Pelvic inflammatory disease

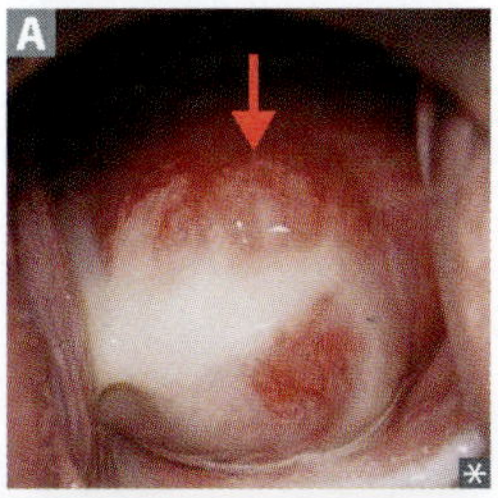

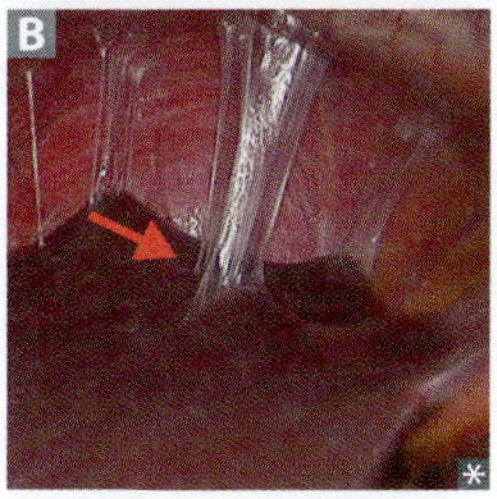

Top bugs—*Chlamydia trachomatis* (subacute, often undiagnosed), *Neisseria gonorrhoeae* (acute). *C trachomatis*—most common bacterial STI in the United States. Cervical motion tenderness (chandelier sign), purulent cervical discharge **A**. PID may include salpingitis, endometritis, hydrosalpinx, and tubo-ovarian abscess.

Salpingitis is a risk factor for ectopic pregnancy, infertility, chronic pelvic pain, and adhesions.
Can lead to **Fitz-Hugh–Curtis syndrome**—infection of the liver capsule and "violin string" adhesions of peritoneum to liver **B**.

Nosocomial infections *E coli* (UTI) and *S aureus* (wound infection) are the two most common causes.

RISK FACTOR	PATHOGEN	UNIQUE SIGNS/SYMPTOMS
Antibiotic use	*Clostridium difficile*	Watery diarrhea, leukocytosis
Aspiration (2° to altered mental status, old age)	Polymicrobial, gram ⊖ bacteria, often anaerobes	Right lower lobe infiltrate or right upper/middle lobe (patient recumbent); purulent malodorous sputum
Decubitus ulcers, surgical wounds, drains	*S aureus* (including MRSA), gram ⊖ anaerobes *(Bacteroides, Prevotella, Fusobacterium)*	Erythema, tenderness, induration, drainage from surgical wound sites
Intravascular catheters	*S aureus* (including MRSA), *S epidermidis* (long term), *Enterobacter*	Erythema, induration, tenderness, drainage from access sites
Mechanical ventilation, endotracheal intubation	Late onset: *P aeruginosa, Klebsiella, Acinetobacter, S aureus*	New infiltrate on CXR, ↑ sputum production; sweet odor *(Pseudomonas)*
Renal dialysis unit, needlestick	HBV	
Urinary catheterization	*E coli, Klebsiella, Proteus* spp.	Dysuria, leukocytosis, flank pain or costovertebral angle tenderness
Water aerosols	*Legionella*	Signs of pneumonia, GI symptoms (nausea, vomiting), neurologic abnormalities

Bugs affecting unvaccinated children

CLINICAL PRESENTATION	FINDINGS/LABS	PATHOGEN
Dermatologic		
Rash	Beginning at head and moving down with postauricular lymphadenopathy	Rubella virus
	Beginning at head and moving down; rash preceded by cough, coryza, conjunctivitis, and blue-white (Koplik) spots on buccal mucosa	Measles virus
Neurologic		
Meningitis	Microbe colonizes nasopharynx	*H influenzae* type B
	Can also lead to myalgia and paralysis	Poliovirus
Respiratory		
Epiglottitis	Fever with dysphagia, drooling, and difficulty breathing due to edematous "cherry red" epiglottis; "thumbprint sign" on x-ray	*H influenzae* type B (also capable of causing epiglottitis in fully immunized children)
Pharyngitis	Grayish oropharyngeal exudate ("pseudomembranes" may obstruct airway); painful throat	*Corynebacterium diphtheriae* (elaborates toxin that causes necrosis in pharynx, cardiac, and CNS tissue)

Bug hints (if all else fails)

CHARACTERISTIC	ORGANISM
Asplenic patient (due to surgical splenectomy or autosplenectomy, eg, chronic sickle cell disease)	Encapsulated microbes, especially **SHiN** (**S** *pneumoniae* >> **H** *influenzae* type B > **N** *meningitidis*)
Branching rods in oral infection, sulfur granules	*Actinomyces israelii*
Chronic granulomatous disease	Catalase ⊕ microbes, especially *S aureus*
"Currant jelly" sputum	*Klebsiella*
Dog or cat bite	*Pasteurella multocida*
Facial nerve palsy	*Borrelia burgdorferi* (Lyme disease)
Fungal infection in diabetic or immunocompromised patient	*Mucor* or *Rhizopus* spp.
Health care provider	HBV (from needlestick)
Neutropenic patients	*Candida albicans* (systemic), *Aspergillus*
Organ transplant recipient	CMV
PAS ⊕	*Tropheryma whipplei* (Whipple disease)
Pediatric infection	*Haemophilus influenzae* (including epiglottitis)
Pneumonia in cystic fibrosis, burn infection	*Pseudomonas aeruginosa*
Pus, empyema, abscess	*S aureus*
Rash on hands and feet	Coxsackie A virus, *Treponema pallidum*, *Rickettsia rickettsii*
Sepsis/meningitis in newborn	Group B strep
Surgical wound	*S aureus*
Traumatic open wound	*Clostridium perfringens*

▶ MICROBIOLOGY—ANTIMICROBIALS

Antimicrobial therapy

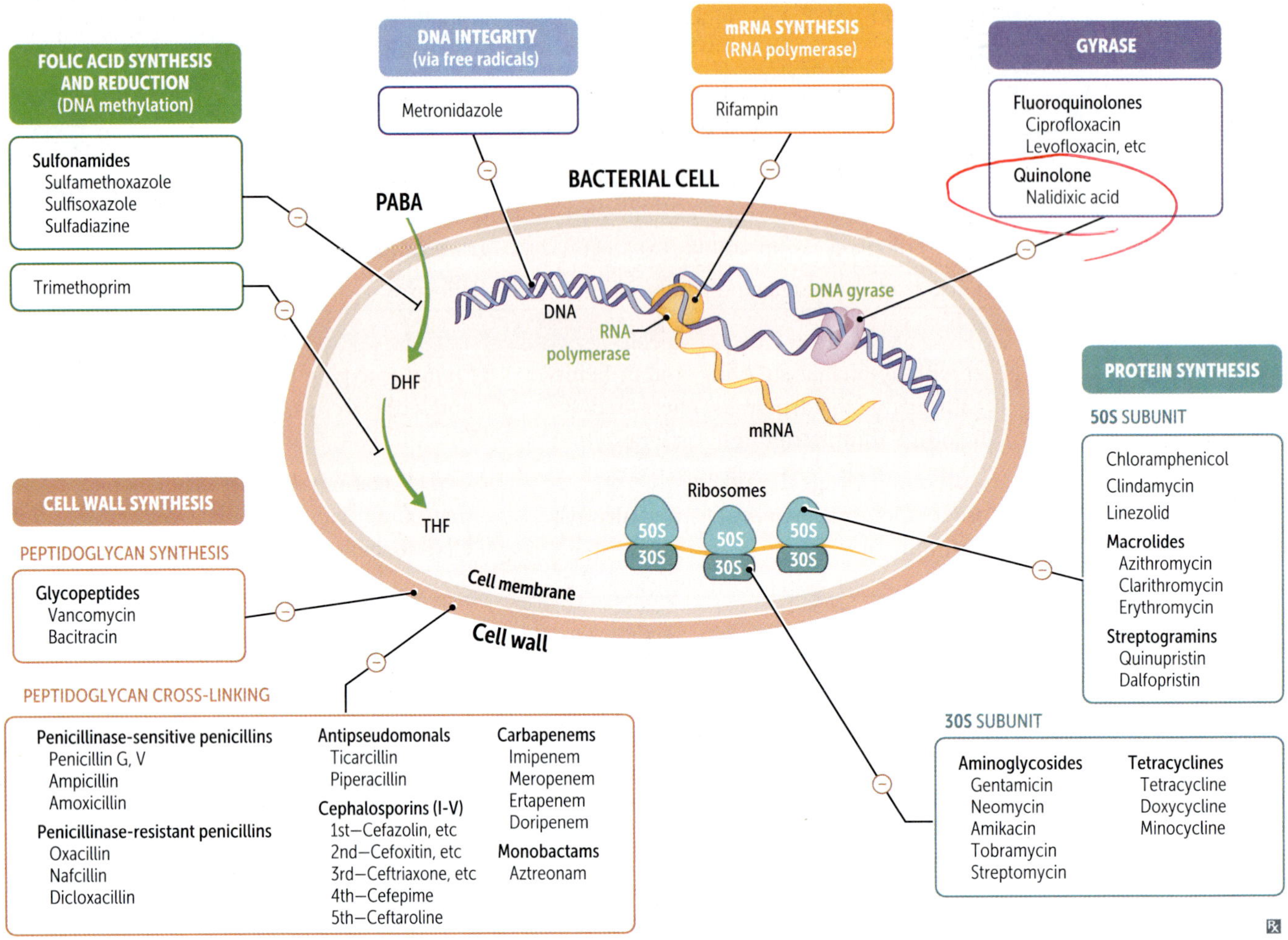

Penicillin G, V	Penicillin G (IV and IM form), penicillin V (oral). Prototype β-lactam antibiotics.
MECHANISM	D-Ala-D-Ala structural analog. Bind penicillin-binding proteins (transpeptidases). Block transpeptidase cross-linking of peptidoglycan in cell wall. Activate autolytic enzymes.
CLINICAL USE	Mostly used for gram ⊕ organisms (*S pneumoniae*, *S pyogenes*, *Actinomyces*). Also used for gram ⊖ cocci (mainly *N meningitidis*) and spirochetes (namely *T pallidum*). Bactericidal for gram ⊕ cocci, gram ⊕ rods, gram ⊖ cocci, and spirochetes. Penicillinase sensitive.
ADVERSE EFFECTS	Hypersensitivity reactions, direct Coombs ⊕ hemolytic anemia.
RESISTANCE	Penicillinase in bacteria (a type of β-lactamase) cleaves β-lactam ring.

Penicillinase-sensitive penicillins	Amoxicillin, ampicillin; aminopenicillins.	
MECHANISM	Same as penicillin. Wider spectrum; penicillinase sensitive. Also combine with clavulanic acid to protect against destruction by β-lactamase.	AMinoPenicillins are AMPed-up penicillin. AmOxicillin has greater Oral bioavailability than ampicillin.
CLINICAL USE	Extended-spectrum penicillin—*H influenzae*, *H pylori*, *E coli*, *Listeria monocytogenes*, *Proteus mirabilis*, *Salmonella*, *Shigella*, enterococci.	Coverage: ampicillin/amoxicillin HHELPSS kill enterococci.
ADVERSE EFFECTS	Hypersensitivity reactions; rash; pseudomembranous colitis.	
MECHANISM OF RESISTANCE	Penicillinase in bacteria (a type of β-lactamase) cleaves β-lactam ring.	

Penicillinase-resistant penicillins	Dicloxacillin, nafcillin, oxacillin.	
MECHANISM	Same as penicillin. Narrow spectrum; penicillinase resistant because bulky R group blocks access of β-lactamase to β-lactam ring.	
CLINICAL USE	*S aureus* (except MRSA; resistant because of altered penicillin-binding protein target site).	"Use naf (nafcillin) for staph."
ADVERSE EFFECTS	Hypersensitivity reactions, interstitial nephritis.	

Antipseudomonal penicillins	Piperacillin, ticarcillin.
MECHANISM	Same as penicillin. Extended spectrum.
CLINICAL USE	*Pseudomonas* spp. and gram ⊖ rods; susceptible to penicillinase; use with β-lactamase inhibitors.
ADVERSE EFFECTS	Hypersensitivity reactions.

β-lactamase inhibitors	Include Clavulanic Acid, Sulbactam, Tazobactam. Often added to penicillin antibiotics to protect the antibiotic from destruction by β-lactamase (penicillinase).	CAST.

Cephalosporins (generations I–V)

MECHANISM	β-lactam drugs that inhibit cell wall synthesis but are less susceptible to penicillinases. Bactericidal.	Organisms typically not covered by 1st–4th generation cephalosporins are **LAME**: ***L**isteria*, **A**typicals (*Chlamydia*, *Mycoplasma*), **M**RSA, and **E**nterococci. Exception: ceftaroline (5th generation cephalosporin) covers MRSA.
CLINICAL USE	1st generation (cefazolin, cephalexin)—gram ⊕ cocci, ***P**roteus mirabilis*, ***E** coli*, ***K**lebsiella pneumoniae*. Cefazolin used prior to surgery to prevent *S aureus* wound infections.	1st generation—**PEcK**.
	2nd generation (ce**fa**clor, ce**fox**itin, ce**fur**oxime)—gram ⊕ cocci, ***H** influenzae*, ***E**nterobacter aerogenes*, ***N**eisseria* spp., ***S**erratia marcescens*, ***P**roteus mirabilis*, ***E** coli*, ***K**lebsiella pneumoniae*.	**Fa**ke **fox fur**. 2nd generation—**HENS PEcK**.
	3rd generation (ceftriaxone, cefotaxime, ceftazidime)—serious gram ⊖ infections resistant to other β-lactams.	Ceftriaxone—meningitis, gonorrhea, disseminated Lyme disease. Ceftazidime—*Pseudomonas*.
	4th generation (cefepime)—gram ⊖ organisms, with ↑ activity against *Pseudomonas* and gram ⊕ organisms.	
	5th generation (ceftaroline)—broad gram ⊕ and gram ⊖ organism coverage, including MRSA; does not cover *Pseudomonas*.	
ADVERSE EFFECTS	Hypersensitivity reactions, autoimmune hemolytic anemia, disulfiram-like reaction, vitamin K deficiency. Exhibit cross-reactivity with penicillins. ↑ nephrotoxicity of aminoglycosides.	
MECHANISM OF RESISTANCE	Structural change in penicillin-binding proteins (transpeptidases).	

Carbapenems	Imipenem, meropenem, ertapenem, doripenem.	
MECHANISM	Imipenem is a broad-spectrum, β-lactamase–resistant carbapenem. Always administered with cilastatin (inhibitor of renal dehydropeptidase I) to ↓ inactivation of drug in renal tubules.	With imipenem, "the kill is **lastin'** with ci**lastatin**." Newer carbapenems include ertapenem (limited *Pseudomonas* coverage) and doripenem.
CLINICAL USE	Gram ⊕ cocci, gram ⊖ rods, and anaerobes. Wide spectrum, but significant side effects limit use to life-threatening infections or after other drugs have failed. Meropenem has a ↓ risk of seizures and is stable to dehydropeptidase I.	
ADVERSE EFFECTS	GI distress, skin rash, and CNS toxicity (seizures) at high plasma levels.	

Monobactams	Aztreonam
MECHANISM	Less susceptible to β-lactamases. Prevents peptidoglycan cross-linking by binding to penicillin-binding protein 3. Synergistic with aminoglycosides. No cross-allergenicity with penicillins.
CLINICAL USE	Gram ⊖ rods only—no activity against gram ⊕ rods or anaerobes. For penicillin-allergic patients and those with renal insufficiency who cannot tolerate aminoglycosides.
ADVERSE EFFECTS	Usually nontoxic; occasional GI upset.

Vancomycin	
MECHANISM	Inhibits cell wall peptidoglycan formation by binding D-ala D-ala portion of cell wall precursors. Bactericidal against most bacteria (bacteriostatic against *C difficile*). Not susceptible to β-lactamases.
CLINICAL USE	Gram ⊕ bugs only—serious, multidrug-resistant organisms, including MRSA, *S epidermidis*, sensitive *Enterococcus* species, and *Clostridium difficile* (oral dose for pseudomembranous colitis).
ADVERSE EFFECTS 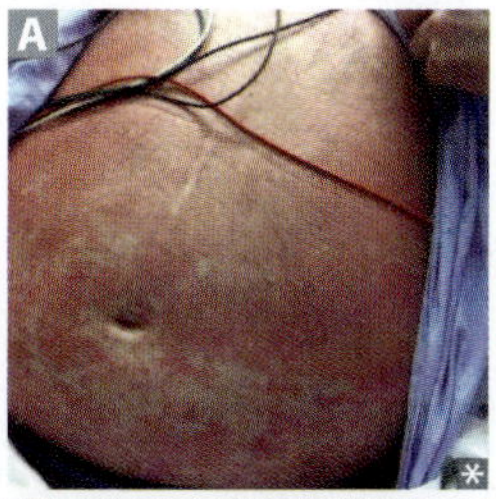	Well tolerated in general—but **NOT** trouble free. **N**ephrotoxicity, **O**totoxicity, **T**hrombophlebitis, diffuse flushing—red man syndrome A (can largely prevent by pretreatment with antihistamines and slow infusion rate).
MECHANISM OF RESISTANCE	Occurs in bacteria via amino acid modification of **D-ala D-ala** to D-ala D-lac. "Pay back **2 D-ala**s (dollars) for **van**dalizing (**van**comycin)."

Protein synthesis inhibitors

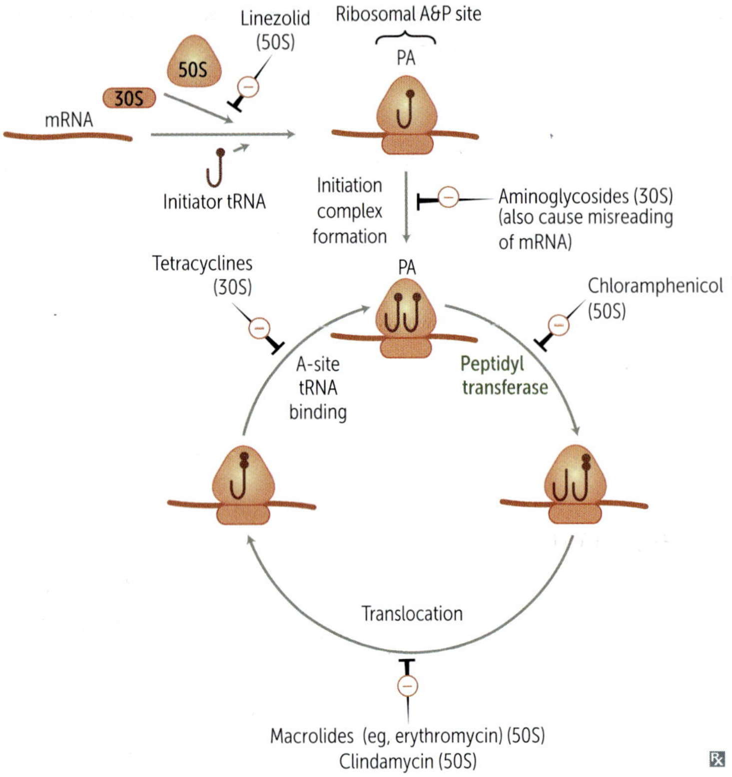

Specifically target smaller bacterial ribosome (70S, made of 30S and 50S subunits), leaving human ribosome (80S) unaffected.

30S inhibitors

A = Aminoglycosides [bactericidal]
T = Tetracyclines [bacteriostatic]

50S inhibitors

C = Chloramphenicol, Clindamycin [bacteriostatic]
E = Erythromycin (macrolides) [bacteriostatic]
L = Linezolid [variable]
"Buy AT 30, CCEL (sell) at 50."

Aminoglycosides	Gentamicin, Neomycin, Amikacin, Tobramycin, Streptomycin.	"Mean" (aminoglycoside) GNATS caNNOT kill anaerobes.
MECHANISM	Bactericidal; irreversible inhibition of initiation complex through binding of the 30S subunit. Can cause misreading of mRNA. Also block translocation. Require O_2 for uptake; therefore ineffective against anaerobes.	
CLINICAL USE	Severe gram ⊖ rod infections. Synergistic with β-lactam antibiotics. Neomycin for bowel surgery.	
ADVERSE EFFECTS	Nephrotoxicity, Neuromuscular blockade, Ototoxicity (especially when used with loop diuretics). Teratogen.	
MECHANISM OF RESISTANCE	Bacterial transferase enzymes inactivate the drug by acetylation, phosphorylation, or adenylation.	

Tetracyclines	Tetracycline, doxycycline, minocycline.
MECHANISM	Bacteriostatic; bind to 30S and prevent attachment of aminoacyl-tRNA; limited CNS penetration. Doxycycline is fecally eliminated and can be used in patients with renal failure. Do not take tetracyclines with milk (Ca^{2+}), antacids (Ca^{2+} or Mg^{2+}), or iron-containing preparations because divalent cations inhibit drugs' absorption in the gut.
CLINICAL USE	*Borrelia burgdorferi*, *M pneumoniae*. Drugs' ability to accumulate intracellularly makes them very effective against *Rickettsia* and *Chlamydia*. Also used to treat acne.
ADVERSE EFFECTS	GI distress, discoloration of teeth and inhibition of bone growth in children, photosensitivity. Contraindicated in pregnancy.
MECHANISM OF RESISTANCE	↓ uptake or ↑ efflux out of bacterial cells by plasmid-encoded transport pumps.

Chloramphenicol	
MECHANISM	Blocks peptidyltransferase at 50S ribosomal subunit. Bacteriostatic.
CLINICAL USE	Meningitis (*Haemophilus influenzae*, *Neisseria meningitidis*, *Streptococcus pneumoniae*) and Rocky Mountain spotted fever (*Rickettsia rickettsii*). Limited use owing to toxicities but often still used in developing countries because of low cost.
ADVERSE EFFECTS	Anemia (dose dependent), aplastic anemia (dose independent), gray baby syndrome (in premature infants because they lack liver UDP-glucuronyl transferase).
MECHANISM OF RESISTANCE	Plasmid-encoded acetyltransferase inactivates the drug.

Clindamycin		
MECHANISM	Blocks peptide transfer (translocation) at 50S ribosomal subunit. Bacteriostatic.	
CLINICAL USE	Anaerobic infections (eg, *Bacteroides* spp., *Clostridium perfringens*) in aspiration pneumonia, lung abscesses, and oral infections. Also effective against invasive group A streptococcal infection.	Treats anaerobic infections **above** the diaphragm vs metronidazole (anaerobic infections **below** diaphragm).
ADVERSE EFFECTS	Pseudomembranous colitis (*C difficile* overgrowth), fever, diarrhea.	

Oxazolidinones	Linezolid.
MECHANISM	Inhibit protein synthesis by binding to 50S subunit and preventing formation of the initiation complex.
CLINICAL USE	Gram ⊕ species including MRSA and VRE.
ADVERSE EFFECTS	Bone marrow suppression (especially thrombocytopenia), peripheral neuropathy, serotonin syndrome.
MECHANISM OF RESISTANCE	Point mutation of ribosomal RNA.

Macrolides	Azithromycin, clarithromycin, erythromycin.
MECHANISM	Inhibit protein synthesis by blocking translocation ("macro**slides**"); bind to the 23S rRNA of the 50S ribosomal subunit. Bacteriostatic.
CLINICAL USE	Atypical pneumonias (*Mycoplasma*, *Chlamydia*, *Legionella*), STIs (*Chlamydia*), gram ⊕ cocci (streptococcal infections in patients allergic to penicillin), and *B pertussis*.
ADVERSE EFFECTS	**MACRO**: Gastrointestinal **M**otility issues, **A**rrhythmia caused by prolonged QT interval, acute **C**holestatic hepatitis, **R**ash, e**O**sinophilia. Increases serum concentration of theophylline, oral anticoagulants. Clarithromycin and erythromycin inhibit cytochrome P-450.
MECHANISM OF RESISTANCE	Methylation of 23S rRNA-binding site prevents binding of drug.

Sulfonamides	Sulfamethoxazole (SMX), sulfisoxazole, sulfadiazine.
MECHANISM	Inhibit dihydropteroate synthase, thus inhibiting folate synthesis. Bacteriostatic (bactericidal when combined with trimethoprim).
CLINICAL USE	Gram-⊕, gram ⊖, *Nocardia*, *Chlamydia*. SMX for simple UTI.
ADVERSE EFFECTS	Hypersensitivity reactions, hemolysis if G6PD deficient, nephrotoxicity (tubulointerstitial nephritis), photosensitivity, kernicterus in infants, displace other drugs from albumin (eg, warfarin).
MECHANISM OF RESISTANCE	Altered enzyme (bacterial dihydropteroate synthase), ↓ uptake, or ↑ PABA synthesis.

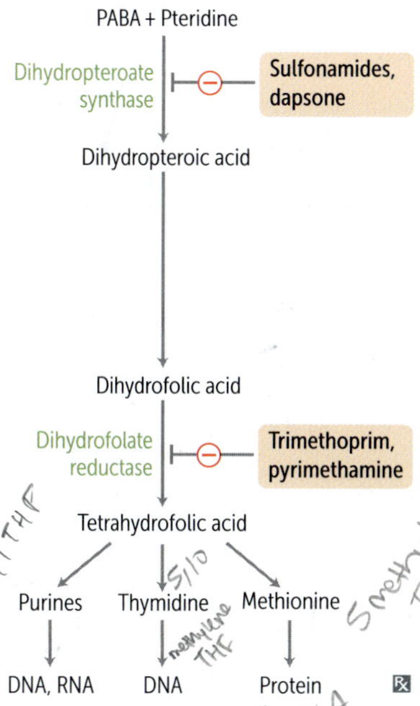

Dapsone	
MECHANISM	Similar to sulfonamides, but structurally distinct agent.
CLINICAL USE	Leprosy (lepromatous and tuberculoid), *Pneumocystis jirovecii* prophylaxis.
ADVERSE EFFECTS	Hemolysis if G6PD deficient.

Trimethoprim	
MECHANISM	Inhibits bacterial dihydrofolate reductase. Bacteriostatic.
CLINICAL USE	Used in combination with sulfonamides (trimethoprim-sulfamethoxazole [TMP-SMX]), causing sequential block of folate synthesis. Combination used for UTIs, *Shigella*, *Salmonella*, *Pneumocystis jirovecii* pneumonia treatment and prophylaxis, toxoplasmosis prophylaxis.
ADVERSE EFFECTS	Megaloblastic anemia, leukopenia, granulocytopenia. (May alleviate with supplemental folinic acid). **TMP T**reats **M**arrow **P**oorly.

Fluoroquinolones

Ciprofloxacin, norfloxacin, levofloxacin, ofloxacin, moxifloxacin, gemifloxacin, enoxacin.

MECHANISM	Inhibit prokaryotic enzymes topoisomerase II (DNA gyrase) and topoisomerase IV. Bactericidal. Must not be taken with antacids.	
CLINICAL USE	Gram ⊖ rods of urinary and GI tracts (including *Pseudomonas*), *Neisseria*, some gram ⊕ organisms.	
ADVERSE EFFECTS	GI upset, superinfections, skin rashes, headache, dizziness. Less commonly, can cause leg cramps and myalgias. Contraindicated in pregnant women, nursing mothers, and children < 18 years old due to possible damage to cartilage. Some may prolong QT interval. May cause tendonitis or tendon rupture in people > 60 years old and in patients taking prednisone.	Fluoroquinolones hurt attachments to your bones.
MECHANISM OF RESISTANCE	Chromosome-encoded mutation in DNA gyrase, plasmid-mediated resistance, efflux pumps.	

Daptomycin

MECHANISM	Lipopeptide that disrupts cell membrane of gram ⊕ cocci.	
CLINICAL USE	*S aureus* skin infections (especially MRSA), bacteremia, endocarditis, VRE.	Not used for pneumonia (avidly binds to and is inactivated by surfactant).
ADVERSE EFFECTS	Myopathy, rhabdomyolysis.	

Metronidazole

MECHANISM	Forms toxic free radical metabolites in the bacterial cell that damage DNA. Bactericidal, antiprotozoal.	
CLINICAL USE	Treats *Giardia*, *Entamoeba*, *Trichomonas*, *Gardnerella vaginalis*, Anaerobes (*Bacteroides*, *C difficile*). Used with a proton pump inhibitor and clarithromycin for "triple therapy" against *H Pylori*.	GET GAP on the Metro with metronidazole! Treats anaerobic infection **below** the diaphragm vs clindamycin (anaerobic infections **above** diaphragm).
ADVERSE EFFECTS	Disulfiram-like reaction (severe flushing, tachycardia, hypotension) with alcohol; headache, metallic taste.	

Antimycobacterial drugs

BACTERIUM	PROPHYLAXIS	TREATMENT
M tuberculosis	Isoniazid	**R**ifampin, **I**soniazid, **P**yrazinamide, **E**thambutol (**RIPE** for treatment)
M avium–intracellulare	Azithromycin, rifabutin	More drug resistant than *M tuberculosis*. Azithromycin or clarithromycin + ethambutol. Can add rifabutin or ciprofloxacin.
M leprae	N/A	Long-term treatment with dapsone and rifampin for tuberculoid form. Add clofazimine for lepromatous form.

MYCOBACTERIAL CELL

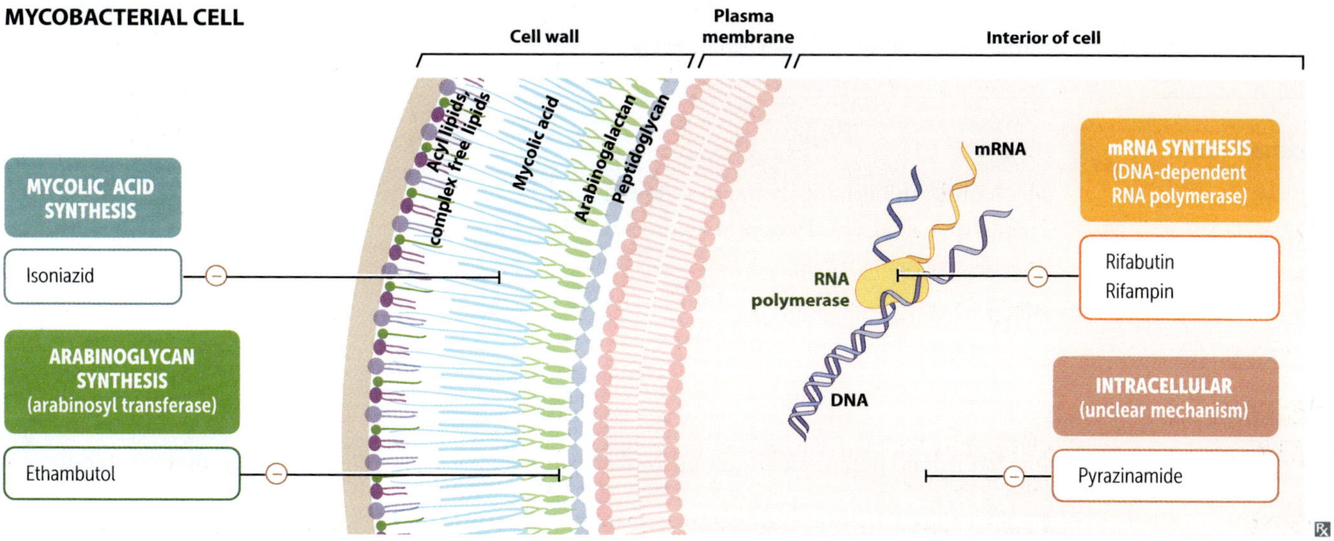

Rifamycins

Rifampin, rifabutin.

MECHANISM	Inhibit DNA-dependent RNA polymerase.	Rifampin's **4 R's**: **R**NA polymerase inhibitor; **R**amps up microsomal cytochrome P-450; **R**ed/orange body fluids; **R**apid resistance if used alone. Rifampin **ramp**s up cytochrome P-450, **but** rifa**but**in does not.
CLINICAL USE	*Mycobacterium tuberculosis*; delay resistance to dapsone when used for leprosy. Used for meningococcal prophylaxis and chemoprophylaxis in contacts of children with *Haemophilus influenzae* type B.	
ADVERSE EFFECTS	Minor hepatotoxicity and drug interactions (↑ cytochrome P-450); orange body fluids (nonhazardous side effect). Rifabutin favored over rifampin in patients with HIV infection due to less cytochrome P-450 stimulation.	
MECHANISM OF RESISTANCE	Mutations reduce drug binding to RNA polymerase. Monotherapy rapidly leads to resistance.	

Isoniazid

MECHANISM	↓ synthesis of mycolic acids. Bacterial catalase-peroxidase (encoded by KatG) needed to convert INH to active metabolite.	
CLINICAL USE	*Mycobacterium tuberculosis.* The only agent used as solo prophylaxis against TB. Also used as monotherapy for latent TB.	Different INH half-lives in fast vs slow acetylators.
ADVERSE EFFECTS	Hepatotoxicity, P-450 inhibition, drug-induced SLE, vitamin B_6 deficiency (peripheral neuropathy, sideroblastic anemia). Administer with pyridoxine (B_6).	**INH I**njures **N**eurons and **H**epatocytes.
MECHANISM OF RESISTANCE	Mutations leading to underexpression of KatG.	

Pyrazinamide

MECHANISM	Mechanism uncertain. Pyrazinamide is a prodrug that is converted to the active compound pyrazinoic acid. Works best at acidic pH (eg, in host phagolysosomes).
CLINICAL USE	*Mycobacterium tuberculosis.*
ADVERSE EFFECTS	Hyperuricemia, hepatotoxicity.

Ethambutol

MECHANISM	↓ carbohydrate polymerization of mycobacterium cell wall by blocking arabinosyltransferase.
CLINICAL USE	*Mycobacterium tuberculosis.*
ADVERSE EFFECTS	**Optic** neuropathy (red-green color blindness). Pronounce "**eye**thambutol."

Streptomycin

MECHANISM	Interferes with 30S component of ribosome.
CLINICAL USE	*Mycobacterium tuberculosis* (2nd line).
ADVERSE EFFECTS	Tinnitus, vertigo, ataxia, nephrotoxicity.

Antimicrobial prophylaxis

CLINICAL SCENARIO	MEDICATION
High risk for endocarditis and undergoing surgical or dental procedures	Amoxicillin
Exposure to gonorrhea	Ceftriaxone
History of recurrent UTIs	TMP-SMX
Exposure to meningococcal infection	Ceftriaxone, ciprofloxacin, or rifampin
Pregnant woman carrying group B strep	Intrapartum penicillin G or ampicillin
Prevention of gonococcal conjunctivitis in newborn	Erythromycin ointment on eyes
Prevention of postsurgical infection due to *S aureus*	Cefazolin
Prophylaxis of strep pharyngitis in child with prior rheumatic fever	Benzathine penicillin G or oral penicillin V
Exposure to syphilis	Benzathine penicillin G

Prophylaxis in HIV patients

CELL COUNT	PROPHYLAXIS	INFECTION
CD4 < 200 cells/mm^3	TMP-SMX	*Pneumocystis* pneumonia
CD4 < 100 cells/mm^3	TMP-SMX	*Pneumocystis* pneumonia and toxoplasmosis
CD4 < 50 cells/mm^3	Azithromycin or clarithromycin	*Mycobacterium avium* complex

Treatment of highly resistant bacteria

MRSA: vancomycin, daptomycin, linezolid, tigecycline, ceftaroline.
VRE: linezolid and streptogramins (quinupristin, dalfopristin).
Multidrug-resistant *P aeruginosa*, multidrug-resistant *Acinetobacter baumannii:* polymyxins B and E (colistin).

Antifungal therapy

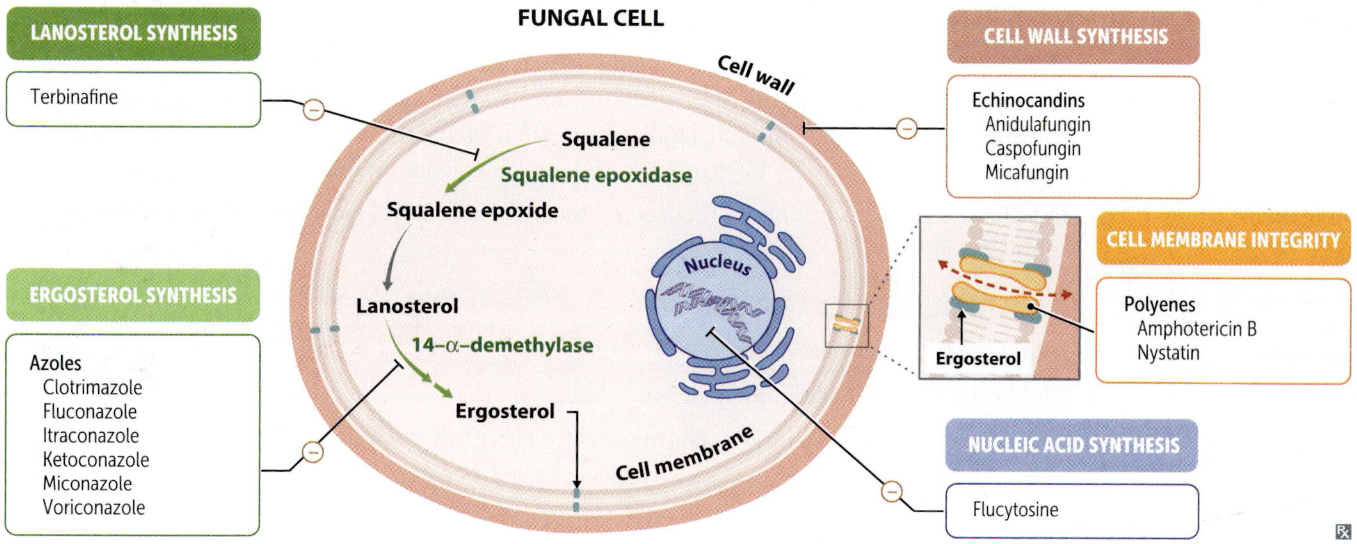

Amphotericin B

MECHANISM	Binds ergosterol (unique to fungi); forms membrane pores that allow leakage of electrolytes.	Amphotericin "**tear**s" holes in the fungal membrane by forming pores.
CLINICAL USE	Serious, systemic mycoses. *Cryptococcus* (amphotericin B with/without flucytosine for cryptococcal meningitis), *Blastomyces*, *Coccidioides*, *Histoplasma*, *Candida*, *Mucor*. Intrathecally for fungal meningitis. Supplement K^+ and Mg^{2+} because of altered renal tubule permeability.	
ADVERSE EFFECTS	Fever/chills ("shake and bake"), hypotension, nephrotoxicity, arrhythmias, anemia, IV phlebitis ("**amphoterri**ble"). Hydration ↓ nephrotoxicity. Liposomal amphotericin ↓ toxicity.	

Nystatin

MECHANISM	Same as amphotericin B. Topical use only as too toxic for systemic use.
CLINICAL USE	"Swish and swallow" for oral candidiasis (thrush); topical for diaper rash or vaginal candidiasis.

Flucytosine

MECHANISM	Inhibits DNA and RNA biosynthesis by conversion to 5-fluorouracil by cytosine deaminase.
CLINICAL USE	Systemic fungal infections (especially meningitis caused by *Cryptococcus*) in combination with amphotericin B.
ADVERSE EFFECTS	Bone marrow suppression.

Azoles

Clotrimazole, fluconazole, itraconazole, ketoconazole, miconazole, voriconazole.

MECHANISM	Inhibit fungal sterol (ergosterol) synthesis by inhibiting the cytochrome P-450 enzyme that converts lanosterol to ergosterol.
CLINICAL USE	Local and less serious systemic mycoses. Fluconazole for chronic suppression of cryptococcal meningitis in AIDS patients and candidal infections of all types. Itraconazole for *Blastomyces*, *Coccidioides*, *Histoplasma*. Clotrimazole and miconazole for topical fungal infections.
ADVERSE EFFECTS	Testosterone synthesis inhibition (gynecomastia, especially with ketoconazole), liver dysfunction (inhibits cytochrome P-450).

Terbinafine

MECHANISM	Inhibits the fungal enzyme squalene epoxidase.
CLINICAL USE	Dermatophytoses (especially onychomycosis—fungal infection of finger or toe nails).
ADVERSE EFFECTS	GI upset, headaches, hepatotoxicity, taste disturbance.

Echinocandins	Anidulafungin, caspofungin, micafungin.
MECHANISM	Inhibit cell wall synthesis by inhibiting synthesis of β-glucan.
CLINICAL USE	Invasive aspergillosis, *Candida*.
ADVERSE EFFECTS	GI upset, flushing (by histamine release).

Griseofulvin	
MECHANISM	Interferes with microtubule function; disrupts mitosis. Deposits in keratin-containing tissues (eg, nails).
CLINICAL USE	Oral treatment of superficial infections; inhibits growth of dermatophytes (tinea, ringworm).
ADVERSE EFFECTS	Teratogenic, carcinogenic, confusion, headaches, ↑ cytochrome P-450 and warfarin metabolism.

Antiprotozoan therapy

Pyrimethamine (toxoplasmosis), suramin and melarsoprol (*Trypanosoma brucei*), nifurtimox (*T cruzi*), sodium stibogluconate (leishmaniasis).

Anti-mite/louse therapy

Permethrin (blocks Na^+ channels → neurotoxicity), malathion (acetylcholinesterase inhibitor), lindane (blocks GABA channels → neurotoxicity). Used to treat scabies (*Sarcoptes scabiei*) and lice (*Pediculus* and *Pthirus*).

Treat **PML** (**P**esty **M**ites and **L**ice) with **PML** (**P**ermethrin, **M**alathion, **L**indane), because they **NAG** you (**N**a, **A**ChE, **G**ABA blockade).

Chloroquine	
MECHANISM	Blocks detoxification of heme into hemozoin. Heme accumulates and is toxic to plasmodia.
CLINICAL USE	Treatment of plasmodial species other than *P falciparum* (frequency of resistance in *P falciparum* is too high). Resistance due to membrane pump that ↓ intracellular concentration of drug. Treat *P falciparum* with artemether/lumefantrine or atovaquone/proguanil. For life-threatening malaria, use quinidine in US (quinine elsewhere) or artesunate.
ADVERSE EFFECTS	Retinopathy; pruritus (especially in dark-skinned individuals).

Antihelminthic therapy

Mebendazole (microtubule inhibitor), pyrantel pamoate, ivermectin, diethylcarbamazine, praziquantel.

Antiviral therapy

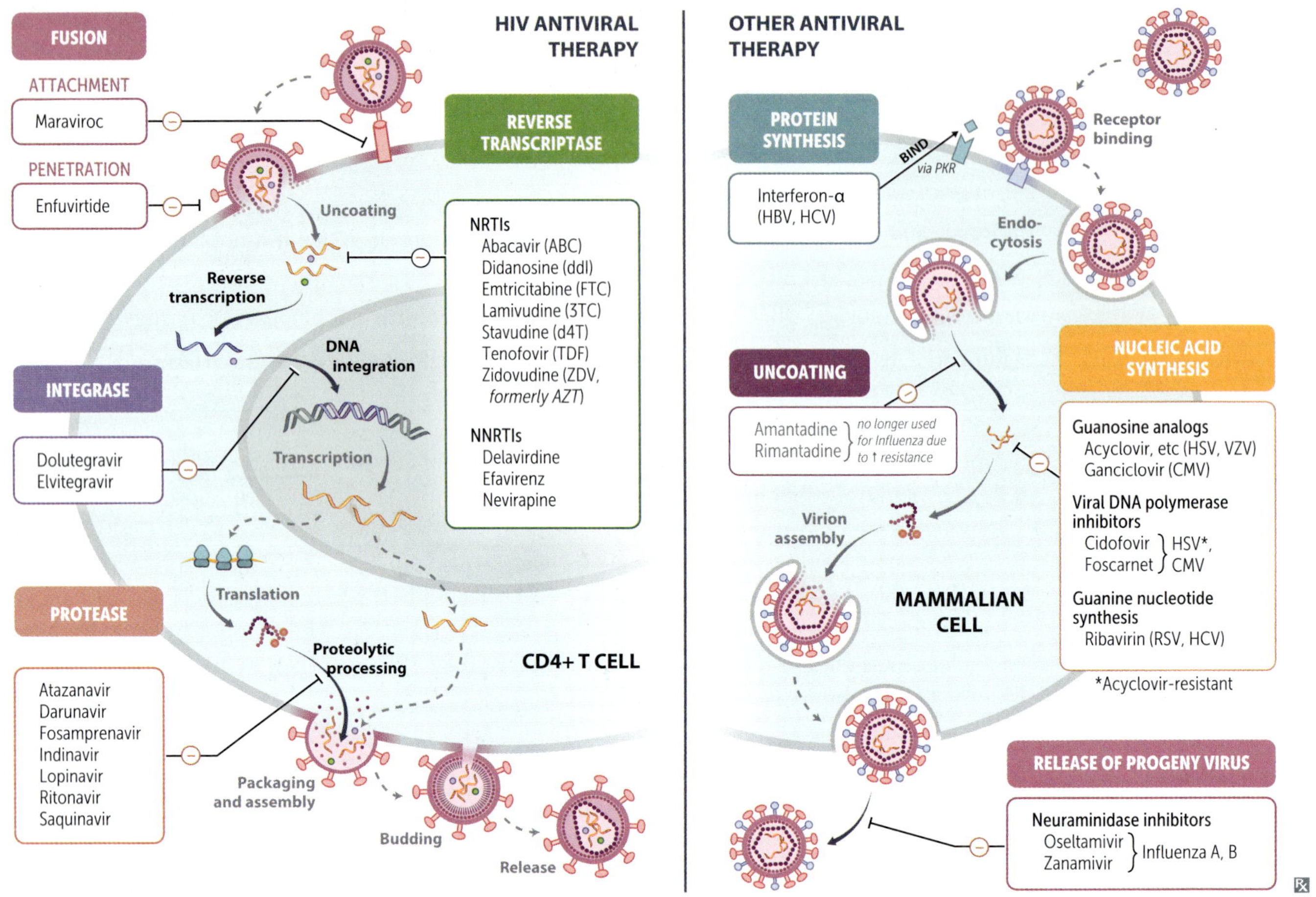

Oseltamivir, zanamivir

MECHANISM	Inhibit influenza neuraminidase → ↓ release of progeny virus.
CLINICAL USE	Treatment and prevention of both influenza A and B.

Acyclovir, famciclovir, valacyclovir

MECHANISM	Guanosine analogs. Monophosphorylated by HSV/VZV thymidine kinase and not phosphorylated in uninfected cells → few adverse effects. Triphosphate formed by cellular enzymes. Preferentially inhibit viral DNA polymerase by chain termination.
CLINICAL USE	HSV and VZV. Weak activity against EBV. No activity against CMV. Used for HSV-induced mucocutaneous and genital lesions as well as for encephalitis. Prophylaxis in immunocompromised patients. No effect on latent forms of HSV and VZV. Valacyclovir, a prodrug of acyclovir, has better oral bioavailability. For herpes zoster, use famciclovir.
ADVERSE EFFECTS	Obstructive crystalline nephropathy and acute renal failure if not adequately hydrated.
MECHANISM OF RESISTANCE	Mutated viral thymidine kinase.

Ganciclovir

MECHANISM	5′-monophosphate formed by a CMV viral kinase. Guanosine analog. Triphosphate formed by cellular kinases. Preferentially inhibits viral DNA polymerase.
CLINICAL USE	CMV, especially in immunocompromised patients. Valganciclovir, a prodrug of ganciclovir, has better oral bioavailability.
ADVERSE EFFECTS	Bone marrow suppression (leukopenia, neutropenia, thrombocytopenia), renal toxicity. More toxic to host enzymes than acyclovir.
MECHANISM OF RESISTANCE	Mutated viral kinase.

Foscarnet

MECHANISM	Viral DNA/RNA polymerase inhibitor and HIV reverse transcriptase inhibitor. Binds to pyrophosphate-binding site of enzyme. Does not require any kinase activation.	**Fos**carnet = pyro**fos**phate analog.
CLINICAL USE	CMV retinitis in immunocompromised patients when ganciclovir fails; acyclovir-resistant HSV.	
ADVERSE EFFECTS	Nephrotoxicity, electrolyte abnormalities (hypo- or hypercalcemia, hypo- or hyperphosphatemia, hypokalemia, hypomagnesemia) can lead to seizures.	
MECHANISM OF RESISTANCE	Mutated DNA polymerase.	

Cidofovir

MECHANISM	Preferentially inhibits viral DNA polymerase. Does not require phosphorylation by viral kinase.
CLINICAL USE	CMV retinitis in immunocompromised patients; acyclovir-resistant HSV. Long half-life.
ADVERSE EFFECTS	Nephrotoxicity (coadminister with probenecid and IV saline to ↓ toxicity).

HIV therapy

Highly active antiretroviral therapy (HAART): often initiated at the time of HIV diagnosis. Strongest indication for patients presenting with AIDS-defining illness, low CD4+ cell counts (< 500 cells/mm^3), or high viral load. Regimen consists of 3 drugs to prevent resistance: 2 NRTIs and preferrably an integrase inhibitor.

DRUG	MECHANISM	TOXICITY
NRTIs		
Abacavir (ABC) Didanosine (ddI) Emtricitabine (FTC) Lamivudine (3TC) Stavudine (d4T) Tenofovir (TDF) Zidovudine (ZDV, formerly AZT)	Competitively inhibit nucleotide binding to reverse transcriptase and terminate the DNA chain (lack a 3′ OH group). Tenofovir is a nucleoTide; the others are nucleosides and need to be phosphorylated to be active. ZDV can be used for general prophylaxis and during pregnancy to ↓ risk of fetal transmission. Have you dined (vudine) with my nuclear (nucleosides) family?	Bone marrow suppression (can be reversed with granulocyte colony-stimulating factor [G-CSF] and erythropoietin), peripheral neuropathy, lactic acidosis (nucleosides), anemia (ZDV), pancreatitis (didanosine). Abacavir contraindicated if patient has HLA-B*5701 mutation.
NNRTIs		
Delavirdine Efavirenz Nevirapine	Bind to reverse transcriptase at site different from NRTIs. Do not require phosphorylation to be active or compete with nucleotides.	Rash and hepatotoxicity are common to all NNRTIs. Vivid dreams and CNS symptoms are common with efavirenz. Delavirdine and efavirenz are contraindicated in pregnancy.
Protease inhibitors		
Atazanavir Darunavir Fosamprenavir Indinavir Lopinavir Ritonavir Saquinavir	Assembly of virions depends on HIV-1 protease (*pol* gene), which cleaves the polypeptide products of HIV mRNA into their functional parts. Thus, protease inhibitors prevent maturation of new viruses. Ritonavir can "boost" other drug concentrations by inhibiting cytochrome P-450. All protease inhibitors end in *-navir.* Navir (never) tease a protease.	Hyperglycemia, GI intolerance (nausea, diarrhea), lipodystrophy (Cushing-like syndrome). Nephropathy, hematuria (indinavir). Rifampin (a potent CYP/UGT inducer) contraindicated with protease inhibitors because it can decrease protease inhibitor concentration.
Integrase inhibitors		
Raltegravir Elvitegravir Dolutegravir	Inhibits HIV genome integration into host cell chromosome by reversibly inhibiting HIV integrase.	↑ creatine kinase.
Fusion inhibitors		
Enfuvirtide	Binds gp41, inhibiting viral entry.	Skin reaction at injection sites.
Maraviroc	Binds CCR-5 on surface of T cells/monocytes, inhibiting interaction with gp120.	

Interferons

MECHANISM	Glycoproteins normally synthesized by virus-infected cells, exhibiting a wide range of antiviral and antitumoral properties.
CLINICAL USE	IFN-α: chronic hepatitis B and C, Kaposi sarcoma, hairy cell leukemia, condyloma acuminatum, renal cell carcinoma, malignant melanoma. IFN-β: multiple sclerosis. IFN-γ: chronic granulomatous disease.
ADVERSE EFFECTS	Flu-like symptoms, depression, neutropenia, myopathy.

Hepatitis C therapy

DRUG	MECHANISM	CLINICAL USE
Ribavirin	Inhibits synthesis of guanine nucleotides by competitively inhibiting inosine monophosphate dehydrogenase.	Chronic HCV; also used in RSV (palivizumab preferred in children) Adverse effects: hemolytic anemia; severe teratogen.
Sofosbuvir	Inhibits HCV RNA-dependent RNA polymerase acting as a chain terminator.	Chronic HCV in combination with ribavirin, +/– peginterferon alfa. Do not use as monotherapy. Adverse effects: fatigue, headache, nausea.
Simeprevir	HCV protease inhibitor; prevents viral replication.	Chronic HCV in combination with ledipasvir (NS5A inhibitor). Do not use as monotherapy. Adverse effects: photosensitivity reactions, rash.

Infection control techniques

Goals include the reduction of pathogenic organism counts to safe levels (disinfection) and the inactivation of self-propagating biological entities (sterilization).

Autoclave	Pressurized steam at > 120°C. May be sporicidal.
Alcohols	Denature proteins and disrupt cell membranes. Not sporicidal.
Chlorhexidine	Denatures proteins and disrupts cell membranes. Not sporicidal.
Hydrogen peroxide	Free radical oxidation. Sporicidal.
Iodine and iodophors	Halogenation of DNA, RNA, and proteins. May be sporicidal.

Antimicrobials to avoid in pregnancy

ANTIMICROBIAL	ADVERSE EFFECT
Sulfonamides	Kernicterus
Aminoglycosides	Ototoxicity
Fluoroquinolones	Cartilage damage
Clarithromycin	Embryotoxic
Tetracyclines	Discolored teeth, inhibition of bone growth
Ribavirin	Teratogenic
Griseofulvin	Teratogenic
Chloramphenicol	Gray baby syndrome

SAFe **C**hildren **T**ake **R**eally **G**ood **C**are.

NOTES

HIGH-YIELD PRINCIPLES IN

Immunology

"I hate to disappoint you, but my rubber lips are immune to your charms."
—Batman & Robin

"No State shall make or enforce any law which shall abridge the privileges or immunities of citizens of the United States . . ."
—The United States Constitution

Mastery of the basic principles and facts in the immunology section will be useful for the Step 1 exam. Cell surface markers are important to know because they are clinically useful (eg, in identifying specific types of immunodeficiency or cancer) and are functionally critical to the jobs immune cells carry out. By spending a little extra effort here, it is possible to turn a traditionally difficult subject into one that is high yield.

▶ IMMUNOLOGY—LYMPHOID STRUCTURES

Lymph node

A 2° lymphoid organ that has many afferents, 1 or more efferents. Encapsulated, with trabeculae. Functions are nonspecific filtration by macrophages, storage of B and T cells, and immune response activation.

Follicle

Site of B-cell localization and proliferation. In outer cortex. 1° follicles are dense and dormant. 2° follicles have pale central germinal centers and are active.

Medulla

Consists of medullary cords (closely packed lymphocytes and plasma cells) and medullary sinuses. Medullary sinuses communicate with efferent lymphatics and contain reticular cells and macrophages.

Paracortex

Houses T cells. Region of cortex between follicles and medulla. Contains high endothelial venules through which T and B cells enter from blood. Not well developed in patients with DiGeorge syndrome.

Paracortex enlarges in an extreme cellular immune response (eg, viral infection).

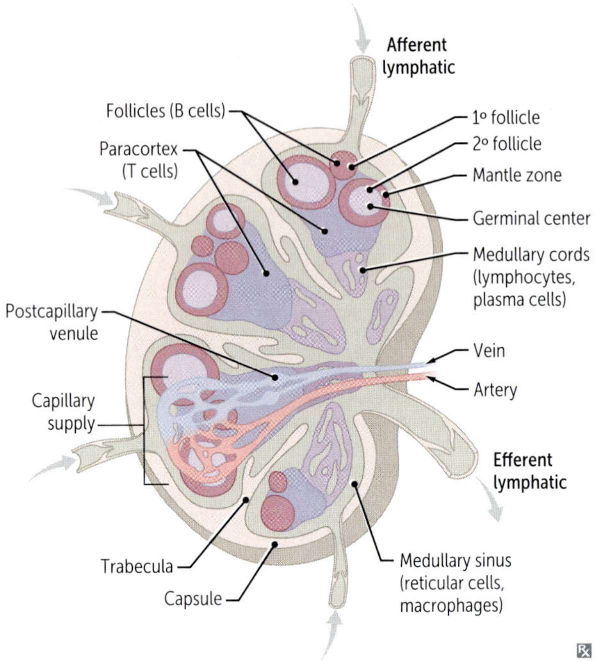

Lymph drainage

LYMPH NODE CLUSTER	AREA OF BODY DRAINED
Cervical	Head and neck
Hilar	Lungs
Mediastinal	Trachea and esophagus
Axillary	Upper limb, breast, skin above umbilicus
Celiac	Liver, stomach, spleen, pancreas, upper duodenum
Superior mesenteric	Lower duodenum, jejunum, ileum, colon to splenic flexure
Inferior mesenteric	Colon from splenic flexure to upper rectum
Internal iliac	Lower rectum to anal canal (above pectinate line), bladder, vagina (middle third), cervix, prostate
Para-aortic	Testes, ovaries, kidneys, uterus
Superficial inguinal	Anal canal (below pectinate line), skin below umbilicus (except popliteal area), scrotum, vulva
Popliteal	Dorsolateral foot, posterior calf

Right lymphatic duct drains right side of body above diaphragm.
Thoracic duct drains everything else into junction of left subclavian and internal jugular veins.

Sinusoids of spleen

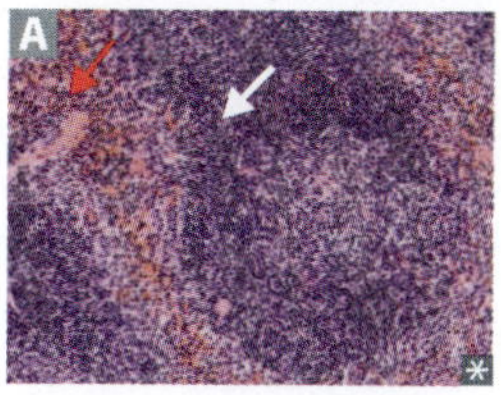

Long, vascular channels in red pulp (red arrow in A) with fenestrated "barrel hoop" basement membrane.
- T cells are found in the periarteriolar lymphatic sheath (PALS) within the white pulp (white arrow in A).
- B cells are found in follicles within the white pulp.
- The marginal zone, in between the red pulp and white pulp, contains macrophages and specialized B cells, and is where antigen-presenting cells (APCs) capture blood-borne antigens for recognition by lymphocytes.

Macrophages found nearby in spleen remove encapsulated bacteria.

Splenic dysfunction (eg, postsplenectomy, sickle cell disease): ↓ IgM → ↓ complement activation → ↓ C3b opsonization → ↑ susceptibility to encapsulated organisms (**Please SHINE my SKiS**):
- ***P**seudomonas aeruginosa*
- ***S**treptococcus pneumoniae*
- ***H**aemophilus **I**nfluenzae* type b
- ***N**eisseria meningitidis*
- ***E**scherichia coli*
- ***S**almonella* spp.
- ***K**lebsiella pneumoniae*
- Group B **S**treptococci

Postsplenectomy:
- Howell-Jolly bodies (nuclear remnants)
- Target cells
- Thrombocytosis (loss of sequestration and removal)
- Lymphocytosis (loss of sequestration)

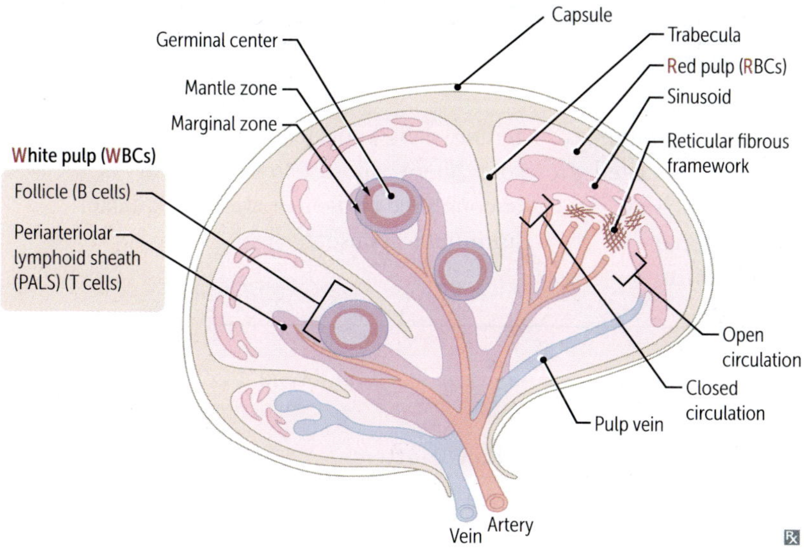

Thymus

Located in the anterosuperior mediastinum. Site of T-cell differentiation and maturation. Encapsulated. **Th**ymus is derived from the **Th**ird pharyngeal pouch. Lymphocytes of mesenchymal origin. Cortex is dense with immature T cells; medulla is pale with mature T cells and Hassall corpuscles containing epithelial reticular cells.

T cells = **T**hymus

B cells = **B**one marrow

Hypoplastic in DiGeorge syndrome and severe combined immunodeficiency (SCID).

Enlarged in myasthenia gravis.

▸ IMMUNOLOGY—LYMPHOCYTES

Innate vs adaptive immunity

	Innate immunity	Adaptive immunity
COMPONENTS	Neutrophils, macrophages, monocytes, dendritic cells, natural killer (NK) cells (lymphoid origin), complement	T cells, B cells, circulating antibodies
MECHANISM	Germline encoded	Variation through V(D)J recombination during lymphocyte development
RESISTANCE	Resistance persists through generations; does not change within an organism's lifetime	Microbial resistance not heritable
RESPONSE TO PATHOGENS	Nonspecific Occurs rapidly (minutes to hours)	Highly specific, refined over time Develops over long periods; memory response is faster and more robust
PHYSICAL BARRIERS	Epithelial tight junctions, mucus	—
SECRETED PROTEINS	Lysozyme, complement, C-reactive protein (CRP), defensins	Immunoglobulins
KEY FEATURES IN PATHOGEN RECOGNITION	Toll-like receptors (TLRs): pattern recognition receptors that recognize pathogen-associated molecular patterns (PAMPs). Examples of PAMPs include LPS (gram ⊖ bacteria), flagellin (bacteria), nucleic acids (viruses).	Memory cells: activated B and T cells; subsequent exposure to a previously encountered antigen → stronger, quicker immune response

MHC I and II

MHC encoded by HLA genes. Present antigen fragments to T cells and bind T-cell receptors (TCRs).

	MHC I (1 letter)	MHC II (2 letters)
LOCI	HLA-A, HLA-B, HLA-C	HLA-DP, HLA-DQ, HLA-DR
BINDING	TCR and CD8	TCR and CD4
EXPRESSION	Expressed on all nucleated cells Not expressed on RBCs	Expressed on APCs
FUNCTION	★ Present **endogenously** synthesized **antigens** (eg, viral or cytosolic proteins) to **CD8+ cytotoxic T cells** every day "check"	Present **exogenously** synthesized **antigens** (eg, bacterial proteins) to **CD4+ helper T cells** new molec check
ANTIGEN LOADING	Antigen peptides loaded onto MHC I in RER after delivery via TAP (transporter associated with antigen processing)	Antigen loaded following release of invariant chain in an acidified endosome
ASSOCIATED PROTEINS	β_2-microglobulin	Invariant chain

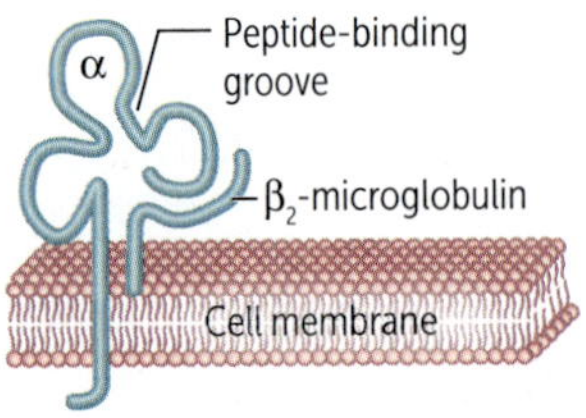

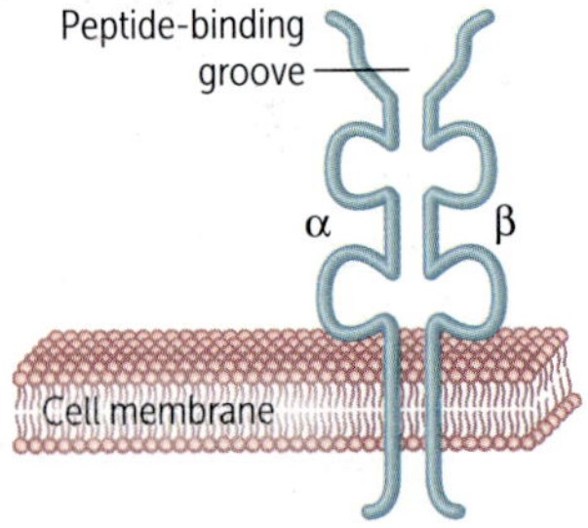

HLA subtypes associated with diseases

A3	Hemochromatosis.	
B8	Addison disease, myasthenia gravis.	
B27	**P**soriatic arthritis, **A**nkylosing spondylitis, **I**BD-associated arthritis, **R**eactive arthritis (formerly Reiter syndrome).	**PAIR.** Also known as seronegative arthropathies.
DQ2/DQ8	Celiac disease.	I ate (8) too (2) much gluten at **D**airy **Q**ueen.
DR2	Multiple sclerosis, hay fever, SLE, Goodpasture syndrome.	
DR3	Diabetes mellitus type 1, SLE, Graves disease, Hashimoto thyroiditis, Addison disease.	
DR4	**Rheum**atoid arthritis, diabetes mellitus type 1, Addison disease.	There are **4** walls in a "**rheum**" (room).
DR5	Pernicious anemia → vitamin B_{12} deficiency, Hashimoto thyroiditis.	

Natural killer cells	Use perforin and granzymes to induce apoptosis of virally infected cells and tumor cells. —like T cells Lymphocyte member of innate immune system. Activity enhanced by IL-2, IL-12, IFN-α, and IFN-β. Induced to kill when exposed to a nonspecific activation signal on target cell and/or to an absence of class I MHC on target cell surface. Also kills via antibody-dependent cell-mediated cytotoxicity (CD16 binds Fc region of bound Ig, activating the NK cell).

Major functions of B and T cells

B-cell functions	Recognize antigen—undergo somatic hypermutation to optimize antigen specificity. Produce antibody—differentiate into plasma cells to secrete specific immunoglobulins. Maintain immunologic memory—memory B cells persist and accelerate future response to antigen.
T-cell functions	CD4+ T cells help B cells make antibodies and produce cytokines to recruit phagocytes and activate other leukocytes. CD8+ T cells directly kill virus-infected cells. Delayed cell-mediated hypersensitivity (type IV). Acute and chronic cellular organ rejection. **Rule of 8**: MHC **II** × CD**4** = **8**; MHC **I** × CD**8** = **8**.

Differentiation of T cells

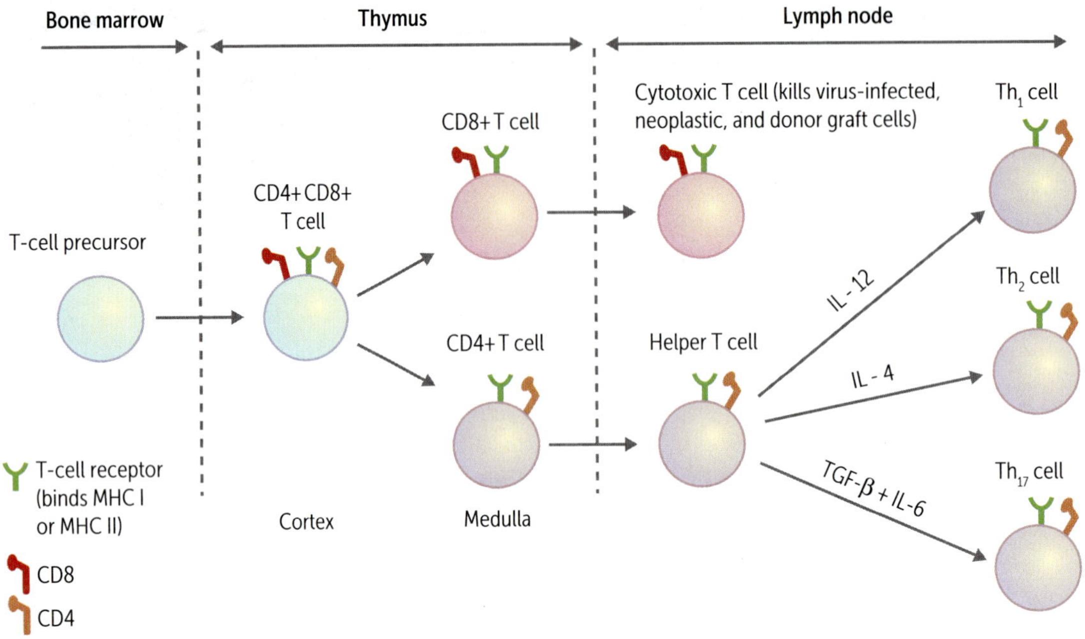

Positive selection	Thymic cortex. T cells expressing TCRs capable of binding self-MHC on cortical epithelial cells survive.
Negative selection	Thymic medulla. T cells expressing TCRs with high affinity for self antigens undergo apoptosis. Tissue-restricted self-antigens are expressed in the thymus due to the action of autoimmune regulator (AIRE); deficiency leads to autoimmune polyendocrine syndrome-1.

Helper T cells

Th1 cell	Th2 cell
Secretes IFN-γ	Secretes IL-4, IL-5, IL-10, IL-13
Activates macrophages and cytotoxic T cells	Recruits eosinophils for parasite defense and promotes IgE production by B cells
Differentiation induced by IFN-γ and IL-12	Differentiation induced by IL-4
Inhibited by IL-4 and IL-10 (from Th2 cell)	Inhibited by IFN-γ (from Th1 cell)

Macrophage-lymphocyte interaction—macrophages and other APCs release IL-12, which stimulates T cells to differentiate into Th1 cells. Th1 cells release IFN-γ to stimulate macrophages.

Helper T cells have CD4, which binds to MHC II on APCs.

Cytotoxic T cells

Kill virus-infected, neoplastic, and donor graft cells by inducing apoptosis.
Release cytotoxic granules containing preformed proteins (eg, perforin, granzyme B).
Cytotoxic T cells have CD8, which binds to MHC I on virus-infected cells.

Regulatory T cells

Help maintain specific immune tolerance by suppressing CD4 and CD8 T-cell effector functions.
Identified by expression of CD3, CD4, CD25, and FOXP3.
Activated regulatory T cells produce anti-inflammatory cytokines (eg, IL-10, TGF-β).

T- and B-cell activation

APCs: B cells, macrophages, dendritic cells.
Two signals are required for T-cell activation, B-cell activation, and class switching.

Naive T-cell activation

1. Dendritic cell (specialized APC) samples and processes antigen.
2. Dendritic cell migrates to the draining lymph node.
3. T-cell activation (signal 1): antigen is presented on MHC II and recognized by TCR on Th (CD4+) cell. Endogenous antigen is presented on MHC I to Tc (CD8+) cell.
4. Proliferation and survival (signal 2): costimulatory signal via interaction of B7 proteins (CD80/86) and CD28.
5. Th cell activates and produces cytokines. Tc cell activates and is able to recognize and kill virus-infected cell. So ext antig presentat → cytok. Internal antig = recog/kill infected cell

B-cell activation and class switching

1. Th-cell activation as above.
2. B-cell receptor–mediated endocytosis; foreign antigen is presented on MHC II and recognized by TCR on Th cell.
3. CD40 receptor on B cell binds CD40 ligand (CD40L) on Th cell.
4. Th cell secretes cytokines that determine Ig class switching of B cell. B cell activates and undergoes class switching, affinity maturation, and antibody production.

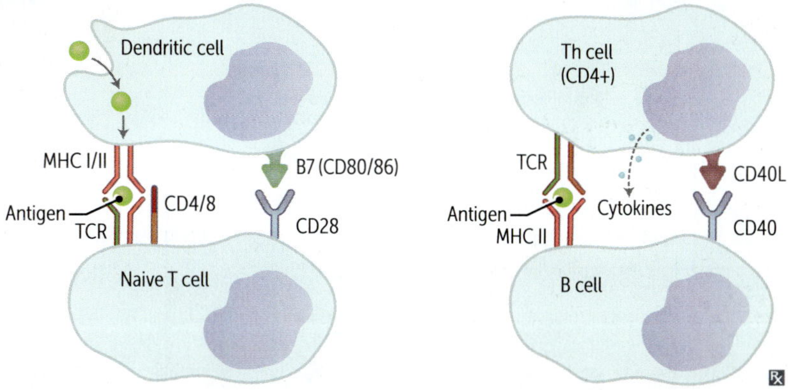

Antibody structure and function

Fab (containing the variable/hypervariable regions) consisting of light (L) and heavy (H) chains recognizes antigens. Fc region of IgM and IgG fixes complement. Heavy chain contributes to Fc and Fab regions. Light chain contributes only to Fab region.

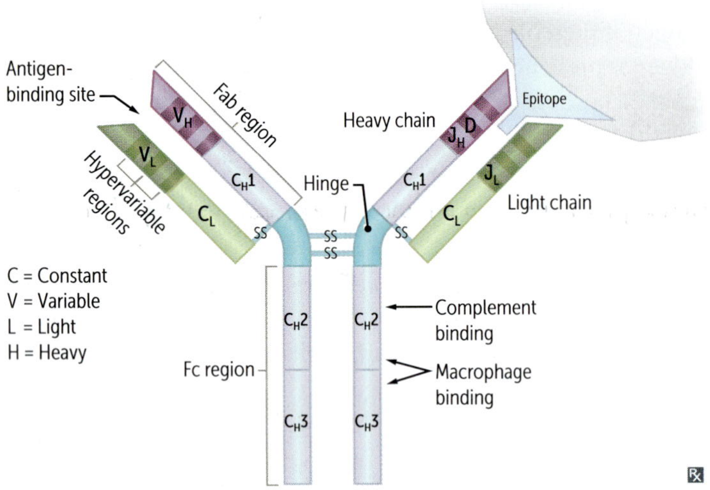

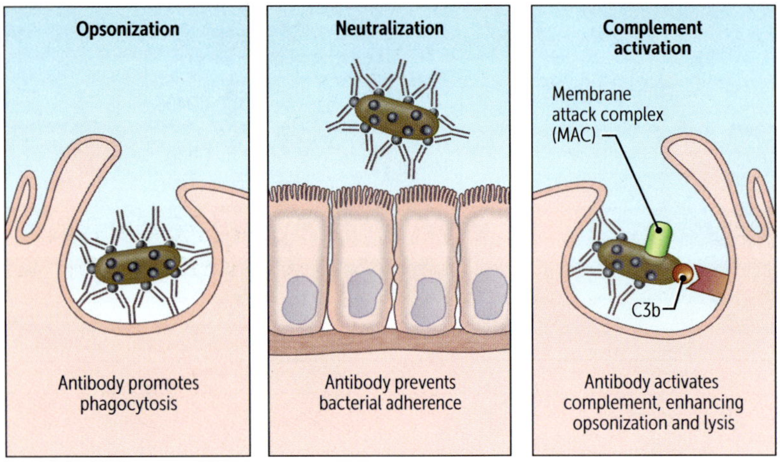

Fab:
- Fragment, antigen binding
- Determines idiotype: unique antigen-binding pocket; only 1 antigenic specificity expressed per B cell

Fc:
- Constant
- Carboxy terminal
- Complement binding
- Carbohydrate side chains
- Determines isotype (IgM, IgD, etc)

Generation of antibody diversity (antigen independent)
1. Random recombination of VJ (light-chain) or V(D)J (heavy-chain) genes
2. Random addition of nucleotides to DNA during recombination by terminal deoxynucleotidyl transferase (TdT)
3. Random combination of heavy chains with light chains

Generation of antibody specificity (antigen dependent)

4. Somatic hypermutation and affinity maturation (variable region)
5. Isotype switching (constant region)

Immunoglobulin isotypes	All isotypes can exist as monomers. Mature, naive B cells prior to activation express IgM and IgD on their surfaces. They may differentiate in germinal centers of lymph nodes by isotype switching (gene rearrangement; mediated by cytokines and CD40L) into plasma cells that secrete IgA, IgE, or IgG.
IgG 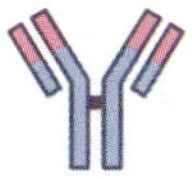	Main antibody in 2° (**delayed**) response to an antigen. Most abundant isotype in serum. Fixes complement, crosses the placenta (provides infants with passive immunity), opsonizes bacteria, neutralizes bacterial toxins and viruses.
IgA 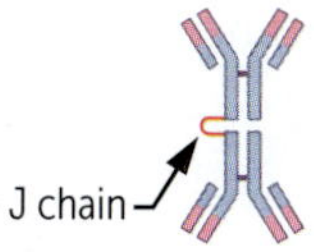	Prevents attachment of bacteria and viruses to mucous membranes; does not fix complement. Monomer (in circulation) or dimer (with J chain when secreted). Crosses epithelial cells by transcytosis. Produced in GI tract (eg, by Peyer patches) and protects against gut infections (eg, *Giardia*). Most produced antibody overall, but has lower serum concentrations. Released into secretions (tears, saliva, mucus) and breast milk. Picks up secretory component from epithelial cells, which protects the Fc portion from luminal proteases.
IgM 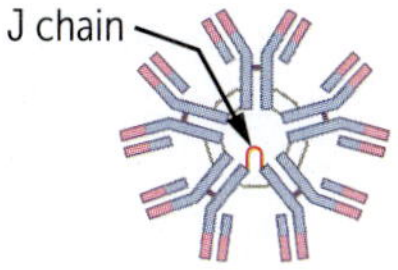	Produced in the 1° (**immediate**) response to an antigen. Fixes complement but does not cross the placenta. Antigen receptor on the surface of B cells. Monomer on B cell, pentamer with J chain when secreted. Pentamer enables avid binding to antigen while humoral response evolves.
IgD 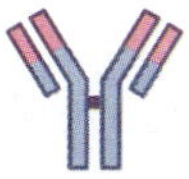	Unclear function. Found on surface of many B cells and in serum.
IgE 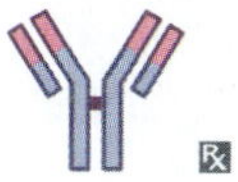	Binds mast cells and basophils; cross-links when exposed to allergen, mediating immediate (type I) hypersensitivity through release of inflammatory mediators such as histamine. Mediates immunity to worms by activating eosinophils. Lowest concentration in serum.

Antigen type and memory

Thymus-independent antigens	Antigens lacking a peptide component (eg, lipopolysaccharides from gram ⊖ bacteria); cannot be presented by MHC to T cells. Weakly immunogenic; vaccines often require boosters and adjuvants (eg, pneumococcal polysaccharide vaccine).
Thymus-dependent antigens	Antigens containing a protein component (eg, diphtheria vaccine). Class switching and immunologic memory occur as a result of direct contact of B cells with Th cells (CD40–CD40L interaction).

▸ IMMUNOLOGY—IMMUNE RESPONSES

Acute-phase reactants	Factors whose serum concentrations change significantly in response to inflammation; produced by the liver in both acute and chronic inflammatory states. Notably induced by IL-6.
POSITIVE (UPREGULATED)	
C-reactive protein	Opsonin; fixes complement and facilitates phagocytosis. Measured clinically as a sign of ongoing inflammation.
Ferritin	Binds and sequesters iron to inhibit microbial iron scavenging.
Fibrinogen	Coagulation factor; promotes endothelial repair; correlates with ESR.
Hepcidin	↓ iron absorption (by degrading ferroportin) and ↓ iron release (from macrophages) → anemia of chronic disease.
Serum amyloid A	Prolonged elevation can lead to amyloidosis.
NEGATIVE (DOWNREGULATED)	
Albumin	Reduction conserves amino acids for positive reactants.
Transferrin	Internalized by macrophages to sequester iron.

Complement

System of hepatically synthesized plasma proteins that play a role in innate immunity and inflammation. Membrane attack complex (MAC) defends against gram ⊖ bacteria.*

ACTIVATION	**Classic** pathway—Ig**G** or Ig**M** mediated. Alternative pathway—microbe surface molecules. Lectin pathway—mannose or other sugars on microbe surface.	**GM** makes **classic** cars.
FUNCTIONS	C3b—opsonization. C3**a**, C4**a**, C5**a**—**a**naphylaxis. C5a—neutrophil chemotaxis. C5b-9—cytolysis by MAC.	C3**b** **b**inds **b**acteria.
	Opsonins—C3b and IgG are the two 1° opsonins in bacterial defense; enhance phagocytosis. C3b also helps clear immune complexes.	*Opsonin* (Greek) = to prepare for eating.
	Inhibitors—decay-accelerating factor (DAF, * (GPI-anchored enz) aka CD55) and C1 esterase inhibitor help prevent complement activation on self cells (eg, RBCs).	

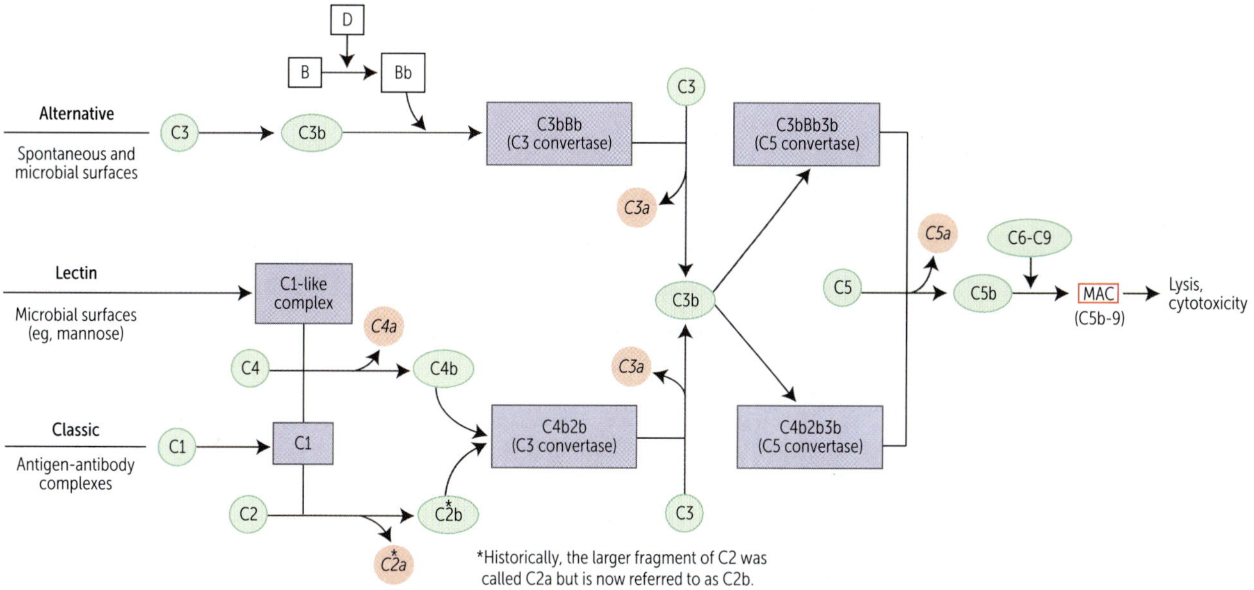

*Historically, the larger fragment of C2 was called C2a but is now referred to as C2b.

Complement disorders

C1 esterase inhibitor deficiency	Causes hereditary angioedema due to unregulated activation of kallikrein → ↑ bradykinin. ACE inhibitors are contraindicated.
C3 deficiency	Increases risk of severe, recurrent pyogenic sinus and respiratory tract infections; ↑ susceptibility to type III hypersensitivity reactions.
C5–C9 deficiencies	Terminal complement deficiency increases susceptibility to recurrent *Neisseria* bacteremia.
DAF (GPI-anchored enzyme) deficiency	Causes complement-mediated lysis of RBCs and paroxysmal nocturnal hemoglobinuria.

Important cytokines

SECRETED BY MACROPHAGES		
IL-1	Also called osteoclast-activating factor. Causes fever, acute inflammation. Activates endothelium to express adhesion molecules. Induces chemokine secretion to recruit WBCs. Fever bye bone sticky endoth hi WBC	"**Hot T-bone stEAK**": IL-1: fever (**hot**). IL-2: stimulates **T** cells. IL-3: stimulates **bone** marrow. IL-4: stimulates Ig**E** production. IL-5: stimulates Ig**A** production. IL-6: stimulates a**K**ute-phase protein production.
IL-6	Causes fever and stimulates production of acute-phase proteins.	
IL-8	Major chemotactic factor for neutrophils.	"**Clean up** on **aisle 8**." Neutrophils are recruited by **IL-8** to **clear** infections.
IL-12	Induces differentiation of T cells into Th1 cells. Activates NK cells.	
TNF-α	Mediates septic shock. Activates endothelium. Causes WBC recruitment, vascular leak.	Causes cachexia in malignancy.
SECRETED BY ALL T CELLS		
IL-2	Stimulates growth of helper, cytotoxic, and regulatory T cells, and NK cells.	
IL-3	Supports growth and differentiation of bone marrow stem cells. Functions like GM-CSF.	
FROM Th1 CELLS		
Interferon-γ	Secreted by NK cells and T cells in response to IL-12 from macrophages; stimulates macrophages to kill phagocytosed pathogens. Inhibits differentiation of Th2 cells.	Also activates NK cells to kill virus-infected cells. Increases MHC expression and antigen presentation by all cells.
FROM Th2 CELLS		
IL-4	Induces differentiation of T cells into Th2 cells. Promotes growth of B cells. Enhances class switching to IgE and IgG.	
IL-5	Promotes growth and differentiation of B cells. Enhances class switching to IgA. Stimulates growth and differentiation of eosinophils.	
IL-10	Attenuates inflammatory response. Decreases expression of MHC class II and Th1 cytokines. Inhibits activated macrophages and dendritic cells. Also secreted by regulatory T cells.	TGF-β and IL-**10** both at**ten**uate the immune response.

Respiratory burst (oxidative burst)

Involves the activation of the phagocyte NADPH oxidase complex (eg, in neutrophils, monocytes), which utilizes O_2 as a substrate. Plays an important role in the immune response → rapid release of reactive oxygen species (ROS). NADPH plays a role in both the creation and neutralization of ROS. Myeloperoxidase is a blue-green heme-containing pigment that gives sputum its color.

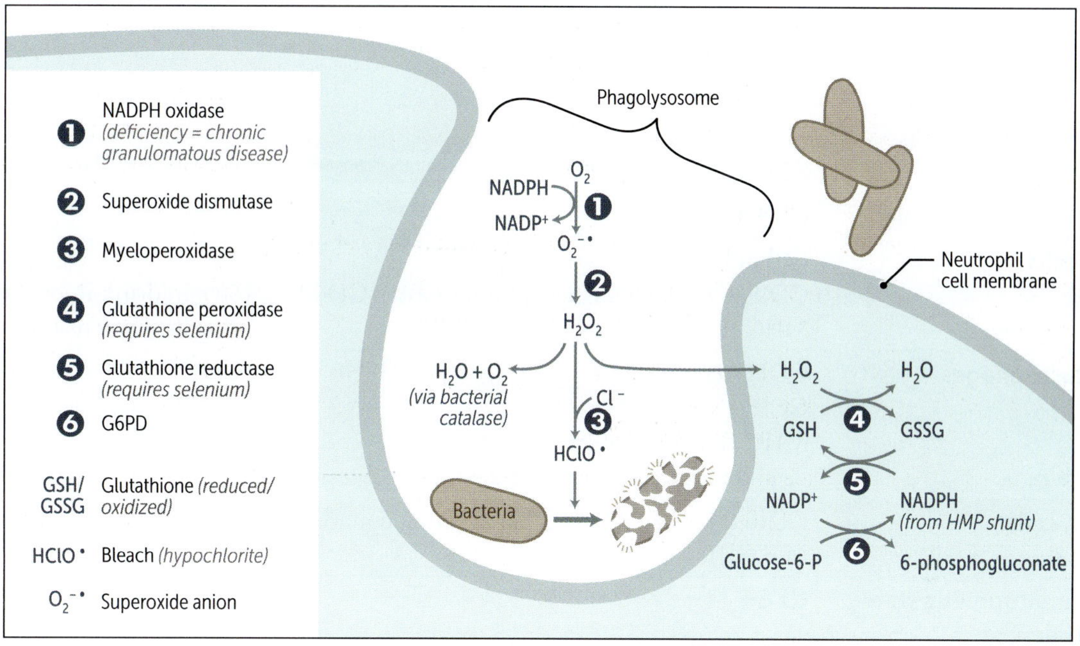

Phagocytes of patients with CGD can utilize H_2O_2 generated by invading organisms and convert it to ROS. Patients are at ↑ risk for infection by catalase ⊕ species (eg, *S aureus*, *Aspergillus*) capable of neutralizing their own H_2O_2, leaving phagocytes without ROS for fighting infections.

Pyocyanin of *P aeruginosa* functions to generate ROS to kill competing microbes. Lactoferrin is a protein found in secretory fluids and neutrophils that inhibits microbial growth via iron chelation.

Interferon-α and -β

A part of innate host defense against both RNA and DNA viruses. Interferons are glycoproteins synthesized by virus-infected cells that act locally on uninfected cells, "priming them" for viral defense by helping to selectively degrade viral nucleic acid and protein.

Interfere with viruses.

Cell surface proteins	MHC I present on all nucleated cells (ie, not mature RBCs).	
T cells	TCR (binds antigen-MHC complex) CD3 (associated with TCR for signal transduction) CD28 (binds B7 on APC) CXCR4/CCR5 (co-receptors for HIV)	
Helper T cells	CD4, CD40L	
Cytotoxic T cells	CD8 CXCR4/CCR5	
Regulatory T cells	CD4, CD25	
B cells	Ig (binds antigen) CD19, CD20, CD21 (receptor for EBV), CD40 MHC II, B7	You can drink **B**eer at the **B**ar when you're **21**: **B** cells, Epstein-**B**arr virus, CD**21**.
Macrophages	CD14 (receptor for PAMPs, eg, LPS), CD40 CCR5 MHC II, B7 (CD80/86) Fc and C3b receptors (enhanced phagocytosis)	
NK cells	CD16 (binds Fc of IgG), CD56 (unique marker for NK)	
Hematopoietic stem cells	CD34	

Anergy

State during which a cell cannot become activated by exposure to its antigen. T and B cells become anergic when exposed to their antigen without costimulatory signal (signal 2). Another mechanism of self-tolerance.

Effects of bacterial toxins

Superantigens (*S pyogenes* and *S aureus*)—cross-link the β region of the T-cell receptor to the MHC class II on APCs. Can activate any CD4+ T cell → massive release of cytokines.
Endotoxins/lipopolysaccharide (gram ⊖ bacteria)—directly stimulate macrophages by binding to endotoxin receptor TLR4/CD14; Th cells are not involved.

Antigenic variation

Classic examples:
- Bacteria—*Salmonella* (2 flagellar variants), *Borrelia recurrentis* (relapsing fever), *N gonorrhoeae* (pilus protein)
- Viruses—influenza, HIV, HCV
- Parasites—trypanosomes

Some mechanisms for variation include DNA rearrangement and RNA segment reassortment (eg, influenza major shift).

Passive vs active immunity

	Passive	Active
MEANS OF ACQUISITION	Receiving preformed antibodies	Exposure to foreign antigens
ONSET	Rapid	Slow
DURATION	Short span of antibodies (half-life = 3 weeks)	Long-lasting protection (memory)
EXAMPLES	IgA in breast milk, maternal IgG crossing placenta, antitoxin, humanized monoclonal antibody	Natural infection, vaccines, toxoid
NOTES	After exposure to **T**etanus toxin, **B**otulinum toxin, **H**BV, **V**aricella, or **R**abies virus, unvaccinated patients are given preformed antibodies (passive)—"**T**o **B**e **H**ealed **V**ery **R**apidly"	Combined passive and active immunizations can be given for hepatitis B or rabies exposure

Vaccination

Induces an active immune response (humoral and/or cellular) to specific pathogens.

VACCINE TYPE	DESCRIPTION	PROS/CONS	EXAMPLES
Live attenuated vaccine	Microorganism loses its pathogenicity but retains capacity for transient growth within inoculated host. Induces **cellular and humoral responses**. MMR is the only live attenuated vaccine given to persons with HIV.	Pro: induces strong, often lifelong immunity. Con: may revert to virulent form. Often contraindicated in pregnancy and immunodeficiency.	BCG, influenza (intranasal), measles, mumps, polio (Sabin), rubella, varicella, yellow fever.
Inactivated or killed vaccine	Pathogen is inactivated by heat or chemicals. Maintaining epitope structure on surface antigens is important for immune response. Mainly induces a **humoral response**.	Pro: safer than live vaccines. Con: weaker immune response; booster shots usually required.	**R**abies, **I**nfluenza (injection), **P**olio (Salk), hepatitis **A** ("**R.I.P. A**lways").

Hypersensitivity types	Four types: **A**naphylactic and **A**topic (type I), **C**ytotoxic (antibody mediated, type II), **I**mmune complex (type III), **D**elayed (cell mediated, type IV) (**ACID**).	
Type I 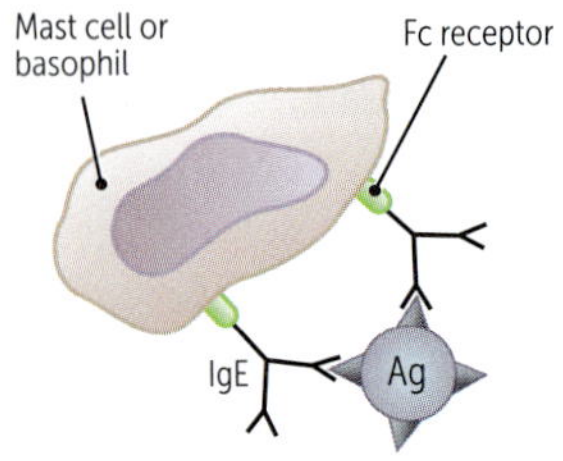 	Anaphylactic and atopic—free antigen cross-links IgE on presensitized mast cells and basophils, triggering immediate release of vasoactive amines that act at postcapillary venules (ie, histamine). Reaction develops rapidly after antigen exposure because of preformed antibody. Delayed response follows due to production of arachidonic acid metabolites (eg, leukotrienes).	**F**irst (type) and **F**ast (anaphylaxis). Types I, II, and III are all antibody mediated. Test: skin test for specific IgE. Examples: ▪ Allergic and atopic disorders (eg, rhinitis, hay fever, eczema, hives, asthma) ▪ Anaphylaxis (eg, bee sting, some food/drug allergies)
Type II 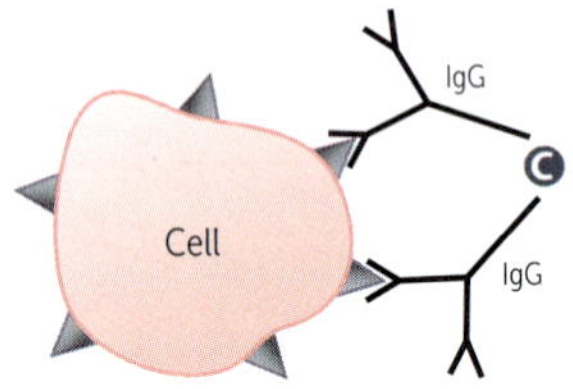 C = complement	Cytotoxic (antibody mediated)—IgM, IgG bind to fixed antigen on "enemy" cell → cellular destruction. Antibody and complement lead to MAC. 3 mechanisms: ▪ Opsonization and phagocytosis ▪ Complement- and Fc receptor–mediated inflammation ▪ Antibody-mediated cellular dysfunction Disease tends to be specific to tissue or site where antigen is found.	Type **II** is cy-**2**-toxic. Direct and indirect Coombs' tests: Direct—detects antibodies that have adhered to patient's RBCs (eg, test an Rh ⊕ infant of an Rh ⊖ mother). Indirect—detects serum antibodies that can adhere to other RBCs (eg, test an Rh ⊖ woman for Rh ⊕ antibodies). Examples: ▪ Acute hemolytic transfusion reactions ▪ Autoimmune hemolytic anemia ▪ Bullous pemphigoid ▪ Erythroblastosis fetalis ▪ Goodpasture syndrome ▪ Graves disease ▪ Guillain-Barré syndrome ▪ Idiopathic thrombocytopenic purpura ▪ Myasthenia gravis ▪ Pemphigus vulgaris ▪ Pernicious anemia ▪ Rheumatic fever

Hypersensitivity types *(continued)*

Type III 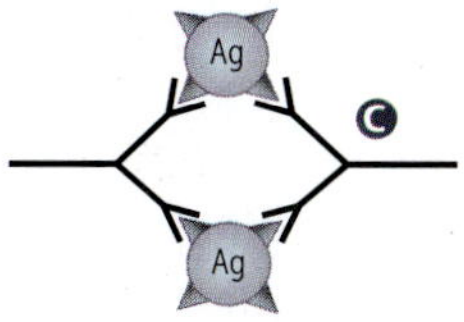	Immune complex—antigen-antibody (IgG) complexes activate complement, which attracts neutrophils; neutrophils release lysosomal enzymes. Can be associated with vasculitis and systemic manifestations.	In type **III** reaction, imagine an immune complex as **3** things stuck together: antigen-antibody-complement. Examples: ▪ Arthus reaction ▪ SLE ▪ Polyarteritis nodosa ▪ Poststreptococcal glomerulonephritis ▪ Serum sickness
	Serum sickness—an immune complex disease in which antibodies to foreign proteins are produced (takes 5 days). Immune complexes form and are deposited in membranes, where they fix complement (leads to tissue damage). More common than Arthus reaction.	Most serum sickness is now caused by drugs (not serum) acting as haptens. Fever, urticaria, arthralgia, proteinuria, lymphadenopathy occur 5–10 days after antigen exposure.
	Arthus reaction—a local subacute antibody-mediated hypersensitivity reaction. Intradermal injection of antigen into a presensitized (has circulating IgG) individual leads to immune complex formation in the skin. Characterized by edema, necrosis, and activation of complement.	Antigen-antibody complexes cause the Arthus reaction. Test: immunofluorescent staining.
Type IV 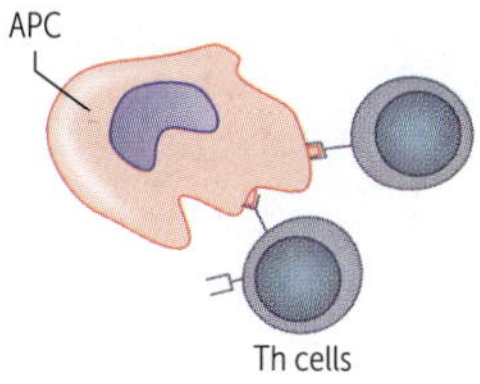	Delayed (T-cell–mediated) type—sensitized T cells encounter antigen and then release cytokines (leads to macrophage activation). Response does **not** involve antibodies (vs types I, II, and III).	**4th** and **last**—delayed. Cell mediated; therefore, it is not transferable by serum. **4 T's** = **T** cells, **T**ransplant rejections, **T**B skin tests, **T**ouching (contact dermatitis). Test: patch test, PPD. Examples: ▪ Contact dermatitis (eg, poison ivy, nickel allergy) ▪ Graft-versus-host disease ▪ Multiple sclerosis

Blood transfusion reactions

TYPE	PATHOGENESIS	CLINICAL PRESENTATION
Allergic reaction	Type I hypersensitivity reaction against plasma proteins in transfused blood.	Urticaria, pruritus, wheezing, fever. Treat with antihistamines.
Anaphylactic reaction	Severe allergic reaction. IgA-deficient individuals must receive blood products without IgA.	Dyspnea, bronchospasm, hypotension, respiratory arrest, shock. Treat with epinephrine.
Febrile nonhemolytic transfusion reaction	Type II hypersensitivity reaction. Host antibodies against donor HLA antigens and WBCs.	Fever, headaches, chills, flushing.
Acute hemolytic transfusion reaction	Type II hypersensitivity reaction. Intravascular hemolysis (ABO blood group incompatibility) or extravascular hemolysis (host antibody reaction against foreign antigen on donor RBCs).	Fever, hypotension, tachypnea, tachycardia, flank pain, hemoglobinuria (intravascular hemolysis), jaundice (extravascular).

Autoantibodies

AUTOANTIBODY	ASSOCIATED DISORDER
Anti-ACh receptor	Myasthenia gravis
Anti-basement membrane	Goodpasture syndrome
Anticardiolipin, lupus anticoagulant	SLE, antiphospholipid syndrome
Anticentromere	Limited scleroderma (CREST syndrome)
Anti-desmoglein (anti-desmosome)	Pemphigus vulgaris
Anti-dsDNA, anti-Smith	SLE
Anti-glutamic acid decarboxylase (GAD-65)	Type 1 diabetes mellitus
Antihemidesmosome	Bullous pemphigoid
Anti-histone	Drug-induced lupus
Anti-Jo-1, anti-SRP, anti-Mi-2	Polymyositis, dermatomyositis
Antimicrosomal, antithyroglobulin	Hashimoto thyroiditis
Antimitochondrial	1° biliary cirrhosis
Antinuclear (ANA)	SLE, nonspecific
Antiparietal cell	Pernicious anemia
Antiphospholipase A_2 receptor	1° membranous nephropathy
Anti-Scl-70 (anti-DNA topoisomerase I)	Scleroderma (diffuse)
Anti-smooth muscle	Autoimmune hepatitis type 1
Anti-SSA, anti-SSB (anti-Ro, anti-La)	Sjögren syndrome
Anti-TSH receptor	Graves disease
Anti-U1 RNP (ribonucleoprotein)	Mixed connective tissue disease
Voltage-gated calcium channel antibodies	Lambert-Eaton syndrome
IgA anti-endomysial, IgA anti-tissue transglutaminase	Celiac disease
MPO-ANCA/p-ANCA	Microscopic polyangiitis, eosinophilic granulomatosis with polyangiitis (Churg-Strauss syndrome)
PR3-ANCA/c-ANCA	Granulomatosis with polyangiitis (Wegener)
Rheumatoid factor (IgM antibody that targets IgG Fc region), anti-CCP (more specific)	Rheumatoid arthritis

Infections in immunodeficiency

PATHOGEN	↓ T CELLS	↓ B CELLS	↓ GRANULOCYTES	↓ COMPLEMENT
Bacteria	Sepsis	Encapsulated: *Pseudomonas aeruginosa*, *Streptococcus pneumoniae*, *Haemophilus Influenzae* type B, *Neisseria meningitidis*, *Escherichia coli*, *Salmonella*, *Klebsiella pneumoniae*, group B Strep (Please SHINE my SKiS)	*Staphylococcus*, *Burkholderia cepacia*, *Pseudomonas aeruginosa*, *Serratia*, *Nocardia*	Encapsulated species with early component deficiencies *Neisseria* with late component (MAC) deficiencies
Viruses	CMV, EBV, JCV, VZV, chronic infection with respiratory/GI viruses	Enteroviral encephalitis, poliovirus (live vaccine contraindicated)	N/A	N/A
Fungi/parasites	*Candida* (local), PCP	GI giardiasis (no IgA)	*Candida* (systemic), *Aspergillus*	N/A

Note: B-cell deficiencies tend to produce recurrent bacterial infections, whereas T-cell deficiencies produce more fungal and viral infections.

Grafts

Autograft	From self.
Syngeneic graft (isograft)	From identical twin or clone.
Allograft	From nonidentical individual of same species.
Xenograft	From different species.

Transplant rejection

TYPE OF REJECTION	ONSET	PATHOGENESIS	FEATURES
Hyperacute	Within minutes	Pre-existing recipient antibodies react to donor antigen (type II hypersensitivity reaction), activate complement.	Widespread thrombosis of graft vessels → ischemia/necrosis. Graft must be removed.
Acute	Weeks to months	Cellular: CD8+ T cells activated against donor MHCs (type IV hypersensitivity reaction). Humoral: similar to hyperacute, except antibodies develop after transplant.	Vasculitis of graft vessels with dense interstitial lymphocytic infiltrate. Prevent/reverse with immunosuppressants.
Chronic	Months to years	CD4+ T cells respond to recipient APCs presenting donor peptides, including allogeneic MHC. Both cellular and humoral components (type II and IV hypersensitivity reactions).	Recipient T cells react and secrete cytokines → proliferation of vascular smooth muscle, parenchymal atrophy, interstitial fibrosis. Dominated by arteriosclerosis. Organ-specific examples: ▪ Bronchiolitis obliterans (lung) ▪ Accelerated atherosclerosis (heart) ▪ Chronic graft nephropathy (kidney) ▪ Vanishing bile duct syndrome (liver)
Graft-versus-host disease	Varies	Grafted immunocompetent T cells proliferate in the immunocompromised host and reject host cells with "foreign" proteins → severe organ dysfunction. Type IV hypersensitivity reaction.	Maculopapular rash, jaundice, diarrhea, hepatosplenomegaly. Usually in bone marrow and liver transplants (rich in lymphocytes). Potentially beneficial in bone marrow transplant for leukemia (graft-versus-tumor effect).

▶ IMMUNOLOGY—IMMUNOSUPPRESSANTS

Immunosuppressants Agents that block lymphocyte activation and proliferation. Reduce acute transplant rejection by suppressing cellular immunity. Frequently combined to achieve greater efficacy with ↓ toxicity. Chronic suppression ↑ risk of infection and malignancy.

DRUG	MECHANISM	USE	TOXICITY	NOTES
Cyclosporine	Calcineurin inhibitor; binds cyclophilin. Blocks T-cell activation by **preventing IL-2 transcription.**	Transplant rejection prophylaxis, psoriasis, rheumatoid arthritis.	**Nephrotoxicity,** hypertension, hyperlipidemia, neurotoxicity, gingival hyperplasia, hirsutism.	Both calcineurin inhibitors are highly nephrotoxic.
Tacrolimus (FK506)	Calcineurin inhibitor; binds FK506 binding protein (FKBP). Blocks T-cell activation by **preventing IL-2 transcription.**	Transplant rejection prophylaxis.	Similar to cyclosporine, ↑ risk of diabetes and neurotoxicity; no gingival hyperplasia or hirsutism.	
Sirolimus (Rapamycin)	mTOR inhibitor; binds FKBP. Blocks T-cell activation and B-cell differentiation by **preventing response to IL-2.**	Kidney transplant rejection prophylaxis.	"PanSirtopenia" (pancytopenia), insulin resistance, hyperlipidemia; **not nephrotoxic.**	Kidney "sir-vives." Synergistic with cyclosporine. Also used in drug-eluting stents.
Daclizumab, basiliximab	Monoclonal antibodies; block IL-2R.	Kidney transplant rejection prophylaxis.	Edema, hypertension, tremor.	
Azathioprine	Antimetabolite precursor of 6-mercaptopurine. Inhibits lymphocyte proliferation by blocking nucleotide synthesis.	Transplant rejection prophylaxis, rheumatoid arthritis, Crohn disease, glomerulonephritis, other autoimmune conditions.	Leukopenia, anemia, thrombocytopenia.	6-MP degraded by xanthine oxidase; toxicity ↑ by allopurinol. Pronounce "azathio-purine."
Mycophenolate mofetil	Reversibly inhibits IMP dehydrogenase, preventing purine synthesis of B and T cells.	Transplant rejection prophylaxis, lupus nephritis.	GI upset, pancytopenia, hypertension, hyperglycemia. Less nephrotoxic and neurotoxic.	Associated with invasive CMV infection.
Corticosteroids	Inhibit NF-κB. Suppress both B- and T-cell function by ↓ transcription of many cytokines. Induce apoptosis of T lymphocytes.	Transplant rejection prophylaxis, many autoimmune and inflammatory disorders.	Hyperglycemia, osteoporosis, central obesity, muscle breakdown, psychosis, acne, hypertension, cataracts, avascular necrosis (femoral head).	Can cause iatrogenic Cushing syndrome.

Immunosuppression targets

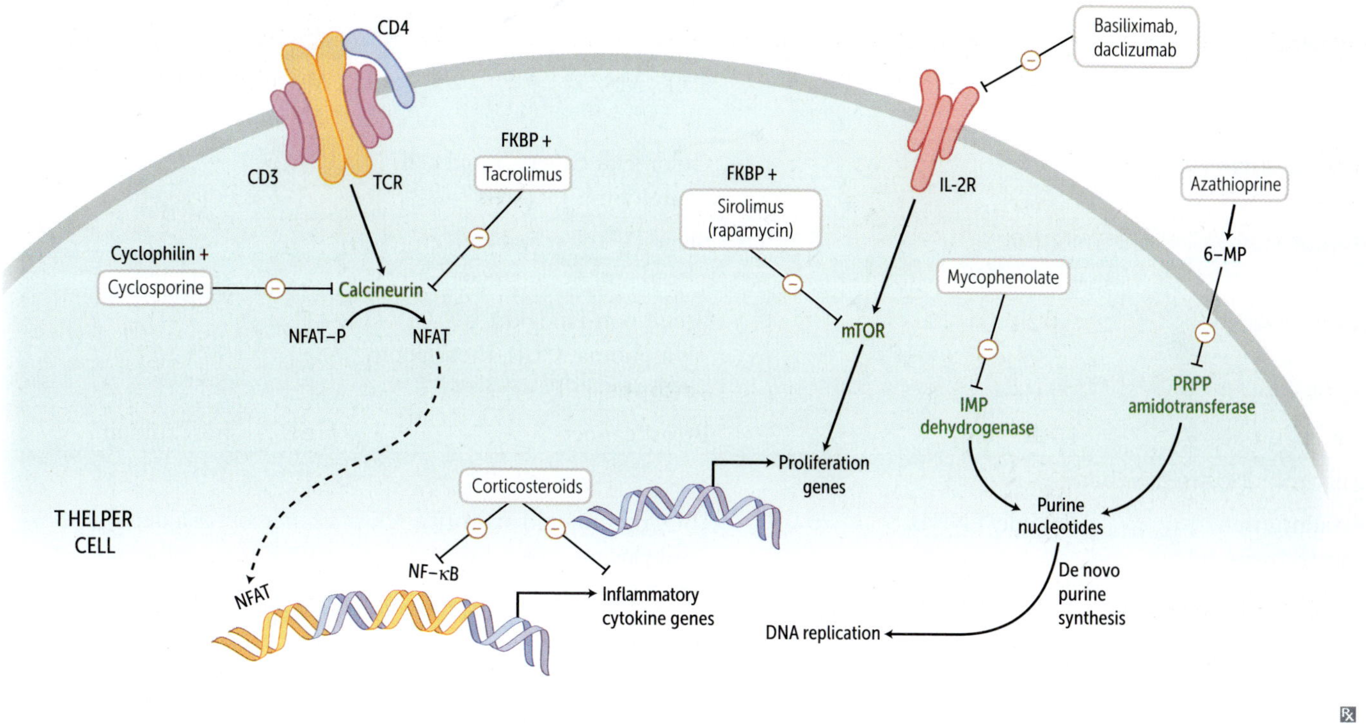

Recombinant cytokines and clinical uses

AGENT	CLINICAL USES
Aldesleukin (IL-2)	Renal cell carcinoma, metastatic melanoma
Epoetin alfa (erythropoietin)	Anemias (especially in renal failure)
Filgrastim (G-CSF)	Recovery of bone marrow
Sargramostim (GM-CSF)	Recovery of bone marrow
IFN-α	Chronic hepatitis B and C, Kaposi sarcoma, malignant melanoma
IFN-β	Multiple sclerosis
IFN-γ	Chronic granulomatous disease
Romiplostim, eltrombopag (thrombopoietin receptor agonists)	Thrombocytopenia
Oprelvekin (IL-11)	Thrombocytopenia

Therapeutic antibodies

AGENT	TARGET	CLINICAL USE	NOTES
Cancer therapy			
Alemtuzumab	CD52	CLL, MS	"Alymtuzumab"—chronic lymphocytic leukemia
Bevacizumab	VEGF	Colorectal cancer, renal cell carcinoma	
Cetuximab	EGFR	Stage IV colorectal cancer, head and neck cancer	
Rituximab	CD20	B-cell non-Hodgkin lymphoma, CLL, rheumatoid arthritis, ITP	
Trastuzumab	HER2/neu	Breast cancer	HER2—"tras2zumab"
Autoimmune disease therapy			
Adalimumab, certolizumab, infliximab	Soluble TNF-α	IBD, rheumatoid arthritis, ankylosing spondylitis, psoriasis	Etanercept is a decoy TNF-α receptor and not a monoclonal antibody
Eculizumab	Complement protein C5	Paroxysmal nocturnal hemoglobinuria	
Natalizumab	α4-integrin	Multiple sclerosis, Crohn disease	α4-integrin: WBC adhesion Risk of PML in patients with JC virus
Other applications			
Abciximab	Platelet glycoproteins **IIb/IIIa**	Antiplatelet agent for prevention of ischemic complications in patients undergoing percutaneous coronary intervention	**IIb** times **IIIa** equals "ab**six**imab"
Denosumab	RANKL	Osteoporosis; inhibits osteoclast maturation (mimics osteoprotegerin)	Den**os**umab affects **os**teoclasts
Digoxin immune Fab	Digoxin	Antidote for digoxin toxicity	
Omalizumab	IgE	Allergic asthma; prevents IgE binding to FcεRI	
Palivizumab	RSV F protein	RSV prophylaxis for high-risk infants	Pali**VI**zumab—**VI**rus
Ranibizumab, bevacizumab	VEGF	Neovascular age-related macular degeneration	

HIGH-YIELD PRINCIPLES IN

Pathology

"Digressions, objections, delight in mockery, carefree mistrust are signs of health; everything unconditional belongs in pathology."

—Friedrich Nietzsche

The fundamental principles of pathology are key to understanding diseases in all organ systems. Major topics such as inflammation and neoplasia appear frequently in questions across different organ systems, and such topics are definitely high yield. For example, the concepts of cell injury and inflammation are key to understanding the inflammatory response that follows myocardial infarction, a very common subject of board questions. Similarly, a familiarity with the early cellular changes that culminate in the development of neoplasias—for example, esophageal or colon cancer—is critical. Finally, make sure you recognize the major tumor-associated genes and are comfortable with key cancer concepts such as tumor staging and metastasis.

▶ PATHOLOGY—INFLAMMATION

Apoptosis

ATP-dependent programmed cell death. Intrinsic or extrinsic pathway; both pathways → activation of cytosolic proteases called caspases that mediate cellular breakdown → cell shrinkage, chromatin condensation, membrane blebbing, and formation of apoptotic bodies, which are then phagocytosed.

Characterized by deeply eosinophilic cytoplasm and basophilic nucleus, pyknosis (nuclear shrinkage), and karyorrhexis (fragmentation caused by endonucleases cleaving at internucleosomal regions). DNA laddering (fragments in multiples of 180 bp) is a sensitive indicator of apoptosis.

Cell membrane typically remains intact without significant inflammation (unlike necrosis).

Intrinsic (mitochondrial) pathway

Involved in tissue remodeling in embryogenesis. Occurs when a regulating factor is withdrawn from a proliferating cell population (eg, ↓ IL-2 after a completed immunologic reaction → apoptosis of proliferating effector cells). Also occurs after exposure to injurious stimuli (eg, radiation, toxins, hypoxia).

Regulated by Bcl-2 family of proteins such as BAX and BAK (proapoptotic) and Bcl-2 (antiapoptotic).

Bcl-2 prevents cytochrome c release by binding to and inhibiting APAF-1. APAF-1 normally binds cytochrome c and induces activation of caspase 9, initiating caspase cascade. If Bcl-2 is overexpressed (eg, follicular lymphoma t[14;18]), then APAF-1 is overly inhibited, → ↓ caspase activation and tumorigenesis.

Extrinsic (death receptor) pathway

2 pathways:

- Ligand receptor interactions (FasL binding to Fas [CD95] or TNF-α binding to TNF)
- Immune cell (cytotoxic T-cell release of perforin and granzyme B)

Fas-FasL interaction is necessary in thymic medullary negative selection. Mutations in Fas ↑ numbers of circulating self-reacting lymphocytes due to failure of clonal deletion.

Defective Fas-FasL interactions cause autoimmune lymphoproliferative syndrome.

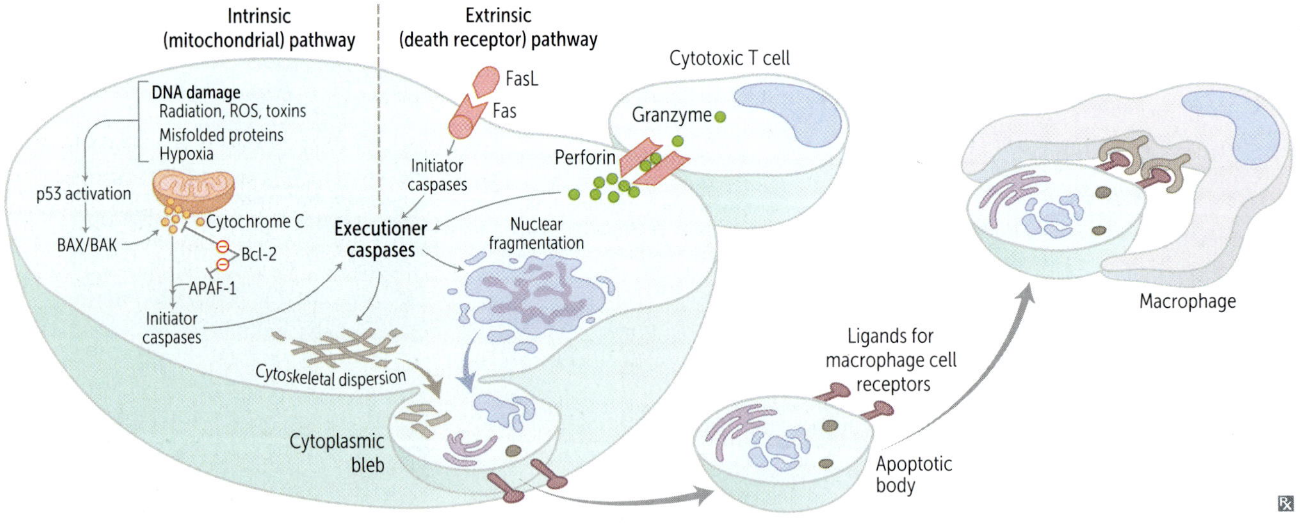

Necrosis

Enzymatic degradation and protein denaturation of cell due to exogenous injury → intracellular components leak. Inflammatory process (unlike apoptosis).

TYPE	SEEN IN	DUE TO	HISTOLOGY
Coagulative	Ischemia/infarcts in most tissues (except brain)	Ischemia or infarction; proteins denature, then enzymatic degradation	Cell outlines preserved; ↑ cytoplasmic binding of acidophilic dyes A
Liquefactive	Bacterial abscesses, brain infarcts (due to ↑ fat content)	Neutrophils release lysosomal enzymes that digest the tissue B; enzymatic degradation first, then proteins denature	Early: cellular debris and macrophages Late: cystic spaces and cavitation (brain) Neutrophils and cell debris seen with bacterial infection
Caseous	TB, systemic fungi (eg, *Histoplasma capsulatum*), *Nocardia*	Macrophages wall off the infecting microorganism → granular debris C	Fragmented cells and debris surrounded by lymphocytes and macrophages
Fat	Enzymatic: acute pancreatitis (saponification of peripancreatic fat) Nonenzymatic: traumatic (eg, breast injury)	Damaged cells release lipase, which breaks down triglycerides in fat cells	Outlines of dead fat cells without peripheral nuclei; saponification of fat (combined with Ca^{2+}) appears dark blue on H&E stain D
Fibrinoid	Immune reactions in vessels (eg, polyarteritis nodosa, giant cell [temporal] arteritis)	Immune complexes combine with fibrin → vessel wall damage	Vessel walls are thick and pink E
Gangrenous	Distal extremity, after chronic ischemia	Dry: ischemia F	Coagulative
		Wet: superinfection	Liquefactive superimposed on coagulative

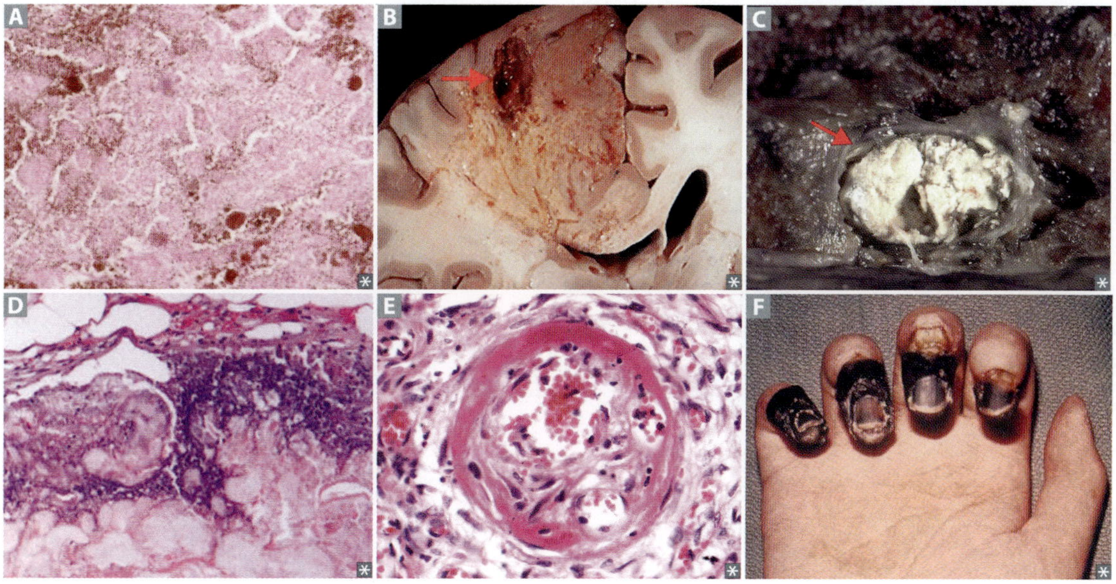

Cell injury

REVERSIBLE WITH O_2	IRREVERSIBLE
Cellular/mitochondrial swelling (↓ ATP → ↓ activity of Na^+/K^+ pumps)	Mitochondrial permeability/vacuolization; phospholipid-containing amorphous densities within mitochondria (swelling alone is reversible)
Nuclear chromatin clumping	Nuclear pyknosis (condensation), karyorrhexis (fragmentation), karyolysis (fading)
Membrane blebbing	Plasma membrane damage (degradation of membrane phospholipid)
↓ glycogen	Lysosomal rupture
Fatty change	
Ribosomal/polysomal detachment (↓ protein synthesis)	

Ischemia

Inadequate blood supply to meet demand.
Regions most vulnerable to hypoxia/ischemia and subsequent infarction:

ORGAN	REGION
Brain	ACA/MCA/PCA boundary areas[a,b]
Heart	Subendocardium (LV)
Kidney	Straight segment of proximal tubule (medulla) Thick ascending limb (medulla)
Liver	Area around central vein (zone III)
Colon	Splenic flexure,[a] rectum[a]

[a]Watershed areas (border zones) receive blood supply from most distal branches of 2 arteries with limited collateral vascularity. These areas are susceptible to ischemia from hypoperfusion.
[b]Neurons most vulnerable to hypoxic-ischemic insults include Purkinje cells of the cerebellum and pyramidal cells of the hippocampus and neocortex.

Infarcts: red vs pale

Red 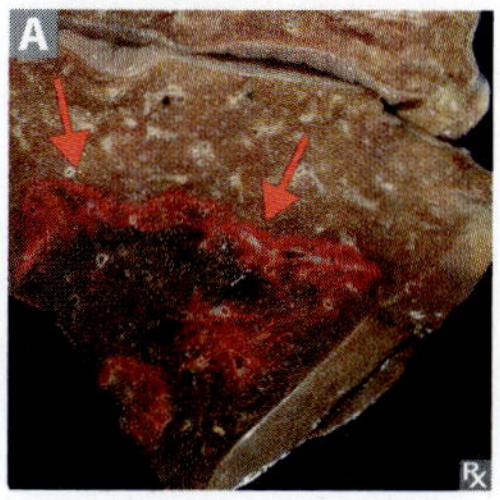	Red (hemorrhagic) infarcts **A** occur in venous occlusion and tissues with multiple blood supplies, such as liver, lung, intestine, testes; reperfusion (eg, after angioplasty). Reperfusion injury is due to damage by free radicals. Red = reperfusion.
Pale 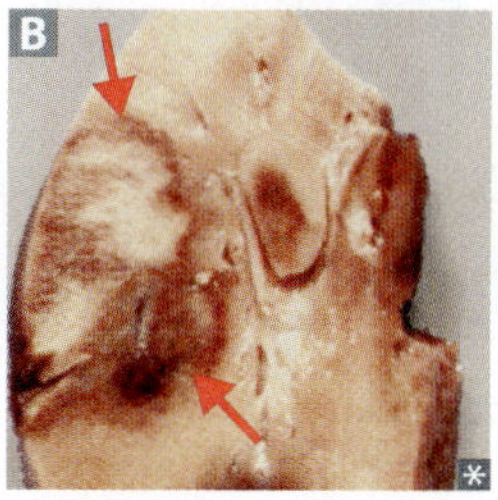	Pale (anemic) infarcts **B** occur in solid organs with a single (end-arterial) blood supply, such as heart, kidney, and spleen.

Inflammation	Characterized by *rubor* (redness), *dolor* (pain), *calor* (heat), *tumor* (swelling), and *functio laesa* (loss of function).
Vascular component	↑ vascular permeability, vasodilation, endothelial injury.
Cellular component	Neutrophils extravasate from circulation to injured tissue to participate in inflammation through phagocytosis, degranulation, and inflammatory mediator release.
Acute	Neutrophil, eosinophil, and antibody mediated. Acute inflammation is rapid onset (seconds to minutes) and of short duration (minutes to days). Outcomes include complete resolution, abscess formation, or progression to chronic inflammation.
Chronic	Mononuclear cell (monocytes/macrophages, lymphocytes, plasma cells) and fibroblast mediated. Characterized by persistent destruction and repair. Associated with blood vessel proliferation, fibrosis. Granuloma: nodular collections of epithelioid macrophages and giant cells. Outcomes include scarring and amyloidosis.

Chromatolysis

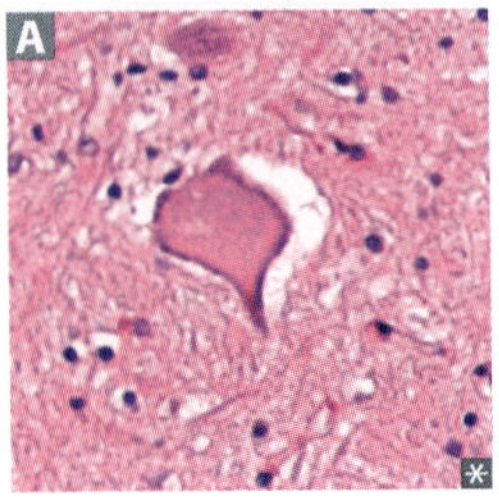

Reaction of neuronal cell body to axonal injury. Changes reflect ↑ protein synthesis in effort to repair the damaged axon. Characterized by:

- Round cellular swelling A
- Displacement of the nucleus to the periphery
- Dispersion of Nissl substance throughout cytoplasm

Concurrent with Wallerian degeneration—degeneration of axon distal to site of injury. Macrophages remove debris and myelin.

Types of calcification

Dystrophic calcification

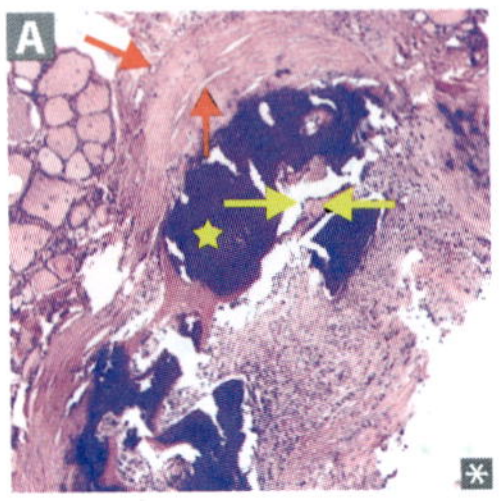

Ca^{2+} deposition in **abnormal tissues** 2° to injury or necrosis.

Tends to be localized (eg, calcific aortic stenosis). A shows dystrophic calcification (yellow star), small bony tissue (yellow arrows), and thick fibrotic wall (red arrows).

Seen in TB (lungs and pericardium), liquefactive necrosis of chronic abscesses, fat necrosis, infarcts, thrombi, schistosomiasis, Mönckeberg arteriolosclerosis, congenital CMV + toxoplasmosis, psammoma bodies.

Is not directly associated with serum Ca^{2+} levels (patients are usually **normocalcemic**).

Metastatic calcification

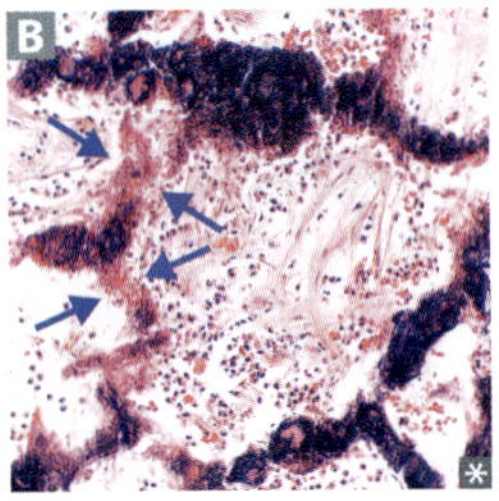

Widespread (ie, diffuse, metastatic) deposition of Ca^{2+} in **normal tissue** 2° to hypercalcemia (eg, 1° hyperparathyroidism, sarcoidosis, hypervitaminosis D) or high calcium-phosphate product levels (eg, chronic renal failure with 2° hyperparathyroidism, long-term dialysis, calciphylaxis, warfarin).

B shows metastatic calcifications of alveolar walls in acute pneumonitis (blue arrows).

Ca^{2+} deposits predominantly in interstitial tissues of kidney, lung, and gastric mucosa (these tissues lose acid quickly; ↑ pH favors deposition).

Patients are usually **not normocalcemic**.

Leukocyte extravasation

Extravasation predominantly occurs at postcapillary venules.
WBCs exit from blood vessels at sites of tissue injury and inflammation in 4 steps:

STEP	VASCULATURE/STROMA	LEUKOCYTE
❶ Margination and rolling—defective in leukocyte adhesion deficiency type 2 (↓ Sialyl-Lewis^X)	E-selectin P-selectin GlyCAM-1, CD34	Sialyl-Lewis^X Sialyl-Lewis^X L-selectin
❷ Tight-binding—defective in leukocyte adhesion deficiency type 1 (↓ CD18 integrin subunit)	ICAM-1 (CD54) VCAM-1 (CD106)	CD11/18 integrins (LFA-1, Mac-1) VLA-4 integrin
❸ Diapedesis—WBC travels between endothelial cells and exits blood vessel	PECAM-1 (CD31)	PECAM-1 (CD31)
❹ Migration—WBC travels through interstitium to site of injury or infection guided by chemotactic signals	Chemotactic products released in response to bacteria: C5a, IL-8, LTB_4, kallikrein, platelet-activating factor	Various

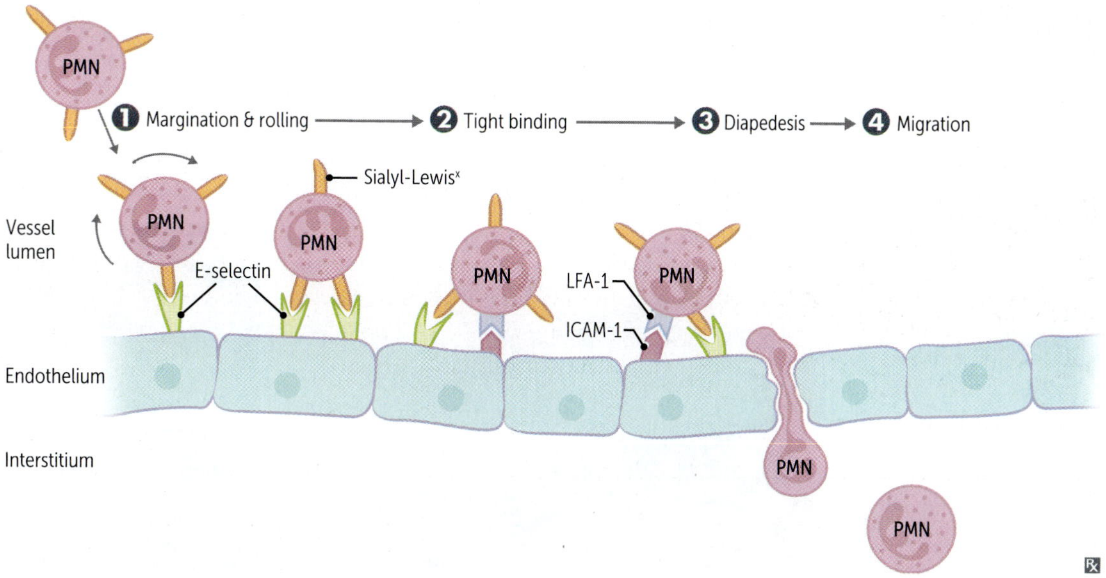

Free radical injury

Free radicals damage cells via membrane lipid peroxidation, protein modification, and DNA breakage.
Initiated via radiation exposure (eg, cancer therapy), metabolism of drugs (phase I), redox reactions, nitric oxide, transition metals, WBC (eg, neutrophils, macrophages) oxidative burst.
Free radicals can be eliminated by scavenging enzymes (eg, catalase, superoxide dismutase, glutathione peroxidase), spontaneous decay, antioxidants (eg, vitamins A, C, E), and certain metal carrier proteins (eg, transferrin, ceruloplasmin).
Examples:
- Oxygen toxicity: retinopathy of prematurity (abnormal vascularization), bronchopulmonary dysplasia
- Drug/chemical toxicity: carbon tetrachloride and acetaminophen overdose (hepatotoxicity)
- Metal storage diseases: hemochromatosis (iron) and Wilson disease (copper)

Inhalational injury and sequelae

Pulmonary complication associated with smoke and fire. Caused by heat, particulates (< 1 μm diameter), or irritants (eg, NH_3) → chemical tracheobronchitis, edema, pneumonia, ARDS. Many patients present 2° to burns, CO inhalation, or arsenic poisoning.

Bronchoscopy shows severe edema, congestion of bronchus, and soot deposition (A, 18 hours after inhalation injury; B, resolution at 11 days after injury).

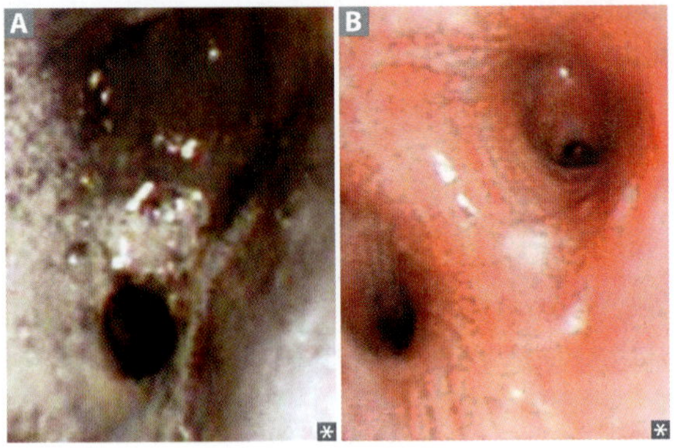

Scar formation

70–80% of tensile strength regained at 3 months; little additional tensile strength will be regained afterward.

SCAR TYPE	Hypertrophic A	Keloid B
COLLAGEN SYNTHESIS	↑	↑↑↑
COLLAGEN ORGANIZATION	Parallel	Disorganized
EXTENT OF SCAR	Confined to borders of original wound	Extends beyond borders of original wound with "clawlike" projections
SCAR EVOLUTION OVER YEARS	Possible spontaneous regression	Possible progressive growth
RECURRENCE	Infrequent	Frequent
PREDISPOSITION	None	↑ incidence in ethnic groups with darker skin

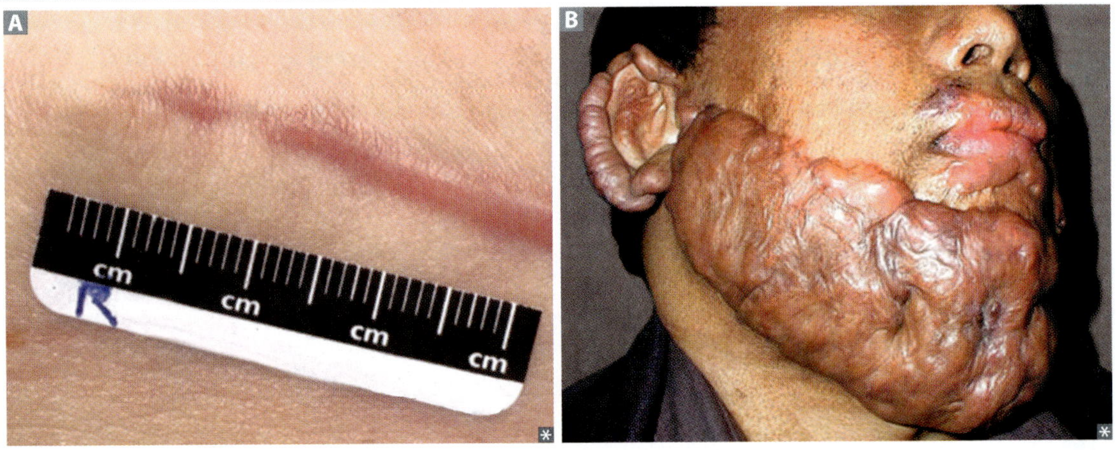

Wound healing

Tissue mediators

MEDIATOR	ROLE
PDGF	Secreted by activated platelets and macrophages Induces vascular remodeling and smooth muscle cell migration Stimulates fibroblast growth for collagen synthesis
FGF	Stimulates angiogenesis
EGF	Stimulates cell growth via tyrosine kinases (eg, EGFR/*ErbB1*)
TGF-β	Angiogenesis, fibrosis, cell cycle arrest
Metalloproteinases	Tissue remodeling
VEGF	Stimulates angiogenesis

PHASE OF WOUND HEALING	EFFECTOR CELLS	CHARACTERISTICS
Inflammatory (up to 3 days after wound)	Platelets, neutrophils, macrophages	Clot formation, ↑ vessel permeability and neutrophil migration into tissue; macrophages clear debris 2 days later
Proliferative (day 3–weeks after wound)	Fibroblasts, myofibroblasts, endothelial cells, keratinocytes, macrophages	Deposition of granulation tissue and type III collagen, angiogenesis, epithelial cell proliferation, dissolution of clot, and wound contraction (mediated by myofibroblasts)
Remodeling (1 week–6+ months after wound)	Fibroblasts	Type III collagen replaced by type I collagen, ↑ tensile strength of tissue

Granulomatous diseases

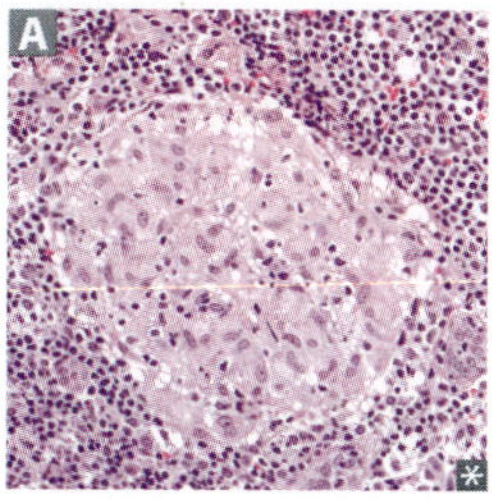

Bacterial:
- *Mycobacteria* (tuberculosis, leprosy)
- *Bartonella henselae* (cat scratch disease)
- *Listeria monocytogenes* (granulomatosis infantiseptica)
- *Treponema pallidum* (3° syphilis)

Fungal: endemic mycoses (eg, histoplasmosis)

Parasitic: schistosomiasis

Chronic granulomatous disease

Autoinflammatory:
- Sarcoidosis A
- Crohn disease
- Primary biliary cirrhosis
- Subacute (de Quervain/granulomatous) thyroiditis
- Granulomatosis with polyangiitis (Wegener)
- Eosinophilic granulomatosis with polyangiitis (Churg-Strauss)
- Giant cell (temporal) arteritis
- Takayasu arteritis

Foreign material: berylliosis, talcosis, hypersensitivity pneumonitis

Th_1 cells secrete IFN-γ, activating macrophages. TNF-α from macrophages induces and maintains granuloma formation. Anti-TNF drugs can, as a side effect, cause sequestering granulomas to break down, leading to disseminated disease. Always test for latent TB before starting anti-TNF therapy.

Associated with hypercalcemia due to calcitriol (1,25-$[OH]_2$ vitamin D_3) production.

Caseating necrosis more common with infectious causes (eg, TB). Diagnosing sarcoidosis requires noncaseating granulomas on biopsy.

Exudate vs transudate

Exudate ("Thick...")	Transudate ("and thin")
Cellular (cloudy)	Hypocellular (clear)
↑ protein, ↑ LDH (vs serum)	↓ protein, ↓ LDH (vs serum)
Specific gravity > 1.020	Specific gravity < 1.012
Due to: ▪ Lymphatic obstruction (chylous) ▪ Inflammation/infection ▪ Malignancy	Due to: ▪ ↑ hydrostatic pressure (eg, HF, Na^+ retention) ▪ ↓ oncotic pressure (eg, cirrhosis, nephrotic syndrome)

Erythrocyte sedimentation rate

Products of inflammation (eg, fibrinogen) coat RBCs and cause aggregation. The denser RBC aggregates fall at a faster rate within a pipette tube. Often co-tested with CRP levels.

↑ ESR	↓ ESR
Most anemias Infections Inflammation (eg, giant cell [temporal] arteritis, polymyalgia rheumatica) Cancer (eg, metastases, multiple myeloma) Renal disease (end-stage or nephrotic syndrome) Pregnancy	Sickle cell anemia (altered shape) Polycythemia (↑ RBCs "dilute" aggregation factors) HF Microcytosis Hypofibrinogenemia

Amyloidosis

Abnormal aggregation of proteins(or their fragments) into β-pleated linear sheets → damage and apoptosis. Amyloid deposits visualized by Congo red stain A, polarized light (apple green birefringence) B, and H&E stain (C shows deposits in glomerular mesangial areas [white arrows], tubular basement membranes [black arrows]).

COMMON TYPES	DESCRIPTION
AL (primary)	Due to deposition of proteins from Ig **L**ight chains. Can occur as a plasma cell disorder or associated with multiple myeloma. Often affects multiple organ systems, including renal (nephrotic syndrome), cardiac (restrictive cardiomyopathy, arrhythmia), hematologic (easy bruising, splenomegaly), GI (hepatomegaly), and neurologic (neuropathy).
AA (secondary)	Seen with chronic inflammatory conditions such as rheumatoid arthritis, IBD, spondyloarthropathy, familial Mediterranean fever, protracted infection. Fibrils composed of serum **A**myloid **A**. Often multisystem like AL amyloidosis.
Dialysis-related	Fibrils composed of β_2-microglobulin in patients with ESRD and/or on long-term dialysis. May present as carpal tunnel syndrome.
Heritable	Heterogeneous group of disorders, including familial amyloid polyneuropathies due to transthyretin gene mutation.
Age-related (senile) systemic	Due to deposition of normal (wild-type) transthyretin (TTR) predominantly in cardiac ventricles. Slower progression of cardiac dysfunction relative to AL amyloidosis.
Organ-specific	Amyloid deposition localized to a single organ. Most important form is amyloidosis in Alzheimer disease due to deposition of β-amyloid protein cleaved from amyloid precursor protein (APP). Islet amyloid polypeptide (IAPP) is commonly seen in diabetes mellitus type 2 and is caused by deposition of amylin in pancreatic islets. Isolated atrial amyloidosis due to atrial natriuretic peptide is common in normal aging.

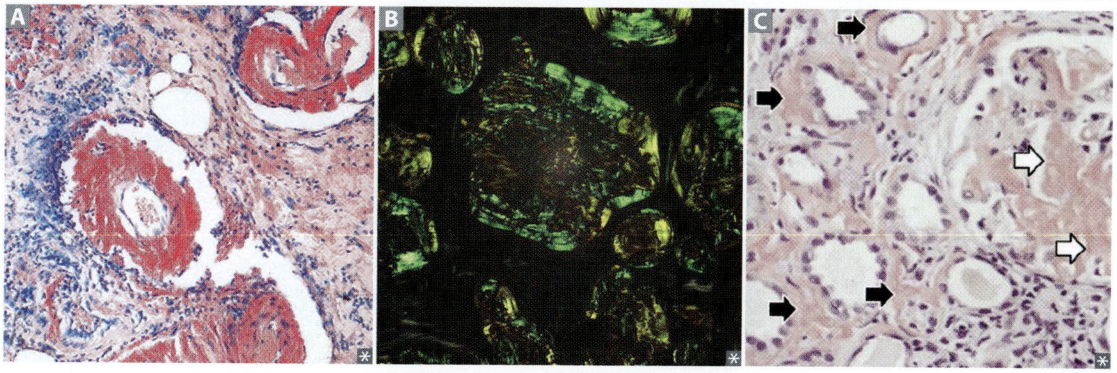

Lipofuscin

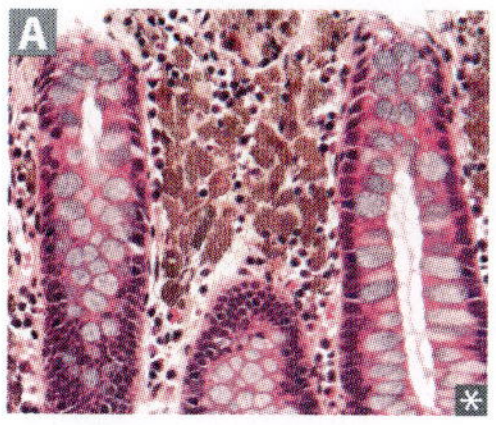

A yellow-brown "wear and tear" pigment associated with normal aging.
Formed by oxidation and polymerization of autophagocytosed organellar membranes.
Autopsy of elderly person will reveal deposits in heart, colon A, liver, kidney, eye, and other organs.

▶ PATHOLOGY—NEOPLASIA

Reactive cellular changes

Atrophy	↓ in tissue mass due to ↓ in size and/or number of cells. Causes include disuse, denervation, loss of blood supply, loss of hormonal stimulation, poor nutrition.
Hypertrophy	↑ in size of cells.
Hyperplasia	↑ in number of cells. May be a risk factor for future malignancy (eg, endometrial hyperplasia) but not considered premalignant.
Metaplasia	Replacement of one cell type by another. Usually due to exposure to an irritant, such as gastric acid or cigarette smoke. Reversible if the irritant is removed but may undergo malignant transformation with persistent insult (eg, Barrett esophagus → esophageal adenocarcinoma).

Preneoplastic and neoplastic cellular changes

Neoplasia	Uncontrolled, clonal proliferation of cells. Can be benign or malignant.
Dysplasia	Disordered, non-neoplastic cell growth. Used only with epithelial cells. Mild dysplasia is usually reversible; severe dysplasia usually progresses to carcinoma in situ.
Differentiation	The degree to which a malignant tumor resembles its tissue of origin. Well-differentiated tumors closely resemble their tissue of origin; poorly differentiated look almost nothing like their tissue of origin.
Anaplasia	Complete lack of differentiation of cells in a malignant neoplasm.

Neoplastic progression

Hallmarks of cancer: evasion of apoptosis, growth signal self-sufficiency, anti-growth signal insensitivity, sustained angiogenesis, limitless replicative potential, tissue invasion, and metastasis.

Normal cells

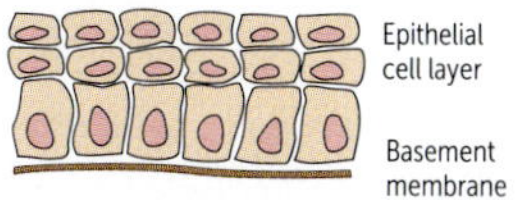

Normal cells with basal → apical differentiation. See cervical example A, which shows normal cells and spectrum of dysplasia, as discussed below.

Dysplasia

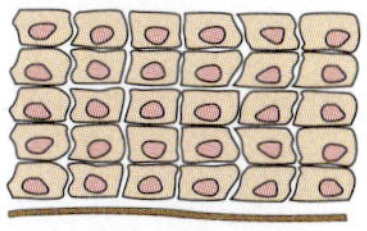

Abnormal proliferation of cells with loss of size, shape, and orientation. Compare vs hyperplasia (cells ↑ in number).

Carcinoma in situ/ preinvasive

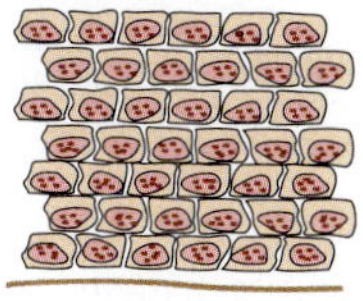

Neoplastic cells have not invaded the intact basement membrane.
↑ nuclear/cytoplasmic (N/C) ratio and clumped chromatin.
Neoplastic cells encompass entire thickness.

Invasive carcinoma

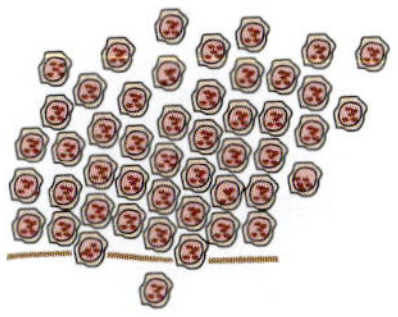

Cells have invaded basement membrane using collagenases and hydrolases (metalloproteinases).
Cell-cell contacts lost by inactivation of E-cadherin.

Metastasis

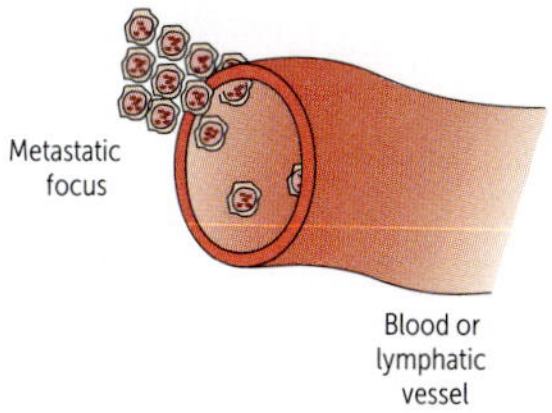

Spread to distant organ, eg, metastatic cells in liver parenchyma.
"Seed and soil" theory of metastasis:

- Seed = tumor embolus.
- Soil = target organ is often the first-encountered capillary bed (eg, liver, lungs, bone, brain, etc).

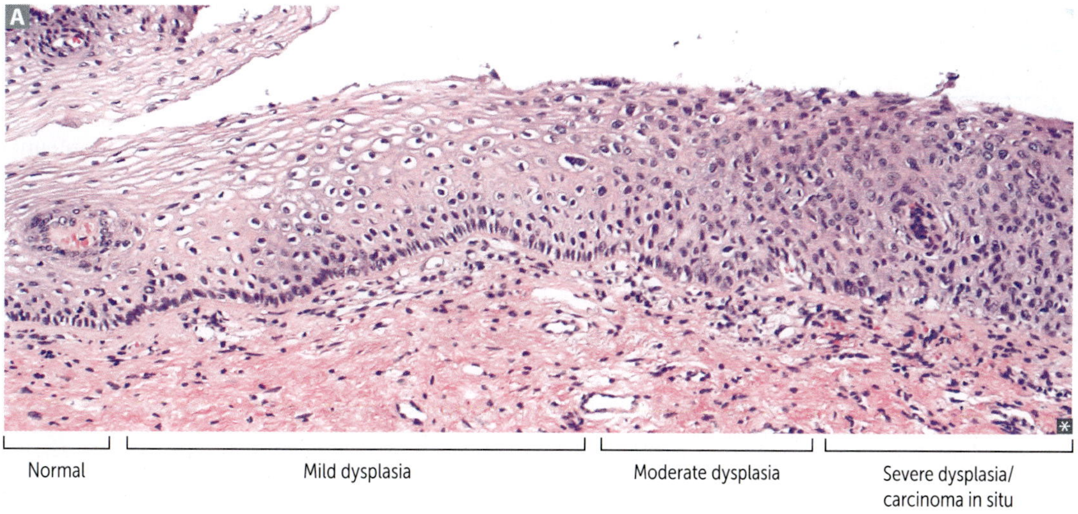

Tumor grade vs stage

Grade	Degree of cellular differentiation and mitotic activity on histology. Range from low grade (well differentiated) to high grade (poorly differentiated, undifferentiated or anaplastic).	Stage almost always has more prognostic value than grade.
Stage	Degree of localization/spread based on site and size of 1° lesion, spread to regional lymph nodes, presence of metastases. Based on clinical (c) or pathology (p) findings. Example: cT3N1M0	TNM staging system (**S**tage = **S**pread): **T** = **T**umor size **N** = **N**ode involvement **M** = **M**etastases Each TNM factor has independent prognostic value; M factor often most important.

Tumor nomenclature

Carcinoma implies epithelial origin, whereas **sarcoma** denotes mesenchymal origin. Both terms imply malignancy.

Terms for non-neoplastic malformations include hamartoma (disorganized overgrowth of tissues in their native location, eg, Peutz-Jeghers polyps) and choristoma (normal tissue in a foreign location, eg, gastric tissue located in distal ileum in Meckel diverticulum).

Benign tumor is usually well differentiated, well demarcated, low mitotic activity, no metastasis, no necrosis.

Malignant tumor may show poor differentiation, erratic growth, local invasion, metastasis, and ↓ apoptosis. Upregulation of telomerase prevents chromosome shortening and cell death.

CELL TYPE	BENIGN	MALIGNANT
Epithelium	Adenoma, papilloma	Adenocarcinoma, papillary carcinoma
Mesenchyme		
Blood cells		Leukemia, lymphoma
Blood vessels	Hemangioma	Angiosarcoma
Smooth muscle	Leiomyoma	Leiomyosarcoma
Striated muscle	Rhabdomyoma	Rhabdomyosarcoma
Connective tissue	Fibroma	Fibrosarcoma
Bone	Osteoma	Osteosarcoma
Fat	Lipoma	Liposarcoma
Melanocyte	Nevus/mole	Melanoma

Cancer epidemiology

Skin cancer (basal > squamous >> melanoma) is the most common cancer (not included in list).

	MALE	FEMALE	NOTES
Incidence	1. Prostate 2. Lung 3. Colon/rectum	1. Breast 2. Lung 3. Colon/rectum	Lung cancer incidence has dropped in men, but has not changed significantly in women.
Mortality	1. Lung 2. Prostate 3. Colon/rectum	1. Lung 2. Breast 3. Colon/rectum	Cancer is the 2nd leading cause of death in the United States (heart disease is 1st).

Paraneoplastic syndromes

MANIFESTATION	DESCRIPTION/MECHANISM	MOST COMMONLY ASSOCIATED CANCER(S)
Cutaneous		
Acanthosis nigricans	Hyperpigmented velvety plaques in axilla and neck	Gastric adenocarcinoma and other visceral malignancies (but more commonly associated with obesity and insulin resistance)
Sign of Leser-Trélat	Sudden onset of multiple seborrheic keratoses	GI adenocarcinomas and other visceral malignancies
Endocrine		
Hypercalcemia	PTHrP	Squamous cell carcinomas of lung, head, and neck; renal, bladder, breast, and ovarian carcinomas
	↑ 1,25-$(OH)_2$ vitamin D_3 (calcitriol)	Lymphoma
Cushing syndrome	↑ ACTH	Small cell lung cancer
Hyponatremia (SIADH)	↑ ADH	Small cell lung cancer
Hematologic		
Polycythemia	↑ Erythropoietin	Renal cell carcinoma, hepatocellular carcinoma, hemangioblastoma, pheochromocytoma, leiomyoma
Pure red cell aplasia	Anemia with low reticulocytes	Thymoma
Good syndrome	Hypogammaglobulinemia	Thymoma
Trousseau syndrome	Migratory superficial thrombophlebitis	Adenocarcinomas, especially pancreatic
Nonbacterial thrombotic (marantic) endocarditis	Deposition of sterile platelet thrombi on heart valves	Adenocarcinomas, especially pancreatic
Neuromuscular		
Anti-NMDA receptor encephalitis	Psychiatric disturbance, memory deficits, seizures, dyskinesias, autonomic instability, language dysfunction	Ovarian teratoma
Opsoclonus-myoclonus ataxia syndrome	"Dancing eyes, dancing feet"	Neuroblastoma (children), small cell lung cancer (adults)
Paraneoplastic cerebellar degeneration	Antibodies against Hu, Yo, and Tr antigens in Purkinje cells	Small cell lung cancer, gynecologic and breast cancers, and Hodgkin lymphoma
Paraneoplastic encephalomyelitis	Antibodies against Hu antigens in neurons	Small cell lung cancer
Lambert-Eaton myasthenic syndrome	Antibodies against presynaptic (P/Q-type) Ca^{2+} channels at NMJ	Small cell lung cancer
Myasthenia gravis	Antibodies against postsynaptic AChR at NMJ	Thymoma

Oncogenes Gain of function → ↑ cancer risk. Need damage to only 1 allele.

GENE	GENE PRODUCT	ASSOCIATED NEOPLASM
ALK	Receptor tyrosine kinase	Lung adenocarcinoma
BCR-ABL	Tyrosine kinase	CML, ALL
BCL-2	Antiapoptotic molecule (inhibits apoptosis)	Follicular and diffuse large B cell lymphomas
BRAF	Serine/threonine kinase	Melanoma, non-Hodgkin lymphoma
c-KIT	Cytokine receptor	Gastrointestinal stromal tumor (GIST)
c-MYC	Transcription factor	Burkitt lymphoma
HER2/neu (c-erbB2)	Tyrosine kinase	Breast and gastric carcinomas
JAK2	Tyrosine kinase	Chronic myeloproliferative disorders
KRAS	GTPase	Colon cancer, lung cancer, pancreatic cancer
MYCL1	Transcription factor	Lung tumor
MYCN	Transcription factor	Neuroblastoma
RET	Tyrosine kinase	MEN 2A and 2B, medullary thyroid cancer

Tumor suppressor genes Loss of function → ↑ cancer risk; both alleles must be lost for expression of disease.

GENE	ASSOCIATED CONDITION	GENE PRODUCT
APC	Colorectal cancer (associated with FAP)	
BRCA1/BRCA2	Breast and ovarian cancer	DNA repair protein
CDKN2A	Melanoma, pancreatic cancer	p16, blocks G_1 → S phase
DCC	Colon cancer	DCC—Deleted in Colon Cancer
DPC4/SMAD4	Pancreatic cancer	DPC—Deleted in Pancreatic Cancer
MEN1	MEN 1	Menin
NF1	NeuroFibromatosis type 1	Ras GTPase activating protein (neurofibromin)
NF2	NeuroFibromatosis type 2	Merlin (schwannomin) protein
PTEN	Breast cancer, prostate cancer, endometrial cancer	
Rb	Retinoblastoma, osteosarcoma	Inhibits E2F; blocks G_1 → S phase
TP53	Most human cancers, Li-Fraumeni syndrome	*p53*, activates p21, blocks G_1 → S phase
TSC1	Tuberous sclerosis	Hamartin protein
TSC2	Tuberous sclerosis	Tuberin protein
VHL	von Hippel-Lindau disease, renal cell carcinoma	Inhibits hypoxia inducible factor 1a
WT1/WT2	Wilms Tumor (nephroblastoma)	

Oncogenic microbes

Microbe	Associated cancer
EBV	Burkitt lymphoma, Hodgkin lymphoma, nasopharyngeal carcinoma, 1° CNS lymphoma (in immunocompromised patients)
HBV, HCV	Hepatocellular carcinoma, lymphoma
HHV-8	Kaposi sarcoma
HPV	Cervical and penile/anal carcinoma (types 16, 18), head and neck cancer
H pylori	Gastric adenocarcinoma and MALT lymphoma
HTLV-1	Adult T-cell leukemia/lymphoma
Liver fluke *(Clonorchis sinensis)*	Cholangiocarcinoma
Schistosoma haematobium	Bladder cancer (squamous cell)

Carcinogens

TOXIN	ORGAN	IMPACT
Aflatoxins (*Aspergillus*)	Liver	Hepatocellular carcinoma
Alkylating agents	Blood	Leukemia/lymphoma
Aromatic amines (eg, benzidine, 2-naphthylamine)	Bladder	Transitional cell carcinoma
Arsenic	Liver Lung Skin	Angiosarcoma Lung cancer Squamous cell carcinoma
Asbestos	Lung	Bronchogenic carcinoma > mesothelioma
Carbon tetrachloride	Liver	Centrilobular necrosis, fatty change
Cigarette smoke	Bladder Cervix Esophagus Kidney Larynx Lung Pancreas	Transitional cell carcinoma Cervical carcinoma Squamous cell carcinoma/adenocarcinoma Renal cell carcinoma Squamous cell carcinoma Squamous cell and small cell carcinoma Pancreatic adenocarcinoma
Ethanol	Esophagus Liver	Squamous cell carcinoma Hepatocellular carcinoma
Ionizing radiation	Thyroid	Papillary thyroid carcinoma
Nitrosamines (smoked foods)	Stomach	Gastric cancer
Radon	Lung	Lung cancer (2nd leading cause after cigarette smoke)
Vinyl chloride	Liver	Angiosarcoma

Psammoma bodies

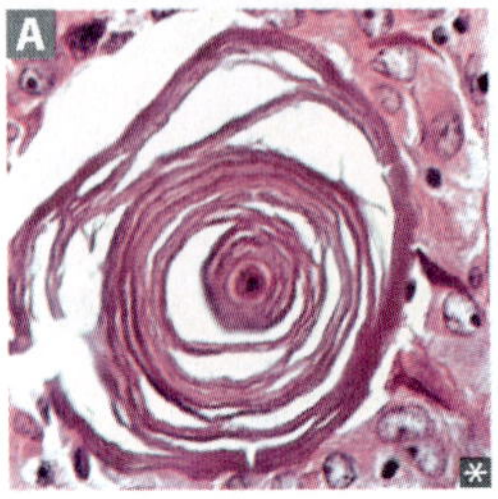

Laminated, concentric spherules with dystrophic calcification A, **PS**a**MM**oma bodies are seen in:
- **P**apillary carcinoma of thyroid
- **S**erous papillary cystadenocarcinoma of ovary
- **M**eningioma
- **M**alignant mesothelioma

Serum tumor markers

Tumor markers should not be used as the 1° tool for cancer diagnosis or screening. They may be used to monitor tumor recurrence and response to therapy, but definitive diagnosis is usually made via biopsy.

Alkaline phosphatase	Metastases to bone or liver, Paget disease of bone, seminoma (placental ALP).	
α-fetoprotein	Hepatocellular carcinoma, hepatoblastoma, yolk sac (endodermal sinus) tumor, mixed germ cell tumor.	Normally made by fetus. Transiently elevated in pregnancy. High levels associated with neural tube and abdominal wall defects, low levels associated with Down syndrome.
β-hCG	**H**ydatidiform moles and **C**horiocarcinomas (**G**estational trophoblastic disease), testicular cancer, mixed germ cell tumor.	Produced by syncytiotrophoblasts of the placenta.
CA 15-3/CA 27-29	Breast cancer.	
CA 19-9	Pancreatic adenocarcinoma.	
CA 125	Ovarian cancer.	
Calcitonin	Medullary thyroid carcinoma.	
CEA	**C**arcino**E**mbryonic **A**ntigen. Very nonspecific but produced by ~ 70% of colorectal and pancreatic cancers; also produced by gastric, breast, and medullary thyroid carcinomas.	
PSA	Prostate-specific antigen. Prostate cancer.	Can also be elevated in BPH and prostatitis. Questionable risk/benefit for screening.

P-glycoprotein

Also known as multidrug resistance protein 1 (MDR1). Classically seen in adrenal cell carcinoma but also expressed by other cancer cells (eg, colon, liver). Used to pump out toxins, including chemotherapeutic agents (one mechanism of ↓ responsiveness or resistance to chemotherapy over time).

Cachexia

Weight loss, muscle atrophy, and fatigue that occur in chronic disease (eg, cancer, AIDS, heart failure, COPD). Mediated by TNF, IFN-γ, IL-1, and IL-6.

Common metastases

Most sarcomas spread hematogenously; most carcinomas spread via lymphatics (except hepatocellular carcinoma, renal cell carcinoma, follicular thyroid carcinoma, and choriocarcinoma).

SITE OF METASTASIS	1° TUMOR	NOTES
Brain	Lung > breast > prostate > melanoma > GI.	50% of brain tumors are from metastases A B. Commonly seen as multiple well-circumscribed tumors at gray/white matter junction.
Liver	Colon >> stomach > pancreas.	Liver C D and lung are the most common sites of metastasis after the regional lymph nodes.
Bone	Prostate, breast > lung, thyroid, kidney.	Bone metastasis E F >> 1° bone tumors (eg, multiple myeloma, lytic). Common mets to bone: breast (mixed), lung (mixed), thyroid (lytic), kidney (lytic), prostate (blastic). Predilection for axial skeleton G.

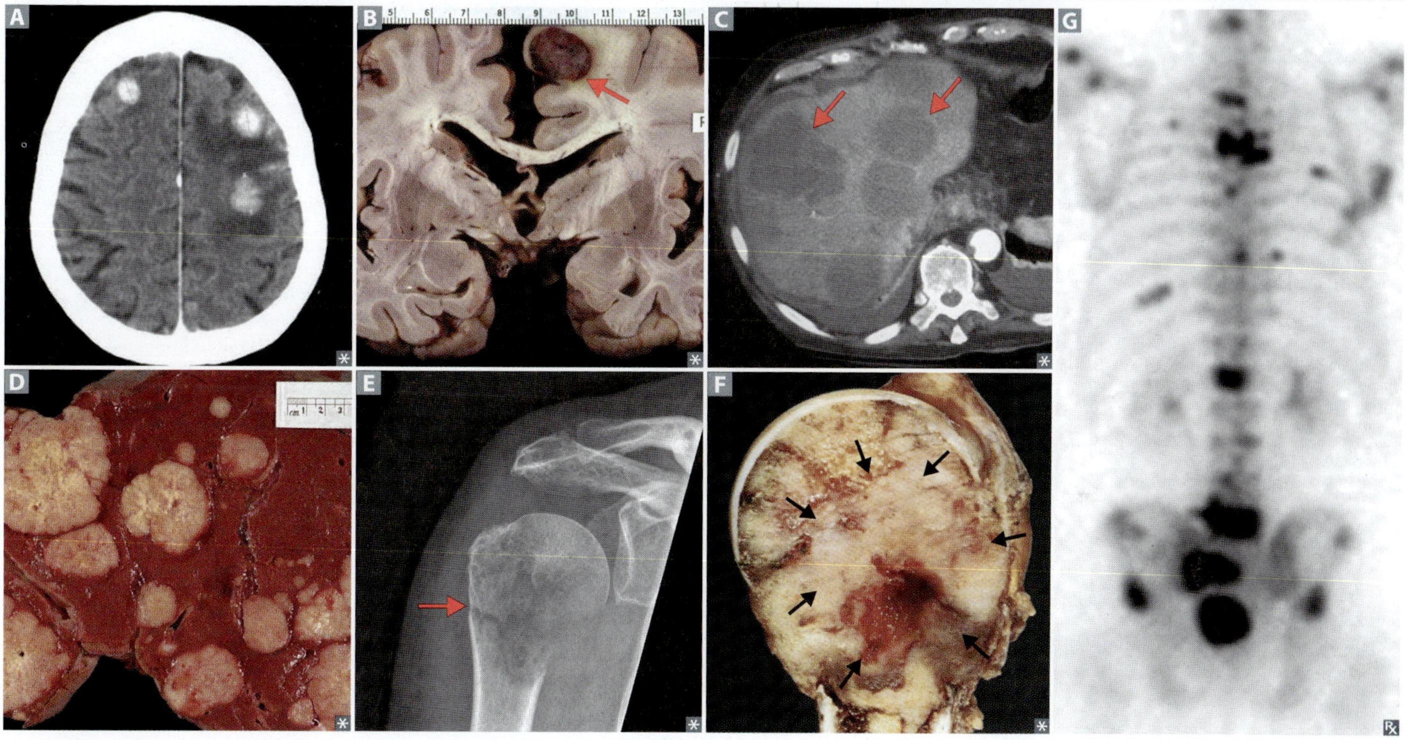

▶ NOTES

HIGH-YIELD PRINCIPLES IN

Pharmacology

"Take me, I am the drug; take me, I am hallucinogenic."

—Salvador Dali

"I was under medication when I made the decision not to burn the tapes."

—Richard Nixon

"I wondher why ye can always read a doctor's bill an' ye niver can read his purscription."

—Finley Peter Dunne

"Once you get locked into a serious drug collection, the tendency is to push it as far as you can."

—Hunter S. Thompson

Preparation for questions on pharmacology is straightforward. Memorizing all the key drugs and their characteristics (eg, mechanisms, clinical use, and important side effects) is high yield. Focus on understanding the prototype drugs in each class. Avoid memorizing obscure derivatives. Learn the "classic" and distinguishing toxicities of the major drugs. Specific drug dosages or trade names are generally not testable. Reviewing associated biochemistry, physiology, and microbiology can be useful while studying pharmacology. There is a strong emphasis on ANS, CNS, antimicrobial, and cardiovascular agents as well as on NSAIDs. Much of the material is clinically relevant. We occasionally mention drugs that are no longer available in the US, but help illustrate high-yield pharmacologic or disease mechanisms. They are highlighted as being of historical significance and should not appear on the USMLE. However, recently approved drugs are fair game for the exam.

so doesn't fill up easily

▶ PHARMACOLOGY—PHARMACOKINETICS & PHARMACODYNAMICS

Enzyme kinetics

↑Km = ↓ affinity. Glucose transp: GLUT2 — 300 (liver) GLUT4 — Fat 90 GLUT1 & 3 — 20 (BBB) & 10 neurons

Michaelis-Menten kinetics

K_m is inversely related to the affinity of the enzyme for its substrate.

V_{max} is directly proportional to the enzyme concentration.

Most enzymatic reactions follow a hyperbolic curve (ie, Michaelis-Menten kinetics); however, enzymatic reactions that exhibit a sigmoid curve usually indicate cooperative kinetics (eg, hemoglobin).

As u bind one it gets easier to bind more. The first step is the hardest then it becomes easy, then it saturates

[S] = concentration of substrate; V = velocity.

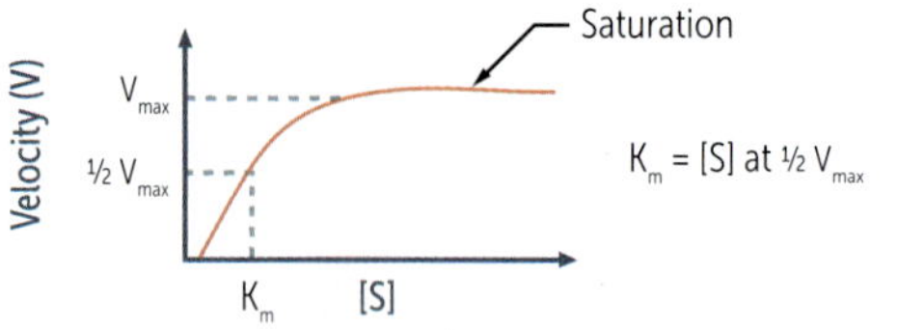

Effects of enzyme inhibition

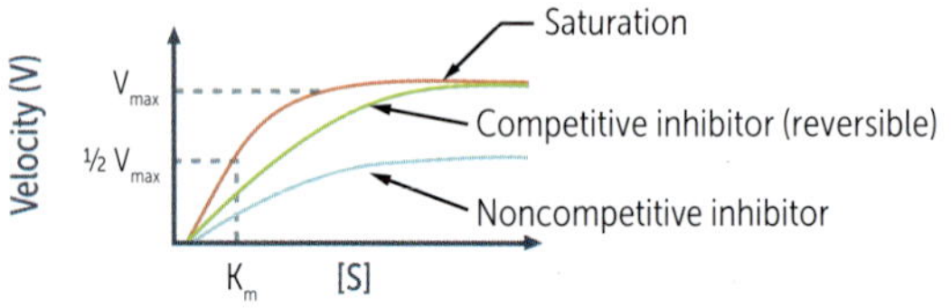

Lineweaver-Burk plot

↑ y-intercept, ↓ V_{max}.

The further to the right the x-intercept (ie, closer to zero), the greater the K_m and the lower the affinity.

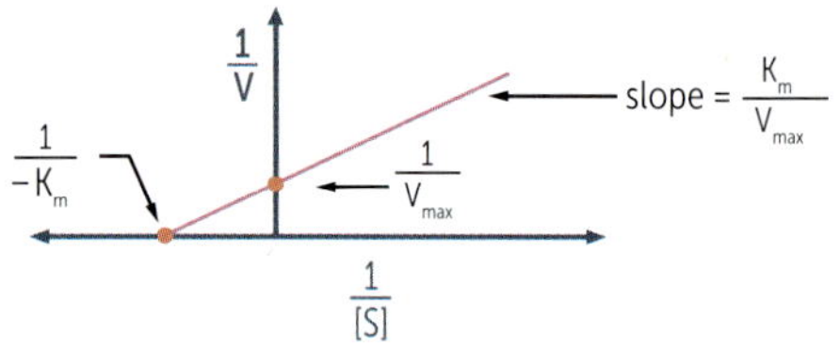

Reversible competitive inhibitors cross each other competitively, whereas noncompetitive inhibitors do not.

Effects of enzyme inhibition

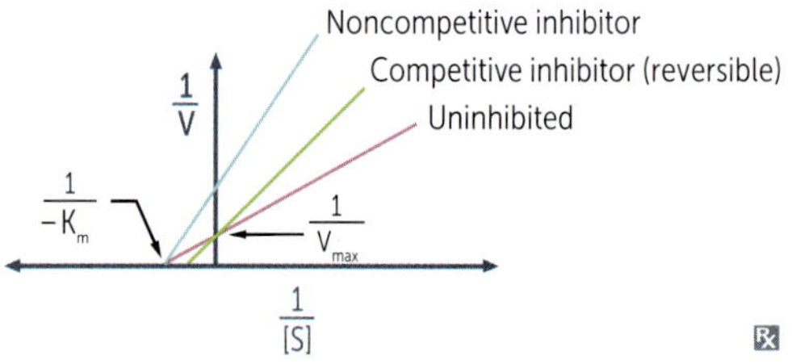

℞

	Competitive inhibitors, reversible	Competitive inhibitors, irreversible	Noncompetitive inhibitors
Resemble substrate	Yes	Yes	No
Overcome by ↑ [S]	Yes	No	No
Bind active site	Yes	Yes	No
Effect on V_{max}	Unchanged	↓	↓
Effect on K_m	↑	Unchanged	Unchanged
Pharmacodynamics	↓ potency	↓ efficacy	↓ efficacy

oh so not even activated?

Pharmacokinetics

Bioavailability (F)

Fraction of administered drug reaching systemic circulation unchanged. For an IV dose, F = 100%. Orally: F typically < 100% due to incomplete absorption and first-pass metabolism.

Volume of distribution (V_d)

Theoretical volume occupied by the total amount of drug in the body relative to its plasma concentration. Apparent V_d of plasma protein–bound drugs can be altered by liver and kidney disease (↓ protein binding, ↑ V_d). Drugs may distribute in more than one compartment.

$$V_d = \frac{\text{amount of drug in the body}}{\text{plasma drug concentration}}$$

V_d	COMPARTMENT	DRUG TYPES
Low	Blood	Large/charged molecules; plasma protein bound
Medium	ECF	Small hydrophilic molecules
High	All tissues including fat	Small lipophilic molecules, especially if bound to tissue protein

Clearance (CL)

The volume of plasma cleared of drug per unit time. Clearance may be impaired with defects in cardiac, hepatic, or renal function.

$$CL = \frac{\text{rate of elimination of drug}}{\text{plasma drug concentration}} = V_d \times K_e \text{ (elimination constant)}$$

Half-life ($t_{1/2}$)

The time required to change the amount of drug in the body by ½ during elimination.

In first-order kinetics, a drug infused at a constant rate takes 4–5 half-lives to reach steady state. It takes 3.3 half-lives to reach 90% of the steady-state level.

$$t_{1/2} = \frac{0.693 \times V_d}{CL} \text{ in first-order elimination}$$

# of half-lives	1	2	3	4
% remaining	50%	25%	12.5%	6.25%

Dosage calculations

$$\text{Loading dose} = \frac{C_p \times V_d}{F}$$

Don't overthink it!

$$\text{Maintenance dose} = \frac{C_p \times CL \times \tau}{F}$$

C_p = target plasma concentration at steady state

τ = dosage interval (time between doses), if not administered continuously

In renal or liver disease, maintenance dose ↓ and loading dose is usually unchanged.

Time to steady state depends primarily on $t_{1/2}$ and is independent of dose and dosing frequency.

Types of drug interactions

TERM	DEFINITION	EXAMPLE
Additive	Effect of substance A and B together is equal to the sum of their individual effects	Aspirin and acetaminophen
Permissive	Presence of substance A is required for the full effects of substance B	Cortisol on catecholamine responsiveness
Synergistic	Effect of substance A and B together is greater than the sum of their individual effects	Clopidogrel with aspirin
Tachyphylactic	Acute decrease in response to a drug after initial/repeated administration	MDMA and LSD

Elimination of drugs

Zero-order elimination	Rate of elimination is constant regardless of C_p (ie, constant **amount** of drug eliminated per unit time). C_p ↓ linearly with time. Examples of drugs—**P**henytoin, **E**thanol, and **A**spirin (at high or toxic concentrations).	Capacity-limited elimination. **PEA.** (A pea is round, shaped like the "0" in **zero**-order.)
First-order elimination	Rate of elimination is directly proportional to the drug concentration (ie, constant **fraction** of drug eliminated per unit time). C_p ↓ exponentially with time. Applies to most drugs.	Flow-dependent elimination.

Zero-order elimination

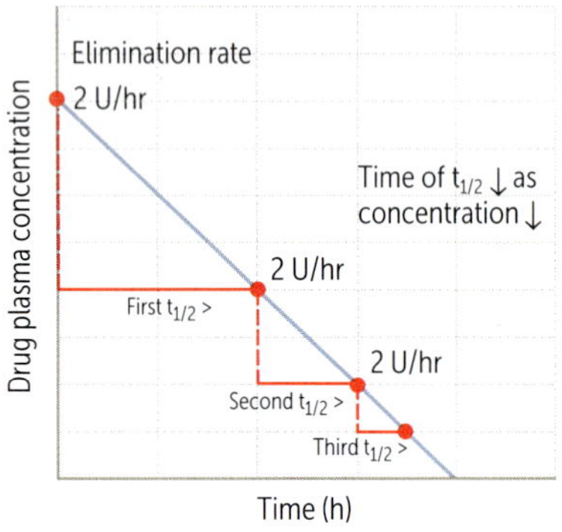

First-order elimination

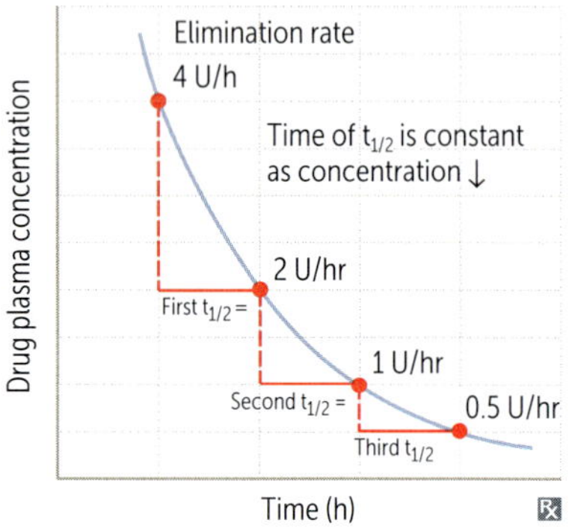

Urine pH and drug elimination

Ionized species are trapped in urine and cleared quickly. Neutral forms can be reabsorbed.

Weak acids	Examples: phenobarbital, methotrexate, aspirin. Trapped in basic environments. Treat overdose with bicarbonate. $RCOOH \rightleftharpoons RCOO^- + H^+$ (lipid soluble) (trapped)
Weak bases	Example: amphetamines, TCAs. Trapped in acidic environments. Treat overdose with ammonium chloride. $RNH_3^+ \rightleftharpoons RNH_2 + H^+$ (trapped) (lipid soluble)

Drug metabolism

Phase I	Reduction, oxidation, hydrolysis with cytochrome P-450 usually yield slightly polar, water-soluble metabolites (often still active).	Geriatric patients lose phase I first.
Phase II	Conjugation (**M**ethylation, **G**lucuronidation, **A**cetylation, **S**ulfation) usually yields very polar, inactive metabolites (renally excreted).	Geriatric patients have **M**ore **GAS** (phase II). Patients who are slow acetylators have ↑ side effects from certain drugs because of ↓ rate of metabolism.

Efficacy vs potency

Efficacy

Maximal effect a drug can produce. Represented by the y-value (V_{max}). ↑ y-value = ↑ V_{max} = ↑ efficacy. Unrelated to potency (ie, efficacious drugs can have high or low potency). Partial agonists have less efficacy than full agonists.

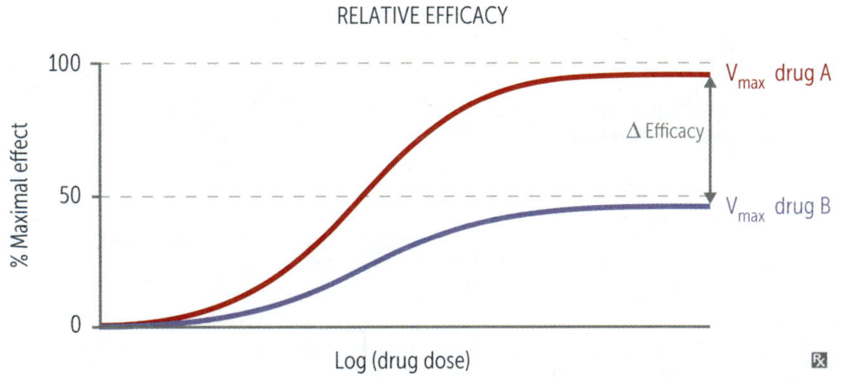

Potency

Amount of drug needed for a given effect. Represented by the x-value (EC_{50}). Left shifting = ↓ EC_{50} = ↑ potency = ↓ drug needed. Unrelated to efficacy (ie, potent drugs can have high or low efficacy).

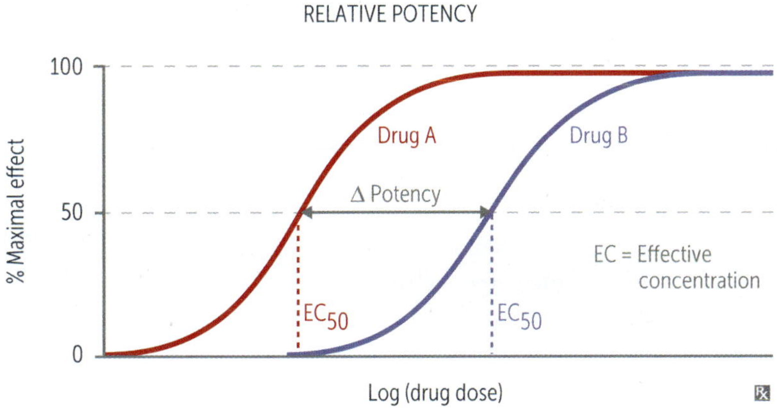

Efficacy = how high does it (effect) go
Potency = how quickly do u need to get to 1/2 tht max.
(much of a dose)

Receptor binding

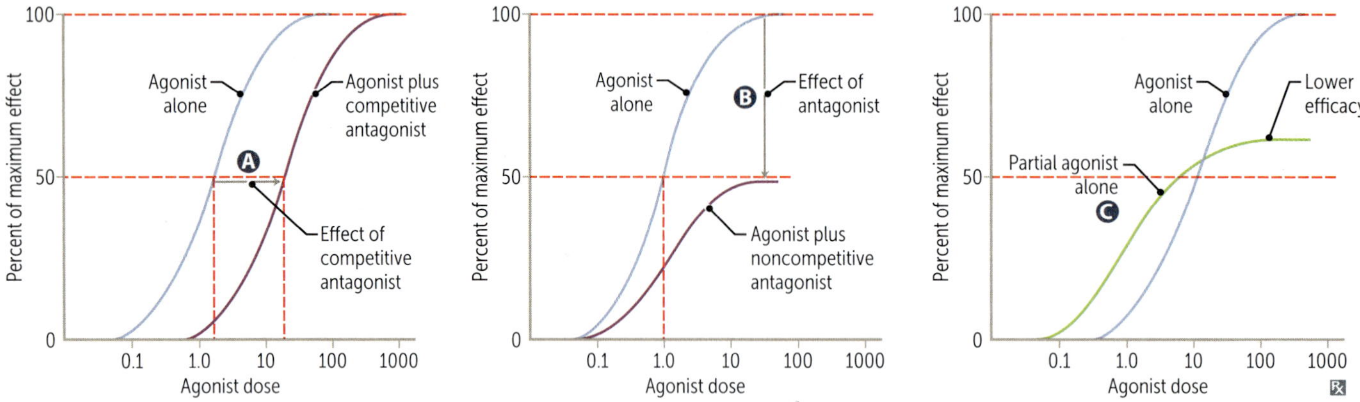

AGONIST WITH	EFFECT	EXAMPLE
Ⓐ Competitive antagonist	Shifts curve right (↓ potency), no change in efficacy. Can be overcome by ↑ the concentration of agonist substrate.	Diazepam (agonist) + **flumazenil** (competitive antagonist) on GABA receptor.
Ⓑ Noncompetitive antagonist	Shifts curve down (↓ efficacy). Cannot be overcome by ↑ agonist substrate concentration.	Norepinephrine (agonist) + **phenoxybenzamine** (noncompetitive antagonist) on α-receptors.
Ⓒ Partial agonist (alone)	Acts at same site as full agonist, but with lower maximal effect (↓ efficacy). Potency is an independent variable.	Morphine (full agonist) vs **buprenorphine** (partial agonist) at opioid μ-receptors.

Therapeutic index

Measurement of drug safety.

$$\frac{TD_{50}}{ED_{50}} = \frac{\text{median toxic dose}}{\text{median effective dose}}$$

Therapeutic window—dosage range that can safely and effectively treat disease.

TITE: Therapeutic Index = TD_{50} / ED_{50}.
Safer drugs have higher TI values. Drugs with lower TI values frequently require monitoring (eg, digoxin, lithium, theophylline, warfarin).
LD_{50} (lethal median dose) often replaces TD_{50} in animal studies.

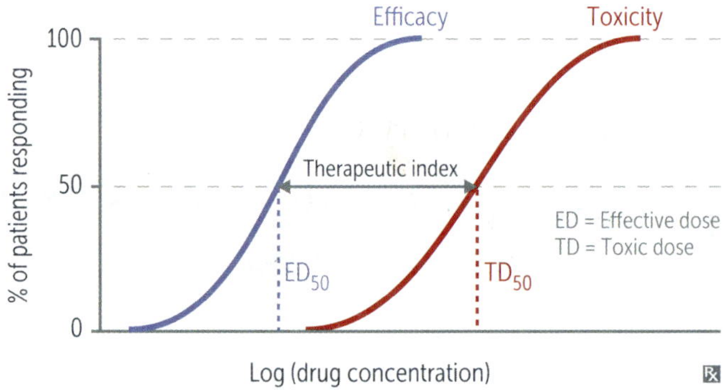

makes sense why phenoxybenz. is used for pheochromo. Bc using a non-competit. block no matter how much NE the tumor makes, it cant displace it & the max eff. of NE is now ↓

▶ PHARMACOLOGY—AUTONOMIC DRUGS

Central and peripheral nervous system

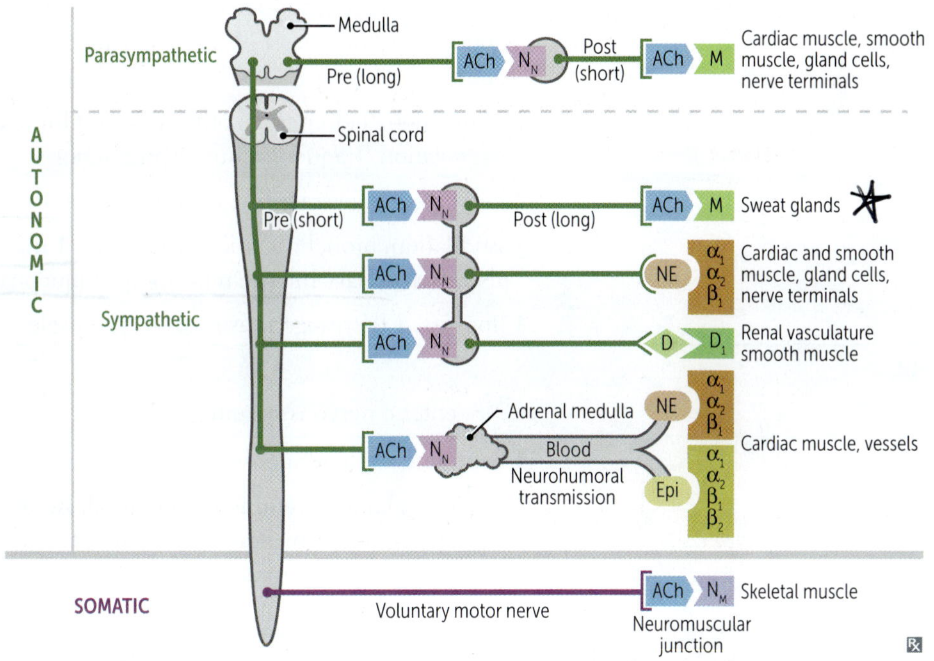

Note that the adrenal medulla and sweat glands are part of the sympathetic nervous system but are innervated by cholinergic fibers.

Botulinum toxin prevents release of acetylcholine at cholinergic terminals.

ACh receptors

Nicotinic ACh receptors are ligand-gated Na^+/K^+ channels. Two subtypes: N_N (found in autonomic ganglia, adrenal medulla) and N_M (found in neuromuscular junction of skeletal muscle).

Muscarinic ACh receptors are G-protein–coupled receptors that usually act through 2nd messengers. 5 subtypes: M_{1-5} found in heart, smooth muscle, brain, exocrine glands, and on sweat glands (cholinergic sympathetic).

Nnerves
Nmuscle] → lig gated Na/K channels

Musc → Gprotein

G-protein–linked 2nd messengers

RECEPTOR	G-PROTEIN CLASS	MAJOR FUNCTIONS
Sympathetic		
α_1	q	↑ vascular smooth muscle contraction, ↑ pupillary dilator muscle contraction (mydriasis), ↑ intestinal and bladder sphincter muscle contraction
α_2	i	↓ sympathetic (adrenergic) outflow, ↓ insulin release, ↓ lipolysis, ↑ platelet aggregation, ↓ aqueous humor production
β_1	s	↑ heart rate, ↑ contractility, ↑ renin release, ↑ lipolysis
β_2	s	Vasodilation, bronchodilation, ↑ lipolysis, ↑ insulin release, ↓ uterine tone (tocolysis), ciliary muscle relaxation, ↑ aqueous humor production
β_3	s	↑ lipolysis, ↑ thermogenesis in skeletal muscle
Parasympathetic		
M_1	q	CNS, enteric nervous system
M_2	i	↓ heart rate and contractility of atria
M_3	q	↑ exocrine gland secretions (eg, lacrimal, sweat, salivary, gastric acid), ↑ gut peristalsis, ↑ bladder contraction, bronchoconstriction, ↑ pupillary sphincter muscle contraction (miosis), ciliary muscle contraction (accommodation)
Dopamine		
D_1	s	Relaxes renal vascular smooth muscle
D_2	i	Modulates transmitter release, especially in brain
Histamine		
H_1	q	↑ nasal and bronchial mucus production, ↑ vascular permeability, contraction of bronchioles, pruritus, pain
H_2	s	↑ gastric acid secretion
Vasopressin		
V_1	q	↑ vascular smooth muscle contraction
V_2	s	↑ H_2O permeability and reabsorption in collecting tubules of kidney (V_2 is found in the 2 kidneys)

"After qisses (kisses), you get a qiq (kick) out of siq (sick) sqs (super qinky sex)."

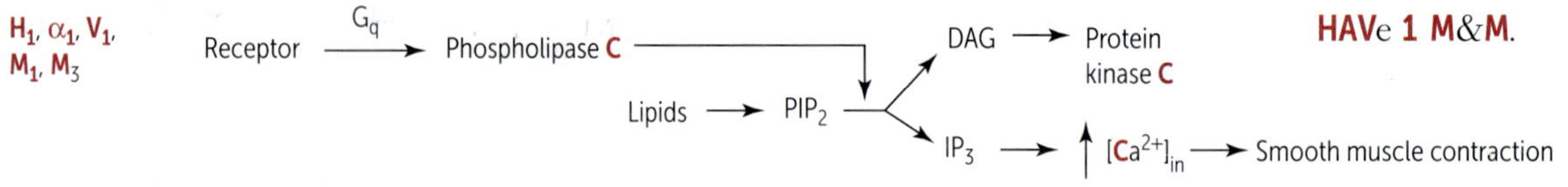

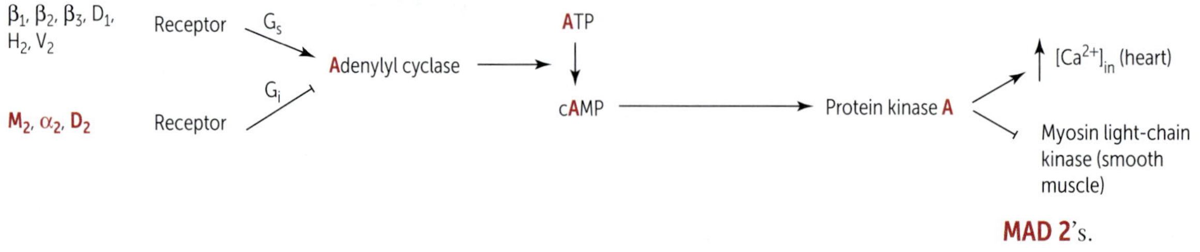

Autonomic drugs

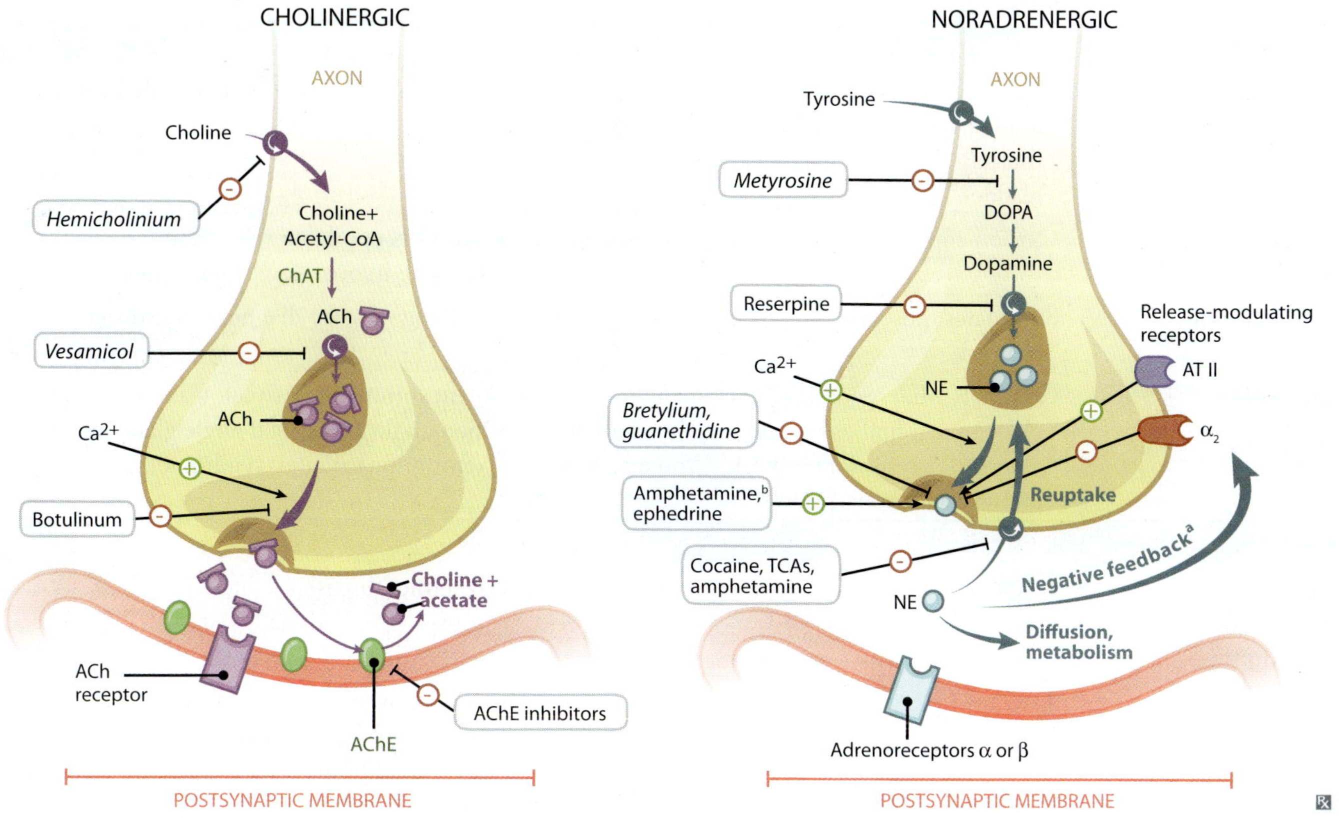

Circles with rotating arrows represent transporters. Drugs in *italics* are of historical significance.

[a]Release of norepinephrine from a sympathetic nerve ending is modulated by norepinephrine itself, acting on presynaptic α_2-autoreceptors.

[b]Amphetamines use the NE transporter (NET) to enter the presynaptic terminal, where they utilize the vesicular monoamine transporter (VMAT) to enter neurosecretory vesicles. This displaces NE from the vesicles. Once NE reaches a concentration threshold within the presynaptic terminal, the action of NET is reversed, and NE is expelled into the synaptic cleft, contributing to the characteristics and effects of ↑ NE observed in patients taking amphetamines.

Tyramine	Normally degraded by monoamine oxidase (MAO). Levels ↑ in patients taking MAO inhibitors who ingest tyramine-rich foods (eg, cheese, wine). Excess tyramine enters presynaptic vesicles and displaces other neurotransmitters (eg, NE) → ↑ active presynaptic neurotransmitters → ↑ diffusion of neurotransmitters into synaptic cleft → ↑ sympathetic stimulation. Classically results in a hypertensive crisis.

Cholinomimetic agents

DRUG	ACTION	APPLICATIONS
Direct agonists		
Bethanechol	Activates bowel and bladder smooth muscle; resistant to AChE. "Bethany, call (bethanechol) me to activate your bowels and bladder."	Postoperative ileus, neurogenic ileus, urinary retention
Carbachol	Carbon copy of acetylcholine.	Constricts pupil and relieves intraocular pressure in open-angle glaucoma
Methacholine	Stimulates muscarinic receptors in airway when inhaled.	Challenge test for diagnosis of asthma
Pilocarpine	Contracts ciliary muscle of eye (open-angle glaucoma), pupillary sphincter (closed-angle glaucoma); resistant to AChE. "You cry, drool, and sweat on your 'pilow.'"	Potent stimulator of sweat, tears, and saliva Open-angle and closed-angle glaucoma, xerostomia (Sjögren syndrome)
Indirect agonists (anticholinesterases)		
Donepezil, galantamine, rivastigmine	↑ ACh.	Alzheimer disease.
Edrophonium	↑ ACh.	Historically, diagnosis of myasthenia gravis (extremely short acting). Myasthenia now diagnosed by anti-AChR Ab (anti-acetylcholine receptor antibody) test.
Neostigmine	↑ ACh. Neo CNS = No CNS penetration (quaternary amine).	Postoperative and neurogenic ileus and urinary retention, myasthenia gravis, reversal of neuromuscular junction blockade (postoperative).
Physostigmine	↑ ACh. Physostigmine "phyxes" atropine overdose.	Anticholinergic toxicity; crosses blood-brain barrier → CNS (tertiary amine).
Pyridostigmine	↑ ACh; ↑ muscle strength. Pyridostigmine gets rid of myasthenia gravis.	Myasthenia gravis (long acting); does not penetrate CNS (quaternary amine).

Note: With all cholinomimetic agents, watch for exacerbation of COPD, asthma, and peptic ulcers when giving to susceptible patients.

Cholinesterase inhibitor poisoning	Often due to organophosphates, such as parathion, that **irreversibly** inhibit AChE. Causes Diarrhea, Urination, Miosis, Bronchospasm, Bradycardia, Excitation of skeletal muscle and CNS, Lacrimation, Sweating, and Salivation. May lead to respiratory failure if untreated.	DUMBBELSS. Organophosphates are often components of insecticides; poisoning usually seen in farmers. Antidote—atropine (competitive inhibitor) + pralidoxime (regenerates AChE if given early).

Muscarinic antagonists

DRUGS	ORGAN SYSTEMS	APPLICATIONS
Atropine, homatropine, tropicamide	Eye	Produce mydriasis and cycloplegia.
Benztropine	CNS	Parkinson disease ("park my Benz"). Acute dystonia.
Glycopyrrolate	GI, respiratory	Parenteral: preoperative use to reduce airway secretions. Oral: drooling, peptic ulcer.
Hyoscyamine, dicyclomine	GI	Antispasmodics for irritable bowel syndrome.
Ipratropium, tiotropium	Respiratory	COPD, asthma ("I pray I can breathe soon!").
Oxybutynin, solifenacin, tolterodine	Genitourinary	Reduce bladder spasms and urge urinary incontinence (overactive bladder).
Scopolamine	CNS	Motion sickness.

Atropine

Muscarinic antagonist. Used to treat bradycardia and for ophthalmic applications.

ORGAN SYSTEM	ACTION	NOTES
Eye	↑ pupil dilation, cycloplegia	Blocks DUMBBeLSS in cholinesterase inhibitor poisoning. Does not block excitation of skeletal muscle and CNS (mediated by nicotinic receptors).
Airway	↓ secretions	
Stomach	↓ acid secretion	
Gut	↓ motility	
Bladder	↓ urgency in cystitis	
ADVERSE EFFECTS	↑ body temperature (due to ↓ sweating); rapid pulse; dry mouth; dry, flushed skin; cycloplegia; constipation; disorientation Can cause acute angle-closure glaucoma in elderly (due to mydriasis), urinary retention in men with prostatic hyperplasia, and hyperthermia in infants	Side effects: Hot as a hare Dry as a bone Red as a beet Blind as a bat Mad as a hatter Jimson weed (*Datura*) → gardener's pupil (mydriasis due to plant alkaloids)

Sympathomimetics

DRUG	ACTION	APPLICATIONS
Direct sympathomimetics		
Albuterol, salmeterol	$\beta_2 > \beta_1$	Albuterol for acute asthma or COPD. Salmeterol for long-term asthma or COPD control.
Dobutamine	$\beta_1 > \beta_2, \alpha$	Heart failure (HF) (inotropic > chronotropic), cardiac stress testing.
Dopamine	$D_1 = D_2 > \beta > \alpha$	Unstable bradycardia, HF, shock; inotropic and chronotropic effects at lower doses due to β effects; vasoconstriction at high doses due to α effects.
Epinephrine	$\beta > \alpha$	Anaphylaxis, asthma, open-angle glaucoma; α effects predominate at high doses. Significantly stronger effect at β_2-receptor than norepinephrine.
Fenoldopam	D_1	Postoperative hypertension, hypertensive crisis. Vasodilator (coronary, peripheral, renal, and splanchnic). Promotes natriuresis. Can cause hypotension and tachycardia.
Isoproterenol	$\beta_1 = \beta_2$	Electrophysiologic evaluation of tachyarrhythmias. Can worsen ischemia.
Midodrine	α_1	Autonomic insufficiency and postural hypotension. May exacerbate supine hypertension.
Norepinephrine	$\alpha_1 > \alpha_2 > \beta_1$	Hypotension, septic shock.
Phenylephrine	$\alpha_1 > \alpha_2$	Hypotension (vasoconstrictor), ocular procedures (mydriatic), rhinitis (decongestant).
Indirect sympathomimetics		
Amphetamine	Indirect general agonist, reuptake inhibitor, also releases stored catecholamines	Narcolepsy, obesity, ADHD.
Cocaine	Indirect general agonist, reuptake inhibitor	Causes vasoconstriction and local anesthesia. Never give β-blockers if cocaine intoxication is suspected (can lead to unopposed α_1 activation and extreme hypertension).
Ephedrine	Indirect general agonist, releases stored catecholamines	Nasal decongestion, urinary incontinence, hypotension.

Norepinephrine vs isoproterenol

Norepinephrine ↑ systolic and diastolic pressures as a result of α_1-mediated vasoconstriction → ↑ mean arterial pressure → reflex bradycardia. However, isoproterenol (no longer commonly used) has little α effect but causes β_2-mediated vasodilation, resulting in ↓ mean arterial pressure and ↑ heart rate through β_1 and reflex activity.

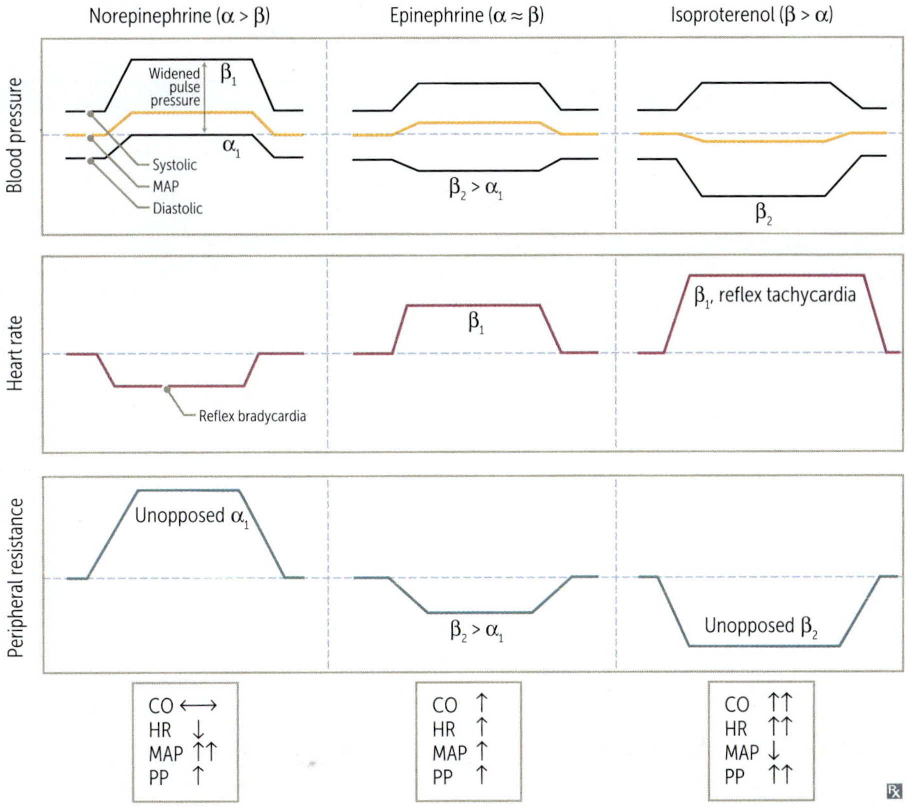

Sympatholytics (α_2-agonists)

DRUG	APPLICATIONS	ADVERSE EFFECTS
Clonidine, guanfacine	Hypertensive urgency (limited situations), ADHD, Tourette syndrome	CNS depression, bradycardia, hypotension, respiratory depression, miosis
α-methyldopa	Hypertension in pregnancy	Direct Coombs ⊕ hemolysis, SLE-like syndrome

α-blockers

DRUG	APPLICATIONS	ADVERSE EFFECTS
Nonselective		
Phenoxybenzamine (irreversible)	Pheochromocytoma (used preoperatively) to prevent catecholamine (hypertensive) crisis	Orthostatic hypotension, reflex tachycardia
Phentolamine (reversible)	Give to patients on MAO inhibitors who eat tyramine-containing foods	
α_1 selective (-osin ending)		
Prazosin, terazosin, doxazosin, tamsulosin	Urinary symptoms of BPH; PTSD (prazosin); hypertension (except tamsulosin)	1st-dose orthostatic hypotension, dizziness, headache
α_2 selective		
Mirtazapine	Depression	Sedation, ↑ serum cholesterol, ↑ appetite

α-blockade of epinephrine vs phenylephrine

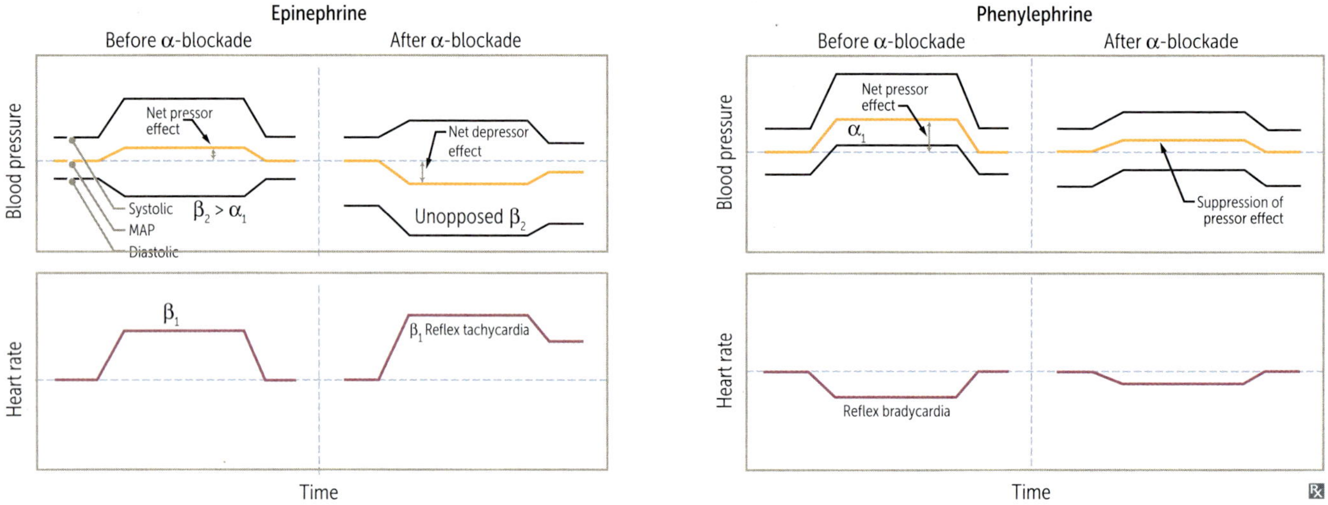

Shown above are the effects of an α-blocker (eg, phentolamine) on blood pressure responses to epinephrine and phenylephrine. The epinephrine response exhibits reversal of the mean blood pressure change, from a net increase (the α response) to a net decrease (the β_2 response). The response to phenylephrine is suppressed but not reversed because phenylephrine is a "pure" α-agonist without β action.

β-blockers	Acebutolol, atenolol, betaxolol, carvedilol, esmolol, labetalol, metoprolol, nadolol, nebivolol, pindolol, propranolol, timolol.	
APPLICATION	ACTIONS	NOTES
Angina pectoris	↓ heart rate and contractility, resulting in ↓ O_2 consumption	
MI	↓ mortality	
SVT (metoprolol, esmolol)	↓ AV conduction velocity (class II antiarrhythmic)	
Hypertension	↓ cardiac output, ↓ renin secretion (due to β_1-receptor blockade on JGA cells)	
HF	↓ mortality (bisoprolol, carvedilol, metoprolol)	
Glaucoma (timolol)	↓ secretion of aqueous humor	
Variceal bleeding (nadolol, propranolol)	↓ hepatic venous pressure gradient and portal hypertension	
ADVERSE EFFECTS	Erectile dysfunction, cardiovascular adverse effects (bradycardia, AV block, HF), CNS adverse effects (seizures, sedation, sleep alterations), dyslipidemia (metoprolol), and asthma/COPD exacerbations	Use with caution in cocaine users due to risk of unopposed α-adrenergic receptor agonist activity Despite theoretical concern of masking hypoglycemia in diabetics, benefits likely outweigh risks; not contraindicated
SELECTIVITY	β_1-selective antagonists ($\beta_1 > \beta_2$)—**a**cebutolol (partial agonist), **a**tenolol, **b**etaxolol, **e**smolol, **m**etoprolol	Selective antagonists mostly go from **A** to **M** (β_1 with **1**st half of alphabet)
	Nonselective antagonists ($\beta_1 = \beta_2$)—**n**adolol, **p**indolol (partial agonist), **p**ropranolol, **t**imolol	**N**onselective antagonists mostly go from **N** to **Z** (β_2 with **2**nd half of alphabet)
	Nonselective α- and β-antagonists—carvedilol, labetalol	Nonselective α- and β-antagonists have modified suffixes (instead of "-olol")
	Nebivolol combines cardiac-selective β_1-adrenergic blockade with stimulation of β_3-receptors, which activate nitric oxide synthase in the vasculature	

Ingested seafood toxins

TOXIN	SOURCE	ACTION	SYMPTOMS	TREATMENT
Tetrodotoxin	Pufferfish.	Highly potent toxin; binds fast voltage-gated Na^+ channels in cardiac/nerve tissue, preventing depolarization.	Nausea, diarrhea, paresthesias, weakness, dizziness, loss of reflexes.	Primarily supportive.
Ciguatoxin	Reef fish such as barracuda, snapper, and moray eel.	Opens Na^+ channels, causing depolarization.	Symptoms mimic cholinergic poisoning.	Primarily supportive.
Histamine (scombroid poisoning)	Spoiled dark-meat fish such as tuna, mahi-mahi, mackerel, and bonito.	Bacterial histidine decarboxylase converts histidine to histamine. Frequently misdiagnosed as fish allergy.	Mimics anaphylaxis: acute burning sensation of mouth, flushing of face, erythema, urticaria, itching. May progress to bronchospasm, angioedema, hypotension.	Antihistamines. Albuterol and epinephrine if needed.

▸ PHARMACOLOGY—TOXICITIES AND SIDE EFFECTS

Specific toxicity treatments

TOXIN	TREATMENT
Acetaminophen	N-acetylcysteine (replenishes glutathione)
AChE inhibitors, organophosphates	Atropine > pralidoxime
Amphetamines (basic)	NH_4Cl (acidify urine)
Antimuscarinic, anticholinergic agents	Physostigmine, control hyperthermia
Arsenic	Dimercaprol, succimer
Benzodiazepines	Flumazenil
β-blockers	Saline, atropine, glucagon
Carbon monoxide	100% O_2, hyperbaric O_2
Copper	Penicillamine, trientine
Cyanide	Nitrite + thiosulfate, hydroxocobalamin
Digitalis (digoxin)	Anti-dig Fab fragments
Gold	Penicillamine, dimercaprol (BAL), succimer
Heparin	Protamine sulfate
Iron	De**fe**roxamine, de**fe**rasirox, de**fe**riprone
Lead	EDTA, dimercaprol, succimer, penicillamine
Mercury	Di**merc**aprol, succimer
Methanol, ethylene glycol (antifreeze)	Fomepizole > ethanol, dialysis
Methemoglobin	**Meth**ylene blue, vitamin C
Opioids	Naloxone
Salicylates	$NaHCO_3$ (alkalinize urine), dialysis
TCAs	$NaHCO_3$
Warfarin	Vitamin K (delayed effect), fresh frozen plasma (immediate)

Drug reactions—cardiovascular

DRUG REACTION	CAUSAL AGENTS
Coronary vasospasm	Cocaine, sumatriptan, ergot alkaloids
Cutaneous flushing	**V**ancomycin, **A**denosine, **N**iacin, **C**a^{2+} channel blockers, **E**chinocandins (**VANCE**)
Dilated cardiomyopathy	Anthracyclines (eg, doxorubicin, daunorubicin); prevent with dexrazoxane
Torsades de pointes	Anti**A**rrhythmics (class IA, III), anti**B**iotics (eg, macrolides), anti"**C**"ychotics (eg, haloperidol), anti**D**epressants (eg, TCAs), anti**E**metics (eg, ondansetron) (**ABCDE**).

Drug reactions—endocrine/reproductive

DRUG REACTION	CAUSAL AGENTS	NOTES
Adrenocortical insufficiency	HPA suppression 2° to glucocorticoid withdrawal	
Hot flashes	Tamoxifen, clomiphene	
Hyperglycemia	Tacrolimus, Protease inhibitors, Niacin, HCTZ, Corticosteroids	Taking Pills Necessitates Having blood Checked
Hypothyroidism	Lithium, amiodarone, sulfonamides	

Drug reactions—GI

DRUG REACTION	CAUSAL AGENTS	NOTES
Acute cholestatic hepatitis, jaundice	Erythromycin	
Diarrhea	Acamprosate, acarbose, cholinesterase inhibitors, colchicine, erythromycin, ezetimibe, metformin, misoprostol, orlistat, pramlintide, quinidine, SSRIs	
Focal to massive hepatic necrosis	Halothane, *Amanita phalloides* (death cap mushroom), Valproic acid, Acetaminophen	Liver "HAVAc"
Hepatitis	Rifampin, isoniazid, pyrazinamide, statins, fibrates	
Pancreatitis	Didanosine, Corticosteroids, Alcohol, Valproic acid, Azathioprine, Diuretics (furosemide, HCTZ)	Drugs Causing A Violent Abdominal Distress
Pill-induced esophagitis	Tetracyclines, bisphosphonates, potassium chloride	Caustic effect minimized with upright posture and adequate water ingestion.
Pseudomembranous colitis	Clindamycin, ampicillin, cephalosporins	Antibiotics predispose to superinfection by resistant *C difficile*

Drug reactions—hematologic

DRUG REACTION	CAUSAL AGENTS	NOTES
Agranulocytosis	Clozapine, Carbamazepine, Propylthiouracil, Methimazole, Colchicine, Ganciclovir	Can Cause Pretty Major Collapse of Granulocytes
Aplastic anemia	Carbamazepine, Methimazole, NSAIDs, Benzene, Chloramphenicol, Propylthiouracil	Can't Make New Blood Cells Properly
Direct Coombs-positive hemolytic anemia	Methyldopa, penicillin	
Gray baby syndrome	Chloramphenicol	
Hemolysis in G6PD deficiency	Isoniazid, Sulfonamides, Dapsone, Primaquine, Aspirin, Ibuprofen, Nitrofurantoin	Hemolysis IS D PAIN
Megaloblastic anemia	Phenytoin, Methotrexate, Sulfa drugs	Having a blast with PMS
Thrombocytopenia	Heparin	
Thrombotic complications	OCPs, hormone replacement therapy	

Drug reactions—musculoskeletal/skin/connective tissue

DRUG REACTION	CAUSAL AGENTS	NOTES
Fat redistribution	Protease inhibitors, Glucocorticoids	Fat PiG
Gingival hyperplasia	Phenytoin, Ca^{2+} channel blockers, cyclosporine	
Hyperuricemia (gout)	Pyrazinamide, Thiazides, Furosemide, Niacin, Cyclosporine	Painful Tophi and Feet Need Care
Myopathy	Fibrates, niacin, colchicine, hydroxychloroquine, interferon-α, penicillamine, statins, glucocorticoids	
Osteoporosis	Corticosteroids, heparin	
Photosensitivity	Sulfonamides, Amiodarone, Tetracyclines, 5-FU	SAT For Photo
Rash (Stevens-Johnson syndrome)	Anti-epileptic drugs (especially lamotrigine), allopurinol, sulfa drugs, penicillin	Steven Johnson has epileptic allergy to sulfa drugs and penicillin
SLE-like syndrome	Sulfa drugs, Hydralazine, Isoniazid, Procainamide, Phenytoin, Etanercept	Having lupus is "SHIPP-E"
Teeth discoloration	Tetracyclines	
Tendonitis, tendon rupture, and cartilage damage	Fluoroquinolones	

Drug reactions—neurologic

DRUG REACTION	CAUSAL AGENTS	NOTES
Cinchonism	Quinidine, quinine	
Parkinson-like syndrome	Antipsychotics, Reserpine, Metoclopramide	Cogwheel rigidity of ARM
Seizures	Isoniazid (vitamin B_6 deficiency), Bupropion, Imipenem/cilastatin, Tramadol, Enflurane	With seizures, I BITE my tongue
Tardive dyskinesia	Antipsychotics, metoclopramide	

Drug reactions—renal/genitourinary

DRUG REACTION	CAUSAL AGENTS	NOTES
Diabetes insipidus	Lithium, demeclocycline	
Fanconi syndrome	Tenofovir, ifosfamide	
Hemorrhagic cystitis	Cyclophosphamide, ifosfamide	Prevent by coadministering with mesna
Interstitial nephritis	Methicillin, NSAIDs, furosemide	
SIADH	Carbamazepine, Cyclophosphamide, SSRIs	Can't Concentrate Serum Sodium

Drug reactions—respiratory

DRUG REACTION	CAUSAL AGENTS	NOTES
Dry cough	ACE inhibitors	
Pulmonary fibrosis	Methotrexate, Nitrofurantoin, Carmustine, Bleomycin, Busulfan, Amiodarone	My Nose Cannot Breathe Bad Air

Drug reactions—multiorgan

DRUG REACTION	CAUSAL AGENTS
Antimuscarinic	Atropine, TCAs, H_1-blockers, antipsychotics
Disulfiram-like reaction	Metronidazole, certain cephalosporins, griseofulvin, procarbazine, 1st-generation sulfonylureas
Nephrotoxicity/ototoxicity	Aminoglycosides, vancomycin, loop diuretics, cisplatin. Cisplatin toxicity may respond to amifostine.

Cytochrome P-450 interactions (selected)

Inducers (+)	Substrates	Inhibitors (–)
Chronic alcohol use	Anti-epileptics	Acute Alcohol Abuse
St. John's wort	Theophylline	Ritonavir
Phenytoin	Warfarin	Amiodarone
Phenobarbital	OCPs	Cimetidine/ciprofloxacin
Nevirapine		Ketoconazole
Rifampin		Sulfonamides
Griseofulvin		Isoniazid (INH)
Carbamazepine		Grapefruit juice
		Quinidine
		Macrolides (except azithromycin)
Chronic alcoholics Steal Phen-Phen and Never Refuse Greasy Carbs	Always Think When Outdoors	AAA RACKS IN GQ Magazine

Sulfa drugs

Sulfonamide antibiotics, Sulfasalazine, Probenecid, Furosemide, Acetazolamide, Celecoxib, Thiazides, Sulfonylureas.

Patients with sulfa allergies may develop fever, urinary tract infection, Stevens-Johnson syndrome, hemolytic anemia, thrombocytopenia, agranulocytosis, and urticaria (hives). Symptoms range from mild to life threatening.

Scary Sulfa Pharm FACTS

▶ PHARMACOLOGY—MISCELLANEOUS

Drug names

ENDING	CATEGORY	EXAMPLE
Antimicrobial		
-azole	Ergosterol synthesis inhibitor	Ketoconazole
-bendazole	Antiparasitic/antihelminthic	Mebendazole
-cillin	Peptidoglycan synthesis inhibitor	Ampicillin
-cycline	Protein synthesis inhibitor	Tetracycline
-ivir	Neuraminidase inhibitor	Oseltamivir
-navir	Protease inhibitor	Ritonavir
-ovir	DNA polymerase inhibitor	Acyclovir
-thromycin	Macrolide antibiotic	Azithromycin
CNS		
-ane	Inhalational general anesthetic	Halothane
-azine	Typical antipsychotic	Thioridazine
-barbital	Barbiturate	Phenobarbital
-caine	Local anesthetic	Lidocaine
-etine	SSRI	Fluoxetine
-ipramine, -triptyline	TCA	Imipramine, amitriptyline
-triptan	5-$HT_{1B/1D}$ agonists	Sumatriptan
-zepam, -zolam	Benzodiazepine	Diazepam, alprazolam
Autonomic		
-chol	Cholinergic agonist	Bethanechol, carbachol
-curium, -curonium	Nondepolarizing paralytic	Atracurium, vecuronium
-olol	β-blocker	Propranolol
-stigmine	AChE inhibitor	Neostigmine
-terol	β_2-agonist	Albuterol
-zosin	α_1-antagonist	Prazosin
Cardiovascular		
-afil	PDE-5 inhibitor	Sildenafil
-dipine	Dihydropyridine Ca^{2+} channel blocker	Amlodipine
-pril	ACE inhibitor	Captopril
-sartan	Angiotensin-II receptor blocker	Losartan
-statin	HMG-CoA reductase inhibitor	Atorvastatin
-xaban	Direct factor Xa inhibitors	Apixaban, edoxaban, rivaroxaban
Other		
-dronate	Bisphosphonate	Alendronate
-glitazone	PPAR-γ activator	Rosiglitazone
-prazole	Proton pump inhibitor	Omeprazole
-prost	Prostaglandin analog	Latanoprost
-tidine	H_2-antagonist	Cimetidine
-tropin	Pituitary hormone	Somatotropin
-ximab	Chimeric monoclonal Ab	Basiliximab
-zumab	Humanized monoclonal Ab	Daclizumab

▶ NOTES

SECTION III

High-Yield Organ Systems

"Symptoms, then, are in reality nothing but the cry from suffering organs."
—Jean-Martin Charcot

"Man is an intelligence in servitude to his organs."
—Aldous Huxley

"Learn that you are a machine, your heart an engine, your lungs a fanning machine and a sieve, your brain with its two lobes an electric battery."
—Andrew T. Still

▶ APPROACHING THE ORGAN SYSTEMS

In this section, we have divided the High-Yield Facts into the major **Organ Systems.** Within each Organ System are several subsections, including **Embryology, Anatomy, Physiology, Pathology,** and **Pharmacology.** As you progress through each Organ System, refer back to information in the previous subsections to organize these basic science subsections into a "vertically integrated" framework for learning. Below is some general advice for studying the organ systems by these subsections.

Embryology

Relevant embryology is included in each organ system subsection. Embryology tends to correspond well with the relevant anatomy, especially with regard to congenital malformations.

Anatomy

Several topics fall under this heading, including gross anatomy, histology, and neuroanatomy. Do not memorize all the small details; however, do not ignore anatomy altogether. Review what you have already learned and what you wish you had learned. Many questions require two or more steps. The first step is to identify a structure on anatomic cross section, electron micrograph, or photomicrograph. The second step may require an understanding of the clinical significance of the structure.

When studying, stress clinically important material. For example, be familiar with gross anatomy and radiologic anatomy related to specific diseases (eg, Pancoast tumor, Horner syndrome), traumatic injuries (eg, fractures, sensory and motor nerve deficits), procedures (eg, lumbar puncture), and common surgeries (eg, cholecystectomy). There are also many questions on the exam involving x-rays, CT scans, and neuro MRI scans. Many students suggest browsing through a general radiology atlas, pathology atlas, and histology atlas. Focus on learning basic anatomy at key levels in the body (eg, sagittal brain MRI; axial CT of the midthorax, abdomen, and pelvis). Basic neuroanatomy (especially pathways, blood supply, and functional anatomy), associated neuropathology, and neurophysiology have good yield. Please note that many of the photographic images in this book are for illustrative purposes and are not necessarily reflective of Step 1 emphasis.

Physiology

The portion of the examination dealing with physiology is broad and concept oriented and thus does not lend itself as well to fact-based review. Diagrams are often the best study aids, especially given the increasing number of questions requiring the interpretation of diagrams. Learn to apply basic physiologic relationships in a variety of ways (eg, the Fick equation, clearance equations). You are seldom asked to perform complex calculations. Hormones are the focus of many questions, so learn their sites of production and action as well as their regulatory mechanisms.

A large portion of the physiology tested on the USMLE Step 1 is clinically relevant and involves understanding physiologic changes associated with pathologic processes (eg, changes in pulmonary function with COPD). Thus, it is worthwhile to review the physiologic changes that are found with common pathologies of the major organ systems (eg, heart, lungs, kidneys, GI tract) and endocrine glands.

Pathology

Questions dealing with this discipline are difficult to prepare for because of the sheer volume of material involved. Review the basic principles and hallmark characteristics of the key diseases. Given the clinical orientation of Step 1, it is no longer sufficient to know only the "buzzword" associations of certain diseases (eg, café-au-lait macules and neurofibromatosis); you must also know the clinical descriptions of these findings.

Given the clinical slant of the USMLE Step 1, it is also important to review the classic presenting signs and symptoms of diseases as well as their associated laboratory findings. Delve into the signs, symptoms, and pathophysiology of major diseases that have a high prevalence in the United States (eg, alcoholism, diabetes, hypertension, heart failure, ischemic heart disease, infectious disease). Be prepared to think one step beyond the simple diagnosis to treatment or complications.

The examination includes a number of color photomicrographs and photographs of gross specimens that are presented in the setting of a brief clinical history. However, read the question and the choices carefully before looking at the illustration, because the history will help you identify the pathologic process. Flip through an illustrated pathology textbook, color atlases, and appropriate Web sites in order to look at the pictures in the days before the exam. Pay attention to potential clues such as age, sex, ethnicity, occupation, recent activities and exposures, and specialized lab tests.

Pharmacology

Preparation for questions on pharmacology is straightforward. Memorizing all the key drugs and their characteristics (eg, mechanisms, clinical use, and important side effects) is high yield. Focus on understanding the prototype drugs in each class. Avoid memorizing obscure derivatives. Learn the "classic" and distinguishing toxicities of the major drugs. Do not bother with drug dosages or trade names. Reviewing associated biochemistry, physiology, and microbiology can be useful while studying pharmacology. There is a strong emphasis on ANS, CNS, antimicrobial, and cardiovascular agents as well as NSAIDs. Much of the material is clinically relevant. Newer drugs on the market are also fair game.

▶ NOTES

HIGH-YIELD SYSTEMS

Cardiovascular

"As for me, except for an occasional heart attack, I feel as young as I ever did."

—Robert Benchley

"Hearts will never be practical until they are made unbreakable."

—The Wizard of Oz

"As the arteries grow hard, the heart grows soft."

—H. L. Mencken

"Nobody has ever measured, not even poets, how much the heart can hold."

—Zelda Fitzgerald

"Only from the heart can you touch the sky."

—Rumi

"It is not the size of the man but the size of his heart that matters."

—Evander Holyfield

▶ CARDIOVASCULAR—EMBRYOLOGY

Heart embryology

EMBRYONIC STRUCTURE	GIVES RISE TO
Truncus arteriosus	Ascending aorta and pulmonary trunk
Bulbus cordis	Smooth parts (outflow tract) of left and right ventricles
Endocardial cushion	Atrial septum, membranous interventricular septum; AV and semilunar valves
Primitive atrium	Trabeculated part of left and right atria
Primitive ventricle	Trabeculated part of left and right ventricles
Primitive pulmonary vein	Smooth part of left atrium
Left horn of sinus venosus	Coronary sinus
Right horn of sinus venosus	Smooth part of right atrium (sinus venarum)
Right common cardinal vein and right anterior cardinal vein	Superior vena cava (SVC)

Heart morphogenesis

First functional organ in vertebrate embryos; beats spontaneously by week 4 of development.

Cardiac looping

Primary heart tube loops to establish left-right polarity; begins in week 4 of gestation.

Defect in left-right dynein (involved in L/R asymmetry) can lead to dextrocardia, as seen in Kartagener syndrome (primary ciliary dyskinesia).

Septation of the chambers

Atria

1. Septum primum grows toward endocardial cushions, narrowing foramen primum.
2. Foramen secundum forms in septum primum (foramen primum disappears).
3. Septum secundum develops as foramen secundum maintains right-to-left shunt.
4. Septum secundum expands and covers most of the foramen secundum. The residual foramen is the foramen ovale.
5. Remaining portion of septum primum forms valve of foramen ovale.
6. (Not shown) Septum secundum and septum primum fuse to form the atrial septum.
7. (Not shown) Foramen ovale usually closes soon after birth because of ↑ LA pressure.

Patent foramen ovale—caused by failure of septum primum and septum secundum to fuse after birth; most are left untreated. Can lead to paradoxical emboli (venous thromboemboli that enter systemic arterial circulation), similar to those resulting from an ASD.

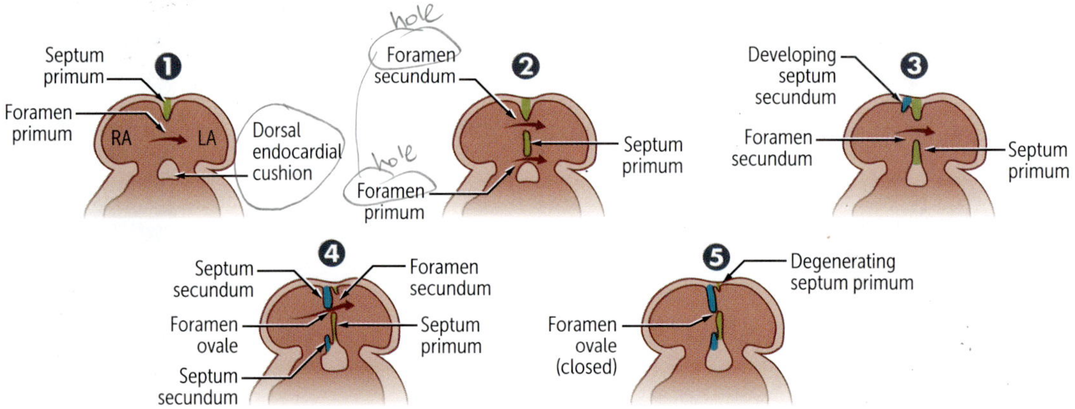

Heart morphogenesis *(continued)*

☆ indiana.edu has a GREAT video

Ventricles	❶ Muscular interventricular septum forms. Opening is called interventricular foramen. ❷ Aorticopulmonary septum rotates and fuses with muscular ventricular septum to form membranous interventricular septum, closing interventricular foramen. ❸ Growth of endocardial cushions separates atria from ventricles and contributes to both atrial septation and membranous portion of the interventricular septum.	Ventricular septal defect (VSD)—most common congenital cardiac anomaly, usually occurs in membranous septum.

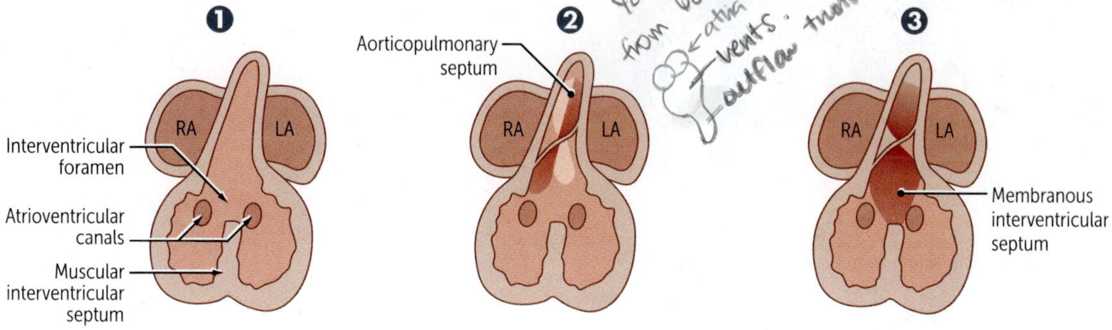

Outflow tract formation	Neural crest and endocardial cell migrations → truncal and bulbar ridges that spiral and fuse to form aorticopulmonary septum → ascending aorta and pulmonary trunk.	Conotruncal abnormalities associated with failure of neural crest cells to migrate: ▪ Transposition of great vessels. ▪ Tetralogy of Fallot. ▪ Persistent truncus arteriosus.
Valve development	Aortic/pulmonary: derived from endocardial cushions of outflow tract. Mitral/tricuspid: derived from fused endocardial cushions of the AV canal.	Valvular anomalies may be stenotic, regurgitant, atretic (eg, tricuspid atresia), or displaced (eg, Ebstein anomaly).

- I guess you need endocard. cushions to make 8 & septum primum, etc to make 8

- embryology events = embryo fold / heart loop = week 4
  heart septation week 5-6 (5 slice)
  remodel outflow tract week 7
  embryonic ends, fetal period begins week 8.

- With the lungs not functional the RA pressure is high & blood flows freely through the foramen ovale. But as the lungs become functional & pressure ↓, the LA pressure is higher in comparison & it forces septum primum on septum secundum & it closes it.

- The aorticopulm septum divides the truncus arteriosus into pulm trunk & aorta

Fetal circulation

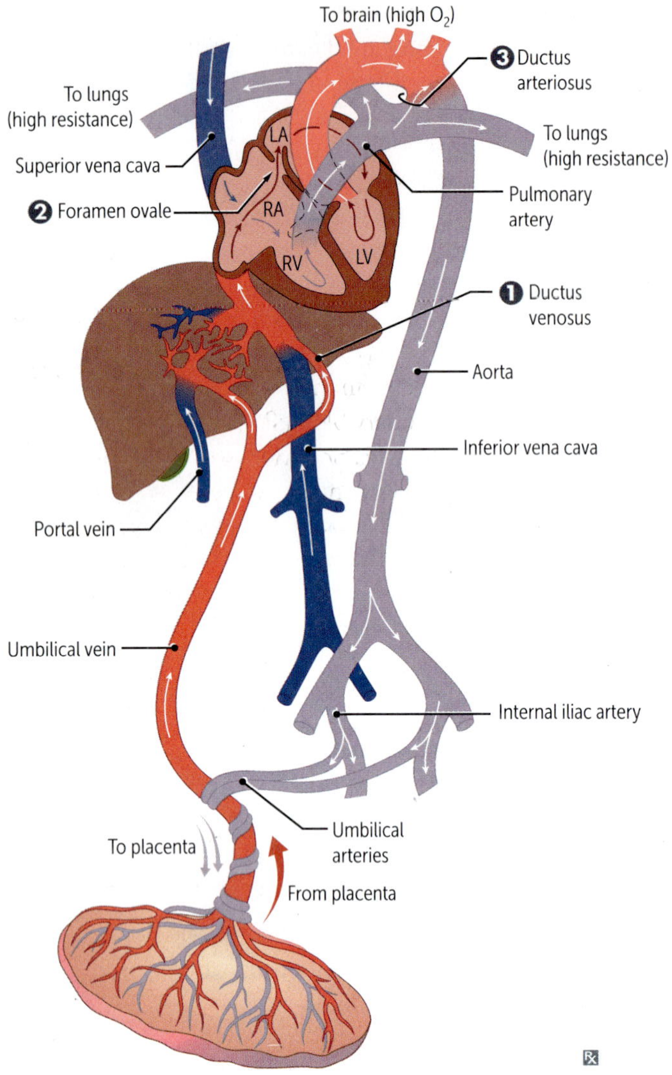

Blood in umbilical vein has a Po_2 of ≈ 30 mm Hg and is ≈ 80% saturated with O_2. Umbilical arteries have low O_2 saturation.

3 important shunts:

1. Blood entering fetus through the umbilical vein is conducted via the **ductus venosus** into the IVC, bypassing hepatic circulation.
2. Most of the highly oxygenated blood reaching the heart via the IVC is directed through the **foramen ovale** and pumped into the aorta to supply the head and body.
3. Deoxygenated blood from the SVC passes through the RA → RV → main pulmonary artery → patent ductus arteriosus → descending aorta; shunt is due to high fetal pulmonary artery resistance (due partly to low O_2 tension).

At birth, infant takes a breath; ↓ resistance in pulmonary vasculature → ↑ left atrial pressure vs right atrial pressure; foramen ovale closes (now called fossa ovalis); ↑ in O_2 (from respiration) and ↓ in prostaglandins (from placental separation) → closure of ductus arteriosus.

Indomethacin helps close PDA → ligamentum arteriosum (remnant of ductus arteriosus).

Prostaglandins E_1 and E_2 kEEp PDA open.

Fetal-postnatal derivatives

AllaNtois → urachus	MediaN umbilical ligament	Urachus is part of allantoic duct between bladder and umbilicus.
Ductus arteriosus	Ligamentum arteriosum	
Ductus venosus	Ligamentum venosum	
Foramen ovale	Fossa ovalis	
Notochord	Nucleus pulposus	
UmbiLical arteries	MediaL umbilical ligaments	
Umbilical vein	Ligamentum teres hepatis	Contained in falciform ligament.

▶ CARDIOVASCULAR—ANATOMY

Coronary artery anatomy

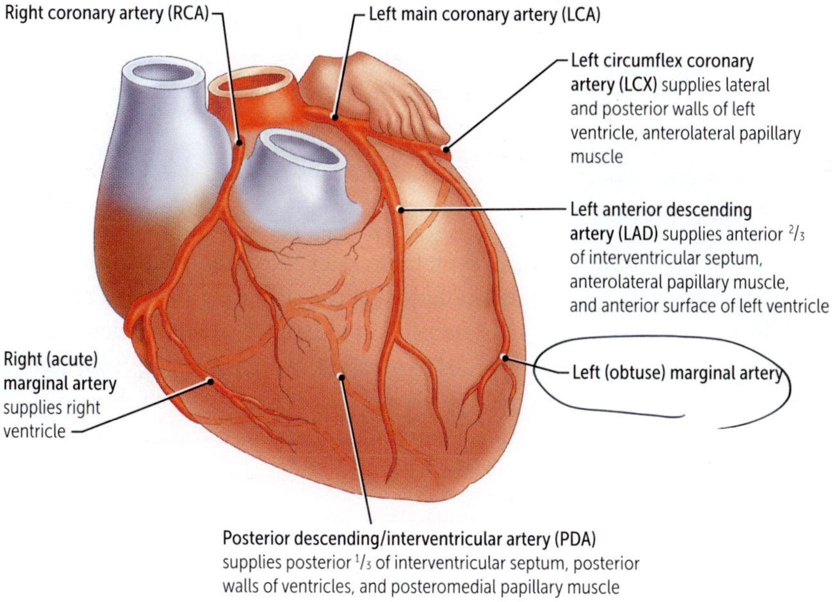

SA and AV nodes are usually supplied by RCA. Infarct may cause nodal dysfunction (bradycardia or heart block).

Right-dominant circulation (85%) = PDA arises from RCA.

Left-dominant circulation (8%) = PDA arises from LCX.

Codominant circulation (7%) = PDA arises from both LCX and RCA.

Coronary artery occlusion most commonly occurs in the LAD.

Coronary blood flow peaks in early diastole.

The most posterior part of the heart is the left atrium; enlargement can cause dysphagia (due to compression of the esophagus) or hoarseness (due to compression of the left recurrent laryngeal nerve, a branch of the vagus).

Pericardium consists of 3 layers (from outer to inner):
- Fibrous pericardium
- Parietal layer of serous pericardium
- Visceral layer of serous pericardium

Pericardial cavity lies between parietal and visceral layers.

▸ CARDIOVASCULAR—PHYSIOLOGY

Cardiac output

CO = stroke volume (SV) × heart rate (HR)

Fick principle:

$$CO = \frac{\text{rate of } O_2 \text{ consumption}}{\text{arterial } O_2 \text{ content} - \text{venous } O_2 \text{ content}}$$

Mean arterial pressure (MAP) = CO × total peripheral resistance (TPR)

During the early stages of exercise, CO is maintained by ↑ HR and ↑ SV. During the late stages of exercise, CO is maintained by ↑ HR only (SV plateaus).

Diastole is preferentially shortened with ↑ HR; less filling time → ↓ CO (eg, ventricular tachycardia).

MAP = ⅔ diastolic pressure + ⅓ systolic pressure

Pulse pressure = systolic pressure – diastolic pressure

Pulse pressure is proportional to SV, inversely proportional to arterial compliance.

SV = end-diastolic volume (EDV) – end-systolic volume (ESV)

↑ pulse pressure in hyperthyroidism, aortic regurgitation, aortic stiffening (isolated systolic hypertension in elderly), obstructive sleep apnea (↑ sympathetic tone), exercise (transient).

↓ pulse pressure in aortic stenosis, cardiogenic shock, cardiac tamponade, advanced heart failure (HF).

Cardiac output variables

Stroke volume	**S**troke **V**olume affected by **C**ontractility, **A**fterload, and **P**reload. ↑ SV with: ▪ ↑ Contractility (eg, anxiety, exercise) ▪ ↑ Preload (eg, early pregnancy) ▪ ↓ Afterload	**SV CAP.** A failing heart has ↓ SV (systolic and/or diastolic dysfunction)
Contractility	Contractility (and SV) ↑ with: ▪ Catecholamines (inhibition of phospholamban → ↑ Ca^{2+} entry into sarcoplasmic reticulum → ↑ Ca^{2+}-induced Ca^{2+} release) ▪ ↑ intracellular Ca^{2+} ▪ ↓ extracellular Na^+ (↓ activity of Na^+/Ca^{2+} exchanger) ▪ Digitalis (blocks Na^+/K^+ pump → ↑ intracellular Na^+ → ↓ Na^+/Ca^{2+} exchanger activity → ↑ intracellular Ca^{2+})	Contractility (and SV) ↓ with: ▪ β_1-blockade (↓ cAMP) ▪ HF with systolic dysfunction ▪ Acidosis ▪ Hypoxia/hypercapnia (↓ Po_2/↑ Pco_2) ▪ Non-dihydropyridine Ca^{2+} channel blockers
Myocardial oxygen demand	↑ Myo**CARD**ial O_2 demand is ↑ by: ▪ ↑ **C**ontractility ▪ ↑ **A**fterload (proportional to arterial pressure) ▪ ↑ heart **R**ate ▪ ↑ **D**iameter of ventricle (↑ wall tension)	Wall tension follows Laplace's law: $\text{Wall tension} = \dfrac{\text{pressure} \times \text{radius}}{2 \times \text{wall thickness}}$ $\dfrac{PR}{2T}$
Preload	Preload approximated by ventricular EDV; depends on venous tone and circulating blood volume.	**VE**nodilators (eg, nitroglycerin) ↓ pr**E**load.
Afterload	Afterload approximated by MAP. ↑ afterload → ↑ pressure → ↑ wall tension per Laplace's law. LV compensates for ↑ afterload by thickening (hypertrophy) in order to ↓ wall tension.	V**A**sodilators (eg, hydr**A**l**A**zine) ↓ **A**fterload (**A**rterial). ACE inhibitors and ARBs ↓ both preload and afterload. Chronic hypertension (↑ MAP) → LV hypertrophy.
Ejection fraction	$EF = \dfrac{SV}{EDV} = \dfrac{EDV - ESV}{EDV}$ Left ventricular EF is an index of ventricular contractility; normal EF is ≥ 55%.	EF ↓ in systolic HF. EF normal in diastolic HF.

Starling curve

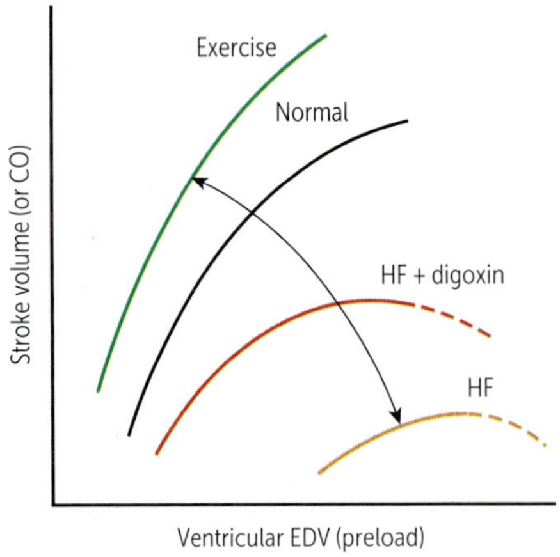

Force of contraction is proportional to end-diastolic length of cardiac muscle fiber (preload).

↑ contractility with catecholamines, positive inotropes (eg, digoxin).

↓ contractility with loss of myocardium (eg, MI), β-blockers (acutely), non-dihydropyridine Ca^{2+} channel blockers, dilated cardiomyopathy.

Resistance, pressure, flow

$\Delta P = Q \times R$

Similar to Ohm's law: $\Delta V = IR$

Volumetric flow rate (Q) = flow velocity (v) × cross-sectional area (A)

Resistance

$$= \frac{\text{driving pressure } (\Delta P)}{\text{flow } (Q)} = \frac{8\eta \text{ (viscosity)} \times \text{length}}{\pi r^4}$$

Total resistance of vessels in series:

$R_T = R_1 + R_2 + R_3 \ldots$

Total resistance of vessels in parallel:

$$\frac{1}{R_T} = \frac{1}{R_1} + \frac{1}{R_2} + \frac{1}{R_3} \ldots$$

Viscosity depends mostly on hematocrit

Viscosity ↑ in hyperproteinemic states (eg, multiple myeloma), polycythemia

Viscosity ↓ in anemia

Capillaries have highest total cross-sectional area and lowest flow velocity.

Removal of organs in parallel arrangement (eg, nephrectomy) → ↓ TPR and ↑ CO.

Pressure gradient drives flow from high pressure to low pressure.

Arterioles account for most of TPR. Veins provide most of blood storage capacity.

Cardiac and vascular function curves

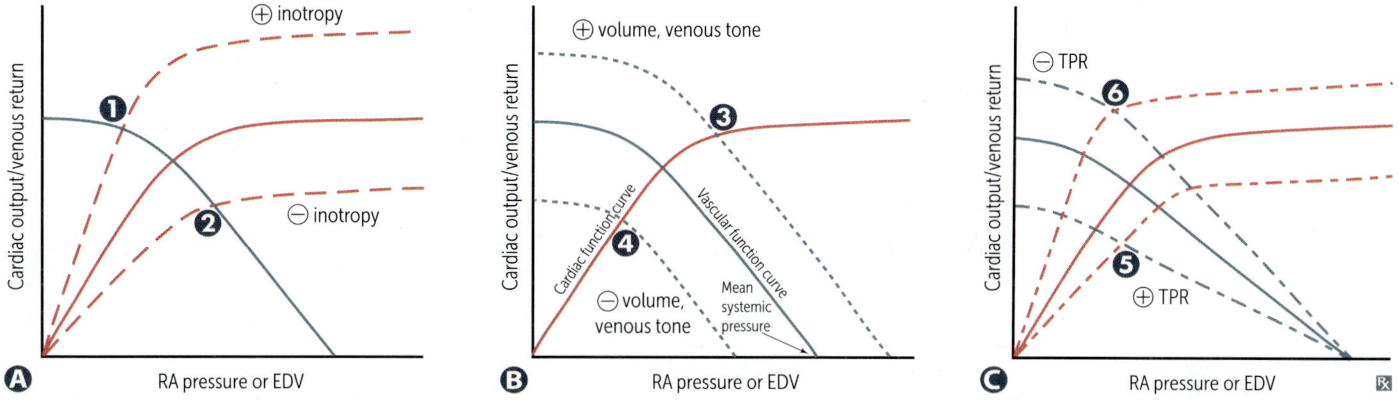

Intersection of curves = operating point of heart (ie, venous return and CO are equal).

CURVE	EFFECT	EXAMPLES
A Inotropy	Changes in contractility → altered CO for a given RA pressure (preload).	❶ Catecholamines, digoxin ⊕ ❷ Uncompensated HF, narcotic overdose ⊖
B Venous return	Changes in circulating volume or venous tone → altered RA pressure for a given CO. Mean systemic pressure (x-intercept) changes with volume/venous tone.	❸ Fluid infusion, sympathetic activity ⊕ ❹ Acute hemorrhage, spinal anesthesia ⊖
C Total peripheral resistance	At a given mean systemic pressure (x-intercept) and RA pressure, changes in TPR → altered CO.	❺ Vasopressors ⊕ ❻ Exercise, AV shunt ⊖

Changes often occur in tandem, and may be reinforcing (eg, exercise ↑ inotropy and ↓ TPR to maximize CO) or compensatory (eg, HF ↓ inotropy → fluid retention to ↑ preload to maintain CO).

Pressure-volume loops and cardiac cycle

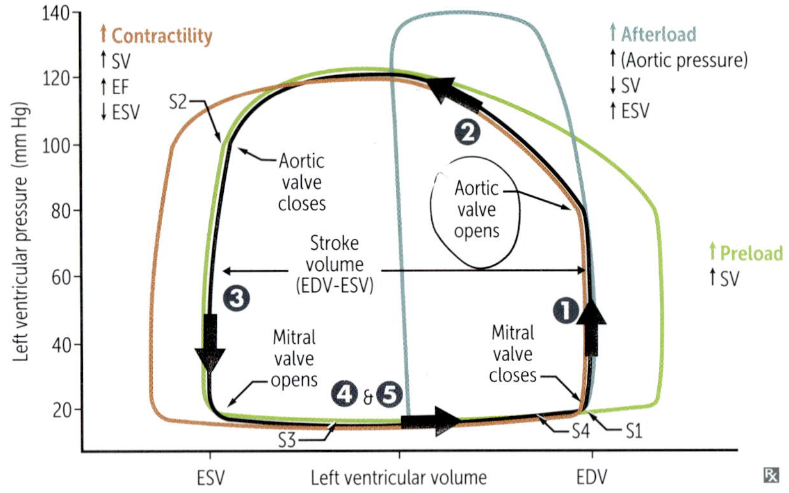

The black loop represents normal cardiac physiology.

Phases—left ventricle:

1. Isovolumetric contraction—period between mitral valve closing and aortic valve opening; period of highest O_2 consumption
2. Systolic ejection—period between aortic valve opening and closing
3. Isovolumetric relaxation—period between aortic valve closing and mitral valve opening
4. Rapid filling—period just after mitral valve opening
5. Reduced filling—period just before mitral valve closing

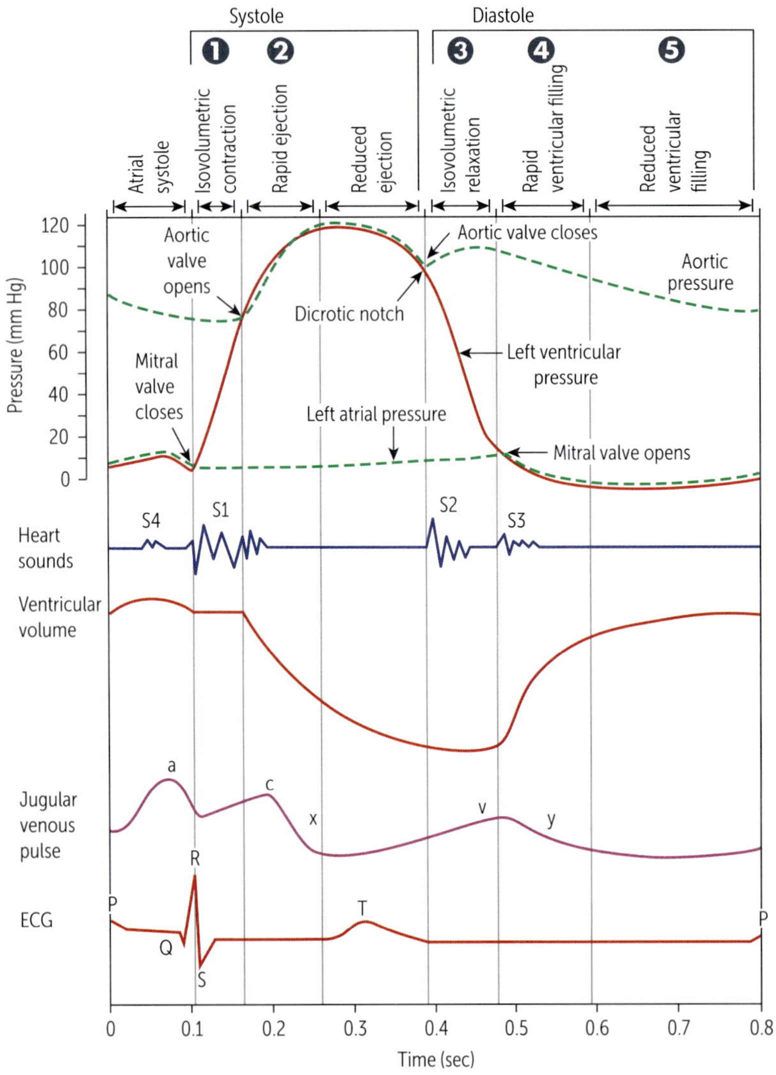

Heart sounds:

S1—mitral and tricuspid valve closure. Loudest at mitral area.

S2—aortic and pulmonary valve closure. Loudest at left upper sternal border.

S3—in early diastole during rapid ventricular filling phase. Associated with ↑ filling pressures (eg, mitral regurgitation, HF) and more common in dilated ventricles (but can be normal in children and young adults).

S4—in late diastole ("atrial kick"). Best heard at apex with patient in left lateral decubitus position. High atrial pressure. Associated with ventricular noncompliance (eg, hypertrophy). Left atrium must push against stiff LV wall. Consider abnormal, regardless of patient age.

Jugular venous pulse (JVP):

a wave—atrial contraction. Absent in atrial fibrillation (AF).

c wave—RV contraction (closed tricuspid valve bulging into atrium).

x descent—atrial relaxation and downward displacement of closed tricuspid valve during ventricular contraction. Absent in tricuspid regurgitation. Prominent in tricuspid insufficiency and right HF.

v wave—↑ right atrial pressure due to filling ("villing") against closed tricuspid valve.

y descent—RA emptying into RV. Prominent in constrictive pericarditis, absent in cardiac tamponade.

Splitting

Normal splitting	Inspiration → drop in intrathoracic pressure → ↑ venous return → ↑ RV filling → ↑ RV stroke volume → ↑ RV ejection time → delayed closure of pulmonic valve. ↓ pulmonary impedance (↑ capacity of the pulmonary circulation) also occurs during inspiration, which contributes to delayed closure of pulmonic valve.	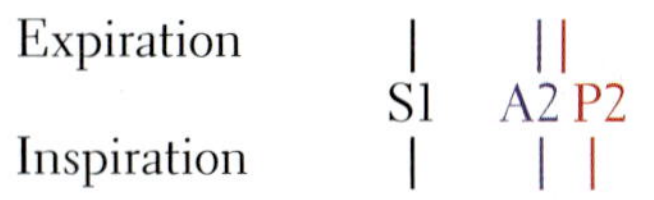
Wide splitting	Seen in conditions that delay RV emptying (eg, pulmonic stenosis, right bundle branch block). Causes delayed pulmonic sound (especially on inspiration). An exaggeration of normal splitting.	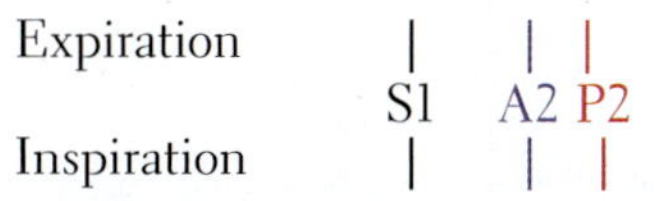
Fixed splitting	Heard in ASD. ASD → left-to-right shunt → ↑ RA and RV volumes → ↑ flow through pulmonic valve such that, regardless of breath, pulmonic closure is greatly delayed.	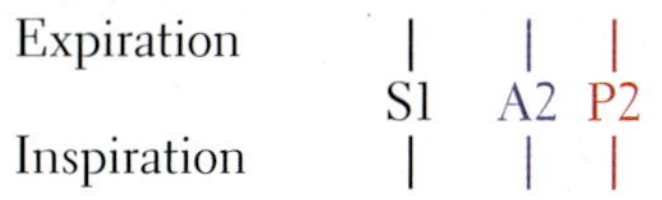
Paradoxical splitting	Heard in conditions that delay aortic valve closure (eg, aortic stenosis, left bundle branch block). Normal order of valve closure is reversed so that P2 sound occurs before delayed A2 sound. Therefore on inspiration, P2 closes later and moves closer to A2, thereby "paradoxically" eliminating the split (usually heard in expiration).	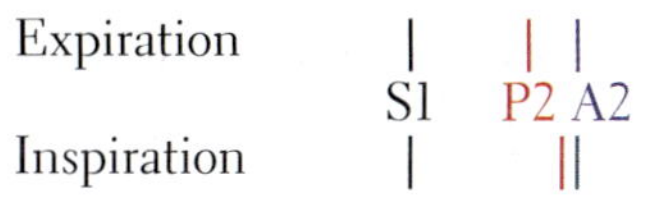

Auscultation of the heart

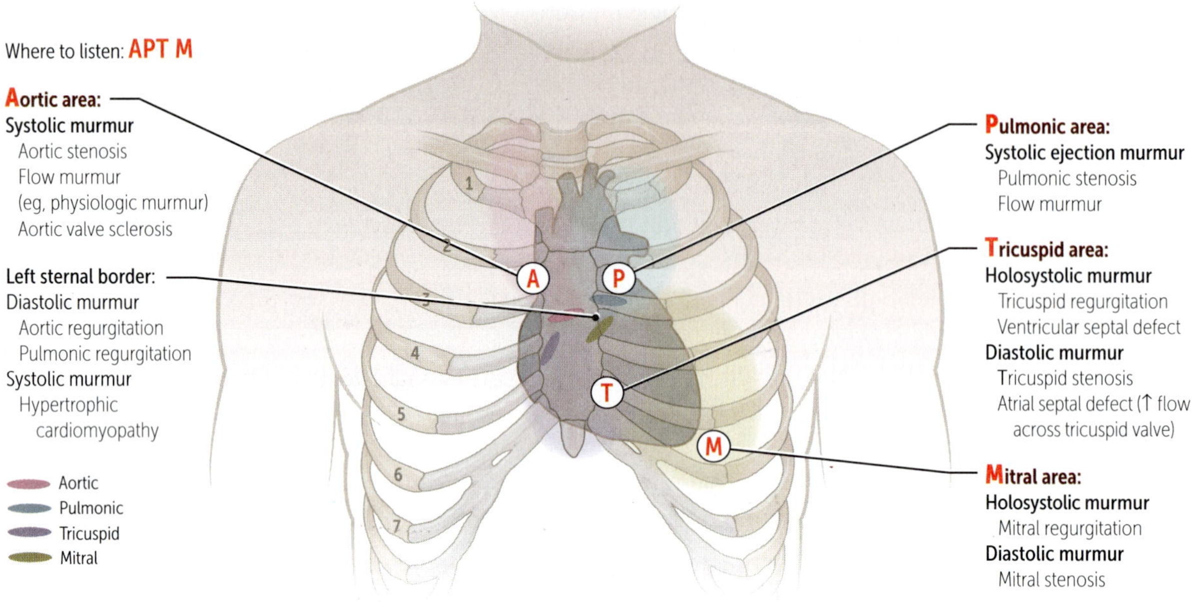

BEDSIDE MANEUVER	EFFECT
Inspiration (↑ venous return to right atrium)	↑ intensity of right heart sounds
Hand grip (↑ afterload)	↑ intensity of MR, AR, VSD murmurs ↓ hypertrophic cardiomyopathy murmurs MVP: later onset of click/murmur
Valsalva (phase II), standing up (↓ preload)	↓ intensity of most murmurs (including AS) ↑ intensity of hypertrophic cardiomyopathy murmur MVP: earlier onset of click/murmur
Rapid squatting (↑ venous return, ↑ preload, ↑ afterload)	↓ intensity of hypertrophic cardiomyopathy murmur ↑ intensity of AS murmur MVP: later onset of click/murmur

Systolic heart sounds include aortic/pulmonic stenosis, mitral/tricuspid regurgitation, VSD, MVP.
Diastolic heart sounds include aortic/pulmonic regurgitation, mitral/tricuspid stenosis.

Heart murmurs

Systolic

Aortic stenosis

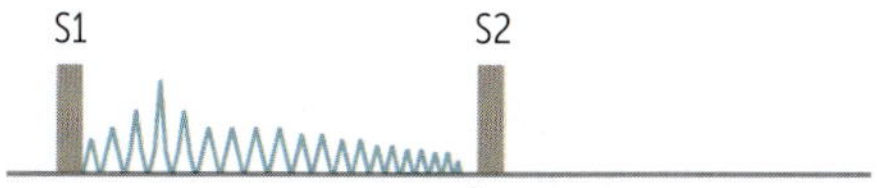

Crescendo-decrescendo systolic ejection murmur (ejection click may be present). LV >> aortic pressure during systole. Loudest at heart base; radiates to carotids. "Pulsus parvus et tardus"—pulses are weak with a delayed peak. Can lead to **S**yncope, **A**ngina, and **D**yspnea on exertion (**SAD**). Most commonly due to age-related calcification in older patients (> 60 years old) or in younger patients with early-onset calcification of bicuspid aortic valve.

Mitral/tricuspid regurgitation

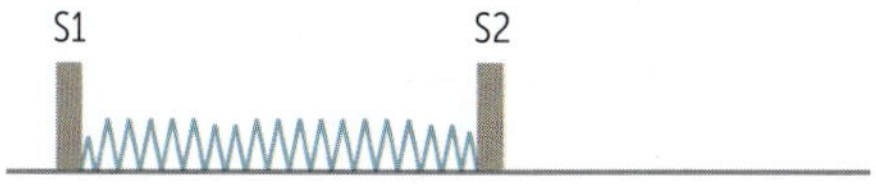

Holosystolic, high-pitched "blowing murmur."

Mitral—loudest at apex and radiates toward axilla. MR is often due to ischemic heart disease (post-MI), MVP, LV dilatation.

Tricuspid—loudest at tricuspid area and radiates to right sternal border. TR commonly caused by RV dilatation.

Rheumatic fever and infective endocarditis can cause either MR or TR.

Mitral valve prolapse

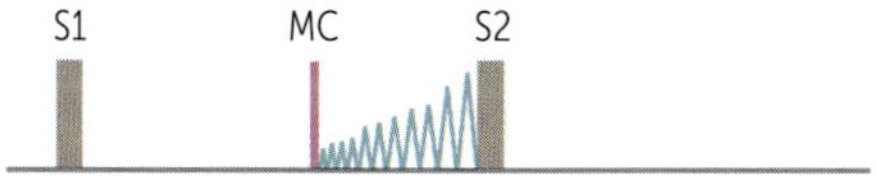

Late systolic crescendo murmur with midsystolic click (MC; due to sudden tensing of chordae tendineae). Most frequent valvular lesion. Best heard over apex. Loudest just before S2. Usually benign. Can predispose to infective endocarditis. Can be caused by myxomatous degeneration (1° or 2° to connective tissue disease such as Marfan or Ehlers-Danlos syndrome), rheumatic fever, chordae rupture.

Ventricular septal defect

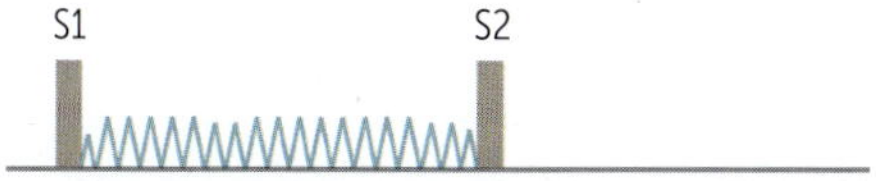

Holosystolic, harsh-sounding murmur. Loudest at tricuspid area.

Diastolic

Aortic regurgitation

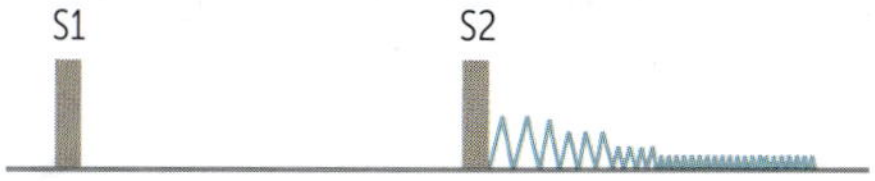

High-pitched "blowing" early diastolic decrescendo murmur. Long diastolic murmur, hyperdynamic pulse, and head bobbing when severe and chronic. Wide pulse pressure. Often due to aortic root dilation, bicuspid aortic valve, endocarditis, rheumatic fever. Progresses to left HF.

Mitral stenosis

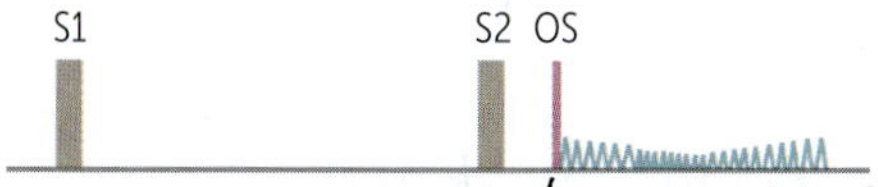

** sounds like S3

Follows opening snap (OS; due to abrupt halt in leaflet motion in diastole, after rapid opening due to fusion at leaflet tips). Delayed rumbling late diastolic murmur (↓ interval between S2 and OS correlates with ↑ severity). LA >> LV pressure during diastole. Often occurs 2° to rheumatic fever. Chronic MS can result in LA dilatation.

Continuous

Patent ductus arteriosus

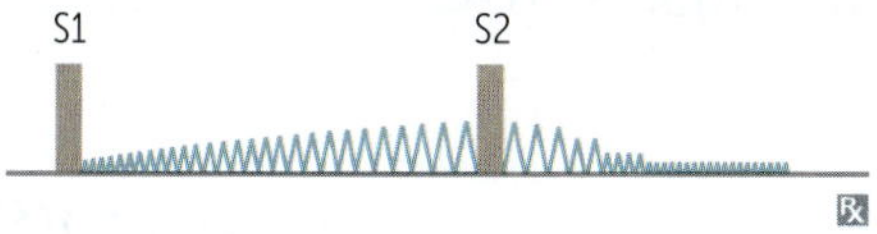

Continuous machine-like murmur. Loudest at S2. Often due to congenital rubella or prematurity. Best heard at left infraclavicular area.

tricus regurg & VSD sound same & in same loc.
- Tricusp may be less harsh

MVP = gets louder so loudest just before S2

Myocardial action potential

Also occurs in bundle of His and Purkinje fibers.

Phase 0 = rapid upstroke and depolarization—voltage-gated Na^+ channels open.

Phase 1 = initial repolarization—inactivation of voltage-gated Na^+ channels. Voltage-gated K^+ channels begin to open.

Phase 2 = plateau—Ca^{2+} influx through voltage-gated Ca^{2+} channels balances K^+ efflux. Ca^{2+} influx triggers Ca^{2+} release from sarcoplasmic reticulum and myocyte contraction.

Phase 3 = rapid repolarization—massive K^+ efflux due to opening of voltage-gated slow K^+ channels and closure of voltage-gated Ca^{2+} channels.

Phase 4 = resting potential—high K^+ permeability through K^+ channels.

In contrast to skeletal muscle:
- Cardiac muscle action potential has a plateau, which is due to Ca^{2+} influx and K^+ efflux.
- Cardiac muscle contraction requires Ca^{2+} influx from ECF to induce Ca^{2+} release from sarcoplasmic reticulum (Ca^{2+}-induced Ca^{2+} release).
- Cardiac myocytes are electrically coupled to each other by gap junctions.

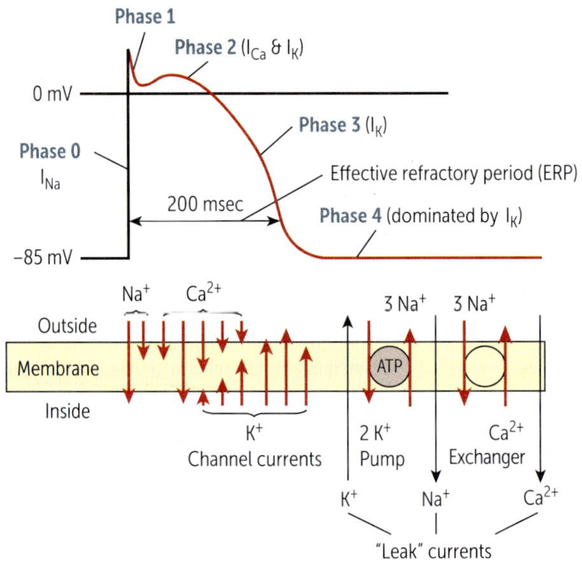

0 = Vg-Na
1 = Ø Vg Na + ↑ K-Vg
2 = ↑ Vg-K + Vg Ca ↑
3 = Vg-K (slow) ↑ + Ø Vg Ca
4 = K permeab ↑

Both cardiac & skel m have troponin C
- cardiac req Ca induced Ca R
- skel. uses ryanodine

Smooth muscle = Hormone / NT — IP3 direct to Ca-I-Ca-R
Vg-Ca (depol) —
- Ca – Calmodul = ↑ MLCK

Pacemaker action potential

Occurs in the SA and AV nodes. Key differences from the ventricular action potential include:

Phase 0 = upstroke—opening of voltage-gated Ca^{2+} channels. Fast voltage-gated Na^+ channels are permanently inactivated because of the less negative resting potential of these cells. Results in a slow conduction velocity that is used by the AV node to prolong transmission from the atria to ventricles.

Phases 1 and 2 are absent.

Phase 3 = inactivation of the Ca^{2+} channels and ↑ activation of K^+ channels → ↑ K^+ efflux.

Phase 4 = slow spontaneous diastolic depolarization due to I_f ("funny current"). I_f channels responsible for a slow, mixed Na^+/K^+ inward current; different from I_{Na} in phase 0 of ventricular action potential. Accounts for automaticity of SA and AV nodes. The slope of phase 4 in the SA node determines HR. ACh/adenosine ↓ the rate of diastolic depolarization and ↓ HR, while catecholamines ↑ depolarization and ↑ HR. Sympathetic stimulation ↑ the chance that I_f channels are open and thus ↑ HR.

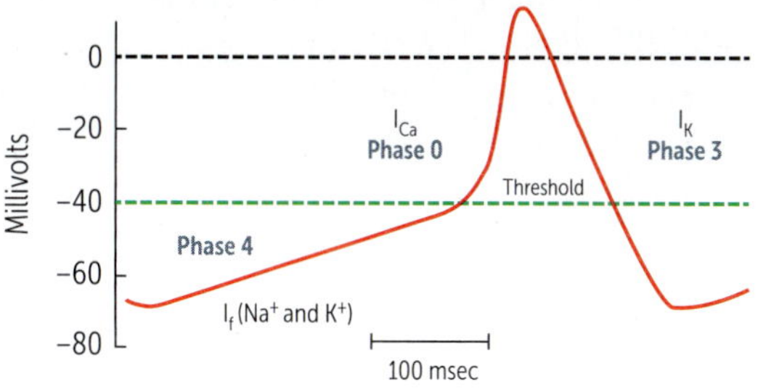

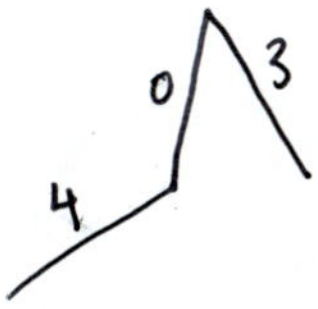

- Phase 4 slope determines HR b/c notice Δx is in time & the quicker you reach threshold = ↑ HR

- I funny = ↑ inward Na & K at hyperpolarizn. bringing it toward depol thresh.
  - so SNS activity ↑ I_f opening

Electrocardiogram

Conduction pathway—SA node → atria → AV node → bundle of His → right and left bundle branches → Purkinje fibers → ventricles; left bundle branch divides into left anterior and posterior fascicles.

SA node "pacemaker" inherent dominance with slow phase of upstroke.

AV node—located in posteroinferior part of interatrial septum. Blood supply usually from RCA. 100-msec delay allows time for ventricular filling.

Pacemaker rates—SA > AV > bundle of His/Purkinje/ventricles.

Speed of conduction—Purkinje > atria > ventricles > AV node.

P wave—atrial depolarization. Atrial repolarization is masked by QRS complex.

PR interval—time from start of atrial depolarization to start of ventricular depolarization (normally < 200 msec).

QRS complex—ventricular depolarization (normally < 120 msec).

QT interval—ventricular depolarization, mechanical contraction of the ventricles, ventricular repolarization.

T wave—ventricular repolarization. T-wave inversion may indicate recent MI.

J point—junction between end of QRS complex and start of ST segment.

ST segment—isoelectric, ventricles depolarized.

U wave—prominent in hypokalemia, bradycardia.

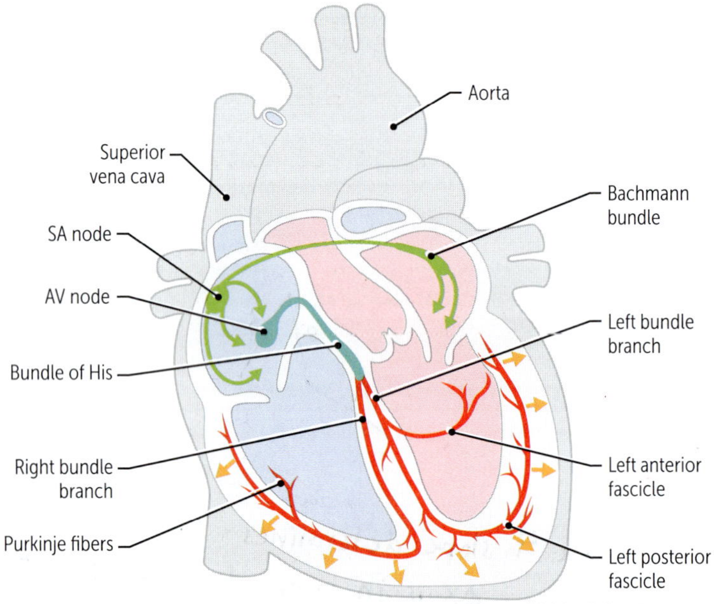

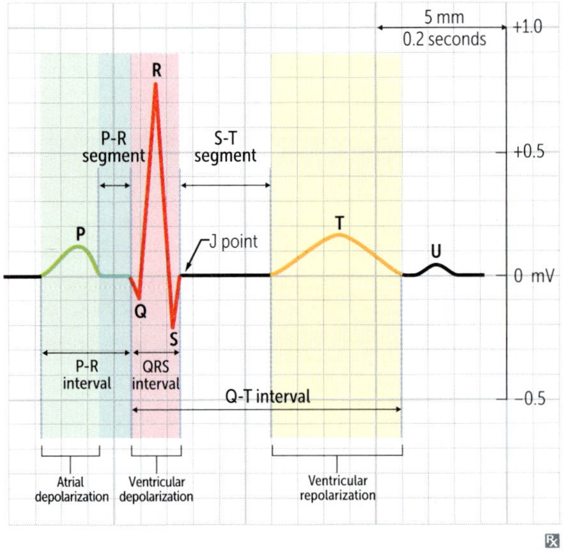

Torsades de pointes

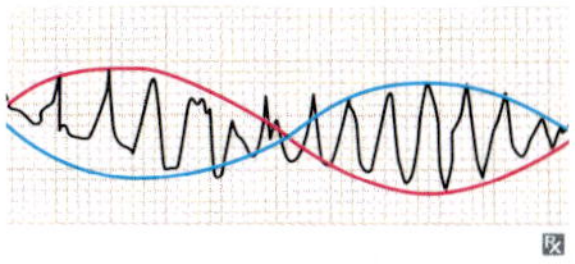

Polymorphic ventricular tachycardia, characterized by shifting sinusoidal waveforms on ECG; can progress to ventricular fibrillation (VF). Long QT interval predisposes to torsades de pointes. Caused by drugs, ↓ K^+, ↓ Mg^{2+}, congenital abnormalities. Treatment includes magnesium sulfate.

Drug-induced long QT (**ABCDE**):
- Anti**A**rrhythmics (class IA, III)
- Anti**B**iotics (eg, macrolides)
- Anti"**C**"ychotics (eg, haloperidol)
- Anti**D**epressants (eg, TCAs)
- Anti**E**metics (eg, ondansetron)

Torsades de pointes = twisting of the points

Congenital long QT syndrome

Inherited disorder of myocardial repolarization, typically due to ion channel defects; ↑ risk of sudden cardiac death (SCD) due to torsades de pointes. Includes:
- Romano-Ward syndrome—autosomal dominant, pure cardiac phenotype (no deafness).
- Jervell and Lange-Nielsen syndrome—autosomal recessive, sensorineural deafness.

*Faint is diff here = NO WARNING.
- often w/ emotion stress, phys.
- wake up sec later = normal
(normal faint = feel tired after)

Brugada syndrome

Autosomal dominant disorder most common in Asian males. ECG pattern of pseudo-right bundle branch block and ST elevations in V_1-V_3. ↑ risk of ventricular tachyarrhythmias and SCD. Prevent SCD with implantable cardioverter-defibrillator (ICD).

Wolff-Parkinson-White syndrome

Most common type of ventricular pre-excitation syndrome. Abnormal fast accessory conduction pathway from atria to ventricle (bundle of Kent) bypasses the rate-slowing AV node → ventricles begin to partially depolarize earlier → characteristic delta wave with widened QRS complex and shortened PR interval on ECG. May result in reentry circuit → supraventricular tachycardia.

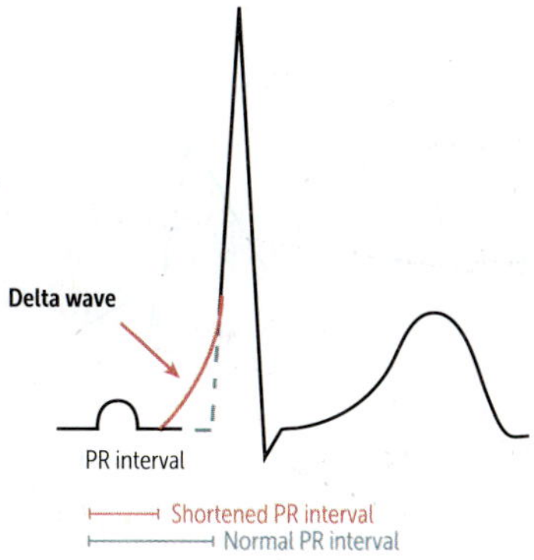

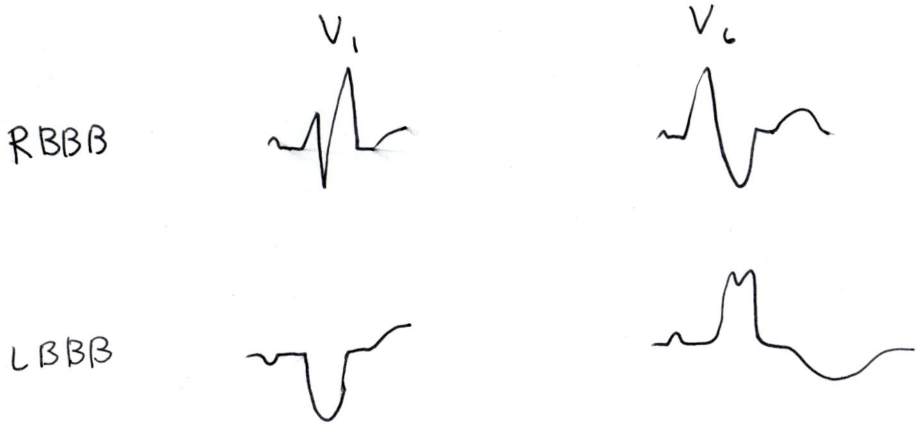

ECG tracings

RHYTHM	DESCRIPTION	EXAMPLE
Atrial fibrillation	Chaotic and erratic baseline with no discrete P waves in between irregularly spaced QRS complexes. Irregularly irregular heartbeat. Most common risk factors include hypertension and coronary artery disease (CAD). Can lead to thromboembolic events, particularly stroke. Treatment includes anticoagulation, rate control, rhythm control, and/or cardioversion.	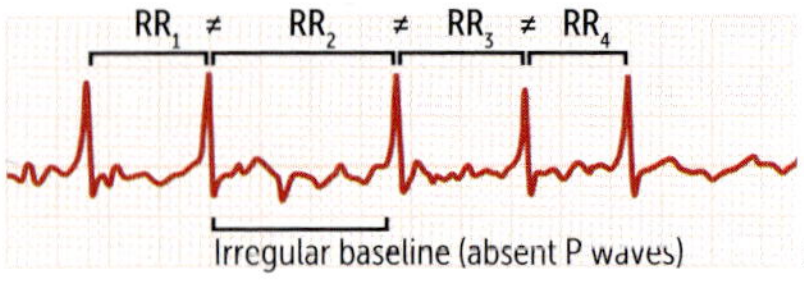
Atrial flutter	A rapid succession of identical, back-to-back atrial depolarization waves. The identical appearance accounts for the "sawtooth" appearance of the flutter waves. Treat like atrial fibrillation. Definitive treatment is catheter ablation.	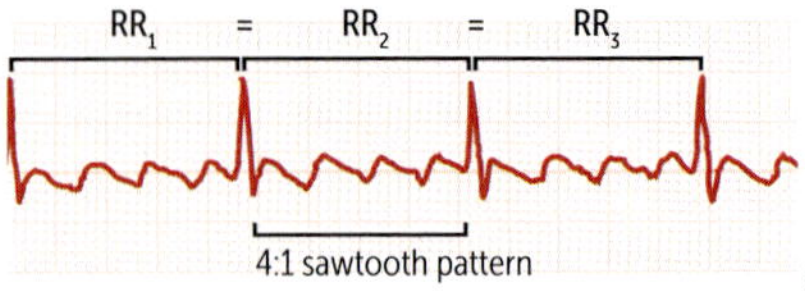
Ventricular fibrillation	A completely erratic rhythm with no identifiable waves. Fatal arrhythmia without immediate CPR and defibrillation.	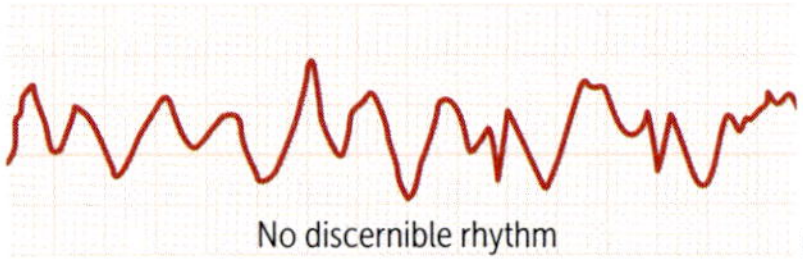
AV block		
1st degree	The PR interval is prolonged (> 200 msec). Benign and asymptomatic. No treatment required.	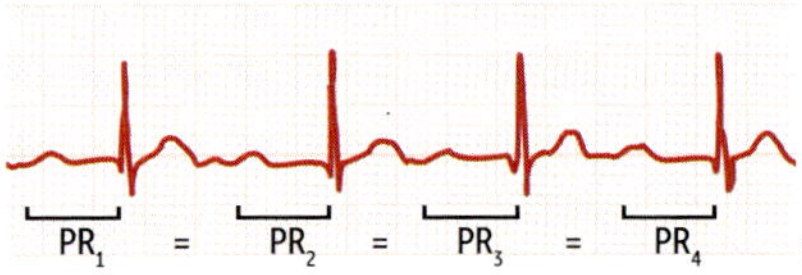
2nd degree		
Mobitz type I (Wenckebach)	Progressive lengthening of PR interval until a beat is "dropped" (a P wave not followed by a QRS complex). Usually asymptomatic. Variable RR interval with a pattern (regularly irregular).	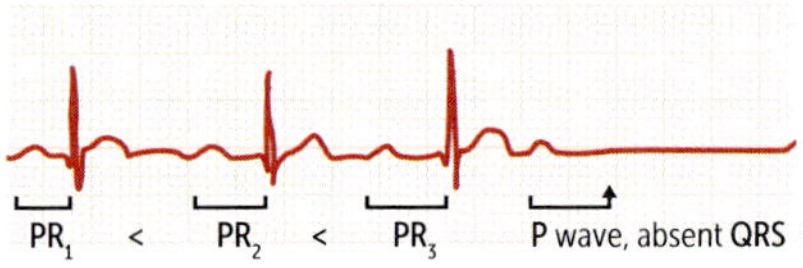
Mobitz type II	Dropped beats that are not preceded by a change in the length of the PR interval (as in type I). May progress to 3rd-degree block. Often treated with pacemaker.	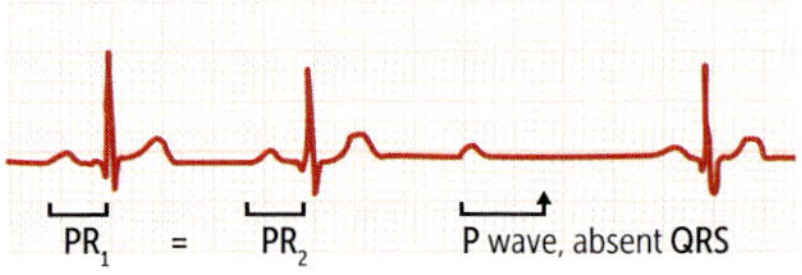
3rd degree (complete)	The atria and ventricles beat independently of each other. P waves and QRS complexes not rhythmically associated. Atrial rate > ventricular rate. Usually treated with pacemaker. Can be caused by Lyme disease.	

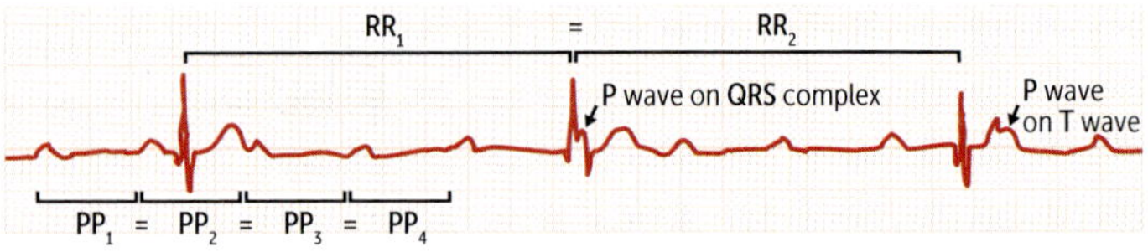

Atrial natriuretic peptide

Released from **atrial myocytes** in response to ↑ blood volume and atrial pressure. Acts via cGMP. Causes vasodilation and ↓ Na^+ reabsorption at the renal collecting tubule. Dilates afferent renal arterioles and constricts efferent arterioles, promoting diuresis and contributing to "aldosterone escape" mechanism.

B-type (brain) natriuretic peptide

Released from **ventricular myocytes** in response to ↑ tension. Similar physiologic action to ANP, with longer half-life. BNP blood test used for diagnosing HF (very good negative predictive value). Available in recombinant form (nesiritide) for treatment of HF.

Baroreceptors and chemoreceptors

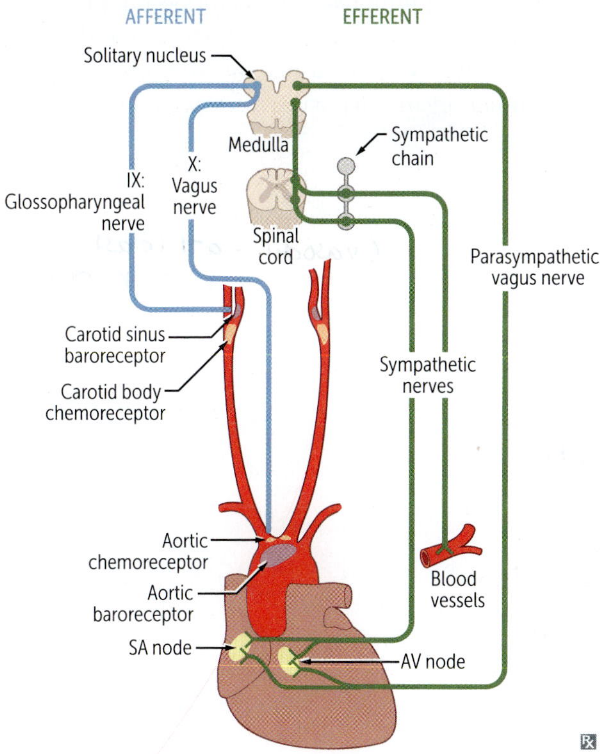

Receptors:

- Aortic arch transmits via vagus nerve to solitary nucleus of medulla (responds to ↓ and ↑ in BP).
- Carotid sinus (dilated region at carotid bifurcation) transmits via glossopharyngeal nerve to solitary nucleus of medulla (responds to ↓ and ↑ in BP).

Baroreceptors:

- Hypotension—↓ arterial pressure → ↓ stretch → ↓ afferent baroreceptor firing → ↑ efferent sympathetic firing and ↓ efferent parasympathetic stimulation → vasoconstriction, ↑ HR, ↑ contractility, ↑ BP. Important in the response to severe hemorrhage.
  - Carotid massage—↑ pressure on carotid sinus → ↑ stretch → ↑ afferent baroreceptor firing → ↑ AV node refractory period → ↓ HR.
  - Contributes to Cushing reaction (triad of hypertension, bradycardia, and respiratory depression)—↑ intracranial pressure constricts arterioles → cerebral ischemia → ↑ pCO_2 and ↓ pH → central reflex sympathetic ↑ in perfusion pressure (hypertension) → ↑ stretch → peripheral reflex baroreceptor–induced bradycardia.

Chemoreceptors:

- Peripheral—carotid and aortic bodies are stimulated by ↓ Po_2 (< 60 mm Hg), ↑ Pco_2, and ↓ pH of blood.
- Central—are stimulated by changes in pH and Pco_2 of brain interstitial fluid, which in turn are influenced by arterial CO_2. Do not directly respond to Po_2.

Normal cardiac pressures

Pulmonary capillary wedge pressure (PCWP; in mm Hg) is a good approximation of left atrial pressure. In mitral stenosis, PCWP > LV end diastolic pressure. PCWP is measured with pulmonary artery catheter (Swan-Ganz catheter).

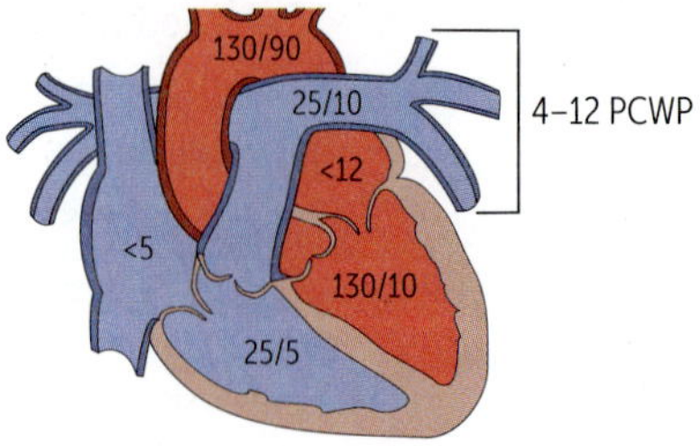

Autoregulation

How blood flow to an organ remains constant over a wide range of perfusion pressures.

ORGAN	FACTORS DETERMINING AUTOREGULATION	
Heart	Local metabolites (vasodilatory): adenosine, NO, CO_2, ↓ O_2	Note: the pulmonary vasculature is unique in that hypoxia causes vasoconstriction so that only well-ventilated areas are perfused. In other organs, hypoxia causes vasodilation.
Brain	Local metabolites (vasodilatory): ✱✱✱ CO_2 (pH)	
Kidneys	Myogenic and tubuloglomerular feedback	
Lungs	Hypoxia causes vasoconstriction	
Skeletal muscle	Local metabolites during exercise: lactate, adenosine, K^+, H^+, CO_2 At rest: sympathetic tone	**C**O_2, **H**$^+$, **A**denosine, **L**actate, **K**$^+$ (**CHALK**) (vasodil. - at least L A K are)
Skin	Sympathetic stimulation most important mechanism: temperature control	

α_1 & β_2 on skelet blood vessels

↑ vasoconst ↑ vasodil.

- heart most imp = ↓ O_2 & adenosine

Capillary fluid exchange

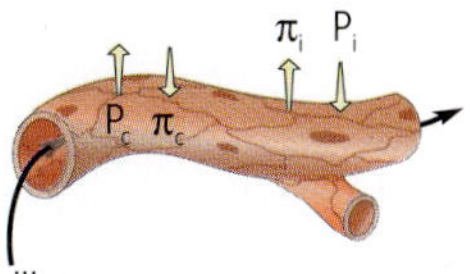

Starling forces determine fluid movement through capillary membranes:
- P_c = capillary pressure—pushes fluid out of capillary
- P_i = interstitial fluid pressure—pushes fluid into capillary
- π_c = plasma colloid osmotic (oncotic) pressure—pulls fluid into capillary
- π_i = interstitial fluid colloid osmotic pressure—pulls fluid out of capillary

J_v = net fluid flow = $K_f\,[(P_c - P_i) - \varsigma(\pi_c - \pi_i)]$

K_f = permeability of capillary to fluid

ς = permeability of capillary to protein

Edema—excess fluid outflow into interstitium commonly caused by:
- ↑ capillary pressure (↑ P_c; eg, HF)
- ↓ plasma proteins (↓ π_c; eg, nephrotic syndrome, liver failure, protein malnutrition)
- ↑ capillary permeability (↑ K_f; eg, toxins, infections, burns)
- ↑ interstitial fluid colloid osmotic pressure (↑ π_i; eg, lymphatic blockage)

▶ CARDIOVASCULAR—PATHOLOGY

Congenital heart diseases

RIGHT-TO-LEFT SHUNTS

Early cyanosis—"blue babies." Often diagnosed prenatally or become evident immediately after birth. Usually require urgent surgical treatment and/or maintenance of a PDA.

The 5 Ts:
1. Truncus arteriosus (1 vessel)
2. Transposition (2 switched vessels)
3. Tricuspid atresia (3 = Tri)
4. Tetralogy of Fallot (4 = Tetra)
5. TAPVR (5 letters in the name)

Persistent truncus arteriosus

Truncus arteriosus fails to divide into pulmonary trunk and aorta due to lack of aorticopulmonary septum formation; most patients have accompanying VSD. ← makes sense embryologically.

D-transposition of great vessels

Aorta leaves RV (anterior) and pulmonary trunk leaves LV (posterior) → separation of systemic and pulmonary circulations. Not compatible with life unless a shunt is present to allow mixing of blood (eg, VSD, PDA, or patent foramen ovale).

Due to failure of the aorticopulmonary septum to spiral.

Without surgical intervention, most infants die within the first few months of life.

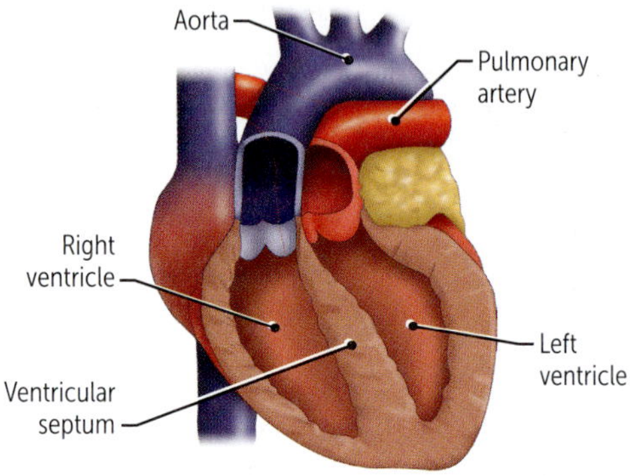

Tricuspid atresia

Absence of tricuspid valve and hypoplastic RV; requires both ASD and VSD for viability.

Tetralogy of Fallot

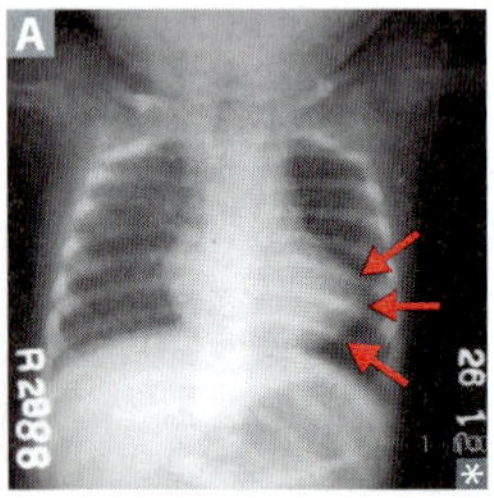

Caused by anterosuperior displacement of the infundibular septum. Most common cause of early childhood cyanosis.

1. Pulmonary infundibular stenosis (most important determinant for prognosis)
2. Right ventricular hypertrophy (RVH)—boot-shaped heart on CXR A
3. Overriding aorta
4. VSD

Pulmonary stenosis forces right-to-left flow across VSD → RVH, "tet spells" (often caused by crying, fever, and exercise due to exacerbation of RV outflow obstruction).

PROVe.

Squatting: ↑ SVR, ↓ right-to-left shunt, improves cyanosis.

Treatment: early surgical correction.

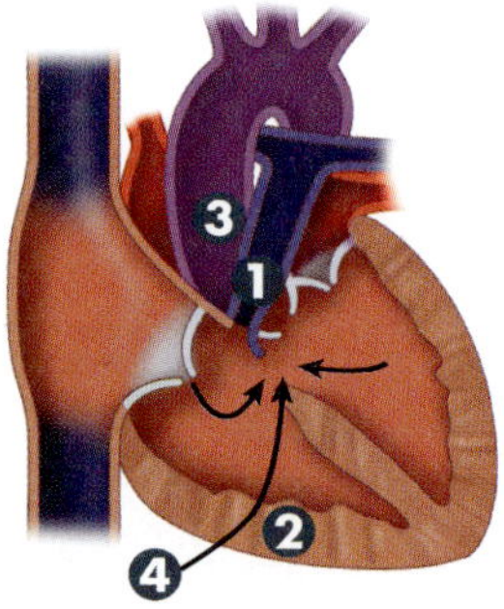

Total anomalous pulmonary venous return

Pulmonary veins drain into right heart circulation (SVC, coronary sinus, etc); associated with ASD and sometimes PDA to allow for right-to-left shunting to maintain CO.

Ebstein anomaly

Characterized by displacement of tricuspid valve leaflets downward into RV, artificially "atrializing" the ventricle. Associated with tricuspid regurgitation and right HF. Can be caused by lithium exposure in utero.

Congenital heart diseases *(continued)*

LEFT-TO-RIGHT SHUNTS	Late cyanosis (2° to Eisenmenger syndrome)—"blue kids." Frequency: VSD > ASD > PDA.	**R**ight-to-**L**eft shunts: ea**RL**y cyanosis. **L**eft-to-**R**ight shunts: "Late**R**" cyanosis.
Ventricular septal defect	Most common congenital cardiac defect. Asymptomatic at birth, may manifest weeks later or remain asymptomatic throughout life. Most self resolve; larger lesions may lead to LV overload and HF.	O_2 saturation ↑ in RV and pulmonary artery. — not right ?? ~~maybe bc the~~ LV has ~~less resistance than~~ pulm art.
Atrial septal defect 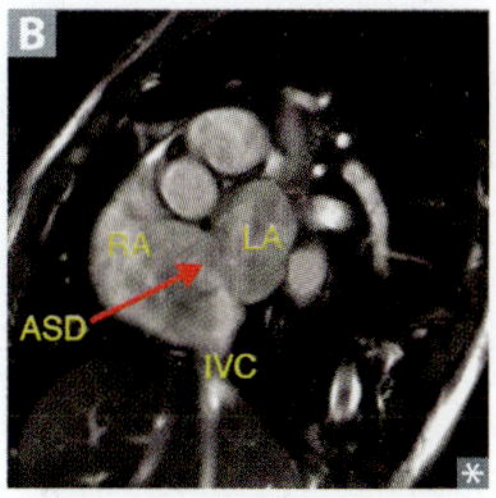	Defect in interatrial septum B; loud S1; wide, fixed split S2. Ostium secundum defects most common and usually occur as isolated findings; ostium primum defects rarer yet usually occur with other cardiac anomalies. Symptoms range from none to HF. Distinct from patent foramen ovale in that septa are missing tissue rather than unfused.	O_2 saturation ↑ in RA, RV, and pulmonary artery.
Patent ductus arteriosus 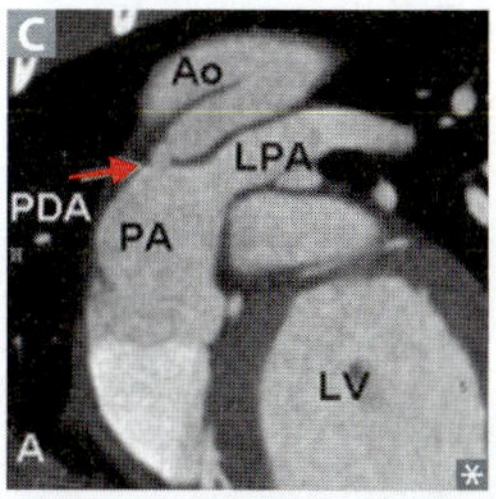	In fetal period, shunt is right to left (normal). In neonatal period, ↓ pulmonary vascular resistance → shunt becomes left to right → progressive RVH and/or LVH and HF. Associated with a continuous, "machine-like" murmur. Patency is maintained by PGE synthesis and low O_2 tension. Uncorrected PDA C can eventually result in late cyanosis in the lower extremities (differential cyanosis).	"**End**omethacin" (indomethacin) **end**s patency of PDA; P**G**E keeps ductus **G**oing (may be necessary to sustain life in conditions such as transposition of the great vessels). PDA is normal in utero and normally closes only after birth.
Eisenmenger syndrome 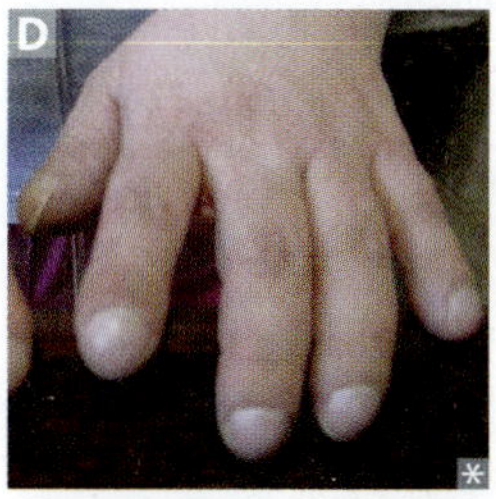	Uncorrected left-to-right shunt (VSD, ASD, PDA) → ↑ pulmonary blood flow → pathologic remodeling of vasculature → pulmonary arterial hypertension. RVH occurs to compensate → shunt becomes right to left. Causes late cyanosis, clubbing D, and polycythemia. Age of onset varies.	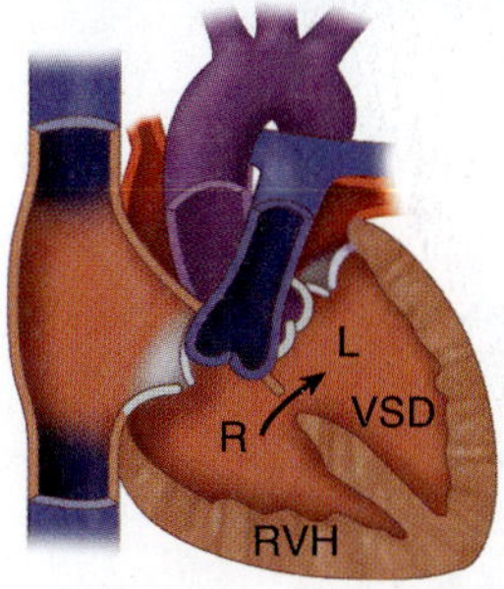
OTHER ANOMALIES		
Coarctation of the aorta	Aortic narrowing near insertion of ductus arteriosus ("juxtaductal"). Associated with bicuspid aortic valve, other heart defects, and Turner syndrome. Hypertension in upper extremities and weak, delayed pulse in lower extremities (brachial-femoral delay). With age, intercostal arteries enlarge due to collateral circulation; arteries erode ribs → notched appearance on CXR. Complications include HF, ↑ risk of cerebral hemorrhage (berry aneurysms), aortic rupture, and possible endocarditis.	

Congenital cardiac defect associations

DISORDER	DEFECT
Alcohol exposure in utero (fetal alcohol syndrome)	VSD, PDA, ASD, tetralogy of Fallot
Congenital rubella	PDA, pulmonary artery stenosis, septal defects
Down syndrome	AV septal defect (endocardial cushion defect), VSD, ASD
Infant of diabetic mother	Transposition of great vessels
Marfan syndrome	MVP, thoracic aortic aneurysm and dissection, aortic regurgitation
Prenatal lithium exposure	Ebstein anomaly
Turner syndrome	Bicuspid aortic valve, coarctation of aorta
Williams syndrome	Supravalvular aortic stenosis
22q11 syndromes	Truncus arteriosus, tetralogy of Fallot

Hypertension

Defined as persistent systolic BP ≥ 140 mm Hg and/or diastolic BP ≥ 90 mm Hg

RISK FACTORS

↑ age, obesity, diabetes, physical inactivity, excess salt intake, excess alcohol intake, family history; African American > Caucasian > Asian.

FEATURES

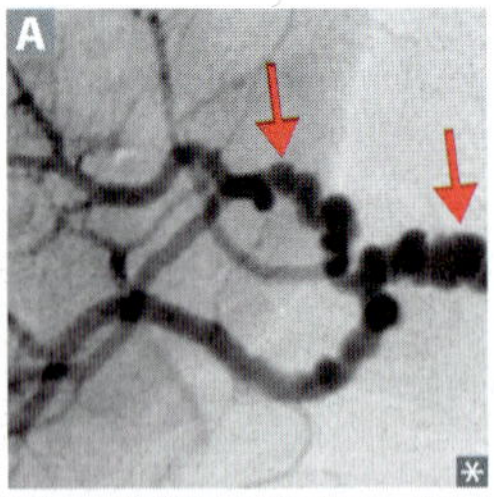

90% of hypertension is 1° (essential) and related to ↑ CO or ↑ TPR; remaining 10% mostly 2° to renal/renovascular disease (eg, fibromuscular dysplasia ["string of beads" appearance A], usually found in younger women) and 1° hyperaldosteronism.

Hypertensive urgency—severe (≥ 180/≥ 120 mm Hg) hypertension without acute end-organ damage.

Hypertensive emergency—severe hypertension with evidence of acute end-organ damage (eg, encephalopathy, stroke, retinal hemorrhages and exudates, papilledema, MI, HF, aortic dissection, kidney injury, microangiopathic hemolytic anemia, eclampsia).

PREDISPOSES TO

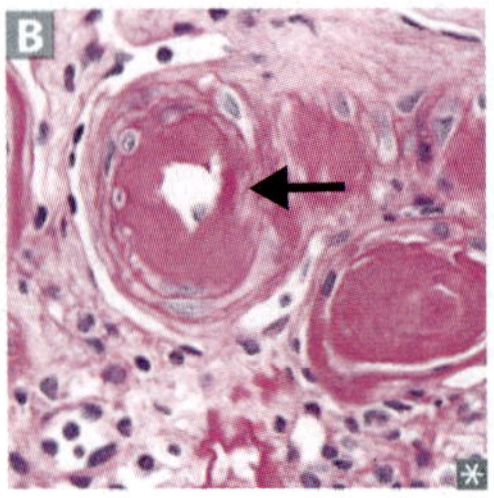

CAD, LVH, HF, AF; aortic dissection, aortic aneurysm; stroke; chronic kidney disease (hypertensive nephropathy) B; retinopathy.

Hyperlipidemia signs

Xanthomas	Plaques or nodules composed of lipid-laden histiocytes in skin A, especially the eyelids (xanthelasma B).
Tendinous xanthoma	Lipid deposit in tendon C, especially Achilles.
Corneal arcus	Lipid deposit in cornea. Common in elderly (arcus senilis D), but appears earlier in life in hypercholesterolemia.

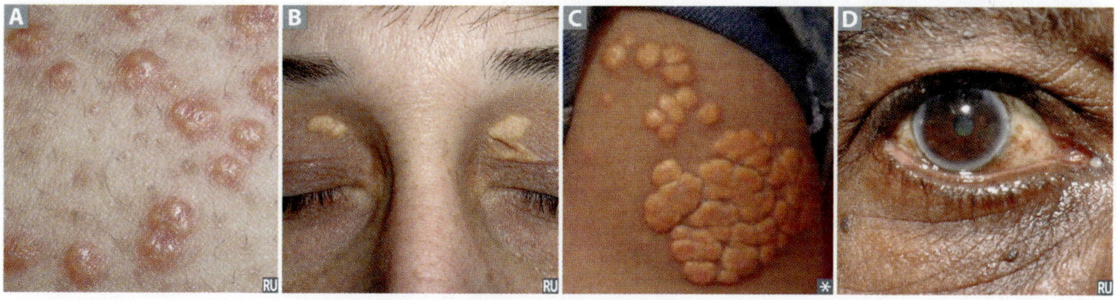

Arteriosclerosis

Arteriosclerosis	Hardening of arteries, with arterial wall thickening and loss of elasticity.
Arteriolosclerosis	Common. Affects small arteries and arterioles. Two types: hyaline (thickening of vessel walls in essential hypertension or diabetes mellitus A) and hyperplastic ("onion skinning" in severe hypertension B with proliferation of smooth muscle cells).
Mönckeberg sclerosis (medial calcific sclerosis)	Uncommon. Affects medium-sized arteries. Calcification of internal elastic lamina and media of arteries → vascular stiffening without obstruction. "Pipestem" appearance on x-ray C. Does not obstruct blood flow; intima not involved.

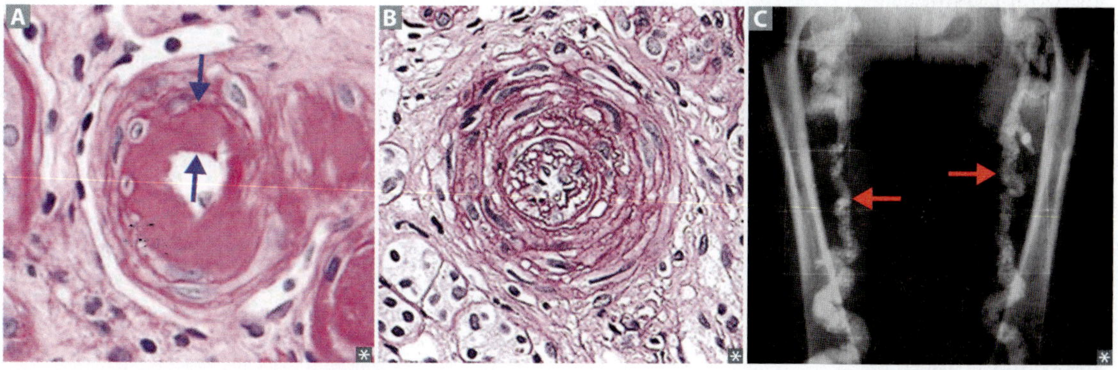

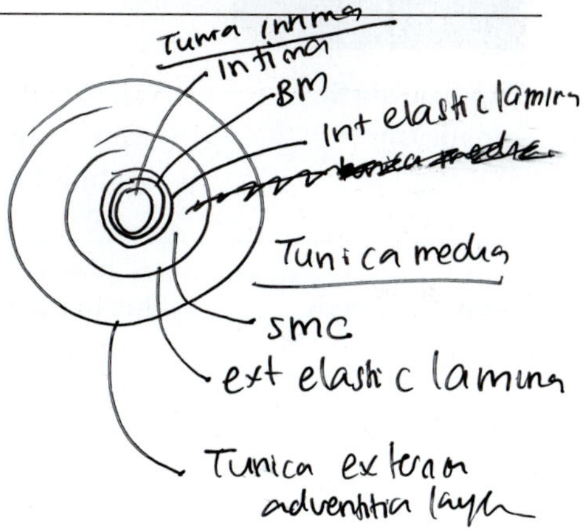

Atherosclerosis	Very common. Disease of elastic arteries and large- and medium-sized muscular arteries; a form of arteriosclerosis caused by buildup of cholesterol plaques.
LOCATION 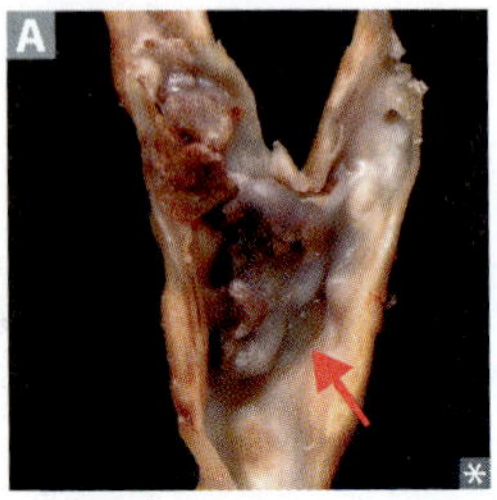	Abdominal aorta > coronary artery > popliteal artery > carotid artery A.
RISK FACTORS	Modifiable: smoking, hypertension, hyperlipidemia (↑ LDL), diabetes. Nonmodifiable: age, sex (↑ in men and postmenopausal women), family history.
SYMPTOMS	Angina, claudication, but can be asymptomatic.
PROGRESSION 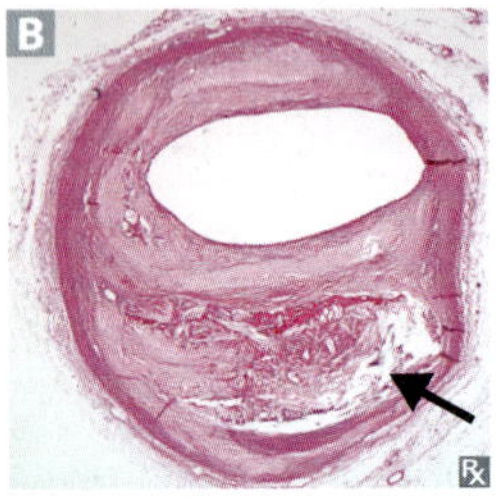	Inflammation important in pathogenesis: endothelial cell dysfunction → macrophage and LDL accumulation → foam cell formation → fatty streaks → smooth muscle cell migration (involves PDGF and FGF), proliferation, and extracellular matrix deposition → fibrous plaque → complex atheromas B.
COMPLICATIONS	Aneurysms, ischemia, infarcts, peripheral vascular disease, thrombus, emboli.

Aortic aneurysm	Localized pathologic dilatation of the aorta. May cause abdominal and/or back pain, which is a sign of leaking, dissection, or imminent rupture.
Abdominal aortic aneurysm 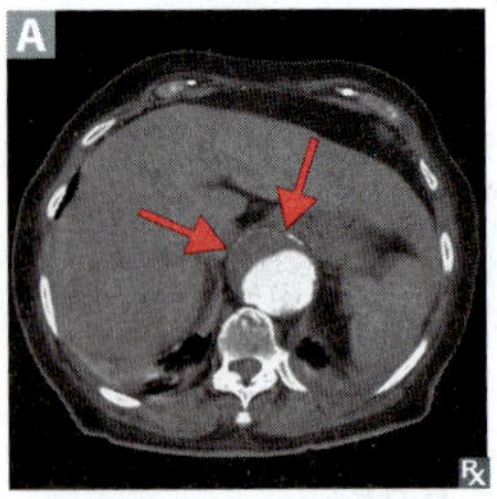	Associated with atherosclerosis. Risk factors include history of tobacco use, ↑ age, male sex, family history. May present as palpable pulsatile abdominal mass A.
Thoracic aortic aneurysm	Associated with cystic medial degeneration. Risk factors include hypertension, bicuspid aortic valve, connective tissue disease (eg, Marfan syndrome). Also historically associated with 3° syphilis (obliterative endarteritis of the vasa vasorum).

Traumatic aortic rupture	Due to trauma and/or deceleration injury, most commonly at aortic isthmus (proximal descending aorta just distal to origin of left subclavian artery).

Bicusp aorta valve – thoracic aneurysm, Aortic dissect.

Aortic dissection

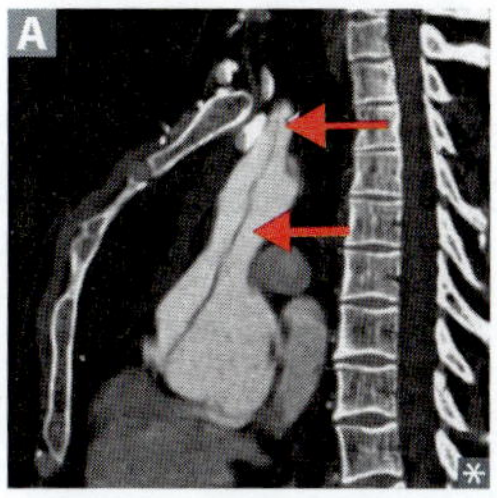

Longitudinal intimal tear forming a false lumen A. Associated with hypertension, bicuspid aortic valve, inherited connective tissue disorders (eg, Marfan syndrome). Can present with tearing chest pain, of sudden onset, radiating to the back +/– markedly unequal BP in arms. CXR shows mediastinal widening. Can result in organ ischemia, aortic rupture, death. Two types:

- Stanford type A (proximal): involves Ascending aorta. May extend to aortic arch or descending aorta. May result in acute aortic regurgitation or cardiac tamponade. Treatment: surgery.
- Stanford type B (distal): involves descending aorta and/or aortic arch. No ascending aorta involvement. Treat medically with β-blockers, then vasodilators.

Ischemic heart disease manifestations

Angina

Chest pain due to ischemic myocardium 2° to coronary artery narrowing or spasm; no myocyte necrosis.

- Stable—usually 2° to atherosclerosis; exertional chest pain in classic distribution (usually with ST depression on ECG), resolving with rest or nitroglycerin.
- Variant (Prinzmetal)—occurs at rest 2° to coronary artery spasm; transient ST elevation on ECG. Known triggers include tobacco, cocaine, and triptans, but trigger is often unknown. Treat with Ca^{2+} channel blockers, nitrates, and smoking cessation (if applicable).
- Unstable—thrombosis with incomplete coronary artery occlusion; +/– ST depression and/or T-wave inversion on ECG but no cardiac biomarker elevation (unlike NSTEMI); ↑ in frequency or intensity of chest pain or any chest pain at rest.

Coronary steal syndrome

Distal to coronary stenosis, vessels are maximally dilated at baseline. Administration of vasodilators (eg, dipyridamole, regadenoson) dilates normal vessels and shunts blood toward well-perfused areas → ↓ flow and ischemia in poststenotic region. Principle behind pharmacologic stress tests.

Sudden cardiac death

Death from cardiac causes within 1 hour of onset of symptoms, most commonly due to a lethal arrhythmia (eg, VF). Associated with CAD (up to 70% of cases), cardiomyopathy (hypertrophic, dilated), and hereditary ion channelopathies (eg, long QT syndrome, Brugada syndrome). Prevent with implantable cardioverter-defibrillator (ICD).

Chronic ischemic heart disease

Progressive onset of HF over many years due to chronic ischemic myocardial damage.

Myocardial infarction

Most often acute thrombosis due to rupture of coronary artery atherosclerotic plaque. ↑ cardiac biomarkers (CK-MB, troponins) are diagnostic.

ST-segment elevation MI (STEMI)

Transmural infarcts
Full thickness of myocardial wall involved
ST elevation on ECG, Q waves

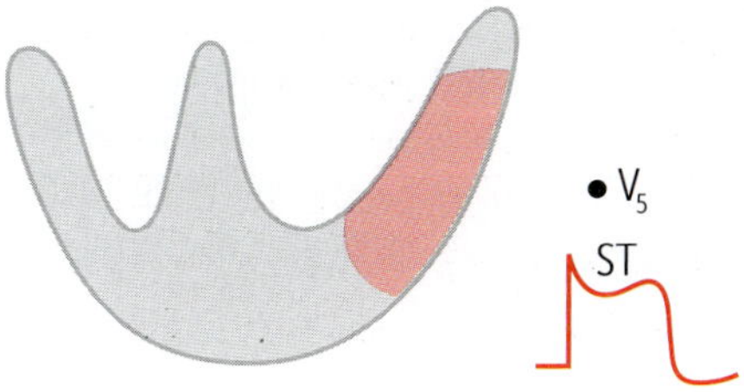

Non–ST-segment elevation MI (NSTEMI)

Subendocardial infarcts
Subendocardium (inner ⅓) especially vulnerable to ischemia
ST depression on ECG

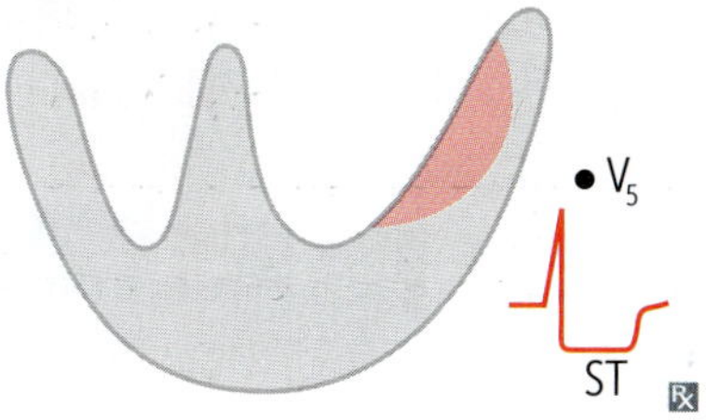

Evolution of myocardial infarction

Commonly occluded coronary arteries: LAD > RCA > circumflex.

Symptoms: diaphoresis, nausea, vomiting, severe retrosternal pain, pain in left arm and/or jaw, shortness of breath, fatigue.

TIME	GROSS	LIGHT MICROSCOPE	COMPLICATIONS
0–24 hr	None 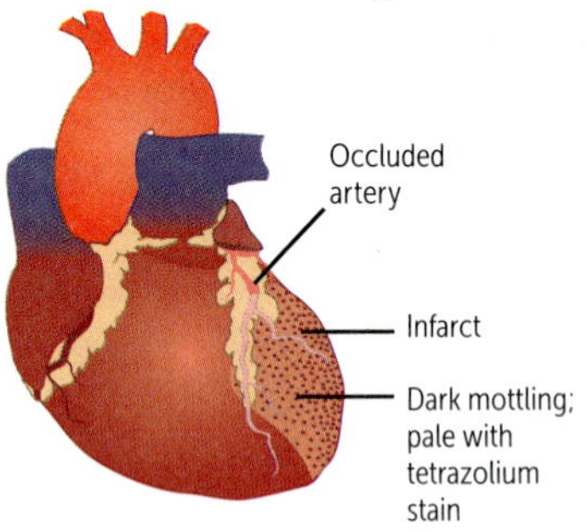	Early coagulative necrosis, release of necrotic cell contents into blood; edema, hemorrhage, wavy fibers. Neutrophils appear. Reperfusion injury, associated with generation of free radicals, leads to hypercontraction of myofibrils through ↑ free calcium influx. 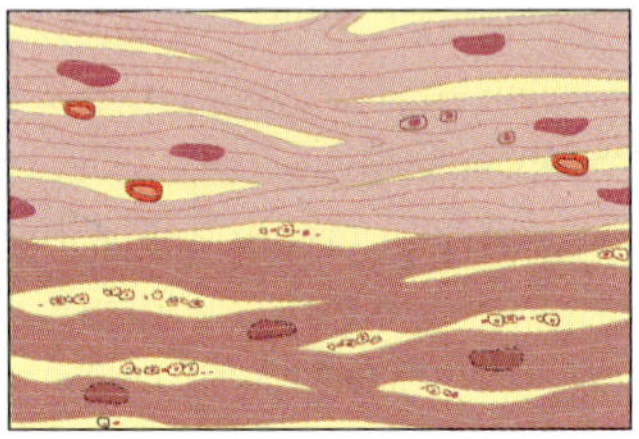	Ventricular arrhythmia, HF, cardiogenic shock.
1–3 days	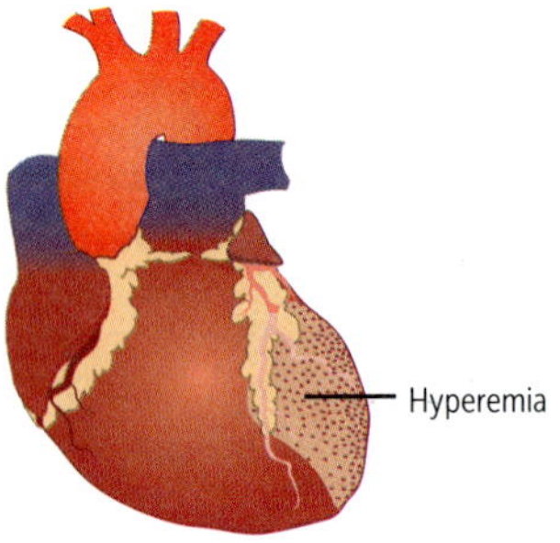	Extensive coagulative necrosis. Tissue surrounding infarct shows acute inflammation with neutrophils. 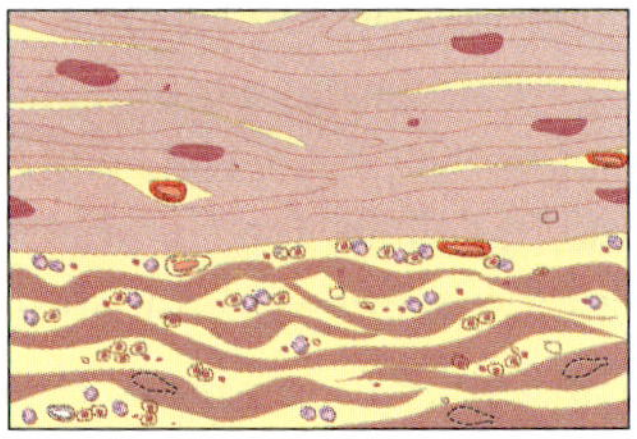	Postinfarction fibrinous pericarditis.
3–14 days	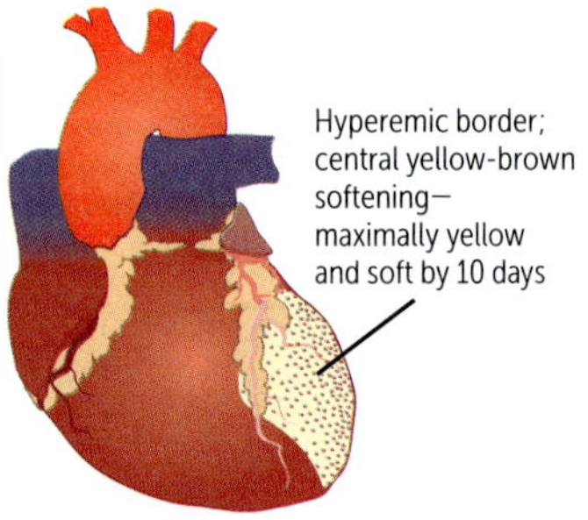	Macrophages, then granulation tissue at margins. 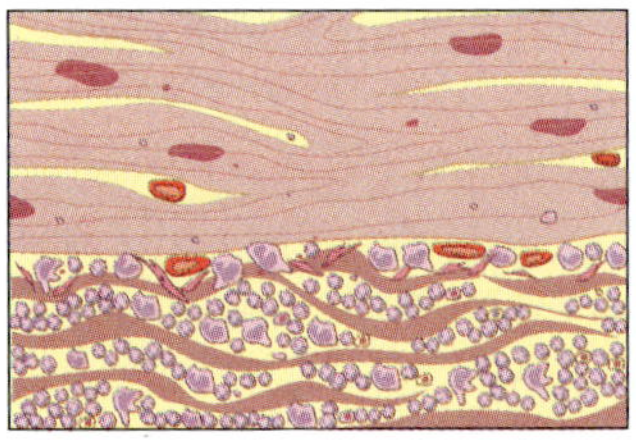	Free wall rupture → tamponade; papillary muscle rupture → mitral regurgitation; interventricular septal rupture due to macrophage-mediated structural degradation. LV pseudoaneurysm (risk of rupture).
2 weeks to several months	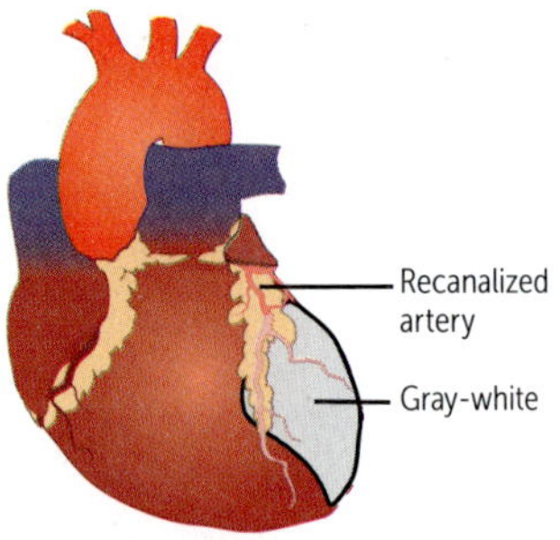	Contracted scar complete. 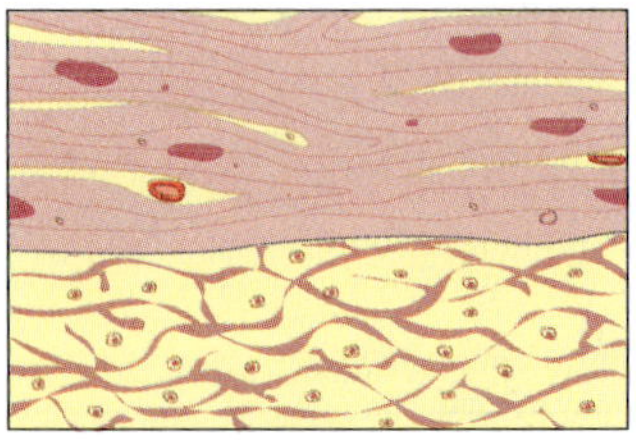	Dressler syndrome, HF, arrhythmias, true ventricular aneurysm (risk of mural thrombus).

Diagnosis of myocardial infarction

In the first 6 hours, ECG is the gold standard.

Cardiac troponin I rises after 4 hours (peaks at 24 hr) and is ↑ for 7–10 days; more specific than other protein markers.

CK-MB rises after 6–12 hours (peaks at 16–24 hr) and is predominantly found in myocardium but can also be released from skeletal muscle. Useful in diagnosing reinfarction following acute MI because levels return to normal after 48 hours.

Large MIs lead to greater elevations in troponin I and CK-MB.

ECG changes can include ST elevation (STEMI, transmural infarct), ST depression (NSTEMI, subendocardial infarct), hyperacute (peaked) T waves, T-wave inversion, new left bundle branch block, and pathologic Q waves or poor R wave progression (evolving or old transmural infarct).

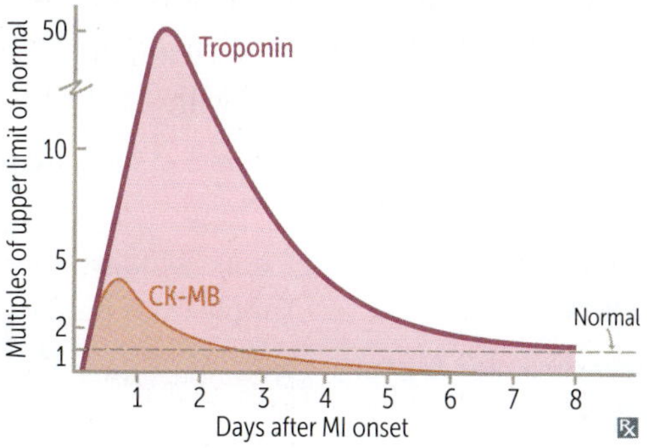

ECG localization of STEMI

INFARCT LOCATION	LEADS WITH ST ELEVATIONS OR Q WAVES
Anteroseptal (LAD)	V_1–V_2
Anteroapical (distal LAD)	V_3–V_4
Anterolateral (LAD or LCX)	V_5–V_6
Lateral (LCX)	I, aV**L**
In**F**erior (RCA)	II, III, aV**F**
Posterior (PDA)	V_7–V_9, ST depression in V_1–V_3 with tall R waves

0-24 hrs coag necrosis (vent arrythm / HF / cardiog shock)
neutrophils
Reperfusion → free radic.
hypercontract. of myofib. thru ↑ free Ca influx

1-3 days more coag necrosis (post infarc. fibrinous pericard)
tissue around = acute inflam w/ neutroph.

3-14 days macroph. / granul tissue at margins (free wall rupture → tamp. cardiac
papillary musc rupture → mitral regurg
IV septum rupture bc of macroph. mediated struct degrad.

2 week-mo Dressler synd / HF
arrythm, true ventricular aneurysm (risk of mural thrombus)
LV pseudoaneu (risk of rupture)

Myocardial infarction complications

Cardiac arrhythmia	Occurs within the first few days after MI. Important cause of death before reaching the hospital and within the first 24 hours post-MI.
Postinfarction fibrinous pericarditis	Occurs 1–3 days after MI. Friction rub.
Papillary muscle rupture	Occurs 2–7 days after MI. Posteromedial papillary muscle rupture A ↑ risk due to single blood supply from posterior descending artery. Can result in severe mitral regurgitation.
Interventricular septal rupture	Occurs 3–5 days after MI. Macrophage-mediated degradation → VSD.
Ventricular pseudoaneurysm formation	Occurs 3–14 days after MI. Contained free wall rupture B; ↓ CO, risk of arrhythmia, embolus from mural thrombus.
Ventricular free wall rupture	Occurs 5–14 days after MI. Free wall rupture C → cardiac tamponade.
True ventricular aneurysm	Occurs 2 weeks to several months after MI. Outward bulge with contraction ("dyskinesia"), associated with fibrosis.
Dressler syndrome	Occurs several weeks after MI. Autoimmune phenomenon resulting in fibrinous pericarditis.
LV failure and pulmonary edema	Can occur 2° to LV infarction, VSD, free wall rupture, papillary muscle rupture with mitral regurgitation.

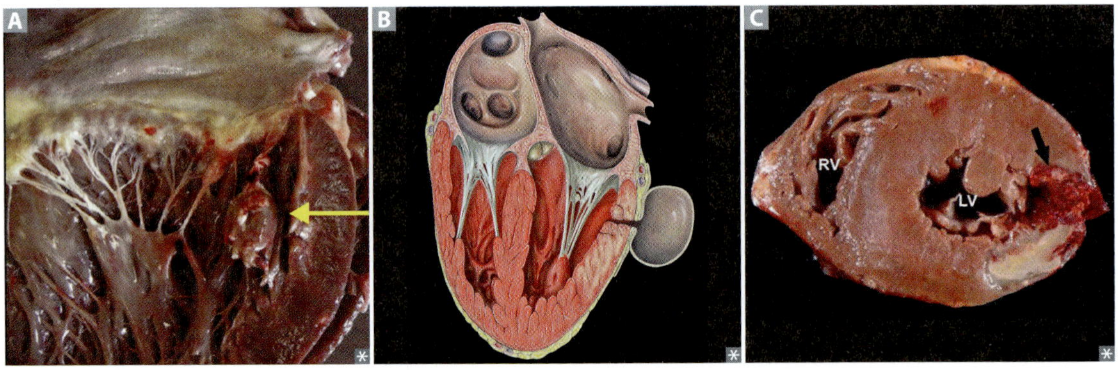

Acute coronary syndrome treatments

Unstable angina/NSTEMI—Anticoagulation (eg, heparin), antiplatelet therapy (eg, aspirin + ADP receptor inhibitors (eg, clopidogrel), β-blockers, ACE inhibitors, statins. Symptom control with nitroglycerin and morphine.

STEMI—In addition to above, reperfusion therapy most important (percutaneous coronary intervention preferred over fibrinolysis).

Cardiomyopathies

Dilated cardiomyopathy 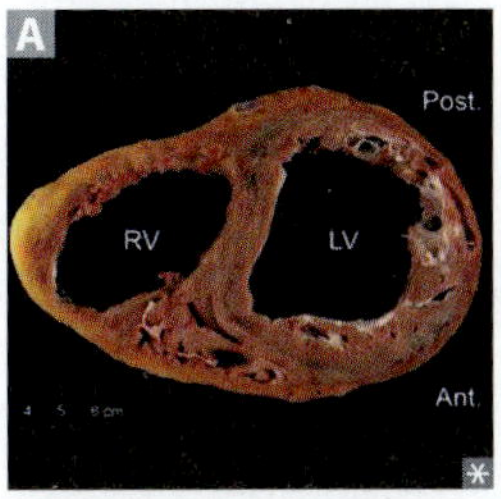	Most common cardiomyopathy (90% of cases). Often idiopathic or familial. Other etiologies include chronic **A**lcohol abuse, wet **B**eriberi, **C**oxsackie B viral myocarditis, chronic **C**ocaine use, **C**hagas disease, **D**oxorubicin toxicity, hemochromatosis, sarcoidosis, peripartum cardiomyopathy. Findings: HF, S3, systolic regurgitant murmur, dilated heart on echocardiogram, balloon appearance of heart on CXR. Treatment: Na^+ restriction, ACE inhibitors, β-blockers, diuretics, digoxin, ICD, heart transplant.	Systolic dysfunction ensues. Eccentric hypertrophy A (sarcomeres added in series). **ABCCCD**.
Hypertrophic cardiomyopathy 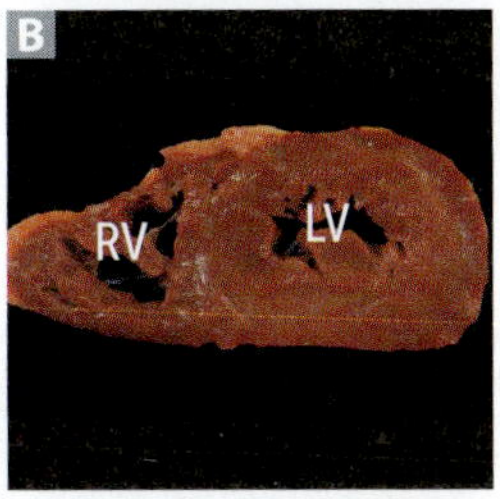	60–70% of cases are familial, autosomal dominant (commonly a β-myosin heavy-chain mutation). Can be associated with Friedreich ataxia. Causes syncope during exercise and may lead to sudden death in young athletes due to ventricular arrhythmia. Findings: S4, systolic murmur. May see mitral regurgitation due to impaired mitral valve closure. Treatment: cessation of high-intensity athletics, use of β-blocker or non-dihydropyridine Ca^{2+} channel blockers (eg, verapamil). ICD if patient is high risk.	Diastolic dysfunction ensues. Marked ventricular hypertrophy B, often septal predominance. Myofibrillar disarray and fibrosis. Obstructive hypertrophic cardiomyopathy (subset)—asymmetric septal hypertrophy and systolic anterior motion of mitral valve → outflow obstruction → dyspnea, possible syncope.
Restrictive/infiltrative cardiomyopathy	Major causes include sarcoidosis, amyloidosis, postradiation fibrosis, endocardial fibroelastosis (thick fibroelastic tissue in endocardium of young children), Löffler syndrome (endomyocardial fibrosis with a prominent eosinophilic infiltrate), and hemochromatosis (although dilated cardiomyopathy is more common).	Diastolic dysfunction ensues. Can have low-voltage ECG despite thick myocardium (especially amyloid).

restrictive HD causes dilated cardiomyop

Heart failure

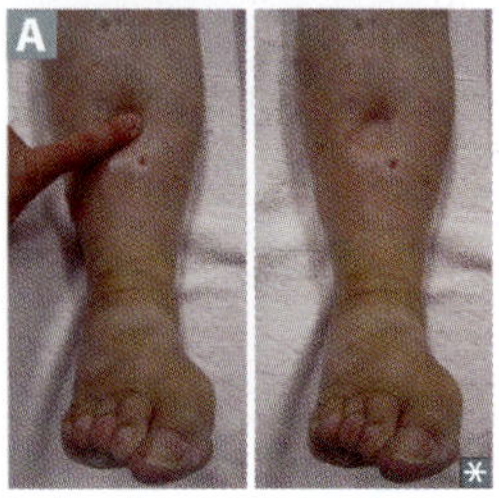

Clinical syndrome of cardiac pump dysfunction → congestion and low perfusion. Symptoms include dyspnea, orthopnea, fatigue; signs include rales, jugular venous distention (JVD), pitting edema A.

Systolic dysfunction—reduced EF, ↑ EDV; ↓ contractility often 2° to ischemia/MI or dilated cardiomyopathy.

Diastolic dysfunction—preserved EF, normal EDV; ↓ compliance often 2° to myocardial hypertrophy.

Right HF most often results from left HF. Cor pulmonale refers to isolated right HF due to pulmonary cause.

ACE inhibitors or angiotensin II receptor blockers, β-blockers (except in acute decompensated HF), and spironolactone ↓ mortality. Thiazide or loop diuretics are used mainly for symptomatic relief. Hydralazine with nitrate therapy improves both symptoms and mortality in select patients.

Left heart failure	
Orthopnea	Shortness of breath when supine: ↑ venous return from redistribution of blood (immediate gravity effect) exacerbates pulmonary vascular congestion.
Paroxysmal nocturnal dyspnea	Breathless awakening from sleep: ↑ venous return from redistribution of blood, reabsorption of peripheral edema, etc.
Pulmonary edema	↑ pulmonary venous pressure → pulmonary venous distention and transudation of fluid. Presence of hemosiderin-laden macrophages ("HF" cells) in lungs.
Right heart failure	
Hepatomegaly (nutmeg liver)	↑ central venous pressure → ↑ resistance to portal flow. Rarely, leads to "cardiac cirrhosis."
Jugular venous distention	↑ venous pressure.
Peripheral edema	↑ venous pressure → fluid transudation.

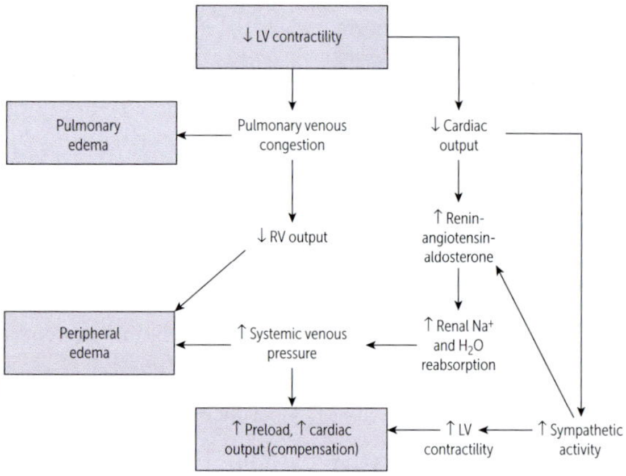

Shock

Inadequate organ perfusion and delivery of nutrients necessary for normal tissue and cellular function. Initially may be reversible but life-threatening if not treated promptly.

<table>
<tr><th></th><th>CAUSED BY</th><th>SKIN</th><th>PCWP (PRELOAD)</th><th>CO</th><th>SVR (AFTERLOAD)</th><th>TREATMENT</th></tr>
<tr><td>Hypovolemic</td><td>Hemorrhage, dehydration, burns</td><td>Cold, clammy</td><td>↓↓</td><td>↓</td><td>↑</td><td>IV fluids</td></tr>
<tr><td>Cardiogenic</td><td>Acute MI, HF, valvular dysfunction, arrhythmia</td><td rowspan="2">Cold, clammy</td><td rowspan="2">↑</td><td rowspan="2">↓↓</td><td rowspan="2">↑</td><td>Inotropes, diuresis</td></tr>
<tr><td>Obstructive</td><td>Cardiac tamponade, pulmonary embolism</td><td>Relieve obstruction</td></tr>
<tr><td rowspan="2">Distributive</td><td>Sepsis, anaphylaxis</td><td>Warm</td><td>↓</td><td>↑</td><td>↓↓</td><td rowspan="2">IV fluids, pressors</td></tr>
<tr><td>CNS injury</td><td>Dry</td><td>↓</td><td>↓</td><td>↓↓</td></tr>
</table>

Bacterial endocarditis

Fever (most common symptom), new murmur, Roth spots (round white spots on retina surrounded by hemorrhage), Osler nodes (tender raised lesions on finger or toe pads), Janeway lesions (small, painless, erythematous lesions on palm or sole) A, glomerulonephritis, septic arterial or pulmonary emboli, splinter hemorrhages B on nail bed. Multiple blood cultures necessary for diagnosis.

- Acute—*S aureus* (high virulence). Large vegetations on previously normal valves C. Rapid onset.
- Subacute—viridans streptococci (low virulence). Smaller vegetations on congenitally abnormal or diseased valves. Sequela of dental procedures. Gradual onset.

S bovis (gallolyticus) is present in colon cancer, *S epidermidis* on prosthetic valves.

Endocarditis may also be nonbacterial (marantic/thrombotic) 2° to malignancy, hypercoagulable state, or lupus.

Mitral valve is most frequently involved.

Tricuspid valve endocarditis is associated with IV **drug** abuse (don't "**tri**" **drugs**). Associated with *S aureus*, *Pseudomonas*, and *Candida*.

Culture ⊖—most likely *Coxiella burnetii*, *Bartonella* spp., HACEK (*Haemophilus*, *Aggregatibacter* (formerly *Actinobacillus*), *Cardiobacterium*, *Eikenella*, *Kingella*)

♥ Bacteria **FROM JANE** ♥:

Fever
Roth spots
Osler nodes
Murmur
Janeway lesions
Anemia
Nail-bed hemorrhage
Emboli

Osler = immune complex depos.

Janeway = septic emboli from valvular veget.

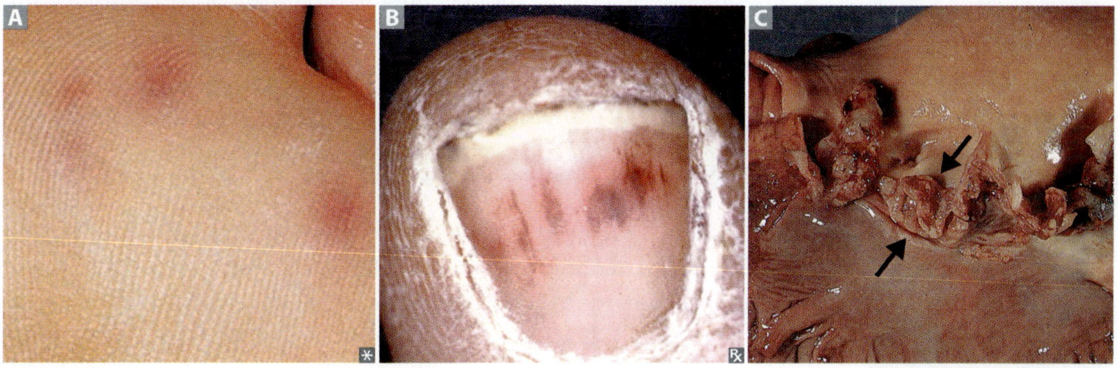

Rheumatic fever

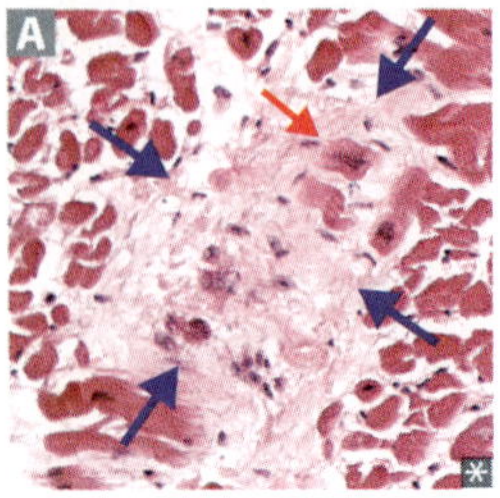

A consequence of pharyngeal infection with group A β-hemolytic streptococci. Late sequelae include rheu**mat**ic heart disease, which affects heart valves—**m**itral > **a**ortic >> **t**ricuspid (high-pressure valves affected most). Early lesion is mitral valve regurgitation; late lesion is mitral stenosis. Associated with Aschoff bodies (granuloma with giant cells [blue arrows in A]), Anitschkow cells (enlarged macrophages with ovoid, wavy, rod-like nucleus [red arrow in A]), ↑ anti-streptolysin O (ASO) titers.

Immune mediated (type II hypersensitivity); not a direct effect of bacteria. Antibodies to M protein cross-react with self antigens (molecular mimicry).

Treatment/prophylaxis: penicillin.

J♥NES (major criteria):
- **J**oint (migratory polyarthritis)
- **♥** (carditis)
- **N**odules in skin (subcutaneous)
- **E**rythema marginatum
- **S**ydenham chorea

Acute pericarditis

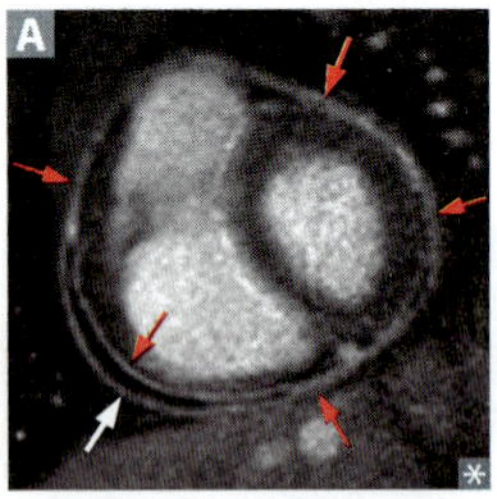

Inflammation of the pericardium [A, arrows]. Commonly presents with sharp pain, aggravated by inspiration, and relieved by sitting up and leaning forward. Often complicated by pericardial effusion [white arrow in A]. Presents with friction rub. ECG changes include widespread ST-segment elevation and/or PR depression.

Causes include idiopathic (most common; presumed viral), confirmed infection (eg, Coxsackievirus), neoplasia, autoimmune (eg, SLE, rheumatoid arthritis), uremia, cardiovascular (acute STEMI or Dressler syndrome), radiation therapy.

Cardiac tamponade

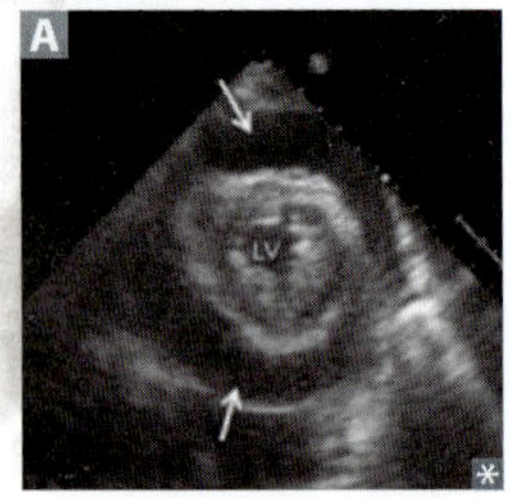

Compression of the heart by fluid (eg, blood, effusions [arrows in A] in pericardial space) → ↓ CO. Equilibration of diastolic pressures in all 4 chambers.

Findings: Beck triad (hypotension, distended neck veins, distant heart sounds), ↑ HR, pulsus paradoxus. ECG shows low-voltage QRS and electrical alternans (due to "swinging" movement of heart in large effusion).

Pulsus paradoxus—↓ in amplitude of systolic BP by > 10 mm Hg during inspiration. Seen in cardiac tamponade, asthma, obstructive sleep apnea, pericarditis, croup.

Syphilitic heart disease

3° syphilis disrupts the vasa vasorum of the aorta with consequent atrophy of vessel wall and dilatation of aorta and valve ring.

May see calcification of aortic root and ascending aortic arch. Leads to "tree bark" appearance of aorta.

Can result in aneurysm of ascending aorta or aortic arch, aortic insufficiency.

Cardiac tumors

Most common heart tumor is a metastasis.

Myxomas

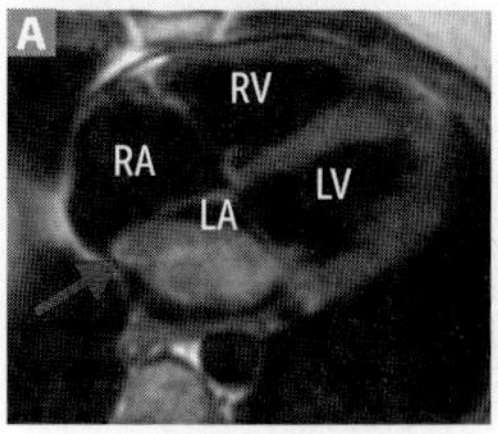

Most common 1° cardiac tumor in adults A. 90% occur in the atria (mostly left atrium). Myxomas are usually described as a "ball valve" obstruction in the left atrium (associated with multiple syncopal episodes). May hear early diastolic "tumor plop" sound.

- myxoma = CT tumor
 - mucus, gelatinous material

Rhabdomyomas

Most frequent 1° cardiac tumor in children (associated with tuberous sclerosis).

Kussmaul sign

↑ in JVP on inspiration instead of a normal ↓.

Inspiration → negative intrathoracic pressure not transmitted to heart → impaired filling of right ventricle → blood backs up into venae cavae → JVD. May be seen with constrictive pericarditis, restrictive cardiomyopathies, right atrial or ventricular tumors.

- rhabdomyoma = benign striated muscle tumor

Vasculitides

	EPIDEMIOLOGY/PRESENTATION	PATHOLOGY/LABS
Large-vessel vasculitis		
Giant cell (temporal) arteritis	Usually elderly females. Unilateral headache (temporal artery), jaw claudication. May lead to irreversible blindness due to ophthalmic artery occlusion. Associated with polymyalgia rheumatica.	Most commonly affects branches of carotid artery. Focal granulomatous inflammation A. ↑ ESR. Treat with high-dose corticosteroids prior to temporal artery biopsy to prevent blindness.
Takayasu arteritis	Usually Asian females < 40 years old. "Pulseless disease" (weak upper extremity pulses), fever, night sweats, arthritis, myalgias, skin nodules, ocular disturbances.	Granulomatous thickening and narrowing of aortic arch B and proximal great vessels. ↑ ESR. Treat with corticosteroids.
Medium-vessel vasculitis		
Polyarteritis nodosa	Young adults. Hepatitis B seropositivity in 30% of patients. Fever, weight loss, malaise, headache. GI: abdominal pain, melena. Hypertension, neurologic dysfunction, cutaneous eruptions, renal damage.	Typically involves renal and visceral vessels, not pulmonary arteries. Immune complex mediated. Transmural inflammation of the arterial wall with fibrinoid necrosis. Different stages of inflammation may coexist in different vessels. Innumerable renal microaneurysms C and spasms on arteriogram. Treat with corticosteroids, cyclophosphamide.
Kawasaki disease (mucocutaneous lymph node syndrome)	Asian children < 4 years old. Conjunctival injection, Rash (polymorphous → desquamating), Adenopathy (cervical), Strawberry tongue (oral mucositis) D, Hand-foot changes (edema, erythema), fever.	CRASH and burn. May develop coronary artery aneurysms E; thrombosis or rupture can cause death. Treat with IV immunoglobulin and aspirin.
Buerger disease (thromboangiitis obliterans)	Heavy smokers, males < 40 years old. Intermittent claudication may lead to gangrene F, autoamputation of digits, superficial nodular phlebitis. Raynaud phenomenon is often present.	Segmental thrombosing vasculitis. Treat with smoking cessation.
Small-vessel vasculitis		
Granulomatosis with polyangiitis (Wegener)	Upper respiratory tract: perforation of nasal septum, chronic sinusitis, otitis media, mastoiditis. Lower respiratory tract: hemoptysis, cough, dyspnea. Renal: hematuria, red cell casts.	Triad: ▪ Focal necrotizing vasculitis ▪ Necrotizing granulomas in the lung and upper airway ▪ Necrotizing glomerulonephritis PR3-ANCA/c-ANCA G (anti-proteinase 3). CXR: large nodular densities. Treat with cyclophosphamide, corticosteroids.
Microscopic polyangiitis	Necrotizing vasculitis commonly involving lung, kidneys, and skin with pauci-immune glomerulonephritis and palpable purpura. Presentation similar to granulomatosis with polyangiitis but without nasopharyngeal involvement.	No granulomas. MPO-ANCA/p-ANCA H (anti-myeloperoxidase). Treat with cyclophosphamide, corticosteroids.

Vasculitides *(continued)*

	EPIDEMIOLOGY/PRESENTATION	PATHOLOGY/LABS
Small-vessel vasculitis *(continued)*		
Eosinophilic granulomatosis with polyangiitis (Churg-Strauss)	Asthma, sinusitis, skin nodules or purpura, peripheral neuropathy (eg, wrist/foot drop). Can also involve heart, GI, kidneys (pauci-immune glomerulonephritis).	Granulomatous, necrotizing vasculitis with eosinophilia I. MPO-ANCA/p-ANCA, ↑ IgE level.
Henoch-Schönlein purpura	Most common childhood systemic vasculitis. Often follows URI. Classic triad: ▪ Skin: palpable purpura on buttocks/legs J ▪ Arthralgias ▪ GI: abdominal pain	Vasculitis 2° to IgA immune complex deposition. Associated with IgA nephropathy (Berger disease).

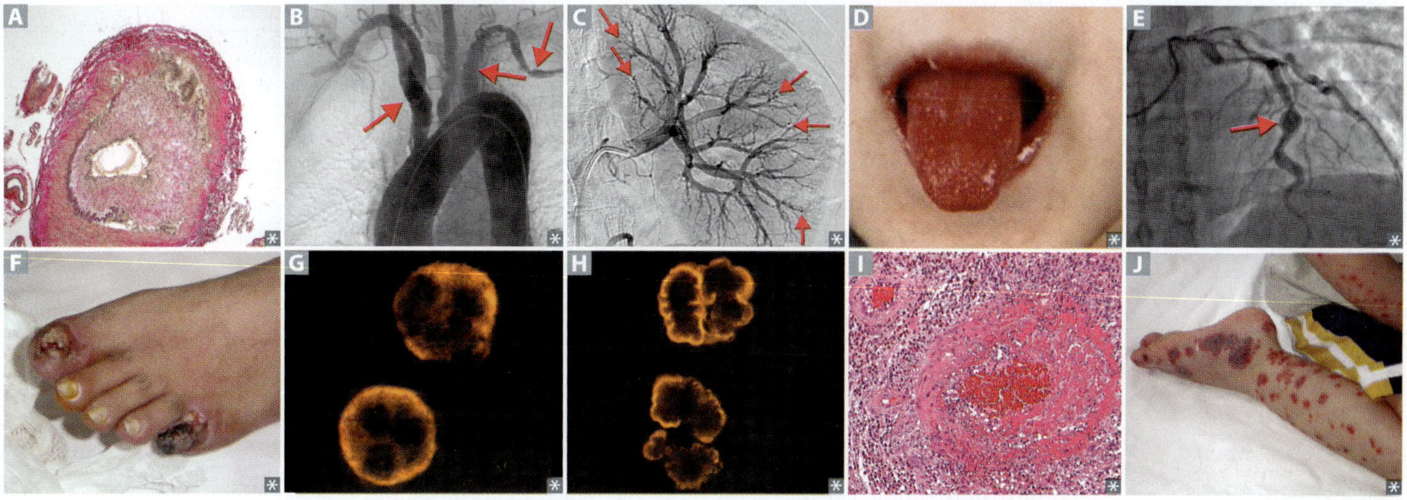

CO = HR × SV

▶ CARDIOVASCULAR—PHARMACOLOGY

Hypertension treatment

Primary (essential) hypertension	Thiazide diuretics, ACE inhibitors, angiotensin II receptor blockers (ARBs), dihydropyridine Ca^{2+} channel blockers.	
Hypertension with heart failure	Diuretics, ACE inhibitors/ARBs, β-blockers (compensated HF), aldosterone antagonists.	β-blockers must be used cautiously in decompensated HF and are contraindicated in cardiogenic shock.
Hypertension with diabetes mellitus	ACE inhibitors/ARBs, Ca^{2+} channel blockers, thiazide diuretics, β-blockers.	ACE inhibitors/ARBs are protective against diabetic nephropathy.
Hypertension in pregnancy	Hydralazine, labetalol, methyldopa, nifedipine.	

Calcium channel blockers

Amlodipine, clevidipine, nicardipine, nifedipine, nimodipine (dihydropyridines, act on vascular smooth muscle); diltiazem, verapamil (non-dihydropyridines, act on heart).

MECHANISM	Block voltage-dependent L-type calcium channels of cardiac and smooth muscle → ↓ muscle contractility. Vascular smooth muscle—amlodipine = nifedipine > diltiazem > verapamil. Heart—verapamil > diltiazem > amlodipine = nifedipine (verapamil = ventricle).
CLINICAL USE	Dihydropyridines (except nimodipine): hypertension, angina (including Prinzmetal), Raynaud phenomenon. Nimodipine: subarachnoid hemorrhage (prevents cerebral vasospasm). Clevidipine: hypertensive urgency or emergency. Non-dihydropyridines: hypertension, angina, atrial fibrillation/flutter.
ADVERSE EFFECTS	Non-dihydropyridine: cardiac depression, AV block, hyperprolactinemia, constipation. Dihydropyridine: peripheral edema, flushing, dizziness, gingival hyperplasia.

Hydralazine

MECHANISM	↑ cGMP → smooth muscle relaxation. Vasodilates arterioles > veins; afterload reduction.
CLINICAL USE	Severe hypertension (particularly acute), HF (with organic nitrate). Safe to use during pregnancy. Frequently coadministered with a β-blocker to prevent reflex tachycardia.
ADVERSE EFFECTS	Compensatory tachycardia (contraindicated in angina/CAD), fluid retention, headache, angina. Lupus-like syndrome.

Hypertensive emergency

Drugs include clevidipine, fenoldopam, labetalol, nicardipine, nitroprusside.

Nitroprusside	Short acting; ↑ cGMP via direct release of NO. Can cause cyanide toxicity (releases cyanide).
Fenoldopam	Dopamine D_1 receptor agonist—coronary, peripheral, renal, and splanchnic vasodilation. ↓ BP, ↑ natriuresis. Also used postoperatively as an antihypertensive. Can cause hypotension and tachycardia.

Nitrates Nitroglycerin, isosorbide dinitrate, isosorbide mononitrate.

MECHANISM	Vasodilate by ↑ NO in vascular smooth muscle → ↑ in cGMP and smooth muscle relaxation. Dilate veins >> arteries. ↓ preload.
CLINICAL USE	Angina, acute coronary syndrome, pulmonary edema.
ADVERSE EFFECTS	Reflex tachycardia (treat with β-blockers), hypotension, flushing, headache, "Monday disease" in industrial exposure: development of tolerance for the vasodilating action during the work week and loss of tolerance over the weekend → tachycardia, dizziness, headache upon reexposure.

Antianginal therapy Goal is reduction of myocardial O_2 consumption (MVO_2) by ↓ 1 or more of the determinants of MVO_2: end-diastolic volume, BP, HR, contractility.

COMPONENT	NITRATES	β-BLOCKERS	NITRATES + β-BLOCKERS
End-diastolic volume	↓	No effect or ↑	No effect or ↓
Blood pressure	↓	↓	↓
Contractility	No effect	↓	Little/no effect
Heart rate	↑ (reflex response)	↓	No effect or ↓
Ejection time	↓	↑	Little/no effect
MVO_2	↓	↓	↓↓

Verapamil is similar to β-blockers in effect.
Pindolol and acebutolol—partial β-agonists contraindicated in angina.

Ranolazine

MECHANISM	Inhibits the late phase of sodium current thereby reducing diastolic wall tension and oxygen consumption. Does not affect heart rate or contractility.
CLINICAL USE	Angina refractory to other medical therapies.
ADVERSE EFFECTS	Constipation, dizziness, headache, nausea, QT prolongation.

- HF
  - compensat = blood isn't reaching tissues so body compensates by ↑ HR/BP etc
    - activate too much = helps less & less (decomp.)
      ↳ more ε req but not enuf blood coming back
  - ↑ SNS, ↑ ADH, ↑ aldost
    ↑ hypertrophy
  - w/ hypertroph = ↓ space for fluid

Lipid-lowering agents

DRUG	LDL	HDL	TRIGLYCERIDES	MECHANISMS OF ACTION	ADVERSE EFFECTS/PROBLEMS
HMG-CoA reductase inhibitors (eg, lovastatin, pravastatin)	↓↓↓	↑	↓	Inhibit conversion of HMG-CoA to mevalonate, a cholesterol precursor; ↓ mortality in CAD patients	Hepatotoxicity (↑ LFTs), myopathy (esp. when used with fibrates or niacin)
Bile acid resins Cholestyramine, colestipol, colesevelam	↓↓	Slightly ↑	Slightly ↑	Prevent intestinal reabsorption of bile acids; liver must use cholesterol to make more	GI upset, ↓ absorption of other drugs and fat-soluble vitamins
Ezetimibe	↓↓	—	—	Prevent cholesterol absorption at small intestine brush border	Rare ↑ LFTs, diarrhea
Fibrates Gemfibrozil, bezafibrate, fenofibrate	↓	↑	↓↓↓	Upregulate LPL → ↑ TG clearance Activates PPAR-α to induce HDL synthesis	Myopathy (↑ risk with statins), cholesterol gallstones
Niacin (vitamin B_3)	↓↓	↑↑	↓	Inhibits lipolysis (hormone-sensitive lipase) in adipose tissue; reduces hepatic VLDL synthesis	Red, flushed face, which is ↓ by NSAIDs or long-term use Hyperglycemia Hyperuricemia

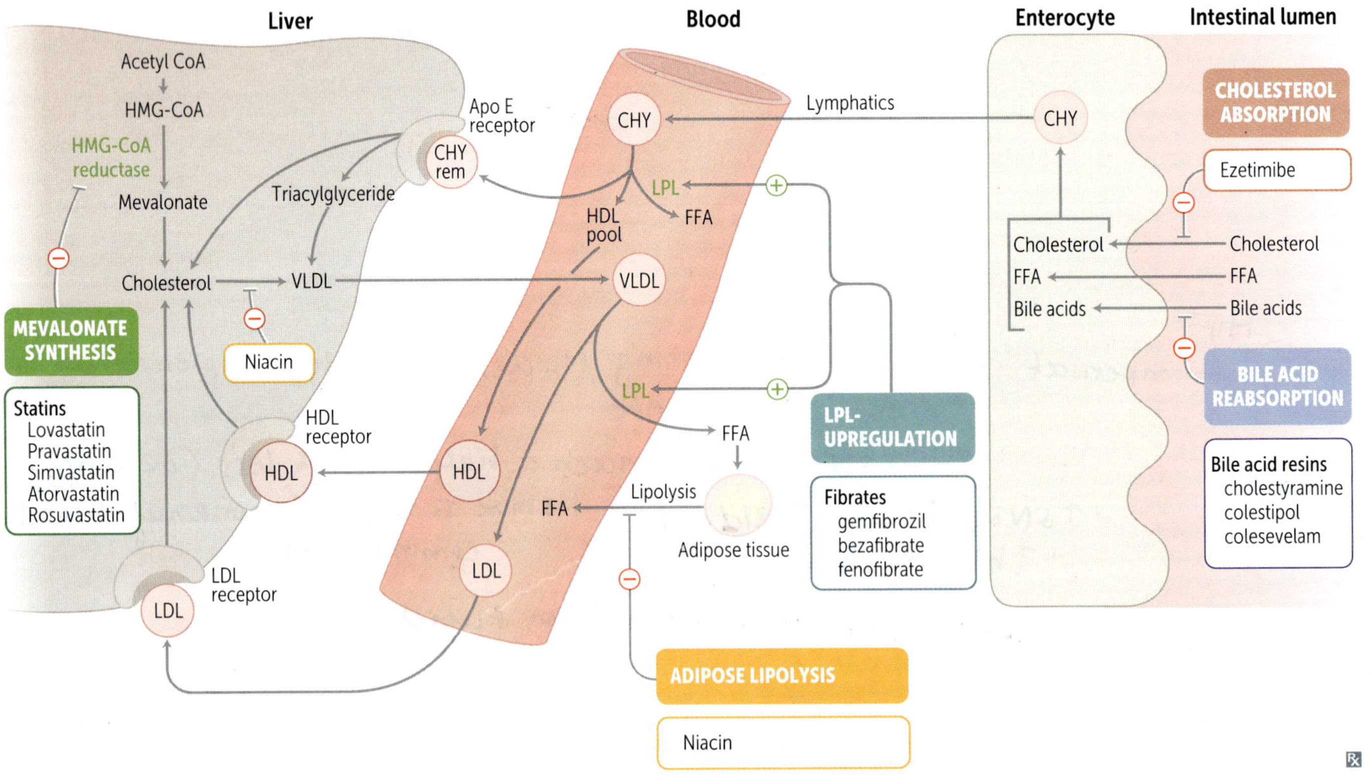

Cardiac glycosides	Digoxin.
MECHANISM	Direct inhibition of Na^+/K^+ ATPase → indirect inhibition of Na^+/Ca^{2+} exchanger. ↑ $[Ca^{2+}]_i$ → positive inotropy. Stimulates vagus nerve → ↓ HR. (force of contraction) ↑force, ↓HR 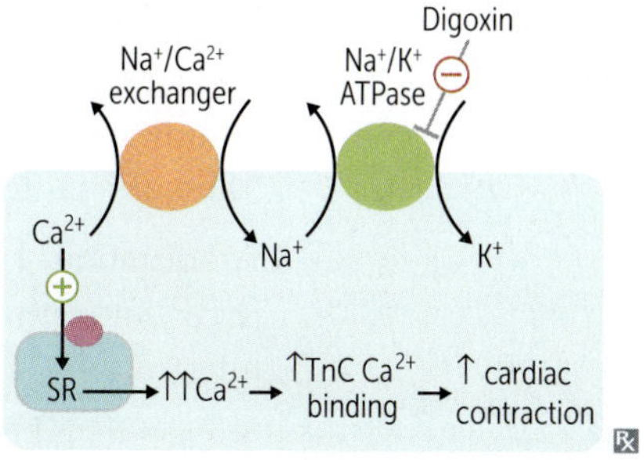
CLINICAL USE	HF (↑ contractility); atrial fibrillation (↓ conduction at AV node and depression of SA node).
ADVERSE EFFECTS	Cholinergic—nausea, vomiting, diarrhea, blurry yellow vision (think van Gogh), arrhythmias, AV block. Can lead to hyperkalemia, which indicates poor prognosis. Factors predisposing to toxicity: renal failure (↓ excretion), hypokalemia (permissive for digoxin binding at K^+-binding site on Na^+/K^+ ATPase), drugs that displace digoxin from tissue-binding sites, and ↓ clearance (eg, verapamil, amiodarone, quinidine).
ANTIDOTE	Slowly normalize K^+, cardiac pacer, anti-digoxin Fab fragments, Mg^{2+}.

LPL = extracell break of fat.

HSL = break adipose

Antiarrhythmics—sodium channel blockers (class I)

Slow or block (↓) conduction (especially in depolarized cells). ↓ slope of phase 0 depolarization. Are state dependent (selectively depress tissue that is frequently depolarized [eg, tachycardia]).

Class IA

Quinidine, Procainamide, Disopyramide. "The Queen Proclaims Diso's pyramid."

MECHANISM	↑ AP duration, ↑ effective refractory period (ERP) in ventricular action potential, ↑ QT interval.
CLINICAL USE	Both atrial and ventricular arrhythmias, especially re-entrant and ectopic SVT and VT.
ADVERSE EFFECTS	Cinchonism (headache, tinnitus with quinidine), reversible SLE-like syndrome (procainamide), heart failure (disopyramide), thrombocytopenia, torsades de pointes due to ↑ QT interval.

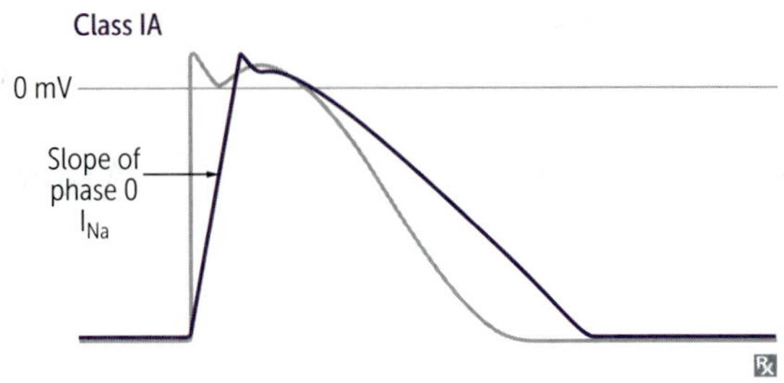

Class IB

Lidocaine, MexileTine. "I'd Buy Liddy's Mexican Tacos."

MECHANISM	↓ AP duration. Preferentially affect ischemic or depolarized Purkinje and ventricular tissue. Phenytoin can also fall into the IB category.
CLINICAL USE	Acute ventricular arrhythmias (especially post-MI), digitalis-induced arrhythmias. IB is Best post-MI.
ADVERSE EFFECTS	CNS stimulation/depression, cardiovascular depression.

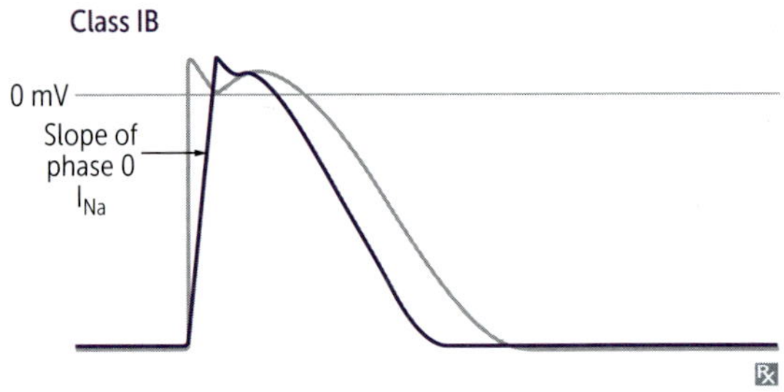

Class IC

Flecainide, Propafenone. "Can I have Fries, Please."

MECHANISM	Significantly prolongs ERP in AV node and accessory bypass tracts. No effect on ERP in Purkinje and ventricular tissue. Minimal effect on AP duration.
CLINICAL USE	SVTs, including atrial fibrillation. Only as a last resort in refractory VT.
ADVERSE EFFECTS	Proarrhythmic, especially post-MI (contraindicated). IC is Contraindicated in structural and ischemic heart disease.

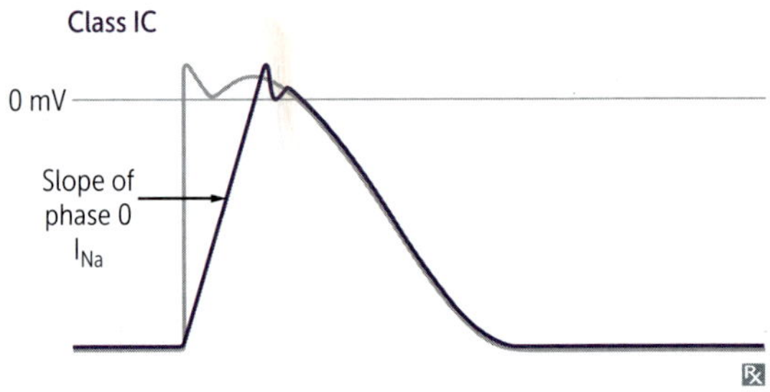

Na
β-block
K-block
Ca-block

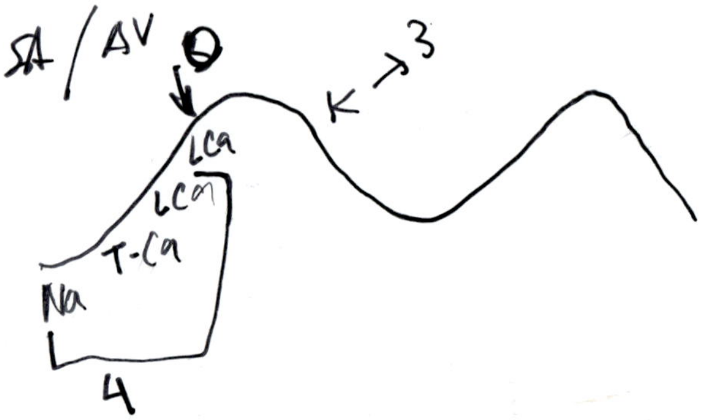

Antiarrhythmics—β-blockers (class II)

Metoprolol, propranolol, esmolol, atenolol, timolol, carvedilol.

MECHANISM

Decrease SA and AV nodal activity by ↓ cAMP, ↓ Ca^{2+} currents. Suppress abnormal pacemakers by ↓ slope of phase 4.

AV node particularly sensitive—↑ PR interval. Esmolol very short acting.

CLINICAL USE

SVT, ventricular rate control for atrial fibrillation and atrial flutter.

ADVERSE EFFECTS

Impotence, exacerbation of COPD and asthma, cardiovascular effects (bradycardia, AV block, HF), CNS effects (sedation, sleep alterations). May mask the signs of hypoglycemia.

Metoprolol can cause dyslipidemia. Propranolol can exacerbate vasospasm in Prinzmetal angina. β-blockers (except the nonselective α- and β-antagonists carvedilol and labetalol) cause unopposed α_1-agonism if given alone for pheochromocytoma or cocaine toxicity. Treat β-blocker overdose with saline, atropine, glucagon.

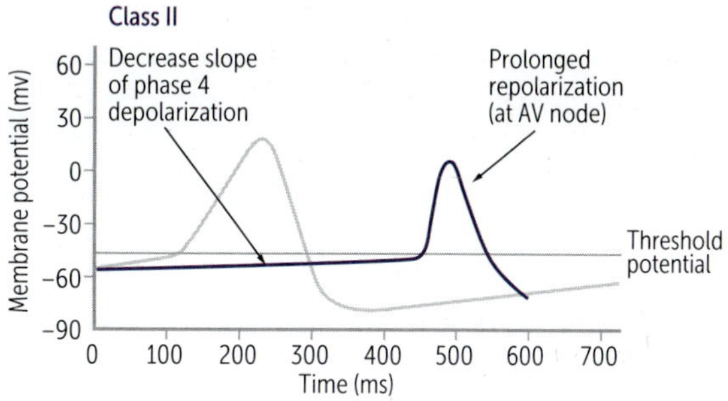

Pacemaker cell action potential

Antiarrhythmics—potassium channel blockers (class III)

Amiodarone, **I**butilide, **D**ofetilide, **S**otalol. **AIDS**.

MECHANISM

↑ AP duration, ↑ ERP, ↑ QT interval.

CLINICAL USE

Atrial fibrillation, atrial flutter; ventricular tachycardia (amiodarone, sotalol).

ADVERSE EFFECTS

Sotalol—torsades de pointes, excessive β blockade.

Ibutilide—torsades de pointes.

Amiodarone—pulmonary fibrosis, hepatotoxicity, hypothyroidism/hyperthyroidism (amiodarone is 40% iodine by weight), acts as hapten (corneal deposits, blue/gray skin deposits resulting in photodermatitis), neurologic effects, constipation, cardiovascular effects (bradycardia, heart block, HF).

Remember to check PFTs, LFTs, and TFTs when using amiodarone.

Amiodarone is lipophilic and has class I, II, III, and IV effects.

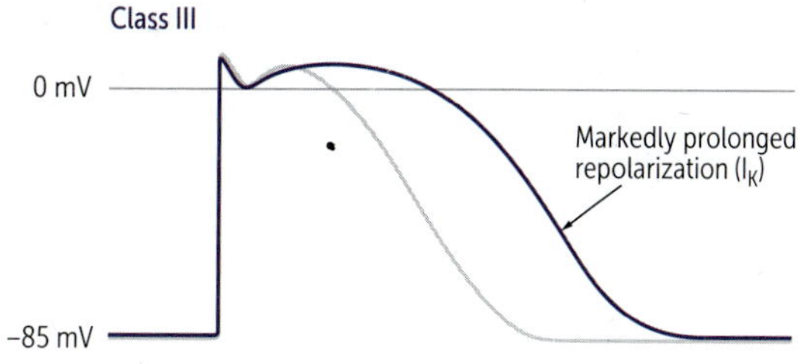

Cell action potential

Antiarrhythmics—calcium channel blockers (class IV)	Verapamil, diltiazem.
MECHANISM	↓ conduction velocity, ↑ ERP, ↑ PR interval.
CLINICAL USE	Prevention of nodal arrhythmias (eg, SVT), rate control in atrial fibrillation.
ADVERSE EFFECTS	Constipation, flushing, edema, cardiovascular effects (HF, AV block, sinus node depression).

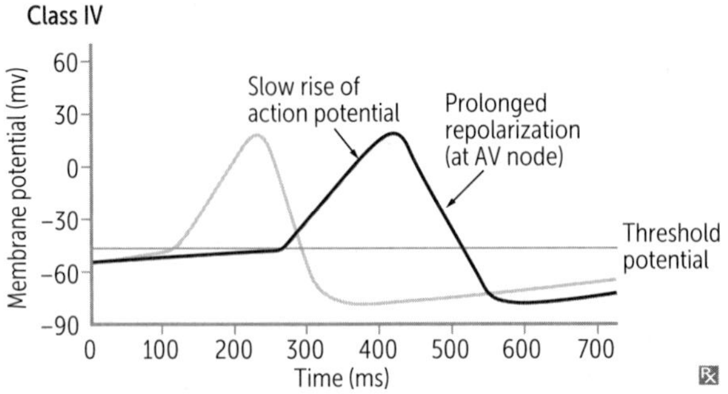

Other antiarrhythmics

Adenosine	↑ K^+ out of cells → hyperpolarizing the cell and ↓ I_{Ca}. Drug of choice in diagnosing/terminating certain forms of SVT. Very short acting (~ 15 sec). Effects blunted by theophylline and caffeine (both are adenosine receptor antagonists). Adverse effects include flushing, hypotension, chest pain, sense of impending doom, bronchospasm.
Mg^{2+}	Effective in torsades de pointes and digoxin toxicity.

Endocrine

"We have learned that there is an endocrinology of elation and despair, a chemistry of mystical insight, and, in relation to the autonomic nervous system, a meteorology and even . . . an astro-physics of changing moods."

—Aldous (Leonard) Huxley

"Chocolate causes certain endocrine glands to secrete hormones that affect your feelings and behavior by making you happy."

—Elaine Sherman, *Book of Divine Indulgences*

▶ ENDOCRINE—EMBRYOLOGY

Thyroid development

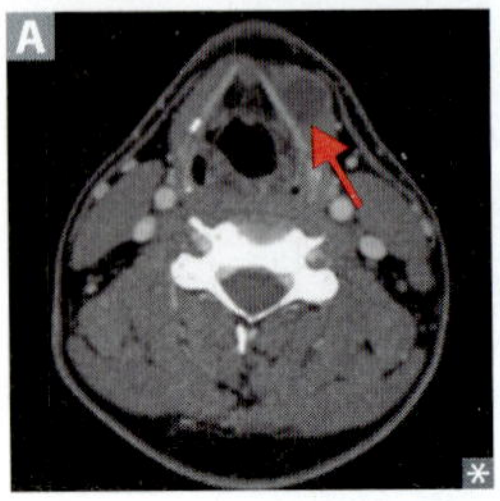

Thyroid diverticulum arises from floor of primitive pharynx and descends into neck. Connected to tongue by thyroglossal duct, which normally disappears but may persist as cysts or the pyramidal lobe of thyroid. Foramen cecum is normal remnant of thyroglossal duct. Most common ectopic thyroid tissue site is the tongue (lingual thyroid). Removal may result in hypothyroidism if it is the only thyroid tissue present.

Thyroglossal duct cyst **A** presents as an anterior midline neck mass that moves with swallowing or protrusion of the tongue (vs persistent cervical sinus leading to branchial cleft cyst in lateral neck).

Thyroid tissue is derived from endoderm. Parafollicular cells (aka, C cells) of the thyroid are derived from neural crest.

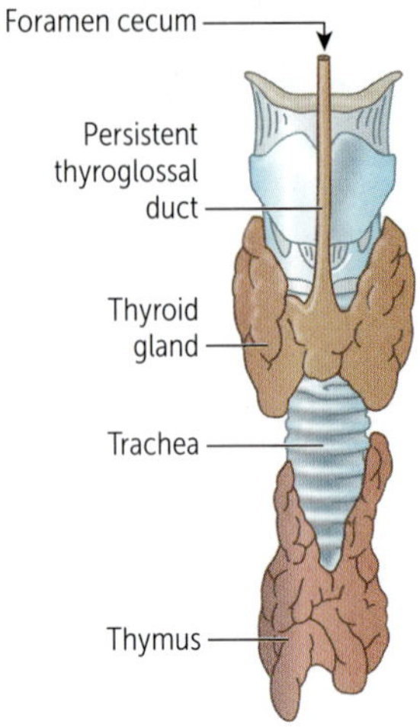

▶ ENDOCRINE—ANATOMY

Adrenal cortex and medulla

Adrenal cortex (derived from mesoderm) and medulla (derived from neural crest).

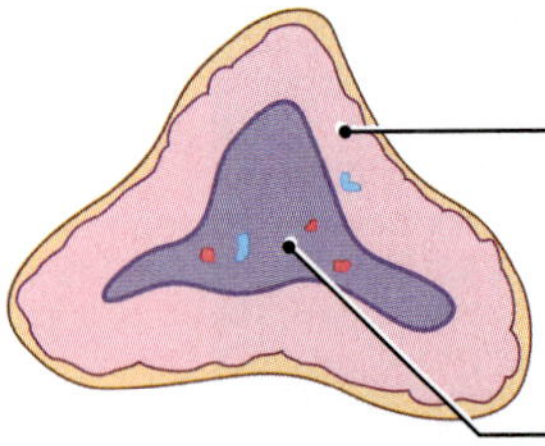

	Anatomy	Primary regulatory control	Secretory products
CORTEX	Zona **G**lomerulosa	Renin-angiotensin	Aldosterone
	Zona **F**asciculata	ACTH, CRH	Cortisol
	Zona **R**eticularis	ACTH, CRH	Sex hormones (eg, androgens)
MEDULLA	Chromaffin cells	Preganglionic sympathetic fibers	Catecholamines (epinephrine, norepinephrine)

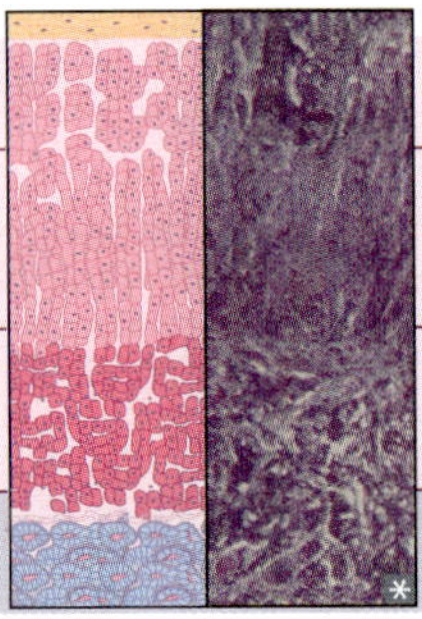

GFR corresponds with **S**alt (Na^+), **S**ugar (glucocorticoids), and **S**ex (androgens). "The deeper you go, **the sweeter it gets**."

Pituitary gland

Anterior pituitary (adenohypophysis)	Secretes FSH, LH, ACTH, TSH, prolactin, GH. Melanotropin (MSH) secreted from intermediate lobe of pituitary. Derived from oral ectoderm (Rathke pouch). ▪ α subunit—hormone subunit common to TSH, LH, FSH, and hCG. ▪ β subunit—determines hormone specificity.	ACTH and MSH are derivatives of proopiomelanocortin (POMC). FLAT PiG: FSH, LH, ACTH, TSH, PRL, GH. B-FLAT: Basophils—FSH, LH, ACTH, TSH. Acidophils: GH, PRL.
Posterior pituitary (neurohypophysis)	Stores and releases vasopressin (antidiuretic hormone, or ADH) and oxytocin, both made in the hypothalamus (supraoptic and paraventricular nuclei) and transported to posterior pituitary via neurophysins (carrier proteins). Derived from neuroectoderm.	

Endocrine pancreas cell types	Islets of Langerhans are collections of α, β, and δ endocrine cells. Islets arise from pancreatic buds. ▪ α = glucagon (peripheral) ▪ β = insulin (central) ▪ δ = somatostatin (interspersed)	Insulin (β cells) inside. 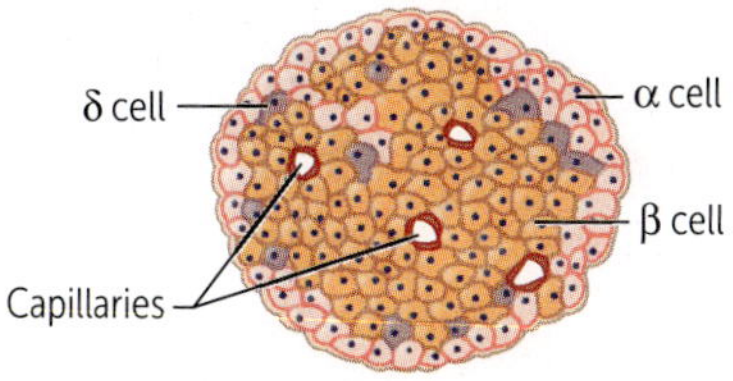

▸ ENDOCRINE—PHYSIOLOGY

Insulin

SYNTHESIS

Preproinsulin (synthesized in RER) → cleavage of "presignal" → proinsulin (stored in secretory granules) → cleavage of proinsulin → exocytosis of insulin and C-peptide equally. Insulin and C-peptide are ↑ in insulinoma and sulfonylurea use, whereas exogenous insulin lacks C-peptide.

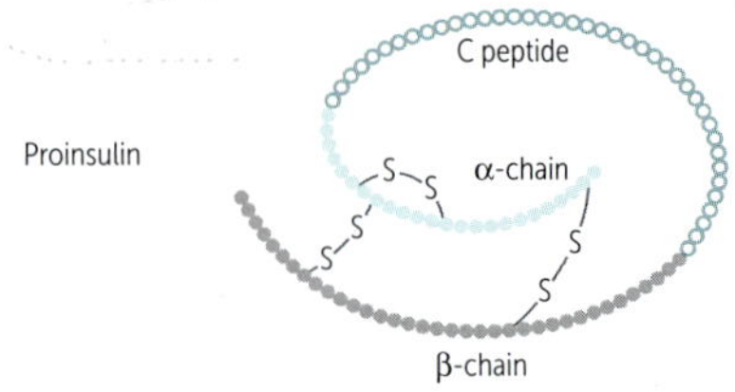

SOURCE

Released from pancreatic β cells.

FUNCTION

Binds **in**sulin receptors (tyrosine kinase activity ❶), **in**ducing glucose uptake (carrier-mediated transport) **in**to insulin-dependent tissue ❷ and gene transcription.

Anabolic effects of insulin:
- ↑ glucose transport in skeletal muscle and adipose tissue
- ↑ glycogen synthesis and storage
- ↑ triglyceride synthesis
- ↑ Na^+ retention (kidneys)
- ↑ protein synthesis (muscles)
- ↑ cellular uptake of K^+ and amino acids
- ↓ glucagon release
- ↓ lipolysis in adipose tissue

Unlike glucose, insulin does not cross placenta.

Insulin-dependent glucose transporters:
- GLUT-4: adipose tissue, striated muscle (exercise can also increase GLUT-4 expression)

Insulin-independent transporters:
- GLUT-1: RBCs, brain, cornea, placenta
- GLUT-2 (bidirectional): β islet cells, liver, kidney, small intestine
- GLUT-3: brain, placenta
- GLUT-5 (fructose): spermatocytes, GI tract

Brain utilizes glucose for metabolism normally and ketone bodies during starvation. RBCs always utilize glucose because they lack mitochondria for aerobic metabolism.

BRICK L (insulin-independent glucose uptake): **B**rain, **R**BCs, **I**ntestine, **C**ornea, **K**idney, **L**iver.

REGULATION

Glucose is the major regulator of insulin release. ↑ insulin response with oral vs IV glucose because of incretins such as glucagon-like peptide 1 (GLP-1), which are released after meals and ↑ β cell sensitivity to glucose.

Glucose enters β cells ❸ → ↑ ATP generated from glucose metabolism ❹ closes K^+ channels (target of sulfonylureas) ❺ and depolarizes β cell membrane ❻. Voltage-gated Ca^{2+} channels open → Ca^{2+} influx ❼ and stimulation of insulin exocytosis ❽.

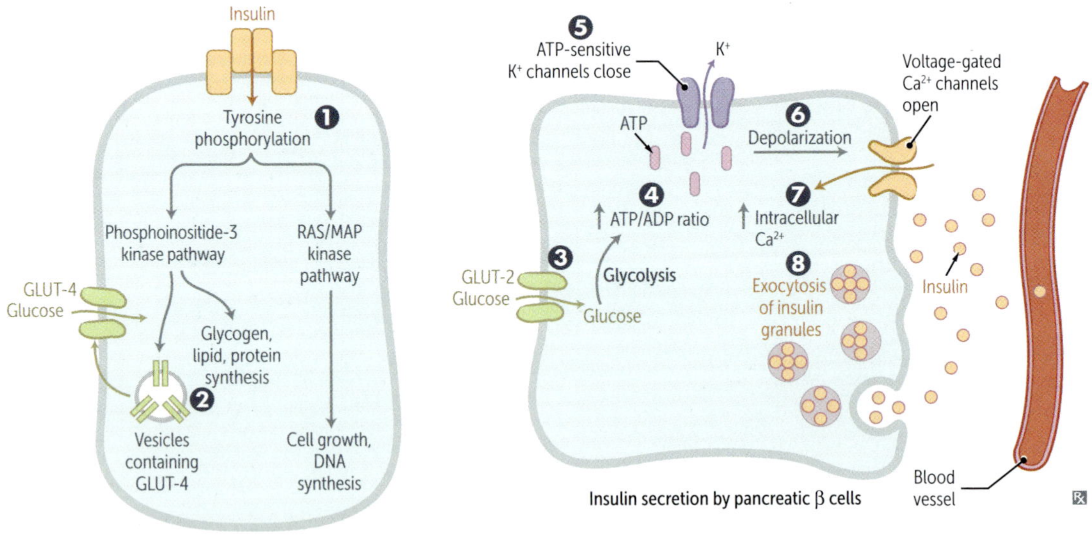

Insulin-dependent glucose uptake

Insulin secretion by pancreatic β cells

Glucagon

SOURCE	Made by α cells of pancreas.
FUNCTION	Catabolic effects of glucagon: ▪ Glycogenolysis, gluconeogenesis ▪ Lipolysis and ketone production
REGULATION	Secreted in response to hypoglycemia. Inhibited by insulin, hyperglycemia, and somatostatin.

Hypothalamic-pituitary hormones

HORMONE	FUNCTION	CLINICAL NOTES
CRH	↑ ACTH, MSH, β-endorphin	↓ in chronic exogenous steroid use
Dopamine	↓ prolactin, TSH	Dopamine antagonists (eg, antipsychotics) can cause galactorrhea due to hyperprolactinemia
GHRH	↑ GH	Analog (tesamorelin) used to treat HIV-associated lipodystrophy
GnRH	↑ FSH, LH	Suppressed by hyperprolactinemia Tonic GnRH suppresses HPG axis Pulsatile GnRH leads to puberty, fertility
Prolactin	↓ GnRH	Pituitary prolactinoma → amenorrhea, osteoporosis, hypogonadism, galactorrhea
Somatostatin	↓ GH, TSH	Analogs used to treat acromegaly
TRH	↑ TSH, prolactin	

Prolactin

SOURCE	Secreted mainly by anterior pituitary.	Structurally homologous to growth hormone.
FUNCTION	Stimulates milk production in breast; inhibits ovulation in females and spermatogenesis in males by inhibiting GnRH synthesis and release.	Excessive amounts of prolactin associated with ↓ libido.
REGULATION	Prolactin secretion from anterior pituitary is tonically inhibited by dopamine from hypothalamus. Prolactin in turn inhibits its own secretion by ↑ dopamine synthesis and secretion from hypothalamus. TRH ↑ prolactin secretion (eg, in 1° or 2° hypothyroidism).	Dopamine agonists (eg, bromocriptine) inhibit prolactin secretion and can be used in treatment of prolactinoma. Dopamine antagonists (eg, most antipsychotics) and estrogens (eg, OCPs, pregnancy) stimulate prolactin secretion.

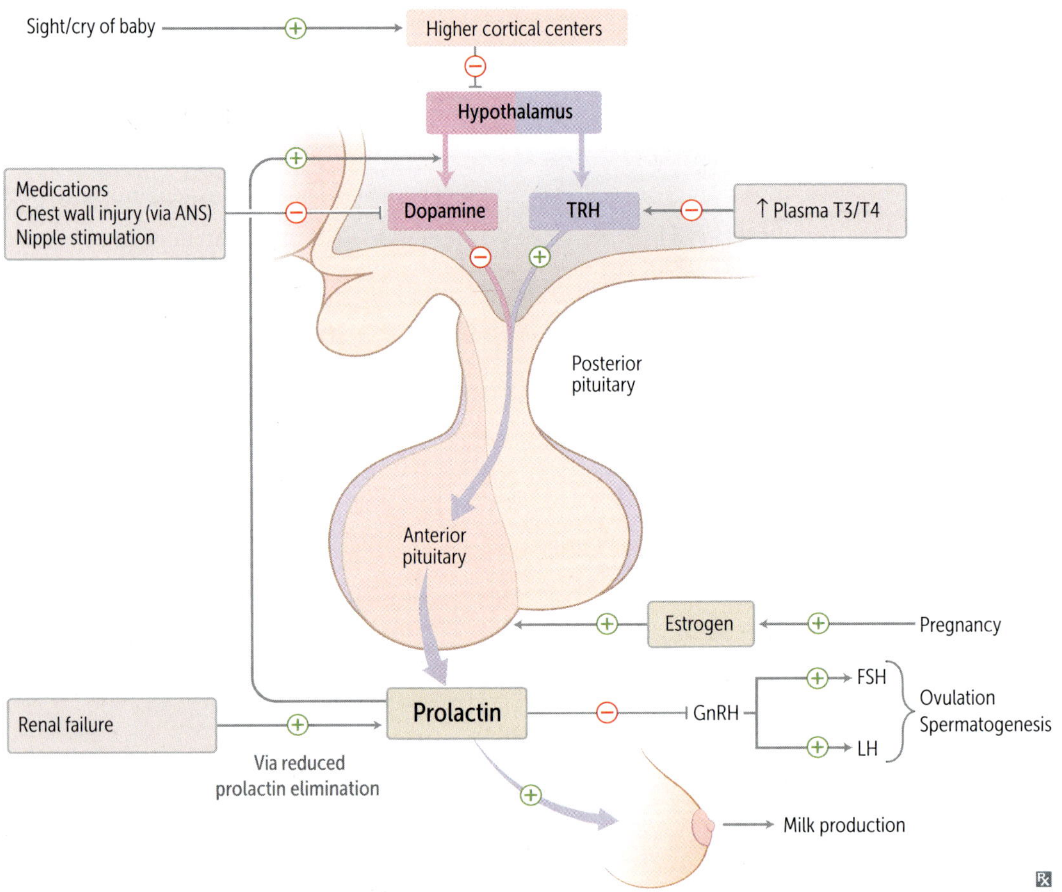

Growth hormone (somatotropin)

SOURCE	Secreted by anterior pituitary.	
FUNCTION	Stimulates linear growth and muscle mass through IGF-1 (somatomedin C) secretion by liver. ↑ insulin resistance (diabetogenic).	
REGULATION	Released in pulses in response to growth hormone–releasing hormone (GHRH). Secretion ↑ during exercise, deep sleep, puberty, hypoglycemia. Secretion inhibited by glucose and somatostatin release via negative feedback by somatomedin.	Excess secretion of GH (eg, pituitary adenoma) may cause acromegaly (adults) or gigantism (children). Treat with somatostatin analogs (eg, octreotide) or surgery.

Appetite regulation

Ghrelin	Stimulates hunger (orexigenic effect) and GH release (via GH secretagog receptor). Produced by stomach. Sleep deprivation or Prader-Willi syndrome → ↑ ghrelin production.	**Ghre**lin makes you hun**ghre**.
Leptin	Satiety hormone. Produced by adipose tissue. Mutation of leptin gene → congenital obesity. Sleep deprivation or starvation → ↓ leptin production.	Lept**in** keeps you th**in**.
Endocannabinoids	Act at cannabinoid receptors in hypothalamus and nucleus accumbens, two key brain areas for the homeostatic and hedonic control of food intake → ↑ appetite.	The munchies.

Antidiuretic hormone

SOURCE	Synthesized in hypothalamus (supraoptic nuclei), stored and secreted by posterior pituitary.	
FUNCTION	Regulates serum osmolarity (V_2-receptors) and blood pressure (V_1-receptors). Primary function is serum osmolarity regulation (ADH ↓ serum osmolarity, ↑ urine osmolarity) via regulation of aquaporin channel insertion in principal cells of renal collecting duct.	ADH level is ↓ in central diabetes insipidus (DI), normal or ↑ in nephrogenic DI. Nephrogenic DI can be caused by mutation in V_2-receptor. Desmopressin acetate (ADH analog) is a treatment for central DI and nocturnal enuresis.
REGULATION	Osmoreceptors in hypothalamus; hypovolemia.	

Adrenal steroids and congenital adrenal hyperplasias

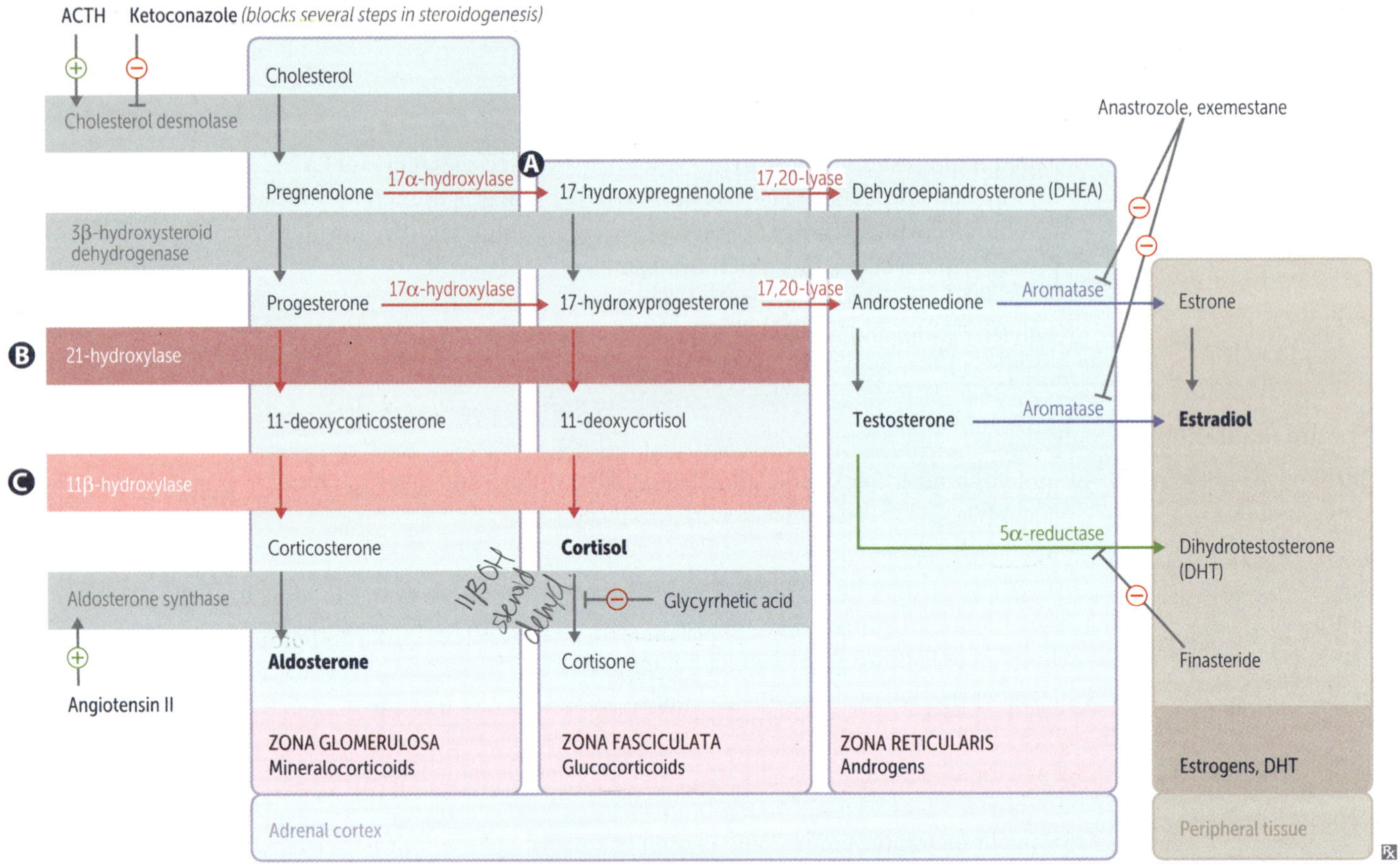

ENZYME DEFICIENCY	MINERALOCORTICOIDS	CORTISOL	SEX HORMONES	BP	[K⁺]	LABS	PRESENTATION
A 17α-hydroxylase[a]	↑	↓	↓	↑	↓	↓ androstenedione	XY: ambiguous genitalia, undescended testes XX: lacks 2° sexual development
B 21-hydroxylase[a]	↓	↓	↑	↓	↑	↑ renin activity ↑ 17-hydroxy-progesterone	Most common Presents in infancy (salt wasting) or childhood (precocious puberty) XX: virilization
C 11β-hydroxylase[a]	↓ aldosterone ↑ 11-deoxycorti-costerone (results in ↑ BP)	↓	↑	↑	↓	↓ renin activity	XX: virilization

[a]All congenital adrenal enzyme deficiencies are characterized by an enlargement of both adrenal glands due to ↑ ACTH stimulation (in response to ↓ cortisol).

Cortisol

SOURCE	Adrenal zona fasciculata.	Bound to corticosteroid-binding globulin.
FUNCTION	↑ **B**lood pressure: ▪ Upregulates α_1-receptors on arterioles → ↑ sensitivity to norepinephrine and epinephrine ▪ At high concentrations, can bind to mineralocorticoid (aldosterone) receptors ↑ **I**nsulin resistance (diabetogenic) ↑ **G**luconeogenesis, lipolysis, and proteolysis ↓ **F**ibroblast activity (causes striae) ↓ **I**nflammatory and **I**mmune responses: ▪ Inhibits production of leukotrienes and prostaglandins ▪ Inhibits WBC adhesion → neutrophilia ▪ Blocks histamine release from mast cells ▪ Reduces eosinophils ▪ Blocks IL-2 production ↓ **B**one formation (↓ osteoblast activity)	Cortisol is a **BIG FIB**. Exogenous corticosteroids can cause reactivation of TB and candidiasis (blocks IL-2 production).
REGULATION	CRH (hypothalamus) stimulates ACTH release (pituitary) → cortisol production in adrenal zona fasciculata. Excess cortisol ↓ CRH, ACTH, and cortisol secretion.	Chronic stress induces prolonged secretion.

Calcium homeostasis	Plasma Ca^{2+} exists in three forms: ▪ Ionized (~ 45%) ▪ Bound to albumin (~ 40%) ▪ Bound to anions (~ 15%)	↑ in pH → ↑ affinity of albumin (↑ negative charge) to bind Ca^{2+} → hypocalcemia (cramps, pain, paresthesias, carpopedal spasm).

Vitamin D (cholecalciferol)

SOURCE	D_3 from exposure of skin to sun, ingestion of fish and plants. D_2 from ingestion of plants, fungi, yeasts. Both converted to 25-OH in liver and to 1,25-$(OH)_2$ (active form) in kidney.	Deficiency → rickets in kids, osteomalacia in adults. Caused by malabsorption, ↓ sunlight, poor diet, chronic kidney failure. 24,25-$(OH)_2$ D_3 is an inactive form of vitamin D. PTH leads to ↑ Ca^{2+} reabsorption and ↓ PO_4^{3-} reabsorption in the kidney, whereas 1,25-$(OH)_2$ D_3 leads to ↑ absorption of both Ca^{2+} and PO_4^{3-} in the gut.
FUNCTION	↑ absorption of dietary Ca^{2+} and PO_4^{3-}. Enhances bone mineralization.	
REGULATION	↑ PTH, ↓ Ca^{2+}, ↓ PO_4^{3-} → ↑ 1,25-$(OH)_2$ production. 1,25-$(OH)_2$ feedback inhibits its own production.	

Parathyroid hormone

SOURCE	Chief cells of parathyroid.	
FUNCTION	↑ bone resorption of Ca^{2+} and PO_4^{3-}. ↑ kidney reabsorption of Ca^{2+} in distal convoluted tubule. ↓ reabsorption of PO_4^{3-} in proximal convoluted tubule. ↑ 1,25-$(OH)_2$ D_3 (calcitriol) production by stimulating kidney 1α-hydroxylase in proximal convoluted tubule.	PTH ↑ serum Ca^{2+}, ↓ serum (PO_4^{3-}), ↑ urine (PO_4^{3-}), ↑ urine cAMP. ↑ RANK-L (receptor activator of NH-κB ligand) secreted by osteoblasts and osteocytes. Binds RANK (receptor) on osteoclasts and their precursors to stimulate osteoclasts and ↑ Ca^{2+} → bone resorption. Intermittent PTH release can also stimulate bone formation. **PTH** = **P**hosphate **T**rashing **H**ormone. PTH-related peptide (PTHrP) functions like PTH and is commonly increased in malignancies (eg, squamous cell carcinoma of the lung, renal cell carcinoma).
REGULATION	↓ serum Ca^{2+} → ↑ PTH secretion. ↑ serum PO_4^{3-} → ↑ PTH secretion. ↓ serum Mg^{2+} → ↑ PTH secretion. ↓↓ serum Mg^{2+} → ↓ PTH secretion. Common causes of ↓ Mg^{2+} include diarrhea, aminoglycosides, diuretics, alcohol abuse.	

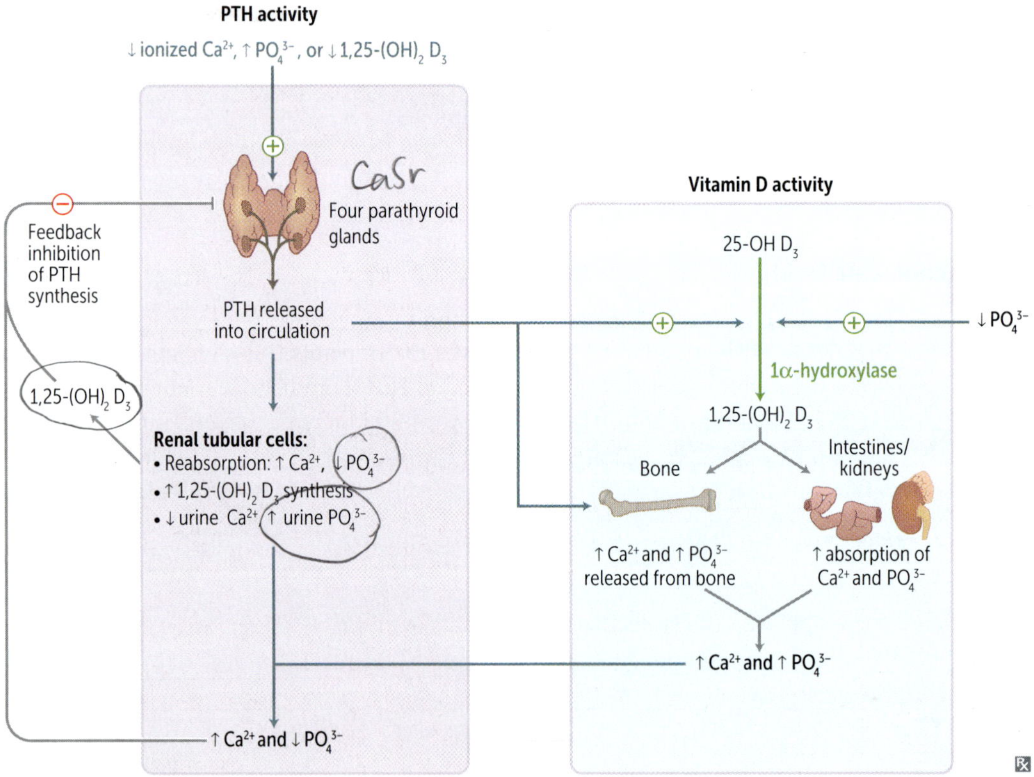

Calcitonin

SOURCE	Parafollicular cells (C cells) of thyroid.	Calcitonin opposes actions of PTH. Not important in normal Ca^{2+} homeostasis. Calcitonin tones down Ca^{2+} levels.
FUNCTION	↓ bone resorption of Ca^{2+}.	
REGULATION	↑ serum Ca^{2+} → calcitonin secretion.	

Thyroid hormones (T_3/T_4)

Iodine-containing hormones that control the body's metabolic rate.

SOURCE	Follicles of thyroid. Most T_3 formed in target tissues.	T_3 functions—**4 B's**: **B**rain maturation **B**one growth **β**-adrenergic effects **B**asal metabolic rate ↑ Thyroxine-binding globulin (TBG) binds most T_3/T_4 in blood; only free hormone is active. ↓ TBG in hepatic failure, steroids; ↑ TBG in pregnancy or OCP use (estrogen ↑ TBG). T_4 is major thyroid product; converted to T_3 in peripheral tissue by 5′-deiodinase. T_3 binds nuclear receptor with greater affinity than T_4. Thyroid peroxidase is the enzyme responsible for oxidation and organification of iodide as well as coupling of monoiodotyrosine (MIT) and di-iodotyrosine (DIT). DIT + DIT = T_4. DIT + MIT = T_3. Propylthiouracil inhibits both thyroid peroxidase and 5′-deiodinase. Methimazole inhibits thyroid peroxidase only.
FUNCTION	Bone growth (synergism with GH) CNS maturation ↑ β_1 receptors in heart = ↑ CO, HR, SV, contractility ↑ basal metabolic rate via ↑ Na^+/K^+-ATPase activity → ↑ O_2 consumption, RR, body temperature ↑ glycogenolysis, gluconeogenesis, lipolysis	
REGULATION	TRH (hypothalamus) stimulates TSH (pituitary), which stimulates follicular cells. May also be stimulated by thyroid-stimulating immunoglobulin (TSI) in Graves disease. Negative feedback by free T_3, T_4 to anterior pituitary ↓ sensitivity to TRH. Wolff-Chaikoff effect—excess iodine temporarily inhibits thyroid peroxidase → ↓ iodine organification → ↓ T_3/T_4 production.	

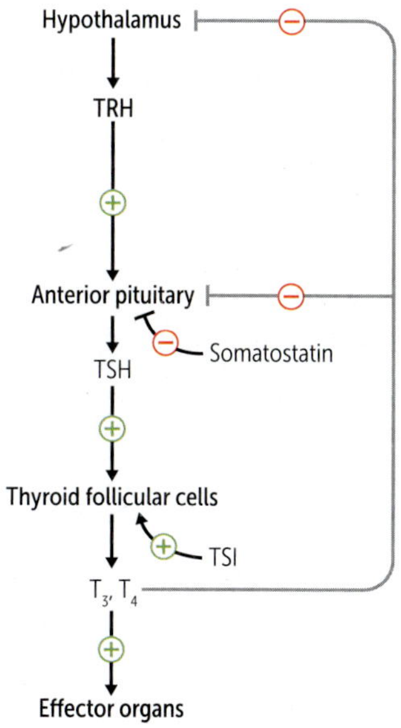

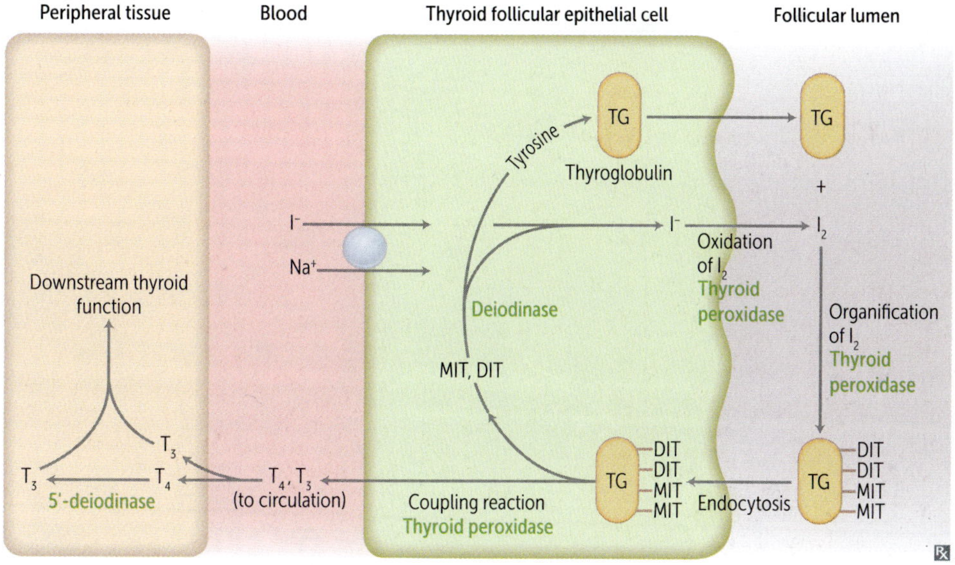

Signaling pathways of endocrine hormones

cAMP	FSH, LH, ACTH, TSH, CRH, hCG, ADH (V_2-receptor), MSH, PTH, calcitonin, GHRH, glucagon	FLAT ChAMP
cGMP	BNP, ANP, EDRF (NO)	BAD GraMPa Think vasodilators
IP_3	GnRH, Oxytocin, ADH (V_1-receptor), TRH, Histamine (H_1-receptor), Angiotensin II, Gastrin	GOAT HAG
Intracellular receptor	Progesterone, Estrogen, Testosterone, Cortisol, Aldosterone, T_3/T_4, Vitamin D	PET CAT on TV
Receptor tyrosine kinase	Insulin, IGF-1, FGF, PDGF, EGF	MAP kinase pathway Think growth factors
Nonreceptor tyrosine kinase	Prolactin, Immunomodulators (eg, cytokines IL-2, IL-6, IFN), GH, G-CSF, Erythropoietin, Thrombopoietin	JAK/STAT pathway Think acidophils and cytokines PIGGLET

Signaling pathway of steroid hormones

Steroid hormones are lipophilic and therefore must circulate bound to specific binding globulins, which ↑ their solubility.

In men, ↑ sex hormone–binding globulin (SHBG) lowers free testosterone → gynecomastia.

In women, ↓ SHBG raises free testosterone → hirsutism.

OCPs, pregnancy → ↑ SHBG.

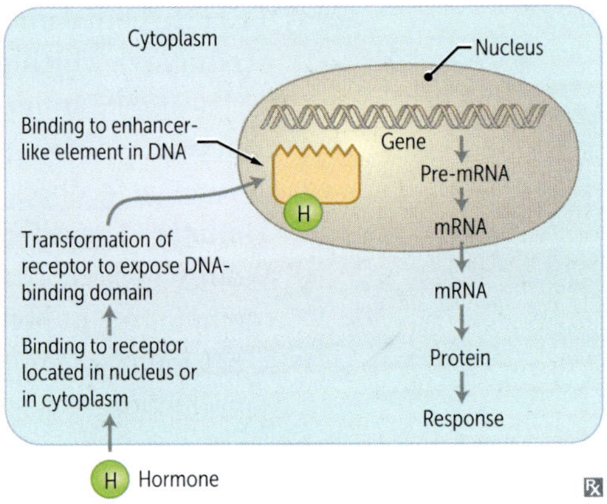

▶ ENDOCRINE—PATHOLOGY

Cushing syndrome

ETIOLOGY

↑ cortisol due to a variety of causes:
- Exogenous corticosteroids—result in ↓ ACTH, bilateral adrenal atrophy. Most common cause.
- Primary adrenal adenoma, hyperplasia, or carcinoma—result in ↓ ACTH, atrophy of uninvolved adrenal gland. Can also present with pseudohyperaldosteronism.
- ACTH-secreting pituitary adenoma (Cushing disease); paraneoplastic ACTH secretion (eg, small cell lung cancer, bronchial carcinoids)—result in ↑ ACTH, bilateral adrenal hyperplasia. Cushing disease is responsible for the majority of endogenous cases of Cushing syndrome.

FINDINGS

Hypertension, weight gain, moon facies A, abdominal striae B and truncal obesity, buffalo hump, skin changes (thinning, striae), osteoporosis, hyperglycemia (insulin resistance), amenorrhea, immunosuppression.

DIAGNOSIS

Screening tests include: ↑ free cortisol on 24-hr urinalysis, ↑ midnight salivary cortisol, and no suppression with overnight low-dose dexamethasone test. Measure serum ACTH. If ↓, suspect adrenal tumor or exogenous glucocorticoids. If ↑, distinguish between Cushing disease and ectopic ACTH secretion with a high-dose (8 mg) dexamethasone suppression test and CRH stimulation test. Ectopic secretion will not decrease with dexamethasone because the source is resistant to negative feedback; ectopic secretion will not increase with CRH because pituitary ACTH is suppressed.

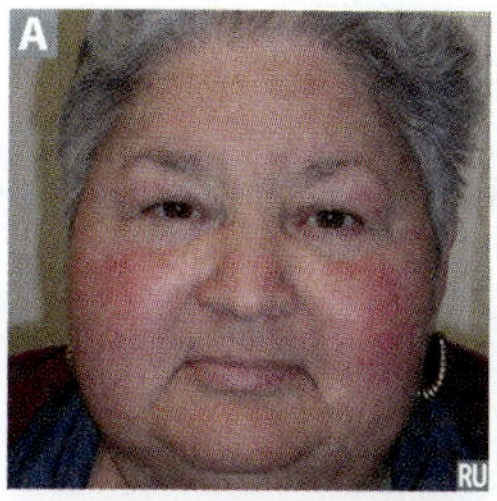

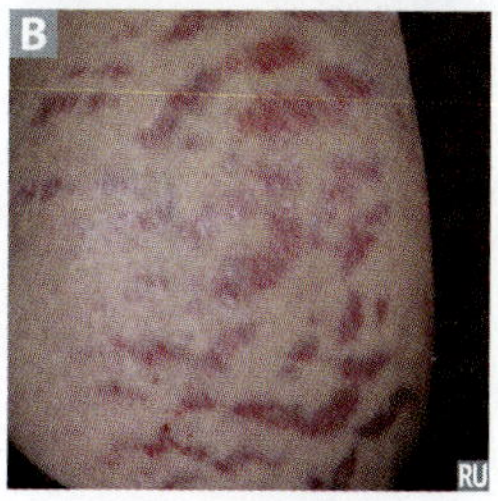

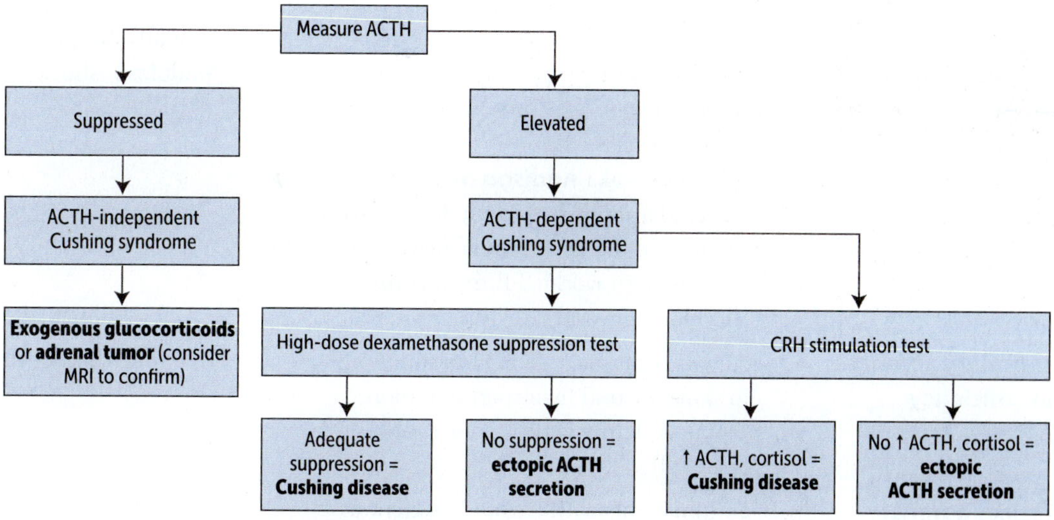

Adrenal insufficiency	Inability of adrenal glands to generate enough glucocorticoids +/– mineralocorticoids for the body's needs. Symptoms include weakness, fatigue, orthostatic hypotension, muscle aches, weight loss, GI disturbances, sugar and/or salt cravings. Treatment: glucocorticoid/mineralocorticoid replacement.	Diagnosis involves measurement of serum electrolytes, morning/random serum cortisol and ACTH (low cortisol, high ACTH in 1° adrenal insufficiency; low cortisol, low ACTH in 2°/3° adrenal insufficiency due to pituitary/hypothalamic disease), and response to ACTH stimulation test. Alternatively, can use metyrapone stimulation test: metyrapone blocks last step of cortisol synthesis (11-deoxycortisol → cortisol). Normal response is ↓ cortisol and compensatory ↑ ACTH and 11-deoxycortisol. In 1° adrenal insufficiency, ACTH is ↑ but 11-deoxycortisol remains ↓ after test. In 2°/3° adrenal insufficiency, both ACTH and 11-deoxycortisol remain ↓ after test.
Primary adrenal insufficiency 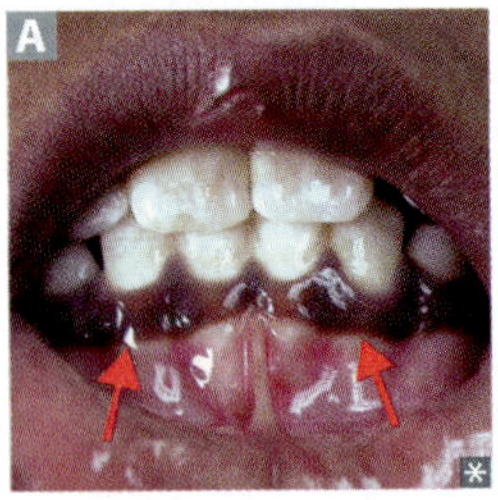	Deficiency of aldosterone and cortisol production due to loss of gland function → hypotension (hyponatremic volume contraction), hyperkalemia, metabolic acidosis, skin and mucosal hyperpigmentation A (due to ↑ MSH, a byproduct of ACTH production from pro-opiomelanocortin [POMC]). ▪ **Acute**—sudden onset (eg, due to massive hemorrhage). May present with shock in acute adrenal crisis. ▪ **Chronic**—aka **Addison disease**. Due to adrenal atrophy or destruction by disease (autoimmune destruction most common in the Western world; TB most common in the developing world).	**P**rimary **P**igments the skin/mucosa. Associated with autoimmune polyglandular syndromes. **Waterhouse-Friderichsen syndrome**—acute 1° adrenal insufficiency due to adrenal hemorrhage associated with septicemia (usually *Neisseria meningitidis*), DIC, endotoxic shock.
Secondary adrenal insufficiency	Seen with ↓ pituitary ACTH production. No skin/mucosal hyperpigmentation, no hyperkalemia (aldosterone synthesis preserved).	**S**econdary **S**pares the skin/mucosa.
Tertiary adrenal insufficiency	Seen in patients with chronic exogenous steroid use, precipitated by abrupt withdrawal. Aldosterone synthesis unaffected.	**T**ertiary from **T**reatment.

Hyperaldosteronism	Increased secretion of aldosterone from adrenal gland. Clinical features include hypertension, ↓ or normal K^+, metabolic alkalosis. No edema due to aldosterone escape mechanism.
Primary hyperaldosteronism	Seen with adrenal adenoma (Conn syndrome) or idiopathic adrenal hyperplasia. ↑ aldosterone, ↓ renin.
Secondary hyperaldosteronism	Seen in patients with renovascular hypertension, juxtaglomerular cell tumor (due to independent activation of renin-angiotensin-aldosterone system). ↑ aldosterone, ↑ renin.

Neuroendocrine tumors

Group of neoplasms originating from Kulchitsky and enterochromaffin-like cells. Occur in various organs (eg, thyroid: medullary carcinoma; lungs: small cell carcinoma; pancreas: islet cell tumor; adrenals: pheochromocytoma). Cells contain amine precursor uptake decarboxylase (APUD) and secrete different hormones (eg, 5-HIAA, neuron-specific enolase [NSE], chromogranin A).

Neuroblastoma

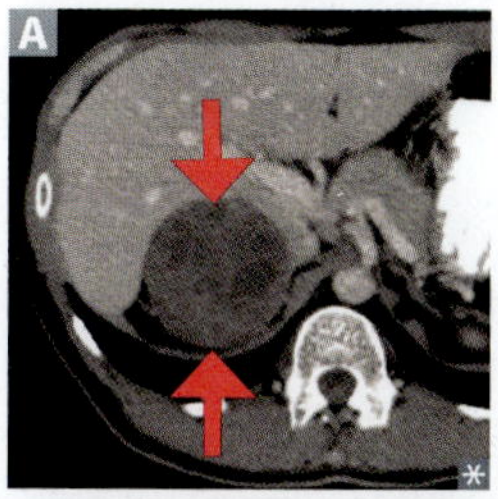

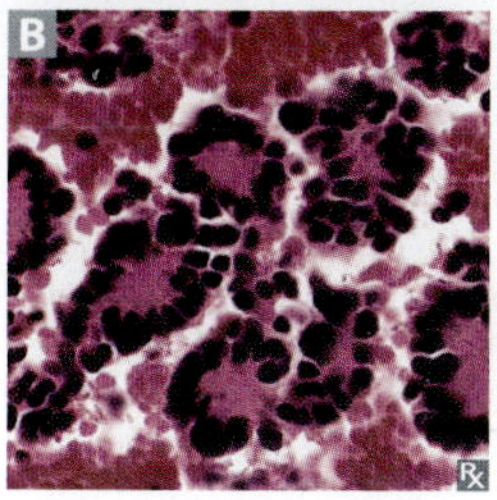

Most common tumor of the adrenal medulla in **children,** usually < 4 years old. Originates from neural crest cells. Occurs anywhere along the sympathetic chain A.

Most common presentation is abdominal distension and a firm, irregular mass that can cross the midline (vs Wilms tumor, which is smooth and unilateral). Less likely to develop hypertension than with pheochromocytoma. Can also present with opsoclonus-myoclonus syndrome ("dancing eyes-dancing feet").

↑ HVA and VMA (catecholamine metabolites) in urine. Homer-Wright rosettes B characteristic of neuroblastoma and medulloblastoma. Bombesin and NSE ⊕. Associated with overexpression of N-*myc* oncogene. Classified as an APUD tumor.

↳ amine precursor uptake decarboxylase.

Pheochromocytoma

ETIOLOGY 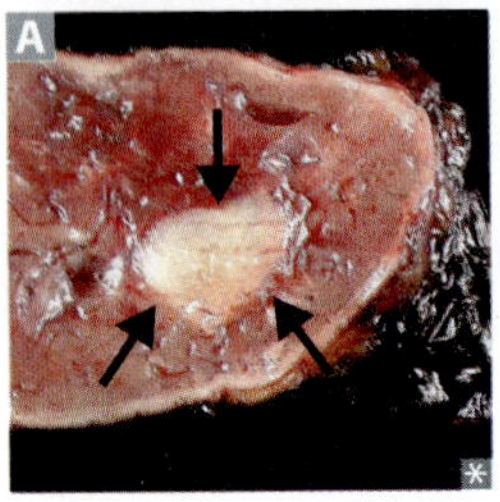	Most common tumor of the adrenal medulla in **adults** A. Derived from chromaffin cells (arise from neural crest). Up to 25% of cases associated with germline mutations (eg, *NF-1*, *VHL*, *RET* [MEN 2A, 2B]).	**Rule of 10's:** 10% malignant 10% bilateral 10% extra-adrenal 10% calcify 10% kids
SYMPTOMS	Most tumors secrete epinephrine, norepinephrine, and dopamine, which can cause episodic hypertension. Symptoms occur in "spells"—relapse and remit.	Episodic hyperadrenergic symptoms (**5 P's**): Pressure (↑ BP) Pain (headache) Perspiration Palpitations (tachycardia) Pallor
FINDINGS	↑ catecholamines and metanephrines in urine and plasma.	
TREATMENT	Irreversible α-antagonists (eg, phenoxybenzamine) followed by β-blockers prior to tumor resection. α-blockade must be achieved before giving β-blockers to avoid a hypertensive crisis.	**Phenoxybenzamine** (16 letters) is given for **pheochromocytoma** (also 16 letters).

Hypothyroidism vs hyperthyroidism

	Hypothyroidism	Hyperthyroidism
SIGNS/SYMPTOMS	Cold intolerance (↓ heat production)	Heat intolerance (↑ heat production)
	Weight gain, ↓ appetite	Weight loss, ↑ appetite
	Hypoactivity, lethargy, fatigue, weakness	Hyperactivity, anxiety, insomnia, hand tremor
	Constipation	Diarrhea
	↓ reflexes (delayed/slow relaxing)	↑ reflexes (brisk)
	Hypothyroid myopathy (proximal muscle weakness, ↑ CK)	Thyrotoxic myopathy (proximal muscle weakness, normal CK)
	Myxedema (facial/periorbital)	Pretibial myxedema (Graves disease), periorbital edema
	Dry, cool skin; coarse, brittle hair	Warm, moist skin; fine hair
	Bradycardia, dyspnea on exertion	Chest pain, palpitations, arrhythmias, ↑ number and sensitivity of β-adrenergic receptors
LAB FINDINGS	↑ TSH (if 1°)	↓ TSH (if 1°)
	↓ free T_3 and T_4	↑ free or total T_3 and T_4
	Hypercholesterolemia (due to ↓ LDL receptor expression)	Hypocholesterolemia (due to ↑ LDL receptor expression)

Causes of goiter

Smooth/diffuse	Nodular
Graves disease Hashimoto thyroiditis Iodine deficiency TSH-secreting pituitary adenoma	Toxic multinodular goiter Thyroid adenoma Thyroid cancer Thyroid cyst

Hypothyroidism

Hashimoto thyroiditis	Most common cause of hypothyroidism in iodine-sufficient regions; an autoimmune disorder with antithyroid peroxidase (antimicrosomal) and antithyroglobulin antibodies. Associated with HLA-DR5. ↑ risk of non-Hodgkin lymphoma (typically of B-cell origin). May be hyperthyroid early in course due to thyrotoxicosis during follicular rupture. Histologic findings: Hürthle cells, lymphoid aggregates with germinal centers A. Findings: moderately enlarged, **nontender** thyroid.
Congenital hypothyroidism (cretinism)	Severe fetal hypothyroidism due to maternal hypothyroidism, thyroid agenesis, thyroid dysgenesis (most common cause in US), iodine deficiency, dyshormonogenetic goiter. Findings: **P**ot-bellied, **P**ale, **P**uffy-faced child with **P**rotruding umbilicus, **P**rotuberant tongue, and **P**oor brain development: the **6 P's** B C.
Subacute granulomatous thyroiditis (de Quervain)	Self-limited disease often following a flu-like illness (eg, viral infection). May be hyperthyroid early in course, followed by hypothyroidism. Histology: granulomatous inflammation. Findings: ↑ ESR, jaw pain, very **tender** thyroid. (de Quer**vain** is associated with **pain**.)
Riedel thyroiditis	Thyroid replaced by fibrous tissue with inflammatory infiltrate D. Fibrosis may extend to local structures (eg, trachea, esophagus), mimicking anaplastic carcinoma. ⅓ are hypothyroid. Considered a manifestation of IgG_4-related systemic disease (eg, autoimmune pancreatitis, retroperitoneal fibrosis, noninfectious aortitis). Findings: fixed, hard (rock-like), **painless** goiter.
Other causes	Iodine deficiency E, goitrogens (eg, amiodarone, lithium), Wolff-Chaikoff effect (thyroid gland downregulation in response to ↑ iodide).

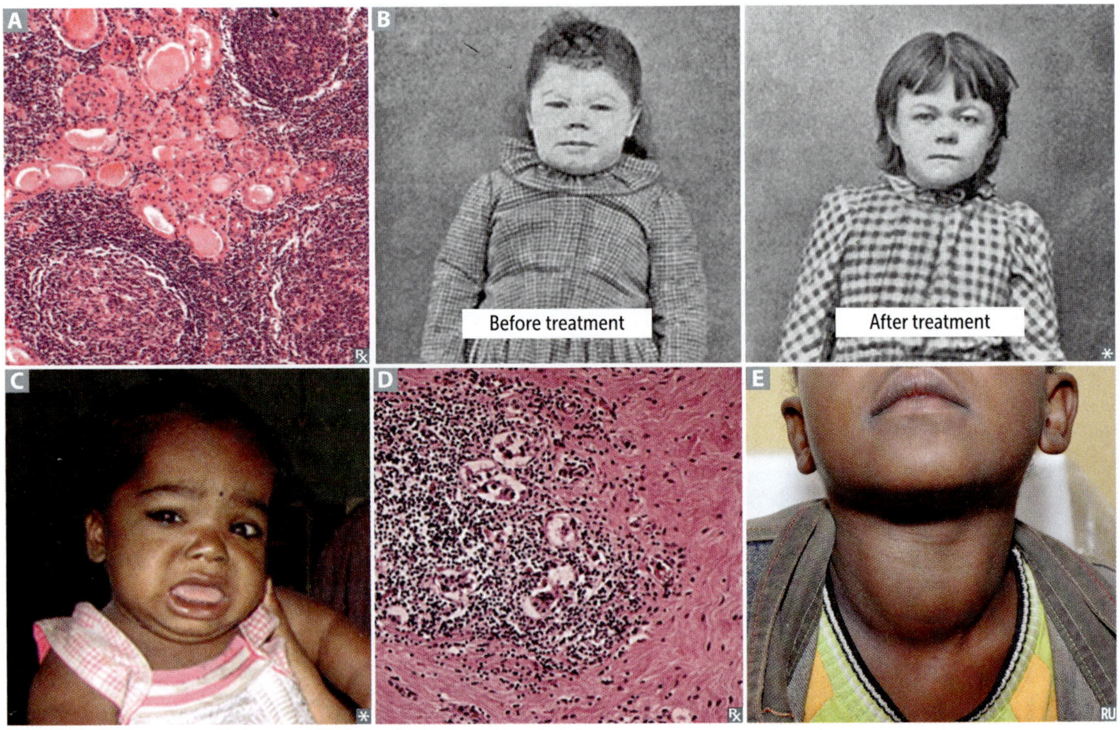

Hyperthyroidism

Graves disease	Most common cause of hyperthyroidism. Thyroid-stimulating immunoglobulin (IgG; type II hypersensitivity) stimulates TSH receptors on thyroid (hyperthyroidism, diffuse goiter) and dermal fibroblasts (pretibial myxedema). Infiltration of retroorbital space by activated T-cells → ↑ cytokines (eg, TNF-α, IFN-γ) → ↑ fibroblast secretion of hydrophilic GAGs → ↑ osmotic muscle swelling, muscle inflammation, and adipocyte count → exophthalmos A. Often presents during stress (eg, pregnancy). Tall, crowded follicular epithelial cells; scalloped colloid B.
Toxic multinodular goiter	Focal patches of hyperfunctioning follicular cells C working independently of TSH (due to TSH receptor mutations in 60% of cases). ↑ release of T_3 and T_4. Hot nodules are rarely malignant.
Thyroid storm	Uncommon but serious complication that occurs when hyperthyroidism is incompletely treated/untreated and then significantly worsens in the setting of acute stress such as infection, trauma, surgery. Presents with agitation, delirium, fever, diarrhea, coma, and tachyarrhythmia (cause of death). May see ↑ LFTs. Treat with the 4 P's: β-blockers (eg, Propranolol), Propylthiouracil, corticosteroids (eg, Prednisolone), Potassium iodide (Lugol iodine).
Jod-Basedow phenomenon	Thyrotoxicosis if a patient with iodine deficiency and partially autonomous thyroid tissue (eg, autonomous nodule) is made iodine replete. Opposite of Wolff-Chaikoff effect.

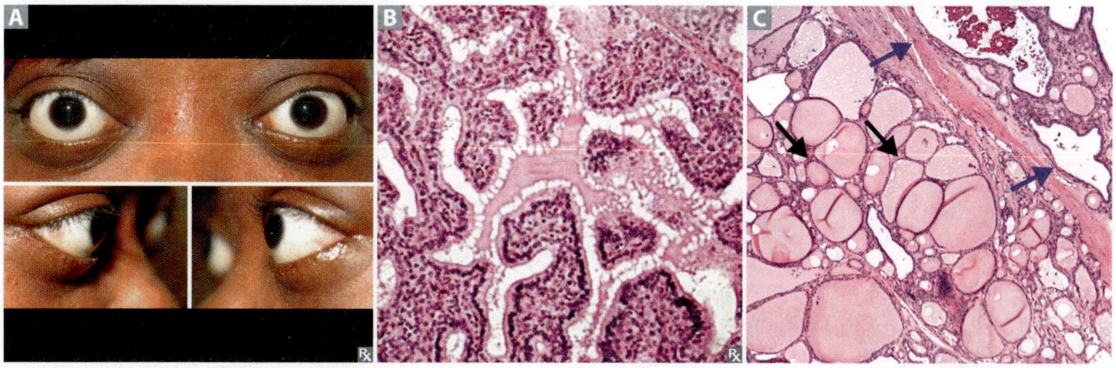

Thyroid adenoma

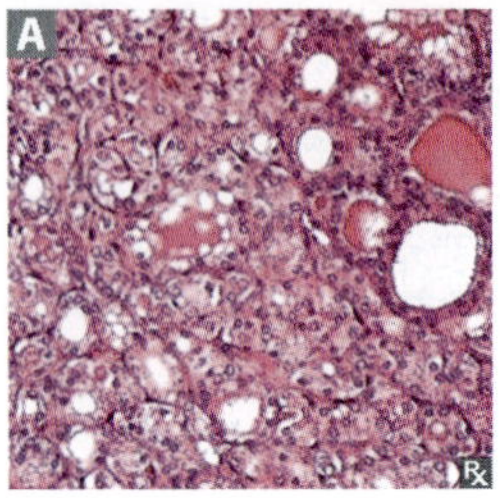

Benign solitary growth of the thyroid. Most are nonfunctional ("cold"), can rarely cause hyperthyroidism via autonomous thyroid hormone production ("hot" or "toxic"). Most common histology is follicular A; absence of capsular or vascular invasion (unlike follicular carcinoma).

Thyroid cancer

Treated with thyroidectomy. Complications of surgery include hoarseness (due to recurrent laryngeal nerve damage), hypocalcemia (due to removal of parathyroid glands), and transection of recurrent and superior laryngeal nerves (during ligation of inferior thyroid artery and superior laryngeal artery, respectively).

Papillary carcinoma

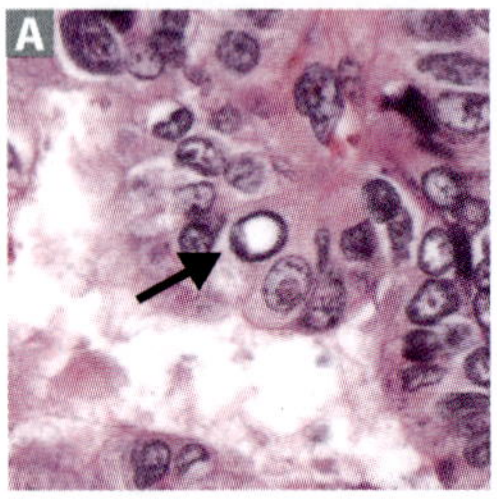

Most common, excellent prognosis. Empty-appearing nuclei with central clearing ("Orphan Annie" eyes) A, psammoma bodies, nuclear grooves. ↑ risk with *RET* and *BRAF* mutations, childhood irradiation.

Follicular carcinoma

Good prognosis, invades thyroid capsule and vasculature (unlike follicular adenoma), uniform follicles; hematogenous spread is common. Associated with *RAS* mutation.

Medullary carcinoma

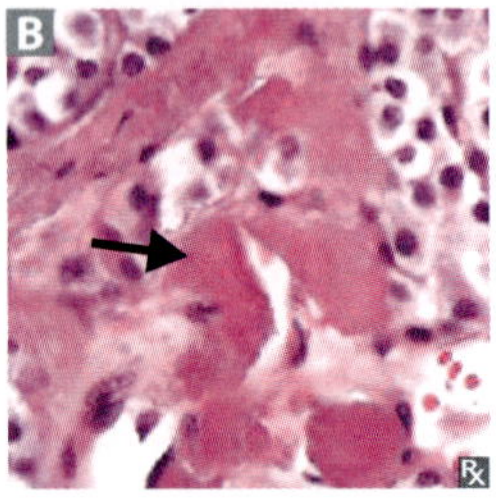

From parafollicular "C cells"; produces calcitonin, sheets of cells in an amyloid stroma (stains with Congo red B). Associated with MEN 2A and 2B (*RET* mutations).

Undifferentiated/ anaplastic carcinoma

Older patients; invades local structures, very poor prognosis.

Lymphoma

Associated with Hashimoto thyroiditis.

Diagnosis of parathyroid disease

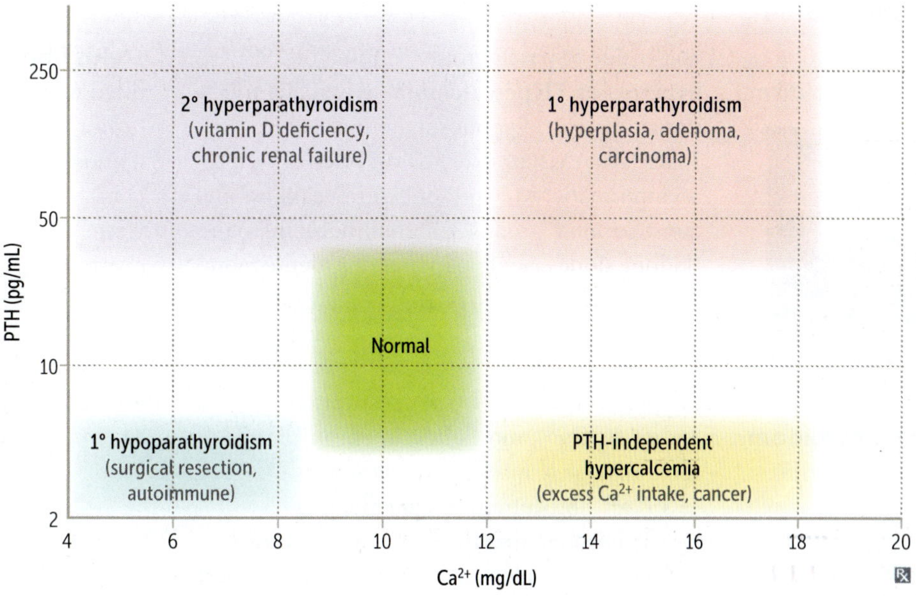

Hypoparathyroidism

Due to accidental surgical excision of parathyroid glands, autoimmune destruction, or DiGeorge syndrome. Findings: tetany, hypocalcemia, hyperphosphatemia.

Chvostek sign—tapping of facial nerve (tap the Cheek) → contraction of facial muscles.

Trousseau sign—occlusion of brachial artery with BP cuff (cuff the Triceps) → carpal spasm.

Pseudohypoparathyroidism type 1A (Albright hereditary osteodystrophy)—unresponsiveness of kidney to PTH → hypocalcemia despite ↑ PTH levels. Characterized by shortened 4th/5th digits, short stature. Autosomal dominant. Due to defective G_s protein α-subunit causing end-organ resistance to PTH. Defect must be inherited from mother due to imprinting.

Pseudopseudohypoparathyroidism—physical exam features of Albright hereditary osteodystrophy but without end-organ PTH resistance. Occurs when defective G_s protein α-subunit is inherited from father.

Familial hypocalciuric hypercalcemia

Defective Ca^{2+}-sensing receptor (CaSR) in multiple tissues (eg, parathyroids, kidneys). Higher than normal Ca^{2+} levels required to suppress PTH. Excessive renal Ca^{2+} reuptake → mild hypercalcemia and hypocalciuria with normal to ↑ PTH levels.

Hyperparathyroidism

Primary hyperparathyroidism

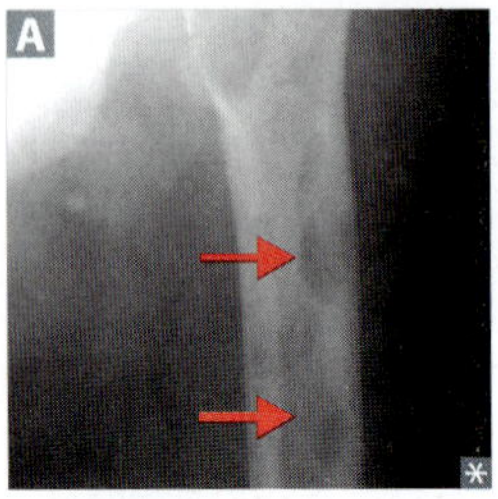

Usually due to parathyroid adenoma or hyperplasia. **Hypercalcemia**, hypercalciuria (renal **stones**), hypophosphatemia, ↑ PTH, ↑ ALP, ↑ cAMP in urine. Most often asymptomatic. May present with weakness and constipation ("**groans**"), abdominal/flank pain (kidney stones, acute pancreatitis), depression ("**psychiatric overtones**").

Osteitis fibrosa cystica—cystic **bone** spaces filled with brown fibrous tissue A ("brown tumor" consisting of osteoclasts and deposited hemosiderin from hemorrhages; causes bone pain).

"**Stones**, **bones**, **groans**, and **psychiatric overtones**."

Secondary hyperparathyroidism

2° hyperplasia due to ↓ Ca^{2+} absorption and/or ↑ PO_4^{3-}, most often in chronic renal disease (causes hypovitaminosis D → ↓ Ca^{2+} absorption). **Hypocalcemia**, hyperphosphatemia in chronic renal failure (vs hypophosphatemia with most other causes), ↑ ALP, ↑ PTH.

Renal osteodystrophy—renal disease → 2° and 3° hyperparathyroidism → bone lesions.

Tertiary hyperparathyroidism

Refractory (autonomous) hyperparathyroidism resulting from chronic renal disease. ↑↑ PTH, ↑ Ca^{2+}.

Pituitary adenoma

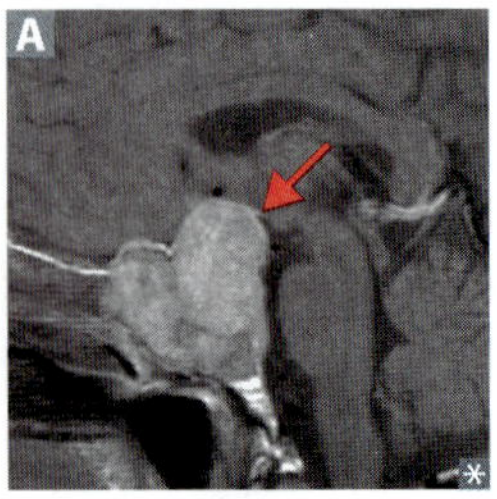

Benign tumor, most commonly prolactinoma (arises from lactotrophs). Adenoma A may be functional (hormone producing) or nonfunctional (silent). Nonfunctional tumors present with mass effect (bitemporal hemianopia, hypopituitarism, headache). Functional tumor presentation is based on the hormone produced.

Treatment for prolactinoma: dopamine agonists (eg, ergot alkaloids such as bromocriptine, cabergoline), transsphenoidal resection.

Nelson syndrome

Enlargement of existing ACTH-secreting pituitary adenoma after bilateral adrenalectomy for refractory Cushing disease (due to removal of cortisol feedback mechanism). Presents with hyperpigmentation, headaches and bitemporal hemianopia. Treatment: pituitary irradiation or surgical resection.

Acromegaly	Excess GH in adults. Typically caused by pituitary adenoma.	
FINDINGS	Large tongue with deep furrows, deep voice, large hands and feet, coarsening of facial features with aging A, frontal bossing, diaphoresis (excessive sweating), impaired glucose tolerance (insulin resistance). ↑ risk of colorectal polyps and cancer.	↑ GH in children → gigantism (↑ linear bone growth). HF most common cause of death. 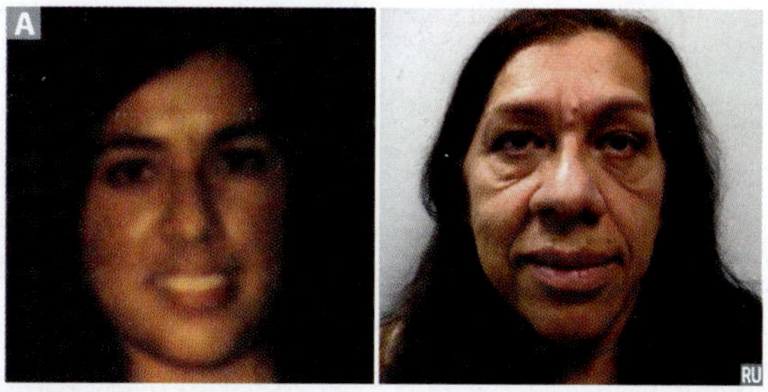
DIAGNOSIS	↑ serum IGF-1; failure to suppress serum GH following oral glucose tolerance test; pituitary mass seen on brain MRI.	
TREATMENT	Pituitary adenoma resection. If not cured, treat with octreotide (somatostatin analog) or pegvisomant (growth hormone receptor antagonist).	

Laron syndrome (dwarfism)	Defective growth hormone receptors → ↓ linear growth. ↑ GH, ↓ IGF-1. Clinical features include short height, small head circumference, characteristic facies with saddle nose and prominent forehead, delayed skeletal maturation, small genitalia.

Diabetes insipidus Characterized by intense thirst and polyuria with inability to concentrate urine due to lack of ADH (central) or failure of response to circulating ADH (nephrogenic).

	Central DI	Nephrogenic DI
ETIOLOGY	Pituitary tumor, autoimmune, trauma, surgery, ischemic encephalopathy, idiopathic	Hereditary (ADH receptor mutation), 2° to hypercalcemia, hypokalemia, lithium, demeclocycline (ADH antagonist)
FINDINGS	↓ ADH Urine specific gravity < 1.006 Serum osmolality > 290 mOsm/kg Hyperosmotic volume contraction	Normal or ↑ ADH levels Urine specific gravity < 1.006 Serum osmolality > 290 mOsm/kg Hyperosmotic volume contraction
WATER DEPRIVATION TEST[a]	> 50% ↑ in urine osmolality only after administration of ADH analog	Minimal change in urine osmolality, even after administration of ADH analog
TREATMENT	Desmopressin acetate Hydration	HCTZ, indomethacin, amiloride Hydration, avoidance of offending agent

[a]No water intake for 2–3 hr followed by hourly measurements of urine volume and osmolarity and plasma Na^+ concentration and osmolarity. ADH analog (desmopressin acetate) is administered if serum osmolality > 295–300 mOsm/kg, plasma $Na^+ \geq 145$, or urine osmolality does not rise despite a rising plasma osmolality.

Syndrome of inappropriate antidiuretic hormone secretion

Characterized by:
- Excessive free water retention
- Euvolemic hyponatremia with continued urinary Na^+ excretion
- Urine osmolality > serum osmolality

Body responds to water retention with ↓ aldosterone and ↑ ANP and BNP → ↑ urinary Na^+ secretion → normalization of extracellular fluid volume → euvolemic hyponatremia. Very low serum Na^+ levels can lead to cerebral edema, seizures. Correct slowly to prevent osmotic demyelination syndrome (formerly known as central pontine myelinolysis).

Causes include:
- Ectopic ADH (eg, small cell lung cancer)
- CNS disorders/head trauma
- Pulmonary disease
- Drugs (eg, cyclophosphamide)

Treatment: fluid restriction, salt tablets, IV hypertonic saline, diuretics, conivaptan, tolvaptan, demeclocycline.

Hypopituitarism

Undersecretion of pituitary hormones due to:
- Nonsecreting pituitary adenoma, craniopharyngioma
- Sheehan syndrome—ischemic infarct of pituitary following postpartum bleeding; pregnancy-induced pituitary growth → ↑ susceptibility to hypoperfusion. Usually presents with failure to lactate, absent menstruation, cold intolerance
- Empty sella syndrome—atrophy or compression of pituitary (which lies in the sella turcica), often idiopathic, common in obese women
- Pituitary apoplexy—sudden hemorrhage of pituitary gland, often in the presence of an existing pituitary adenoma. Usually presents with sudden onset severe headache, visual impairment (eg, bitemporal hemianopia, diplopia due to CN III palsy), and features of hypopituitarism.
- Brain injury
- Radiation

Treatment: hormone replacement therapy (corticosteroids, thyroxine, sex steroids, human growth hormone).

Diabetes mellitus

ACUTE MANIFESTATIONS

Polydipsia, polyuria, polyphagia, weight loss, DKA (type 1), hyperosmolar coma (type 2). Rarely, can be caused by unopposed secretion of GH and epinephrine. Also seen in patients on glucocorticoid therapy (steroid diabetes).

CHRONIC COMPLICATIONS

Nonenzymatic glycation:

- Small vessel disease (diffuse thickening of basement membrane) → retinopathy (hemorrhage, exudates, microaneurysms, vessel proliferation), glaucoma, neuropathy, nephropathy (nodular glomerulosclerosis, aka Kimmelstiel-Wilson nodules → progressive proteinuria [initially microalbuminuria; ACE inhibitors are renoprotective] and arteriolosclerosis → hypertension; both lead to chronic renal failure).
- Large vessel atherosclerosis, CAD, peripheral vascular occlusive disease, gangrene → limb loss, cerebrovascular disease. MI most common cause of death.

Osmotic damage (sorbitol accumulation in organs with aldose reductase and ↓ or absent sorbitol dehydrogenase):

- Neuropathy (motor, sensory [glove and stocking distribution], and autonomic degeneration)
- Cataracts

DIAGNOSIS

TEST	DIAGNOSTIC CUTOFF	NOTES
HbA_{1c}	≥ 6.5%	Reflects average blood glucose over prior 3 months
Fasting plasma glucose	≥ 126 mg/dL	Fasting for > 8 hours
2-hour oral glucose tolerance test	≥ 200 mg/dL	2 hours after consumption of 75 g of glucose in water

Insulin deficiency

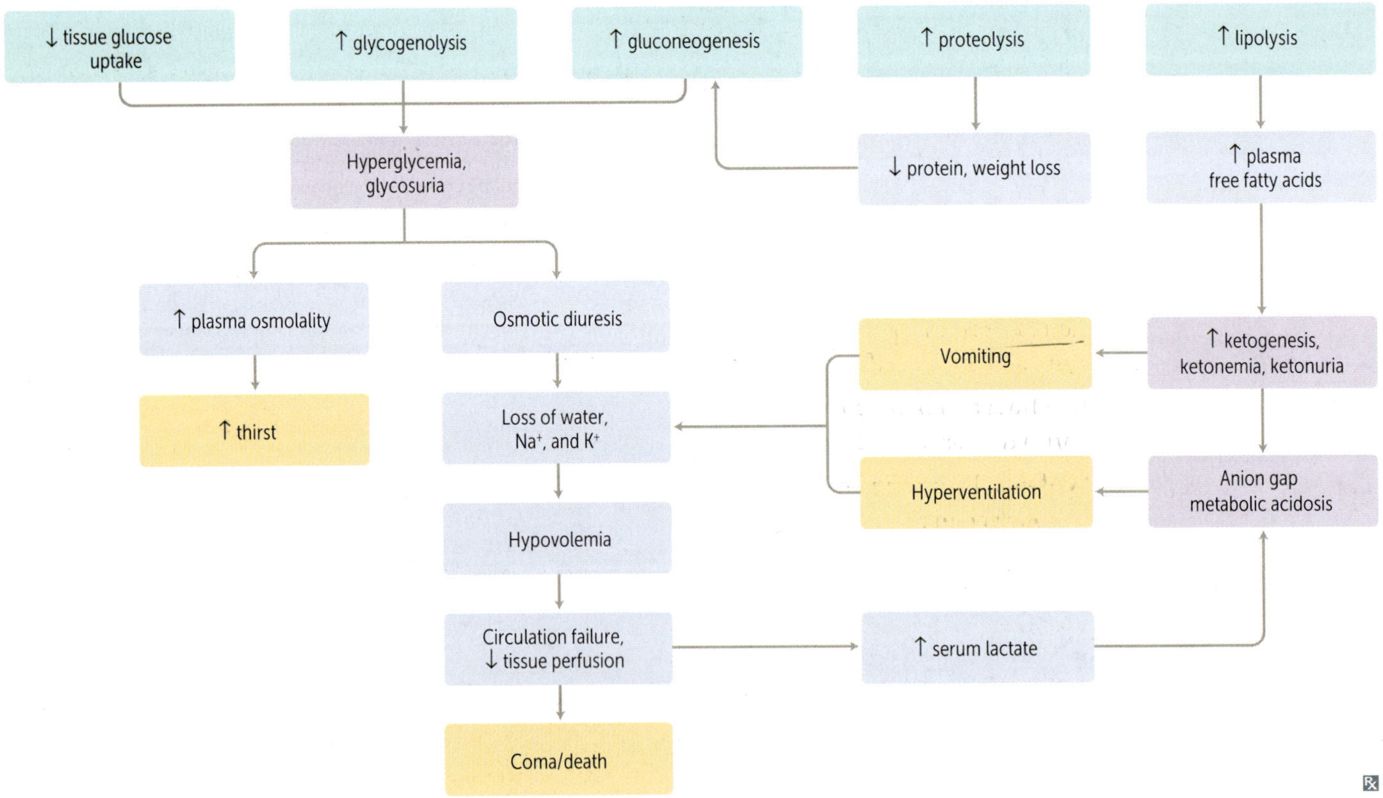

Type 1 vs type 2 diabetes mellitus

Variable	Type 1	Type 2
1° DEFECT	Autoimmune destruction of β cells (eg, due to glutamic acid decarboxylase antibodies)	↑ resistance to insulin, progressive pancreatic β-cell failure
INSULIN NECESSARY IN TREATMENT	Always	Sometimes
AGE (EXCEPTIONS COMMONLY OCCUR)	< 30 yr	> 40 yr
ASSOCIATION WITH OBESITY	No	Yes
GENETIC PREDISPOSITION	Relatively weak (50% concordance in identical twins), polygenic	Relatively strong (90% concordance in identical twins), polygenic
ASSOCIATION WITH HLA SYSTEM	Yes (HLA-DR3 and -DR4)	No
GLUCOSE INTOLERANCE	Severe	Mild to moderate
INSULIN SENSITIVITY	High	Low
KETOACIDOSIS	Common	Rare
β-CELL NUMBERS IN THE ISLETS	↓	Variable (with amyloid deposits)
SERUM INSULIN LEVEL	↓	Variable
CLASSIC SYMPTOMS OF POLYURIA, POLYDIPSIA, POLYPHAGIA, WEIGHT LOSS	Common	Sometimes
HISTOLOGY	Islet leukocytic infiltrate	Islet amyloid polypeptide (IAPP) deposits

Diabetic ketoacidosis

One of the most feared complications of diabetes. Usually due to insulin noncompliance or ↑ insulin requirements from ↑ stress (eg, infection). Excess fat breakdown and ↑ ketogenesis from ↑ free fatty acids, which are then made into ketone bodies (β-hydroxybutyrate > acetoacetate). Usually occurs in type 1 diabetes, as endogenous insulin in type 2 diabetes usually prevents lipolysis.

SIGNS/SYMPTOMS	DKA is Deadly: Delirium/psychosis, Kussmaul respirations (rapid/deep breathing), Abdominal pain/nausea/vomiting, Dehydration. Fruity breath odor (due to exhaled acetone).
LABS	Hyperglycemia, ↑ H^+, ↓ HCO_3^- (↑ anion gap metabolic acidosis), ↑ blood ketone levels, leukocytosis. Hyperkalemia, but depleted intracellular K^+ due to transcellular shift from ↓ insulin and acidosis (therefore total body K^+ is depleted).
COMPLICATIONS	Life-threatening mucormycosis (usually caused by *Rhizopus* infection), cerebral edema, cardiac arrhythmias, heart failure.
TREATMENT	IV fluids, IV insulin, and K^+ (to replete intracellular stores); glucose if necessary to prevent hypoglycemia.

Hyperosmolar hyperglycemia nonketotic syndrome

State of profound hyperglycemia-induced dehydration and ↑ serum osmolarity, classically seen in elderly type 2 diabetics with limited ability to drink. Hyperglycemia → excessive osmotic diuresis → dehydration → eventual onset of HHNS. Symptoms: thirst, polyuria, lethargy, focal neurological deficits (eg, seizures), can progress to coma and death if left untreated. Labs: hyperglycemia (often > 600 mg/dL), ↑ serum osmolarity (> 320 mOsm/kg), no acidosis (pH > 7.3, ketone production inhibited by presence of insulin). Treatment: aggressive IV fluids, insulin therapy.

Glucagonoma

Tumor of pancreatic α cells → overproduction of glucagon. Presents with **d**ermatitis (necrolytic migratory erythema), **d**iabetes (hyperglycemia), **D**VT, **d**eclining weight, **d**epression. Treatment: octreotide, surgery.

Insulinoma

Tumor of pancreatic β cells → overproduction of insulin → hypoglycemia. May see Whipple triad: low blood glucose, symptoms of hypoglycemia (eg, lethargy, syncope, diplopia), and resolution of symptoms after normalization of glucose levels. Symptomatic patients have ↓ blood glucose and ↑ C-peptide levels (vs exogenous insulin use). ~ 10% of cases associated with MEN 1 syndrome. Treatment: surgical resection.

Somatostatinoma

Tumor of pancreatic δ cells → overproduction of somatostatin → ↓ secretion of secretin, cholecystokinin, glucagon, insulin, gastrin. May present with diabetes/glucose intolerance, steatorrhea, gallstones. Treatment: surgical resection; somatostatin analogs (eg, octreotide) for symptom control.

Carcinoid syndrome

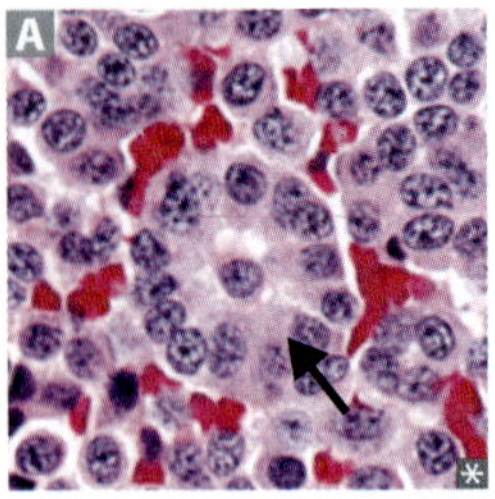

Rare syndrome caused by carcinoid tumors (neuroendocrine cells A; note prominent rosettes [arrow]), especially metastatic small bowel tumors, which secrete high levels of serotonin (5-HT). Not seen if tumor is limited to GI tract (5-HT undergoes first-pass metabolism in liver). Results in recurrent diarrhea, cutaneous flushing, asthmatic wheezing, right-sided valvular heart disease (tricuspid regurgitation, pulmonic stenosis). ↑ 5-hydroxyindoleacetic acid (5-HIAA) in urine, niacin deficiency (pellagra).
Treatment: surgical resection, somatostatin analog (eg, octreotide).

Rule of 1/3s:
- 1/3 metastasize
- 1/3 present with 2nd malignancy
- 1/3 are multiple

Most common malignancy in the small intestine.

Zollinger-Ellison syndrome

Gastrin-secreting tumor (gastrinoma) of pancreas or duodenum. Acid hypersecretion causes recurrent ulcers in duodenum and jejunum. Presents with abdominal pain (peptic ulcer disease, distal ulcers), diarrhea (malabsorption). Positive secretin stimulation test: gastrin levels remain elevated after administration of secretin, which normally inhibits gastrin release. May be associated with MEN 1.

VIP = relaxes GI SMCs + esoph.
↑ HCO_3 from pancreas
↓ gastrin H+ secret. (like secretin)

Multiple endocrine neoplasias

All **MEN** syndromes have autosomal **dominant** inheritance.
"All **MEN** are **dominant**" (or so they think).

SUBTYPE	CHARACTERISTICS	COMMENTS
MEN 1	**P**ituitary tumors (prolactin or GH) **P**ancreatic endocrine tumors—Zollinger-Ellison syndrome, insulinomas, VIPomas, glucagonomas (rare) (→ panc. islet cells) **P**arathyroid adenomas Associated with mutation of *MEN1* (menin, a tumor suppressor, chromosome 11)	
MEN 2A	**P**arathyroid hyperplasia Medullary thyroid carcinoma—neoplasm of parafollicular or C cells; secretes calcitonin; prophylactic thyroidectomy required **P**heochromocytoma (secretes catecholamines) Associated with mutation in *RET* (codes for receptor tyrosine kinase) in cells of neural crest origin	
MEN 2B	Medullary thyroid carcinoma **P**heochromocytoma Mucosal neuromas (oral/intestinal ganglioneuromatosis) Associated with marfanoid habitus; mutation in *RET* gene	

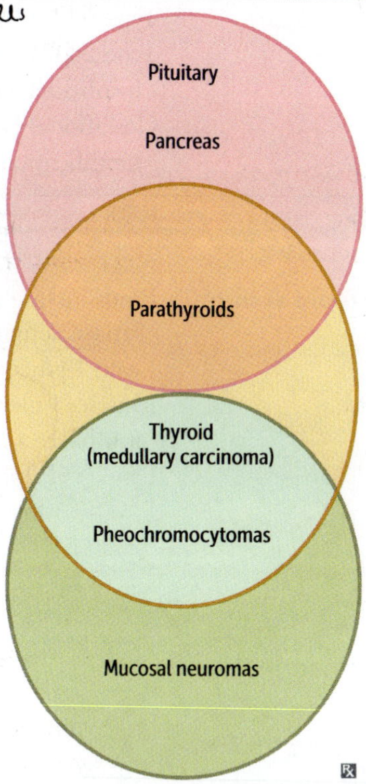

MEN 1 = **3 P's**: **P**ituitary, **P**arathyroid, and **P**ancreas
MEN 2A = **2 P's**: **P**arathyroids and **P**heochromocytoma
MEN 2B = **1 P**: **P**heochromocytoma

▶ ENDOCRINE—PHARMACOLOGY

Diabetes mellitus drugs

Treatment strategies:

Type 1 DM—low-carbohydrate diet, insulin replacement

Type 2 DM—dietary modification and exercise for weight loss; oral agents, non-insulin injectables, insulin replacement

Gestational DM (GDM)—dietary modifications, exercise, insulin replacement if lifestyle modification fails

DRUG CLASSES	ACTION	CLINICAL USE	RISKS/CONCERNS
Insulin preparations			
Insulin, rapid acting Lispro, Aspart, Glulisine	Binds insulin receptor (tyrosine kinase activity) rapidly, no LAG. Liver: ↑ glucose stored as glycogen. Muscle: ↑ glycogen, protein synthesis; ↑ K^+ uptake. Fat: ↑ TG storage.	Type 1 DM, type 2 DM, GDM (postprandial glucose control).	Hypoglycemia, lipodystrophy, rare hypersensitivity reactions.
Insulin, short acting Regular		Type 1 DM, type 2 DM, GDM, DKA (IV), hyperkalemia (+ glucose), stress hyperglycemia.	
Insulin, intermediate acting NPH		Type 1 DM, type 2 DM, GDM.	
Insulin, long acting Detemir, glargine		Type 1 DM, type 2 DM, GDM (basal glucose control).	
Oral hypoglycemic drugs			
Biguanides Metformin	Exact mechanism unknown. ↓ gluconeogenesis, ↑ glycolysis, ↑ peripheral glucose uptake (↑ insulin sensitivity).	Oral. First-line therapy in type 2 DM, causes modest weight loss. Can be used in patients without islet function.	GI upset; most serious adverse effect is lactic acidosis (thus contraindicated in renal insufficiency).
Sulfonylureas First generation: chlorpropamide, tolbutamide Second generation: glimepiride, glipizide, glyburide	Close K^+ channel in β-cell membrane → cell depolarizes → insulin release via ↑ Ca^{2+} influx.	Stimulate release of endogenous insulin in type 2 DM. Require some islet function, so useless in type 1 DM.	Risk of hypoglycemia ↑ in renal failure, weight gain. First generation: disulfiram-like effects. Second generation: hypoglycemia.
Glitazones/ thiazolidinediones Pioglitazone, rosiglitazone	↑ insulin sensitivity in peripheral tissue. Binds to PPAR-γ nuclear transcription regulator.[a]	Used as monotherapy in type 2 DM or combined with above agents. Safe to use in renal impairment.	Weight gain, edema. Hepatotoxicity, HF, ↑ risk of fractures.

Diabetes mellitus drugs *(continued)*

DRUG CLASSES	ACTION	CLINICAL USE	RISKS/CONCERNS
Oral hypoglycemic drugs *(continued)*			
Meglitinides Nateglinide, repaglinide	Stimulate postprandial insulin release by binding to K^+ channels on β-cell membranes (site differs from sulfonylureas).	Used as monotherapy in type 2 DM or combined with metformin.	Hypoglycemia (↑ risk with renal failure), weight gain.
GLP-1 analogs Exenatide, liraglutide (sc injection)	↑ glucose-dependent insulin release, ↓ glucagon release, ↓ gastric emptying, ↑ satiety.	Type 2 DM.	Nausea, vomiting, pancreatitis; modest weight loss.
DPP-4 inhibitors Linagliptin, saxagliptin, sitagliptin	Inhibits DPP-4 enzyme that deactivates GLP-1, thereby ↑ glucose-dependent insulin release, ↓ glucagon release, ↓ gastric emptying, ↑ satiety.	Type 2 DM.	Mild urinary or respiratory infections; weight neutral.
Amylin analogs Pramlintide (sc injection)	↓ gastric emptying, ↓ glucagon.	Type 1 DM, type 2 DM.	Hypoglycemia (in setting of mistimed prandial insulin), nausea.
Sodium-glucose co-transporter 2 (SGLT-2) inhibitors Canagliflozin, dapagliflozin, empagliflozin	Block reabsorption of glucose in PCT.	Type 2 DM.	Glucosuria, UTIs, vaginal yeast infections, hyperkalemia, dehydration (orthostatic hypotension).
α-glucosidase inhibitors Acarbose, miglitol	Inhibit intestinal brush-border α-glucosidases. Delayed carbohydrate hydrolysis and glucose absorption → ↓ postprandial hyperglycemia.	Type 2 DM.	GI disturbances.

[a]Genes activated by PPAR-γ regulate fatty acid storage and glucose metabolism. Activation of PPAR-γ ↑ insulin sensitivity and levels of adiponectin.

Thionamides	Propylthiouracil (PTU), methimazole.
MECHANISM	Block thyroid peroxidase, inhibiting the oxidation of iodide and the organification (coupling) of iodine → inhibition of thyroid hormone synthesis. Propylthiouracil also blocks 5′-deiodinase → ↓ peripheral conversion of T_4 to T_3.
CLINICAL USE	Hyperthyroidism. PTU blocks Peripheral conversion and is used in Pregnancy.
ADVERSE EFFECTS	Skin rash, agranulocytosis (rare), aplastic anemia, hepatotoxicity. Methimazole is a possible teratogen (can cause aplasia cutis).

Levothyroxine (T_4), triiodothyronine (T_3)

MECHANISM	Thyroid hormone replacement.
CLINICAL USE	Hypothyroidism, myxedema. Used off-label as weight loss supplements.
ADVERSE EFFECTS	Tachycardia, heat intolerance, tremors, arrhythmias.

Hypothalamic/pituitary drugs

DRUG	CLINICAL USE
ADH antagonists (conivaptan, tolvaptan)	SIADH, block action of ADH at V_2-receptor.
Desmopressin acetate	Central (not nephrogenic) DI.
GH	GH deficiency, Turner syndrome.
Oxytocin	Stimulates labor, uterine contractions, milk let-down; controls uterine hemorrhage.
Somatostatin (octreotide)	Acromegaly, carcinoid syndrome, gastrinoma, glucagonoma, esophageal varices.

Demeclocycline

MECHANISM	ADH antagonist (member of tetracycline family).
CLINICAL USE	SIADH.
ADVERSE EFFECTS	Nephrogenic DI, photosensitivity, abnormalities of bone and teeth.

Glucocorticoids

Beclomethasone, dexamethasone, hydrocortisone, methylprednisolone, prednisone, triamcinolone.

MECHANISM	Metabolic, catabolic, anti-inflammatory, and immunosuppressive effects mediated by interactions with glucocorticoid response elements, inhibition of phospholipase A_2, and inhibition of transcription factors such as NF-κB.
CLINICAL USE	Adrenal insufficiency, inflammation, immunosuppression, asthma.
ADVERSE EFFECTS	Iatrogenic Cushing syndrome (hypertension, weight gain, moon facies, truncal obesity, buffalo hump, thinning of skin, striae, acne, osteoporosis, hyperglycemia, amenorrhea, immunosuppression), adrenocortical atrophy, peptic ulcers, steroid diabetes, steroid psychosis, cataracts. Adrenal insufficiency when drug stopped abruptly after chronic use.

Fludrocortisone

MECHANISM	Synthetic analog of aldosterone with little glucocorticoid effects.
CLINICAL USE	Mineralocorticoid replacement in 1° adrenal insufficiency.
ADVERSE EFFECTS	Similar to glucocorticoids; also edema, exacerbation of heart failure, hyperpigmentation.

Cinacalcet

MECHANISM	Sensitizes Ca^{2+}-sensing receptor (CaSR) in parathyroid gland to circulating Ca^{2+} → ↓ PTH.
CLINICAL USE	1° or 2° hyperparathyroidism.
ADVERSE EFFECTS	Hypocalcemia.

HIGH-YIELD SYSTEMS

Gastrointestinal

"A good set of bowels is worth more to a man than any quantity of brains."
—Josh Billings

"Man should strive to have his intestines relaxed all the days of his life."
—Moses Maimonides

"Is life worth living? It all depends on the liver."
—William James

▸ GASTROINTESTINAL—EMBRYOLOGY

Normal gastrointestinal embryology

Foregut—pharynx to duodenum.
Midgut—duodenum to proximal 2/3 of transverse colon.
Hindgut—distal 1/3 of transverse colon to anal canal above pectinate line.
Midgut development:
- 6th week—physiologic midgut herniates through umbilical ring
- 10th week—returns to abdominal cavity + rotates around superior mesenteric artery (SMA), total 270° counterclockwise

---

Ventral wall defects

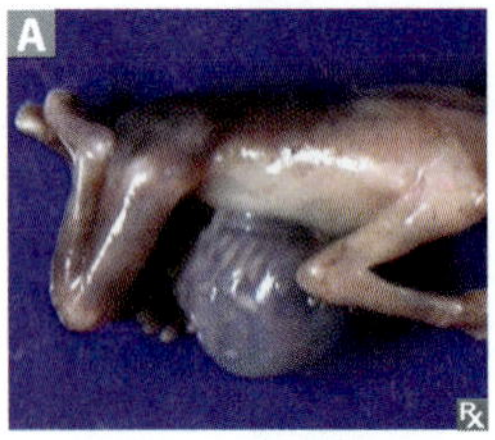

Developmental defects due to failure of:
- Rostral fold closure—sternal defects
- Lateral fold closure—omphalocele, gastroschisis
- Caudal fold closure—bladder exstrophy

Gastroschisis—extrusion of abdominal contents through abdominal folds (typically right of umbilicus); not covered by peritoneum.

Omphalocele—persistence of herniation of abdominal contents into umbilical cord, **sealed** by peritoneum A.

Tracheoesophageal anomalies

Esophageal atresia (EA) with distal tracheoesophageal fistula (TEF) is the most common (85%). Polyhydramnios in utero. Neonates drool, choke, and vomit with first feeding. TEF allows air to enter stomach (visible on CXR). Cyanosis is 2° to laryngospasm (to avoid reflux-related aspiration). Clinical test: failure to pass nasogastric tube into stomach.
In **H**-type, the fistula resembles the letter **H**. In pure EA the CXR shows gasless abdomen.

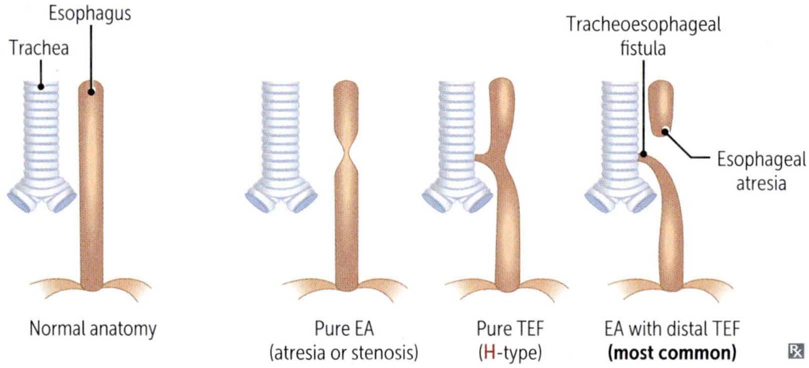

Intestinal atresia

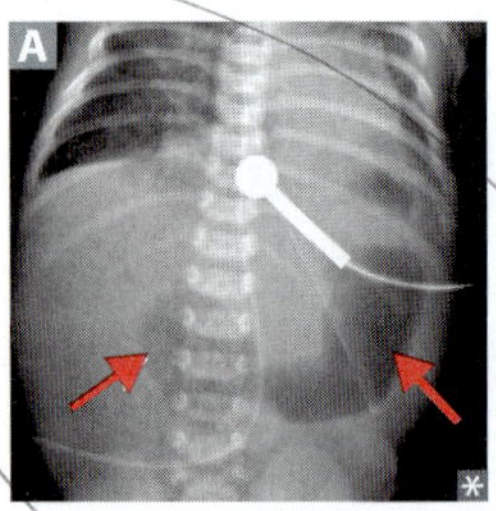

Presents with bilious vomiting and abdominal distension within first 1–2 days of life.
Duodenal atresia—failure to recanalize → dilation of stomach and proximal duodenum ("double bubble" on x-ray A). Associated with Down syndrome.
Jejunal and ileal atresia—disruption of mesenteric vessels → ischemic necrosis → segmental resorption (bowel discontinuity or "apple peel").

Hypertrophic pyloric stenosis

Most common cause of gastric outlet obstruction in infants (1:600). Palpable "olive" mass in epigastric region and nonbilious projectile vomiting at ~ 2–6 weeks old. More common in firstborn males; associated with exposure to macrolides. Results in hypokalemic hypochloremic metabolic alkalosis (2° to vomiting of gastric acid and subsequent volume contraction). Treatment is surgical incision (pyloromyotomy).

Pancreas and spleen embryology

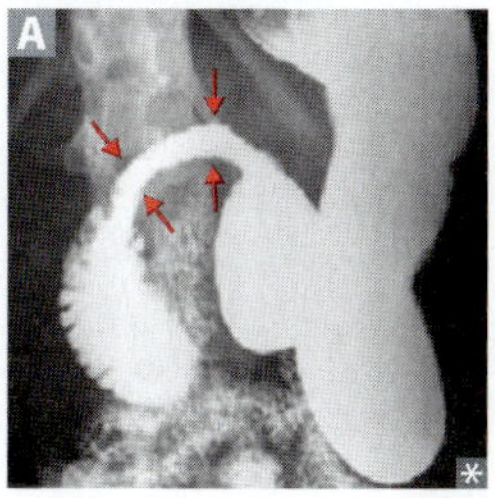

Pancreas—derived from foregut. Ventral pancreatic buds contribute to uncinate process and main pancreatic duct. The dorsal pancreatic bud alone becomes the body, tail, isthmus, and accessory pancreatic duct. Both the ventral and dorsal buds contribute to pancreatic head.

Annular pancreas—ventral pancreatic bud abnormally encircles 2nd part of duodenum; forms a ring of pancreatic tissue that may cause duodenal narrowing **A** and nonbilious vomiting.

Pancreas divisum—ventral and dorsal parts fail to fuse at 8 weeks. Common anomaly; mostly asymptomatic, but may cause chronic abdominal pain and/or pancreatitis.

Spleen—arises in mesentery of stomach (hence is mesodermal) but has foregut supply (celiac trunk → splenic artery).

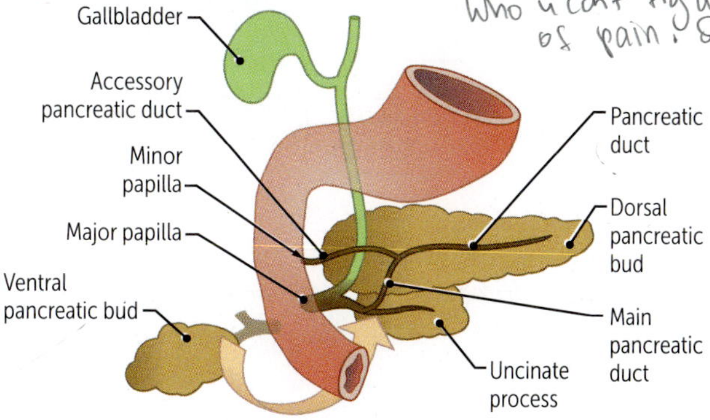

▸ GASTROINTESTINAL—ANATOMY

Retroperitoneal structures

Retroperitoneal structures include GI structures that lack a mesentery and non-GI structures. Injuries to retroperitoneal structures can cause blood or gas accumulation in retroperitoneal space.

SAD PUCKER:
- **S**uprarenal (adrenal) glands [not shown]
- **A**orta and IVC
- **D**uodenum (2nd through 4th parts)
- **P**ancreas (except tail)
- **U**reters [not shown]
- **C**olon (descending and ascending)
- **K**idneys
- **E**sophagus (thoracic portion) [not shown]
- **R**ectum (partially) [not shown]

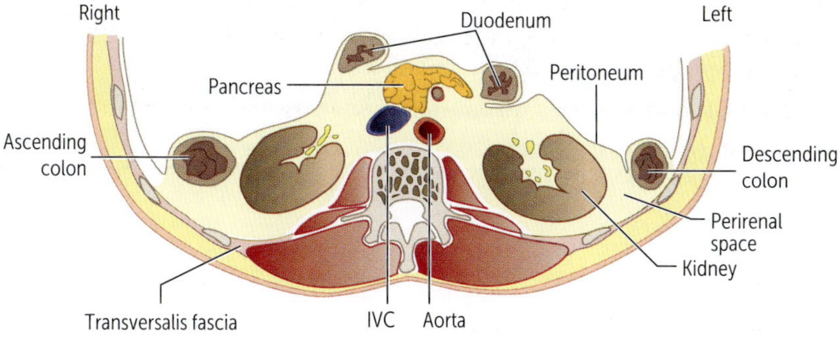

Important gastrointestinal ligaments

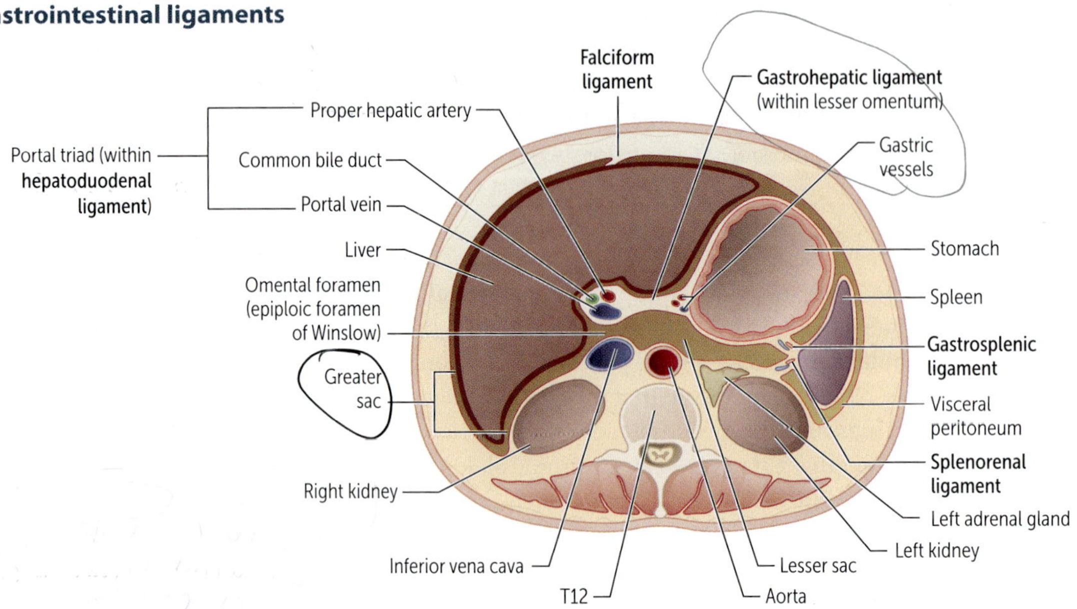

LIGAMENT	CONNECTS	STRUCTURES CONTAINED	NOTES
Falciform	Liver to anterior abdominal wall	Ligamentum teres hepatis (derivative of fetal umbilical vein)	Derivative of ventral mesentery
Hepatoduodenal	Liver to duodenum	Portal triad: proper hepatic artery, portal vein, common bile duct	Pringle maneuver—ligament may be compressed between thumb and index finger placed in omental foramen to control bleeding Borders the omental foramen, which connects the greater and lesser sacs
Gastrohepatic	Liver to lesser curvature of stomach	Gastric arteries	Separates greater and lesser sacs on the right May be cut during surgery to access lesser sac
Gastrocolic (not shown)	Greater curvature and transverse colon	Gastroepiploic arteries	Part of greater omentum
Gastrosplenic	Greater curvature and spleen	Short gastrics, left gastroepiploic vessels	Separates greater and lesser sacs on the left Part of greater omentum
Splenorenal	Spleen to posterior abdominal wall	Splenic artery and vein, tail of pancreas	

Digestive tract anatomy

Layers of gut wall (inside to outside—MSMS):
- Mucosa—epithelium, lamina propria, muscularis mucosa
- Submucosa—includes Submucosal nerve plexus (Meissner), Secretes fluid
- Muscularis externa—includes Myenteric nerve plexus (Auerbach), Motility
- Serosa (when intraperitoneal), adventitia (when retroperitoneal)

Ulcers can extend into submucosa, inner or outer muscular layer. Erosions are in the mucosa only.

Frequencies of basal electric rhythm (slow waves):
- Stomach—3 waves/min
- Duodenum—12 waves/min
- Ileum—8–9 waves/min

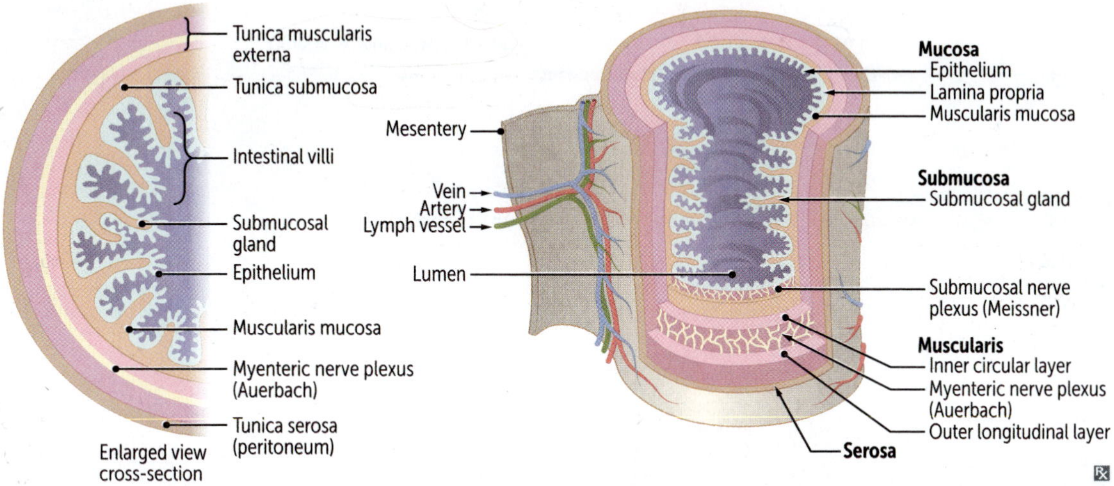

Digestive tract histology

Esophagus	Nonkeratinized stratified squamous epithelium.
Stomach	Gastric glands.
Duodenum	Villi and microvilli ↑ absorptive surface. Brunner glands (HCO_3^--secreting cells of submucosa) and crypts of Lieberkühn.
Jejunum	Plicae circulares and crypts of Lieberkühn.
Ileum	Peyer patches (lymphoid aggregates in lamina propria, submucosa), plicae circulares (proximal ileum), and crypts of Lieberkühn. Largest number of goblet cells in the small intestine.
Colon	Crypts of Lieberkühn but no villi; abundant goblet cells.

Abdominal aorta and branches

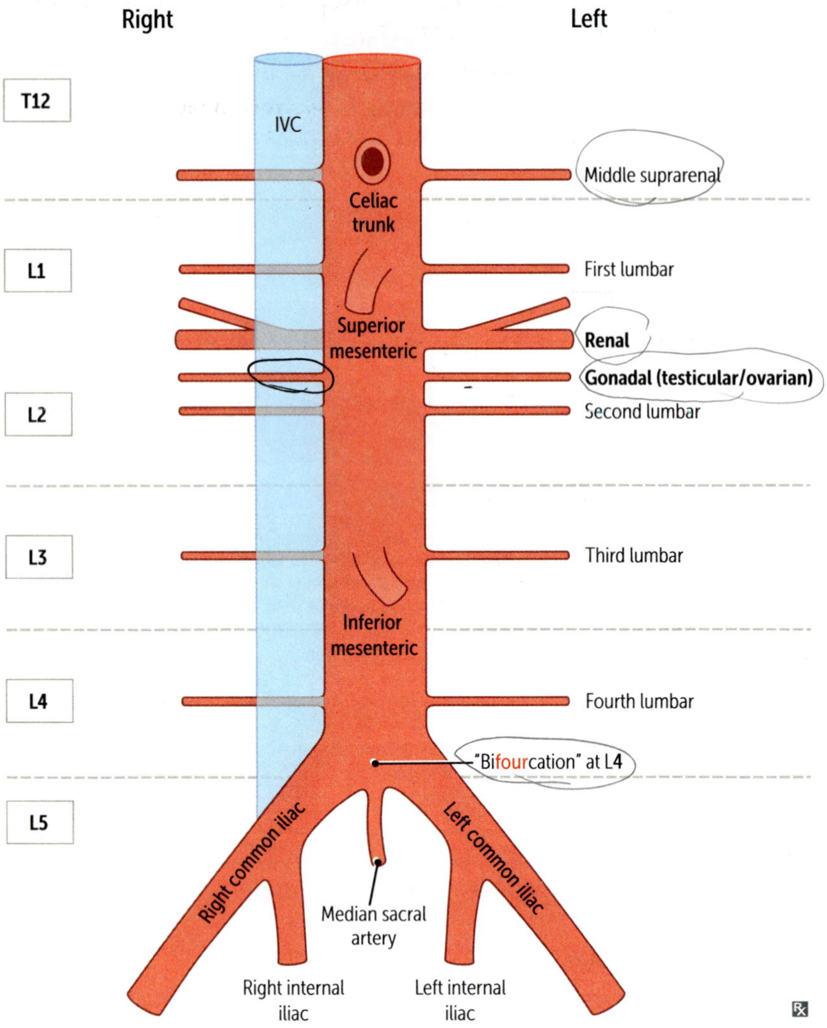

Arteries supplying GI structures branch **anteriorly**. Arteries supplying non-GI structures branch **laterally** and **posteriorly**.

Superior mesenteric artery syndrome

Characterized by intermittent intestinal obstruction symptoms (primarily postprandial pain) when transverse (third) portion of duodenum is compressed between SMA and aorta. Typically occurs in conditions associated with diminished mesenteric fat (eg, low body weight/malnutrition).

Gastrointestinal blood supply and innervation

EMBRYONIC GUT REGION	ARTERY	PARASYMPATHETIC INNERVATION	VERTEBRAL LEVEL	STRUCTURES SUPPLIED
Foregut	Celiac	Vagus	T12/L1	Pharynx (vagus nerve only) and lower esophagus (celiac artery only) to proximal duodenum; liver, gallbladder, pancreas, spleen (mesoderm)
Midgut	SMA	Vagus	L1	Distal duodenum to proximal $^2/_3$ of transverse colon
Hindgut	IMA	Pelvic	L3	Distal $^1/_3$ of transverse colon to upper portion of rectum

Celiac trunk

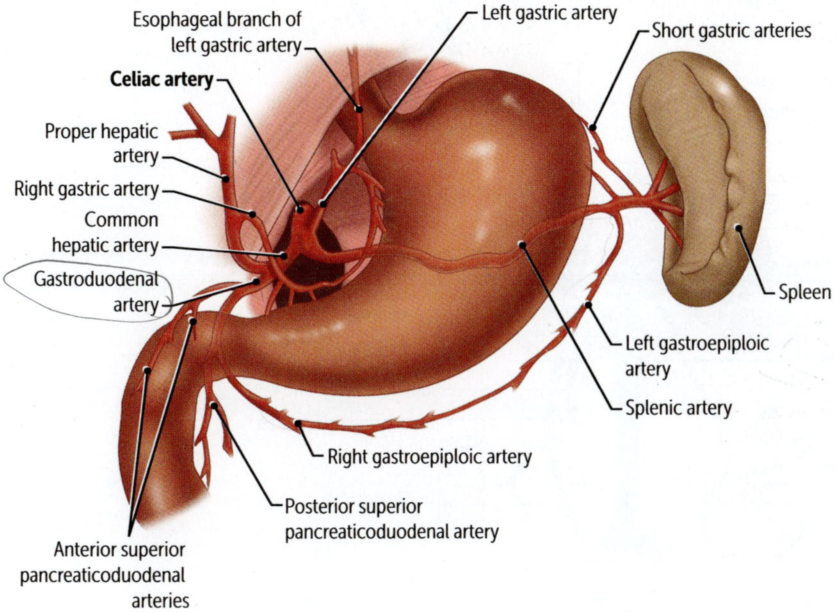

Branches of celiac trunk: common hepatic, splenic, and left gastric. These constitute the main blood supply of the stomach.

Strong anastomoses exist between:

- Left and right gastroepiploics
- Left and right gastrics

Portosystemic anastomoses

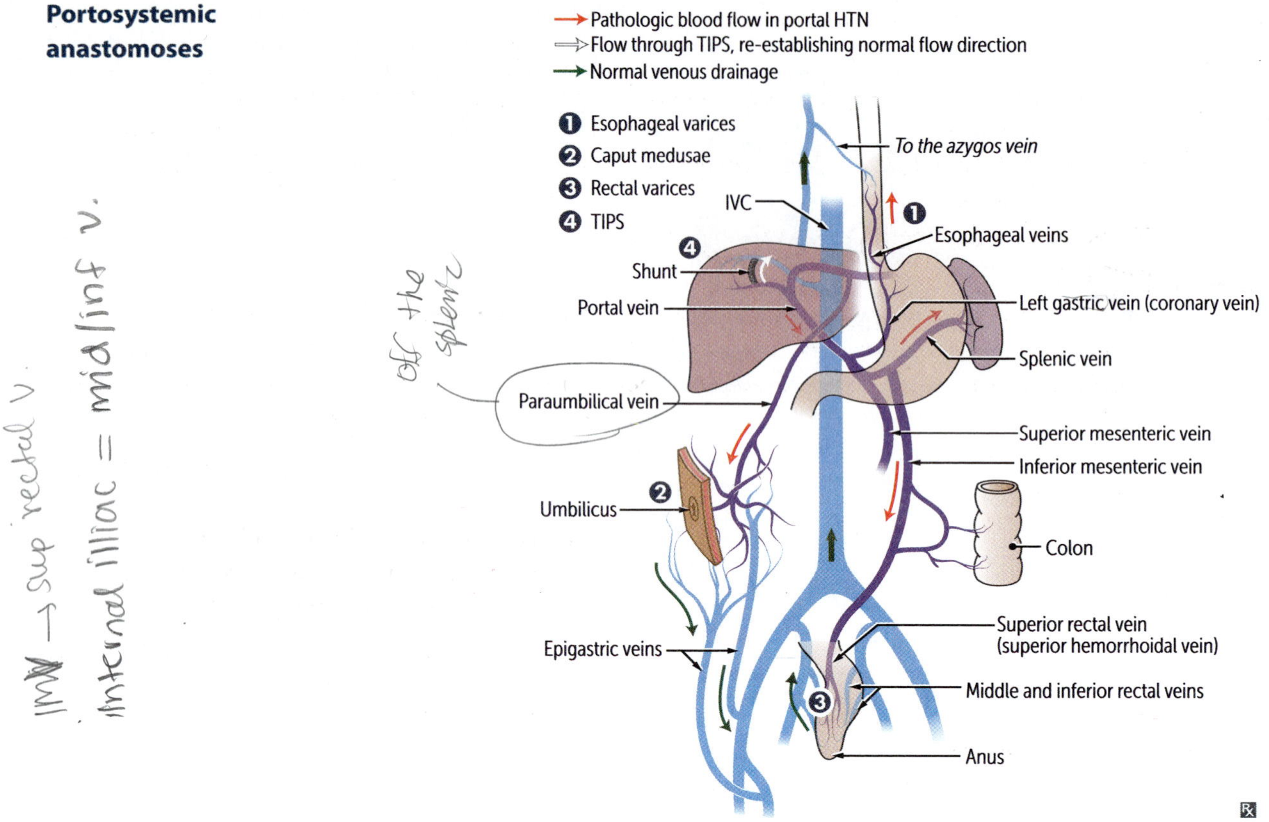

SITE OF ANASTOMOSIS	CLINICAL SIGN	PORTAL ↔ SYSTEMIC
❶ Esophagus	Esophageal varices	Left gastric ↔ azygos
❷ Umbilicus	Caput medusae	Paraumbilical ↔ small epigastric veins of the anterior abdominal wall.
❸ Rectum	Anorectal varices	Superior rectal ↔ middle and inferior rectal

Varices of gut, butt, and caput (medusae) are commonly seen with portal hypertension.

Treatment with a transjugular intrahepatic portosystemic shunt (TIPS) ❹ between the portal vein and hepatic vein relieves portal hypertension by shunting blood to the systemic circulation, bypassing the liver.

Pectinate (dentate) line

Formed where endoderm (hindgut) meets ectoderm.

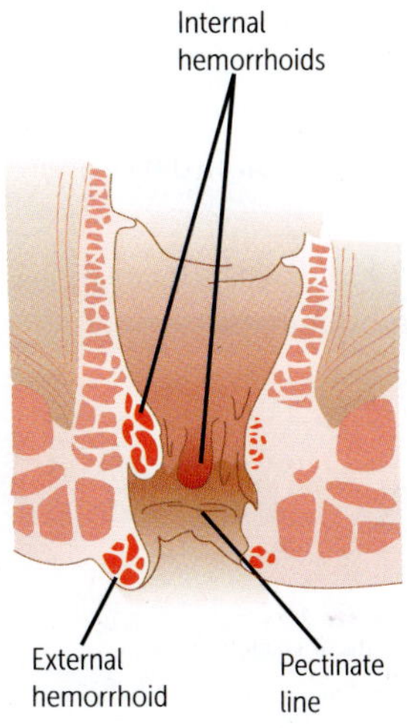

Above pectinate line—internal hemorrhoids, adenocarcinoma.

Arterial supply from superior rectal artery (branch of IMA).

Venous drainage: superior rectal vein → inferior mesenteric vein → portal system.

Internal hemorrhoids receive visceral innervation and are therefore **not painful**.

Lymphatic drainage to internal iliac lymph nodes.

Below pectinate line—external hemorrhoids, anal fissures, squamous cell carcinoma.

Arterial supply from inferior rectal artery (branch of internal pudendal artery).

Venous drainage: inferior rectal vein → internal pudendal vein → internal iliac vein → common iliac vein → IVC.

External hemorrhoids receive somatic innervation (inferior rectal branch of pudendal nerve) and are therefore **painful** if thrombosed.

Lymphatic drainage to superficial inguinal nodes.

Anal fissure—tear in the anal mucosa below the Pectinate line. Pain while Pooping; blood on toilet Paper. Located Posteriorly because this area is Poorly Perfused. Associated with low-fiber diets and constipation.

A: IMA → sup rectal
V: IMV → sup rectal
portal

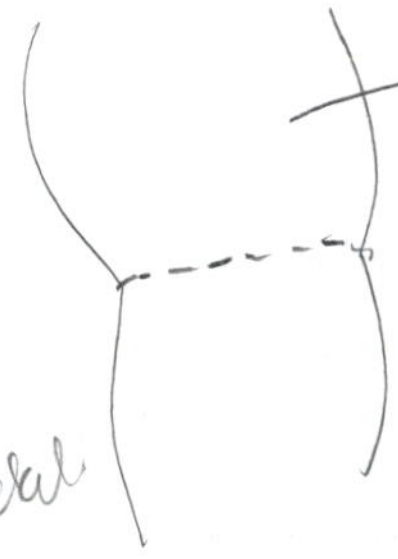

Int illiac
A: Int. pudend → Inf rectal
V: Int illiac → intern pudend → inf rectal

Liver tissue architecture

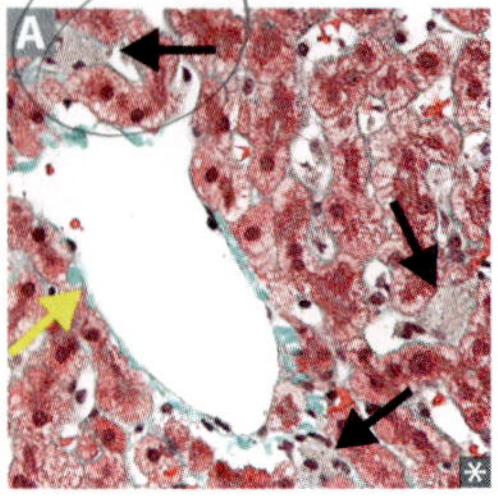

Apical surface of hepatocytes faces bile canaliculi. Basolateral surface faces sinusoids.

Kupffer cells, which are specialized macrophages, form the lining of these sinusoids (black arrows in A; yellow arrow shows hepatic venule).

Hepatic stellate (Ito) cells in space of Disse store vitamin A (when quiescent) and produce extracellular matrix (when activated).

Zone I—periportal zone:
- Affected 1st by viral hepatitis
- Ingested toxins (eg, cocaine)

Zone II—intermediate zone:
- Yellow fever

Zone III—pericentral vein (centrilobular) zone:
- Affected 1st by ischemia
- Contains cytochrome P-450 system
- Most sensitive to metabolic toxins
- Site of alcoholic hepatitis

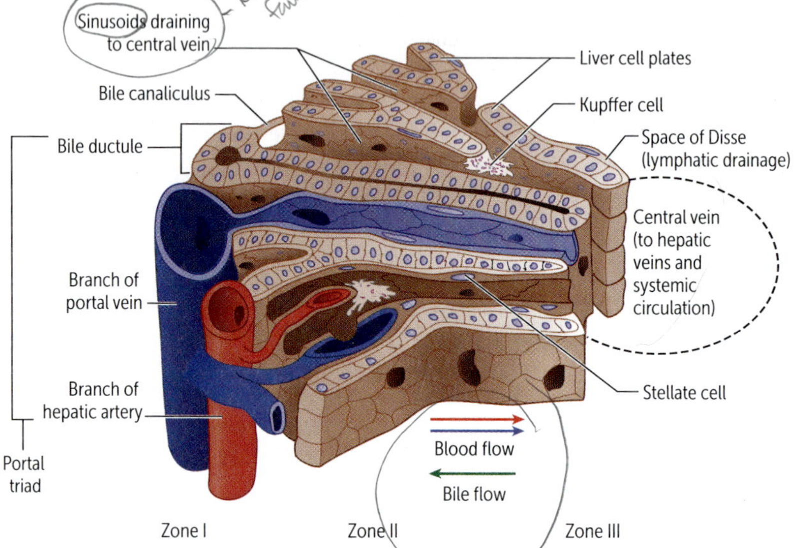

Biliary structures

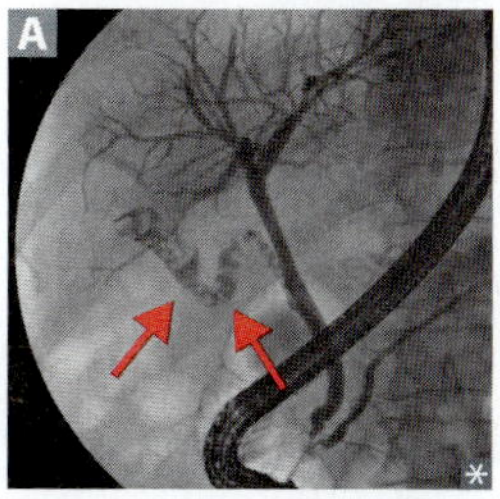

Gallstones (filling defects, red arrows in A) that reach the confluence of the common bile and pancreatic ducts at the ampulla of Vater can block both the common bile and pancreatic ducts (double duct sign), causing both cholangitis and pancreatitis, respectively.

Tumors that arise in head of pancreas (usually ductal adenocarcinoma) can cause obstruction of common bile duct → painless jaundice.

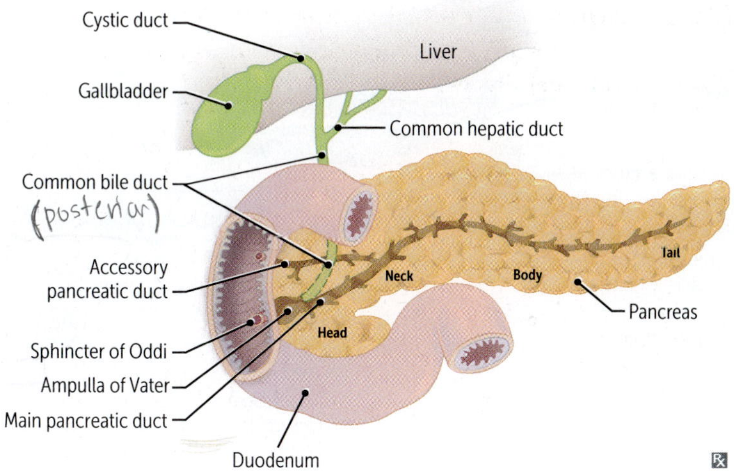

Femoral region

ORGANIZATION	**Lateral to medial**: **N**erve-**A**rtery-**V**ein-**L**ymphatics.	You go from **lateral to medial** to find your **NAVeL**.
Femoral triangle	Contains femoral nerve, artery, vein.	**Venous** near the **penis**.
Femoral sheath	Fascial tube 3–4 cm below inguinal ligament. Contains femoral vein, artery, and canal (deep inguinal lymph nodes) but not femoral nerve.	

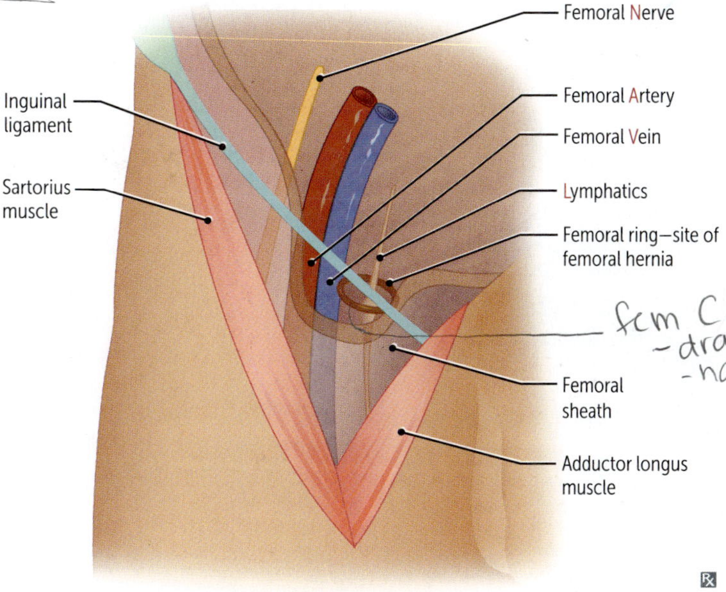

Inguinal canal

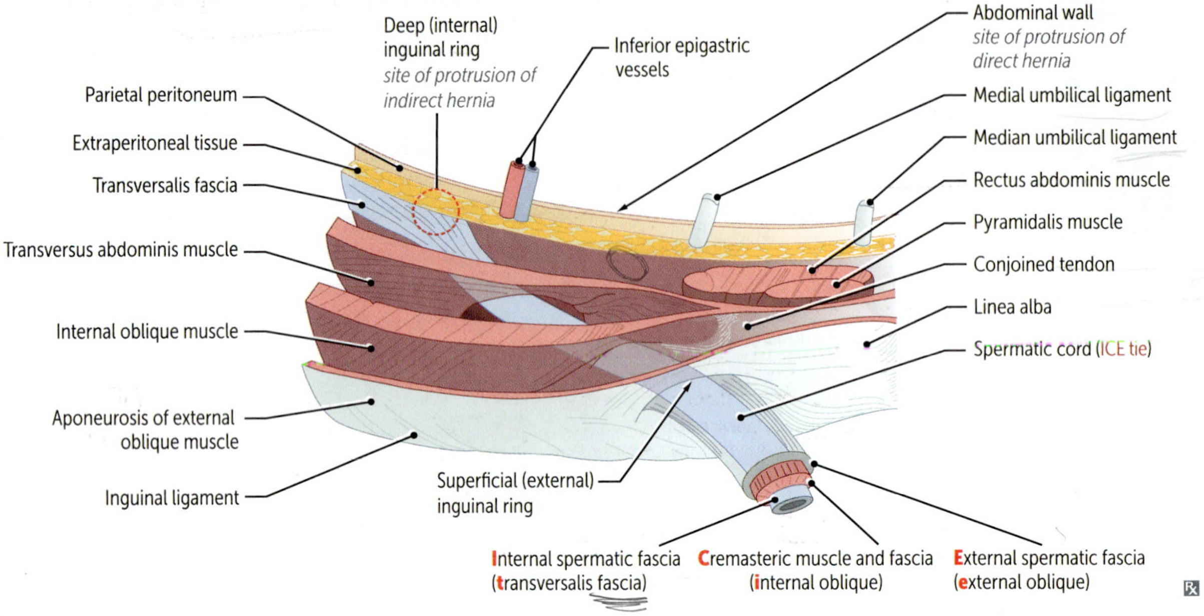

Hernias	A protrusion of peritoneum through an opening, usually at a site of weakness. Contents may be at risk for incarceration (not reducible back into abdomen/pelvis) and strangulation (ischemia and necrosis). Complicated hernias can present with tenderness, erythema, fever.	
Diaphragmatic hernia 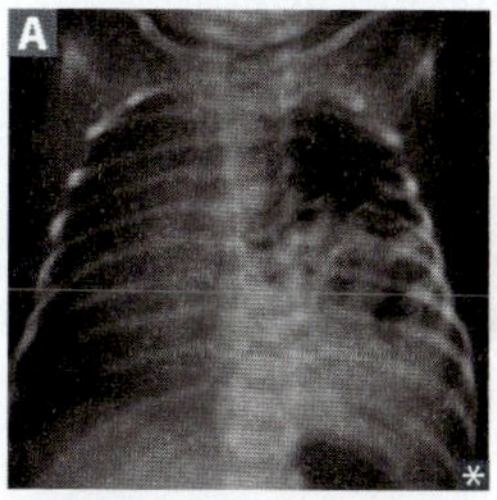	Abdominal structures enter the thorax; may occur due to congenital defect of pleuroperitoneal membrane **A**, or as a result of trauma. Commonly occurs on left side due to relative protection of right hemidiaphragm by liver. Most commonly a **hiatal hernia**, in which stomach herniates upward through the esophageal hiatus of the diaphragm.	**Sliding hiatal hernia** is most common. Gastroesophageal junction is displaced upward; "hourglass stomach." **Paraesophageal hernia**—gastroesophageal junction is usually normal. Fundus protrudes into the thorax.
Indirect inguinal hernia 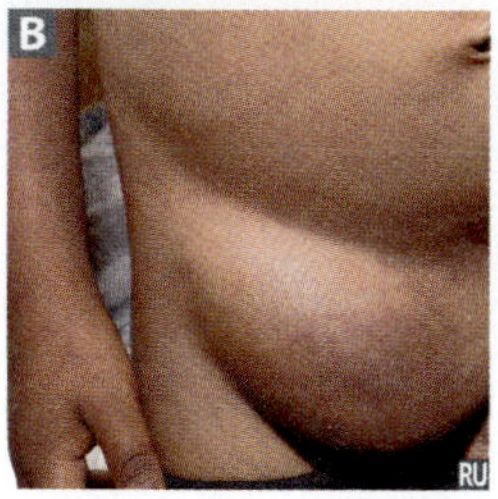	Goes through the **in**ternal (deep) inguinal ring, external (superficial) inguinal ring, and **in**to the scrotum. Enters internal inguinal ring lateral to inferior epigastric vessels. Occurs in **in**fants owing to failure of processus vaginalis to close (can form hydrocele). Much more common in males **B**.	An indirect inguinal hernia follows the path of descent of the testes. Covered by all 3 layers of spermatic fascia.
Direct inguinal hernia	Protrudes through the inguinal (Hesselbach) triangle. Bulges directly through abdominal wall medial to inferior epigastric vessels. Goes through the external (superficial) inguinal ring only. Covered by external spermatic fascia. Usually in older men.	**MD**s don't **LI**e: **M**edial to inferior epigastric vessels = **D**irect hernia. **L**ateral to inferior epigastric vessels = **I**ndirect hernia.
Femoral hernia	Protrudes below inguinal ligament through femoral canal below and lateral to pubic tubercle. More common in **fem**ales.	More likely to present with incarceration or strangulation than inguinal hernias.

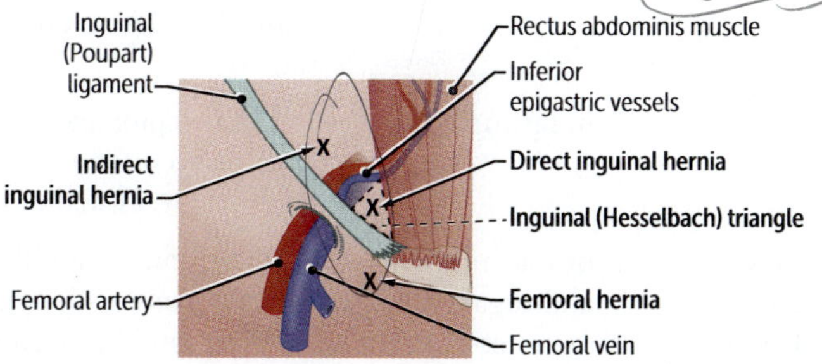

Inguinal (Hesselbach) triangle:
- Inferior epigastric vessels
- Lateral border of rectus abdominis
- Inguinal ligament

▶ GASTROINTESTINAL—PHYSIOLOGY

Gastrointestinal regulatory substances

REGULATORY SUBSTANCE	SOURCE	ACTION	REGULATION	NOTES
Gastrin	G cells (antrum of stomach, duodenum)	↑ gastric H^+ secretion ↑ growth of gastric mucosa ↑ gastric motility	↑ by stomach distention/alkalinization, amino acids, peptides, vagal stimulation via gastrin-releasing peptide (GRP) ↓ by pH < 1.5	↑ by chronic PPI use. ↑ in chronic atrophic gastritis (eg, *H pylori*). ↑↑ in Zollinger-Ellison syndrome (gastrinoma).
Somatostatin	D cells (pancreatic islets, GI mucosa)	↓ gastric acid and pepsinogen secretion ↓ pancreatic and small intestine fluid secretion ↓ gallbladder contraction ↓ insulin and glucagon release	↑ by acid ↓ by vagal stimulation	Inhibits secretion of various hormones (encourages somato-stasis). Octreotide is an analog used to treat acromegaly, carcinoid syndrome, and variceal bleeding.
Cholecystokinin	I cells (duodenum, jejunum)	↑ pancreatic secretion ↑ gallbladder contraction ↓ gastric emptying ↑ sphincter of Oddi relaxation	↑ by fatty acids, amino acids	Acts on neural muscarinic pathways to cause pancreatic secretion.
Secretin	S cells (duodenum)	↑ pancreatic HCO_3^- secretion ↓ gastric acid secretion ↑ bile secretion	↑ by acid, fatty acids in lumen of duodenum	↑ HCO_3^- neutralizes gastric acid in duodenum, allowing pancreatic enzymes to function.
Glucose-dependent insulinotropic peptide	K cells (duodenum, jejunum)	Exocrine: ↓ gastric H^+ secretion Endocrine: ↑ insulin release	↑ by fatty acids, amino acids, oral glucose	Also known as gastric inhibitory peptide (GIP). Oral glucose load leads to ↑ insulin compared to IV equivalent due to GIP secretion.
Motilin	Small intestine	Produces migrating motor complexes (MMCs)	↑ in fasting state	Motilin receptor agonists (eg, erythromycin) are used to stimulate intestinal peristalsis.
Vasoactive intestinal polypeptide	Parasympathetic ganglia in sphincters, gallbladder, small intestine	↑ intestinal water and electrolyte secretion ↑ relaxation of intestinal smooth muscle and sphincters	↑ by distention and vagal stimulation ↓ by adrenergic input	VIPoma—non-α, non-β islet cell pancreatic tumor that secretes VIP. Watery Diarrhea, Hypokalemia, and Achlorhydria (WDHA syndrome).
Nitric oxide		↑ smooth muscle relaxation, including lower esophageal sphincter (LES)		Loss of NO secretion is implicated in ↑ LES tone of achalasia.
Ghrelin	Stomach	↑ appetite	↑ in fasting state ↓ by food	↑ in Prader-Willi syndrome. ↓ after gastric bypass surgery.

Gastrointestinal secretory products

PRODUCT	SOURCE	ACTION	REGULATION	NOTES
Intrinsic factor	Parietal cells (stomach)	Vitamin B_{12}–binding protein (required for B_{12} uptake in terminal ileum)		Autoimmune destruction of parietal cells → chronic gastritis and pernicious anemia.
Gastric acid	Parietal cells (stomach)	↓ stomach pH	↑ by histamine, ACh, gastrin ↓ by somatostatin, GIP, prostaglandin, secretin	
Pepsin	Chief cells (stomach)	Protein digestion	↑ by vagal stimulation, local acid	Pepsinogen (inactive) is converted to pepsin (active) in the presence of H^+.
Bicarbonate	Mucosal cells (stomach, duodenum, salivary glands, pancreas) and Brunner glands (duodenum)	Neutralizes acid	↑ by pancreatic and biliary secretion with secretin	Trapped in mucus that covers the gastric epithelium.

Locations of gastrointestinal secretory cells

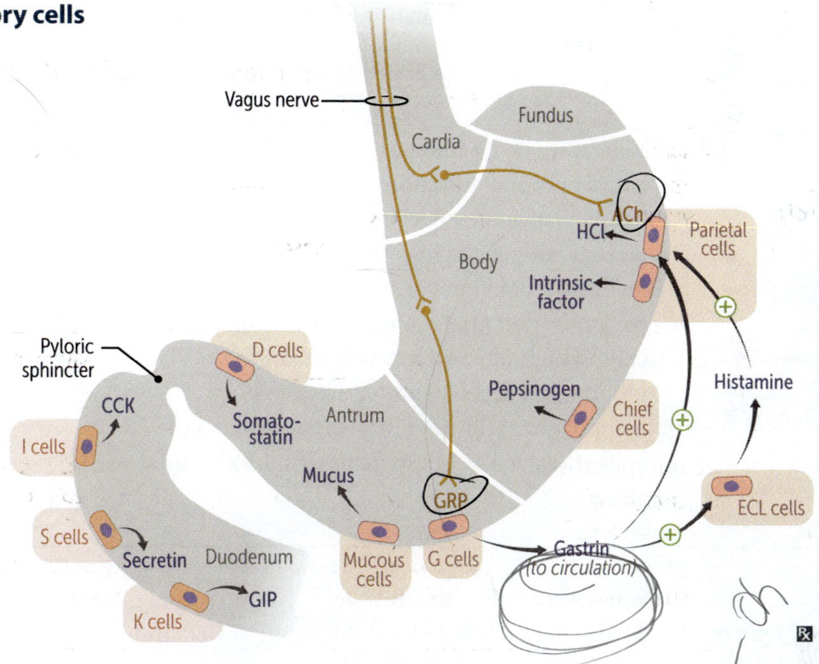

Gastrin ↑ acid secretion primarily through its effects on enterochromaffin-like (ECL) cells (leading to histamine release) rather than through its direct effect on parietal cells.

Pancreatic secretions

Isotonic fluid; low flow → high Cl^-, high flow → high HCO_3^-.

ENZYME	ROLE	NOTES
α-amylase	Starch digestion	Secreted in active form
Lipases	Fat digestion	
Proteases	Protein digestion	Includes trypsin, chymotrypsin, elastase, carboxypeptidases Secreted as proenzymes also known as zymogens
Trypsinogen	Converted to active enzyme trypsin → activation of other proenzymes and cleaving of additional trypsinogen molecules into active trypsin (positive feedback loop)	Converted to trypsin by enterokinase/enteropeptidase, a brush-border enzyme on duodenal and jejunal mucosa

Carbohydrate absorption

Only monosaccharides (glucose, galactose, fructose) are absorbed by enterocytes. Glucose and galactose are taken up by SGLT1 (Na^+ dependent). Fructose is taken up by facilitated diffusion by GLUT-5. All are transported to blood by GLUT-2.

D-xylose absorption test: distinguishes GI mucosal damage from other causes of malabsorption.

Vitamin/mineral absorption

Iron	Absorbed as Fe^{2+} in duodenum.	Iron Fist, Bro
Folate	Absorbed in small bowel.	Clinically relevant in patients with small bowel disease or after resection.
B_{12}	Absorbed in terminal ileum along with bile salts, requires intrinsic factor.	

Peyer patches

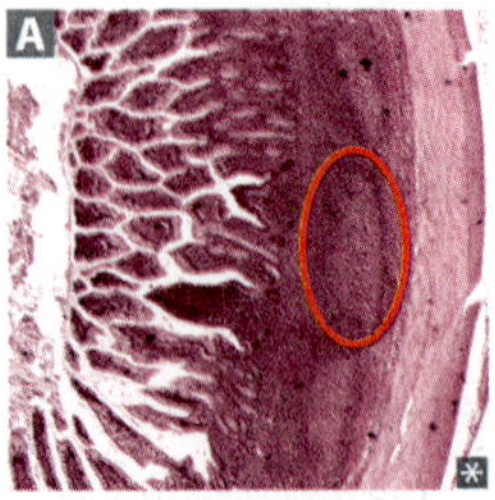

Unencapsulated lymphoid tissue **A** found in lamina propria and submucosa of ileum.

Contain specialized M cells that sample and present antigens to immune cells.

B cells stimulated in germinal centers of Peyer patches differentiate into IgA-secreting plasma cells, which ultimately reside in lamina propria. IgA receives protective secretory component and is then transported across the epithelium to the gut to deal with intraluminal antigen.

Think of IgA, the Intra-gut Antibody. And always say "secretory IgA."

Bile

Composed of bile salts (bile acids conjugated to glycine or taurine, making them water soluble), phospholipids, cholesterol, bilirubin, water, and ions. Cholesterol 7α-hydroxylase catalyzes rate-limiting step of bile acid synthesis.

Functions:

- Digestion and absorption of lipids and fat-soluble vitamins
- Cholesterol excretion (body's only means of eliminating cholesterol)
- Antimicrobial activity (via membrane disruption)

Bilirubin

Heme is metabolized by heme oxygenase to biliverdin, which is subsequently reduced to bilirubin. Unconjugated bilirubin is removed from blood by liver, conjugated with glucuronate, and excreted in bile.

Direct bilirubin—conjugated with glucuronic acid; water soluble.

Indirect bilirubin—unconjugated; water **in**soluble.

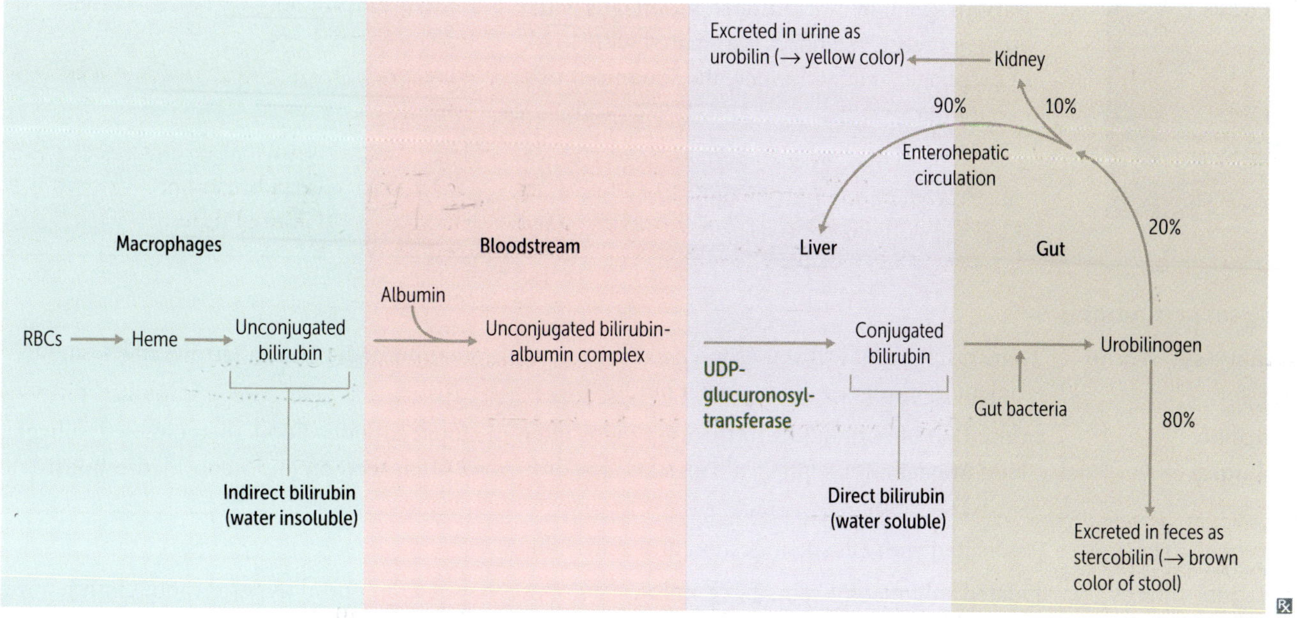

▶ GASTROINTESTINAL—PATHOLOGY

Salivary gland tumors

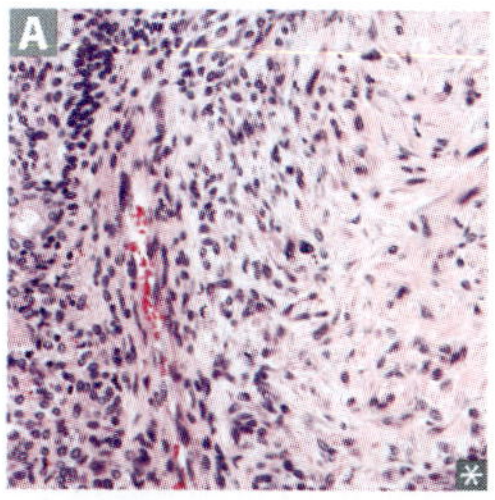

Most commonly benign and in parotid gland. Tumors in smaller glands more likely malignant. Typically present as painless mass/swelling. Facial pain or paralysis suggests malignant involvement of CN VII.

- Pleomorphic adenoma (benign mixed tumor)—most common salivary gland tumor A. Composed of chondromyxoid stroma and epithelium and recurs if incompletely excised or ruptured intraoperatively. "10yr mass now w/ facial n prob." otherwise painless
- Mucoepidermoid carcinoma—most common malignant tumor, has mucinous and squamous components. involves CN 7
- Warthin tumor (papillary cystadenoma lymphomatosum)—benign cystic tumor with germinal centers. & abund lymphoc

Achalasia

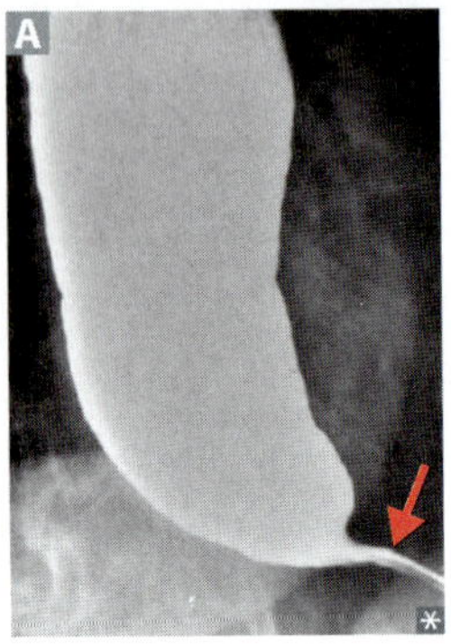

Failure of relaxation of LES due to loss of myenteric (Auerbach) plexus. High LES resting pressure and uncoordinated or absent peristalsis → progressive dysphagia to solids and liquids (vs obstruction—solids only). Barium swallow shows dilated esophagus with an area of distal stenosis. Associated with ↑ risk of esophageal cancer, especially squamous cell carcinoma.

A-*chalasia* = absence of relaxation.
"Bird's beak" on barium swallow A.
2° achalasia may arise from Chagas disease (*T cruzi* infection) or extraesophageal malignancies (mass effect or paraneoplastic).

Esophageal pathologies

Boerhaave syndrome	Transmural, usually distal esophageal rupture with pneumomediastinum (arrows in A) due to violent retching; surgical emergency.
Eosinophilic esophagitis	Infiltration of eosinophils in the esophagus often in atopic patients. Food allergens → dysphagia, food impaction. Esophageal rings and linear furrows often seen on endoscopy. Unresponsive to GERD therapy.
Esophageal strictures	Associated with caustic ingestion and acid reflux.
Esophageal varices	Dilated submucosal veins B C in lower ⅓ of esophagus 2° to portal hypertension. Common in cirrhotics, may be source of life-threatening hematemesis.
Esophagitis	Associated with reflux, infection in immunocompromised (*Candida*: white pseudomembrane; HSV-1: punched-out ulcers; CMV: linear ulcers), caustic ingestion, or medications.
Gastroesophageal reflux disease	Commonly presents as heartburn, regurgitation, dysphagia. May also present as chronic cough, hoarseness (laryngopharyngeal reflux). Associated with asthma. Transient decreases in LES tone.
Mallory-Weiss syndrome	Mucosal lacerations at the gastroesophageal junction due to severe vomiting. Leads to hematemesis that can be painful. Usually found in alcoholics and bulimics.
Plummer-Vinson syndrome	Triad of Dysphagia, Iron deficiency anemia, and Esophageal webs. May be associated with glossitis. Increased risk of esophageal squamous cell carcinoma ("Plumbers" DIE).
Sclerodermal esophageal dysmotility	Esophageal smooth muscle atrophy → ↓ LES pressure and dysmotility → acid reflux and dysphagia → stricture, Barrett esophagus, and aspiration. Part of CREST syndrome.

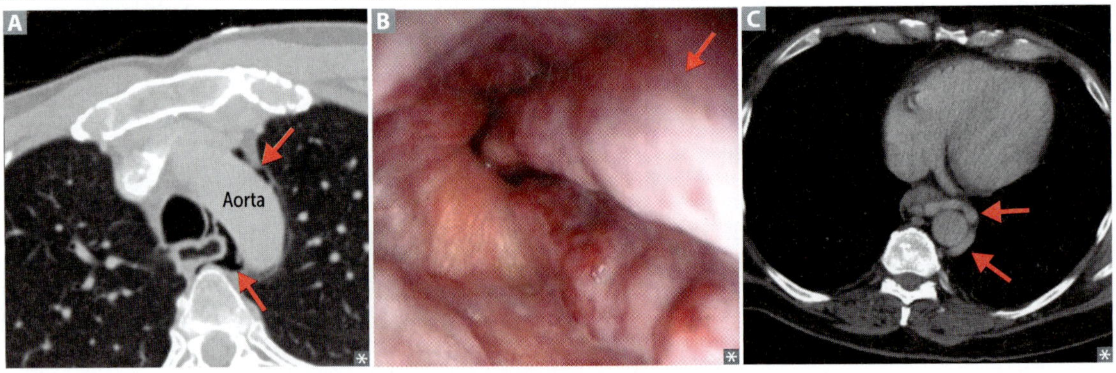

Barrett esophagus

Specialized intestinal metaplasia A —replacement of nonkeratinized stratified squamous epithelium with intestinal epithelium (nonciliated columnar with goblet cells [stained blue in B]) in distal esophagus. Due to chronic reflux esophagitis (GERD). Associated with ↑ risk of esophageal adenocarcinoma.

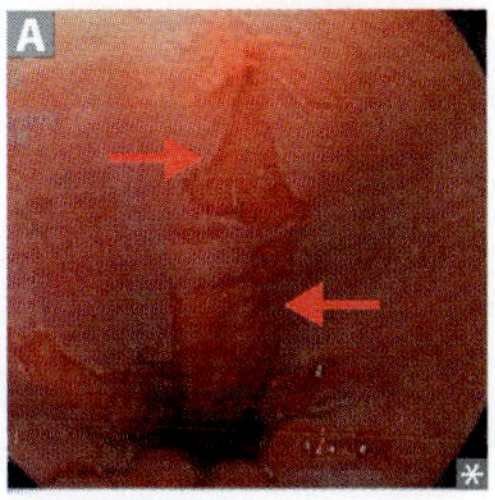

B

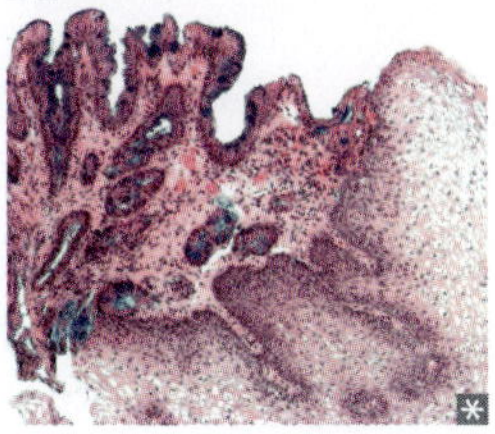

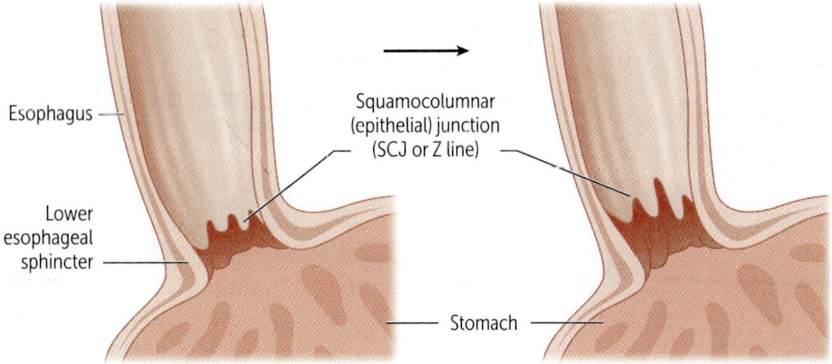

Esophageal cancer

Typically presents with progressive dysphagia (first solids, then liquids) and weight loss; poor prognosis.

CANCER	PART OF ESOPHAGUS AFFECTED	RISK FACTORS	PREVALENCE
Squamous cell carcinoma	Upper 2/3	Alcohol, hot liquids, caustic strictures, smoking, achalasia	More common worldwide
Adenocarcinoma	Lower 1/3	Chronic GERD, Barrett esophagus, obesity, smoking, achalasia	More common in America

Gastritis

Acute gastritis	Erosions can be caused by: ▪ NSAIDs—↓ PGE_2 → ↓ gastric mucosa protection ▪ Burns (Curling ulcer)—hypovolemia → mucosal ischemia ▪ Brain injury (Cushing ulcer)—↑ vagal stimulation → ↑ ACh → ↑ H^+ production	Especially common among alcoholics and patients taking daily NSAIDs (eg, patients with rheumatoid arthritis). **Burn**ed by the **Curling** iron. Always **Cush**ion the **brain**.
Chronic gastritis	Mucosal inflammation, often leading to atrophy (hypochlorhydria → hypergastrinemia) and intestinal metaplasia (↑ risk of gastric cancers).	
H pylori	Most common. ↑ risk of peptic ulcer disease, MALT lymphoma.	Affects antrum first and spreads to body of stomach.
Autoimmune	Autoantibodies to parietal cells and intrinsic factor. ↑ risk of pernicious anemia.	Affects body/fundus of stomach.

Ménétrier disease

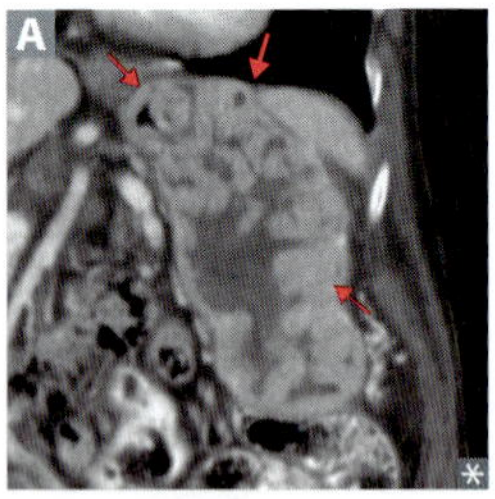

Gastric hyperplasia of mucosa → hypertrophied rugae (looking like brain gyri A), excess mucus production with resultant protein loss and parietal cell atrophy with ↓ acid production. Precancerous.

Gastric cancer

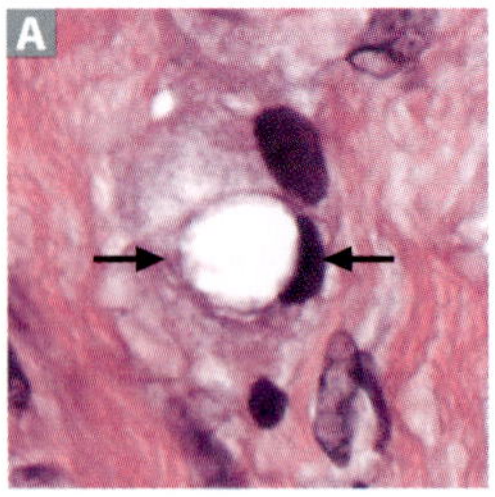

Most commonly gastric adenocarcinoma; lymphoma, GI stromal tumor, carcinoid (rare). Early aggressive local spread with node/liver metastases. Often presents late, with weight loss, early satiety, and in some cases acanthosis nigricans or Leser-Trélat sign.

- **Intestinal**—associated with *H pylori*, dietary nitrosamines (smoked foods), tobacco smoking, achlorhydria, chronic gastritis. Commonly on lesser curvature; looks like ulcer with raised margins.
- **Diffuse**—not associated with *H pylori*; signet ring cells (mucin-filled cells with peripheral nuclei) A; stomach wall grossly thickened and leathery (linitis plastica).

Virchow node—involvement of left supraclavicular node by metastasis from stomach.

Krukenberg tumor—bilateral metastases to ovaries. Abundant mucin-secreting, signet ring cells.

Sister Mary Joseph nodule—subcutaneous periumbilical metastasis.

Peptic ulcer disease

	Gastric ulcer	Duodenal ulcer
PAIN	Can be **G**reater with meals—weight loss	**D**ecreases with meals—weight gain
H PYLORI INFECTION	~ 70%	~ 90%
MECHANISM	↓ mucosal protection against gastric acid	↓ mucosal protection or ↑ gastric acid secretion
OTHER CAUSES	NSAIDs	Zollinger-Ellison syndrome
RISK OF CARCINOMA	↑ any time u see stom ulcer u MUST rule out cancer	Generally benign remember, small GI canc are rare
OTHER	Biopsy margins to rule out malignancy on lesser curve (can look like cancer)	Hypertrophy of Brunner glands

Ulcer complications

Hemorrhage	Gastric, duodenal (posterior > anterior). Most common complication. But ant ulcer > post for locat. Ruptured gastric ulcer on the lesser curvature of stomach → bleeding from left gastric artery. An ulcer on the posterior wall of duodenum → bleeding from gastroduodenal artery.
Obstruction	Pyloric channel, duodenal
Perforation	Duodenal (anterior > posterior). May see free air under diaphragm **A** with referred pain to the shoulder via phrenic nerve.

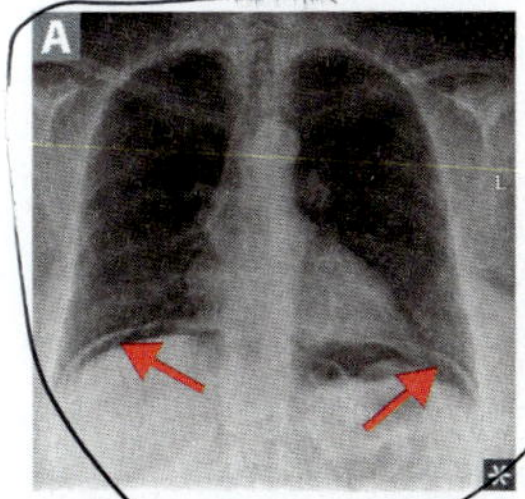

stomach doesnt normally have inflam cells (unlike ukus/GI)

stomach cancer vs ulcer
- large
- pile, crimp around/heaped up (intestinal)
- small
- punched out, margins flat

Malabsorption syndromes	Can cause diarrhea, steatorrhea, weight loss, weakness, vitamin and mineral deficiencies. Screen for fecal fat (eg, Sudan stain).	
Celiac disease A 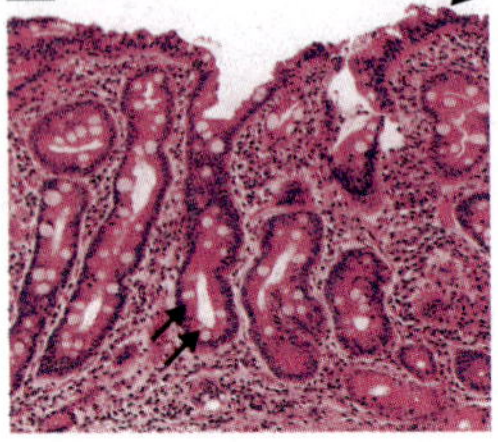	Gluten-sensitive enteropathy, celiac sprue. Autoimmune-mediated intolerance of gliadin (gluten protein found in wheat) → malabsorption and steatorrhea. Associated with HLA-DQ2, HLA-DQ8, northern European descent, dermatitis herpetiformis, ↓ bone density. Findings: IgA anti-tissue transglutaminase, anti-endomysial, anti-deamidated gliadin peptide antibodies; villous atrophy (arrow in A shows blunting), crypt hyperplasia (double arrows in A), and intraepithelial lymphocytosis. Moderately ↑ risk of malignancy (eg, T-cell lymphoma).	↓ mucosal absorption primarily affects distal duodenum and/or proximal jejunum. D-xylose test: passively absorbed in proximal small intestine; blood and urine levels ↓ with mucosa defects or bacterial overgrowth, normal in pancreatic insufficiency. Treatment: gluten-free diet.
Lactose intolerance	Lactase deficiency. Normal-appearing villi, except when 2° to injury at tips of villi (eg, viral enteritis). Osmotic diarrhea with ↓ stool pH (colonic bacteria ferment lactose).	Lactose hydrogen breath test: ⊕ for lactose malabsorption if postlactose breath hydrogen value rises > 20 ppm compared with baseline.
Pancreatic insufficiency	Due to chronic pancreatitis, cystic fibrosis, obstructing cancer. Causes malabsorption of fat and fat-soluble vitamins (A, D, E, K) as well as vitamin B_{12}.	↓ duodenal pH (bicarbonate) and fecal elastase.
Tropical sprue	Similar findings as celiac sprue (affects small bowel), but responds to antibiotics. Cause is unknown, but seen in residents of or recent visitors to tropics.	↓ mucosal absorption affecting duodenum and jejunum but can involve ileum with time. Associated with megaloblastic anemia due to folate deficiency and, later, B_{12} deficiency.
Whipple disease B 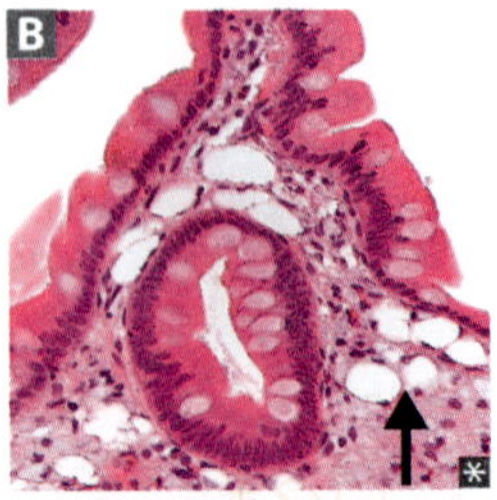	Infection with *Tropheryma whipplei* (intracellular gram ⊕); PAS ⊕ foamy macrophages in intestinal lamina propria B, mesenteric nodes. Cardiac symptoms, Arthralgias, and Neurologic symptoms are common. Most often occurs in older men.	Foamy Whipped cream in a CAN.

Inflammatory bowel diseases

	Crohn disease	Ulcerative colitis
LOCATION	Any portion of the GI tract, usually the terminal ileum and colon. Skip lesions, rectal sparing.	Colitis = colon inflammation. Continuous colonic lesions, always with rectal involvement.
GROSS MORPHOLOGY	Transmural inflammation → fistulas. Cobblestone mucosa, creeping fat, bowel wall thickening ("string sign" on barium swallow x-ray A), linear ulcers, fissures.	Mucosal and submucosal inflammation only. Friable mucosal pseudopolyps (compare normal B with diseased C) with freely hanging mesentery. Loss of haustra → "lead pipe" appearance on imaging.
MICROSCOPIC MORPHOLOGY	Noncaseating granulomas and lymphoid aggregates.	Crypt abscesses and ulcers, bleeding, no granulomas.
COMPLICATIONS	Malabsorption/malnutrition, colorectal cancer (↑ risk with pancolitis). Fistulas (eg, enterovesical fistulae, which can cause recurrent UTI and pneumaturia), phlegmon/abscess, strictures (causing obstruction), perianal disease.	Malabsorption/malnutrition, colorectal cancer (↑ risk with pancolitis). Fulminant colitis, toxic megacolon, perforation.
INTESTINAL MANIFESTATION	Diarrhea that may or may not be bloody.	Bloody diarrhea.
EXTRAINTESTINAL MANIFESTATIONS	Rash (pyoderma gangrenosum, erythema nodosum), eye inflammation (episcleritis, uveitis), oral ulcerations (aphthous stomatitis), arthritis (peripheral, spondylitis).	
	Kidney stones (usually calcium oxalate), gallstones.	1° sclerosing cholangitis. Associated with p-ANCA.
TREATMENT	Corticosteroids, azathioprine, antibiotics (eg, ciprofloxacin, metronidazole), infliximab, adalimumab.	5-aminosalicylic preparations (eg, mesalamine), 6-mercaptopurine, infliximab, colectomy.
	For Crohn, think of a fat granny and an old crone skipping down a cobblestone road away from the wreck (rectal sparing).	Ulcerative colitis causes ULCCCERS: Ulcers; Large intestine; Continuous, Colorectal carcinoma, Crypt abscesses; Extends proximally; Red diarrhea; Sclerosing cholangitis

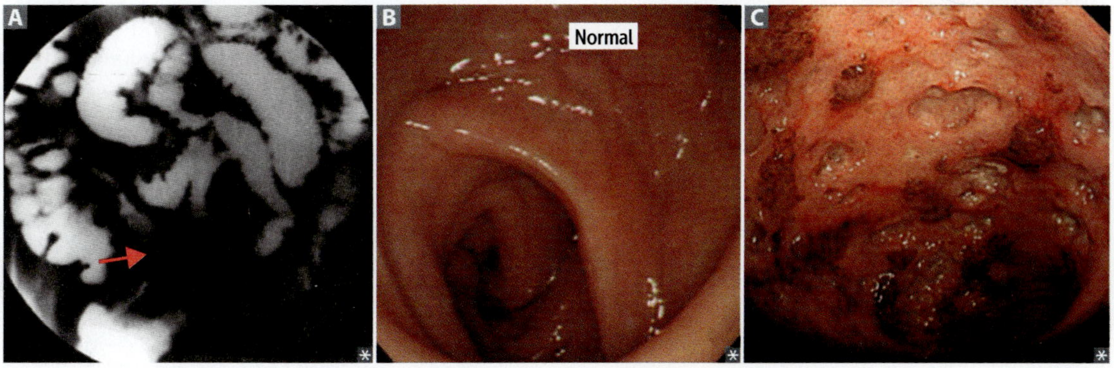

Irritable bowel syndrome

Recurrent abdominal pain associated with ≥ 2 of the following:
- Pain improves with defecation
- Change in stool frequency
- Change in appearance of stool

No structural abnormalities. Most common in middle-aged women. Chronic symptoms may be diarrhea-predominant, constipation-predominant, or mixed. Pathophysiology is multifaceted.

Appendicitis

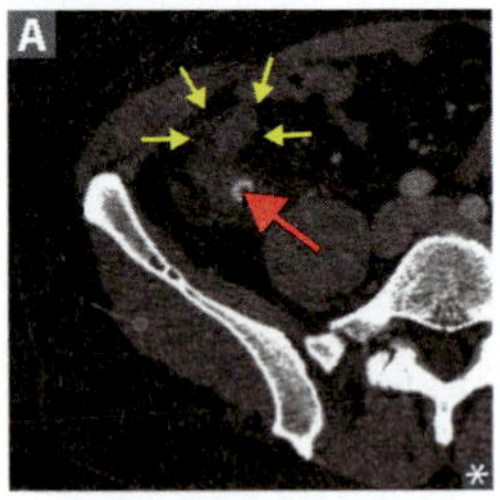

Acute inflammation of the appendix (yellow arrows in A), can be due to obstruction by fecalith (red arrow in A) (in adults) or lymphoid hyperplasia (in children).

Initial diffuse periumbilical pain migrates to McBurney point (1/3 the distance from right anterior superior iliac spine to umbilicus). Nausea, fever; may perforate → peritonitis; may elicit psoas, obturator, and Rovsing signs, guarding and rebound tenderness on exam.

Differential: diverticulitis (elderly), ectopic pregnancy (use β-hCG to rule out).

Treatment: appendectomy.

Diverticula of the GI tract

Diverticulum

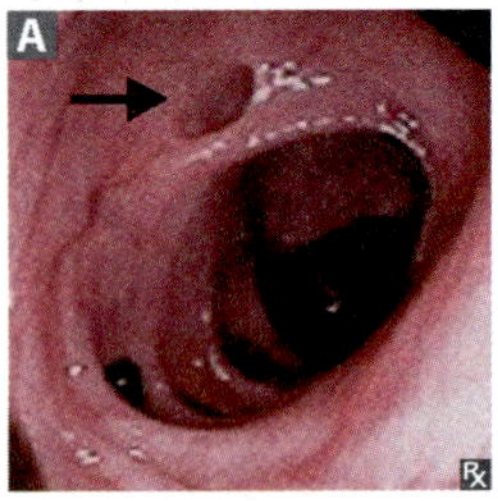

Blind pouch A protruding from the alimentary tract that communicates with the lumen of the gut. Most diverticula (esophagus, stomach, duodenum, colon) are acquired and are termed "false" in that they lack or have an attenuated muscularis externa. Most often in sigmoid colon.

"True" diverticulum—all 3 gut wall layers outpouch (eg, Meckel).

"False" diverticulum or pseudodiverticulum—only mucosa and submucosa outpouch. Occur especially where vasa recta perforate muscularis externa.

Diverticulosis

Many false diverticula of the colon, commonly sigmoid. Common (in ~ 50% of people > 60 years). Caused by ↑ intraluminal pressure and focal weakness in colonic wall. Associated with low-fiber diets.

Often asymptomatic or associated with vague discomfort.

Complications include diverticular bleeding (painless hematochezia), diverticulitis.

Diverticulitis

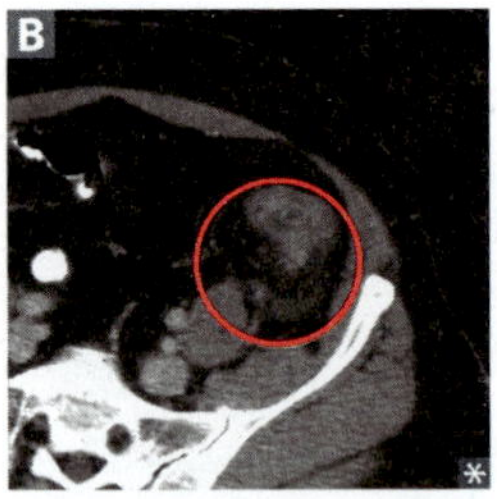

Diverticulosis with inflamed microperforations B classically causing LLQ pain, fever, leukocytosis. Treat with antibiotics.

Complications: abscess, fistula (colovesical fistula → pneumaturia), obstruction (inflammatory stenosis), perforation (→ peritonitis). Treat with percutaneous drainage or surgery.

Zenker diverticulum

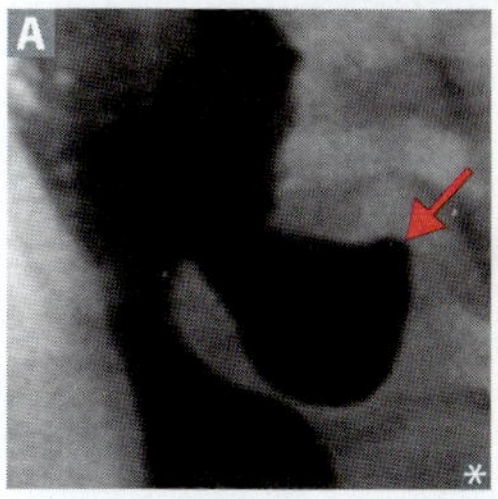

Pharyngoesophageal **false** diverticulum A. Esophageal dysmotility causes herniation of mucosal tissue at Killian triangle between the thyropharyngeal and cricopharyngeal parts of the inferior pharyngeal constrictor. Presenting symptoms: dysphagia, obstruction, gurgling, aspiration, foul breath, neck mass. Most common in elderly males.

Elder MIKE has **bad breath**.
- **Elder**ly
- **M**ales
- **I**nferior pharyngeal constrictor
- **K**illian triangle
- **E**sophageal dysmotility
- **Halitosis**

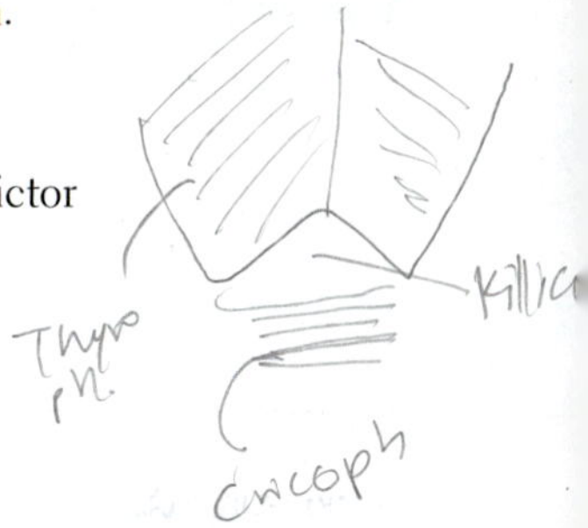

Meckel diverticulum

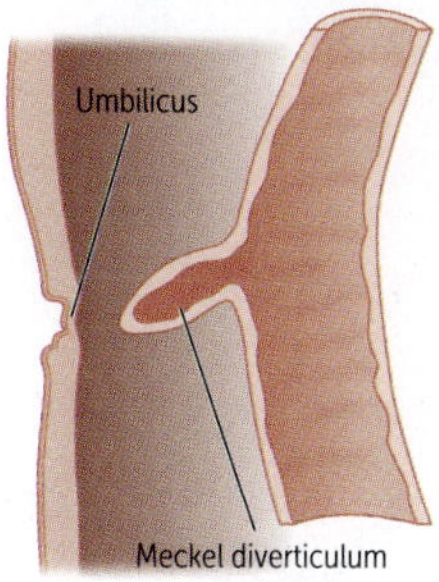

True diverticulum. Persistence of the vitelline duct. May contain ectopic acid–secreting gastric mucosa and/or pancreatic tissue. Most common congenital anomaly of GI tract. Can cause melena, RLQ pain, intussusception, volvulus, or obstruction near terminal ileum. Contrast with omphalomesenteric cyst = cystic dilation of vitelline duct.

Diagnosis: pertechnetate study for uptake by ectopic gastric mucosa.

The **six 2's**:
- 2 times as likely in males.
- 2 inches long.
- 2 feet from the ileocecal valve.
- 2% of population.
- Commonly presents in first 2 years of life.
- May have 2 types of epithelia (gastric/pancreatic).

Hirschsprung disease

Congenital megacolon characterized by lack of ganglion cells/enteric nervous plexuses (Auerbach and Meissner plexuses) in distal segment of colon. Due to failure of neural crest cell migration. Associated with mutations in RET.

Presents with bilious emesis, abdominal distention, and failure to pass meconium within 48 hours → chronic constipation. Normal portion of the colon proximal to the aganglionic segment is dilated, resulting in a "transition zone."

Think of Hirsch**sprung** as a giant spring that has **sprung** in the colon. Risk ↑ with Down syndrome.

Diagnosed by rectal suction biopsy.

Treatment: resection.

Malrotation

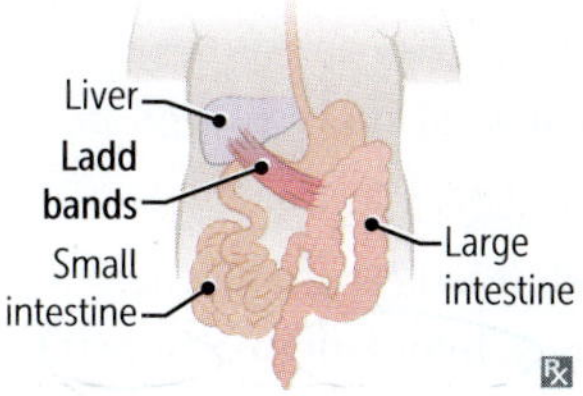

Anomaly of midgut rotation during fetal development → improper positioning of bowel, formation of fibrous bands (Ladd bands). Can lead to volvulus, duodenal obstruction.

Volvulus

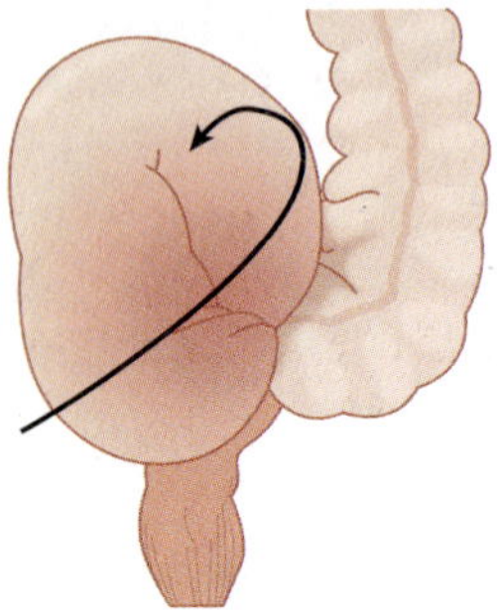

Twisting of portion of bowel around its mesentery; can lead to obstruction and infarction A. Can occur throughout the GI tract. Midgut volvulus more common in infants and children. Sigmoid volvulus more common in elderly.

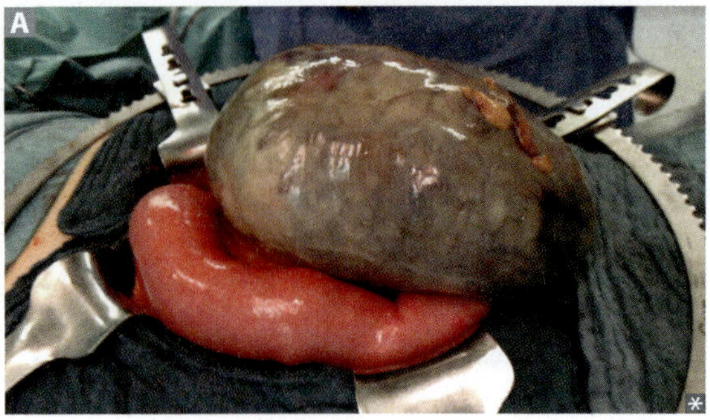

Intussusception

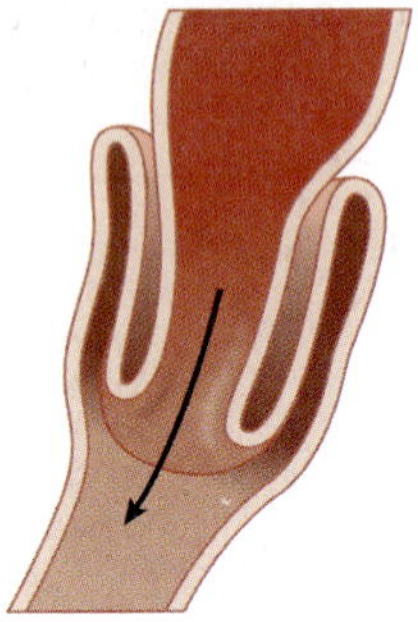

Telescoping A of proximal bowel segment into distal segment, commonly at ileocecal junction. Compromised blood supply → intermittent abdominal pain often with "currant jelly" stools. Unusual in adults (associated with intraluminal mass or tumor that acts as lead point that is pulled into the lumen). Majority of cases occur in children (usually idiopathic; may be associated with recent viral infection, such as adenovirus → Peyer patch hypertrophy → lead point; most common pathologic lead point is Meckel diverticulum). Abdominal emergency in early childhood, with bull's-eye appearance on ultrasound.

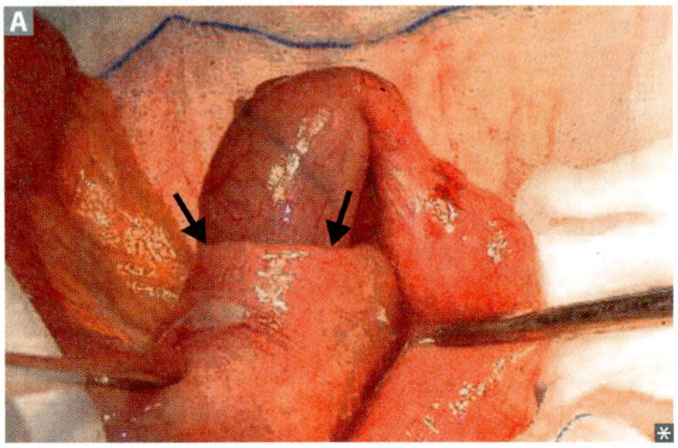

Other intestinal disorders

Acute mesenteric ischemia	Critical blockage of intestinal blood flow (often embolic occlusion of SMA) → small bowel necrosis → abdominal pain out of proportion to physical findings. May see red "currant jelly" stools.
Chronic mesenteric ischemia	"Intestinal angina": atherosclerosis of celiac artery, SMA, or IMA → intestinal hypoperfusion → postprandial epigastric pain → food aversion and weight loss.
Colonic ischemia	Reduction in intestinal blood flow causes ischemia. Crampy abdominal pain followed by hematochezia. Commonly occurs at watershed areas (splenic flexure, distal colon). Typically affects elderly.
Angiodysplasia	Tortuous dilation of vessels → hematochezia. Most often found in cecum, terminal ileum, ascending colon. More common in older patients. Confirmed by angiography.
Adhesion	Fibrous band of scar tissue; commonly forms after surgery; most common cause of small bowel obstruction. Can have well-demarcated necrotic zones.
Ileus	Intestinal hypomotility without obstruction → constipation and ↓ flatus; distended/tympanic abdomen with ↓ bowel sounds. Associated with abdominal surgeries, opiates, hypokalemia, sepsis. Treatment: bowel rest, electrolyte correction, cholinergic drugs (stimulate intestinal motility).
Meconium ileus	In cystic fibrosis, meconium plug obstructs intestine, preventing stool passage at birth.
Necrotizing enterocolitis	Seen in premature, formula-fed infants with immature immune system. Necrosis of intestinal mucosa (primarily colonic) with possible perforation, which can lead to pneumatosis intestinalis, free air in abdomen, portal venous gas.

Colonic polyps	Growths of tissue within the colon A. May be neoplastic or non-neoplastic. Grossly characterized as flat, sessile, or pedunculated (on a stalk) on the basis of protrusion into colonic lumen. Generally classified by histologic type.
HISTOLOGIC TYPE	CHARACTERISTICS
Hyperplastic	Non-neoplastic. Generally smaller and majority located in rectosigmoid area.
Hamartomatous	Generally non-neoplastic; solitary lesions do not have a significant risk of malignant transformation. Growths of normal colonic tissue with distorted architecture. Associated with Peutz-Jeghers syndrome and juvenile polyposis.
Adenomatous	Neoplastic, via chromosomal instability pathway with mutations in *APC* and *KRAS*. Tubular B histology has less malignant potential than villous C; tubulovillous has intermediate malignant potential. Usually asymptomatic; may present with occult bleeding.
Serrated	Premalignant, via CpG hypermethylation phenotype pathway with microsatellite instability and mutations in *BRAF*. "Saw-tooth" pattern of crypts on biopsy. Up to 20% of cases of sporadic CRC.

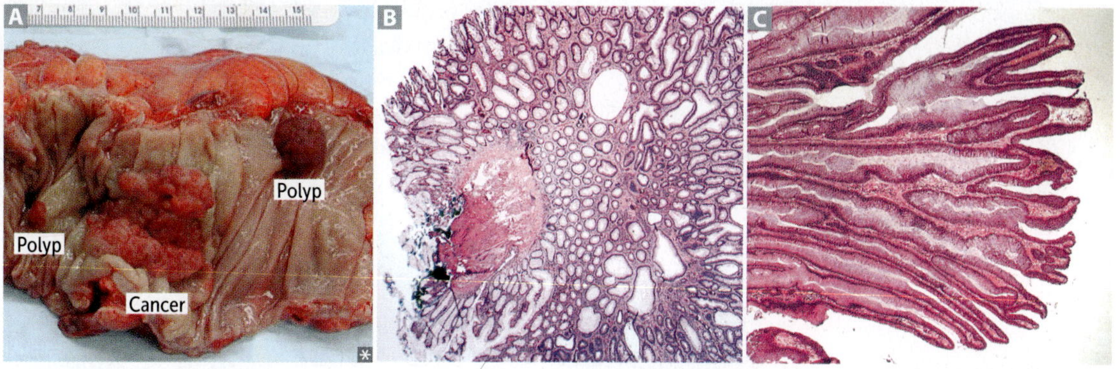

Polyposis syndromes	
Familial adenomatous polyposis	Autosomal dominant mutation of *APC* tumor suppressor gene on chromosome 5q. 2-hit hypothesis. Thousands of polyps arise starting after puberty; pancolonic; always involves rectum. Prophylactic colectomy or else 100% progress to CRC.
Gardner syndrome	FAP + osseous and soft tissue tumors, congenital hypertrophy of retinal pigment epithelium, impacted/supernumerary teeth.
Turcot syndrome	FAP + malignant CNS tumor. **Tur**cot = **Tur**ban.
Peutz-Jeghers syndrome	Autosomal dominant syndrome featuring numerous hamartomas throughout GI tract, along with hyperpigmented mouth, lips, hands, genitalia. Associated with ↑ risk of breast and GI cancers (eg, colorectal, stomach, small bowel, pancreatic).
Juvenile polyposis syndrome	Autosomal dominant syndrome in children (typically < 5 years old) featuring numerous hamartomatous polyps in the colon, stomach, small bowel. Associated with ↑ risk of CRC.

Lynch syndrome	Previously known as hereditary nonpolyposis colorectal cancer (HNPCC). Autosomal dominant mutation of DNA mismatch repair genes with subsequent microsatellite instability. ~ 80% progress to CRC. Proximal colon is always involved. Associated with endometrial, ovarian, and skin cancers.

Colorectal cancer

EPIDEMIOLOGY	Most patients are > 50 years old. ~ 25% have a family history.	
RISK FACTORS	Adenomatous and serrated polyps, familial cancer syndromes, IBD, tobacco use, diet of processed meat with low fiber.	
PRESENTATION	Rectosigmoid > ascending > descending. Ascending—exophytic mass, iron deficiency anemia, weight loss. Descending—infiltrating mass, partial obstruction, colicky pain, hematochezia. Rarely, presents with *Streptococcus bovis* bacteremia.	Right side bleeds; left side obstructs.
DIAGNOSIS	Iron deficiency anemia in males (especially > 50 years old) and postmenopausal females raises suspicion. Screen patients > 50 years old with colonoscopy A, flexible sigmoidoscopy, fecal occult blood test, or fecal DNA test. "Apple core" lesion seen on barium enema x-ray B. CEA tumor marker: good for monitoring recurrence, should not be used for screening.	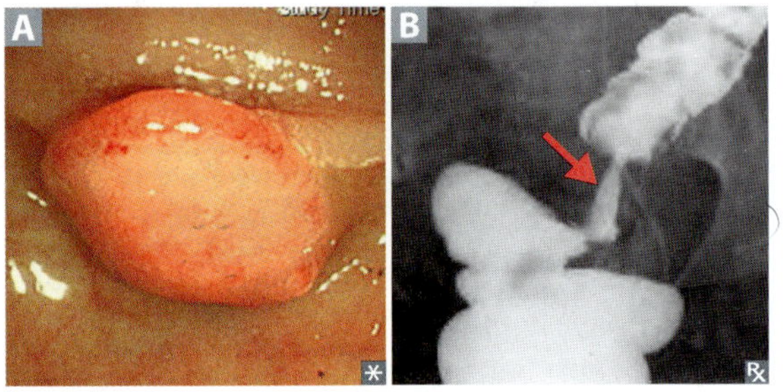

Molecular pathogenesis of colorectal cancer

Chromosomal instability pathway: mutations in *APC* cause FAP and most sporadic CRC (via adenoma-carcinoma sequence; (**firing**) order of events is **AK-53**).
Microsatellite instability pathway: mutations or methylation of mismatch repair genes (eg, *MLH1*) cause Lynch syndrome and some sporadic CRC (via serrated polyp pathway).

Chromosomal instability pathway

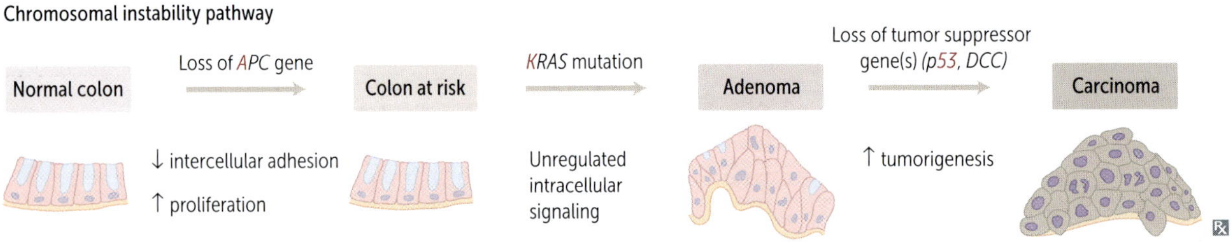

Cirrhosis and portal hypertension

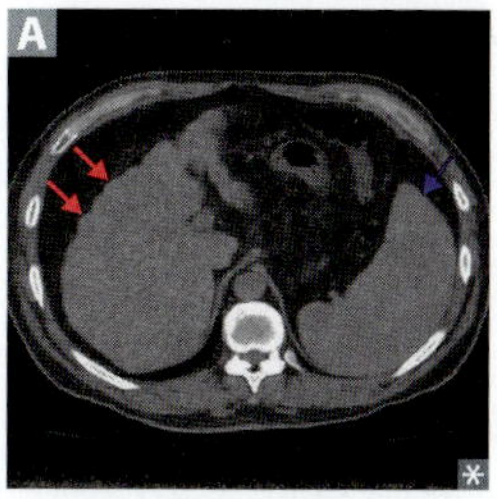

Cirrhosis—diffuse bridging fibrosis (via stellate cells) and regenerative nodules (red arrows in A; blue arrow shows splenomegaly) disrupt normal architecture of liver; ↑ risk for hepatocellular carcinoma (HCC). Etiologies include alcohol (60–70% of cases in the US), nonalcoholic steatohepatitis, chronic viral hepatitis, autoimmune hepatitis, biliary disease, genetic/metabolic disorders.

Portal hypertension—↑ pressure in portal venous system. Etiologies include cirrhosis (most common cause in Western countries), vascular obstruction (eg, portal vein thrombosis, Budd-Chiari syndrome), schistosomiasis.

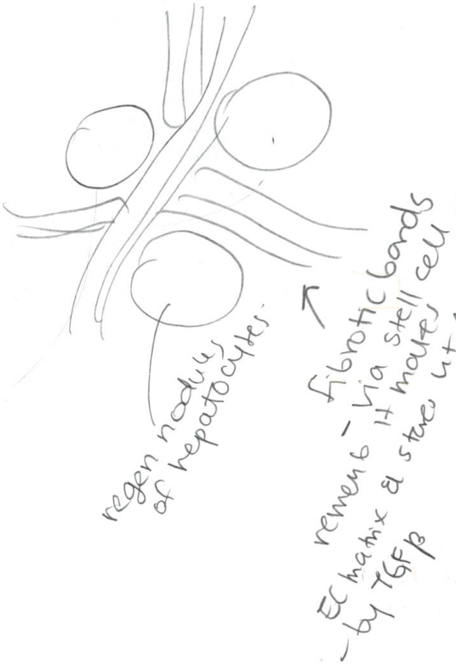

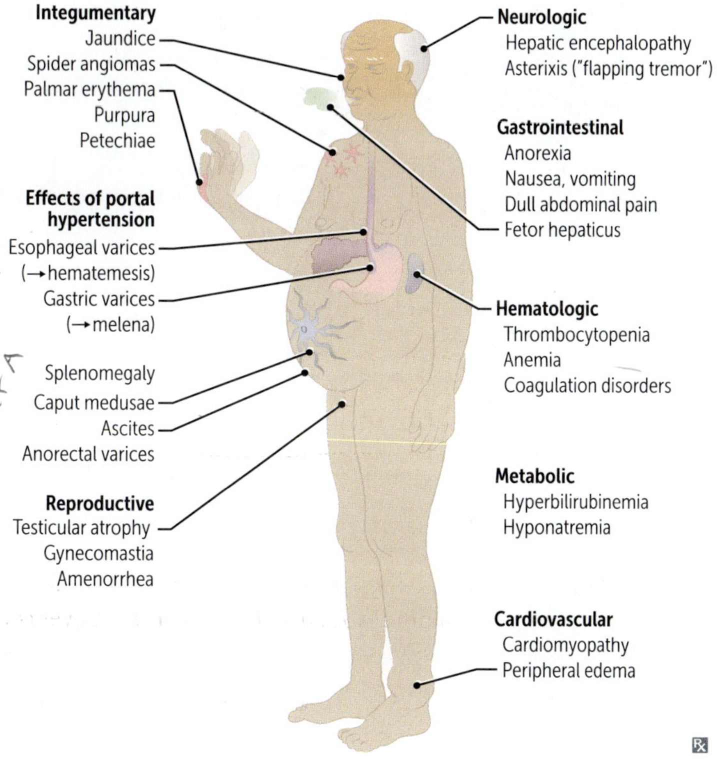

Serum markers of liver pathology

ENZYMES RELEASED IN LIVER DAMAGE	
Aspartate aminotransferase and alanine aminotransferase	↑ in most liver disease: ALT > AST ↑ in alcoholic liver disease: AST > ALT AST > ALT in nonalcoholic liver disease suggests progression to advanced fibrosis or cirrhosis
Alkaline phosphatase	↑ in cholestasis (eg, biliary obstruction), infiltrative disorders, bone disease
γ-glutamyl transpeptidase	↑ in various liver and biliary diseases (just as ALP can), but not in bone disease; associated with alcohol use
FUNCTIONAL LIVER MARKERS	
Bilirubin	↑ in various liver diseases (eg, biliary obstruction, alcoholic or viral hepatitis, cirrhosis), hemolysis
Albumin	↓ in advanced liver disease
Prothrombin	↑ in advanced liver disease (↓ production of clotting factors)
Platelets	↓ in advanced liver disease (↓ thrombopoietin, liver sequestration) and portal hypertension (splenomegaly/splenic sequestration)

Reye syndrome	Rare, often fatal childhood hepatic encephalopathy. Findings: mitochondrial abnormalities, fatty liver (microvesicular fatty change), hypoglycemia, vomiting, hepatomegaly, coma. Associated with viral infection (especially VZV and influenza B) that has been treated with aspirin. Mechanism: aspirin metabolites ↓ β-oxidation by reversible inhibition of mitochondrial enzymes. Avoid aspirin in children, except in those with Kawasaki disease.

Alcoholic liver disease

Hepatic steatosis	Macrovesicular fatty change A that may be reversible with alcohol cessation.	
Alcoholic hepatitis	Requires sustained, long-term consumption. Swollen and necrotic hepatocytes with neutrophilic infiltration. Mallory bodies B (intracytoplasmic eosinophilic inclusions of damaged keratin filaments).	Make a toAST with alcohol: AST > ALT (ratio usually > 2:1).
Alcoholic cirrhosis	Final and irreversible form. Micronodular, irregularly shrunken liver with "hobnail" appearance. Sclerosis (arrows in C) around central vein (zone III). Manifestations of chronic liver disease (eg, jaundice, hypoalbuminemia).	

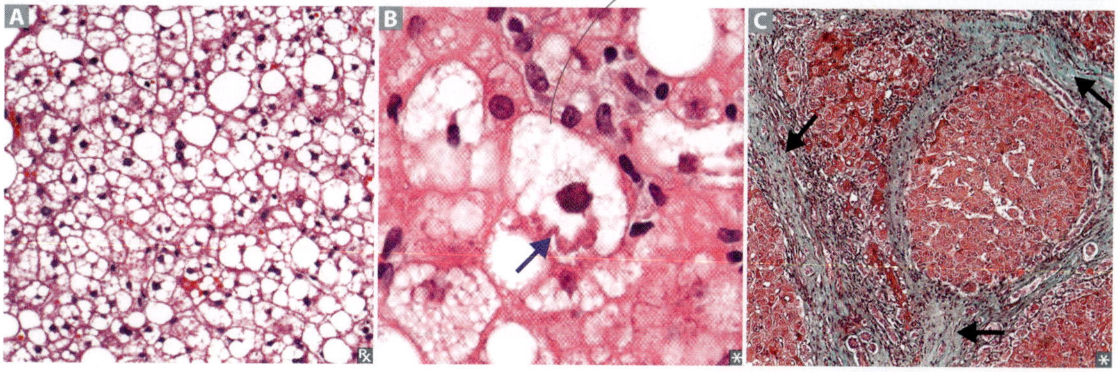

Non-alcoholic fatty liver disease	Metabolic syndrome (insulin resistance); obesity → fatty infiltration of hepatocytes A → cellular "ballooning" and eventual necrosis. May cause cirrhosis and HCC. Independent of alcohol use.	ALT > AST (Lipids)

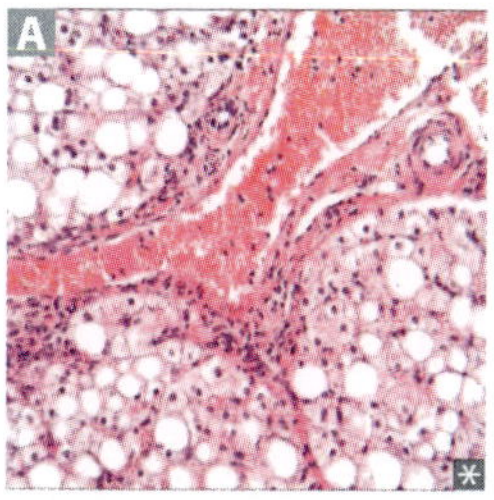

Hepatic encephalopathy	Cirrhosis → portosystemic shunts → ↓ NH_3 metabolism → neuropsychiatric dysfunction. Spectrum from disorientation/asterixis (mild) to difficult arousal or coma (severe). Triggers: ▪ ↑ NH_3 production and absorption (due to dietary protein, GI bleed, constipation, infection). ▪ ↓ NH_3 removal (due to renal failure, diuretics, bypassed hepatic blood flow post-TIPS). Treatment: lactulose (↑ NH_4^+ generation) and rifaximin or neomycin (↓ NH_4^+ producing gut bacteria).

Hepatocellular carcinoma/hepatoma

Most common 1° malignant tumor of liver in adults A. Associated with HBV (+/– cirrhosis) and all other causes of cirrhosis (including HCV, alcoholic and non-alcoholic fatty liver disease, autoimmune disease, hemochromatosis, α_1-antitrypsin deficiency) and specific carcinogens (eg, aflatoxin from *Aspergillus*). May lead to Budd-Chiari syndrome.

Findings: jaundice, tender hepatomegaly, ascites, polycythemia, anorexia. Spreads hematogenously.

Diagnosis: ↑ α-fetoprotein; ultrasound or contrast CT/MRI B, biopsy.

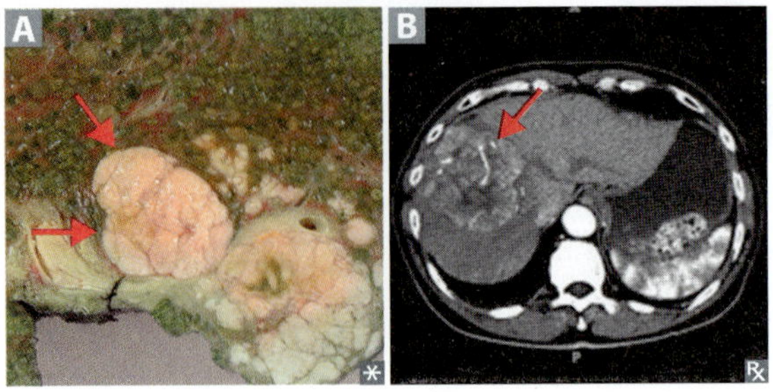

Other liver tumors

Cavernous hemangioma

Common, benign liver tumor A; typically occurs at age 30–50 years. Biopsy contraindicated because of risk of hemorrhage.

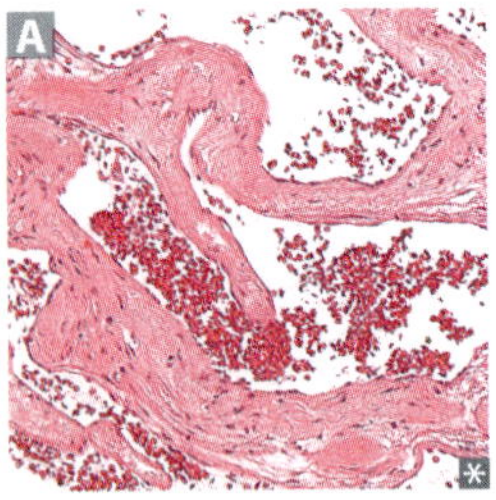

Hepatic adenoma

Rare, benign liver tumor, often related to oral contraceptive or anabolic steroid use; may regress spontaneously or rupture (abdominal pain and shock).

Angiosarcoma

Malignant tumor of endothelial origin; associated with exposure to arsenic, vinyl chloride.

Metastases

GI malignancies, breast and lung cancer. Most common overall.

Budd-Chiari syndrome

Thrombosis or compression of hepatic veins with centrilobular congestion and necrosis → congestive liver disease (hepatomegaly, ascites, varices, abdominal pain, liver failure). Absence of JVD. Associated with hypercoagulable states, polycythemia vera, postpartum state, HCC. May cause nutmeg liver (mottled appearance).

α_1-antitrypsin deficiency 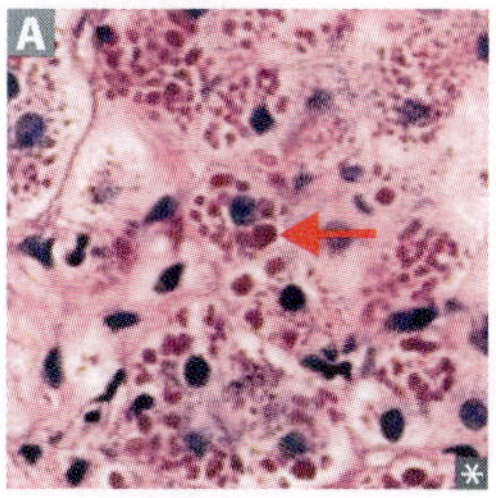	Misfolded gene product protein aggregates in hepatocellular ER → cirrhosis with PAS ⊕ globules A in liver. Codominant trait.	In lungs, ↓ α_1-antitrypsin → uninhibited elastase in alveoli → ↓ elastic tissue → panacinar emphysema.

Jaundice 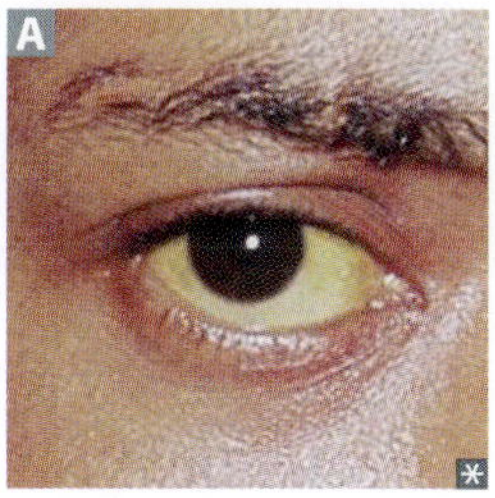	Abnormal yellowing of the skin and/or sclera A due to bilirubin deposition. Hyperbilirubinemia 2° to ↑ production or ↓ disposition (impaired hepatic uptake, conjugation, excretion).
Unconjugated (indirect) hyperbilirubinemia	Hemolytic, physiologic (newborns), Crigler-Najjar, Gilbert syndrome.
Conjugated (direct) hyperbilirubinemia	Biliary tract obstruction: gallstones, cholangiocarcinoma, pancreatic or liver cancer, liver fluke. Biliary tract disease: ▪ 1° sclerosing cholangitis ▪ 1° biliary cirrhosis Excretion defect: Dubin-Johnson syndrome, Rotor syndrome.
Mixed (direct and indirect) hyperbilirubinemia	Hepatitis, cirrhosis.

Physiologic neonatal jaundice	At birth, immature UDP-glucuronosyltransferase → unconjugated hyperbilirubinemia → jaundice/kernicterus (bilirubin deposition in brain, particularly basal ganglia). Occurs after first 24 hours of life and usually resolves without treatment in 1–2 weeks. Treatment: phototherapy (non-UV) isomerizes unconjugated bilirubin to water-soluble form.

Hereditary hyperbilirubinemias	All autosomal recessive.	
❶ Gilbert syndrome	Mildly ↓ UDP-glucuronosyltransferase conjugation and impaired bilirubin uptake. Asymptomatic or mild jaundice. ↑ unconjugated bilirubin without overt hemolysis. Bilirubin ↑ with fasting and stress.	Very common. No clinical consequences.
❷ Crigler-Najjar syndrome, type I	Absent UDP-glucuronosyltransferase. Presents early in life; patients die within a few years. Findings: jaundice, kernicterus (bilirubin deposition in brain), ↑ unconjugated bilirubin. Treatment: plasmapheresis and phototherapy.	Type II is less severe and responds to phenobarbital, which ↑ liver enzyme synthesis.
❸ Dubin-Johnson syndrome	Conjugated hyperbilirubinemia due to defective liver excretion. Grossly black liver. Benign.	❹ Rotor syndrome is similar, but milder in presentation without black liver. Due to impaired hepatic uptake and excretion.

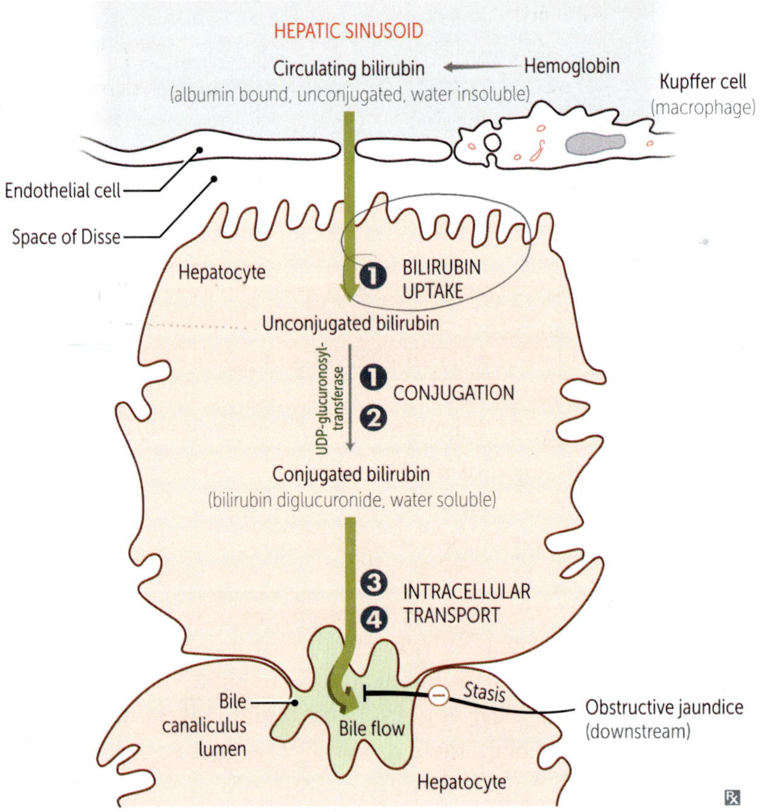

Wilson disease (hepatolenticular degeneration)

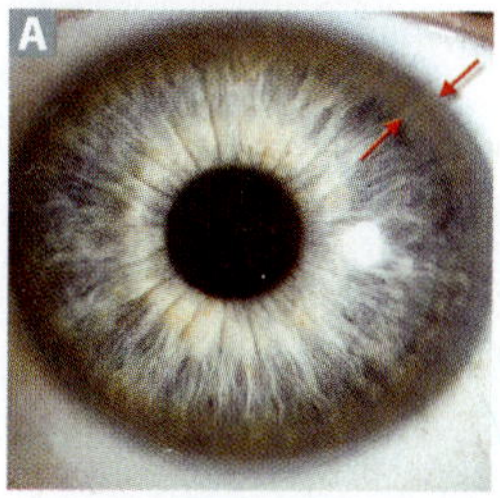

Recessive mutations in hepatocyte copper-transporting ATPase (*ATP7B* gene; chromosome 13) → inadequate copper excretion into bile and blood (↓ serum ceruloplasmin, ↑ urine copper). Copper accumulates, especially in liver, brain, cornea, kidneys, joints.

Presents before age 40 with liver disease (eg, hepatitis, acute liver failure, cirrhosis), neurologic disease (eg, dysarthria, dystonia, tremor, parkinsonism), psychiatric disease, Kayser-Fleischer rings (deposits in Descemet membrane of cornea) A, hemolytic anemia, renal disease (eg, Fanconi syndrome).

Treatment: chelation with penicillamine or trientine, oral zinc.

Hemochromatosis

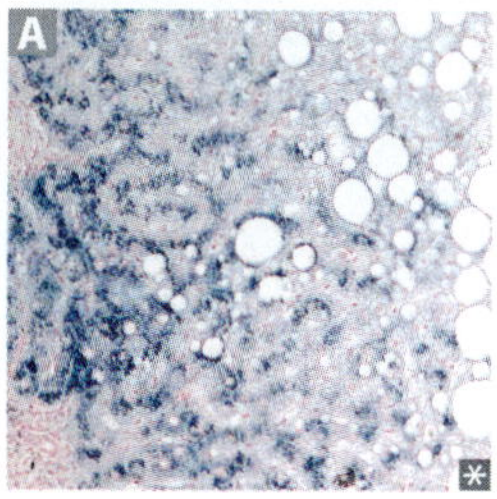

Recessive mutations in *HFE* gene (C282Y > H63D, chromosome 6) → abnormal iron sensing and ↑ intestinal absorption (↑ ferritin, ↑ iron, ↓ TIBC → ↑ transferrin saturation). Iron overload can also be 2° to chronic transfusion therapy (eg, β-thalassemia major). Iron accumulates, especially in liver, pancreas, skin, heart, pituitary, joints. Hemosiderin (iron) can be identified on liver MRI or biopsy with Prussian blue stain A.

Presents after age 40 when total body iron > 20 g; iron loss through menstruation slows progression in women. Classic triad of cirrhosis, diabetes mellitus, skin pigmentation ("bronze diabetes"). Also causes dilated cardiomyopathy (reversible), hypogonadism, arthropathy (calcium pyrophosphate deposition; especially metacarpophalangeal joints). HCC is common cause of death.

Treatment: repeated phlebotomy, chelation with deferasirox, deferoxamine, oral deferiprone.

Biliary tract disease

May present with pruritus, jaundice, dark urine, light-colored stool, hepatosplenomegaly. Typically with cholestatic pattern of LFTs (↑ conjugated bilirubin, ↑ cholesterol, ↑ ALP).

	PATHOLOGY	EPIDEMIOLOGY	ADDITIONAL FEATURES
Primary sclerosing cholangitis	Unknown cause of concentric "onion skin" bile duct fibrosis → alternating strictures and dilation with "beading" of intra- and extrahepatic bile ducts on ERCP, magnetic resonance cholangiopancreatography (MRCP).	Classically in middle-aged men with IBD.	Associated with ulcerative colitis. p-ANCA ⊕. ↑ IgM. Can lead to 2° biliary cirrhosis. ↑ risk of cholangiocarcinoma and gallbladder cancer.
Primary biliary cirrhosis	Autoimmune reaction → lymphocytic infiltrate + granulomas → destruction of intralobular bile ducts.	Classically in middle-aged women.	Anti-mitochondrial antibody ⊕, ↑ IgM. Associated with other autoimmune conditions (eg, Sjögren syndrome, Hashimoto thyroiditis, CREST, rheumatoid arthritis, celiac disease).
Secondary biliary cirrhosis	Extrahepatic biliary obstruction → ↑ pressure in intrahepatic ducts → injury/ fibrosis and bile stasis.	Patients with known obstructive lesions (gallstones, biliary strictures, pancreatic carcinoma).	May be complicated by ascending cholangitis.

Gallstones (cholelithiasis)

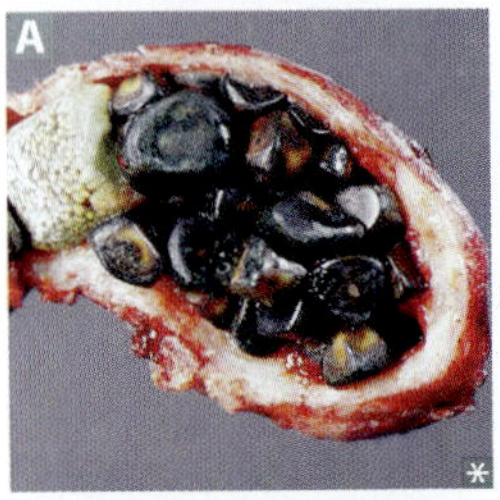

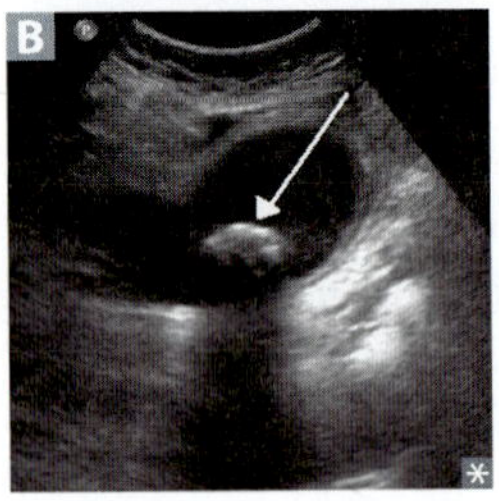

↑ cholesterol and/or bilirubin, ↓ bile salts, and gallbladder stasis all cause stones A.

2 types of stones:

- Cholesterol stones (radiolucent with 10–20% opaque due to calcifications)—80% of stones. Associated with obesity, Crohn disease, advanced age, estrogen therapy, multiparity, rapid weight loss, Native American origin.
- Pigment stones (black = radiopaque, Ca^{2+} bilirubinate, hemolysis; brown = radiolucent, infection)—seen in patients with Crohn disease, chronic hemolysis, alcoholic cirrhosis, advanced age, biliary infections, total parenteral nutrition (TPN).

Uncomplicated disease manifests as **biliary colic**—neurohormonal activation (eg, by CCK after a fatty meal) triggers contraction of gallbladder, forcing a stone into the cystic duct. May present without pain (eg, in diabetics).

Diagnose with ultrasound B. Treat with cholecystectomy if symptomatic.

Risk factors (4 **F**'s):

1. **F**emale
2. **F**at
3. **F**ertile (pregnant)
4. **F**orty

Most common complication is cholecystitis; also acute pancreatitis, ascending cholangitis.

Charcot triad of cholangitis:

- Jaundice
- Fever
- RUQ pain

Can cause fistula between gallbladder and gastrointestinal tract → air in biliary tree (pneumobilia) → passage of gallstones into intestinal tract → obstruction of ileocecal valve (gallstone ileus).

Cholecystitis

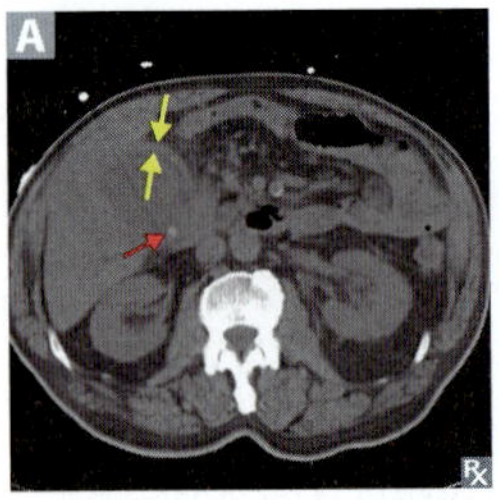

Acute or chronic inflammation of gallbladder usually from cholelithiasis (stone at neck of gallbladder [red arrow in A] with gallbladder wall thickening [yellow arrows]). Gallstones most commonly blocking the cystic duct → 2° infection; rarely acalculous due to ischemia and stasis, or 1° infection (CMV). Murphy sign ⊕: inspiratory arrest on RUQ palpation due to pain. ↑ ALP if bile duct becomes involved (eg, ascending cholangitis).

Diagnose with ultrasound or cholescintigraphy (HIDA, or hepatobiliary iminodiacetic acid scan).

Porcelain gallbladder

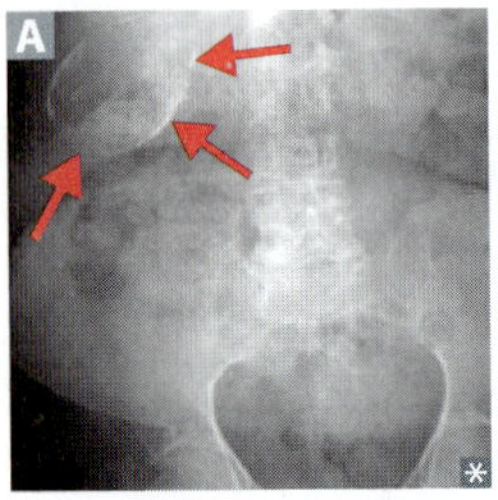

Calcified gallbladder due to chronic cholecystitis; usually found incidentally on imaging A. Treatment: prophylactic cholecystectomy due to high rates of gallbladder cancer (mostly adenocarcinoma).

Acute pancreatitis

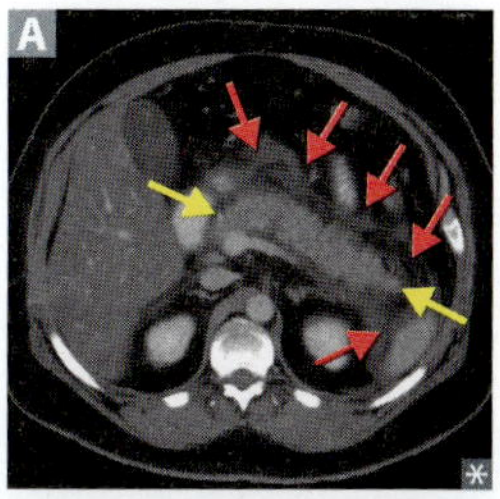

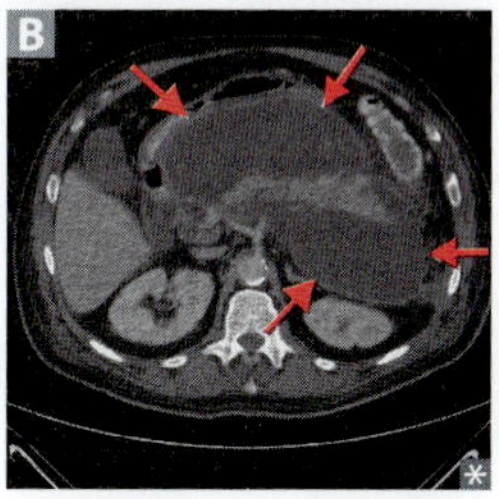

Autodigestion of pancreas by pancreatic enzymes (A shows pancreas [yellow arrows] surrounded by edema [red arrows]).

Causes: Idiopathic, Gallstones, Ethanol, Trauma, Steroids, Mumps, Autoimmune disease, Scorpion sting, Hypercalcemia/Hypertriglyceridemia (> 1000 mg/dL), ERCP, Drugs (eg, sulfa drugs, NRTIs, protease inhibitors). I GET SMASHED.

Diagnosis by 2 of 3 criteria: acute epigastric pain often radiating to the back, ↑ serum amylase or lipase (more specific) to 3× upper limit of normal, or characteristic imaging findings.

Complications: pseudocyst B (lined by granulation tissue, not epithelium), necrosis, hemorrhage, infection, organ failure (ARDS, shock, renal failure), hypocalcemia (precipitation of Ca^{2+} soaps).

Chronic pancreatitis

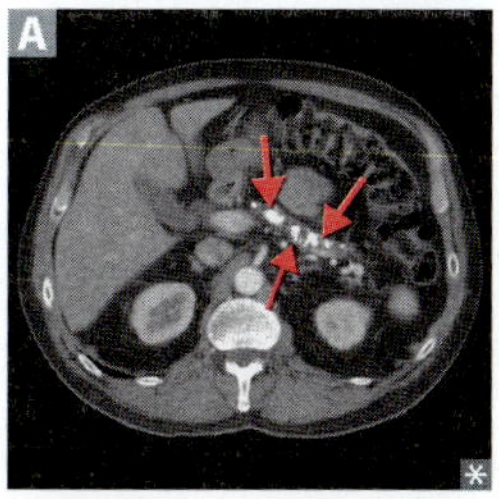

Chronic inflammation, atrophy, calcification of the pancreas A. Major causes are alcohol abuse and idiopathic. Mutations in *CFTR* (cystic fibrosis) can cause chronic pancreatic insufficiency.

Can lead to pancreatic insufficiency → steatorrhea, fat-soluble vitamin deficiency, diabetes mellitus.

Amylase and lipase may or may not be elevated (almost always elevated in acute pancreatitis).

Pancreatic adenocarcinoma

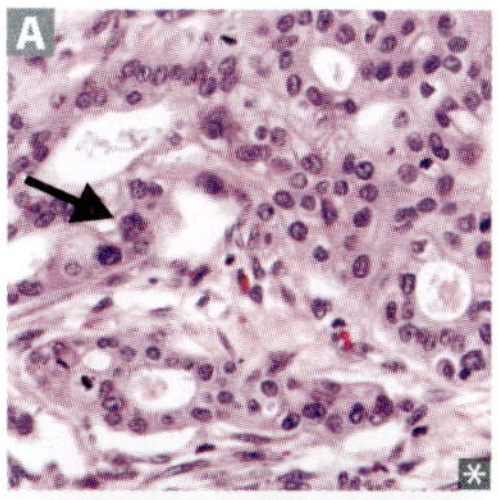

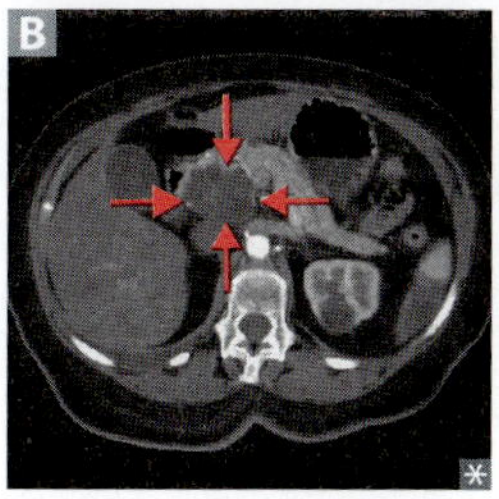

Very aggressive tumor arising from pancreatic ducts (disorganized glandular structure with cellular infiltration A); often metastatic at presentation, with average survival ~ 1 year after diagnosis.

Tumors more common in pancreatic head B (→ obstructive jaundice). Associated with CA 19-9 tumor marker (also CEA, less specific).

Risk factors:
- Tobacco use
- Chronic pancreatitis (especially > 20 years)
- Diabetes
- Age > 50 years
- Jewish and African-American males

Often presents with:
- Abdominal pain radiating to back
- Weight loss (due to malabsorption and anorexia)
- Migratory thrombophlebitis—redness and tenderness on palpation of extremities (Trousseau syndrome)
- Obstructive jaundice with palpable, nontender gallbladder (Courvoisier sign)

Treatment: Whipple procedure, chemotherapy, radiation therapy.

▶ GASTROINTESTINAL—PHARMACOLOGY

Acid suppression therapy

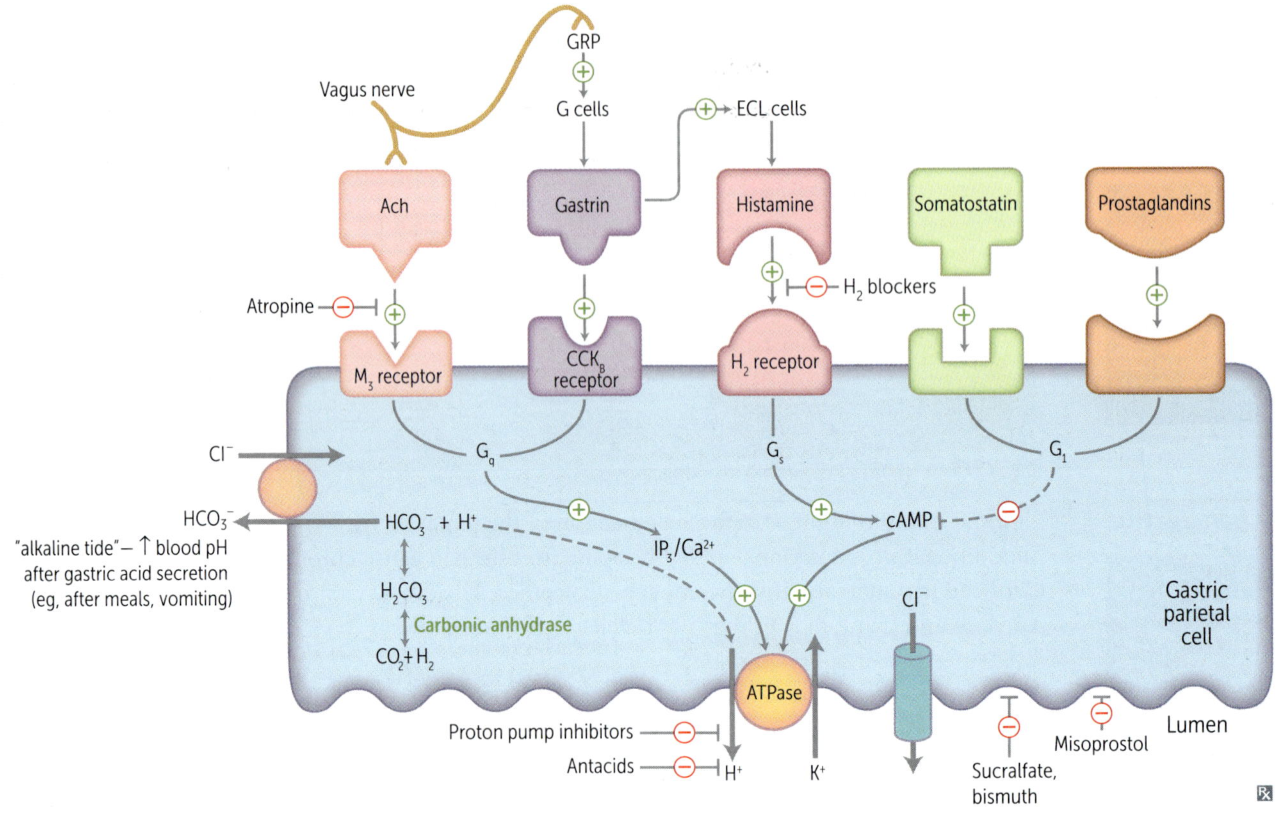

H_2 blockers	Cimetidine, ranitidine, famotidine, nizatidine.	Take H_2 blockers before you **dine**. Think "**table for 2**" to remember **H_2**.
MECHANISM	Reversible block of histamine H_2-receptors → ↓ H^+ secretion by parietal cells.	
CLINICAL USE	Peptic ulcer, gastritis, mild esophageal reflux.	
ADVERSE EFFECTS	Cimetidine is a potent inhibitor of cytochrome P-450 (multiple drug interactions); it also has antiandrogenic effects (prolactin release, gynecomastia, impotence, ↓ libido in males); can cross blood-brain barrier (confusion, dizziness, headaches) and placenta. Both cimetidine and ranitidine ↓ renal excretion of creatinine. Other H_2 blockers are relatively free of these effects.	

Proton pump inhibitors	Omeprazole, lansoprazole, esomeprazole, pantoprazole, dexlansoprazole.
MECHANISM	Irreversibly inhibit H^+/K^+ ATPase in stomach parietal cells.
CLINICAL USE	Peptic ulcer, gastritis, esophageal reflux, Zollinger-Ellison syndrome.
ADVERSE EFFECTS	↑ risk of *C difficile* infection, pneumonia. ↓ serum Mg^{2+} with long-term use.

Antacid use	Can affect absorption, bioavailability, or urinary excretion of other drugs by altering gastric and urinary pH or by delaying gastric emptying. All can cause hypokalemia. Overuse can also cause the following problems.	
Aluminum hydroxide	Constipation and hypophosphatemia; proximal muscle weakness, osteodystrophy, seizures	Aluminimum amount of feces.
Calcium carbonate	Hypercalcemia (milk-alkali syndrome), rebound acid ↑	Can chelate and ↓ effectiveness of other drugs (eg, tetracycline).
Magnesium hydroxide	Diarrhea, hyporeflexia, hypotension, cardiac arrest	Mg^{2+} = Must go to the bathroom.

Bismuth, sucralfate

MECHANISM	Bind to ulcer base, providing physical protection and allowing HCO_3^- secretion to reestablish pH gradient in the mucous layer.
CLINICAL USE	↑ ulcer healing, travelers' diarrhea.

Misoprostol

MECHANISM	A PGE_1 analog. ↑ production and secretion of gastric mucous barrier, ↓ acid production.
CLINICAL USE	Prevention of NSAID-induced peptic ulcers (NSAIDs block PGE_1 production); maintenance of a PDA. Also used off-label for induction of labor (ripens cervix).
ADVERSE EFFECTS	Diarrhea. Contraindicated in women of childbearing potential (abortifacient).

Octreotide

MECHANISM	Long-acting somatostatin analog; inhibits secretion of various splanchnic vasodilatory hormones.
CLINICAL USE	Acute variceal bleeds, acromegaly, VIPoma, carcinoid tumors.
ADVERSE EFFECTS	Nausea, cramps, steatorrhea. ↑ risk of cholelithiasis due to CCK inhibition.

Osmotic laxatives

Magnesium hydroxide, magnesium citrate, polyethylene glycol, lactulose.

MECHANISM	Provide osmotic load to draw water into the GI lumen.
CLINICAL USE	Constipation. Lactulose also treats hepatic encephalopathy since gut flora degrade it into metabolites (lactic acid and acetic acid) that promote nitrogen excretion as NH_4^+.
ADVERSE EFFECTS	Diarrhea, dehydration; may be abused by bulimics.

Sulfasalazine

MECHANISM	A combination of sulfapyridine (antibacterial) and 5-aminosalicylic acid (anti-inflammatory). Activated by colonic bacteria.
CLINICAL USE	Ulcerative colitis, Crohn disease (colitis component).
ADVERSE EFFECTS	Malaise, nausea, sulfonamide toxicity, reversible oligospermia.

Loperamide

MECHANISM	Agonist at μ-opioid receptors; slows gut motility. Poor CNS penetration (low addictive potential).
CLINICAL USE	Diarrhea.
ADVERSE EFFECTS	Constipation, nausea.

Ondansetron

MECHANISM	5-HT_3 antagonist; ↓ vagal stimulation. Powerful central-acting antiemetic.	At a party but feeling queasy? Keep **on dancing** with **ondans**etron!
CLINICAL USE	Control vomiting postoperatively and in patients undergoing cancer chemotherapy.	
ADVERSE EFFECTS	Headache, constipation, QT interval prolongation.	

Metoclopramide

MECHANISM	D_2 receptor antagonist. ↑ resting tone, contractility, LES tone, motility. Does not influence colon transport time.
CLINICAL USE	Diabetic and postsurgery gastroparesis, antiemetic.
ADVERSE EFFECTS	↑ parkinsonian effects, tardive dyskinesia. Restlessness, drowsiness, fatigue, depression, diarrhea. Drug interaction with digoxin and diabetic agents. Contraindicated in patients with small bowel obstruction or Parkinson disease (due to D_2-receptor blockade).

Orlistat

MECHANISM	Inhibits gastric and pancreatic lipase → ↓ breakdown and absorption of dietary fats.
CLINICAL USE	Weight loss.
ADVERSE EFFECTS	Steatorrhea, ↓ absorption of fat-soluble vitamins.

Ursodiol (ursodeoxycholic acid)

MECHANISM	Nontoxic bile acid. ↑ bile secretion, ↓ cholesterol secretion and reabsorption.
CLINICAL USE	Primary biliary cirrhosis, gallstone prevention or dissolution.

HIGH-YIELD SYSTEMS

Hematology and Oncology

"Of all that is written, I love only what a person has written with his own blood."

—Friedrich Nietzsche

"I used to get stressed out, but my cancer has put everything into perspective."

—Delta Goodrem

"The best blood will at some time get into a fool or a mosquito."

—Austin O'Malley

"Carcinoma works cunningly from the inside out. Detection and treatment often work more slowly and gropingly, from the outside in."

—Christopher Hitchens

Study tip: When reviewing oncologic drugs, focus on mechanisms and side effects rather than details of clinical uses, which may be lower yield.

▶ HEMATOLOGY AND ONCOLOGY—ANATOMY

Erythrocyte

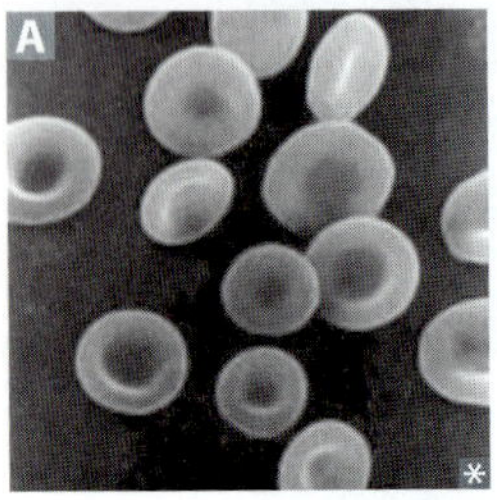

Carries O_2 to tissues and CO_2 to lungs. Anucleate and lacks organelles; biconcave A, with large surface area-to-volume ratio for rapid gas exchange. Life span of 120 days. Source of energy is glucose (90% used in glycolysis, 10% used in HMP shunt). Membrane contains Cl^-/HCO_3^- antiporter, which allows RBCs to export HCO_3^- and transport CO_2 from the periphery to the lungs for elimination.

Eryth = red; *cyte* = cell.

Erythrocytosis = polycythemia = ↑ hematocrit.
Anisocytosis = varying sizes.
Poikilocytosis = varying shapes.

Reticulocyte = immature RBC; reflects erythroid proliferation.
Bluish color on Wright-Giemsa stain of reticulocytes represents residual ribosomal RNA.

Thrombocyte (platelet)

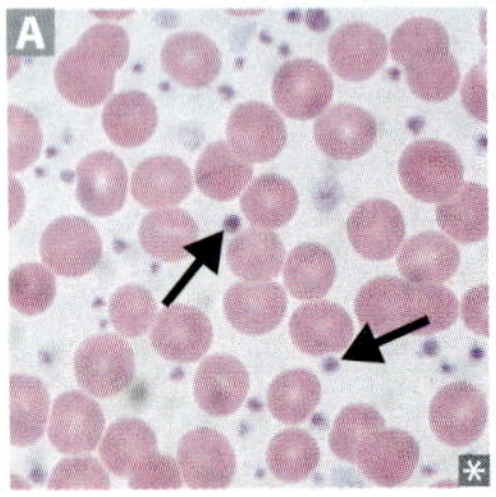

Involved in 1° hemostasis. Small cytoplasmic fragment A derived from megakaryocytes. Life span of 8–10 days. When activated by endothelial injury, aggregates with other platelets and interacts with fibrinogen to form platelet plug. Contains dense granules (ADP, Ca^{2+}) and α granules (vWF, fibrinogen, fibronectin). Approximately ⅓ of platelet pool is stored in the spleen.

Thrombocytopenia or ↓ platelet function results in petechiae.
vWF receptor: GpIb.
Fibrinogen receptor: GpIIb/IIIa.

Leukocyte

Divided into granulocytes (neutrophil, eosinophil, basophil) and mononuclear cells (monocytes, lymphocytes).
WBC differential from highest to lowest (normal ranges per USMLE):
- **N**eutrophils (54–62%)
- **L**ymphocytes (25–33%)
- **M**onocytes (3–7%)
- **E**osinophils (1–3%)
- **B**asophils (0–0.75%)

Leuk = white; *cyte* = cell.

Neutrophils **L**ike **M**aking **E**verything **B**etter.

Neutrophil

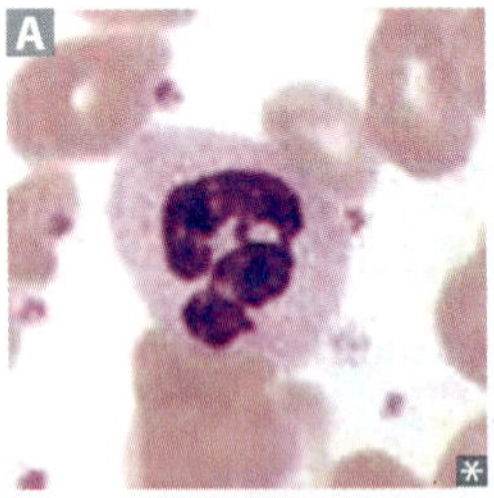

Acute inflammatory response cell. Increased in bacterial infections. Phagocytic. Multilobed nucleus A. Specific granules contain leukocyte alkaline phosphatase (LAP), collagenase, lysozyme, and lactoferrin. Azurophilic granules (lysosomes) contain proteinases, acid phosphatase, myeloperoxidase, and β-glucuronidase.

Hypersegmented neutrophils (nucleus has 6+ lobes) are seen in vitamin B_{12}/folate deficiency.
↑ band cells (immature neutrophils) reflect states of ↑ myeloid proliferation (bacterial infections, CML).
Important neutrophil chemotactic agents: C5a, IL-8, LTB_4, kallikrein, platelet-activating factor.

Monocyte

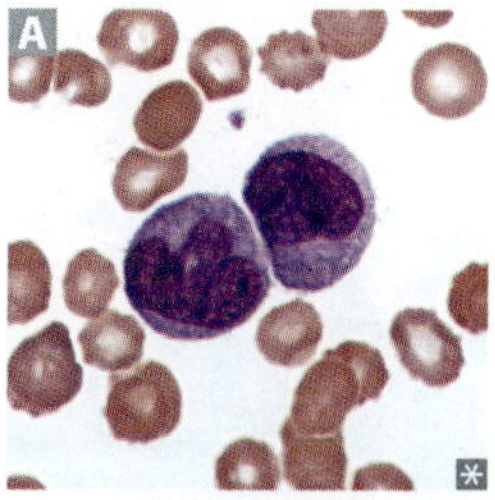

Differentiates into macrophage in tissues. Large, kidney-shaped nucleus A. Extensive "frosted glass" cytoplasm.

Mono = one (nucleus); *cyte* = cell.
Monocyte: in the blood.

Macrophage

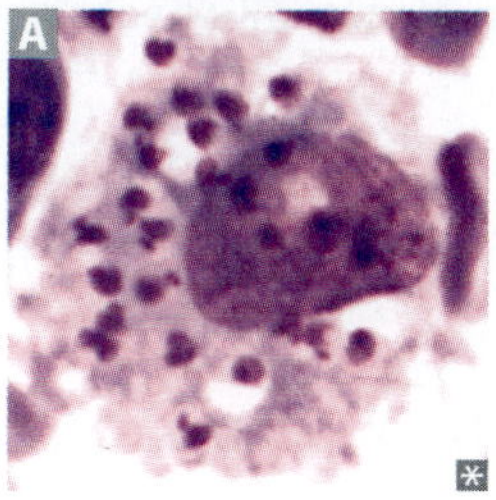

Phagocytoses bacteria, cellular debris, and senescent RBCs. Long life in tissues. Macrophages differentiate from circulating blood monocytes A. Activated by γ-interferon. Can function as antigen-presenting cell via MHC II.

Macro = large; *phage* = eater.
Macrophage: in the tissue.
Important component of granuloma formation (eg, TB, sarcoidosis).
Lipid A from bacterial LPS binds CD14 on macrophages to initiate septic shock.

Eosinophil

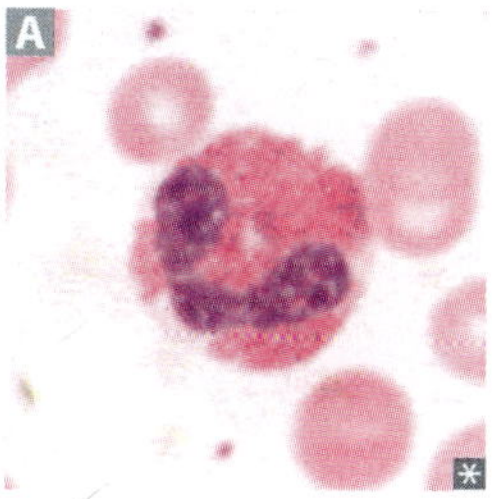

Defends against helminthic infections (major basic protein). Bilobate nucleus. Packed with large eosinophilic granules of uniform size A. Highly phagocytic for antigen-antibody complexes.
Produces histaminase and major basic protein (MBP, a helminthotoxin).

Eosin = pink dye; *philic* = loving.
Causes of eosinophilia = **NAACP**:
- **N**eoplasia
- **A**sthma
- **A**llergic processes
- **C**hronic adrenal insufficiency
- **P**arasites (invasive)

Basophil

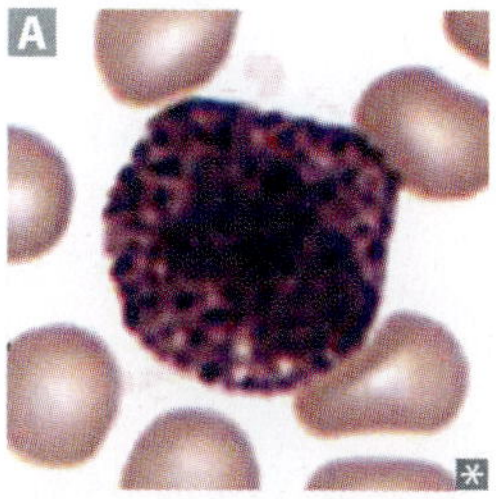

Mediates allergic reaction. Densely basophilic granules A contain heparin (anticoagulant) and histamine (vasodilator). Leukotrienes synthesized and released on demand.

Basophilic—staining readily with **basic** stains.
Basophilia is uncommon, but can be a sign of myeloproliferative disease, particularly CML.

- circulate in blood (mast cells are in tissues only - skin, GI/resp mucosa)
- have IgE-R

Mast cell

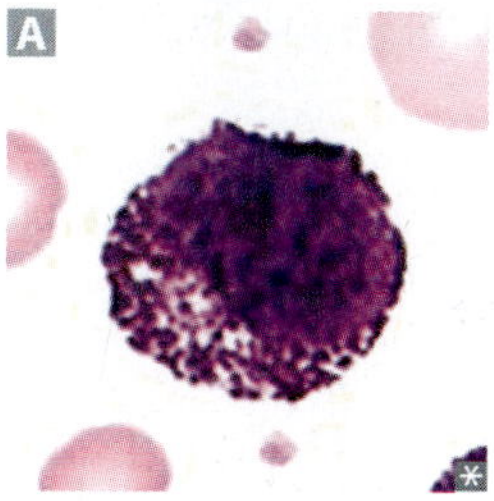

Mediates allergic reaction in local tissues. Mast cells contain basophilic granules A and originate from the same precursor as basophils but are not the same cell type. Can bind the Fc portion of IgE to membrane. IgE cross-links upon antigen binding → degranulation → release of histamine, heparin, tryptase, and eosinophil chemotactic factors.

- Have TLRs*

Involved in type I hypersensitivity reactions.
Cromolyn sodium prevents mast cell degranulation (used for asthma prophylaxis).

Dendritic cell

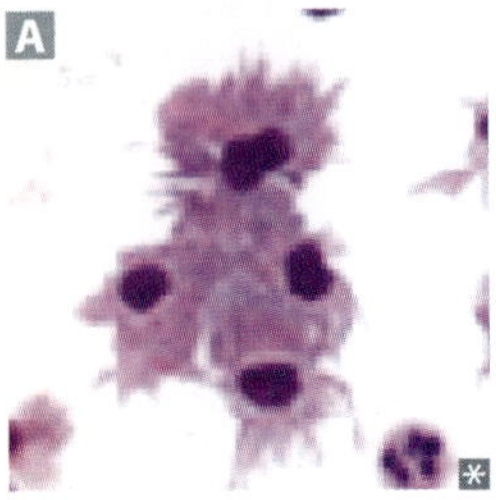

Highly phagocytic APC A. Functions as link between innate and adaptive immune systems. Expresses MHC class II and Fc receptors on surface. Called Langerhans cell in the skin.

Lymphocyte

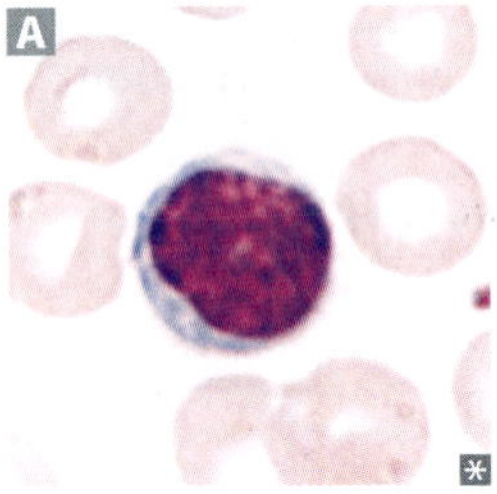

Refers to B cells, T cells, and NK cells. B cells and T cells mediate adaptive immunity. NK cells are part of the innate immune response. Round, densely staining nucleus with small amount of pale cytoplasm A.

B cell

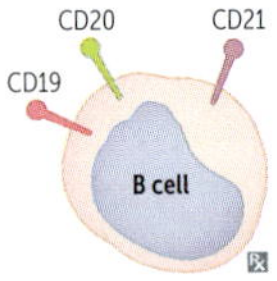

Part of humoral immune response. Originates from stem cells in bone marrow and matures in marrow. Migrates to peripheral lymphoid tissue (follicles of lymph nodes, white pulp of spleen, unencapsulated lymphoid tissue). When antigen is encountered, B cells differentiate into plasma cells (which produce antibodies) and memory cells. Can function as an APC via MHC II.

B = **B**one marrow.

T cell

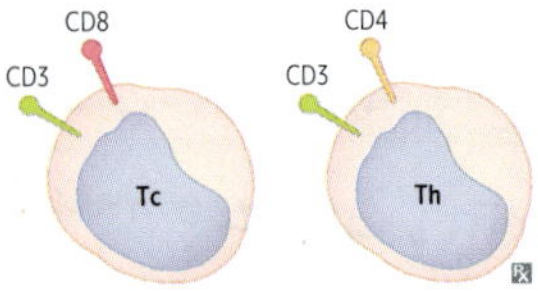

Mediates cellular immune response. Originates from stem cells in the bone marrow, but matures in the thymus. T cells differentiate into cytotoxic T cells (express CD8, recognize MHC I), helper T cells (express CD4, recognize MHC II), and regulatory T cells. CD28 (costimulatory signal) necessary for T-cell activation. The majority of circulating lymphocytes are T cells (80%).

T is for **T**hymus.

CD4+ helper T cells are the primary target of HIV.

MHC × CD = 8 (eg, MHC 2 × CD4 = 8, and MHC 1 × CD8 = 8).

Plasma cell

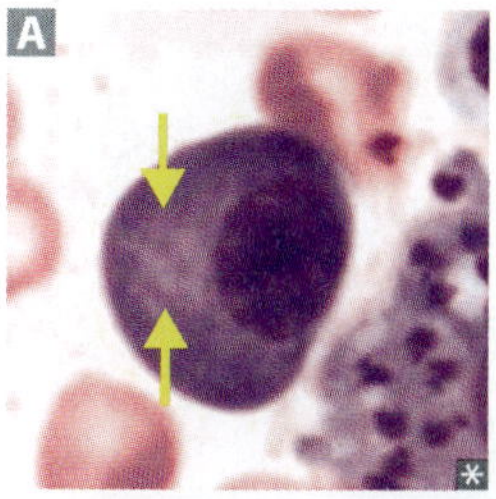

Produces large amounts of antibody specific to a particular antigen. "Clock-face" chromatin distribution and eccentric nucleus, abundant RER, and well-developed Golgi apparatus (yellow arrows in A). Found in bone marrow and normally do not circulate in peripheral blood.

Multiple myeloma is a plasma cell cancer.

▶ HEMATOLOGY AND ONCOLOGY—PHYSIOLOGY

Fetal erythropoiesis

Fetal erythropoiesis occurs in:
- **Y**olk sac (3–8 weeks)
- **L**iver (6 weeks–birth)
- **S**pleen (10–28 weeks)
- **B**one marrow (18 weeks to adult)

Young **L**iver **S**ynthesizes **B**lood.

Hemoglobin development

Embryonic globins: ζ and ε.
Fetal hemoglobin (HbF) = $\alpha_2\gamma_2$.
Adult hemoglobin (HbA_1) = $\alpha_2\beta_2$.
HbF has higher affinity for O_2 due to less avid binding of 2,3-BPG, allowing HbF to extract O_2 from maternal hemoglobin (HbA_1 and HbA_2) across the placenta.

From fetal to adult hemoglobin:
Alpha **A**lways; **G**amma **G**oes, **B**ecomes **B**eta.

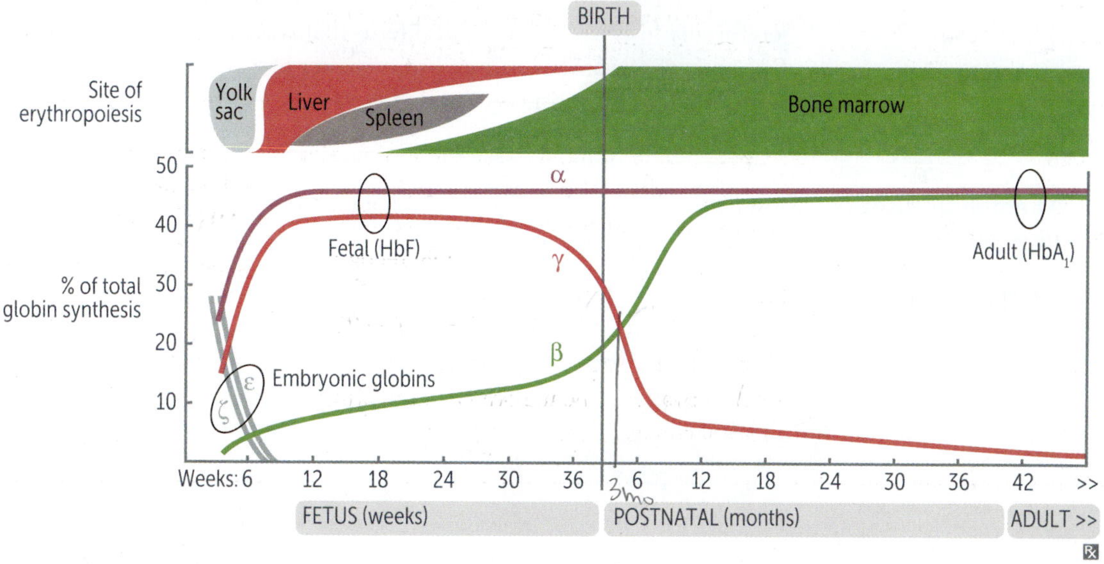

Blood groups

	ABO classification				Rh classification	
	A	B	AB	O	Rh⊕	Rh⊖
RBC type	A	B	AB	O		
Group antigens on RBC surface	A	B	A & B	None	Rh (D)	None
Antibodies in plasma	Anti-B IgM	Anti-A IgM	None	Anti-A Anti-B IgM	None	Anti-D IgG
Clinical relevance	Receive B or AB → hemolytic reaction	Receive A or AB → hemolytic reaction	Universal recipient of RBCs; universal donor of plasma	Receive any non-O → hemolytic reaction Universal donor of RBCs; universal recipient of plasma	Universal recipient of RBCs	Treat mother with anti-D Ig (RhoGAM) during and after each pregnancy to prevent anti-D IgG formation

IgM – A/B
IgG – Rh (can but preg prob)

Rh hemolytic disease of the newborn

IgM does not cross placenta; IgG does cross placenta.
Rh⊖ mothers exposed to fetal Rh⊕ blood (often during delivery) may make anti-D IgG. In subsequent pregnancies, anti-D IgG crosses the placenta → hemolytic disease of the newborn (erythroblastosis fetalis) in the next fetus that is Rh⊕. Administration of anti-D IgG (RhoGAM) to Rh⊖ pregnant women during third trimester prevents maternal anti-D IgG production.
Rh⊖ mothers have anti-D IgG only if previously exposed to Rh⊕ blood.

ABO hemolytic disease of the newborn

Most common form. Usually occurs in a type O mother with a type A, B, or AB fetus. Can occur in a first pregnancy as maternal anti-A and/or anti-B IgG antibodies are formed early in life. Does not worsen with future pregnancies. Presents as mild jaundice in the neonate within 24 hours of birth; treatment is phototherapy or exchange transfusion.

I guess anti-ABO are preformed but anti-Rh are not until a preg/transfus exposes u

- anti A & B in O ppl tend to be IgG (cross placenta)
& in anti B only or anti-A only = IgM

Hemoglobin electrophoresis

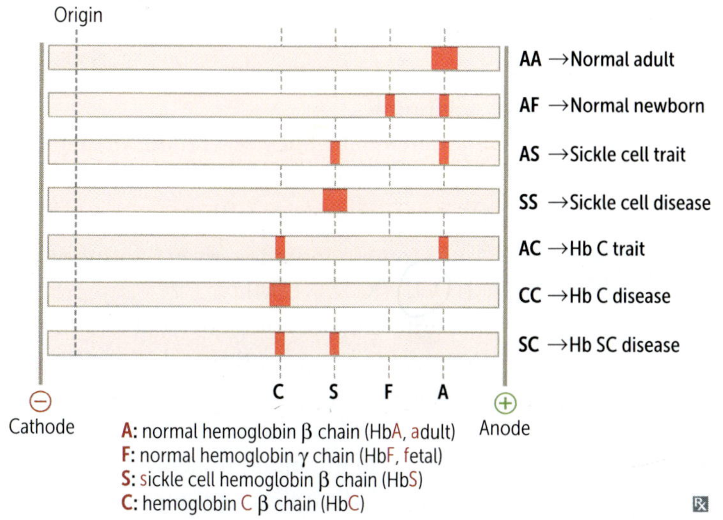

On a gel, hemoglobin migrates from the negatively charged cathode to the positively charged anode. HbA migrates the farthest, followed by HbS, followed by HbC. This is because the missense mutations in HbS and HbC replace glutamic acid ⊖ with valine (neutral) and lysine ⊕, respectively, impacting the net protein charge.

A Fat Santa Claus

Coagulation and kinin pathways

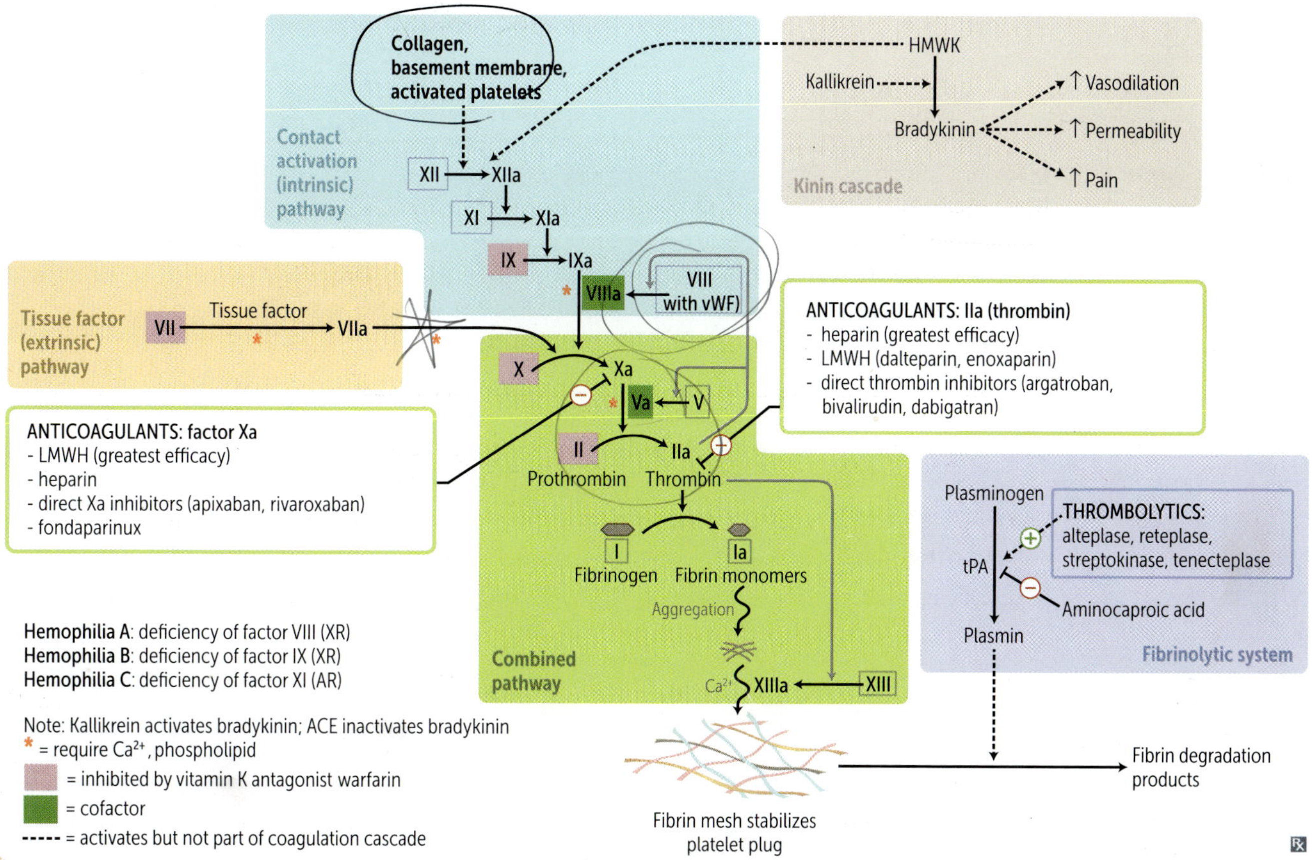

Coagulation cascade components

Procoagulation

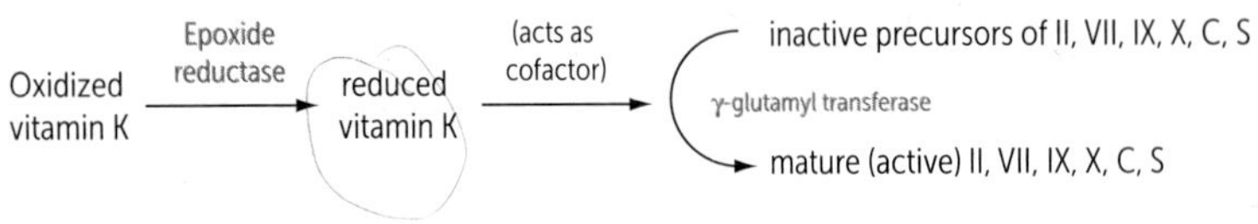

Warfarin inhibits the enzyme vitamin K epoxide reductase.
Neonates lack enteric bacteria, which produce vitamin K.
Vitamin K deficiency: ↓ synthesis of factors II, VII, IX, X, protein C, protein S.
vWF carries/protects VIII.

Anticoagulation

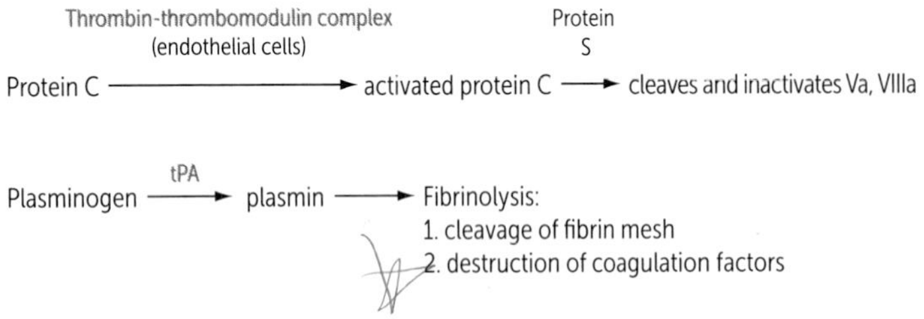

Antithrombin inhibits activated forms of factors II, VII, IX, X, XI, XII.
Heparin enhances the activity of antithrombin.
Principal targets of antithrombin: thrombin and factor Xa.
Factor V Leiden mutation produces a factor V resistant to inhibition by activated protein C.
tPA is used clinically as a thrombolytic.

Platelet plug formation (primary hemostasis)

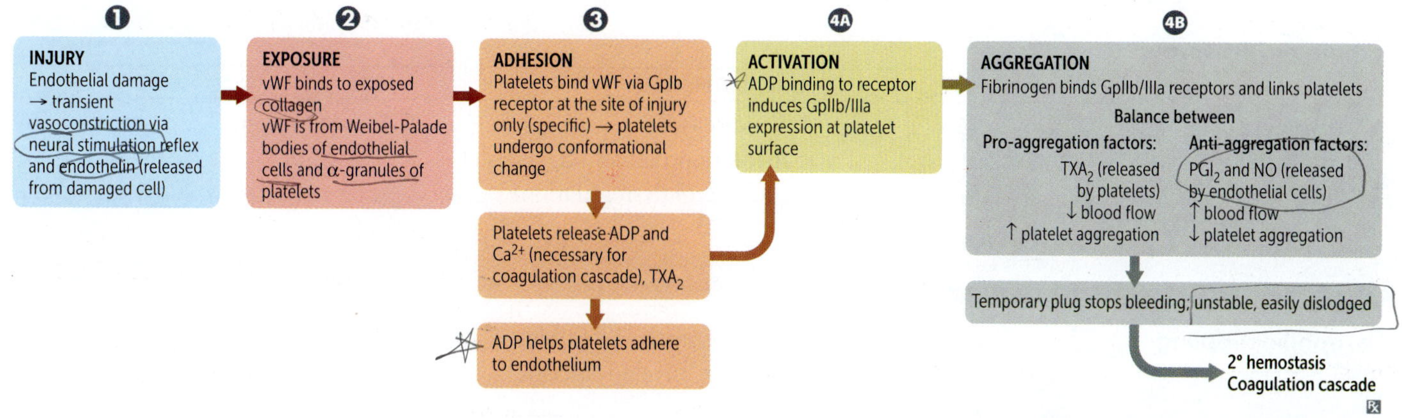

Thrombogenesis

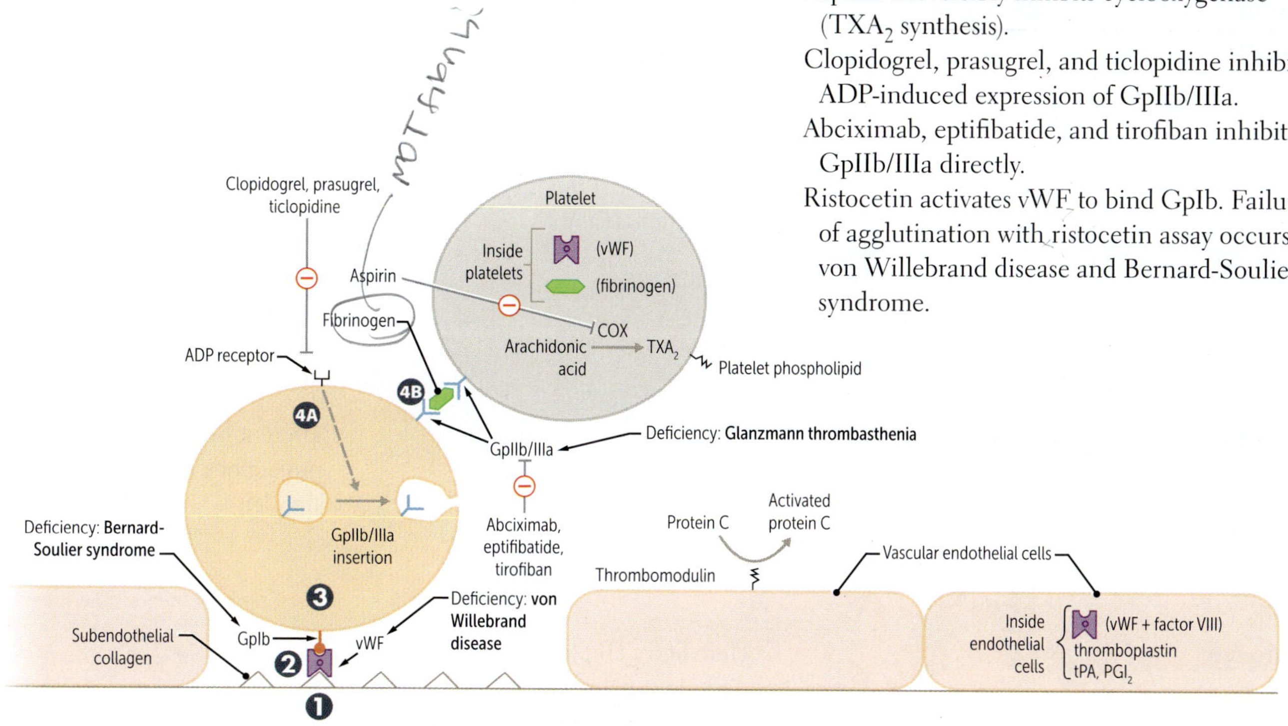

Formation of insoluble fibrin mesh.

Aspirin irreversibly inhibits cyclooxygenase (TXA_2 synthesis).

Clopidogrel, prasugrel, and ticlopidine inhibit ADP-induced expression of GpIIb/IIIa.

Abciximab, eptifibatide, and tirofiban inhibit GpIIb/IIIa directly.

Ristocetin activates vWF to bind GpIb. Failure of agglutination with ristocetin assay occurs in von Willebrand disease and Bernard-Soulier syndrome.

▸ HEMATOLOGY AND ONCOLOGY—PATHOLOGY

Pathologic RBC forms

TYPE	EXAMPLE	ASSOCIATED PATHOLOGY	NOTES
Acanthocyte ("spur cell")	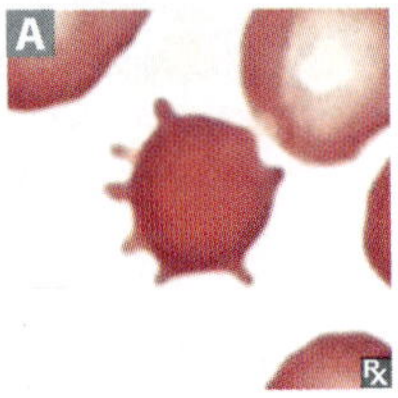	Liver disease, abetalipoproteinemia (states of cholesterol dysregulation).	*Acantho* = spiny.
Basophilic stippling	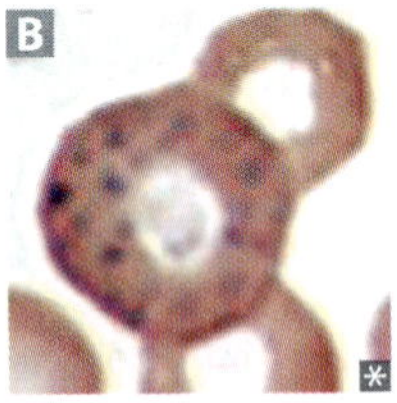	Lead poisoning, sideroblastic anemias, myelodysplastic syndromes.	
Dacrocyte ("teardrop cell")	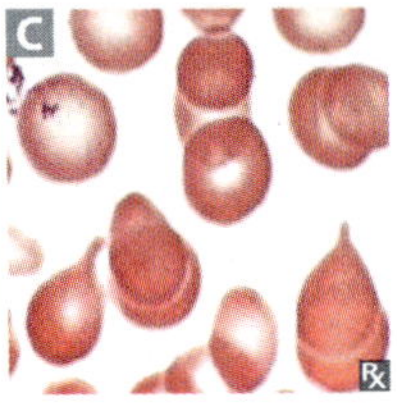	Bone marrow infiltration (eg, myelofibrosis).	RBC "sheds a **tear**" because it's mechanically squeezed out of its home in the bone marrow.
Degmacyte ("bite cell")	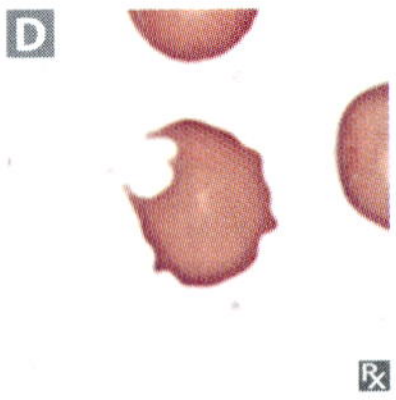	G6PD deficiency.	
Echinocyte ("burr cell")	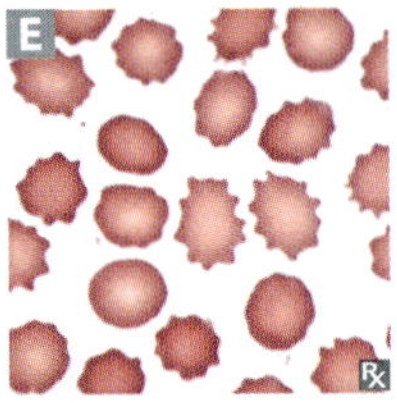	End-stage renal disease, liver disease, pyruvate kinase deficiency.	Different from acanthocyte; its projections are more uniform and smaller.
Elliptocyte	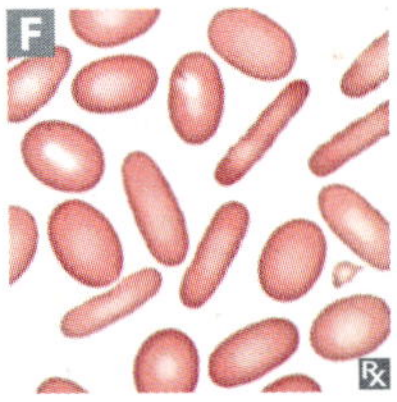	Hereditary elliptocytosis, usually asymptomatic; caused by mutation in genes encoding RBC membrane proteins (eg, spectrin).	
Macro-ovalocyte	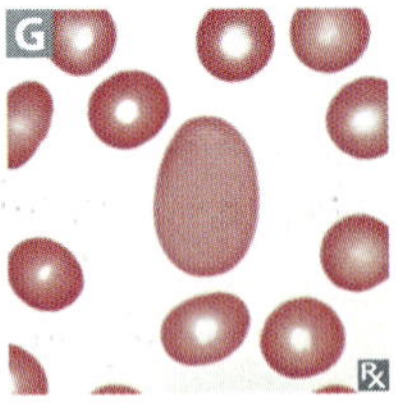	Megaloblastic anemia (also hypersegmented PMNs), marrow failure.	

Pathologic RBC forms *(continued)*

TYPE	EXAMPLE	ASSOCIATED PATHOLOGY	NOTES
Ringed sideroblast	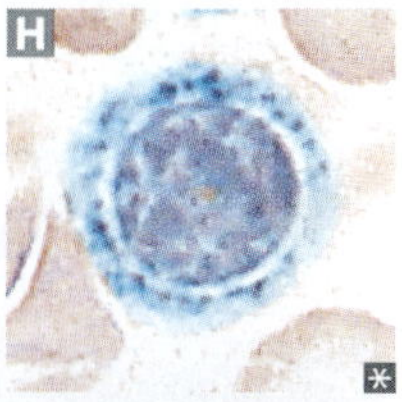	Sideroblastic anemia. Excess iron in mitochondria.	
Schistocyte	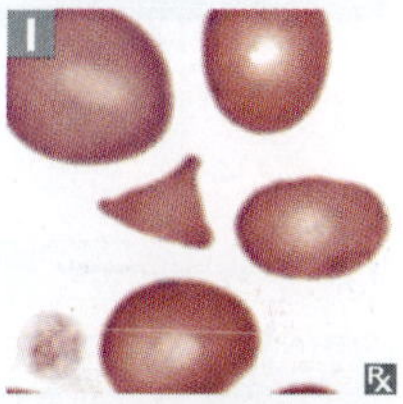	DIC, TTP/HUS, HELLP syndrome, mechanical hemolysis (eg, heart valve prosthesis).	Examples include helmet cell.
Sickle cell	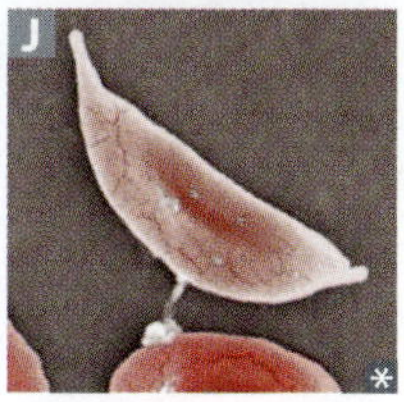	Sickle cell anemia.	Sickling occurs with dehydration, deoxygenation, and at high altitude.
Spherocyte	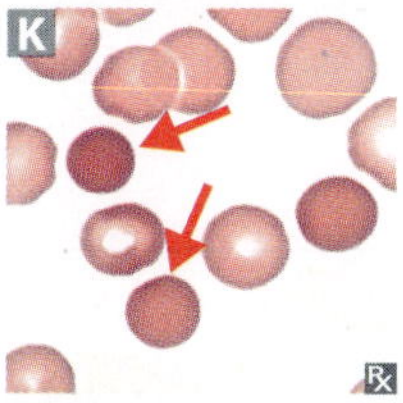	Hereditary spherocytosis, drug- and infection-induced hemolytic anemia.	
Target cell	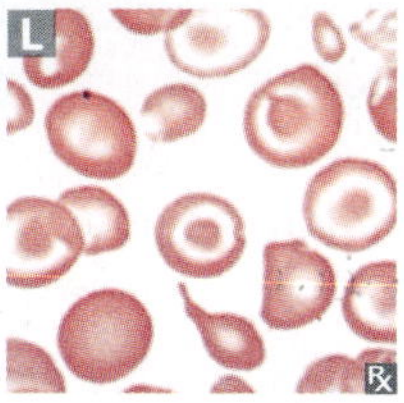	**H**bC disease, **A**splenia, **L**iver disease, **T**halassemia.	"**HALT**," said the hunter to his **target**.

Other RBC abnormalities

TYPE	EXAMPLE	ASSOCIATED PATHOLOGY	NOTES
Heinz bodies	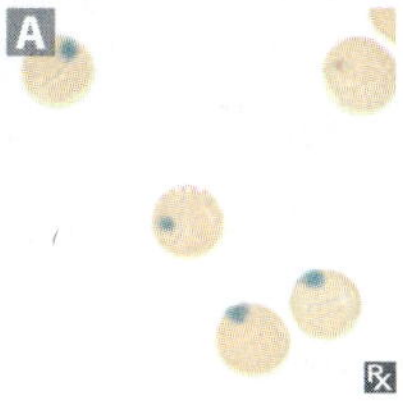	Seen in G6PD deficiency.	Oxidation of Hb -SH groups to -S—S- → Hb precipitation (Heinz bodies), with subsequent phagocytic damage to RBC membrane → bite cells.
Howell-Jolly bodies	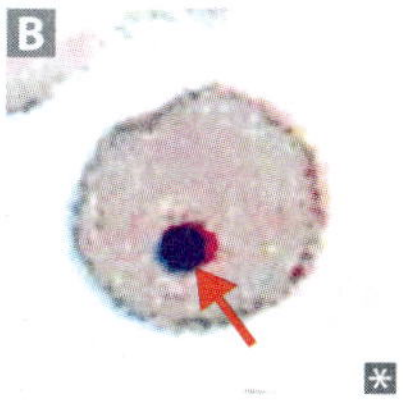	Seen in patients with functional hyposplenia or asplenia.	Basophilic nuclear remnants found in RBCs. Howell-Jolly bodies are normally removed from RBCs by splenic macrophages.

Anemias

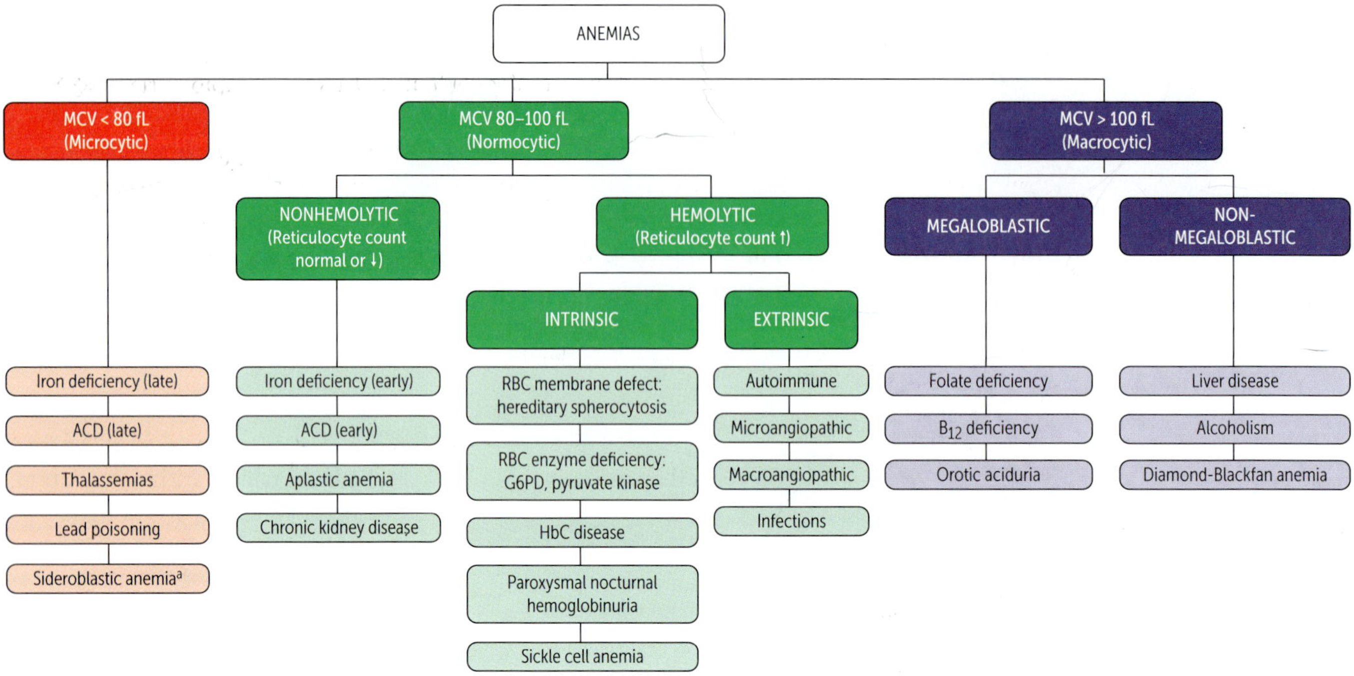

On a peripheral blood smear, a lymphocyte nucleus is approximately the same size as a normocytic RBC. If RBC is larger than lymphocyte nucleus, consider macrocytosis; if RBC is smaller, consider microcytosis.

[a] Copper deficiency can cause a microcytic sideroblastic anemia.

Microcytic (MCV < 80 fL), hypochromic anemia

Iron deficiency

↓ iron due to chronic bleeding (eg, GI loss, menorrhagia), malnutrition, absorption disorders, or ↑ demand (eg, pregnancy) → ↓ final step in heme synthesis.

Labs: ↓ iron, ↑ TIBC, ↓ ferritin. Microcytosis and hypochromasia (central pallor) A.

Symptoms: fatigue, conjunctival pallor B, pica (consumption of nonfood substances), spoon nails (koilonychia). Restless legs, glossitis, angular chelitis

May manifest as Plummer-Vinson syndrome (triad of iron deficiency anemia, esophageal webs, and dysphagia).

α-thalassemia AR

Defect: α-globin gene deletions → ↓ α-globin synthesis. *cis* deletion (both deletions occur on same chromosome) prevalent in Asian populations; *trans* deletion (deletions occur on separate chromosomes) prevalent in African populations.

4 allele deletion: No α-globin. Excess γ-globin forms γ_4 (Hb Barts). Incompatible with life (causes hydrops fetalis).

3 allele deletion: inheritance of chromosome with *cis* deletion + a chromosome with 1 allele deleted → HbH disease. Very little α-globin. Excess β-globin forms β_4 (HbH).

2 allele deletion: less clinically severe anemia.

1 allele deletion: no anemia (clinically silent).

x x | | Asian (cis) | x | x African (trans) # β doesnt aggreg as much as α

x x | | x = HbH disease w/ β4

x x | | x x = hydrops fetalis (all γ = HbBarts = death)

Microcytic (MCV < 80 fL), hypochromic anemia *(continued)*

β-thalassemia	Point mutations in splice sites and promoter sequences → ↓ β-globin synthesis. Prevalent in Mediterranean populations. β-thalassemia minor (heterozygote): β chain is underproduced. Usually asymptomatic. Diagnosis confirmed by ↑ HbA_2 (> 3.5%) on electrophoresis. β-thalassemia major (homozygote): β chain is absent → severe microcytic, hypochromic anemia with target cells and increased anisopoikilocytosis **C** requiring blood transfusion (2° hemochromatosis). Marrow expansion ("crew cut" on skull x-ray) → skeletal deformities. "Chipmunk" facies. Extramedullary hematopoiesis → hepatosplenomegaly. ↑ risk of parvovirus B19–induced aplastic crisis. ↑ HbF ($\alpha_2\gamma_2$). HbF is protective in the infant and disease becomes symptomatic only after 6 months, when fetal hemoglobin declines. HbS/β-thalassemia heterozygote: mild to moderate sickle cell disease depending on amount of β-globin production.
Lead poisoning	Lead inhibits ferrochelatase and ALA dehydratase → ↓ heme synthesis and ↑ RBC protoporphyrin. Also inhibits rRNA degradation → RBCs retain aggregates of rRNA (basophilic stippling). Symptoms of LEAD poisoning: ▪ **L**ead **L**ines on gingivae (Burton lines) and on metaphyses of long bones **D** on x-ray. ▪ **E**ncephalopathy and **E**rythrocyte basophilic stippling. ▪ **A**bdominal colic and sideroblastic **A**nemia. ▪ **D**rops—wrist and foot drop. **D**imercaprol and E**D**TA are 1st line of treatment. **Succ**imer used for chelation for kids (It "**suc**ks" to be a kid who eats lead). Exposure risk ↑ in old houses with chipped paint.
Sideroblastic anemia	Defect in heme synthesis due to X-linked defect in δ-ALA synthase gene. Causes: genetic, acquired (myelodysplastic syndromes), and reversible (alcohol is most common; also lead, vitamin B_6 deficiency, copper deficiency, isoniazid). Lab findings: ↑ iron, normal/↓ TIBC, ↑ ferritin. Ringed sideroblasts (with iron-laden, Prussian blue–stained mitochondria) seen in bone marrow **E**. Peripheral blood smear: basophilic stippling of RBCs. Treatment: pyridoxine (B_6, cofactor for δ-ALA synthase).

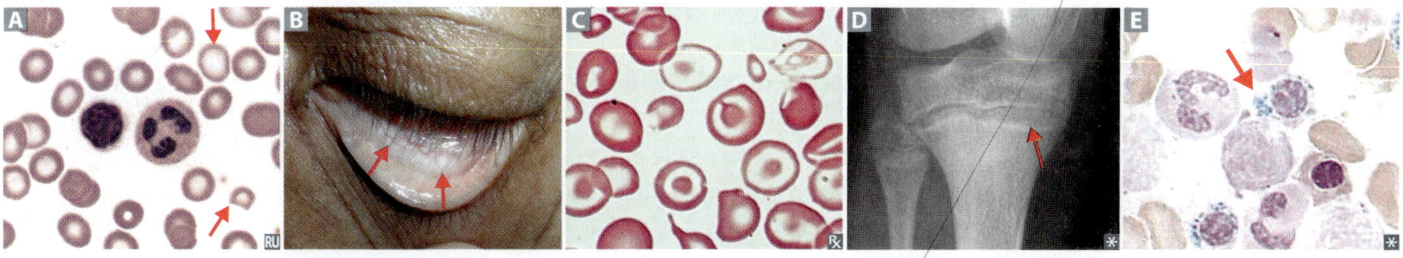

Macrocytic (MCV > 100 fL) anemia

	DESCRIPTION	FINDINGS
Megaloblastic anemia A 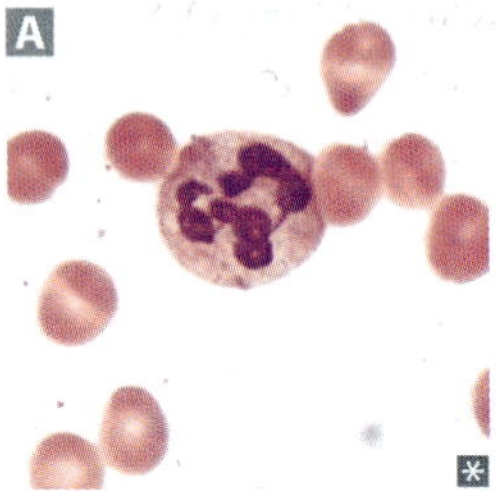	Impaired DNA synthesis → maturation of nucleus of precursor cells in bone marrow delayed relative to maturation of cytoplasm.	RBC macrocytosis, hypersegmented neutrophils A, glossitis.
Folate deficiency	Causes: malnutrition (eg, alcoholics), malabsorption, drugs (eg, methotrexate, trimethoprim, phenytoin), ↑ requirement (eg, hemolytic anemia, pregnancy).	↑ homocysteine, normal methylmalonic acid. **No neurologic symptoms** (vs B_{12} deficiency).
Vitamin B_{12} (cobalamin) deficiency	Causes: insufficient intake (eg, veganism), malabsorption (eg, Crohn disease), pernicious anemia, *Diphyllobothrium latum* (fish tapeworm), gastrectomy.	↑ homocysteine, ↑ methylmalonic acid. **Neurologic symptoms:** subacute combined degeneration (due to involvement of B_{12} in fatty acid pathways and myelin synthesis): spinocerebellar tract, lateral corticospinal tract, dorsal column dysfunction. Historically diagnosed with the Schilling test, a 4-stage test that determines if the cause is dietary insufficiency vs malabsorption.
Orotic aciduria	Inability to convert orotic acid to UMP (de novo pyrimidine synthesis pathway) because of defect in UMP synthase. Autosomal recessive. Presents in children as failure to thrive, developmental delay, and megaloblastic anemia refractory to folate and B_{12}. No hyperammonemia (vs ornithine transcarbamylase deficiency—↑ orotic acid with hyperammonemia).	Orotic acid in urine. Treatment: uridine monophosphate to bypass mutated enzyme.
Diamond-Blackfan anemia	Rapid-onset anemia within 1st year of life due to intrinsic defect in erythroid progenitor cells.	↑ % HbF (but ↓ total Hb). Short stature, craniofacial abnormalities, and upper extremity malformations (triphalangeal thumbs) in up to 50% of cases.
Nonmegaloblastic anemia	Macrocytic anemia in which DNA synthesis is unimpaired. Causes: alcoholism, liver disease.	RBC macrocytosis without hypersegmented neutrophils.

Normocytic, normochromic anemia	Normocytic, normochromic anemias are classified as nonhemolytic or hemolytic. The hemolytic anemias are further classified according to the cause of the hemolysis (intrinsic vs extrinsic to the RBC) and by the location of the hemolysis (intravascular vs extravascular).
Intravascular hemolysis	Findings: ↓ haptoglobin, ↑ LDH, schistocytes and ↑ reticulocytes on blood smear. Characteristic hemoglobinuria, hemosiderinuria, and urobilinogen in urine. May also see ↑ unconjugated bilirubin. Notable causes are mechanical hemolysis (eg, prosthetic valve), paroxysmal nocturnal hemoglobinuria, microangiopathic hemolytic anemias.
Extravascular hemolysis	Findings: macrophages in spleen clear RBCs. Spherocytes in peripheral smear, ↑ LDH, no hemoglobinuria/hemosiderinuria, ↑ unconjugated bilirubin, which can cause jaundice. Can present with urobilinogen in urine.

Nonhemolytic, normocytic anemia

	DESCRIPTION	FINDINGS
Anemia of chronic disease	Inflammation → ↑ hepcidin (released by liver, binds ferroportin on intestinal mucosal cells and macrophages, thus inhibiting iron transport) → ↓ release of iron from macrophages and ↓ iron absorption from gut. Associated with conditions such as rheumatoid arthritis, SLE, neoplastic disorders, and chronic kidney disease.	↓ iron, ↓ TIBC, ↑ ferritin. Normocytic, but can become microcytic. Treatment: EPO (chronic kidney disease only). #Notice how a pt can have anemia w/ normal RBCs.
Aplastic anemia 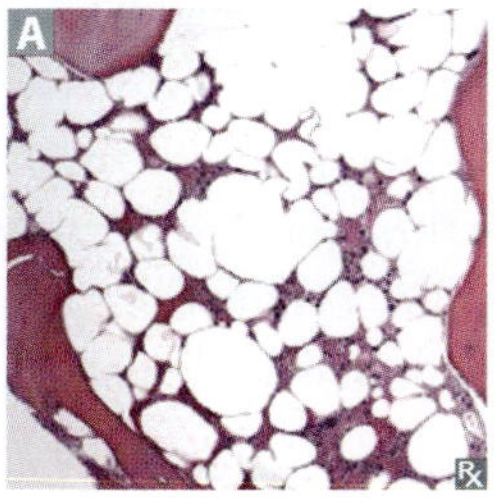	Caused by failure or destruction of myeloid stem cells due to: ▪ Radiation and drugs (benzene, chloramphenicol, alkylating agents, antimetabolites) ▪ Viral agents (parvovirus B19, EBV, HIV, hepatitis viruses) ▪ Fanconi anemia (DNA repair defect causing bone marrow failure); also short stature, ↑ incidence of tumors/leukemia, café-au-lait spots, thumb/radial defects ▪ Idiopathic (immune mediated, 1° stem cell defect); may follow acute hepatitis	↓ reticulocyte count, ↑ EPO. Pancytopenia characterized by severe anemia, leukopenia, and thrombocytopenia. Normal cell morphology, but hypocellular bone marrow with fatty infiltration A (dry bone marrow tap). Symptoms: fatigue, malaise, pallor, purpura, mucosal bleeding, petechiae, infection. Treatment: withdrawal of offending agent, immunosuppressive regimens (eg, antithymocyte globulin, cyclosporine), bone marrow allograft, RBC/platelet transfusion, bone marrow stimulation (eg, GM-CSF).

TIBC = apo (2/3) + holo (full) (1/3)

Serum Fe = holo

Serum Fe / TIBC = % bound

Intrinsic hemolytic anemia

	DESCRIPTION	FINDINGS
Hereditary spherocytosis	Extravascular hemolysis due to defect in proteins interacting with RBC membrane skeleton and plasma membrane (eg, ankyrin, band 3, protein 4.2, spectrin). Results in small, round RBCs with less surface area and no central pallor (↑ MCHC) → premature removal by spleen.	Splenomegaly, aplastic crisis (parvovirus B19 infection). Labs: osmotic fragility test ⊕. Normal to ↓ MCV with abundance of cells. Treatment: splenectomy.
G6PD deficiency	Most common enzymatic disorder of RBCs. Causes extravascular and intravascular hemolysis. X-linked recessive. Defect in G6PD → ↓ glutathione → ↑ RBC susceptibility to oxidant stress. Hemolytic anemia following oxidant stress (eg, sulfa drugs, antimalarials, infections, **fava beans**).	Back pain, hemoglobinuria a few days after oxidant **stress**. Labs: blood smear shows RBCs with **Heinz** bodies and **bite** cells. "**Stress** makes me eat **bites** of **fava beans** with **Heinz** ketchup."
Pyruvate kinase deficiency	Autosomal recessive. Defect in pyruvate kinase → ↓ ATP → rigid RBCs → extravascular hemolysis.	Hemolytic anemia in a newborn.
HbC disease	Glutamic acid–to-lysine mutation in β-globin. Causes extravascular hemolysis.	Patients with HbSC (1 of each mutant gene) have milder disease than HbSS patients. Labs (homozygotes): blood smear shows hemoglobin crystals inside RBCs and target cells.
Paroxysmal nocturnal hemoglobinuria	↑ complement-mediated intravascular RBC lysis (impaired synthesis of GPI anchor for decay-accelerating factor that protects RBC membrane from complement). Acquired mutation in a hematopoietic stem cell. ↑ incidence of acute leukemias.	Triad: Coombs ⊖ hemolytic anemia, pancytopenia, and venous thrombosis. Labs: CD55/59 ⊖ RBCs on flow cytometry. Treatment: eculizumab (terminal complement inhibitor).
Sickle cell anemia A 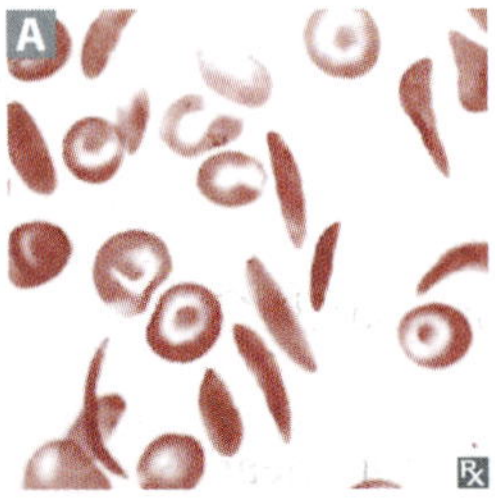 B 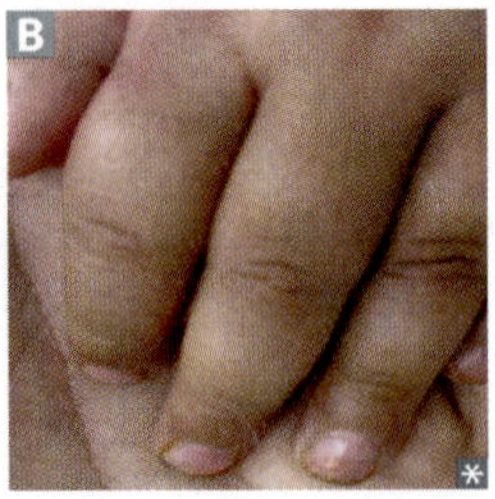	HbS point mutation causes a single amino acid replacement in β chain (substitution of glutamic acid with valine). Causes extravascular and intravascular hemolysis. Pathogenesis: low O_2, high altitude, or acidosis precipitates sickling (deoxygenated HbS polymerizes) → anemia and vaso-occlusive disease. Newborns are initially asymptomatic because of ↑ HbF and ↓ HbS. Heterozygotes (sickle cell trait) also have resistance to malaria. 8% of African Americans carry an HbS allele. Sickle cells are crescent-shaped RBCs A. "Crew cut" on skull x-ray due to marrow expansion from ↑ erythropoiesis (also seen in thalassemias).	Complications in sickle cell disease: ▪ Aplastic crisis (due to parvovirus B19). ▪ Autosplenectomy (Howell-Jolly bodies) → ↑ risk of infection by encapsulated organisms (eg, *S pneumoniae*). ▪ Splenic infarct/sequestration crisis. ▪ *Salmonella* osteomyelitis. ▪ Painful crises (vaso-occlusive): dactylitis B (painful swelling of hands/feet), priapism, acute chest syndrome, avascular necrosis, stroke. ▪ Renal papillary necrosis (↓ Po_2 in papilla) and microhematuria (medullary infarcts). Diagnosis: hemoglobin electrophoresis. Treatment: hydroxyurea (↑ HbF), hydration.

Extrinsic hemolytic anemia

	DESCRIPTION	FINDINGS
Autoimmune hemolytic anemia 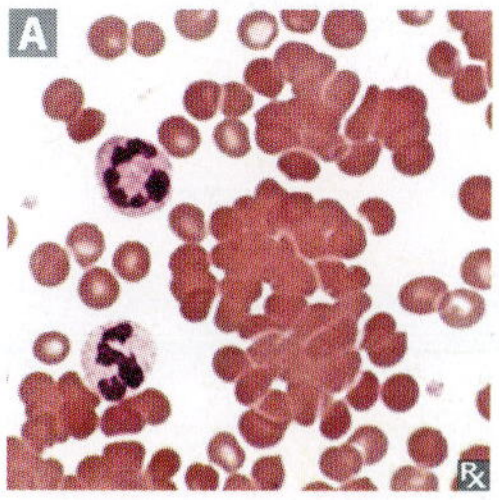	**Warm** (IgG)—chronic anemia seen in SLE and CLL and with certain drugs (eg, α-methyldopa) ("**warm** weather is **G**reat"). **Cold** (Ig**M** and complement)—acute anemia triggered by cold; seen in CLL, ***M**ycoplasma pneumonia* infections, and infectious **M**ononucleosis ("**cold** weather is **MMM**iserable"). RBC agglutinates **A** may cause painful, blue fingers and toes with cold exposure. Many warm and cold AIHAs are idiopathic in etiology.	Autoimmune hemolytic anemias are usually Coombs ⊕. Direct Coombs test—anti-Ig antibody (Coombs reagent) added to patient's blood. RBCs agglutinate if RBCs are coated with Ig. Indirect Coombs test—normal RBCs added to patient's serum. If serum has anti-RBC surface Ig, RBCs agglutinate when Coombs reagent added.

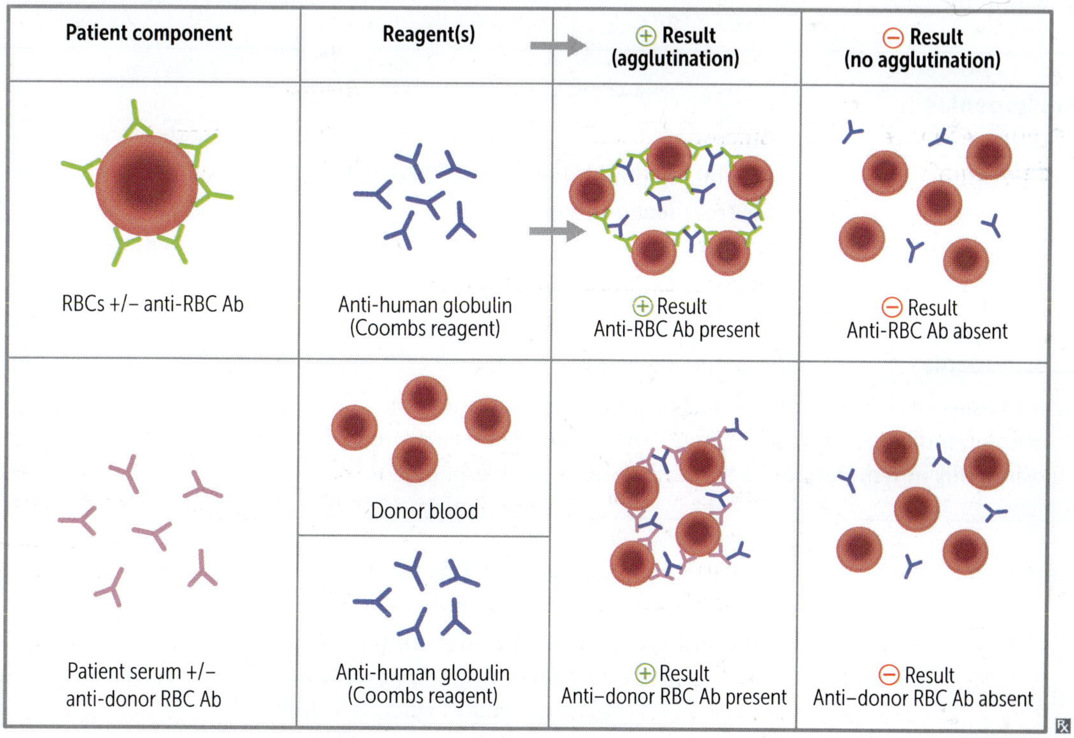

Microangiopathic anemia	Pathogenesis: RBCs are damaged when passing through obstructed or narrowed vessel lumina. Seen in DIC, TTP/HUS, SLE, and malignant hypertension.	**Schisto**cytes (eg, "helmet cells") are seen on peripheral blood smear due to mechanical destruction (***schisto*** = to split) of RBCs.
Macroangiopathic anemia	Prosthetic heart valves and aortic stenosis may also cause hemolytic anemia 2° to mechanical destruction of RBCs.	Schistocytes on peripheral blood smear.
Infections	↑ destruction of RBCs (eg, malaria, *Babesia*).	

Lab values in anemia

	Iron deficiency	Chronic disease	Hemochromatosis	Pregnancy/OCP use
Serum iron	↓ (1°)	↓	↑ (1°)	—
Transferrin or TIBC	↑	↓[a]	↓	↑ (1°)
Ferritin	↓	↑ (1°)	↑	—
% transferrin saturation (serum iron/TIBC)	↓↓	—	↑↑	↓

Transferrin—**trans**ports iron in blood.
TIBC—indirectly measures transferrin.
Ferritin—1° iron storage protein of body.
[a] Evolutionary reasoning—pathogens use circulating iron to thrive. The body has adapted a system in which iron is stored within the cells of the body and prevents pathogens from acquiring circulating iron.

Leukopenias

CELL TYPE	CELL COUNT	CAUSES
Neutropenia	Absolute neutrophil count < 1500 cells/mm^3. Severe infections typical when < 500 cells/mm^3.	Sepsis/postinfection, drugs (including chemotherapy), aplastic anemia, SLE, radiation
Lymphopenia	Absolute lymphocyte count < 1500 cells/mm^3 (< 3000 cells/mm^3 in children)	HIV, DiGeorge syndrome, SCID, SLE, corticosteroids,[a] radiation, sepsis, postoperative
Eosinopenia	Absolute eosinophil count < 30 cells/mm^3	Cushing syndrome, corticosteroids[a]

[a] Corticosteroids cause neutrophilia, despite causing eosinopenia and lymphopenia. Corticosteroids ↓ activation of neutrophil adhesion molecules, impairing migration out of the vasculature to sites of inflammation. In contrast, corticosteroids sequester eosinophils in lymph nodes and cause apoptosis of lymphocytes.

Left shift

↑ neutrophil precursors, such as band cells and metamyelocytes, in peripheral blood. Usually seen with neutrophilia in the acute response to infection or inflammation. Called **leukoerythroblastic reaction** when left shift is seen with immature RBCs; occurs with severe anemia (physiologic response) or marrow response (eg, fibrosis, tumor taking up space in marrow).

A **left shift** is a shift to a more **immature** cell in the maturation process.

TIBC = bound & unbound transferrin
serum Fe = bound transferrin
Transf Fe Sat = serum Fe / TIBC

↑ neut = Ep, Corticost, Lithium, CSFs

Acute Intermitt Porphyria

Abd pain, back, leg, arm
vague pain - toothache like in bones
WORSE w/ drugs of P450.
Then paralysis - fing/toes going up even to lungs
Nausea/constip

Heme synthesis, porphyrias, and lead poisoning

The porphyrias are hereditary or acquired con… accumulation of heme precursors. Lead inhi… leading to a similar condition.

CONDITION	AFFECTED ENZYME	ACCUMULATED SUBSTRATE
Lead poisoning 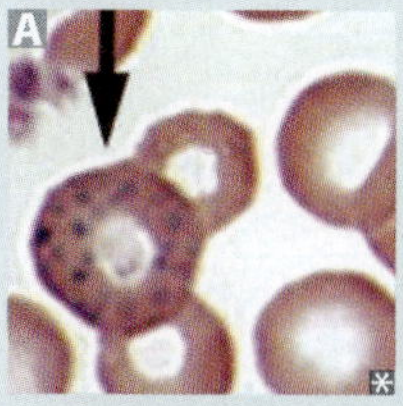	Ferrochelatase and ALA dehydratase ↳ ↓ porphobilinogen	Protoporphyrin, δ-A… (blood)
Acute intermittent porphyria AD	Porphobilinogen deaminase	Porphobilinogen, δ-ALA, coporphobilin… (urine)
Porphyria cutanea tarda AD 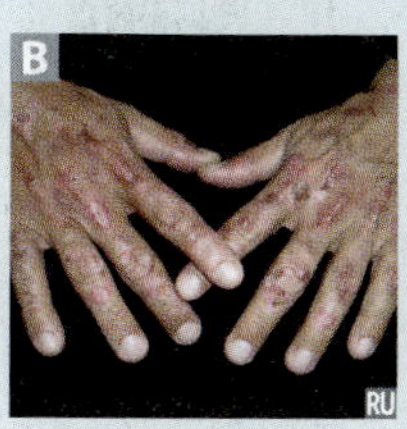	Uroporphyrinogen decarboxylase	Uroporphyrin (… colored urine)

Cutanea tarda
Presents: middle age
skin blisters/burning (extreme) on sun exp. areas.
urine can be any color

Youtube girl had congen erythrop porphyr. (BM & skin porph)
- can lose nose/lips

Any urine color change, psych prob, skin change/bliste consider porphyrias
& esp if its worse w/ meds, she

1. sideroblastic XL (BM) like lead pois this why abd hurts
2. ALA dehyd defic - AR
Acute Intermitt - AD] hepatic + nervous syst
Hepatoerythropoeh. - AR
3. congen Erythropoeitic protop - AR
4. Heredit coproporphyria - AD] hep nerv skin
Variegate porphyria - AD
5. Cutanea Tarda

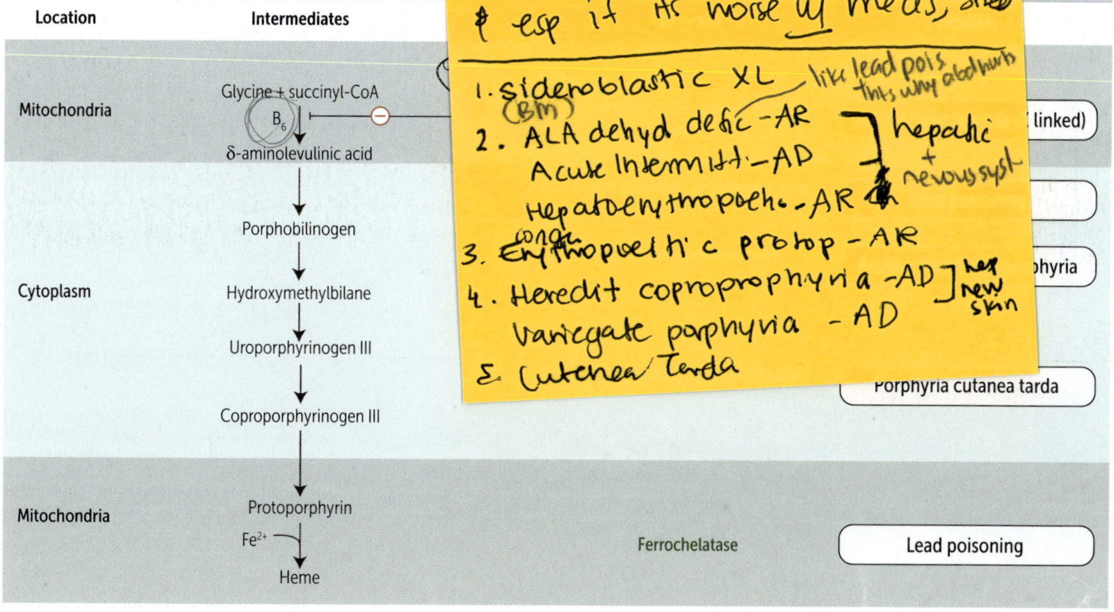

↓ heme → ↑ ALA synthase activity
↑ heme → ↓ ALA synthase activity

Iron poisoning	High mortality rate with accidental ingestion by children (adult iron tablets may look like candy).
MECHANISM	Cell death due to peroxidation of membrane lipids.
SYMPTOMS/SIGNS	Nausea, vomiting, gastric bleeding, lethargy, scarring leading to GI obstruction.
TREATMENT	Chelation (eg, IV deferoxamine, oral deferasirox) and dialysis.

Coagulation disorders

PT—tests function of common and extrinsic pathway (factors I, II, V, VII, and X). Defect → ↑ PT.

INR (international normalized ratio)—calculated from PT. 1 = normal, > 1 = prolonged. Most common test used to follow patients on warfarin.

PTT—tests function of common and intrinsic pathway (all factors except VII and XIII). Defect → ↑ PTT.

DISORDER	PT	PTT	MECHANISM AND COMMENTS
Hemophilia A, B, or C 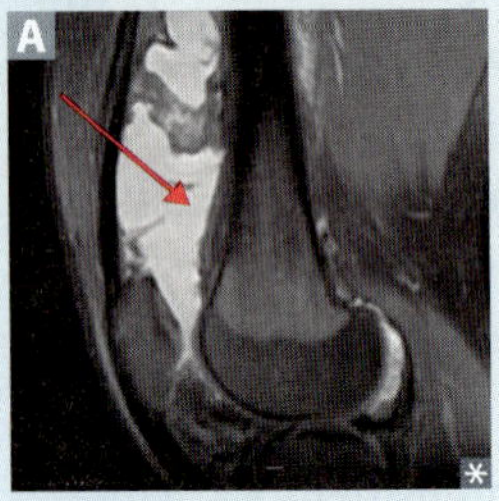	—	↑	Intrinsic pathway coagulation defect. ▪ A: deficiency of factor VIII → ↑ PTT; X-linked recessive. ▪ B: deficiency of factor IX → ↑ PTT; X-linked recessive. ▪ C: deficiency of factor XI → ↑ PTT; autosomal recessive. Macrohemorrhage in hemophilia—hemarthroses (bleeding into joints, such as knee A), easy bruising, bleeding after trauma or surgery (eg, dental procedures). Treatment: desmopressin + factor VIII concentrate (A); factor IX concentrate (B); factor XI concentrate (C).
Vitamin K deficiency	↑	↑	General coagulation defect. Bleeding time normal. ↓ activity of factors II, VII, IX, X, protein C, protein S.

Platelet disorders

Defects in platelet plug formation → ↑ bleeding time (BT).
Platelet abnormalities → microhemorrhage: mucous membrane bleeding, epistaxis, petechiae, purpura, ↑ bleeding time, possibly decreased platelet count (PC).

DISORDER	PC	BT	MECHANISM AND COMMENTS
Bernard-Soulier syndrome	–/↓	↑	Defect in platelet plug formation. Large platelets. ↓ GpIb → defect in platelet-to-vWF adhesion.
Glanzmann thrombasthenia	–	↑	Defect in platelet plug formation. ↓ GpIIb/IIIa → defect in platelet-to-platelet aggregation. Labs: blood smear shows no platelet clumping.
Hemolytic-uremic syndrome	↓	↑	Characterized by thrombocytopenia, microangiopathic hemolytic anemia, and acute renal failure. Typical HUS is seen in children, accompanied by diarrhea and commonly caused by Shiga toxin-producing *E coli* (STEC) (eg, O157:H7). HUS in adults does not present with diarrhea; STEC infection not required. Same spectrum as TTP, with a similar clinical presentation and same initial treatment of plasmapheresis.
Immune thrombocytopenia	↓	↑	Anti-GpIIb/IIIa antibodies → splenic macrophage consumption of platelet-antibody complex. Commonly due to viral illness. Labs: ↑ megakaryocytes on bone marrow biopsy. Treatment: steroids, IVIG, splenectomy (for refractory ITP).
Thrombotic thrombocytopenic purpura	↓	↑	Inhibition or deficiency of ADAMTS 13 (vWF metalloprotease) → ↓ degradation of vWF multimers. Pathogenesis: ↑ large vWF multimers → ↑ platelet adhesion → ↑ platelet aggregation and thrombosis. Labs: schistocytes, ↑ LDH. Symptoms: pentad of neurologic and renal symptoms, fever, thrombocytopenia, and microangiopathic hemolytic anemia. Treatment: plasmapheresis, steroids.

Mixed platelet and coagulation disorders

DISORDER	PC	BT	PT	PTT	MECHANISM AND COMMENTS
von Willebrand disease AD	—	↑	—	↑[a]	Intrinsic pathway coagulation defect: ↓ vWF → ↑ PTT (vWF acts to carry/protect factor VIII). Defect in platelet plug formation: ↓ vWF → defect in platelet-to-vWF adhesion. Autosomal dominant. Mild but most common inherited bleeding disorder. No platelet aggregation with ristocetin cofactor assay. Treatment: desmopressin, which releases vWF stored in endothelium.
Disseminated intravascular coagulation	↓	↑	↑	↑	Widespread activation of clotting → deficiency in clotting factors → bleeding state. Causes: **S**epsis (gram ⊖), **T**rauma, **O**bstetric complications, acute **P**ancreatitis, **M**alignancy, **N**ephrotic syndrome, **T**ransfusion (**STOP M**aking **N**ew **T**hrombi). Labs: schistocytes, ↑ fibrin degradation products (D-dimers), ↓ fibrinogen, ↓ factors V and VIII.

[a]PTT may also be normal in von Willebrand disease.

Hereditary thrombosis syndromes leading to hypercoagulability

DISEASE	DESCRIPTION
Antithrombin deficiency	Inherited deficiency of antithrombin: has no direct effect on the PT, PTT, or thrombin time but diminishes the increase in PTT following heparin administration. Can also be acquired: renal failure/nephrotic syndrome → antithrombin loss in urine → ↓ inhibition of factors IIa and Xa.
Factor V Leiden	Production of mutant factor V (G → A DNA point mutation → Arg506Gln mutation near the cleavage site) that is resistant to degradation by activated protein C. Most common cause of inherited hypercoagulability in Caucasians. Complications include DVT, cerebral vein thromboses, recurrent pregnancy loss.
Protein C or S deficiency	↓ ability to inactivate factors Va and VIIIa. ↑ risk of thrombotic skin necrosis with hemorrhage after administration of warfarin. If this occurs, think protein C deficiency. Together, protein **C** **C**ancels, and protein **S** **S**tops, **C**oagulation.
Prothrombin gene mutation	Mutation in 3′ untranslated region → ↑ production of prothrombin → ↑ plasma levels and venous clots.

Blood transfusion therapy

COMPONENT	DOSAGE EFFECT	CLINICAL USE
Packed RBCs	↑ Hb and O_2 carrying capacity	Acute blood loss, severe anemia
Platelets	↑ platelet count (↑ ~ 5000/mm^3/unit)	Stop significant bleeding (thrombocytopenia, qualitative platelet defects)
Fresh frozen plasma	↑ coagulation factor levels	DIC, cirrhosis, immediate warfarin reversal
Cryoprecipitate	Contains fibrinogen, factor VIII, factor XIII, vWF, and fibronectin	Coagulation factor deficiencies involving fibrinogen and factor VIII

Blood transfusion risks include infection transmission (low), transfusion reactions, iron overload (may lead to 2° hemochromatosis), hypocalcemia (citrate is a Ca^{2+} chelator), and hyperkalemia (RBCs may lyse in old blood units).

Leukemia vs lymphoma

Leukemia	Lymphoid or myeloid neoplasm with widespread involvement of bone marrow. Tumor cells are usually found in peripheral blood.
Lymphoma	Discrete tumor mass arising from lymph nodes. Presentations often blur definitions.

Hodgkin vs non-Hodgkin lymphoma

Hodgkin	Non-Hodgkin
Localized, single group of nodes; contiguous spread (stage is strongest predictor of prognosis). Many patients have a relatively good prognosis.	Multiple lymph nodes involved; extranodal involvement common; noncontiguous spread.
Characterized by Reed-Sternberg cells.	Majority involve B cells; a few are of T-cell lineage.
Bimodal distribution–young adulthood and > 55 years; more common in men except for nodular sclerosing type.	Can occur in children and adults.
Associated with EBV.	May be associated with HIV and autoimmune diseases.
Constitutional ("B") signs/symptoms: low-grade fever, night sweats, weight loss.	May present with constitutional signs/symptoms.

Reed-Sternberg cells

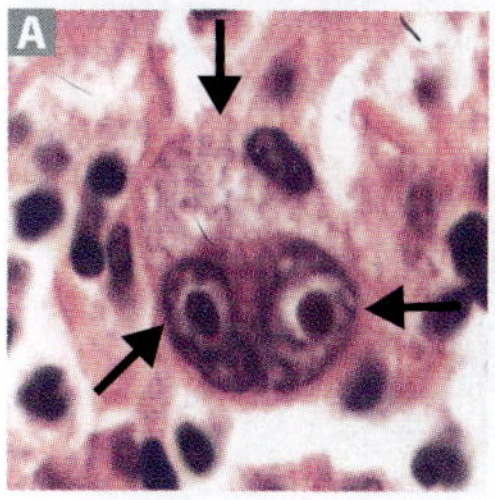

Distinctive tumor giant cell seen in Hodgkin lymphoma; binucleate or bilobed with the 2 halves as mirror images ("owl eyes" A). 2 owl eyes × 15 = 30. RS cells are CD15+ and CD30+ B-cell origin. Necessary but not sufficient for a diagnosis of Hodgkin lymphoma.

Non-Hodgkin lymphoma

TYPE	OCCURS IN	GENETICS	COMMENTS
Neoplasms of mature B cells			
Burkitt lymphoma	Adolescents or young adults	t(8;14)—translocation of c-*myc* (8) and heavy-chain Ig (14)	"Starry sky" appearance, sheets of lymphocytes with interspersed "tingible body" macrophages (arrows in A). Associated with EBV. Jaw lesion B in endemic form in Africa; pelvis or abdomen in sporadic form.
Diffuse large B-cell lymphoma	Usually older adults, but 20% in children		Most common type of non-Hodgkin lymphoma in adults.
Follicular lymphoma	Adults	t(14;18)—translocation of heavy-chain Ig (14) and *BCL-2* (18)	Indolent course; Bcl-2 inhibits apoptosis. Presents with painless "waxing and waning" lymphadenopathy. Follicular architecture: small cleaved cells (grade 1), large cells (grade 3), or mixture (grade 2).
Mantle cell lymphoma	Adult males	t(11;14)—translocation of cyclin D1 (11) and heavy-chain Ig (14)	Very aggressive, patients typically present with late-stage disease.
Primary central nervous system lymphoma	Adults	Most commonly associated with HIV/AIDS	Considered an AIDS-defining illness. Variable presentation: confusion, memory loss, seizures. Mass lesion(s) on MRI, needs to be distinguished from toxoplasmosis via CSF analysis or other lab tests.
Neoplasms of mature T cells			
Adult T-cell lymphoma	Adults	Caused by HTLV (associated with IV drug abuse)	Adults present with cutaneous lesions; especially affects populations in Japan, West Africa, and the Caribbean. Lytic bone lesions, hypercalcemia.
Mycosis fungoides/ Sézary syndrome	Adults		Mycosis fungoides presents with skin patches C/ plaques (cutaneous T-cell lymphoma), characterized by atypical CD4+ cells with "cerebriform" nuclei. May progress to Sézary syndrome (T-cell leukemia).

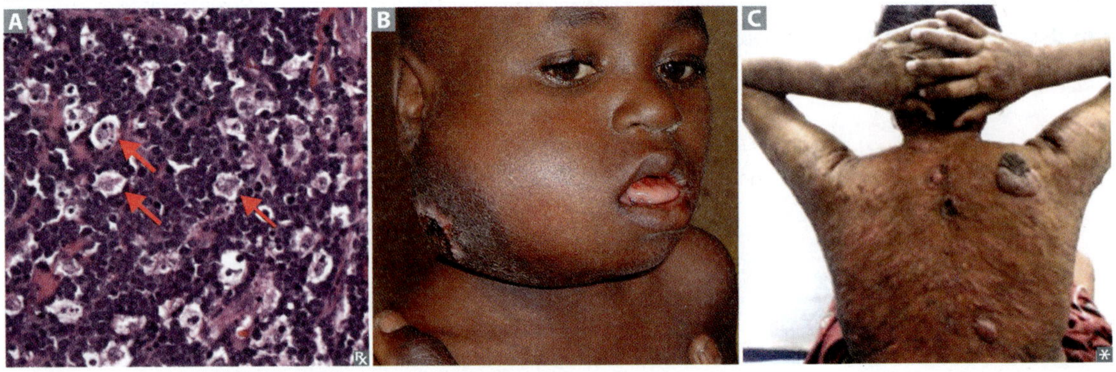

Multiple myeloma

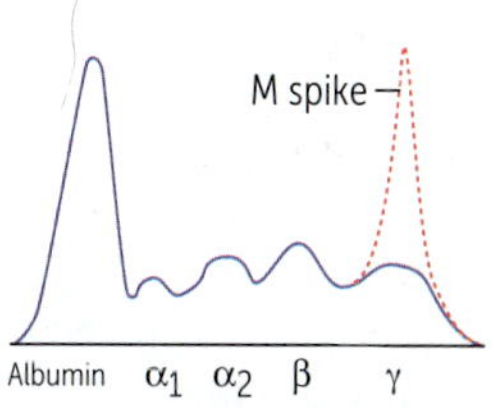

Monoclonal plasma cell ("fried egg" 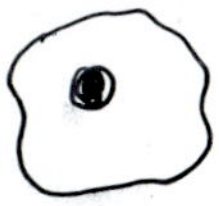 appearance) cancer that arises in the marrow and produces large amounts of IgG (55%) or IgA (25%). Most common 1° tumor arising within bone in people > 40–50 years old.

Associated with:

- ↑ susceptibility to infection
- Primary amyloidosis (AL)
- Punched-out lytic bone lesions on x-ray A
- M spike on serum protein electrophoresis
- Ig light chains in urine (Bence Jones protein)
- Rouleaux formation B (RBCs stacked like poker chips in blood smear)

Numerous plasma cells C with "clock-face" chromatin and intracytoplasmic inclusions containing immunoglobulin.

Monoclonal gammopathy of undetermined significance (MGUS)—monoclonal expansion of plasma cells, asymptomatic, may lead to multiple myeloma. No "**CRAB**" findings. Patients with MGUS develop multiple myeloma at a rate of 1–2% per year.

Think **CRAB**:
- Hyper**C**alcemia
- **R**enal involvement
- **A**nemia
- **B**one lytic lesions/**B**ack pain

Multiple **M**yeloma: **M**onoclonal **M** protein spike

Distinguish from **Waldenström macroglobulinemia** → M spike = IgM → hyperviscosity syndrome (eg, blurred vision, Raynaud phenomenon); no "**CRAB**" findings.

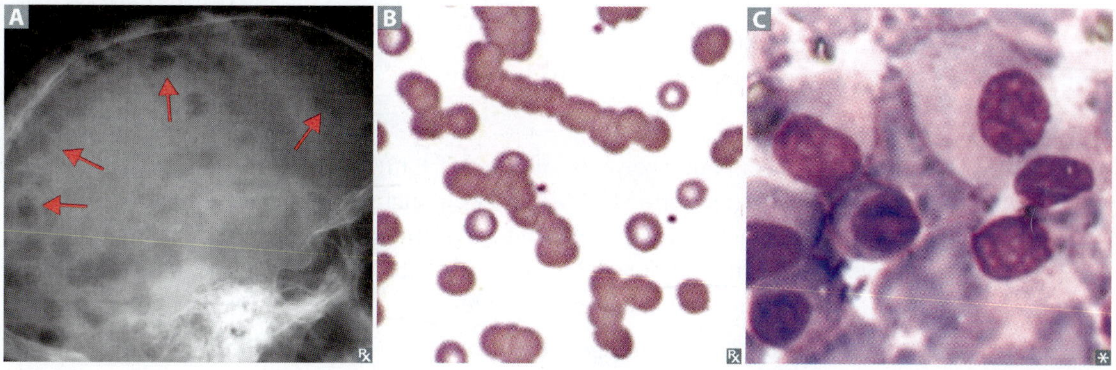

Myelodysplastic syndromes

Stem-cell disorders involving ineffective hematopoiesis → defects in cell maturation of all nonlymphoid lineages. Caused by de novo mutations or environmental exposure (eg, radiation, benzene, chemotherapy). Risk of transformation to AML.

Pseudo-Pelger-Huet anomaly—neutrophils with bilobed nuclei. Typically seen after chemotherapy.

Leukemias

Unregulated growth and differentiation of WBCs in bone marrow → marrow failure → anemia (↓ RBCs), infections (↓ mature WBCs), and hemorrhage (↓ platelets). Usually presents with ↑ circulating WBCs (malignant leukocytes in blood); rare cases present with normal/↓ WBCs.
Leukemic cell infiltration of liver, spleen, lymph nodes, and skin (leukemia cutis) possible.

TYPE	NOTES
Lymphoid neoplasms	
Acute lymphoblastic leukemia/lymphoma	Most frequently occurs in children; less common in adults (worse prognosis). T-cell ALL can present as mediastinal mass (presenting as SVC-like syndrome). Associated with Down syndrome. Peripheral blood and bone marrow have ↑↑↑ lymphoblasts A. TdT+ (marker of pre-T and pre-B cells), CD10+ (marker of pre-B cells). Most responsive to therapy. May spread to CNS and testes. t(12;21) → better prognosis.
Chronic lymphocytic leukemia/small lymphocytic lymphoma	Age: > 60 years. Most common adult leukemia. CD20+, CD5+ B-cell neoplasm. Often asymptomatic, progresses slowly; smudge cells B in peripheral blood smear; autoimmune hemolytic anemia. CLL = Crushed Little Lymphocytes (smudge cells). Richter transformation—SLL/CLL transformation into an aggressive lymphoma, most commonly diffuse large B-cell lymphoma (DLBCL).
Hairy cell leukemia	Age: Adult males. Mature B-cell tumor. Cells have filamentous, hair-like projections (fuzzy appearing on LM C). Causes marrow fibrosis → dry tap on aspiration. Patients usually present with massive splenomegaly. Stains TRAP (tartrate-resistant acid phosphatase) ⊕. TRAP stain largely replaced with flow cytometry. Treatment: cladribine, pentostatin.
Myeloid neoplasms	
Acute myelogenous leukemiaa	Median onset 65 years. Auer rods D; myeloperoxidase ⊕ cytoplasmic inclusions seen mostly in APL (formerly M3 AML); ↑↑↑ circulating myeloblasts on peripheral smear; adults. Risk factors: prior exposure to alkylating chemotherapy, radiation, myeloproliferative disorders, Down syndrome. t(15;17) → APL subtype responds to all-*trans* retinoic acid (vitamin A), inducing differentiation of promyelocytes; DIC is a common presentation.
Chronic myelogenous leukemia	Occurs across the age spectrum with peak incidence 45–85 years, median age at diagnosis 64 years. Defined by the Philadelphia chromosome (t[9;22], *BCR-ABL*) and myeloid stem cell proliferation. Presents with dysregulated production of mature and maturing granulocytes (eg, neutrophils, metamyelocytes, myelocytes, basophils E) and splenomegaly. May accelerate and transform to AML or ALL ("blast crisis"). Very low LAP as a result of low activity in malignant neutrophils (vs benign neutrophilia [leukemoid reaction], in which LAP is ↑). Responds to *bcr-abl* tyrosine kinase inhibitors (eg, imatinib).

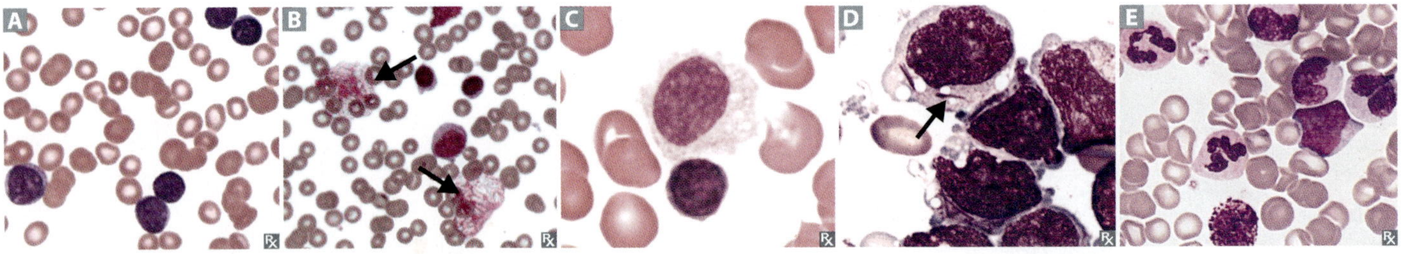

Chromosomal translocations

TRANSLOCATION	ASSOCIATED DISORDER	
t(8;14)	Burkitt lymphoma (c-*myc* activation)	
t(9;22) (**Philadelphia** chromosome)	**CML** (*BCR-ABL* hybrid), rarely ALL	**Philadelphia CreaML** cheese. The Ig heavy chain genes on chromosome 14 are constitutively expressed. When other genes (eg, *c-myc* and *BCL-2*) are translocated next to this heavy chain gene region, they are overexpressed.
t(11;14)	Mantle cell lymphoma (cyclin D1 activation)	
t(14;18)	Follicular lymphoma (*BCL-2* activation)	
t(15;17)	APL (M3 type of AML)	Responds to all-*trans* retinoic acid.

Langerhans cell histiocytosis

Collective group of proliferative disorders of dendritic (Langerhans) cells. Presents in a child as lytic bone lesions A and skin rash or as recurrent otitis media with a mass involving the mastoid bone. Cells are functionally immature and do not effectively stimulate primary T cells via antigen presentation. Cells express S-100 (mesodermal origin) and CD1a. Birbeck granules ("tennis rackets" or rod shaped on EM) are characteristic B.

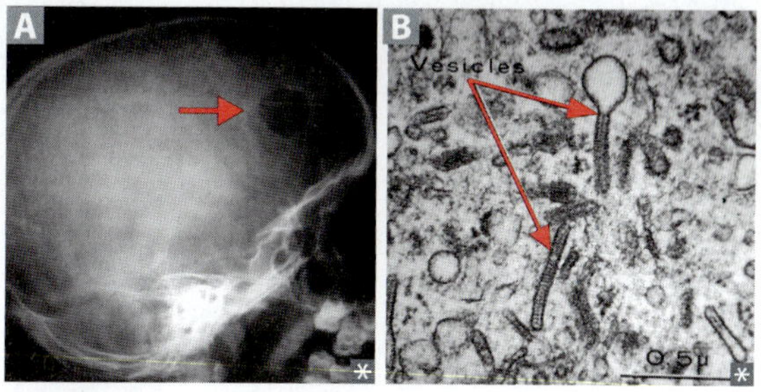

Lytic bone lesion = ① MM
OR
② Langerhan cell histo.

Chronic myeloproliferative disorders — The myeloproliferative disorders (polycythemia vera, essential thrombocythemia, myelofibrosis, and CML) are malignant hematopoietic neoplasms with varying impacts on WBCs and myeloid cell lines. Associated with V617F *JAK2* mutation.

Polycythemia vera — A form of 1° polycythemia. Disorder of ↑ hematocrit. May present as intense itching after hot shower. Rare but classic symptom is erythromelalgia (severe, burning pain and red-blue coloration) due to episodic blood clots in vessels of the extremities A. Responds to aspirin. ↓ EPO (vs 2° polycythemia, which presents with endogenous or artificially ↑ EPO).

Essential thrombocythemia — Characterized by massive proliferation of megakaryocytes and platelets. Symptoms include bleeding and thrombosis. Blood smear shows markedly increased number of platelets, which may be large or otherwise abnormally formed B. Erythromelalgia may occur. — Severe burning/red feet/hand

Myelofibrosis — Obliteration of bone marrow with fibrosis C due to ↑ fibroblast activity. Often associated with massive splenomegaly and "**teardrop**" RBCs D. "Bone marrow is **crying** because it's fibrosed and is a dry tap."

	RBCs	WBCs	PLATELETS	PHILADELPHIA CHROMOSOME	*JAK2* MUTATIONS
Polycythemia vera	↑	↑	↑	⊖	⊕
Essential thrombocythemia	–	–	↑	⊖	⊕ (30–50%)
Myelofibrosis	↓	Variable	Variable	⊖	⊕ (30–50%)
CML	↓	↑	↑	⊕	⊖

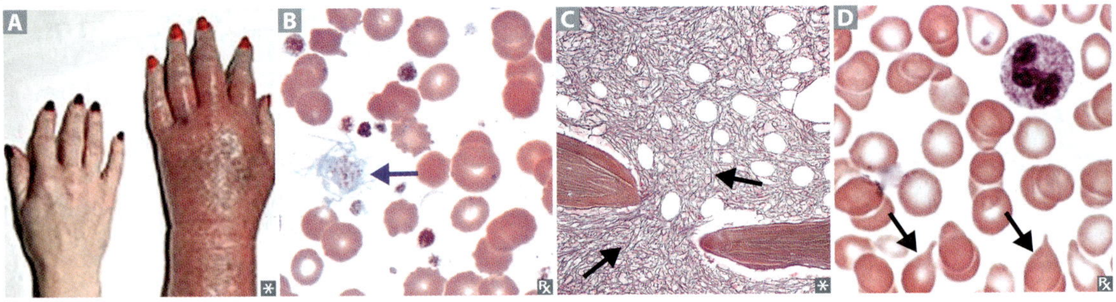

Polycythemia

	PLASMA VOLUME	RBC MASS	O_2 SATURATION	EPO LEVELS	ASSOCIATIONS
Relative	↓	–	–	–	Dehydration, burns.
Appropriate absolute	–	↑	↓	↑	Lung disease, congenital heart disease, high altitude.
Inappropriate absolute	–	↑	–	↑	Malignancy (eg, renal cell carcinoma, hepatocellular carcinoma), hydronephrosis. Due to ectopic EPO secretion.
Polycythemia vera	↑	↑↑	–	↓	EPO ↓ in PCV due to negative feedback suppressing renal EPO production.

▶ HEMATOLOGY AND ONCOLOGY—PHARMACOLOGY

Heparin

MECHANISM	Lowers the activity of thrombin and factor Xa. Short half-life.
CLINICAL USE	Immediate anticoagulation for pulmonary embolism (PE), acute coronary syndrome, MI, deep venous thrombosis (DVT). Used during pregnancy (does not cross placenta). Follow PTT.
ADVERSE EFFECTS	Bleeding, thrombocytopenia (HIT), osteoporosis, drug-drug interactions. For rapid reversal (antidote), use protamine sulfate (positively charged molecule that binds negatively charged heparin).
NOTES	Low-molecular-weight heparins (eg, enoxaparin, dalteparin) and fondaparinux act more on factor Xa, have better bioavailability, and 2–4 times longer half-life; can be administered subcutaneously and without laboratory monitoring. Not easily reversible. **Heparin-induced thrombocytopenia** (HIT)—development of IgG antibodies against heparin-bound platelet factor 4 (PF4). Antibody-heparin-PF4 complex activates platelets → thrombosis and thrombocytopenia.

Direct thrombin inhibitors	Bivalirudin (related to hirudin, the anticoagulant used by leeches).
MECHANISM	Directly inhibits activity of free and clot-associated thrombin.
CLINICAL USE	Venous thromboembolism, atrial fibrillation. Can be used in HIT. Does not require lab monitoring.
ADVERSE EFFECTS	Bleeding; no specific reversal agent. Can attempt to use activated prothrombin complex concentrates (PCC) and/or fibrinolytics (eg, tranexamic acid).

Warfarin

MECHANISM	Interferes with γ-carboxylation of vitamin K–dependent clotting factors II, VII, IX, and X, and proteins C and S. Metabolism affected by polymorphisms in the gene for vitamin K epoxide reductase complex (*VKORC1*). In laboratory assay, has effect on **EX**trinsic pathway and ↑ **PT**. Long half-life.	The **EX-P**residen**T** went to **war**(farin).
CLINICAL USE	Chronic anticoagulation (eg, venous thromboembolism prophylaxis, and prevention of stroke in atrial fibrillation). Not used in pregnant women (because warfarin, unlike heparin, crosses placenta). Follow PT/INR.	
ADVERSE EFFECTS 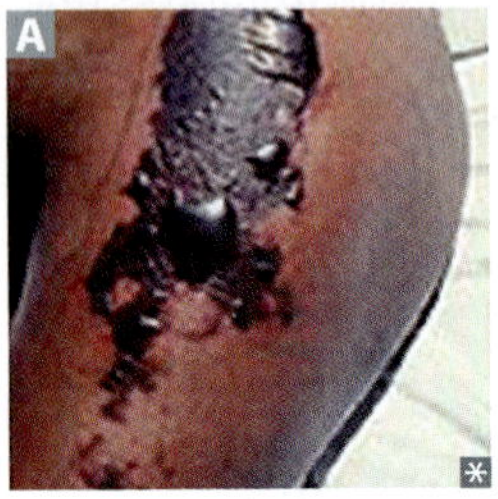	Bleeding, teratogenic, skin/tissue necrosis A, drug-drug interactions. Proteins C and S have shorter half-lives than clotting factors II, VII, IX, and X, resulting in early transient hypercoagulability with warfarin use. Skin/tissue necrosis within first few days of large doses believed to be due to small vessel microthromboses.	For reversal of warfarin, give vitamin K. For rapid reversal, give fresh frozen plasma. Heparin "bridging": heparin frequently used when starting warfarin. Heparin's activation of antithrombin enables anticoagulation during initial, transient hypercoagulable state caused by warfarin. Initial heparin therapy reduces risk of recurrent venous thromboembolism and skin/tissue necrosis.

Heparin vs warfarin

	Heparin	Warfarin
STRUCTURE	Large, anionic, acidic polymer	Small, amphipathic molecule
ROUTE OF ADMINISTRATION	Parenteral (IV, SC)	Oral
SITE OF ACTION	Blood	Liver
ONSET OF ACTION	Rapid (seconds)	Slow, limited by half-lives of normal clotting factors
MECHANISM OF ACTION	Activates antithrombin, which ↓ the action of IIa (thrombin) and factor Xa	Impairs synthesis of vitamin K–dependent clotting factors II, VII, IX, and X, and anti-clotting proteins C and S
DURATION OF ACTION	Acute (hours)	Chronic (days)
INHIBITS COAGULATION IN VITRO	Yes	No
AGENTS FOR REVERSAL	Protamine sulfate	Vitamin K, fresh frozen plasma
MONITORING	PTT (intrinsic pathway)	PT/INR (extrinsic pathway)
CROSSES PLACENTA	No	Yes (teratogenic)

Direct factor Xa inhibitors	ApiXaban, rivaroXaban.
MECHANISM	Bind to and directly inhibit factor Xa.
CLINICAL USE	Treatment and prophylaxis for DVT and PE (rivaroxaban); stroke prophylaxis in patients with atrial fibrillation. Oral agents do not usually require coagulation monitoring.
ADVERSE EFFECTS	Bleeding (no reversal agent available).

Thrombolytics	Alteplase (tPA), reteplase (rPA), streptokinase, tenecteplase (TNK-tPA).
MECHANISM	Directly or indirectly aid conversion of plasminogen to plasmin, which cleaves thrombin and fibrin clots. ↑ PT, ↑ PTT, no change in platelet count.
CLINICAL USE	Early MI, early ischemic stroke, direct thrombolysis of severe PE.
ADVERSE EFFECTS	Bleeding. Contraindicated in patients with active bleeding, history of intracranial bleeding, recent surgery, known bleeding diatheses, or severe hypertension. Treat toxicity with aminocaproic acid, an inhibitor of fibrinolysis. Fresh frozen plasma and cryoprecipitate can also be used to correct factor deficiencies.

ADP receptor inhibitors	Clopidogrel, prasugrel, ticagrelor (reversible), ticlopidine.
MECHANISM	Inhibit platelet aggregation by irreversibly blocking ADP receptors. Prevent expression of glycoproteins IIb/IIIa on platelet surface.
CLINICAL USE	Acute coronary syndrome; coronary stenting. ↓ incidence or recurrence of thrombotic stroke.
ADVERSE EFFECTS	Neutropenia (ticlopidine). TTP may be seen.

Cilostazol, dipyridamole	
MECHANISM	Phosphodiesterase III inhibitor; ↑ cAMP in platelets, resulting in inhibition of platelet aggregation; vasodilators.
CLINICAL USE	Intermittent claudication, coronary vasodilation, prevention of stroke or TIAs (combined with aspirin), angina prophylaxis.
ADVERSE EFFECTS	Nausea, headache, facial flushing, hypotension, abdominal pain.

Glycoprotein IIb/IIIa inhibitors	Abciximab, eptifibatide, tirofiban.
MECHANISM	Bind to the glycoprotein receptor IIb/IIIa on activated platelets, preventing aggregation. Abciximab is made from monoclonal antibody Fab fragments.
CLINICAL USE	Unstable angina, percutaneous transluminal coronary angioplasty.
ADVERSE EFFECTS	Bleeding, thrombocytopenia.

Cancer drugs—cell cycle

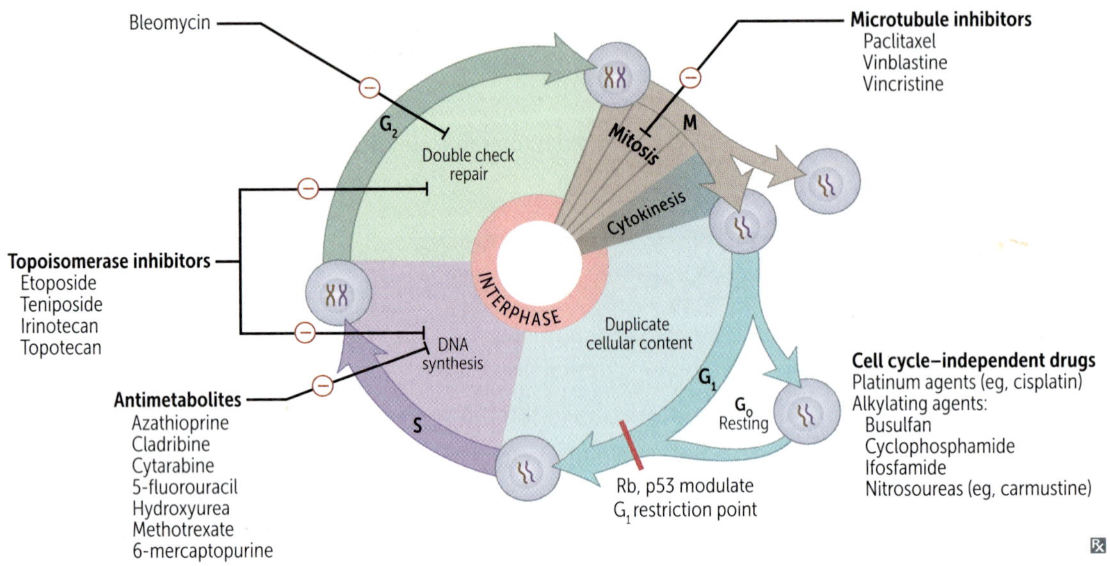

Cancer drugs—targets

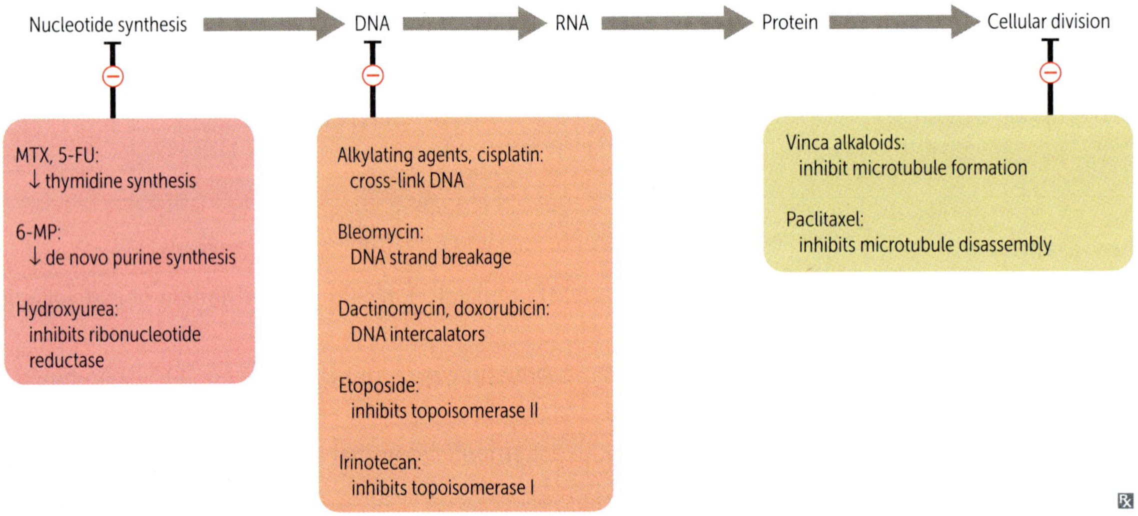

Antimetabolites

DRUG	MECHANISM[a]	CLINICAL USE	ADVERSE EFFECTS
Azathioprine, 6-mercaptopurine	Purine (thiol) analogs → ↓ de novo purine synthesis. Activated by HGPRT. Azathioprine is metabolized into 6-MP.	Preventing organ rejection, rheumatoid arthritis, IBD, SLE; used to wean patients off steroids in chronic disease and to treat steroid-refractory chronic disease.	Myelosuppression, GI, liver. Azathioprine and 6-MP are metabolized by xanthine oxidase; thus both have ↑ toxicity with allopurinol or febuxostat.
Cladribine	Purine analog → multiple mechanisms (eg, inhibition of DNA polymerase, DNA strand breaks).	Hairy cell leukemia.	Myelosuppression, nephrotoxicity, and neurotoxicity.
Cytarabine (arabinofuranosyl cytidine)	Pyrimidine analog → inhibition of DNA polymerase.	Leukemias (AML), lymphomas.	Myelosuppression with megaloblastic anemia. CYTarabine causes panCYTopenia.
5-fluorouracil	Pyrimidine analog bioactivated to 5-FdUMP, which covalently complexes folic acid. This complex inhibits thymidylate synthase → ↓ dTMP → ↓ DNA synthesis.	Colon cancer, pancreatic cancer, basal cell carcinoma (topical). Effects enhanced with the addition of leucovorin.	Myelosuppression—worsened with the addition of leucovorin (folinic acid).
Methotrexate	Folic acid analog that competitively inhibits dihydrofolate reductase → ↓ dTMP → ↓ DNA synthesis.	Cancers: leukemias (ALL), lymphomas, choriocarcinoma, sarcomas. Non-neoplastic: ectopic pregnancy, medical abortion (with misoprostol), rheumatoid arthritis, psoriasis, IBD, vasculitis.	Myelosuppression, which is reversible with leucovorin "rescue." Hepatotoxicity. Mucositis (eg, mouth ulcers). Pulmonary fibrosis.

[a]All are S-phase specific.

Antitumor antibiotics

DRUG	MECHANISM	CLINICAL USE	ADVERSE EFFECTS
Bleomycin	Induces free radical formation → breaks in DNA strands.	Testicular cancer, Hodgkin lymphoma.	Pulmonary fibrosis, skin hyperpigmentation. Minimal myelosuppression.
Dactinomycin (actinomycin D)	Intercalates in DNA.	Wilms tumor, Ewing sarcoma, rhabdomyosarcoma. Used for childhood tumors ("children act out").	Myelosuppression.
Doxorubicin, daunorubicin	Generate free radicals. Intercalate in DNA → breaks in DNA → ↓ replication.	Solid tumors, leukemias, lymphomas.	Cardiotoxicity (dilated cardiomyopathy), myelosuppression, alopecia. Dexrazoxane (iron chelating agent), used to prevent cardiotoxicity.

Alkylating agents

DRUG	MECHANISM	CLINICAL USE	ADVERSE EFFECTS
Busulfan	Cross-links DNA.	CML. Also used to ablate patient's bone marrow before bone marrow transplantation.	Severe myelosuppression (in almost all cases), pulmonary fibrosis, hyperpigmentation.
Cyclophosphamide, ifosfamide	Cross-link DNA at guanine N-7. Require bioactivation by liver.	Solid tumors, leukemia, lymphomas.	Myelosuppression; hemorrhagic cystitis, prevented with mesna (thiol group of mesna binds toxic metabolites) or N-acetylcysteine.
Nitrosoureas Carmustine, lomustine, semustine, streptozocin)	Require bioactivation. Cross blood-brain barrier → CNS. Cross-link DNA.	Brain tumors (including glioblastoma multiforme).	CNS toxicity (convulsions, dizziness, ataxia).

Microtubule inhibitors

DRUG	MECHANISM	CLINICAL USE	ADVERSE EFFECTS
Paclitaxel, other taxols	Hyperstabilize polymerized microtubules in M phase so that mitotic spindle cannot break down (anaphase cannot occur).	Ovarian and breast carcinomas.	Myelosuppression, neuropathy, hypersensitivity.
Vincristine, vinblastine	Vinca alkaloids that bind β-tubulin and inhibit its polymerization into microtubules → prevent mitotic spindle formation (M-phase arrest).	Solid tumors, leukemias, Hodgkin (vinblastine) and non-Hodgkin (vincristine) lymphomas.	Vincristine: neurotoxicity (areflexia, peripheral neuritis), constipation (including paralytic ileus).

Cisplatin, carboplatin

MECHANISM	Cross-link DNA.
CLINICAL USE	Testicular, bladder, ovary, and lung carcinomas.
ADVERSE EFFECTS	Nephrotoxicity, peripheral neuropathy, ototoxicity. Prevent nephrotoxicity with amifostine (free radical scavenger) and chloride (saline) diuresis.

Etoposide, teniposide

MECHANISM	Etoposide inhibits topoisomerase II → ↑ DNA degradation.
CLINICAL USE	Solid tumors (particularly testicular and small cell lung cancer), leukemias, lymphomas.
ADVERSE EFFECTS	Myelosuppression, alopecia.

Irinotecan, topotecan

MECHANISM	Inhibit topoisomerase I and prevent DNA unwinding and replication.
CLINICAL USE	Colon cancer (irinotecan); ovarian and small cell lung cancers (topotecan).
ADVERSE EFFECTS	Severe myelosuppression, diarrhea.

Hydroxyurea

MECHANISM	Inhibits ribonucleotide reductase → ↓ DNA Synthesis (S-phase specific).
CLINICAL USE	Melanoma, CML, sickle cell disease (↑ HbF).
ADVERSE EFFECTS	Severe myelosuppression.

Prednisone, prednisolone

MECHANISM	Various; bind intracytoplasmic steroid receptor; alter gene transcription.
CLINICAL USE	Most commonly used glucocorticoids in cancer chemotherapy. Used in CLL, non-Hodgkin lymphoma (part of combination chemotherapy regimen). Also used as immunosuppressants (eg, in autoimmune diseases).
ADVERSE EFFECTS	Cushing-like symptoms; weight gain, central obesity, muscle breakdown, cataracts, acne, osteoporosis, hypertension, peptic ulcers, hyperglycemia, psychosis.

Bevacizumab

MECHANISM	Monoclonal antibody against VEGF. Inhibits angiogenesis.
CLINICAL USE	Solid tumors (colorectal cancer, renal cell carcinoma).
ADVERSE EFFECTS	Hemorrhage, blood clots, and impaired wound healing.

Erlotinib

MECHANISM	EGFR tyrosine kinase inhibitor.
CLINICAL USE	Non-small cell lung carcinoma.
ADVERSE EFFECTS	Rash.

Cetuximab

MECHANISM	Monoclonal antibody against EGFR.
CLINICAL USE	Stage IV colorectal cancer (wild-type *KRAS*), head and neck cancer.
ADVERSE EFFECTS	Rash, elevated LFTs, diarrhea.

Imatinib

MECHANISM	Tyrosine kinase inhibitor of *BCR-ABL* (Philadelphia chromosome fusion gene in CML) and c-*kit* (common in GI stromal tumors).
CLINICAL USE	CML, GI stromal tumors.
ADVERSE EFFECTS	Fluid retention.

Rituximab

MECHANISM	Monoclonal antibody against CD20, which is found on most B-cell neoplasms.
CLINICAL USE	Non-Hodgkin lymphoma, CLL, ITP, rheumatoid arthritis.
ADVERSE EFFECTS	↑ risk of progressive multifocal leukoencephalopathy.

Tamoxifen, raloxifene

MECHANISM	Selective estrogen receptor modulators (SERMs)—receptor antagonists in breast and agonists in bone. Block the binding of estrogen to ER ⊕ cells.
CLINICAL USE	Breast cancer treatment (tamoxifen only) and prevention. Raloxifene also useful to prevent osteoporosis.
ADVERSE EFFECTS	Tamoxifen—partial agonist in endometrium, which ↑ the risk of endometrial cancer; "hot flashes." Raloxifene—no ↑ in endometrial carcinoma because it is an estrogen receptor antagonist in endometrial tissue. Both ↑ risk of thromboembolic events (eg, DVT, PE).

Trastuzumab (Herceptin)

MECHANISM	Monoclonal antibody against HER-2 (*c-erbB2*), a tyrosine kinase receptor. Helps kill cancer cells that overexpress HER-2, through inhibition of HER2-initiated cellular signaling and antibody-dependent cytotoxicity.
CLINICAL USE	HER-**2** ⊕ breast cancer and gastric cancer (tras**2**zumab).
ADVERSE EFFECTS	Cardiotoxicity. "**Heart**ceptin" damages the **heart**.

Vemurafenib

MECHANISM	Small molecule inhibitor of *BRAF* oncogene ⊕ melanoma. **VEmuRAF-enib** is for **V600E-mu**tated ***BRAF* inhib**ition.
CLINICAL USE	Metastatic melanoma.

Common chemotoxicities

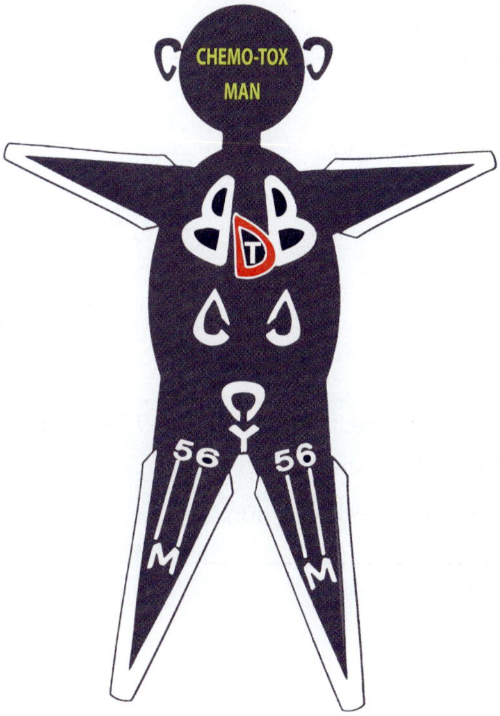

Cisplatin/**C**arboplatin → ototoxicity (and nephrotoxicity)

Vincristine → peripheral neuropathy
Bleomycin, **B**usulfan → pulmonary fibrosis
Doxorubicin → cardiotoxicity
Trastuzumab → cardiotoxicity
Cisplatin/**C**arboplatin → nephrotoxic (and acoustic nerve damage)

CYclophosphamide → hemorrhagic cystitis

5-FU → myelosuppression
6-MP → myelosuppression

Methotrexate → myelosuppression

▶ NOTES

HIGH-YIELD SYSTEMS

Musculoskeletal, Skin, and Connective Tissue

"Rigid, the skeleton of habit alone upholds the human frame."

—Virginia Woolf

"Beauty may be skin deep, but ugly goes clear to the bone."

—Redd Foxx

"The function of muscle is to pull and not to push, except in the case of the genitals and the tongue."

—Leonardo da Vinci

▶ MUSCULOSKELETAL, SKIN, AND CONNECTIVE TISSUE—ANATOMY AND PHYSIOLOGY

Knee exam

ACL: extends from lateral femoral condyle to anterior tibia.
PCL: extends from medial femoral condyle to posterior tibia.
Perform knee exam with patient supine.

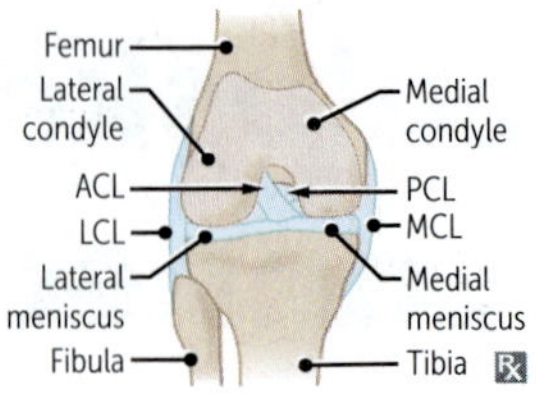

TEST	PROCEDURE	
Anterior drawer sign	Bending knee at 90° angle, ↑ anterior gliding of tibia due to ACL injury. Lachman test is similar, but at 30° angle.	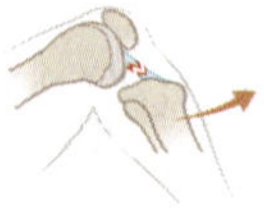 ACL tear Anterior drawer sign
Posterior drawer sign	Bending knee at 90° angle, ↑ posterior gliding of tibia due to PCL injury.	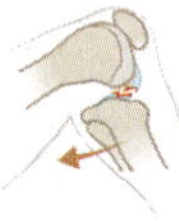 PCL tear Posterior drawer sign
Abnormal passive abduction	Knee either extended or at ~ 30° angle, lateral (valgus) force → medial space widening of tibia → MCL injury.	External rotation 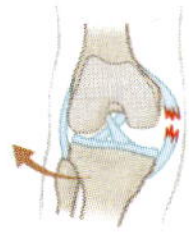 MCL tear
Abnormal passive adduction	Knee either extended or at ~ 30° angle, medial (varus) force → lateral space widening of tibia → LCL injury.	Internal rotation 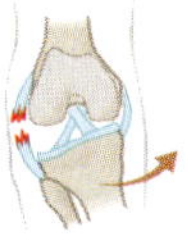 LCL tear
McMurray test	During flexion and extension of knee with rotation of tibia/foot: ▪ Pain, "popping" on external rotation → medial meniscal tear ▪ Pain, "popping" on internal rotation → lateral meniscal tear	External rotation 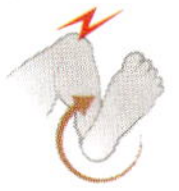 Medial tear Internal rotation 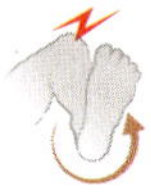 Lateral tear

Common knee conditions

"Unhappy triad"	Common injury in contact sports due to lateral force applied to a planted leg. Classically, consists of damage to the ACL **A**, MCL, and medial meniscus (attached to MCL); however, lateral meniscus injury is more common. Presents with acute knee pain and signs of joint injury/instability.
Prepatellar bursitis	Inflammation of knee's largest sac of synovial fluid **B**. Can be caused by repeated trauma or pressure from excessive kneeling.
Baker cyst	Popliteal fluid collection in gastrocnemius-semimembranous bursa **C** commonly communicating with synovial space and related to chronic joint disease.

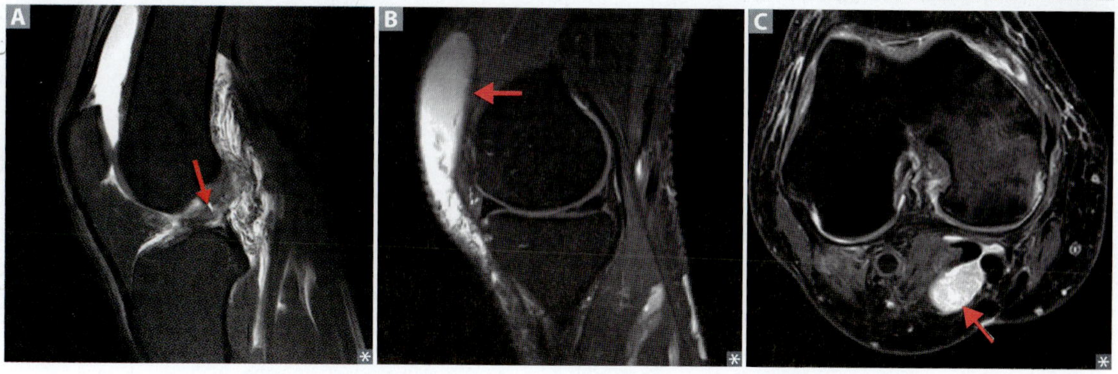

Rotator cuff muscles

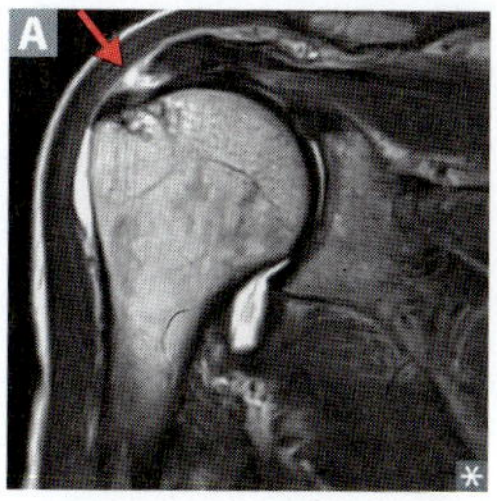

Shoulder muscles that form the rotator cuff:
- Supraspinatus (suprascapular nerve)—abducts arm initially (before the action of the deltoid); most common rotator cuff injury **A** (trauma or degeneration and impingement → tendinopathy or tear), assessed by "empty/full can" test.
- Infraspinatus (suprascapular nerve)—laterally rotates arm; pitching injury.
- teres minor (axillary nerve)—adducts and laterally rotates arm.
- Subscapularis (upper and lower subscapular nerves)—medially rotates and adducts arm.

Innervated primarily by C5-C6.

SItS (small t is for teres minor).

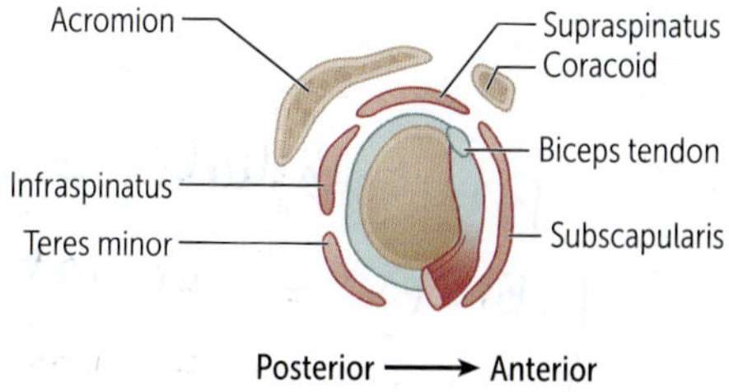

Overuse injuries of the elbow

Medial epicondylitis (golfer's elbow)	Repetitive flexion (forehand shots) or idiopathic → pain near medial epicondyle.
Lateral epicondylitis (tennis elbow)	Repetitive extension (backhand shots) or idiopathic → pain near lateral epicondyle.

Wrist bones	Scaphoid, Lunate, Triquetrum, Pisiform, Hamate, Capitate, Trapezoid, Trapezium **A**. (So Long To Pinky, Here Comes The Thumb). Scaphoid (palpated in anatomic snuff box) is the most commonly fractured carpal bone (typically from a fall on an outstretched hand) and is prone to avascular necrosis owing to retrograde blood supply. Dislocation of lunate may cause acute carpal tunnel syndrome. A fall on an outstretched hand that damages the hook of the hamate can cause ulnar nerve injury.
Carpal tunnel syndrome	Entrapment of median nerve in carpal tunnel; nerve compression → paresthesia, pain, and numbness in distribution of median nerve (thenar eminence atrophies but sensation spared, because palmar cutaneous branch enters the hand external to carpal tunnel). Associated with pregnancy, rheumatoid arthritis, hypothyroidism, diabetes, dialysis-related amyloidosis; may be associated with repetitive use.
Guyon canal syndrome	Compression of ulnar nerve at wrist or hand. Classically seen in cyclists due to pressure from handlebars.

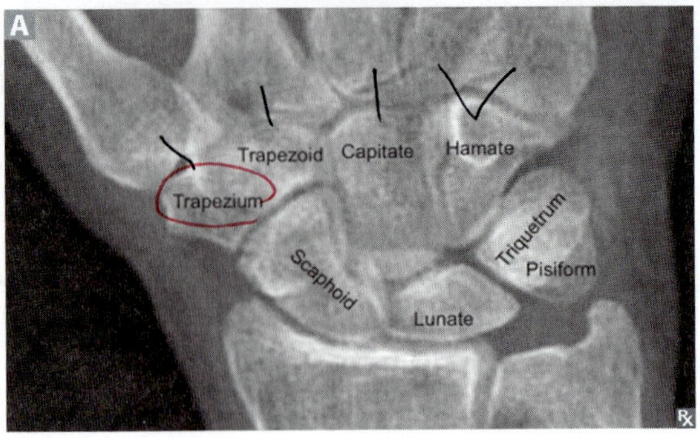

Brachioradialis = Flex + midprone

musc-cutaneous n.
Biceps = supinat + flex
brachialis = Flex
coracobracialis = flex + weak add.

Upper extremity nerves

NERVE	CAUSES OF INJURY	PRESENTATION
Axillary (C5-C6)	Fractured surgical neck of humerus; anterior dislocation of humerus	Flattened deltoid Loss of arm abduction at shoulder (> 15 degrees) Loss of sensation over deltoid muscle and lateral arm
Musculocutaneous (C5-C7)	Upper trunk compression	Loss of forearm flexion and supination Loss of sensation over lateral forearm
Radial (C5-T1)	Midshaft fracture of humerus; compression of axilla, eg, due to crutches or sleeping with arm over chair ("Saturday night palsy")	Wrist drop: loss of elbow, wrist, and finger extension ↓ grip strength (wrist extension necessary for maximal action of flexors) Loss of sensation over posterior arm/forearm and dorsal hand
Median (C5-T1)	Supracondylar fracture of humerus (proximal lesion); carpal tunnel syndrome and wrist laceration (distal lesion)	"Ape hand" and "Pope's blessing" Loss of wrist flexion, flexion of lateral fingers, thumb opposition, lumbricals of 2nd and 3rd digits Loss of sensation over thenar eminence and dorsal and palmar aspects of lateral 3½ fingers with proximal lesion Tinel sign (tingling on percussion) in carpal tunnel syndrome
Ulnar (C8-T1)	Fracture of medial epicondyle of humerus "funny bone" (proximal lesion); fractured hook of hamate (distal lesion)	"Ulnar claw" on digit extension Radial deviation of wrist upon flexion (proximal lesion) Loss of wrist flexion, flexion of medial fingers, abduction and adduction of fingers (interossei), actions of medial 2 lumbrical muscles Loss of sensation over medial 1½ fingers including hypothenar eminence
Recurrent branch of median nerve (C5-T1)	Superficial laceration of palm	"Ape hand" Loss of thenar muscle group: opposition, abduction, and flexion of thumb No loss of sensation

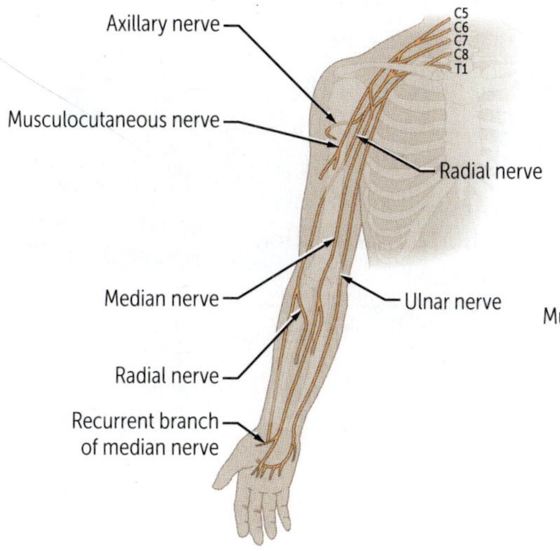

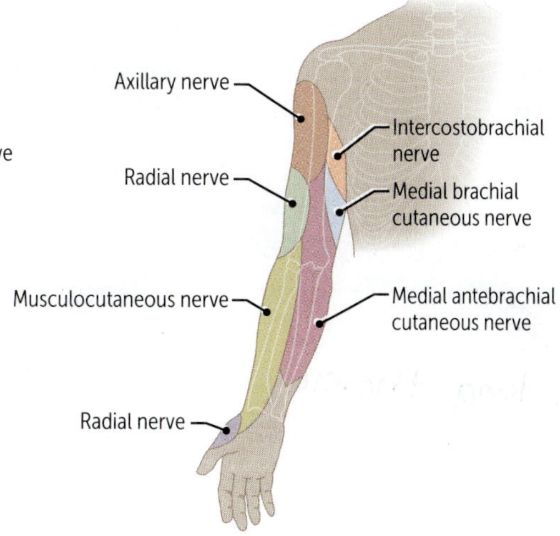

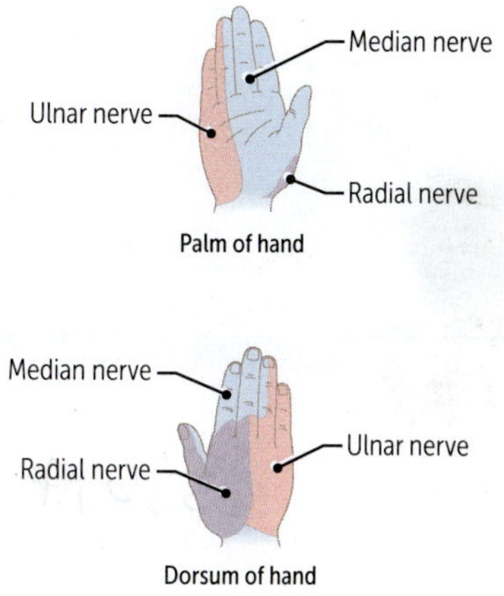

Brachial plexus lesions

1. Erb palsy ("waiter's tip")
2. Claw hand (Klumpke palsy)
3. Wrist drop
4. Winged scapula
5. Deltoid paralysis
6. "Saturday night palsy" (wrist drop)
7. Difficulty flexing elbow, variable sensory loss
8. Decreased thumb function, "Pope's blessing"
9. Intrinsic muscles of hand, claw hand

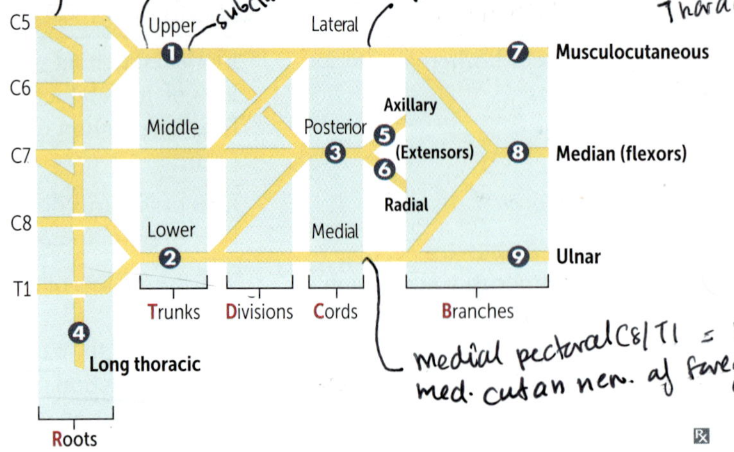

Randy
Travis
Drinks
Cold
Beer

CONDITION	INJURY	CAUSES	MUSCLE DEFICIT	FUNCTIONAL DEFICIT	PRESENTATION
Erb palsy ("waiter's tip")	Traction or tear of **upper** ("**Erb**-er") trunk: C5-C6 roots	Infants—lateral traction on neck during delivery Adults—trauma	Deltoid, supraspinatus	Abduction (arm hangs by side)	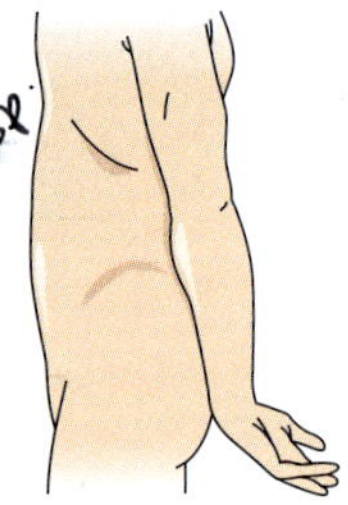
			Infraspinatus	Lateral rotation (arm medially rotated)	
			Biceps brachii	Flexion, supination (arm extended and pronated)	
Klumpke palsy	Traction or tear of **lower** trunk: C8-T1 root	Infants—upward force on arm during delivery Adults—trauma (eg, grabbing a tree branch to break a fall)	Intrinsic hand muscles: lumbricals, interossei, thenar, hypothenar	Total claw hand: lumbricals normally flex MCP joints and extend DIP and PIP joints	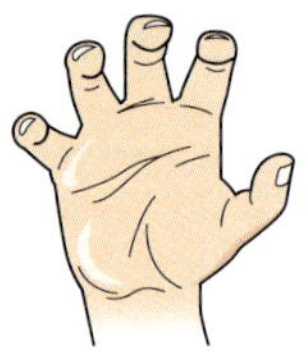
Thoracic outlet syndrome	Compression of **lower** trunk and subclavian vessels	Cervical rib, Pancoast tumor	Same as Klumpke palsy	Atrophy of intrinsic hand muscles; ischemia, pain, and edema due to vascular compression	
Winged scapula	Lesion of long thoracic nerve	Axillary node dissection after mastectomy, stab wounds	Serratus anterior	Inability to anchor scapula to thoracic cage → cannot abduct arm above horizontal position	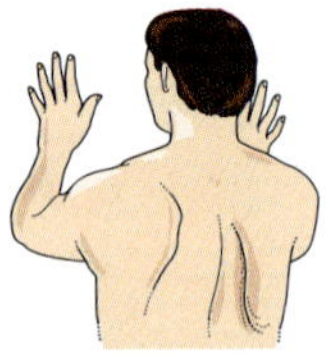

C5,6,7 = long thoracic

Distortions of the hand

At rest, a balance exists between the extrinsic flexors and extensors of the hand, as well as the intrinsic muscles of the hand—particularly the lumbrical muscles (flexion of MCP, extension of DIP and PIP joints).

"Clawing"—seen best with **distal** lesions of median or ulnar nerves. Remaining extrinsic flexors of the digits exaggerate the loss of the lumbricals → fingers extend at MCP, flex at DIP and PIP joints.

Deficits less pronounced in **proximal** lesions; deficits present during voluntary flexion of the digits.

PRESENTATION	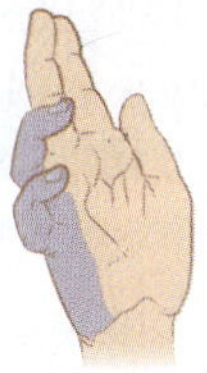	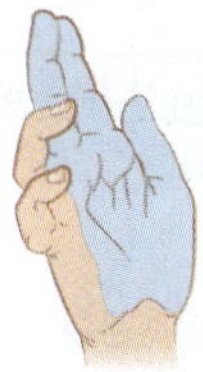	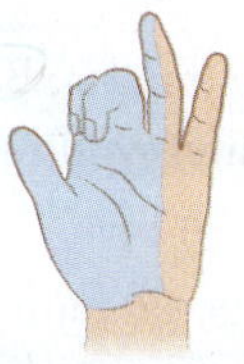	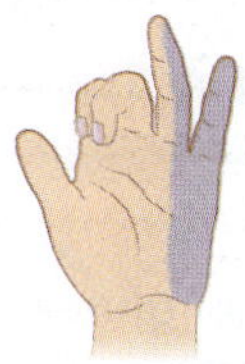
CONTEXT	Extending fingers/at rest	Making a fist	Extending fingers/at rest	Making a fist
LOCATION OF LESION	Distal ulnar nerve	Proximal median nerve	Distal median nerve	Proximal ulnar nerve
SIGN	"Ulnar claw"	"Pope's blessing"	"Median claw"	"OK gesture" (with digits 1–3 flexed)

Note: Atrophy of the thenar eminence (unopposable thumb → "ape hand") can be seen in median nerve lesions, while atrophy of the hypothenar eminence can be seen in ulnar nerve lesions.

Hand muscles

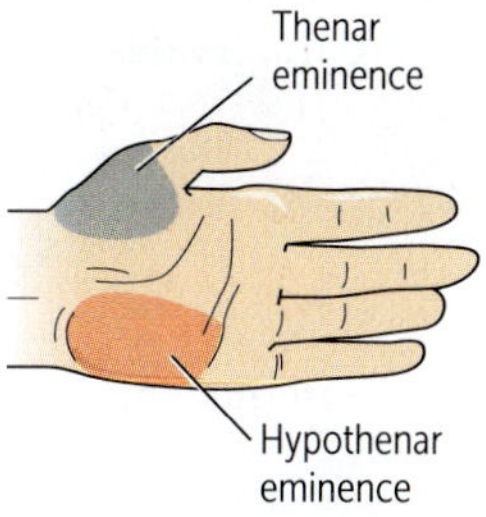

Thenar (median)—**O**pponens pollicis, **A**bductor pollicis brevis, **F**lexor pollicis brevis, superficial head (deep head by ulnar nerve).

Hypothenar (ulnar)—**O**pponens digiti minimi, **A**bductor digiti minimi, **F**lexor digiti minimi brevis.

Both groups perform the same functions: **O**ppose, **A**bduct, and **F**lex (**OAF**).

Dorsal interossei—abduct the fingers. **DAB** = **D**orsals **AB**duct.

Palmar interossei—adduct the fingers. **PAD** = **P**almars **AD**duct.

Lumbricals—flex at the MCP joint, extend PIP and DIP joints.

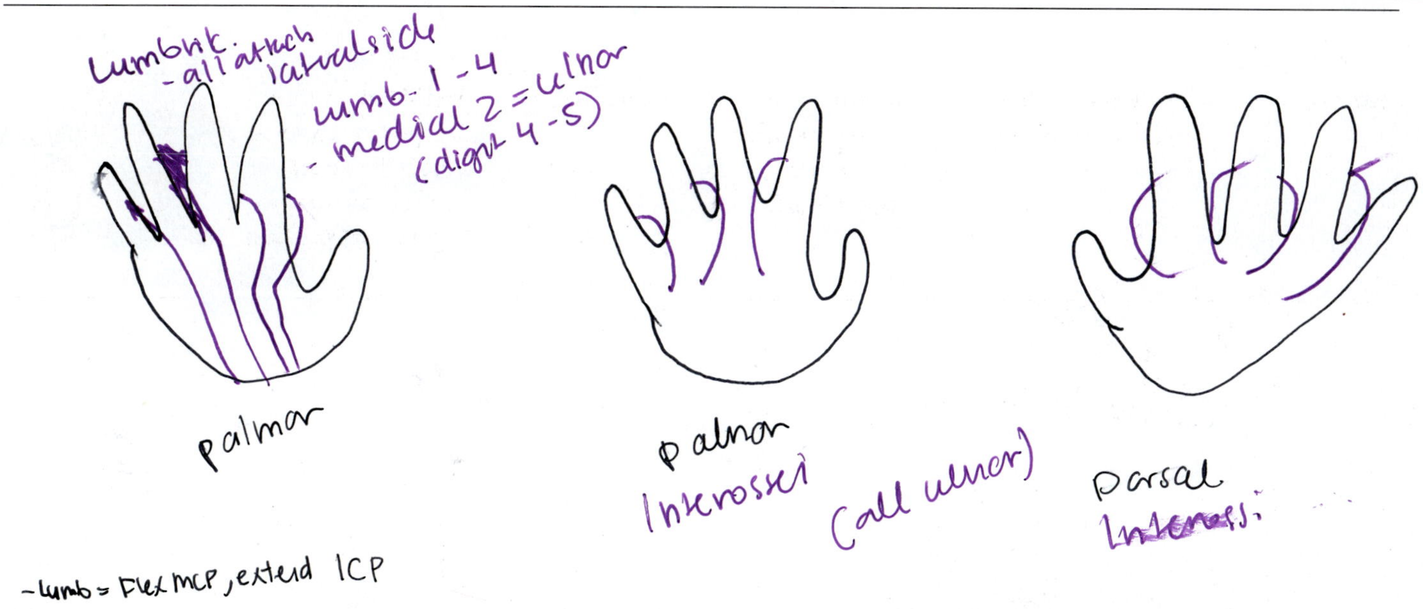

Lower extremity nerves

NERVE	CAUSE OF INJURY	PRESENTATION
Obturator (L2–L4)	Pelvic surgery	↓ thigh sensation (medial) and ↓ adduction.
Femoral (L2–L4)	Pelvic fracture	↓ thigh flexion and leg extension.
Common peroneal (L4–S2)	Trauma or compression of lateral aspect of leg, fibular neck fracture	Foot drop—inverted and plantarflexed at rest, loss of eversion and dorsiflexion. "Steppage gait." Loss of sensation on dorsum of foot.
Tibial (L4–S3)	Knee trauma, Baker cyst (proximal lesion); tarsal tunnel syndrome (distal lesion)	Inability to curl toes and loss of sensation on sole of foot. In proximal lesions, foot everted at rest with loss of inversion and plantarflexion.
Superior gluteal (L4–S1) 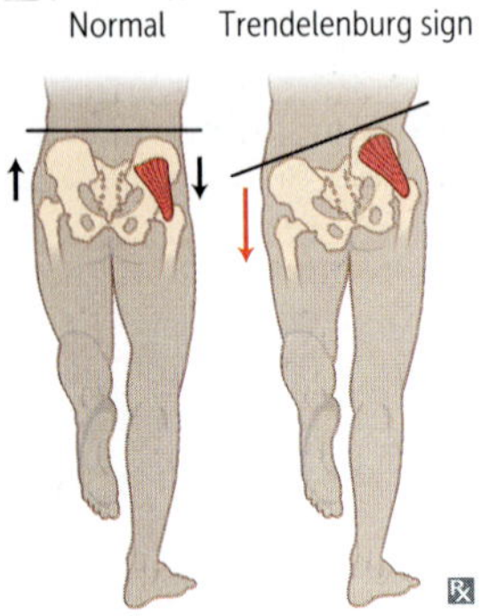	Iatrogenic injury during intramuscular injection to upper medial gluteal region	Trendelenburg sign/gait—pelvis tilts because weight-bearing leg cannot maintain alignment of pelvis through hip abduction. Lesion is contralateral to the side of the hip that drops, ipsilateral to extremity on which the patient stands.
Inferior gluteal (L5–S2)	Posterior hip dislocation	Difficulty climbing stairs, rising from seated position. Loss of hip extension.

Superior gluteal nerve innervates gluteus medius, gluteus minimus, and tensor fascia latae. Inferior gluteal nerve innervates gluteus maximus.

PED = Peroneal Everts and Dorsiflexes; if injured, foot dropPED.

TIP = Tibial Inverts and Plantarflexes; if injured, can't stand on TIPtoes.

Sciatic nerve (L4–S3) innervates posterior thigh, splits into common peroneal and tibial nerves.

Pudendal nerve (S2–S4) innervates perineum. Can be blocked with local anesthetic during childbirth using the ischial spine as a landmark for injection.

Choose superolateral gluteal quadrant as intramuscular injection site to avoid nerve injury.

Signs of lumbosacral radiculopathy

Paresthesias and weakness in distribution of specific lumbar or sacral spinal nerves. Often due to intervertebral disc herniation in which the nerve associated with the inferior vertebral body is impinged (eg, herniation of L3–L4 disc affects the L4 spinal nerve).

Intervertebral discs generally herniate posterolaterally, due to the thin posterior longitudinal ligament and thicker anterior longitudinal ligament along the midline of the vertebral bodies.

DISC LEVEL	FINDINGS
L3–L4	Weakness of knee extension, ↓ patellar reflex
L4–L5	Weakness of dorsiflexion, difficulty in heel-walking
L5–S1	Weakness of plantarflexion, difficulty in toe-walking, ↓ Achilles reflex

Neurovascular pairing

Nerves and arteries are frequently named together by the bones/regions with which they are associated. The following are exceptions to this naming convention.

LOCATION	NERVE	ARTERY
Axilla/lateral thorax	Long thoracic	Lateral thoracic
Surgical neck of humerus	Axillary	Posterior circumflex
Midshaft of humerus	Radial	Deep brachial
Distal humerus/ cubital fossa	Median	Brachial
Popliteal fossa	Tibial	Popliteal
Posterior to medial malleolus	Tibial	Posterior tibial

I didn't know cardiac m has cisterna

Muscle conduction to contraction

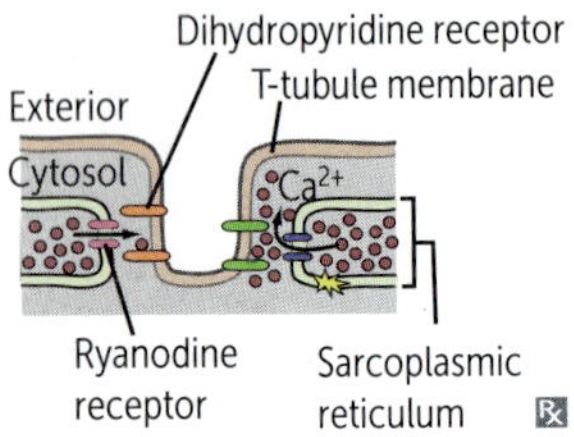

T-tubules are extensions of plasma membrane juxtaposed with terminal cisternae of the sarcoplasmic reticulum.

In skeletal muscle, 1 T-tubule + 2 terminal cisternae = triad.

In cardiac muscle, 1 T-tubule + 1 terminal cisterna = dyad.

1. Action potential depolarization opens presynaptic voltage-gated Ca^{2+} channels, inducing neurotransmitter release.
2. Postsynaptic ligand binding leads to muscle cell depolarization in the motor end plate.
3. Depolarization travels along muscle cell and down the T-tubule.
4. Depolarization of the voltage-sensitive dihydropyridine receptor, mechanically coupled to the ryanodine receptor on the sarcoplasmic reticulum, induces a conformational change in both receptors, causing Ca^{2+} release from sarcoplasmic reticulum.
5. Released Ca^{2+} binds to troponin C, causing a conformational change that moves tropomyosin out of the myosin-binding groove on actin filaments.
6. Myosin releases bound ADP and P_i → displacement of myosin on the actin filament (power stroke). Contraction results in shortening of **H** and **I** bands and between **Z** lines (**HIZ** shrinkage), but the A band remains the same length (**A** band is **A**lways the same length) A.
7. Binding of a new ATP molecule causes detachment of myosin head from actin filament. Hydrolysis of bound ATP → ADP, myosin head adopts high-energy position ("cocked") for the next contraction cycle.

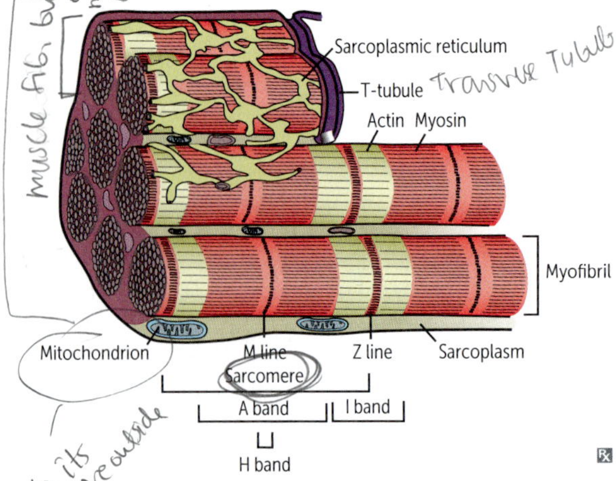

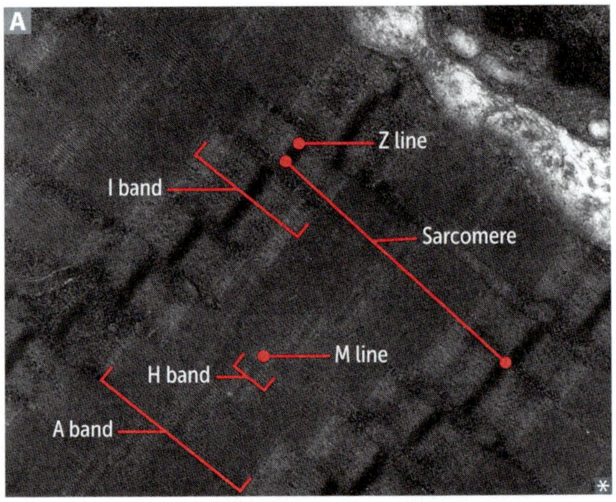

Types of muscle fibers

Type 1 muscle	**Slow** twitch; **red** fibers resulting from ↑ mitochondria and myoglobin concentration (↑ **ox**idative phosphorylation) → sustained contraction. Proportion ↑ after endurance training.	Think "**1 slow red ox.**"
Type 2 muscle	Fast twitch; white fibers resulting from ↓ mitochondria and myoglobin concentration (↑ anaerobic glycolysis). Proportion ↑ after weight/resistance training.	

ATP very labile (reactive) so E is stored as ATP in organs that use it quickly — Type 2. (Cr. Phosph too)

Type 1 stores E as TRIGLYC.

Smooth muscle contraction

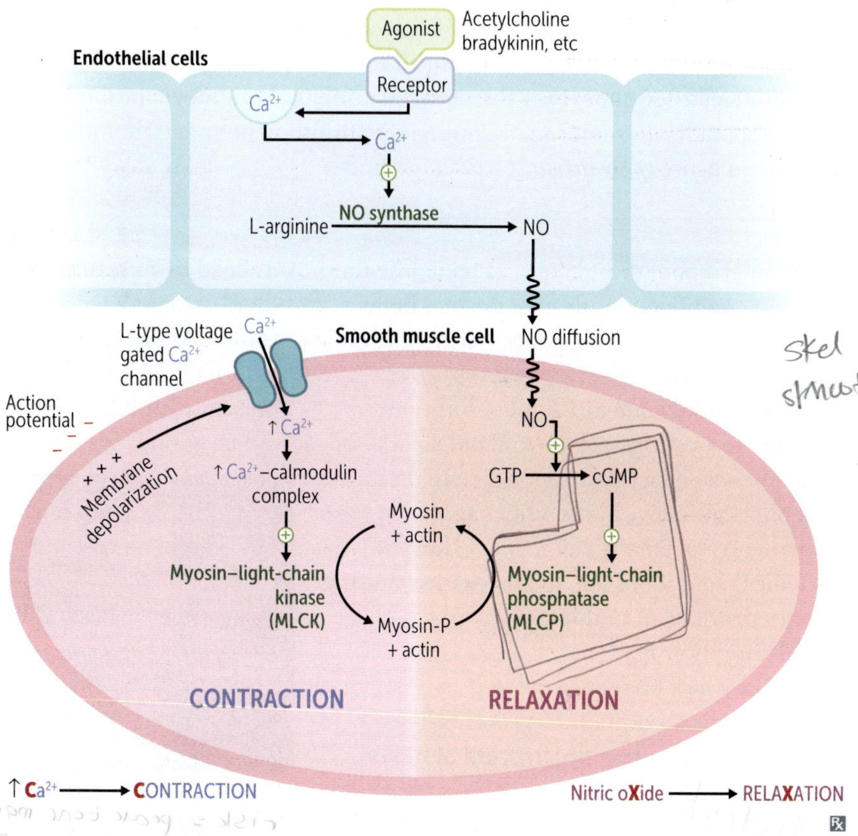

Bone formation

Endochondral ossification	Bones of axial skeleton, appendicular skeleton, and base of skull. Cartilaginous model of bone is first made by chondrocytes. Osteoclasts and osteoblasts later replace with woven bone and then remodel to lamellar bone. In adults, woven bone occurs after fractures and in Paget disease. Defective in achondroplasia.
Membranous ossification	Bones of calvarium and facial bones. Woven bone formed directly without cartilage. Later remodeled to lamellar bone.

Cell biology of bone

Osteoblast	**B**uilds **b**one by secreting collagen and catalyzing mineralization in alkaline environment via ALP. Differentiates from mesenchymal stem cells in periosteum.
Osteoclast	Dissolves bone by secreting H^+ and collagenases. Differentiates from a fusion of monocyte/macrophage lineage precursors.
Parathyroid hormone	At low, intermittent levels, exerts anabolic effects (building bone) on osteoblasts and osteoclasts (indirect). Chronically ↑ PTH levels (1° hyperparathyroidism) cause catabolic effects (osteitis fibrosa cystica).
Estrogen	Inhibits apoptosis in bone-forming osteoblasts and induces apoptosis in bone-resorbing osteoclasts. Estrogen deficiency (surgical or postmenopausal), excess cycles of remodeling, and bone resorption lead to osteoporosis.

▶ MUSCULOSKELETAL, SKIN, AND CONNECTIVE TISSUE—PATHOLOGY

Achondroplasia

Failure of longitudinal bone growth (endochondral ossification) → short limbs. Membranous ossification is not affected → large head relative to limbs. Constitutive activation of fibroblast growth factor receptor (FGFR3) actually inhibits chondrocyte proliferation. > 85% of mutations occur sporadically; autosomal dominant with full penetrance (homozygosity is lethal). Most common cause of dwarfism.

Osteoporosis

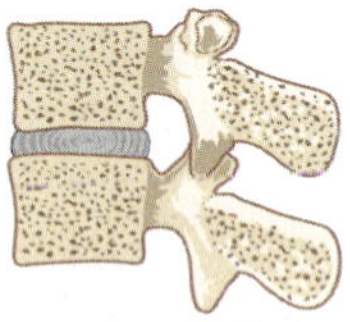

Normal vertebrae

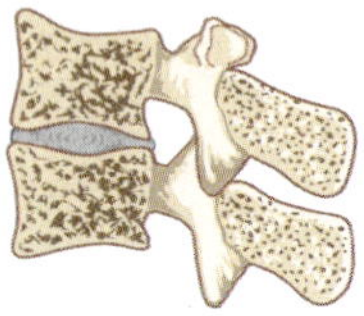

Mild compression fracture

Trabecular (spongy) and cortical bone lose mass and interconnections despite normal bone mineralization and lab values (serum Ca^{2+} and PO_4^{3-}).

Most commonly due to ↑ bone resorption related to ↓ estrogen levels and old age. Can be secondary to drugs (eg, steroids, alcohol, anticonvulsants, anticoagulants, thyroid replacement therapy) or other medical conditions (eg, hyperparathyroidism, hyperthyroidism, multiple myeloma, malabsorption syndromes).

Diagnosed by a bone mineral density scan (dual-energy x-ray absorptiometry) with a T-score of ≤ −2.5 or by a fragility fracture of hip or vertebra.

Prophylaxis: regular weight-bearing exercise and adequate Ca^{2+} and vitamin D intake throughout adulthood.

Treatment: bisphosphonates, teriparatide, SERMs, rarely calcitonin; denosumab (monoclonal antibody against RANKL).

Can lead to vertebral compression fractures (A, small arrows; large arrows show normal-for-age vertebral body height for comparison)—acute back pain, loss of height, kyphosis. Also can present with fractures of femoral neck, distal radius (Colles fracture).

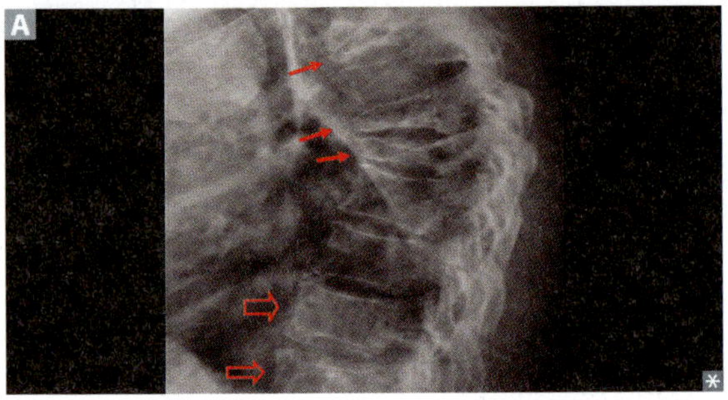

Osteopetrosis (marble bone disease)

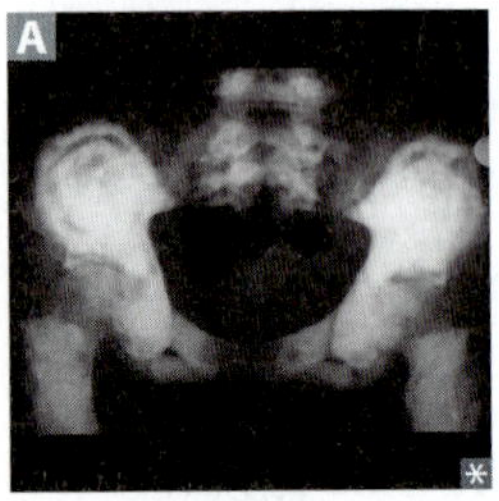

Failure of normal bone resorption due to defective osteoclasts → thickened, dense bones that are prone to fracture. Bone fills marrow space → pancytopenia, extramedullary hematopoiesis. Mutations (eg, carbonic anhydrase II) impair ability of osteoclast to generate acidic environment necessary for bone resorption. X-rays show bone-in-bone ("stone" bone) appearance A. Can result in cranial nerve impingement and palsies as a result of narrowed foramina. Bone marrow transplant is potentially curative as osteoclasts are derived from monocytes.

Osteomalacia/rickets

Defective mineralization of osteoid (osteomalacia) or cartilaginous growth plates (rickets, only in children). Most commonly due to vitamin D deficiency.

X-rays show osteopenia and "Looser zones" (pseudofractures) in osteomalacia, epiphyseal widening and metaphyseal cupping/fraying in rickets. Children with rickets have bow legs **A**, bead-like costochondral junctions (rachitic rosary), craniotabes (soft skull).

↓ vitamin D → ↓ serum Ca^{2+} → ↑ PTH secretion → ↓ serum PO_4^{3-}.

Hyperactivity of osteoblasts → ↑ ALP.

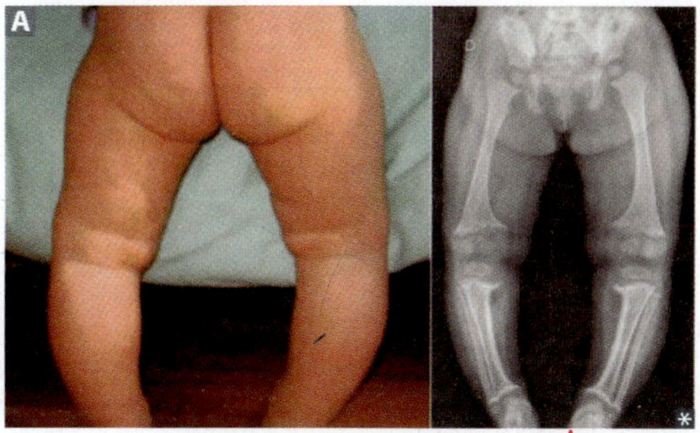

Paget disease of bone (osteitis deformans)

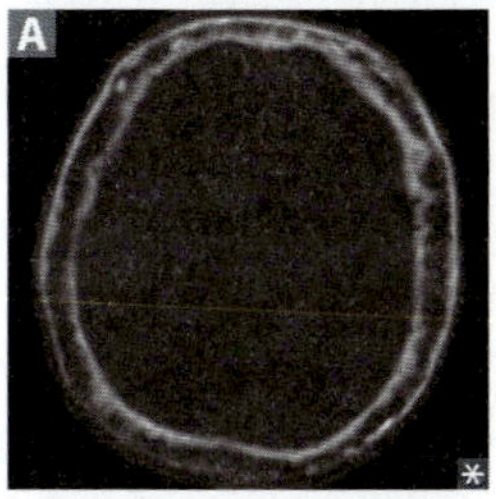

Common, localized disorder of bone remodeling caused by ↑ osteoclastic activity followed by ↑ osteoblastic activity that forms poor-quality bone. Serum Ca^{2+}, phosphorus, and PTH levels are normal. ↑ ALP. Mosaic pattern of woven and lamellar bone (osteocytes with lacunae in chaotic juxtapositions); long bone chalk-stick fractures. ↑ blood flow from ↑ arteriovenous shunts may cause high-output heart failure. ↑ risk of osteogenic sarcoma.

Hat size can be increased due to skull thickening **A**; hearing loss is common due to auditory foramen narrowing.

Stages of Paget disease:

- Lytic—osteoclasts
- Mixed—osteoclasts + osteoblasts
- Sclerotic—osteoblasts
- Quiescent—minimal osteoclast/osteoblast activity

Osteonecrosis (avascular necrosis)

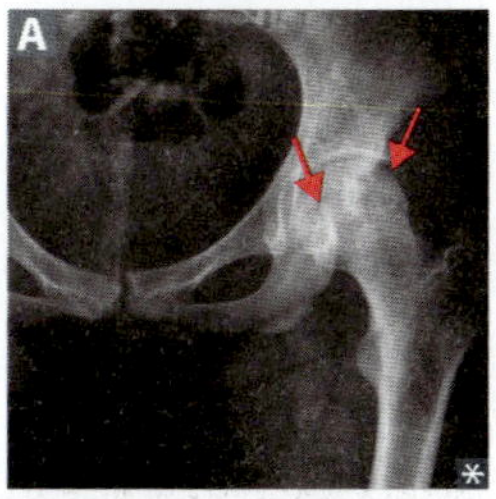

Infarction of bone and marrow, usually very painful. Most common site is femoral head **A** (due to insufficiency of medial circumflex femoral artery). Causes include Corticosteroids, Alcoholism, Sickle cell disease, Trauma, "the Bends" (caisson/decompression disease), LEgg-Calvé-Perthes disease (idiopathic), Gaucher disease, Slipped capital femoral epiphysis—CAST Bent LEGS.

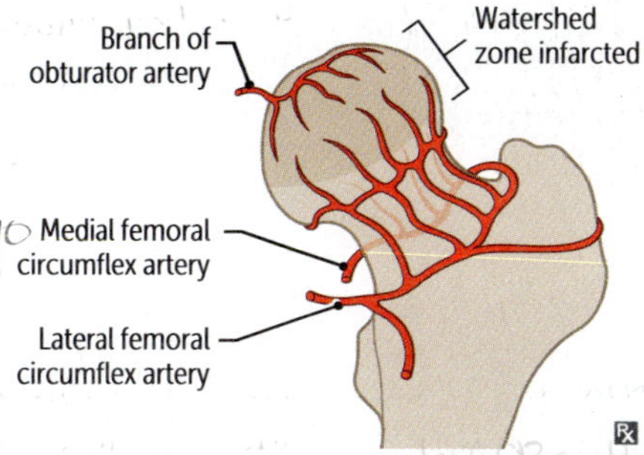

Lab values in bone disorders

DISORDER	SERUM Ca^{2+}	PO_4^{3-}	ALP	PTH	COMMENTS
Osteoporosis	—	—	—	—	↓ bone mass
Osteopetrosis	—/↓	—	—	—	Dense, brittle bones. Ca^{2+} ↓ in severe, malignant disease
Paget disease of bone	—	—	↑	—	Abnormal "mosaic" bone architecture
Osteitis fibrosa cystica					"Brown tumors" due to fibrous replacement of bone, subperiosteal thinning
Primary hyperparathyroidism	↑	↓	↑	↑	Idiopathic or parathyroid hyperplasia, adenoma, carcinoma
Secondary hyperparathyroidism	↓	↑	↑	↑	Often as compensation for CKD (↓ PO_4^{3-} excretion and production of activated vitamin D)
Osteomalacia/rickets	↓	↓	↑	↑	Soft bones; vitamin D deficiency also causes 2° hyperparathyroidism
Hypervitaminosis D	↑	↑	—	↓	Caused by oversupplementation or granulomatous disease (eg, sarcoidosis)

- bacteremia = kids — metaph; adult — epiphys

Primary bone tumors

TUMOR TYPE	EPIDEMIOLOGY/LOCATION	CHARACTERISTICS
Benign tumors		
Osteochondroma	Most common benign bone tumor. Males < 25 years old.	Bony exostosis with cartilaginous (chondroid) cap A. Rarely transforms to chondrosarcoma.
Giant cell tumor	20–40 years old. Epiphyseal end of long bones. Often around knee. "Osteoclastoma."	Locally aggressive benign tumor. "Soap bubble" appearance on x-ray B. Multinucleated giant cells.
Malignant tumors		
Osteosarcoma (osteogenic sarcoma)	2nd most common 1° malignant bone tumor (after multiple myeloma). Bimodal distribution: 10–20 years old (1°), > 65 (2°). Predisposing factors: Paget disease of bone, bone infarcts, radiation, familial retinoblastoma, Li-Fraumeni syndrome (germline *p53* mutation). Metaphysis of long bones, often around knee C.	Codman triangle (from elevation of periosteum) or sunburst pattern on x-ray. Aggressive. Treat with surgical en bloc resection (with limb salvage) and chemotherapy.
Ewing sarcoma	Boys < 15 years old. Commonly appears in diaphysis of long bones, pelvis, scapula, ribs.	Anaplastic small blue cell malignant tumor D. Extremely aggressive with early metastases, but responsive to chemotherapy. "Onion skin" periosteal reaction in bone. Associated with t(11;22) translocation causing fusion protein EWS-FLI 1. 11 + 22 = 33 (Patrick Ewing's jersey number).

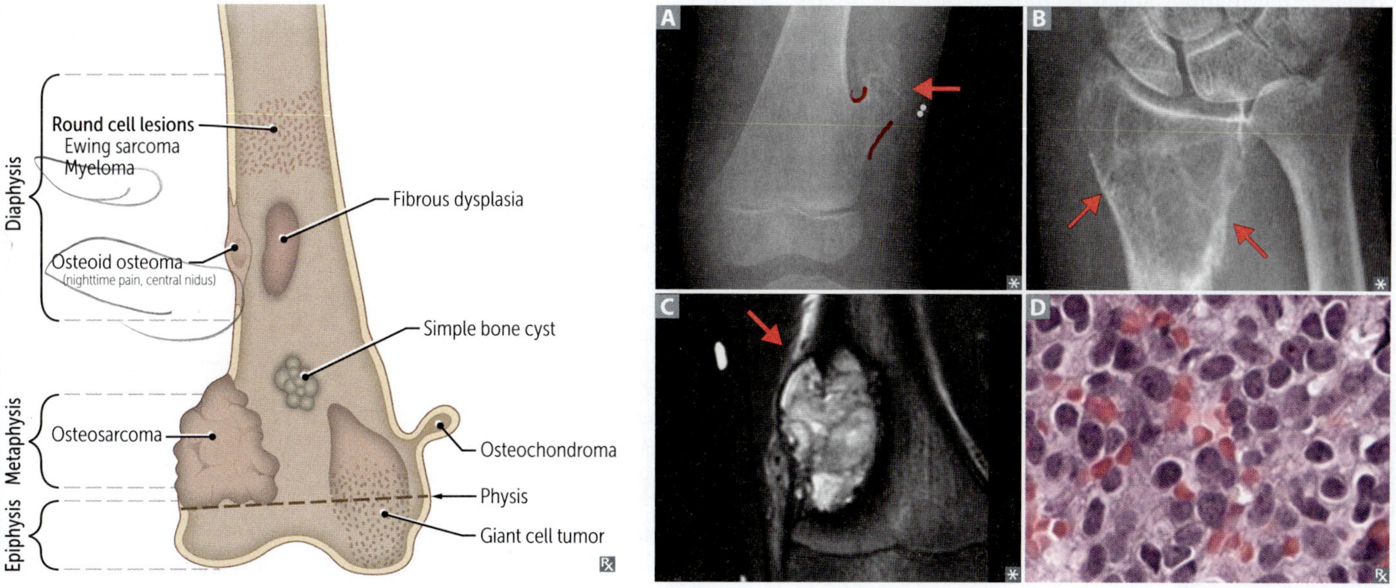

Osteoarthritis and rheumatoid arthritis

	Osteoarthritis	Rheumatoid arthritis
PATHOGENESIS	Mechanical—wear and tear destroys articular cartilage ("degenerative joint disease"). Chondrocytes mediate degradation and inadequate repair.	Autoimmune—inflammatory cytokines and cells induce pannus (proliferative granulation tissue) formation, which erodes articular cartilage and bone.
PREDISPOSING FACTORS	Age, female, obesity, joint trauma.	Female, HLA-DR4, smoking, silica exposure. ⊕ rheumatoid factor (anti-IgG antibody; in 80%), anti-cyclic citrullinated peptide antibody (more specific).
PRESENTATION	Pain in weight-bearing joints after use (eg, at the end of the day), improving with rest. Asymmetric joint involvement. Knee cartilage loss begins medially ("bowlegged"). No systemic symptoms.	Pain, swelling, and morning stiffness lasting > 1 hour, improving with use. Symmetric joint involvement. Systemic symptoms (fever, fatigue, weight loss). Extraarticular manifestations common.*
JOINT FINDINGS	Osteophytes (bone spurs), joint space narrowing, subchondral sclerosis and cysts. Synovial fluid non-inflammatory (WBC < 2000/mm^3). Involves DIP (Heberden nodes A) and PIP (Bouchard nodes), and 1st CMC; not MCP.	Erosions, juxtaarticular osteopenia, joint space narrowing, soft tissue swelling, subchondral cysts. Deformities include subluxation, fingers with ulnar deviation, swan neck B, and boutonniere. Synovial fluid inflammatory (WBC > 2000/mm^3). Involves MCP, PIP, wrist; not DIP or 1st CMC.
TREATMENT	Acetaminophen, NSAIDs, intra-articular glucocorticoids.	NSAIDs, glucocorticoids, disease-modifying agents (methotrexate, sulfasalazine, hydroxychloroquine, leflunomide), biologic agents (eg, TNF-α inhibitors).

*Extraarticular manifestations include rheumatoid nodules (fibrinoid necrosis with palisading histiocytes) in subcutaneous tissue and lung (+ pneumoconiosis → Caplan syndrome), interstitial lung disease, pleuritis, pericarditis, anemia of chronic disease, neutropenia + splenomegaly (Felty syndrome), AA amyloidosis, Sjögren syndrome, scleritis, carpal tunnel syndrome.

A
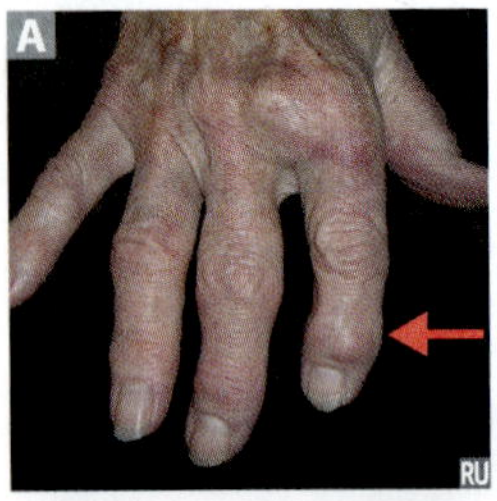

B
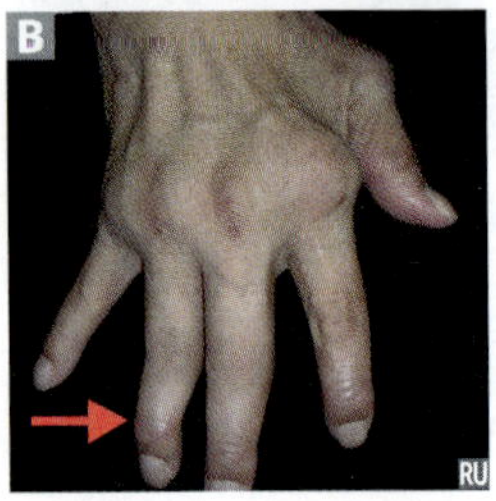

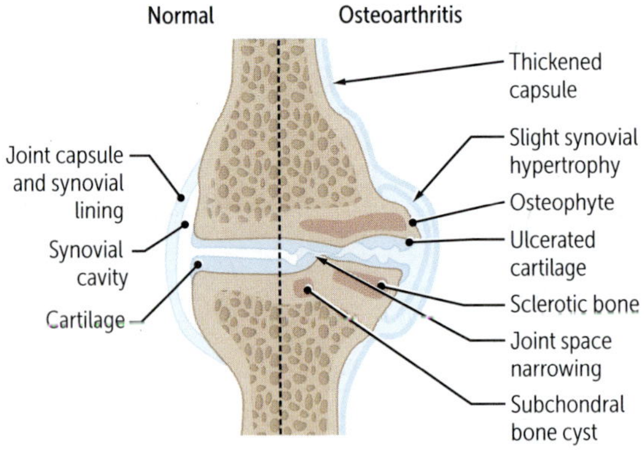

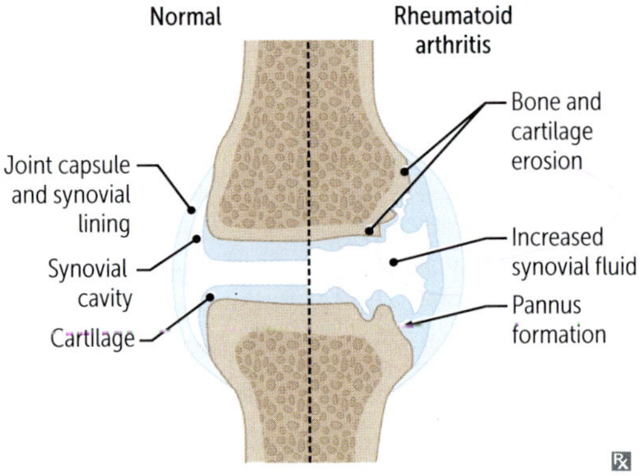

Gout

FINDINGS	Acute inflammatory monoarthritis caused by precipitation of monosodium urate crystals in joints A. More common in males. Associated with hyperuricemia, which can be caused by: ▪ Underexcretion of uric acid (90% of patients)—largely idiopathic; can be exacerbated by certain medications (eg, thiazide diuretics). ▪ Overproduction of uric acid (10% of patients)—Lesch-Nyhan syndrome, PRPP excess, ↑ cell turnover (eg, tumor lysis syndrome), von Gierke disease. Crystals are needle shaped and ⊖ birefringent under polarized light (yellow under parallel light, blue under perpendicular light B).
SYMPTOMS	Asymmetric joint distribution. Joint is swollen, red, and painful. Classic manifestation is painful MTP joint of big toe (podagra). Tophus formation C (often on external ear, olecranon bursa, or Achilles tendon). Acute attack tends to occur after a large meal or alcohol consumption (alcohol metabolites compete for same excretion sites in kidney as uric acid → ↓ uric acid secretion and subsequent buildup in blood).
TREATMENT	Acute: NSAIDs (eg, indomethacin), glucocorticoids, colchicine. Chronic (preventive): xanthine oxidase inhibitors (eg, allopurinol, febuxostat).

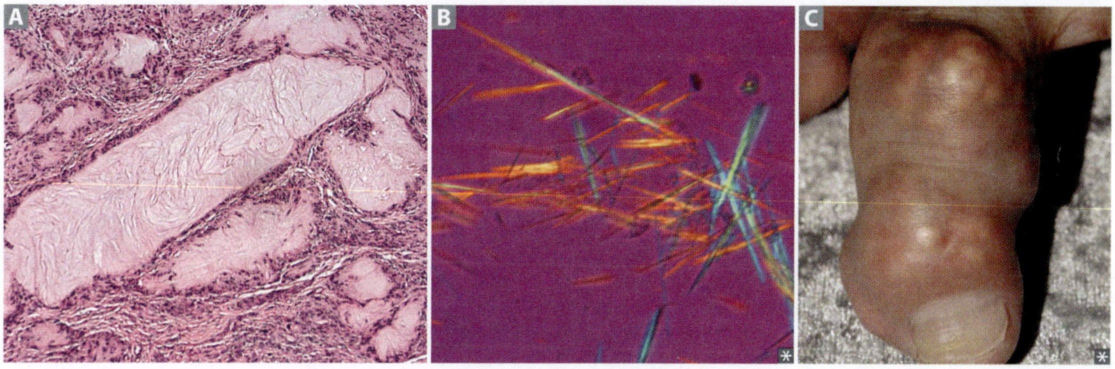

Calcium pyrophosphate deposition disease

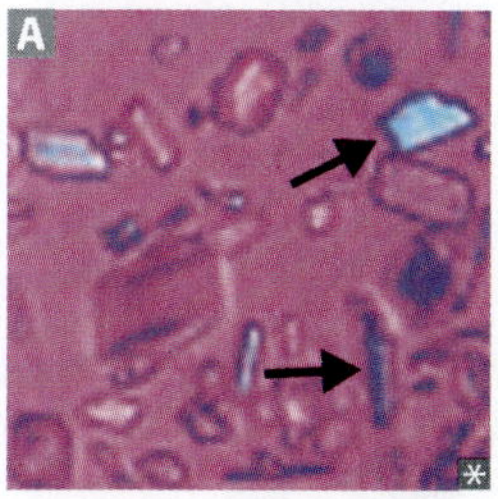

Deposition of calcium pyrophosphate crystals within the joint space. Occurs in patients > 50 years old; both sexes affected equally. Usually idiopathic, sometimes associated with hemochromatosis, hyperparathyroidism, joint trauma.

Pain and swelling with acute inflammation (pseudogout) and/or chronic degeneration (pseudo-osteoarthritis). Knee most commonly affected joint.

Chondrocalcinosis (cartilage calcification) on x-ray.

Crystals are rhomboid and weakly ⊕ birefringent under polarized light (blue when parallel to light) A.

Acute treatment: NSAIDs, colchicine, glucocorticoids.

Prophylaxis: colchicine.

Sjögren syndrome

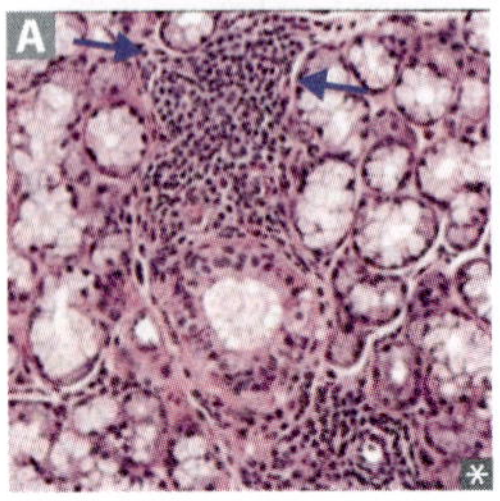

Autoimmune disorder characterized by destruction of exocrine glands (especially lacrimal and salivary) by lymphocytic infiltrates A. Predominantly affects females 40–60 years old.

Findings:

- Inflammatory joint pain
- Keratoconjunctivitis sicca (↓ tear production and subsequent corneal damage)
- Xerostomia (↓ saliva production)
- Presence of antinuclear antibodies: SS-A (anti-Ro) and/or SS-B (anti-La)
- Bilateral parotid enlargement

A common 1° disorder or a 2° syndrome associated with other autoimmune disorders (eg, rheumatoid arthritis, SLE, systemic sclerosis).

Complications: dental caries; mucosa-associated lymphoid tissue (MALT) lymphoma (may present as parotid enlargement).

Septic arthritis

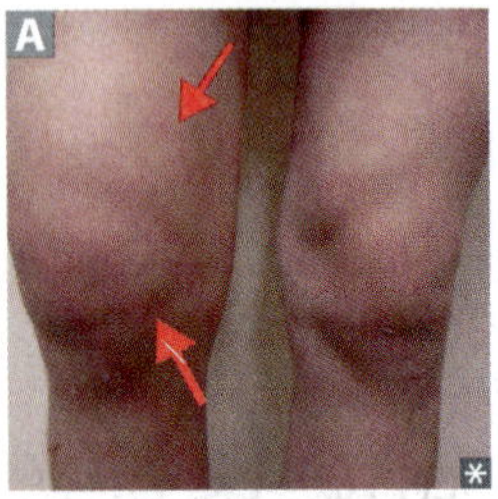

S aureus, *Streptococcus*, and *Neisseria gonorrhoeae* are common causes. Affected joint is swollen A, red, and painful. Synovial fluid purulent (WBC > 50,000/mm^3). Autoim was >2000

Gonococcal arthritis—STI that presents as either purulent arthritis (eg, knee) or triad of polyarthralgias, tenosynovitis (eg, hand), dermatitis (eg, pustules).

Seronegative spondyloarthritis	Arthritis without rheumatoid factor (no anti-IgG antibody). Strong association with HLA-B27 (MHC class I serotype). Subtypes (**PAIR**) share variable occurrence of inflammatory back pain (associated with morning stiffness, improves with exercise), peripheral arthritis, enthesitis (inflamed insertion sites of tendons, eg, Achilles), dactylitis ("sausage fingers"), uveitis.	
Psoriatic arthritis	Associated with skin psoriasis and nail lesions. Asymmetric and patchy involvement A. Dactylitis and "pencil-in-cup" deformity of DIP on x-ray B.	Seen in fewer than ⅓ of patients with psoriasis.
Ankylosing spondylitis	Symmetric involvement of spine and sacroiliac joints → ankylosis (joint fusion), uveitis, aortic regurgitation.	Bamboo spine (vertebral fusion) C. More common in males.
Inflammatory bowel disease	Crohn disease and ulcerative colitis are often associated with spondyloarthritis.	
Reactive arthritis	Formerly known as Reiter syndrome. Classic triad: ▪ **Conjunctivitis** ▪ **Urethritis** ▪ **Arthritis**	**"Can't see, can't pee, can't bend my knee."** Post-GI (*Shigella, Salmonella, Yersinia, Campylobacter*) or *Chlamydia* infections.

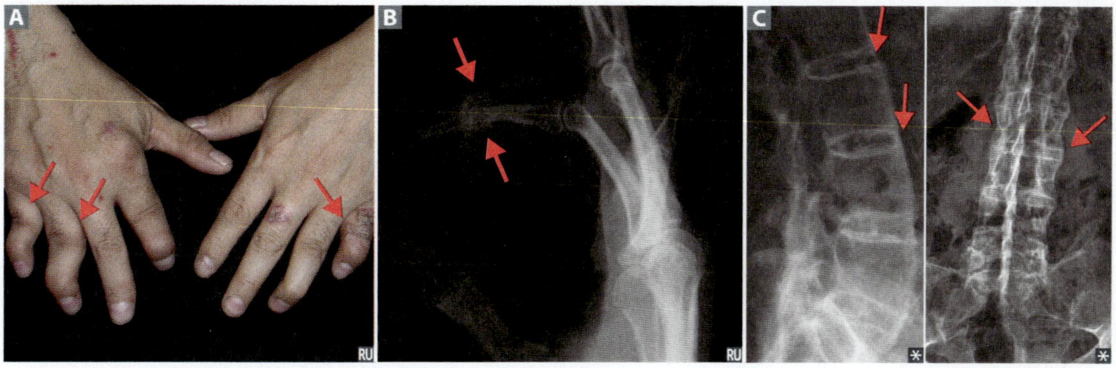

Systemic lupus erythematosus

SYMPTOMS

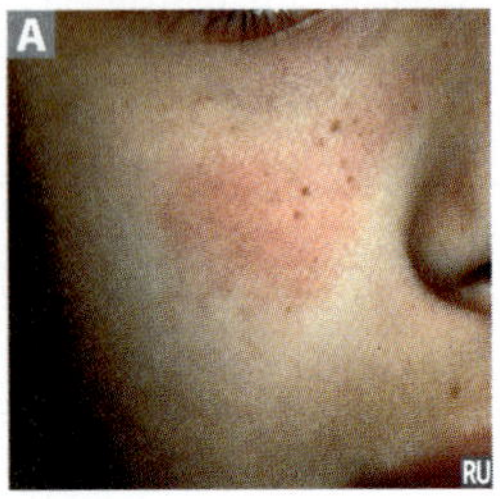

Classic presentation: rash, joint pain, and fever, most commonly in a female of reproductive age and African-American descent.

Libman-Sacks Endocarditis—nonbacterial, verrucous thrombi usually on mitral or aortic valve (LSE in SLE).

Lupus nephritis (glomerular deposition of anti-DNA immune complexes) can be nephritic or nephrotic (hematuria or proteinuria). Most common and severe type is diffuse proliferative.

Common causes of death in SLE:

- Cardiovascular disease
- Infections
- Renal disease

RASH OR PAIN:

- **R**ash (malar **A** or discoid)
- **A**rthritis (nonerosive)
- **S**erositis
- **H**ematologic disorders (eg, cytopenias)
- **O**ral/nasopharyngeal ulcers
- **R**enal disease
- **P**hotosensitivity
- **A**ntinuclear antibodies
- **I**mmunologic disorder (anti-dsDNA, anti-Sm, antiphospholipid)
- **N**eurologic disorders (eg, seizures, psychosis)

FINDINGS

Antinuclear antibodies (ANA)	Sensitive, not specific
Anti-dsDNA antibodies	Specific, poor prognosis (renal disease)
Anti-Smith antibodies	Specific, not prognostic (directed against snRNPs)
Antihistone antibodies	Sensitive for drug-induced lupus (eg, hydralazine, procainamide)
↓ C3, C4, and CH_{50} due to immune complex formation.	

TREATMENT

NSAIDs, steroids, immunosuppressants, hydroxychloroquine.

Antiphospholipid syndrome

1° or 2° autoimmune disorder (most commonly in SLE).

Diagnose based on clinical criteria including history of thrombosis (arterial or venous) or spontaneous abortion along with laboratory findings of lupus anticoagulant, anticardiolipin, anti-β_2 glycoprotein antibodies.

Treat with systemic anticoagulation.

Anticardiolipin antibodies and lupus anticoagulant can cause false-positive VDRL/RPR and prolonged PTT.

Mixed connective tissue disease

Features of SLE, systemic sclerosis, and/or polymyositis. Associated with anti-U1 RNP antibodies (speckled ANA).

Sarcoidosis

Characterized by immune-mediated, widespread noncaseating granulomas **A**, elevated serum ACE levels, and elevated CD4+/CD8+ ratio in bronchoalveolar lavage fluid. More common in African-American females. Often asymptomatic except for enlarged lymph nodes. Findings on CXR of bilateral adenopathy and coarse reticular opacities **B**; CT of the chest better demonstrates the extensive hilar and mediastinal adenopathy **C**.

Associated with restrictive lung disease (interstitial fibrosis), erythema nodosum, lupus pernio (skin lesions on face resembling lupus), Bell palsy, epithelioid granulomas containing microscopic Schaumann and asteroid bodies, uveitis, hypercalcemia (due to ↑ 1α-hydroxylase–mediated vitamin D activation in macrophages).

Treatment: steroids (if symptomatic).

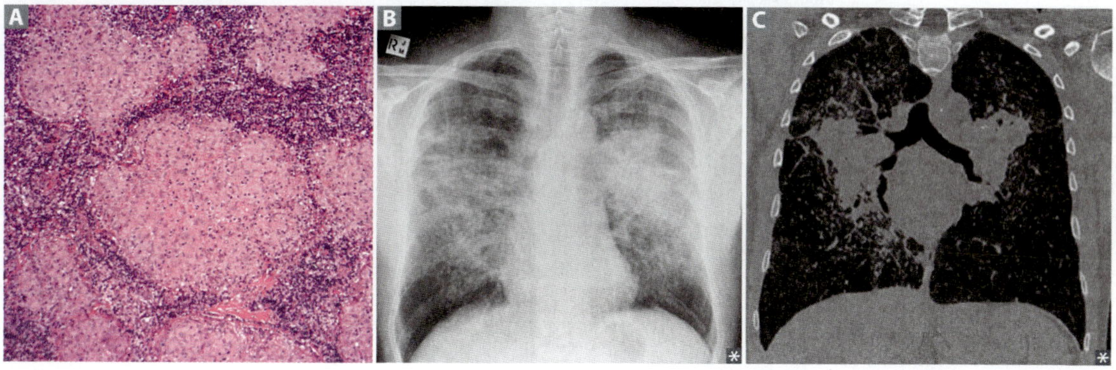

Polymyalgia rheumatica

SYMPTOMS	Pain and stiffness in shoulders and hips, often with fever, malaise, weight loss. Does not cause muscular weakness. More common in women > 50 years old; associated with giant cell (temporal) arteritis.
FINDINGS	↑ ESR, ↑ CRP, normal CK.
TREATMENT	Rapid response to low-dose corticosteroids.

Fibromyalgia

Most commonly seen in females 20–50 years old. Chronic, widespread musculoskeletal pain associated with stiffness, paresthesias, poor sleep, fatigue, cognitive disturbance ("fibro fog"). Treatment: regular exercise, antidepressants (TCAs, SNRIs), anticonvulsants.

Polymyositis/ dermatomyositis	↑ CK, ⊕ ANA, ⊕ anti-Jo-1, ⊕ anti-SRP, ⊕ anti-Mi-2 antibodies. Treatment: steroids followed by long-term immunosuppressant therapy (eg, methotrexate).
Polymyositis	Progressive symmetric proximal muscle weakness, characterized by endomysial inflammation with CD8+ T cells. Most often involves shoulders.
Dermatomyositis	Similar to polymyositis, but also involves malar rash (similar to SLE), Gottron papules **A**, heliotrope (erythematous periorbital) rash **B**, "shawl and face" rash **C**, "mechanic's hands." ↑ risk of occult malignancy. Perimysial inflammation and atrophy with CD4+ T cells.

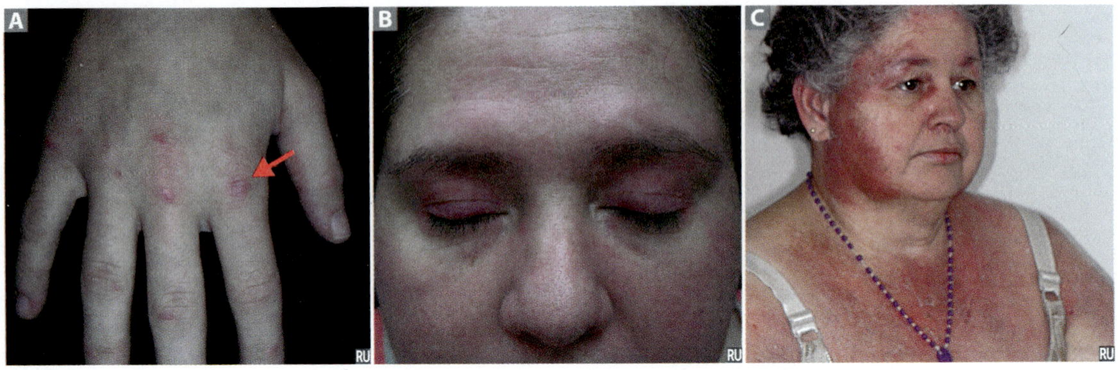

Neuromuscular junction diseases

	Myasthenia gravis	Lambert-Eaton myasthenic syndrome
FREQUENCY	Most common NMJ disorder	Uncommon
PATHOPHYSIOLOGY	Autoantibodies to postsynaptic ACh receptor	Autoantibodies to presynaptic Ca^{2+} channel → ↓ ACh release
CLINICAL	Ptosis, diplopia, weakness Worsens with muscle use	Proximal muscle weakness, autonomic symptoms (dry mouth, impotence) Improves with muscle use
ASSOCIATED WITH	Thymoma, thymic hyperplasia	Small cell lung cancer
AChE INHIBITOR ADMINISTRATION	Reverses symptoms (edrophonium to diagnose, pyridostigmine to treat)	Minimal effect

Myositis ossificans

Heterotopic ossification of skeletal muscle following muscular trauma **A**. Most often seen in upper or lower extremity. May present as suspicious "mass" at site of known trauma or as incidental finding on radiography.

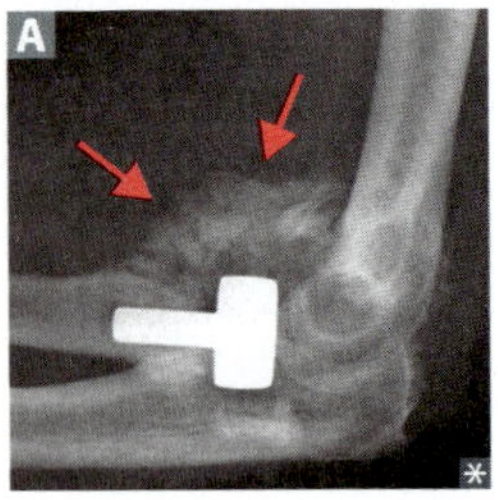

Scleroderma (systemic sclerosis)

Triad of autoimmunity, noninflammatory vasculopathy, and collagen deposition with fibrosis. Commonly sclerosis of skin, manifesting as puffy, taut skin A without wrinkles, fingertip pitting B. Also sclerosis of renal, pulmonary (most common cause of death), cardiovascular, GI systems. 75% female. 2 major types:

- **Diffuse scleroderma**—widespread skin involvement, rapid progression, early visceral involvement. Associated with anti-Scl-70 antibody (anti-DNA topoisomerase I antibody).
- **Limited scleroderma**—limited skin involvement confined to fingers and face. Also with CREST syndrome: Calcinosis C, Raynaud phenomenon, Esophageal dysmotility, Sclerodactyly, and Telangiectasia. More benign clinical course. Associated with anti-centromere antibody.

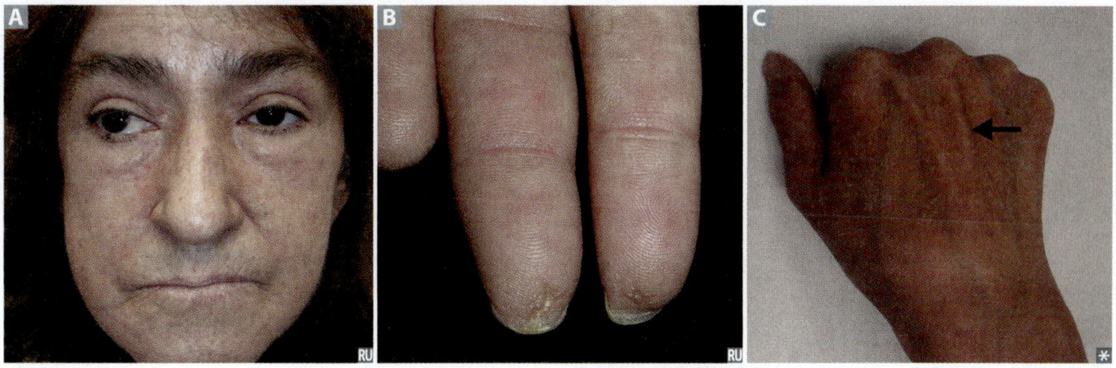

Raynaud phenomenon

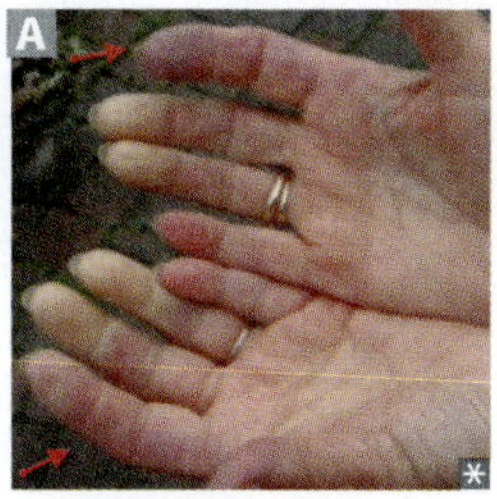

↓ blood flow to the skin due to arteriolar (small vessel) vasospasm in response to cold or stress: color change from white (ischemia) to blue (hypoxia) to red (reperfusion). Most often in the fingers A and toes. Called Raynaud disease when 1° (idiopathic), Raynaud syndrome when 2° to a disease process such as mixed connective tissue disease, SLE, or CREST (limited form of systemic sclerosis) syndrome. Digital ulceration (critical ischemia) seen in 2° Raynaud syndrome. Treat with Ca^{2+} channel blockers.

▶ MUSCULOSKELETAL, SKIN, AND CONNECTIVE TISSUE—DERMATOLOGY

Skin layers

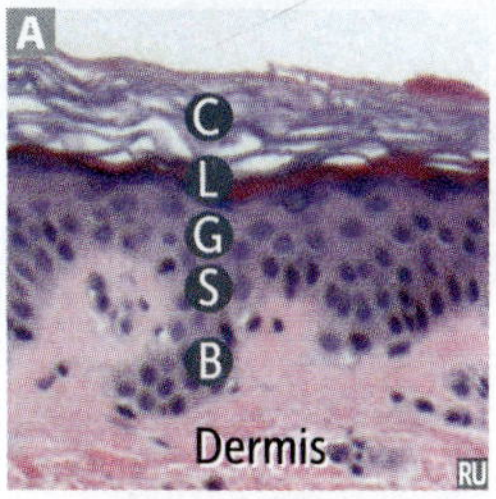

Skin has 3 layers: epidermis, dermis, subcutaneous fat (hypodermis, subcutis).

Epidermis layers from surface to base A:

- Stratum Corneum (keratin)
- Stratum Lucidum
- Stratum Granulosum
- Stratum Spinosum (desmosomes)
- Stratum Basale (stem cell site)

Californians Like Girls in String Bikinis.

Epithelial cell junctions

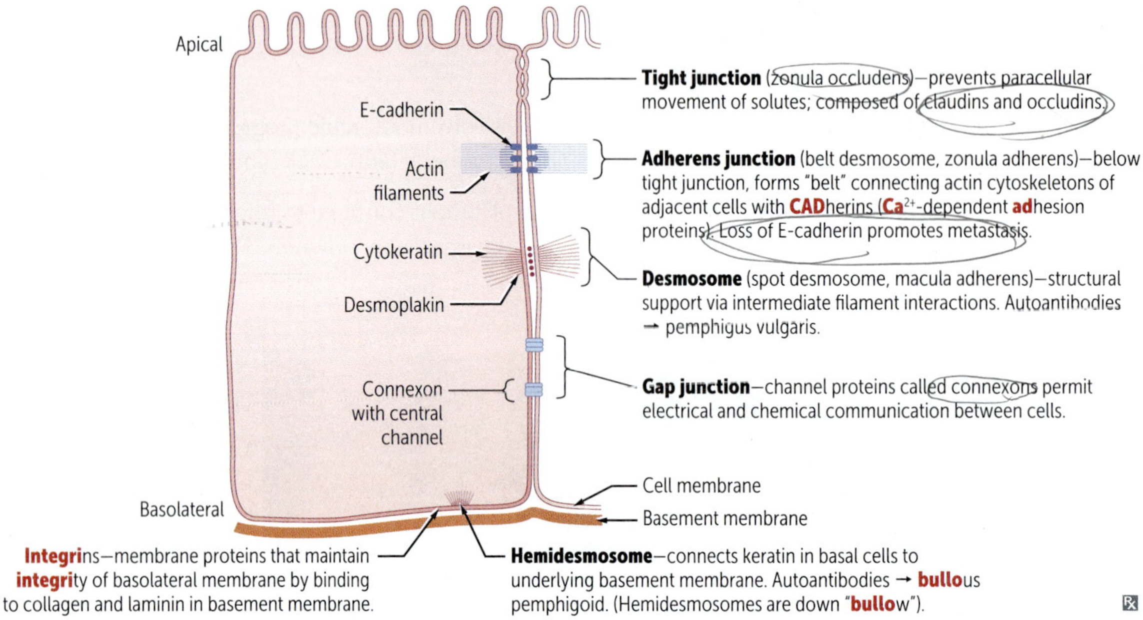

Dermatologic macroscopic terms (morphology)

LESION	CHARACTERISTICS	EXAMPLES
Macule	Flat lesion with well-circumscribed change in skin color < 1 cm	Freckle, labial macule A
Patch	Macule > 1 cm	Large birthmark (congenital nevus) B
Papule	Elevated solid skin lesion < 1 cm	Mole (nevus) C, acne
Plaque	Papule > 1 cm	Psoriasis D
Vesicle	Small fluid-containing blister < 1 cm	Chickenpox (varicella), shingles (zoster) E
Bulla	Large fluid-containing blister > 1 cm	Bullous pemphigoid F
Pustule	Vesicle containing pus	Pustular psoriasis G
Wheal	Transient smooth papule or plaque	Hives (urticaria) H
Scale	Flaking off of stratum corneum	Eczema, psoriasis, SCC I
Crust	Dry exudate	Impetigo J

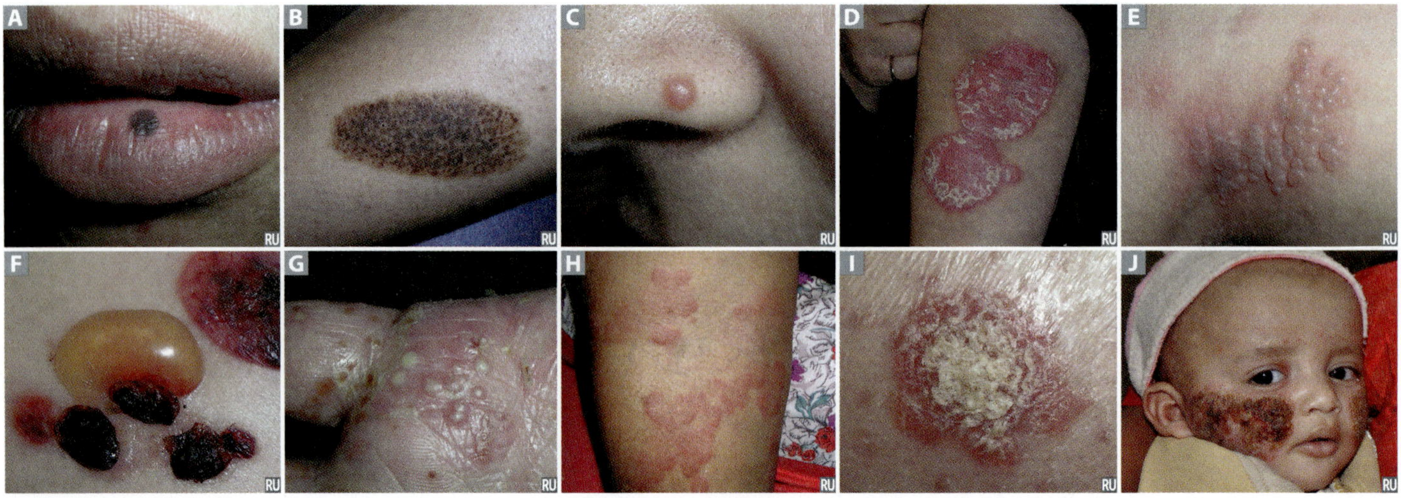

Dermatologic microscopic terms

LESION	CHARACTERISTICS	EXAMPLES
Hyperkeratosis	↑ thickness of stratum corneum	Psoriasis, calluses
Parakeratosis	Hyperkeratosis with retention of nuclei in stratum corneum	Psoriasis
Hypergranulosis	↑ thickness of stratum granulosum	Lichen planus
Spongiosis	Epidermal accumulation of edematous fluid in intercellular spaces	Eczematous dermatitis
Acantholysis	Separation of epidermal cells	Pemphigus vulgaris
Acanthosis	Epidermal hyperplasia (↑ spinosum)	Acanthosis nigricans

Pigmented skin disorders

Albinism	Normal melanocyte number with ↓ melanin production A due to ↓ tyrosinase activity or defective tyrosine transport. ↑ risk of skin cancer.
Melasma (chloasma)	Hyperpigmentation associated with pregnancy ("mask of pregnancy" B) or OCP use.
Vitiligo	Irregular areas of complete depigmentation C. Caused by autoimmune destruction of melanocytes.

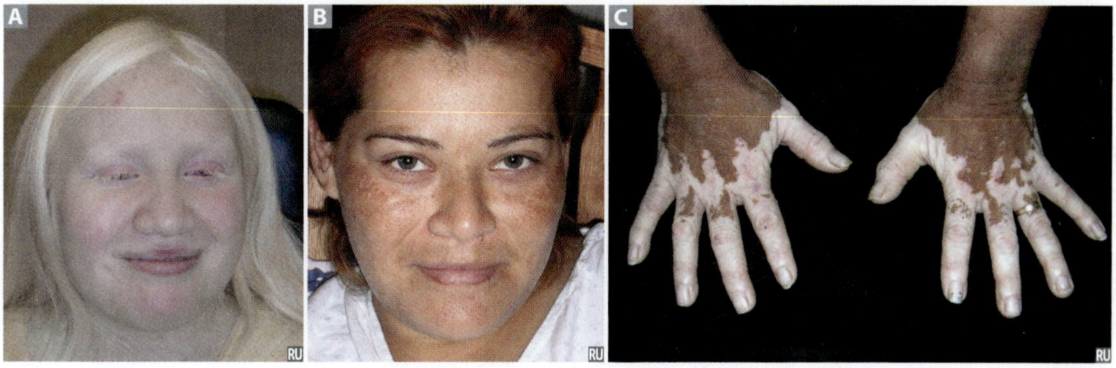

Common skin disorders

Acne	Pilosebaceous follicles with ↑ sebum, keratin, *Propionibacterium acnes* → obstruction (comedones) and inflammation (papules/pustules A, nodules, cysts). Treatment includes retinoids, benzoyl peroxide, antibiotics.
Atopic dermatitis (eczema)	Pruritic eruption, commonly on skin flexures. Often associated with other atopic diseases (asthma, allergic rhinitis, food allergies); ↑ serum IgE. Usually appears on face in infancy B and then antecubital fossae C.
Allergic contact dermatitis	Type IV hypersensitivity reaction that follows exposure to allergen. Lesions occur at site of contact (eg, nickel D, poison ivy, neomycin E).
Melanocytic nevus	Common mole. Benign, but melanoma can arise in congenital or atypical moles. Intradermal nevi are papular F. Junctional nevi are flat macules G.
Psoriasis	Papules and plaques with silvery scaling H, especially on knees and elbows. Acanthosis with parakeratotic scaling (nuclei still in stratum corneum), Munro microabscesses. ↑ stratum spinosum, ↓ stratum granulosum. Auspitz sign (arrow in I)—pinpoint bleeding spots from exposure of dermal papillae when scales are scraped off. Can be associated with nail pitting and psoriatic arthritis.
Rosacea	Inflammatory facial skin disorder characterized by erythematous papules and pustules J, but no comedones. May be associated with facial flushing in response to external stimuli (eg, alcohol, heat). Phymatous rosacea can cause rhinophyma (bulbous deformation of nose).
Seborrheic keratosis	Flat, greasy, pigmented squamous epithelial proliferation with keratin-filled cysts (horn cysts) K. Looks "stuck on." Lesions occur on head, trunk, and extremities. Common benign neoplasm of older persons. Leser-Trélat sign L—sudden appearance of multiple seborrheic keratoses, indicating an underlying malignancy (eg, GI, lymphoid).
Verrucae	Warts; caused by HPV. Soft, tan-colored, cauliflower-like papules M. Epidermal hyperplasia, hyperkeratosis, koilocytosis. Condyloma acuminatum on genitals N.
Urticaria	Hives. Pruritic wheals that form after mast cell degranulation O. Characterized by superficial dermal edema and lymphatic channel dilation.

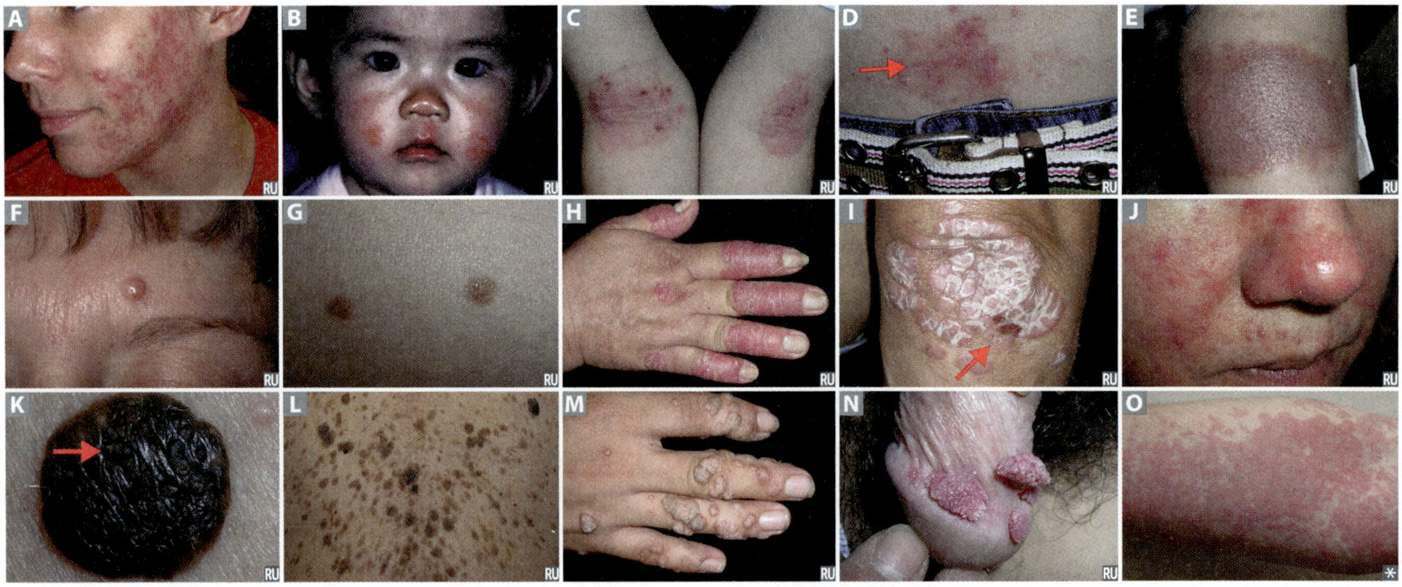

Vascular tumors of skin

Angiosarcoma	Rare blood vessel malignancy typically occurring in the head, neck, and breast areas. Usually in elderly, on sun-exposed areas. Associated with radiation therapy and chronic postmastectomy lymphedema. Hepatic angiosarcoma associated with vinyl chloride and arsenic exposures. Very aggressive and difficult to resect due to delay in diagnosis.
Bacillary angiomatosis	Benign capillary skin papules **A** found in AIDS patients. Caused by *Bartonella henselae* infections. Frequently mistaken for Kaposi sarcoma, but has neutrophilic infiltrate.
Cherry hemangioma	Benign capillary hemangioma of the elderly **B**. Does not regress. Frequency ↑ with age.
Cystic hygroma	Cavernous lymphangioma of the neck **C**. Associated with Turner syndrome.
Glomus tumor	Benign, painful, red-blue tumor, commonly under fingernails. Arises from modified smooth muscle cells of the thermoregulatory glomus body.
Kaposi sarcoma	Endothelial malignancy most commonly of the skin, but also mouth, GI tract, and respiratory tract. Associated with HHV-8 and HIV. Frequently mistaken for bacillary angiomatosis, but has lymphocytic infiltrate.
Pyogenic granuloma	Polypoid lobulated capillary hemangioma **D** that can ulcerate and bleed. Associated with trauma and pregnancy.
Strawberry hemangioma	Benign capillary hemangioma of infancy **E**. Appears in first few weeks of life (1/200 births); grows rapidly and regresses spontaneously by 5–8 years old.

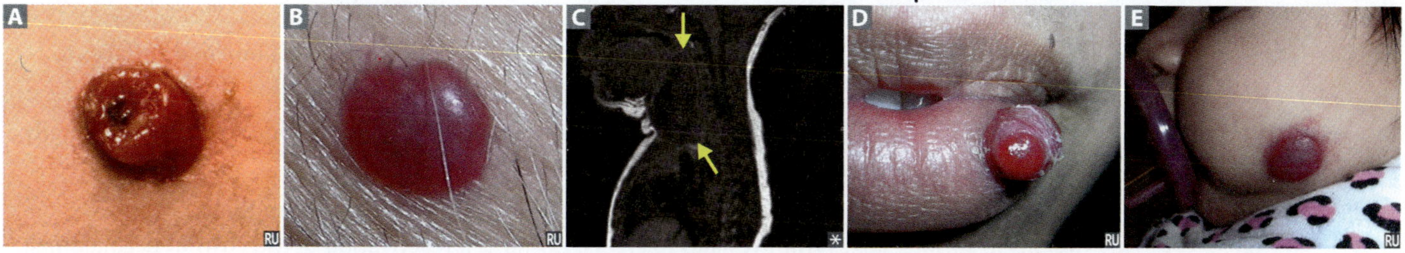

Skin infections

Bacterial infections	
Impetigo	Very superficial skin infection. Usually from *S aureus* or *S pyogenes*. Highly contagious. Honey-colored crusting **A**. Bullous impetigo **B** has bullae and is usually caused by *S aureus*.
Erysipelas	Infection involving upper dermis and superficial lymphatics, usually from *S pyogenes*. Presents with well-defined demarcation between infected and normal skin **C**.
Cellulitis	Acute, painful, spreading infection of deeper dermis and subcutaneous tissues. Usually from *S pyogenes* or *S aureus*. Often starts with a break in skin from trauma or another infection **D**.
Abscess	Collection of pus from a walled-off infection within deeper layers of skin **E**. Offending organism is almost always *S aureus*.
Necrotizing fasciitis	Deeper tissue injury, usually from anaerobic bacteria or *S pyogenes*. Results in crepitus from methane and CO_2 production. "Flesh-eating bacteria." Causes bullae and a purple color to the skin **F**.
Staphylococcal scalded skin syndrome	Exotoxin destroys keratinocyte attachments in stratum granulosum only (vs toxic epidermal necrolysis, which destroys epidermal-dermal junction). Characterized by fever and generalized erythematous rash with sloughing of the upper layers of the epidermis **G** that heals completely. ⊕ Nikolsky sign. Seen in newborns and children, adults with renal insufficiency.
Viral infections	
Herpes	Herpes virus infections (HSV1 and HSV2) of skin can occur anywhere from mucosal surfaces to normal skin. These include herpes labialis, herpes genitalis, herpetic whitlow **H** (finger).
Molluscum contagiosum	Umbilicated papules **I** caused by a poxvirus. While frequently seen in children, it may be sexually transmitted in adults.
Varicella zoster virus	Causes varicella (chickenpox) and zoster (shingles). Varicella presents with multiple crops of lesions in various stages from vesicles to crusts. Zoster is a reactivation of the virus in dermatomal distribution (unless it is disseminated).
Hairy leukoplakia	Irregular, white, painless plaques on lateral tongue that cannot be scraped off **J**. EBV mediated. Occurs in HIV-positive patients, organ transplant recipients. Contrast with thrush (scrapable) and leukoplakia (precancerous).

exfoliat. toxin
= ∅ strat granulos.

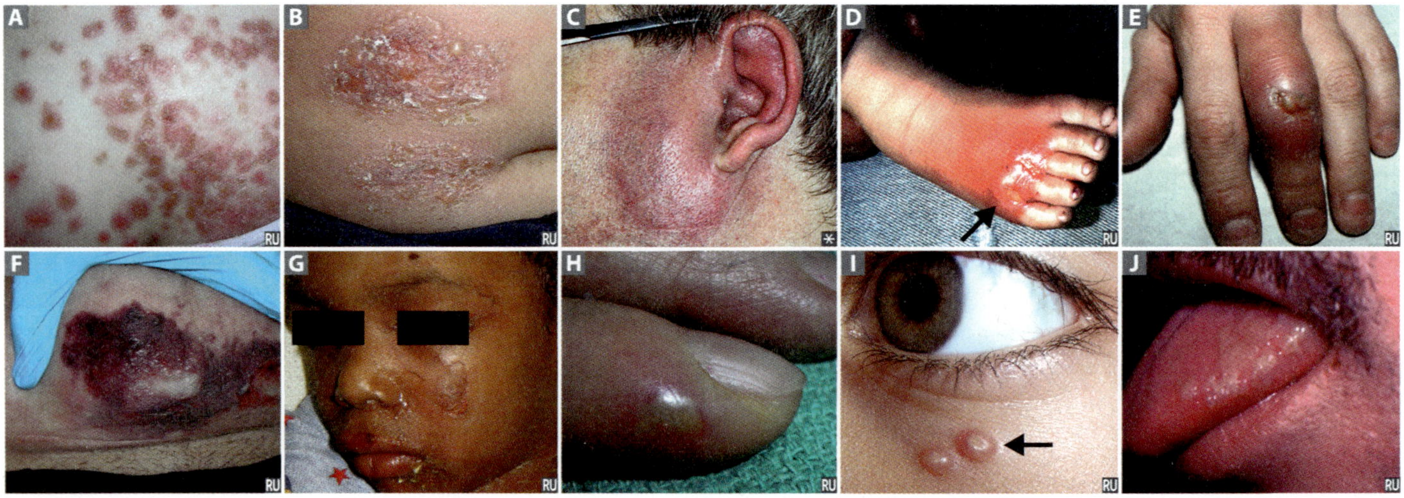

Blistering skin disorders

Pemphigus vulgaris	Potentially fatal autoimmune skin disorder with IgG antibody against desmoglein (component of desmosomes). Flaccid intraepidermal bullae **A** caused by acantholysis (keratinocytes in stratum spinosum are connected by desmosomes); oral mucosa also involved. Immunofluorescence reveals antibodies around epidermal cells in a reticular (net-like) pattern **B**. Nikolsky sign $\oplus$ (separation of epidermis upon manual stroking of skin).
Bullous pemphigoid	Less severe than pemphigus vulgaris. Involves IgG antibody against hemidesmosomes (epidermal basement membrane; antibodies are "bullow" the epidermis). Tense blisters **C** containing eosinophils affect skin but spare oral mucosa. Immunofluorescence reveals linear pattern at epidermal-dermal junction **D**. Nikolsky sign $\ominus$.
Dermatitis herpetiformis	Pruritic papules, vesicles, and bullae (often found on elbows) **E**. Deposits of IgA at tips of dermal papillae. Associated with celiac disease. Treatment: dapsone, gluten-free diet.
Erythema multiforme	Associated with infections (eg, *Mycoplasma pneumoniae*, HSV), drugs (eg, sulfa drugs, β-lactams, phenytoin), cancers, autoimmune disease. Presents with multiple types of lesions—macules, papules, vesicles, target lesions (look like targets with multiple rings and dusky center showing epithelial disruption) **F**.
Stevens-Johnson syndrome	Characterized by fever, bullae formation and necrosis, sloughing of skin at dermal-epidermal junction, high mortality rate. Typically 2 mucous membranes are involved **G** **H**, and targetoid skin lesions may appear, as seen in erythema multiforme. Usually associated with adverse drug reaction. A more severe form of Stevens-Johnson syndrome (SJS) with > 30% of the body surface area involved is toxic epidermal necrolysis **I** **J** (TEN). 10–30% involvement denotes SJS-TEN.

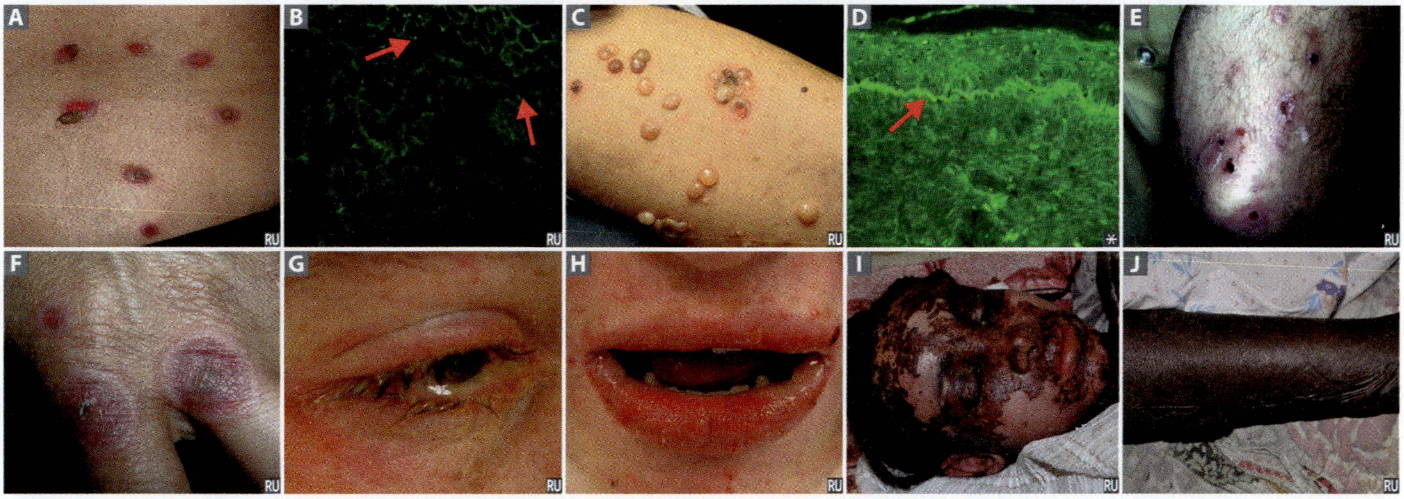

Miscellaneous skin disorders

Acanthosis nigricans	Epidermal hyperplasia causing symmetric, hyperpigmented thickening of skin, especially in axilla or on neck A B. Associated with insulin resistance (eg, diabetes, obesity, Cushing syndrome), visceral malignancy (eg, gastric adenocarcinoma).
Actinic keratosis	Premalignant lesions caused by sun exposure. Small, rough, erythematous or brownish papules or plaques C D. Risk of squamous cell carcinoma is proportional to degree of epithelial dysplasia.
Erythema nodosum	Painful inflammatory lesions of subcutaneous fat, usually on anterior shins. Often idiopathic, but can be associated with sarcoidosis, coccidioidomycosis, histoplasmosis, TB, streptococcal infections E, leprosy F, inflammatory bowel disease.
Lichen Planus	Pruritic, Purple, Polygonal Planar Papules and Plaques are the 6 P's of lichen Planus G H. Mucosal involvement manifests as Wickham striae (reticular white lines). Sawtooth infiltrate of lymphocytes at dermal-epidermal junction. Associated with hepatitis C.
Pityriasis rosea	"Herald patch" I followed days later by other scaly erythematous plaques, often in a "Christmas tree" distribution on trunk J. Multiple plaques with collarette scale. Self-resolving in 6–8 weeks.
Sunburn	Acute cutaneous inflammatory reaction due to excessive UV irradiation. Causes DNA mutations, inducing apoptosis of keratinocytes. UVB is dominant in sunBurn, UVA in tAnning and photoAging. Can lead to impetigo, skin cancers (basal cell carcinoma, squamous cell carcinoma, melanoma).

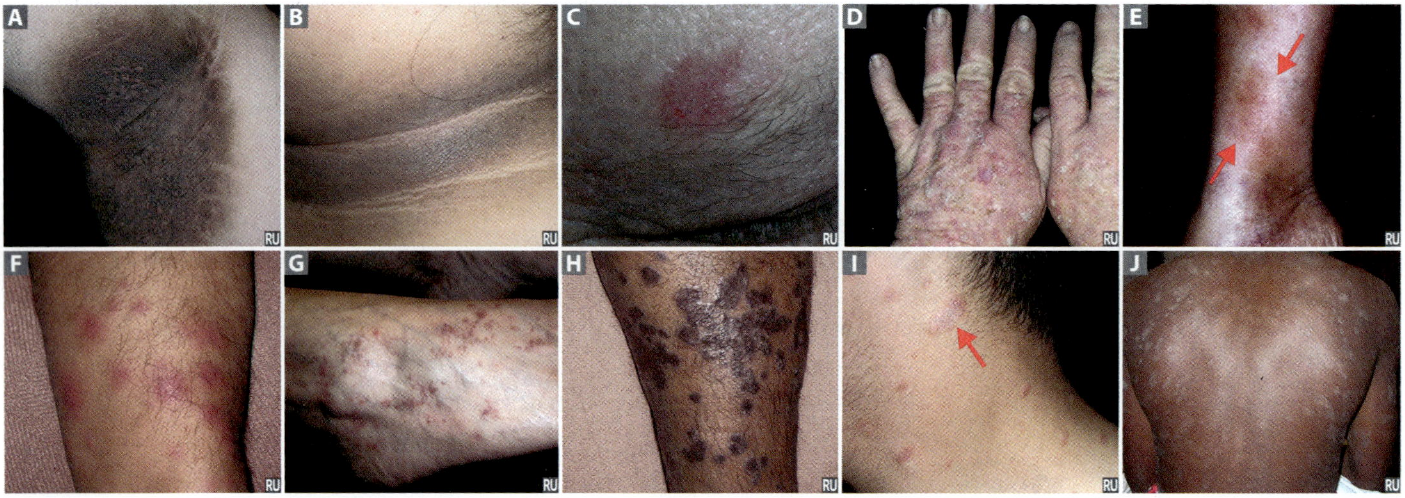

Skin cancer

Basal cell carcinoma

Most common skin cancer. Found in sun-exposed areas of body (eg, face). Locally invasive, but rarely metastasizes. Pink, pearly nodules, commonly with telangiectasias, rolled borders, central crusting or ulceration A. BCCs also appear as nonhealing ulcers with infiltrating growth B or as a scaling plaque (superficial BCC) C. Basal cell tumors have "palisading" nuclei D.

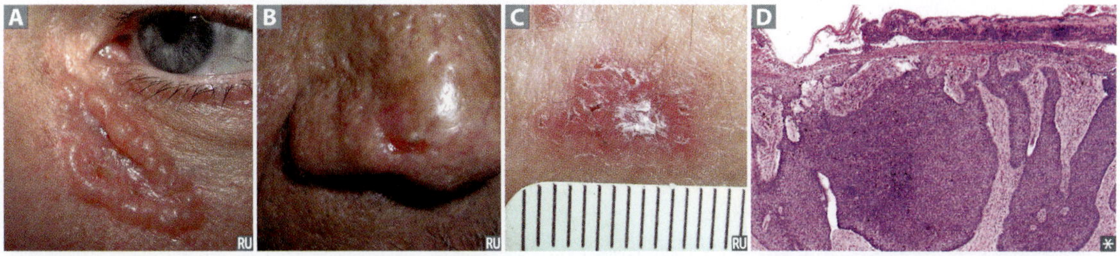

Squamous cell carcinoma

Second most common skin cancer. Associated with excessive exposure to sunlight, immunosuppression, and occasionally arsenic exposure. Commonly appears on face E, lower lip F, ears, hands. Locally invasive, may spread to lymph nodes, and will rarely metastasize. Ulcerative red lesions with frequent scale. Associated with chronic draining sinuses. Histopathology: keratin "pearls" G.

Actinic keratosis, a scaly plaque, is a precursor to squamous cell carcinoma.

Keratoacanthoma is a variant that grows rapidly (4–6 weeks) and may regress spontaneously over months H.

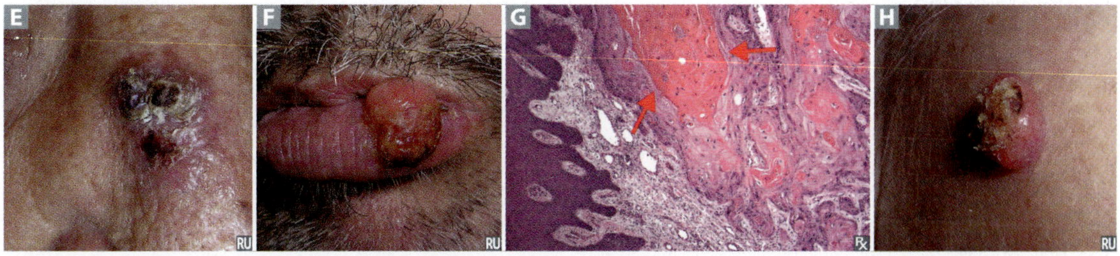

Melanoma

Common tumor with significant risk of metastasis. S-100 tumor marker. Associated with sunlight exposure; fair-skinned persons are at ↑ risk. Depth of tumor correlates with risk of metastasis. Look for the ABCDEs: Asymmetry, Border irregularity, Color variation, Diameter > 6 mm, and Evolution over time. At least 4 different types of melanoma, including superficial spreading I, nodular J, lentigo maligna K, and acral lentiginous L. Often driven by activating mutation in BRAF kinase. Primary treatment is excision with appropriately wide margins. Metastatic or unresectable melanoma in patients with *BRAF* V600E mutation may benefit from vemurafenib, a BRAF kinase inhibitor.

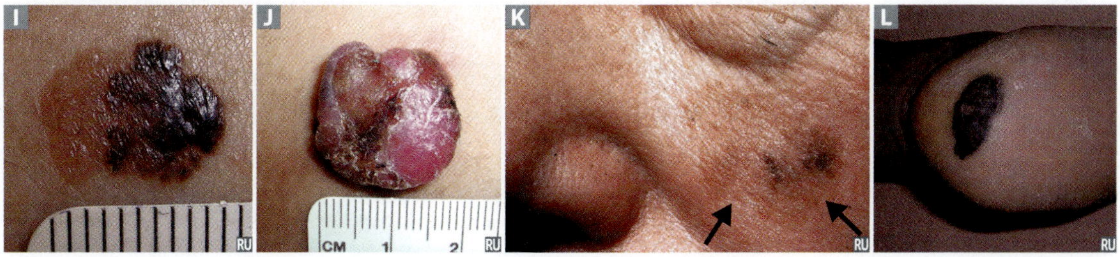

▶ MUSCULOSKELETAL, SKIN, AND CONNECTIVE TISSUE—PHARMACOLOGY

Arachidonic acid pathway

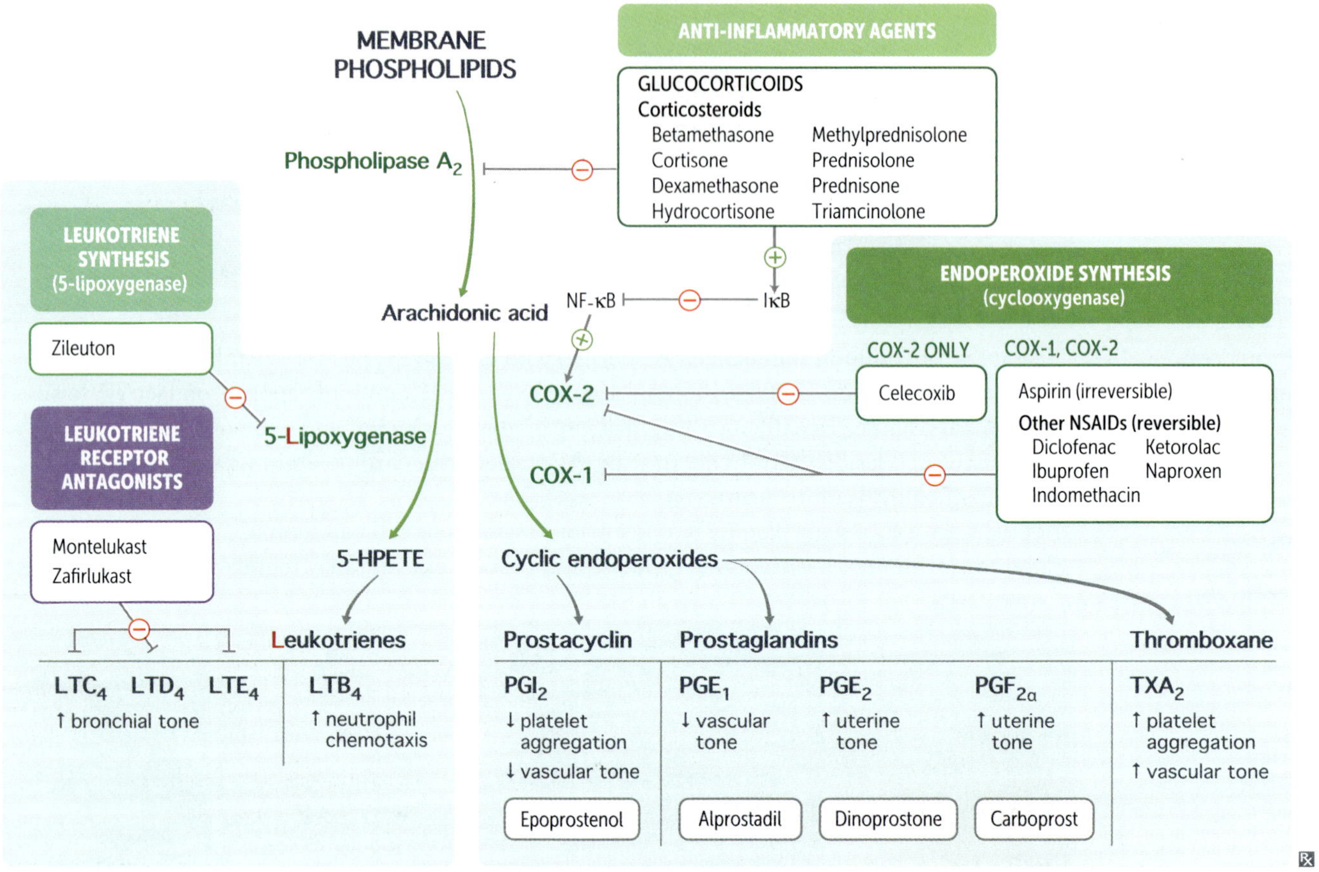

LTB_4 is a **neutrophil** chemotactic agent. **Neutrophils** arrive "**B4**" others.

PGI_2 inhibits platelet aggregation and promotes vasodilation. **P**latelet-**G**athering **I**nhibitor.

Acetaminophen

MECHANISM	Reversibly inhibits cyclooxygenase, mostly in CNS. Inactivated peripherally.
CLINICAL USE	Antipyretic, analgesic, but not anti-inflammatory. Used instead of aspirin to avoid Reye syndrome in children with viral infection.
ADVERSE EFFECTS	Overdose produces hepatic necrosis; acetaminophen metabolite (NAPQI) depletes glutathione and forms toxic tissue byproducts in liver. N-acetylcysteine is antidote—regenerates glutathione.

Aspirin

MECHANISM	NSAID that irreversibly inhibits cyclooxygenase (both COX-1 and COX-2) by covalent acetylation → ↓ synthesis of TXA_2 and prostaglandins. ↑ bleeding time. No effect on PT, PTT. Effect lasts until new platelets are produced.
CLINICAL USE	Low dose (< 300 mg/day): ↓ platelet aggregation. Intermediate dose (300–2400 mg/day): antipyretic and analgesic. High dose (2400–4000 mg/day): anti-inflammatory.
ADVERSE EFFECTS	Gastric ulceration, tinnitus (CN VIII). Chronic use can lead to acute renal failure, interstitial nephritis, GI bleeding. Risk of Reye syndrome in children treated with aspirin for viral infection. Causes respiratory alkalosis early, but transitions to mixed metabolic acidosis-respiratory alkalosis.

Celecoxib

MECHANISM	Reversibly inhibits specifically the cyclooxygenase (COX) isoform 2, which is found in inflammatory cells and vascular endothelium and mediates inflammation and pain; spares COX-1, which helps maintain gastric mucosa. Thus, does not have the corrosive effects of other NSAIDs on the GI lining. Spares platelet function as TXA_2 production is dependent on COX-1.
CLINICAL USE	Rheumatoid arthritis, osteoarthritis.
ADVERSE EFFECTS	↑ risk of thrombosis. Sulfa allergy.

NSAIDs

NSAIDs	Ibuprofen, naproxen, indomethacin, ketorolac, diclofenac, meloxicam, piroxicam.
MECHANISM	Reversibly inhibit cyclooxygenase (both COX-1 and COX-2). Block prostaglandin synthesis.
CLINICAL USE	Antipyretic, analgesic, anti-inflammatory. Indomethacin is used to close a PDA.
ADVERSE EFFECTS	Interstitial nephritis, gastric ulcer (prostaglandins protect gastric mucosa), renal ischemia (prostaglandins vasodilate afferent arteriole).

Leflunomide

MECHANISM	Reversibly inhibits dihydroorotate dehydrogenase, preventing pyrimidine synthesis. Suppresses T-cell proliferation.
CLINICAL USE	Rheumatoid arthritis, psoriatic arthritis.
ADVERSE EFFECTS	Diarrhea, hypertension, hepatotoxicity, teratogenicity.

Bisphosphonates

Bisphosphonates	Alendronate, ibandronate, risedronate, zoledronate.
MECHANISM	Pyrophosphate analogs; bind hydroxyapatite in bone, inhibiting osteoclast activity.
CLINICAL USE	Osteoporosis, hypercalcemia, Paget disease of bone, metastatic bone disease, osteogenesis imperfecta.
ADVERSE EFFECTS	Esophagitis (if taken orally, patients are advised to take with water and remain upright for 30 minutes), osteonecrosis of jaw, atypical stress fractures.

Teriparatide

MECHANISM	Recombinant PTH analog given subcutaneously daily. ↑ osteoblastic activity.
CLINICAL USE	Osteoporosis. Causes ↑ bone growth compared to antiresorptive therapies (eg, bisphosphonates).
ADVERSE EFFECTS	Transient hypercalcemia.

Gout drugs

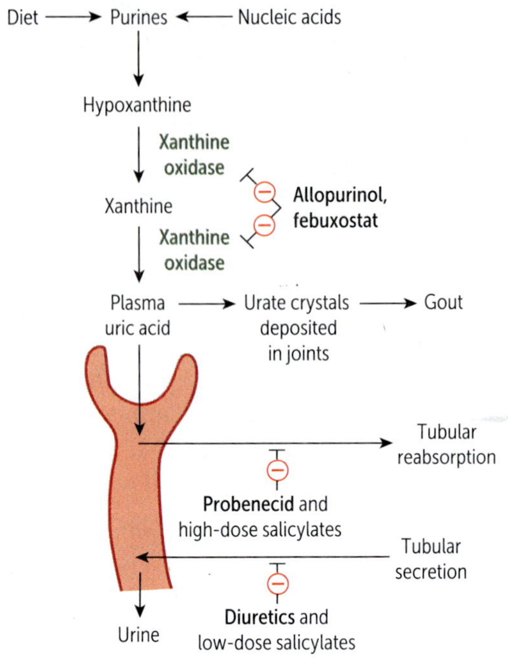

Chronic gout drugs (preventive)	
Allopurinol	Competitive inhibitor of xanthine oxidase. ↓ conversion of hypoxanthine and xanthine to urate. Also used in lymphoma and leukemia to prevent tumor lysis–associated urate nephropathy. ↑ concentrations of azathioprine and 6-MP (both normally metabolized by xanthine oxidase).
Febuxostat	Inhibits xanthine oxidase.
Pegloticase	Recombinant uricase that catalyzes metabolism of uric acid to allantoin (a more water-soluble product).
Probenecid Pro-at pro-ximal tubule	Inhibits reabsorption of uric acid in proximal convoluted tubule (also inhibits secretion of penicillin). Can precipitate uric acid calculi.
Acute gout drugs	
NSAIDs	Naproxen, indomethacin. Do not give salicylates; all but the highest doses depress uric acid clearance. Even high doses (5–6 g/day) have only minor uricosuric activity.
Glucocorticoids	Oral, intra-articular, or parenteral.
Colchicine	Binds and stabilizes tubulin to inhibit microtubule polymerization, impairing neutrophil chemotaxis and degranulation. Acute and prophylactic value. GI side effects.

TNF-α inhibitors

All TNF-α inhibitors predispose to infection, including reactivation of latent TB, since TNF is important in granuloma formation and stabilization.

DRUG	MECHANISM	CLINICAL USE
Etanercept	Fusion protein (receptor for TNF-α + IgG_1 Fc), produced by recombinant DNA. Etanercept is a TNF decoy receptor.	Rheumatoid arthritis, psoriasis, ankylosing spondylitis
Infliximab, adalimumab	Anti-TNF-α monoclonal antibody.	Inflammatory bowel disease, rheumatoid arthritis, ankylosing spondylitis, psoriasis

Rasburicase

MECHANISM	Recombinant uricase that catalyzes metabolism of uric acid to allantoin.
CLINICAL USE	Prevention and treatment of tumor lysis syndrome.

Neurology

"Estimated amount of glucose used by an adult human brain each day, expressed in M&Ms: 250."

—Harper's Index

"He has two neurons held together by a spirochete."

—Anonymous

"Anything's possible if you've got enough nerve."

—J.K. Rowling, *Harry Potter and the Order of the Phoenix*

"I like nonsense; it wakes up the brain cells."

—Dr. Seuss

▸ NEUROLOGY—EMBRYOLOGY

Neural development

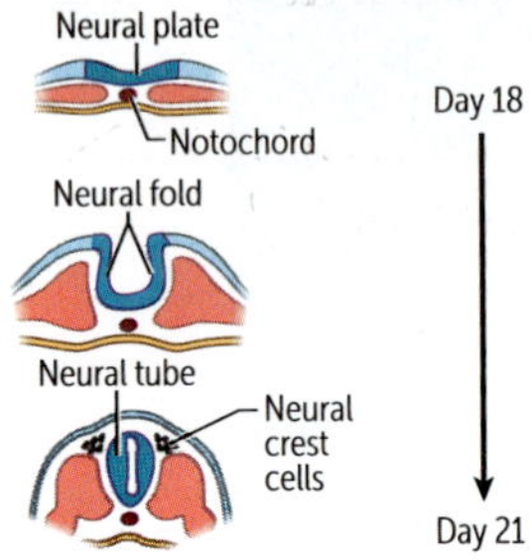

Notochord induces overlying ectoderm to differentiate into neuroectoderm and form neural plate.
Neural plate gives rise to neural tube and neural crest cells.
Notochord becomes nucleus pulposus of intervertebral disc in adults.

Alar plate (dorsal): sensory ⎤
Basal plate (ventral): motor ⎦ Same orientation as spinal cord.

Regional specification of developing brain

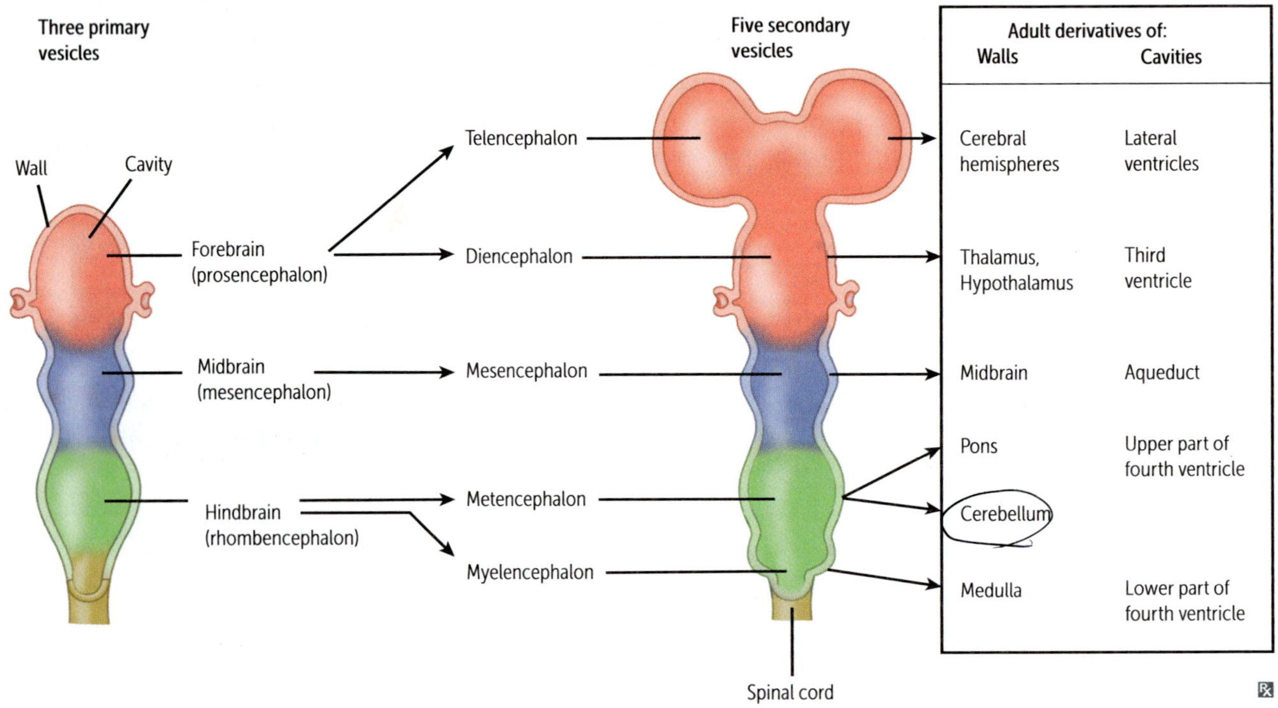

CNS/PNS origins

Neuroectoderm—CNS neurons, ependymal cells (inner lining of ventricles, make CSF), oligodendroglia, astrocytes.
Neural crest—PNS neurons, Schwann cells.
Mesoderm—**M**icroglia (like **M**acrophages).

Neural tube defects	Neuropores fail to fuse (4th week) → persistent connection between amniotic cavity and spinal canal. Associated with low folic acid intake before conception and during pregnancy. ↑ α-fetoprotein (AFP) in amniotic fluid and maternal serum (except spina bifida occulta). ↑ acetylcholinesterase (AChE) in amniotic fluid is a helpful confirmatory test (fetal AChE in CSF flows through defect into amniotic fluid).
Spina bifida occulta	Failure of bony spinal canal to close, but no herniation. Usually seen at lower vertebral levels. Dura is intact. Associated with tuft of hair or skin dimple at level of bony defect. Normal AFP.
Meningocele	Meninges (but no neural tissue) herniate through bony defect.
Meningomyelocele	Meninges and neural tissue (eg, cauda equina) herniate through bony defect.

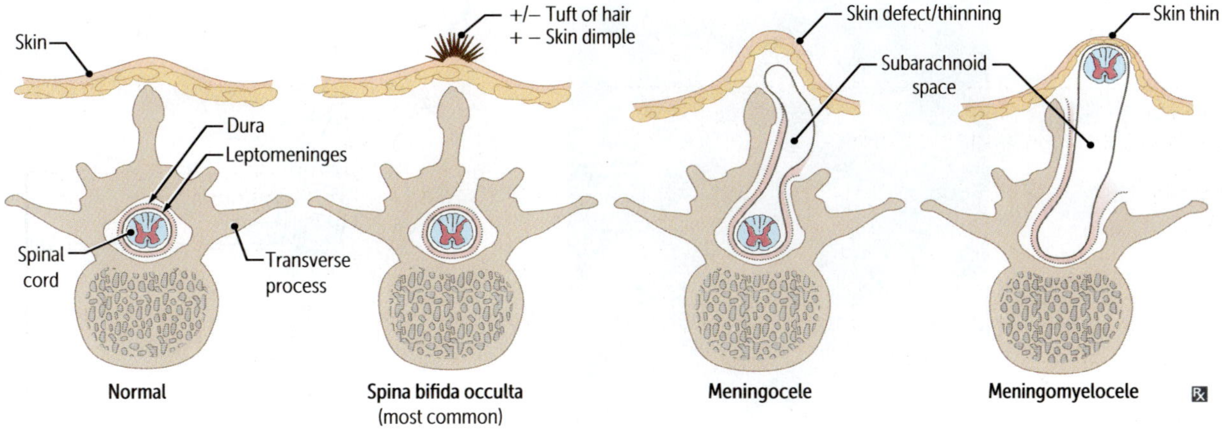

Forebrain anomalies

Anencephaly	Malformation of anterior neural tube → no forebrain, open calvarium. Clinical findings: ↑ AFP, polyhydramnios (no swallowing center in brain). Associated with maternal type 1 diabetes. Maternal folate supplementation ↓ risk.
Holoprosencephaly	Failure of left and right hemispheres to separate; usually occurs during weeks 5–6. May be related to mutations in sonic hedgehog signaling pathway. Moderate form has cleft lip/palate, most severe form results in cyclopia. Seen in Patau syndrome and fetal alcohol syndrome.

Posterior fossa malformations

Chiari II malformation	Herniation of low-lying cerebellar vermis through foramen magnum with aqueductal stenosis → hydrocephalus. Usually associated with lumbosacral meningomyelocele (paralysis/sensory loss at and below the level of the lesion).
Dandy-Walker syndrome	Agenesis of cerebellar vermis with cystic enlargement of 4th ventricle (fills the enlarged posterior fossa A). Associated with noncommunicating hydrocephalus, spina bifida.

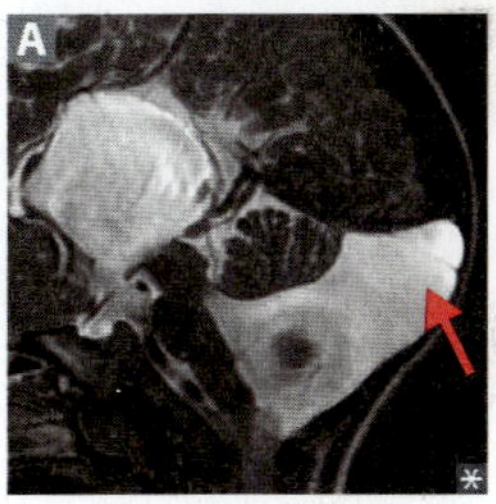

SX = 20-30 y°

Syringomyelia

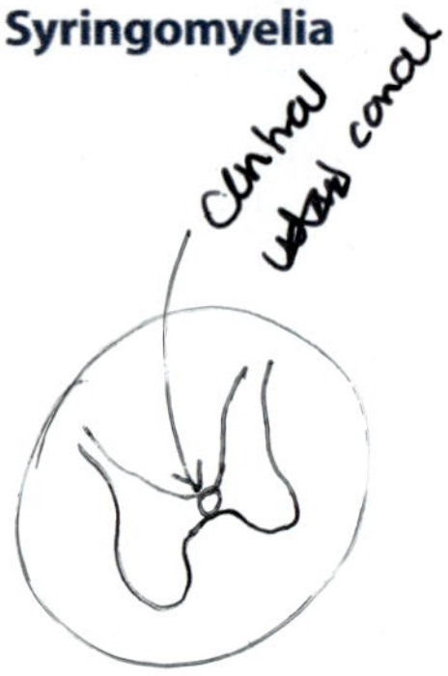

Cystic cavity (syrinx) within central canal of spinal cord (yellow arrow in A). Fibers crossing in anterior white commissure (spinothalamic tract) are typically damaged first. Results in a "cape-like," bilateral loss of pain and temperature sensation in upper extremities (fine touch sensation is preserved). Associated with Chiari malformations (red arrow in A), trauma, and tumors.

Syrinx = tube, as in syringe.
Most common at C8–T1.
Chiari I malformation—cerebellar tonsillar ectopia > 3–5 mm; congenital, usually asymptomatic in childhood, manifests with headaches and cerebellar symptoms.

Extend into brainstem = syringobulbia

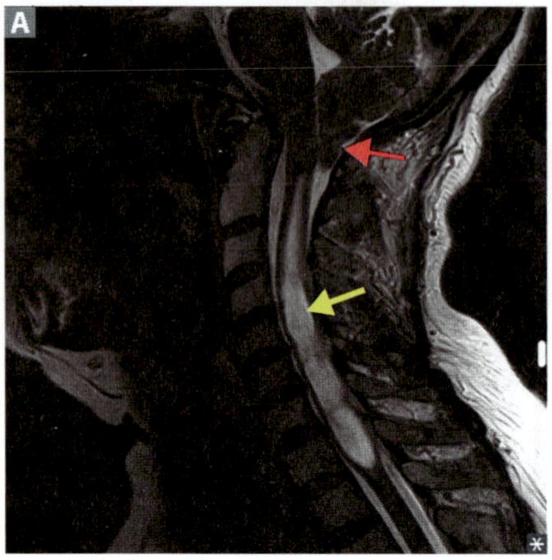

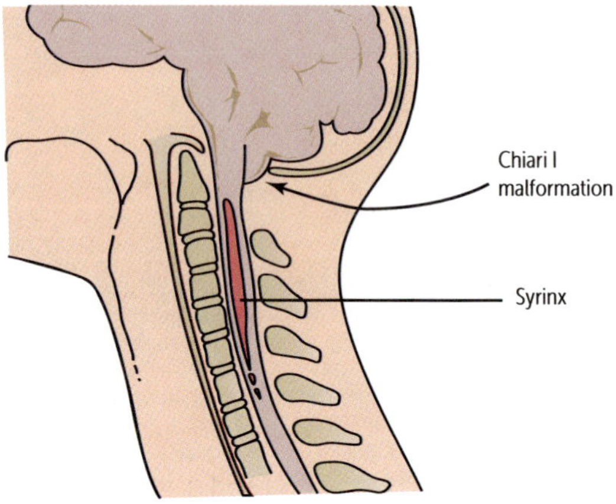

Tongue development

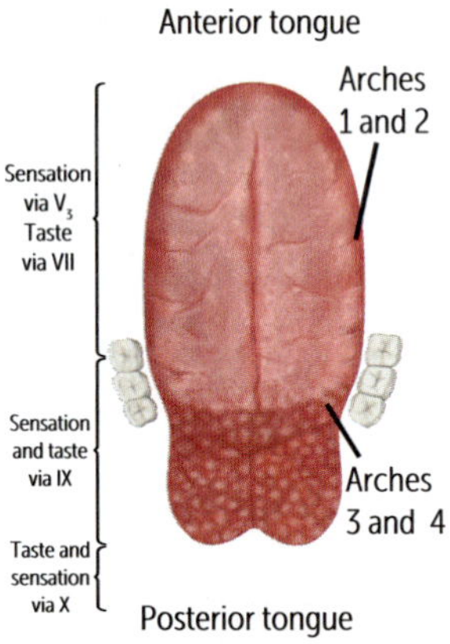

1st and 2nd branchial arches form anterior 2/3 (thus sensation via CN V_3, taste via CN VII).
3rd and 4th branchial arches form posterior 1/3 (thus sensation and taste mainly via CN IX, extreme posterior via CN X).
Motor innervation is via CN XII to hyoglossus (retracts and depresses tongue), genioglossus (protrudes tongue), and styloglossus (draws sides of tongue upward to create a trough for swallowing).
Motor innervation is via CN X to palatoglossus (elevates posterior tongue during swallowing).

Taste—CN VII, IX, X (solitary nucleus).
Pain—CN V_3, IX, X.
Motor—CN X, XII.

▶ NEUROLOGY—ANATOMY AND PHYSIOLOGY

Neurons

Signal-transmitting cells of the nervous system. Permanent cells—do not divide in adulthood.

Signal-relaying cells with dendrites (receive input), cell bodies, and axons (send output). Cell bodies and dendrites can be seen on Nissl staining (stains RER). RER is not present in the axon.

Injury to axon → Wallerian degeneration—degeneration distal to injury and axonal retraction proximally; allows for potential regeneration of axon (if in PNS).

Astrocytes

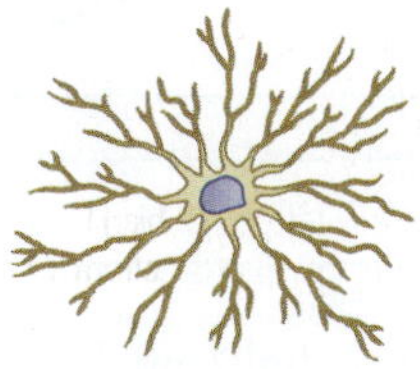

Physical support, repair, K^+ metabolism, removal of excess neurotransmitter, component of blood-brain barrier, glycogen fuel reserve buffer. Reactive gliosis in response to neural injury. Astrocyte marker: GFAP. Derived from neuroectoderm.

④ BBB
① "scaffold" - a lot of the space in brain & SC
② w/ injury the arms prolif. / hypertrophy, "walls off"
- gliosis is that ↑. walling off
③ Homeostasis of CSF fluid esp K.
- can have glycogen & secrete as lactate for fuel!!

Microglia

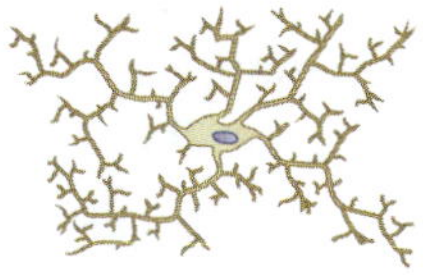

Phagocytic scavenger cells of CNS (mesodermal, mononuclear origin). Activated in response to tissue damage. Not readily discernible by Nissl stain.

HIV-infected microglia fuse to form multinucleated giant cells in CNS.

Myelin

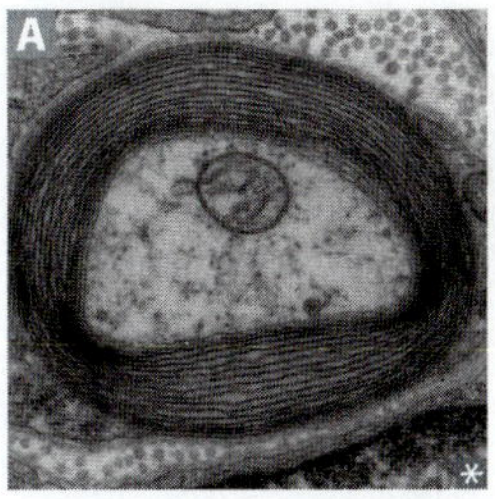

↑ conduction velocity of signals transmitted down axons → saltatory conduction of action potential at the nodes of Ranvier, where there are high concentrations of Na^+ channels. CNS—oligodendrocytes; PNS—Schwann cells.

Wraps and insulates axons A: ↑ space constant and ↑ conduction velocity.

Schwann cells

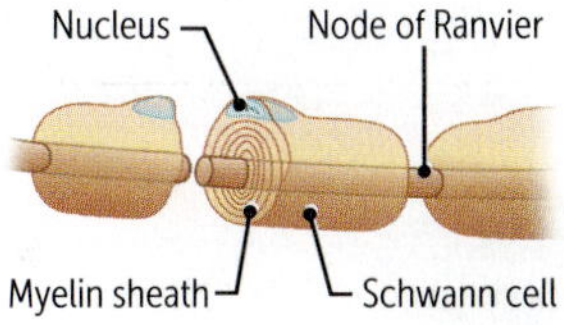

Each Schwann cell myelinates only 1 PNS axon. Also promote axonal regeneration. Derived from neural crest.

↑ conduction velocity via saltatory conduction at the nodes of Ranvier, where there is a high concentration of Na^+ channels.

May be injured in Guillain-Barré syndrome.

Vestibular schwannoma—typically located on CN VIII in internal acoustic meatus, may extend to cerebellopontine angle.

- glial cells = support & "glue" cells
CNS is 50% neuron, 50% glial tiss.
= astrocytes of BBB — the "mom" — most of the glia
ependym cells of ventricles.
oligod. myelin axons

Oligodendroglia

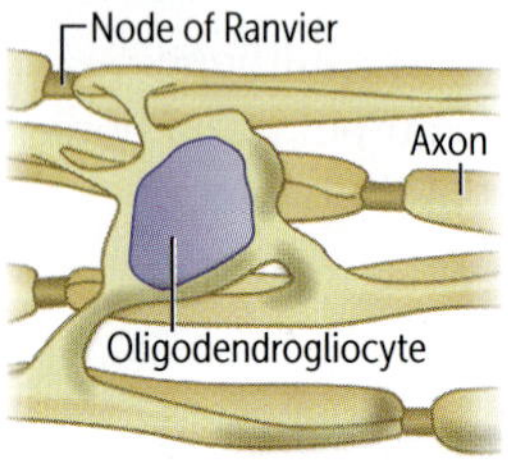

Myelinates axons of neurons in CNS. Each oligodendrocyte can myelinate many axons (~ 30). Predominant type of glial cell in white matter.

Derived from neuroectoderm.
"Fried egg" appearance histologically.
Injured in multiple sclerosis, progressive multifocal leukoencephalopathy (PML), leukodystrophies.

Sensory receptors

RECEPTOR TYPE	SENSORY NEURON FIBER TYPE	LOCATION	SENSES
Free nerve endings	C—slow, unmyelinated fibers Aδ—fast, myelinated fibers	All skin, epidermis, some viscera	Pain, temperature
Meissner corpuscles	Large, myelinated fibers; adapt quickly	Glabrous (hairless) skin	Dynamic, fine/light touch, position sense
Pacinian corpuscles	Large, myelinated fibers; adapt quickly	Deep skin layers, ligaments, joints	Vibration, pressure
Merkel discs	Large, myelinated fibers; adapt slowly	Finger tips, superficial skin	Pressure, deep static touch (eg, shapes, edges), position sense
Ruffini corpuscles	Dendritic endings with capsule; adapt slowly	Finger tips, joints	Pressure, slippage of objects along surface of skin, joint angle change

Peripheral nerve

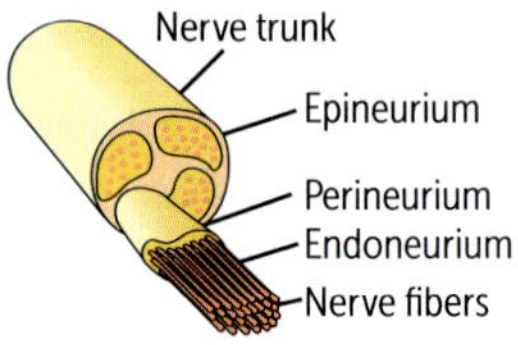

Endoneurium—invests single nerve fiber layers (inflammatory infiltrate in Guillain-Barré syndrome).
Perineurium (Permeability barrier)—surrounds a fascicle of nerve fibers. Must be rejoined in microsurgery for limb reattachment.
Epineurium—dense connective tissue that surrounds entire nerve (fascicles and blood vessels).

Endo = inner.
Peri = around.
Epi = outer.

Neurotransmitters

	LOCATION OF SYNTHESIS	ANXIETY	DEPRESSION	SCHIZOPHRENIA	ALZHEIMER DISEASE	HUNTINGTON DISEASE	PARKINSON DISEASE
Acetylcholine	Basal nucleus of Meynert				↓	↓	↑
Dopamine	Ventral tegmentum, SNpc		↓	↑		↑	↓
GABA	Nucleus accumbens	↓				↓	
Norepinephrine	Locus ceruleus	↑	↓				
Serotonin	Raphe nucleus	↓	↓				↑

Blood-brain barrier

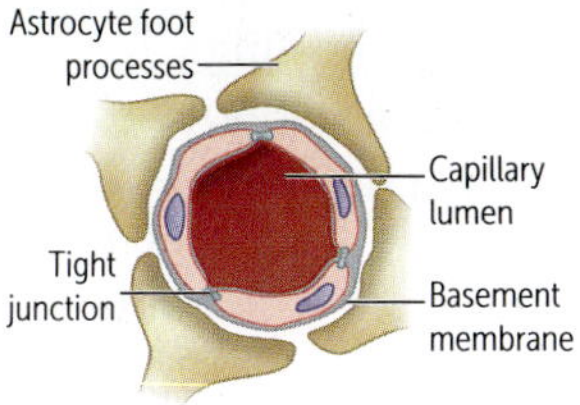

Prevents circulating blood substances (eg, bacteria, drugs) from reaching the CSF/CNS. Formed by 3 structures:

- Tight junctions between nonfenestrated capillary endothelial cells
- Basement membrane
- Astrocyte foot processes

Glucose and amino acids cross slowly by carrier-mediated transport mechanisms.

Nonpolar/lipid-soluble substances cross rapidly via diffusion.

A few specialized brain regions with fenestrated capillaries and no blood-brain barrier allow molecules in blood to affect brain function (eg, area postrema—vomiting after chemo; OVLT—osmotic sensing) or neurosecretory products to enter circulation (eg, neurohypophysis—ADH release).

Infarction and/or neoplasm destroys endothelial cell tight junctions → vasogenic edema.

Other notable barriers include:

- Blood-testis barrier
- Maternal-fetal blood barrier of placenta

Hypothalamus

The hypothalamus wears **TAN HATS**—**T**hirst and water balance, **A**denohypophysis control (regulates anterior pituitary), **N**eurohypophysis releases hormones produced in the hypothalamus, **H**unger, **A**utonomic regulation, **T**emperature regulation, **S**exual urges.

Inputs (areas not protected by blood-brain barrier): OVLT (organum vasculosum of the lamina terminalis; senses change in osmolarity), area postrema (found in medulla, responds to emetics).

Supraoptic nucleus primarily makes ADH.

Paraventricular nucleus primarily makes oxytocin.

Hypothalamus makes ADH and oxytocin. They are carried by neurophysins down axons to posterior pituitary, where they are stored and released.

Lateral area	Hunger. Destruction → anorexia, failure to thrive (infants). Stimulated by ghrelin, inhibited by leptin.	If you zap your **lateral** area, you shrink **lateral**ly.
Ventromedial area	Satiety. Destruction (eg, craniopharyngioma) → hyperphagia. Stimulated by leptin.	If you zap your **ventromedial** area, you grow **ventral**ly and **medial**ly.
Anterior hypothalamus	Cooling, parasympathetic.	**Anterior** nucleus = cool off (**cooling**, p**A**rasympathetic). **A/C** = **anterior cooling**.
Posterior hypothalamus	Heating, sympathetic.	Posterior nucleus = get fired up (heating, sympathetic). If you zap your **p**osterior hypothalamus, you become a **p**oikilotherm (cold-blooded, like a snake).
Suprachiasmatic nucleus	Circadian rhythm.	You need **sleep** to be **charismatic** (chiasmatic).

Sleep physiology

Sleep cycle is regulated by the circadian rhythm, which is driven by suprachiasmatic nucleus (SCN) of hypothalamus. Circadian rhythm controls nocturnal release of ACTH, prolactin, melatonin, norepinephrine: SCN → norepinephrine release → pineal gland → melatonin. SCN is regulated by environment (eg, light).

Two stages: rapid-eye movement (REM) and non-REM. Extraocular movements during REM sleep due to activity of PPRF (paramedian pontine reticular formation/conjugate gaze center). REM sleep occurs every 90 minutes, and duration ↑ through the night. ↑ ACh in REM.

Alcohol, benzodiazepines, and barbiturates are associated with ↓ REM sleep and delta wave sleep; norepinephrine also ↓ REM sleep.

Treat bedwetting (sleep enuresis) with oral desmopressin (ADH analog); preferred over imipramine because of the latter's adverse effects.

Benzodiazepines are useful for night terrors and sleepwalking.

SLEEP STAGE (% OF TOTAL SLEEP TIME IN YOUNG ADULTS)	DESCRIPTION	EEG WAVEFORM
Awake (eyes open)	Alert, active mental concentration	Beta (highest frequency, lowest amplitude)
Awake (eyes closed)		Alpha
Non-REM sleep		
Stage N1 (5%)	Light sleep	Theta
Stage N2 (45%)	Deeper sleep; when bruxism occurs	Sleep spindles and K complexes
Stage N3 (25%)	Deepest non-REM sleep (slow-wave sleep); when sleepwalking, night terrors, and bedwetting occur	Delta (lowest frequency, highest amplitude)
REM sleep (25%)	Loss of motor tone, ↑ brain O_2 use, ↑ and variable pulse and blood pressure; when dreaming, nightmares, and penile/clitoral tumescence occur; may serve memory processing function	Beta At night, BATS Drink Blood

Thalamus Major relay for all ascending sensory information except olfaction.

NUCLEUS	INPUT	SENSES	DESTINATION	MNEMONIC
Ventral postero-lateral nucleus	Spinothalamic and dorsal columns/medial lemniscus	Pain, temperature; pressure, touch, vibration, proprioception	1° somatosensory cortex	
Ventral postero-Medial nucleus	Trigeminal and gustatory pathway	Face sensation, taste	1° somatosensory cortex	Makeup goes on the face (VPM)
Lateral geniculate nucleus	CN II	Vision	Calcarine sulcus	Lateral = Light
Medial geniculate nucleus	Superior olive and inferior colliculus of tectum	Hearing	Auditory cortex of temporal lobe	Medial = Music
Ventral lateral nucleus	Basal ganglia, cerebellum	Motor	Motor cortex	

Limbic system

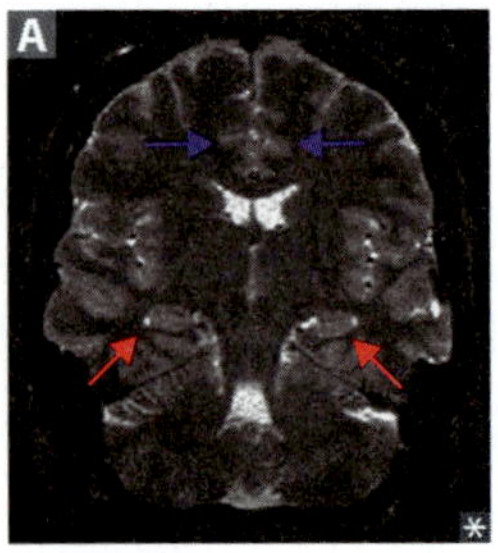

Collection of neural structures involved in emotion, long-term memory, olfaction, behavior modulation, ANS function.

Structures include hippocampus (red arrows in A), amygdala, fornix, mammillary bodies, cingulate gyrus (blue arrows in A).

Responsible for Feeding, Fleeing, Fighting, Feeling, and Sex.

The famous 5 F's.

Dopaminergic pathways Commonly altered by drugs (eg, antipsychotics) and movement disorders (eg, Parkinson disease).

PATHWAY	SYMPTOMS OF ALTERED ACTIVITY	NOTES
Mesocortical	↓ activity → "negative" symptoms (eg, flat affect, limited speech).	Antipsychotic drugs have limited effect.
Mesolimbic	↑ activity → "positive" symptoms (eg, delusions, hallucinations).	Primary therapeutic target of antipsychotic drugs → ↓ positive symptoms (eg, in schizophrenia).
Nigrostriatal	↓ activity → extrapyramidal symptoms (eg, dystonia, akathisia, parkinsonism, tardive dyskinesia).	Major dopaminergic pathway in brain. Significantly affected by movement disorders and antipsychotic drugs.
Tuberoinfundibular	↓ activity → ↑ prolactin → ↓ libido, sexual dysfunction, galactorrhea, gynecomastia (in men).	

Cerebellum

Modulates movement; aids in coordination and balance.

Input:

- Contralateral cortex via middle cerebellar peduncle.
- Ipsilateral proprioceptive information via inferior cerebellar peduncle from spinal cord.

Output:

- Sends information to contralateral cortex to modulate movement. Output nerves = Purkinje cells → deep nuclei of cerebellum → contralateral cortex via superior cerebellar peduncle.
- Deep nuclei (lateral → medial)—**D**entate, **E**mboliform, **G**lobose, **F**astigial ("**D**on't **E**at **G**reasy **F**oods").

Lateral lesions—affect voluntary movement of extremities; when injured, propensity to fall toward injured (ipsilateral) side.

Medial lesions—involvement of midline structures (vermal cortex, fastigial nuclei) and/or flocculonodular lobe → truncal ataxia (wide-based cerebellar gait), nystagmus, head tilting. Generally result in bilateral motor deficits affecting axial and proximal limb musculature.

Taste — CN7/9/Ten → NTS (medulla) → central tegment. tract (medul to thal. tract) → VPM of thal → Gust cortex in parietal/ deep insula (all same side)

Smell — Bipol olf cells → specif. glomeruli synapse → olf bulb → → piriform cortex ↓ MDN ↓ orbitofrontal cortex for discrim

Hear — Inner hair cells → glutamate → → coch nuc rost/vent/d medulla → oppos superior olive nuc.

↳ lat leminisc tract → oppos infer collic → MGN → Aud cortex

Basal ganglia

Important in voluntary movements and making postural adjustments.

Receives cortical input, provides negative feedback to cortex to modulate movement.

Striatum = putamen (motor) + caudate (cognitive).

Lentiform = putamen + globus pallidus.

D_1-Receptor = **D1Rect** pathway.

Indirect = **In**hibitory.

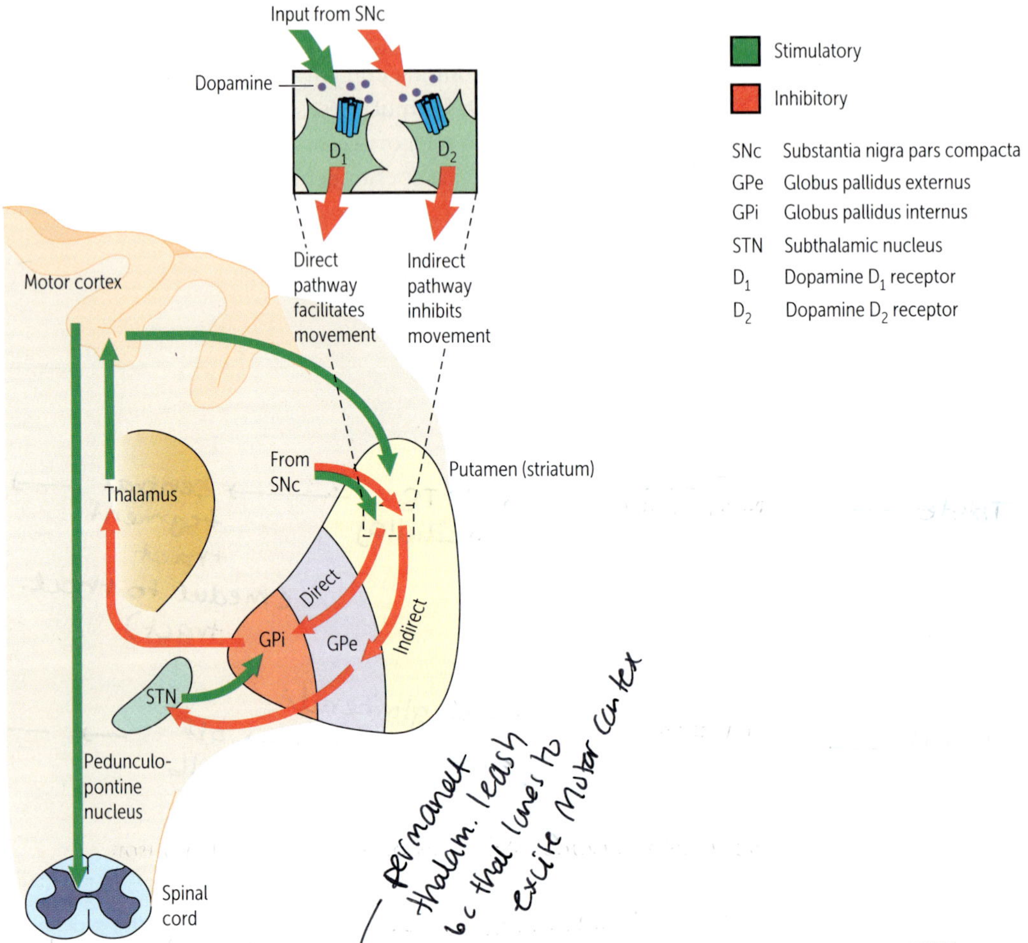

Excitatory pathway—cortical inputs stimulate the striatum, stimulating the release of GABA, which inhibits GABA release from the GPi, disinhibiting the thalamus via the GPi (↑ motion).

Inhibitory pathway—cortical inputs stimulate the striatum, releasing GABA that disinhibits STN via GPe inhibition, and STN stimulates GPi to inhibit the thalamus (↓ motion).

Dopamine binds to D_1, stimulating the excitatory pathway, and to D_2, inhibiting the inhibitory pathway → ↑ motion.

- Activating globus pal internus means ↓ signals from Thal to motor cortex. The Direct path inhibits GPI (↑ transm to cortex). The indirect activ GPI = ↓ transm.
- striatum inhib GPI in direct & inhib GPE in indirect (& so ↗)

Direct D_1 = Mot. cortex → striat ∅→ GPI take off / inhibit → Thal → MC (move)

(subthal nuc → subst nigra)

DA on D_1 = ↑direct, on D_2 = ↓indirect

Indirect D_2 = MC → striatum ↓∅ GPE ∅→ subthal nuc → GPI ∅→ Thal ∅→ no signal MC

* subthal nuc → SN → striatum (Direct)

Movement disorders

DISORDER	PRESENTATION	CHARACTERISTIC LESION	NOTES
Athetosis	Slow, writhing movements; especially seen in fingers	Basal ganglia (eg, Huntington)	Writhing, snake-like movement.
Chorea	Sudden, jerky, purposeless movements	Basal ganglia (eg, Huntington)	*Chorea* = dancing.
Dystonia	Sustained, involuntary muscle contractions		Writer's cramp; blepharospasm (sustained eyelid twitch).
Essential tremor	High-frequency tremor with sustained posture (eg, outstretched arms), worsened with movement or when anxious		Often familial. Patients often self-medicate with alcohol, which ↓ tremor amplitude. Treatment: nonselective β-blockers (eg, propranolol), primidone.
Hemiballismus	Sudden, wild flailing of 1 arm +/– ipsilateral leg	Contralateral subthalamic nucleus (eg, lacunar stroke)	Pronounce "**Half**-of-body **ball**istic." Contralateral lesion.
Intention tremor	Slow, zigzag motion when pointing/extending toward a target	Cerebellar dysfunction	
Myoclonus	Sudden, brief, uncontrolled muscle contraction		Jerks; hiccups; common in metabolic abnormalities such as renal and liver failure.
Resting tremor	Uncontrolled movement of distal appendages (most noticeable in hands); tremor alleviated by intentional movement	Parkinson disease	Occurs at rest; "pill-rolling tremor" of Parkinson disease.

Parkinson disease

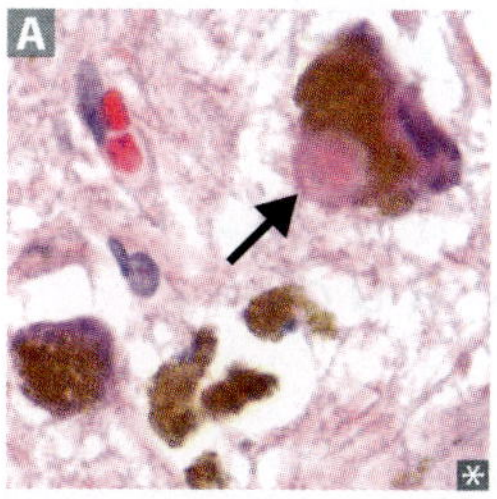

Degenerative disorder of CNS associated with Lewy bodies (composed of α-synuclein—intracellular eosinophilic inclusions A) and loss of dopaminergic neurons (ie, depigmentation) of substantia nigra pars compacta.

Parkinson **TRAPS** your body:
- **T**remor (pill-rolling tremor at rest)
- **R**igidity (cogwheel)
- **A**kinesia (or bradykinesia)
- **P**ostural instability
- **S**huffling gait

Huntington disease

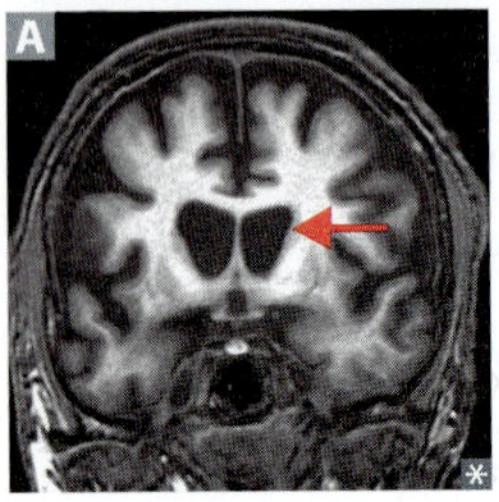

Autosomal dominant trinucleotide repeat disorder on chromosome 4. Symptoms manifest between ages 20 and 50; characterized by choreiform movements, aggression, depression, dementia (sometimes initially mistaken for substance abuse). ↑ dopamine, ↓ GABA, ↓ ACh in brain. Neuronal death via NMDA-R binding and glutamate excitotoxicity. Atrophy of caudate and putamen with hydrocephalus ex vacuo A.

Expansion of CAG repeats (anticipation). Caudate loses ACh and GABA.

Cerebral cortex functions

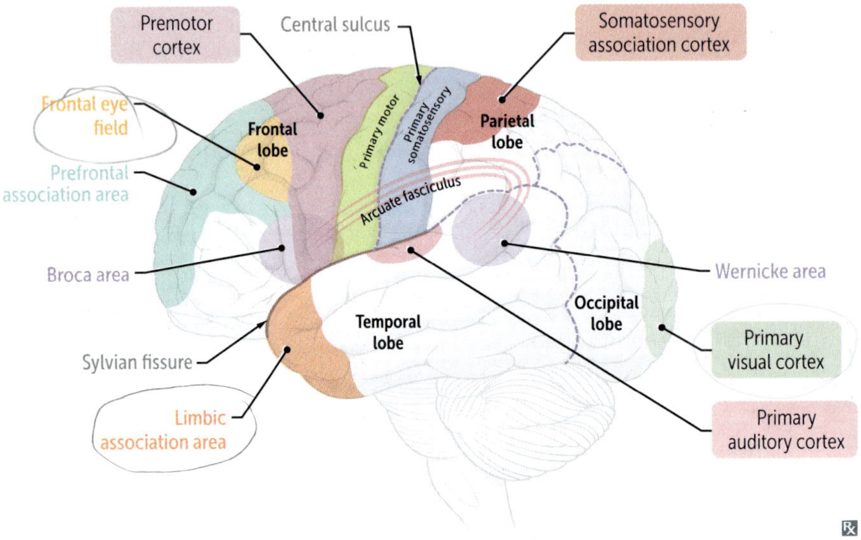

The frontal eye fields evoke saccadic eye movements

voluntary eye movements occur in jumps or "saccades"

- R frontal field tells eyes to look left
  this info goes to paramed pontine retic format near CN 6 nucleus
  this crucial for horiz. saccade
- No L PPRF = no left movement.
- R front field ⟶ L PPRF ⟶ L Med long Fascic → Contralat occulom nuc.
  L CN 6 nuc (1st)

*MLF links medial movement w/ 1 eye to lat movem of the other

"Language"

Aphasia

Aphasia—higher-order language deficit (inability to understand/speak/read/write).
Dysarthria—motor inability to speak (movement deficit).

TYPE	SPEECH FLUIDITY	COMPREHENSION	REPETITION	COMMENTS
Broca	Nonfluent	Intact	Impaired	**B**roca = **B**roken **B**oca (*boca* = mouth in Spanish). Broca area in inferior frontal gyrus of frontal lobe.
Wernicke "Fluent aphas"	Fluent	Impaired	Impaired	**W**ernicke is **W**ordy but makes no sense. Wernicke area in superior temporal gyrus of temporal lobe.
Conduction	Fluent	Intact	Impaired	Can be caused by damage to arcuate fasciculus.
Global	Nonfluent	Impaired	Impaired	Arcuate fasciculus; Broca and Wernicke areas affected.
Transcortical motor	Nonfluent	Intact	Intact	Affects frontal lobe around Broca area, but Broca area is spared.
Transcortical sensory	Fluent	Impaired	Intact	Affects temporal lobe around Wernicke area, but Wernicke area is spared.
Transcortical, mixed	Nonfluent	Impaired	Intact	Broca and Wernicke areas and arcuate fasciculus remain intact; surrounding watershed areas affected.

R handed — lang. in L lobe usually.

Global = Wern + Broca. Cant understand. Repeat same phrase over & over

Wern. & Broca connected by arcuate fasciculus

- when this is damaged, conduction b/w listening & speak is affected → "conduct. aphas"
  - underst but cant repeat

- conduct aphas — "count 1-10" after 4 starts naming animals (disconnect of what she heard/says)
-

Common brain lesions

AREA OF LESION	CONSEQUENCE	NOTES
Amygdala (bilateral)	Klüver-Bucy syndrome—disinhibited behavior (eg, hyperphagia, hypersexuality, hyperorality).	Associated with HSV-1 encephalitis. not afraid too
Frontal lobe	Disinhibition and deficits in concentration, orientation, judgment; may have reemergence of primitive reflexes.	
Nondominant parietal cortex	Hemispatial neglect syndrome (agnosia of the contralateral side of the world).	
Dominant parietal cortex	Agraphia, acalculia, finger agnosia, left-right disorientation.	Gerstmann syndrome.
Reticular activating system (midbrain)	Reduced levels of arousal and wakefulness (eg, coma).	
Mammillary bodies (bilateral)	Wernicke-Korsakoff syndrome—confusion, ophthalmoplegia, ataxia; memory loss (anterograde and retrograde amnesia), confabulation, personality changes.	Associated with thiamine (B_1) deficiency and excessive alcohol use; can be precipitated by giving glucose without B_1 to a B_1-deficient patient. Wernicke problems come in a **CAN** of beer: **C**onfusion, **A**taxia, **N**ystagmus.
Basal ganglia	May result in tremor at rest, chorea, athetosis.	Parkinson disease, Huntington disease.
Cerebellar hemisphere	Intention tremor, limb ataxia, loss of balance; damage to cerebellum → ipsilateral deficits; fall toward side of lesion.	Degeneration associated with chronic alcohol use. Cerebellar hemispheres are **lateral**ly located—affect **lateral** limbs.
Cerebellar vermis	Truncal ataxia, dysarthria.	Vermis is **central**ly located—affects **central** body.
Subthalamic nucleus	Contralateral hemiballismus.	
Hippocampus (bilateral)	Anterograde amnesia—inability to make new memories.	
Paramedian pontine reticular formation	Eyes look away from side of lesion.	
Frontal eye fields	Eyes look toward lesion.	

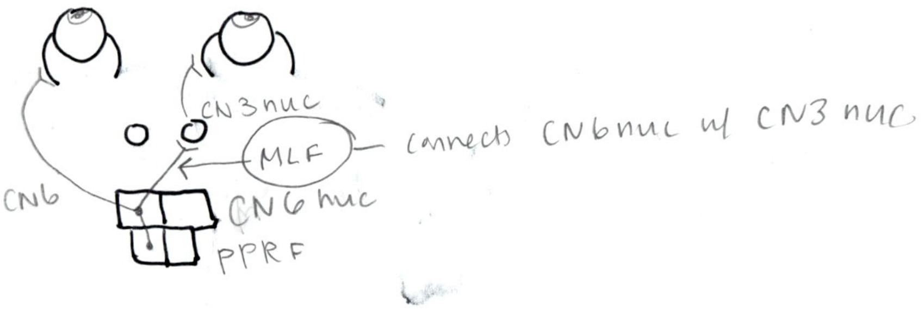

Homunculus

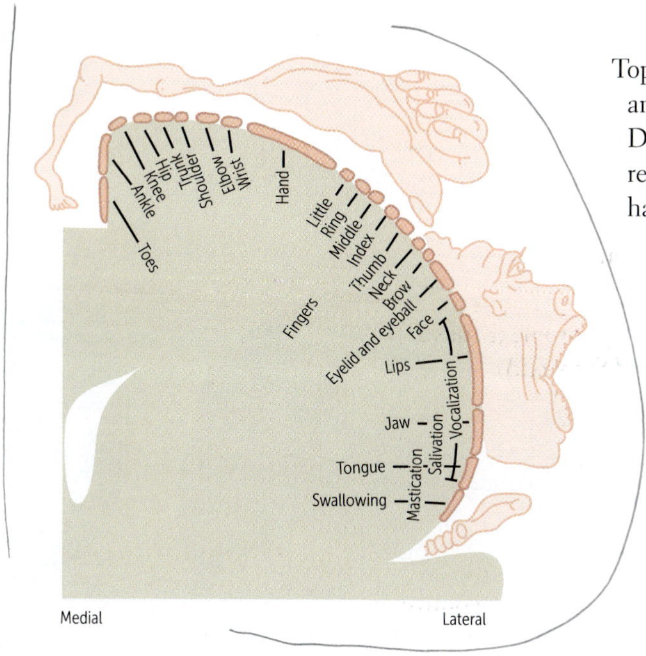

Topographic representation of motor (shown) and sensory areas in the cerebral cortex. Distorted appearance is due to certain body regions being more richly innervated and thus having ↑ cortical representation.

Cerebral perfusion

Brain perfusion relies on tight autoregulation. Cerebral perfusion is primarily driven by P_{CO_2} (P_{O_2} also modulates perfusion in severe hypoxia).

Cerebral perfusion relies on a pressure gradient between mean arterial pressure (MAP) and ICP. ↓ blood pressure or ↑ ICP → ↓ cerebral perfusion pressure (CPP).

Therapeutic hyperventilation → ↓ P_{CO_2} → vasoconstriction → ↓ cerebral blood flow → ↓ intracranial pressure (ICP). May be used to treat acute cerebral edema (eg, 2° to stroke) unresponsive to other interventions.

CPP = MAP – ICP. If CPP = 0, there is no cerebral perfusion → brain death.

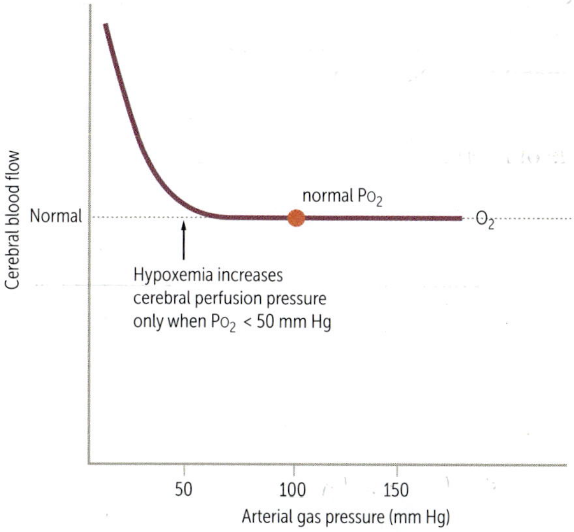

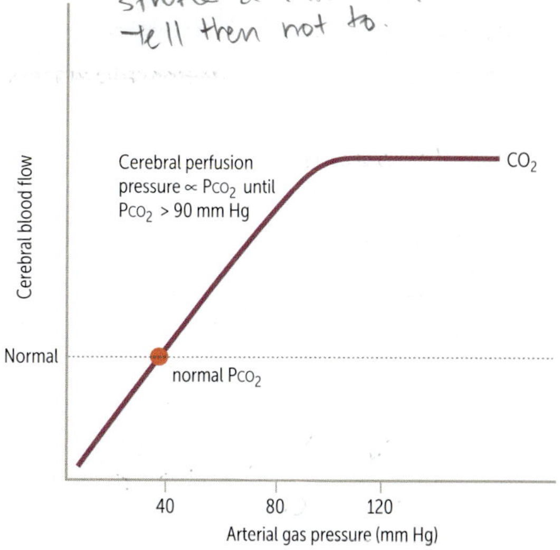

Cerebral arteries—cortical distribution

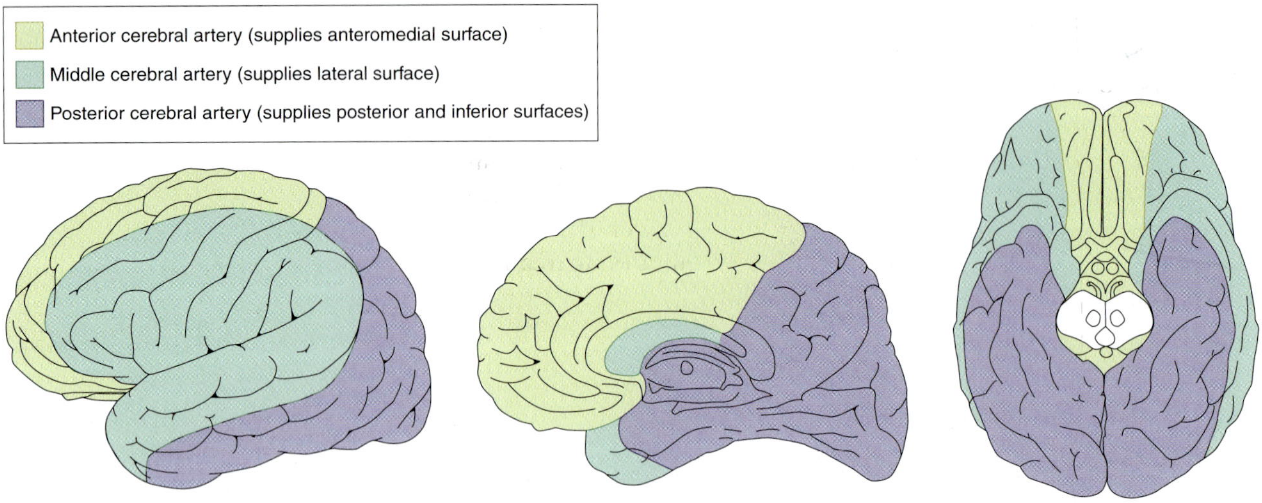

Watershed zones Between anterior cerebral/middle cerebral, posterior cerebral/middle cerebral arteries. Damage by severe hypotension → upper leg/upper arm weakness, defects in higher-order visual processing.

Circle of Willis System of anastomoses between anterior and posterior blood supplies to brain.

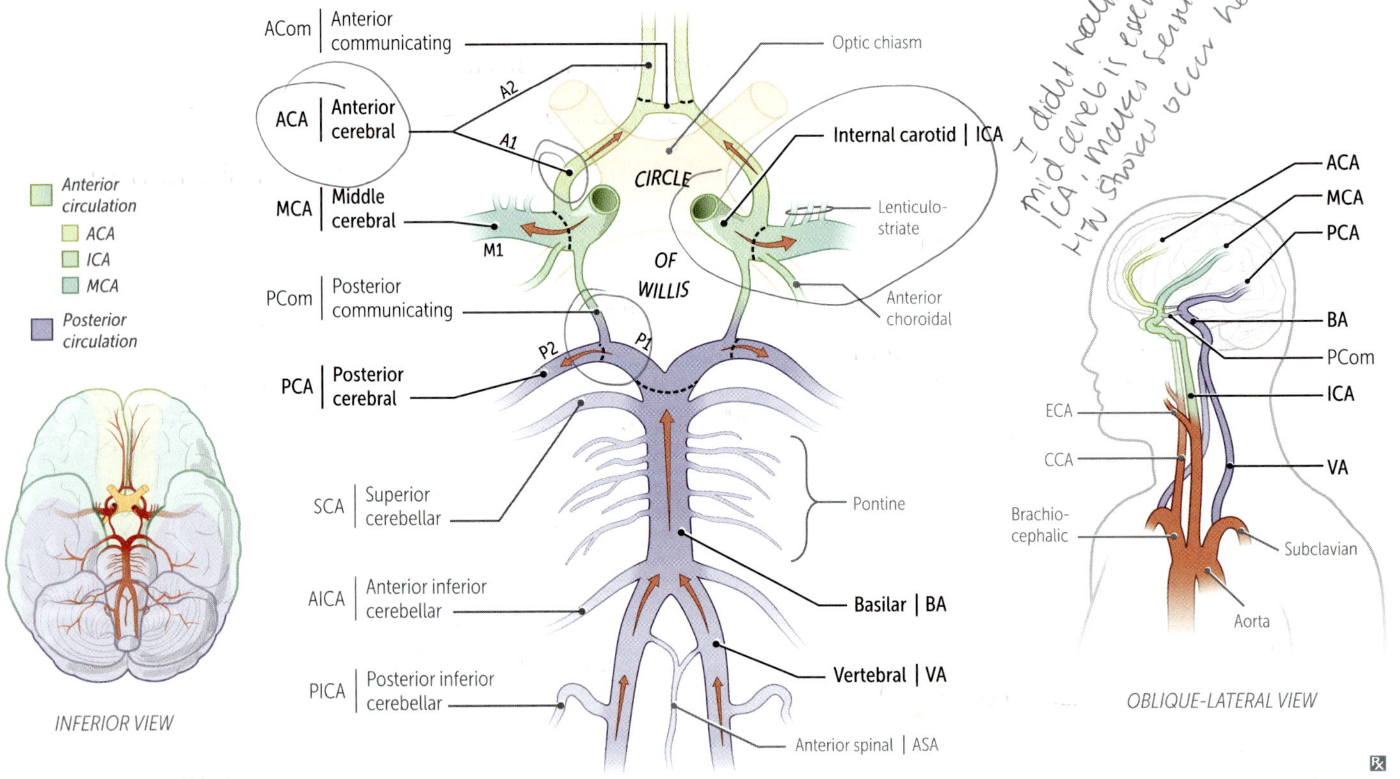

Effects of strokes

ARTERY	AREA OF LESION	SYMPTOMS	NOTES
Anterior circulation			
Middle cerebral artery	Motor and sensory cortices—upper limb and face. Temporal lobe (Wernicke area); frontal lobe (Broca area).	Contralateral paralysis and sensory loss—face and upper limb. Aphasia if in dominant (usually left) hemisphere. Hemineglect if lesion affects nondominant (usually right) side.	
Anterior cerebral artery	Motor and sensory cortices—lower limb.	Contralateral paralysis and sensory loss—lower limb.	
Lenticulo-striate artery	Striatum, internal capsule.	Contralateral paralysis and/or sensory loss—face and body. Absence of cortical signs (eg, neglect, aphasia, visual field loss).	Common location of lacunar infarcts, 2° to unmanaged hypertension.
Posterior circulation			
Anterior spinal artery	Lateral corticospinal tract. Medial lemniscus. Caudal medulla—hypoglossal nerve.	Contralateral paralysis—upper and lower limbs. ↓ contralateral proprioception. Ipsilateral hypoglossal dysfunction (tongue deviates ipsilaterally).	Medial medullary syndrome—caused by infarct of paramedian branches of ASA and/or vertebral arteries.
Posterior inferior cerebellar artery	Lateral medulla—vestibular nuclei, lateral spinothalamic tract, spinal trigeminal nucleus, nucleus ambiguus, sympathetic fibers, inferior cerebellar peduncle.	Vomiting, vertigo, nystagmus; ↓ pain and temperature sensation from ipsilateral face and contralateral body; **dysphagia**, **hoarseness**, ↓ gag reflex; ipsilateral Horner syndrome; ataxia, dysmetria.	Lateral medullary (Wallenberg) syndrome. Nucleus ambiguus effects are specific to PICA lesions. "Don't **pick a** (**PICA**) **horse** (hoarseness) that **can't eat** (dysphagia)."
Anterior inferior cerebellar artery	Lateral pons—cranial nerve nuclei (vestibular nuclei, facial nucleus, spinal trigeminal nucleus, cochlear nuclei), spinothalamic tract, corticospinal tract, sympathetic fibers. Middle and inferior cerebellar peduncles.	Vomiting, vertigo, nystagmus. **Paralysis of face**, ↓ lacrimation, salivation, ↓ taste from anterior ⅔ of tongue. Ipsilateral ↓ pain and temperature of the face, contralateral ↓ pain and temperature of the body. Ataxia, dysmetria.	Lateral pontine syndrome. Facial nucleus effects are specific to AICA lesions. "**Facial droop** means AICA's **pooped**."
Basilar artery	Pons, medulla, lower midbrain, corticospinal and corticobulbar tracts, ocular cranial nerve nuclei, paramedian pontine reticular formation.	Preserved consciousness, vertical eye movement, blinking; quadriplegia, loss of voluntary facial, mouth, and tongue movements.	"Locked-in syndrome."
Posterior cerebral artery	Occipital cortex, visual cortex.	Contralateral hemianopia with macular sparing.	

Aneurysms	Abnormal dilation of an artery due to weakening of vessel wall.
Saccular (berry) aneurysm	Occurs at bifurcations in the circle of Willis. Most common site is junction of anterior communicating artery and anterior cerebral artery. Rupture (most common complication) → subarachnoid hemorrhage ("worst headache of my life") or hemorrhagic stroke. Associated with ADPKD, Ehlers-Danlos syndrome. Other risk factors: advanced age, hypertension, smoking, race (↑ risk in blacks).
Charcot-Bouchard microaneurysm (Intraparenchym)	Common, associated with chronic hypertension; affects small vessels (eg, in basal ganglia, thalamus); not seen on angiogram. CharcBouch = chronic BP ↑

Effects of saccular aneurysms	Usually clinically silent until rupture → subarachnoid hemorrhage (eg, thunderclap headache). Can also cause symptoms via direct compression on surrounding structures by growing aneurysm.
ARTERY	ASSOCIATED SYMPTOMS
Anterior communicating artery	Compression may cause bitemporal hemianopia (compression of optic chiasm); visual acuity deficits. Rupture may cause ischemia in ACA distribution → contralateral lower extremity hemiparesis, sensory deficits.
Posterior communicating artery	Compression may cause ipsilateral CN III palsy → mydriasis ("blown pupil"); may also see ptosis, "down and out" eye.
Middle cerebral artery	Rupture may cause ischemia in MCA distribution → contralateral upper extremity and facial hemiparesis, sensory deficits. So it'll be hard to tell b/w stroke vs hemor for MCA

Central post-stroke pain syndrome	Neuropathic pain due to thalamic lesions. Initial paresthesias followed in weeks to months by allodynia (ordinarily painless stimuli cause pain) and dysesthesia. Occurs in 10% of stroke patients.

- most common stroke area = Midd. cereb.
- most " aneurysm " = ① b/w ant comm & ant cereb.
  ② Lenticulostriat / MCA
  ③ b/w ICA & middle cereb.

Intracranial hemorrhage

Epidural hematoma	Rupture of middle meningeal artery (branch of maxillary artery), often 2° to skull fracture A. Lucid interval. Rapid expansion under systemic arterial pressure → transtentorial herniation, CN III palsy. CT shows biconvex (lentiform), hyperdense blood collection B **not crossing suture lines.**
Subdural hematoma	Rupture of bridging veins. Can be acute (traumatic, high-energy impact → hyperdense on CT) or chronic (associated with mild trauma, cerebral atrophy, elderly, alcoholism → hypodense on CT). Also seen in shaken babies. Predisposing factors: brain atrophy, trauma. Crescent-shaped hemorrhage that **crosses suture lines** (red arrows in C and D). Can cause midline shift (blue arrow in C), findings of "acute on chronic" hemorrhage (blue arrow in D).
Subarachnoid hemorrhage	Rupture of an aneurysm (such as a saccular aneurysm E) or arteriovenous malformation. Rapid time course. Patients complain of "worst headache of my life." Bloody or yellow (xanthochromic) spinal tap. 4–10 days after hemorrhage, vasospasm (narrowing of blood vessels) can occur → ischemic infarct; nimodipine used for prevention F. ↑ risk of developing communicating and/or obstructive hydrocephalus.
Intraparenchymal hemorrhage	Most commonly caused by systemic hypertension. Also seen with amyloid angiopathy (recurrent lobar hemorrhagic stroke in elderly), vasculitis, neoplasm. May be 2° to reperfusion injury in ischemic stroke. Typically occurs in basal ganglia G and internal capsule (Charcot-Bouchard aneurysm of lenticulostriate vessels), but can be lobar H.

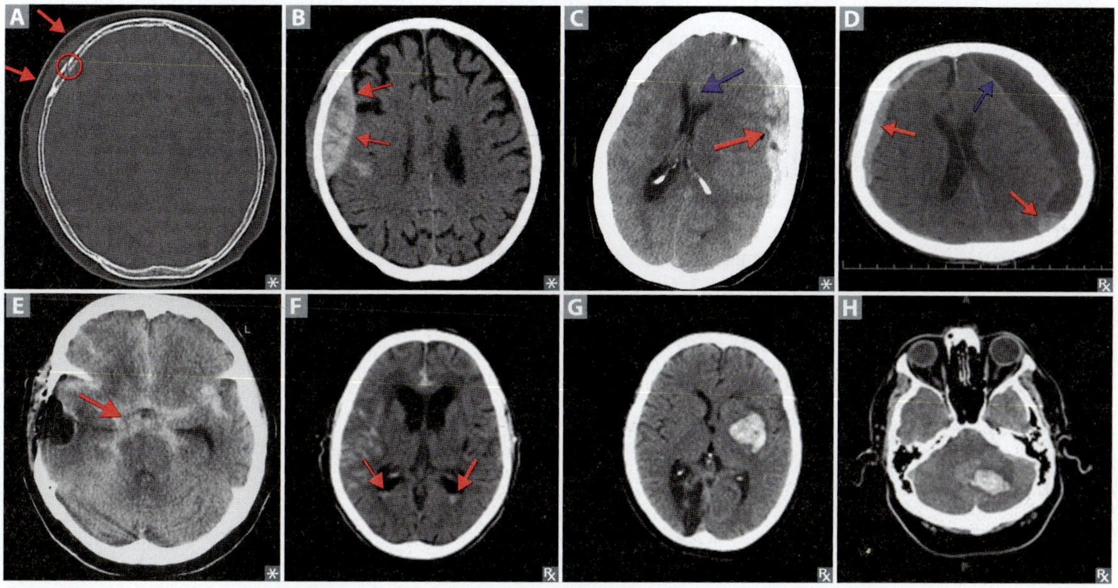

Ischemic brain disease/stroke

Irreversible damage begins after 5 minutes of hypoxia. Most vulnerable: hippocampus, neocortex, cerebellum, watershed areas. Irreversible neuronal injury. Ischemic **hypo**xia—"**hypo**campus" is most vulnerable.

Stroke imaging: Noncontrast CT to exclude hemorrhage (before tPA can be given). CT detects ischemic changes in 6–24 hr. Diffusion-weighted MRI can detect ischemia within 3–30 min.

TIME SINCE ISCHEMIC EVENT	12–48 HOURS	24–72 HOURS	3–5 DAYS	1–2 WEEKS	> 2 WEEKS
Histologic features	Red neurons	Necrosis + neutrophils	Macrophages (microglia)	Reactive gliosis + vascular proliferation	Glial scar

Ischemic stroke

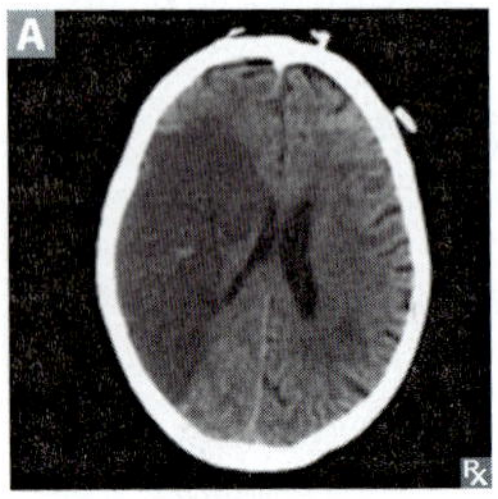

Acute blockage of vessels → disruption of blood flow and subsequent ischemia → liquefactive necrosis.

3 types:

- Thrombotic—due to a clot forming directly at site of infarction (commonly the MCA A), usually over an atherosclerotic plaque.
- Embolic—embolus from another part of the body obstructs vessel. Can affect multiple vascular territories. Examples: atrial fibrillation; DVT with patent foramen ovale.
- Hypoxic—due to hypoperfusion or hypoxemia. Common during cardiovascular surgeries, tends to affect watershed areas.

Treatment: tPA (if within 3–4.5 hr of onset and no hemorrhage/risk of hemorrhage). Reduce risk with medical therapy (eg, aspirin, clopidogrel); optimum control of blood pressure, blood sugars, lipids; and treat conditions that ↑ risk (eg, atrial fibrillation).

Transient ischemic attack

Brief, reversible episode of focal neurologic dysfunction without acute infarction (⊖ MRI), with the majority resolving in < 15 minutes; deficits due to focal ischemia.

Dural venous sinuses

Large venous channels that run through the dura. Drain blood from cerebral veins and receive CSF from arachnoid granulations. Empty into internal jugular vein.

Venous sinus thrombosis—presents with signs/symptoms of ↑ ICP (eg, headache, seizures, focal neurologic deficits). May lead to venous hemorrhage. Associated with hypercoagulable states (eg, pregnancy, OCP use, factor V Leiden).

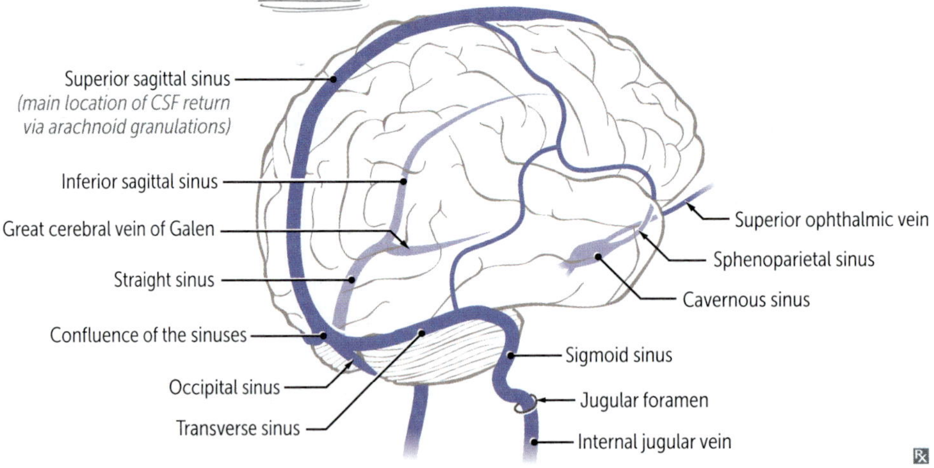

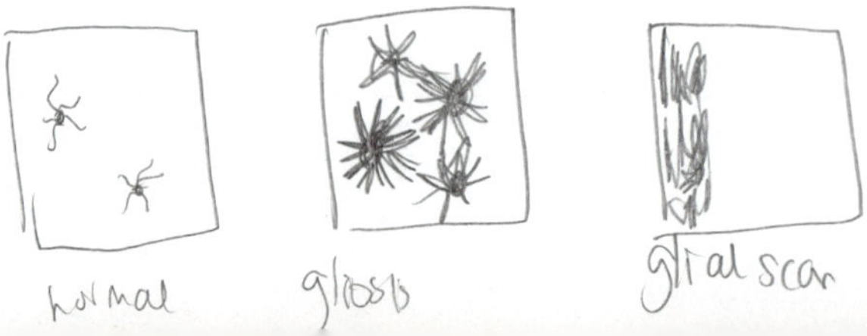

Ventricular system

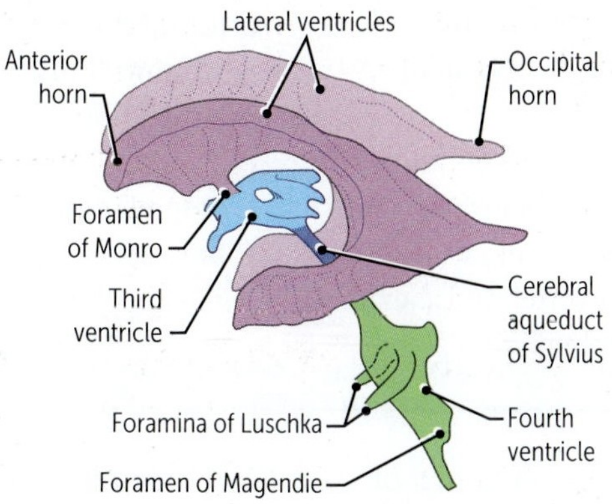

Lateral ventricle → 3rd ventricle via right and left interventricular foramina of Monro.

3rd ventricle → 4th ventricle via cerebral aqueduct (of Sylvius).

4th ventricle → subarachnoid space via:

- Foramina of **L**uschka = **L**ateral.
- Foramen of **M**agendie = **M**edial.

CSF is made by ependymal cells of choroid plexus; it is reabsorbed by arachnoid granulations and then drains into dural venous sinuses.

CSF flows b/w pia & arach

Idiopathic intracranial hypertension (pseudotumor cerebri)

↑ ICP with no apparent cause on imaging (eg, hydrocephalus, obstruction of CSF outflow). Risk factors include being a woman of childbearing age, vitamin A excess, danazol, tetracycline.

Findings: headache, diplopia (usually from CN VI palsy), without change in mental status. Papilledema seen on fundoscopy. Lumbar puncture reveals ↑ opening pressure and provides headache relief.

easily stretched

Treatment: weight loss, acetazolamide, topiramate, invasive procedures for refractory cases (eg, repeat lumbar puncture, CSF shunt placement, optic nerve fenestration surgery).

Hydrocephalus

↑ CSF volume → ventricular dilation +/– ↑ ICP.

Communicating

Communicating hydrocephalus: ↓ CSF absorption by arachnoid granulations (eg, arachnoid scarring post-meningitis) → ↑ ICP, papilledema, herniation.

Normal pressure hydrocephalus: Affects the elderly; idiopathic; CSF pressure elevated only episodically; does not result in increased subarachnoid space volume. Expansion of ventricles **A** distorts the fibers of the corona radiata → triad of **urinary incontinence**, **ataxia**, and **cognitive dysfunction** (sometimes reversible). "**Wet**, **wobbly**, and **wacky**." Characteristic magnetic gait (feet appear stuck to floor).

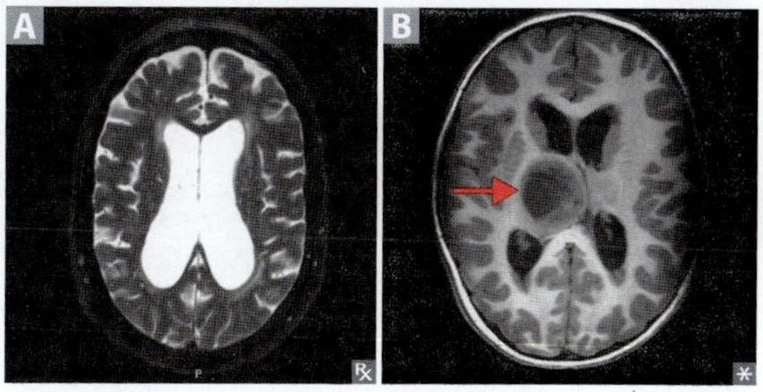

Δ = urinary I
dementia
gait prob

Noncommunicating (obstructive)

Noncommunicating hydrocephalus: Caused by structural blockage of CSF circulation within ventricular system (eg, stenosis of aqueduct of Sylvius; colloid cyst blocking foramen of Monro; tumors **B**).

Hydrocephalus mimics

Ex vacuo ventriculomegaly: Appearance of ↑ CSF on imaging, but is actually due to decreased brain tissue (neuronal atrophy) (eg, Alzheimer disease, advanced HIV, Pick disease). ICP is normal; triad is not seen.

Spinal nerves

There are 31 pairs of spinal nerves in total: 8 cervical, 12 thoracic, 5 lumbar, 5 sacral, 1 coccygeal.

Nerves C1–C7 exit above the corresponding vertebra. C8 spinal nerve exits below C7 and above T1. All other nerves exit below (eg, C3 exits above the 3rd cervical vertebra; L2 exits below the 2nd lumbar vertebra).

Vertebral disc herniation—nucleus pulposus (soft central disc) herniates through annulus fibrosus (outer ring); usually occurs posterolaterally at L4–L5 or L5–S1. Compression of S1 nerve root → absent ankle reflex.

Spinal cord—lower extent

In adults, spinal cord ends at lower border of L1–L2 vertebrae. Subarachnoid space (which contains the CSF) extends to lower border of S2 vertebra. Lumbar puncture is usually performed between L3–L4 or L4–L5 (level of cauda equina).

Goal of lumbar puncture is to obtain sample of CSF without damaging spinal cord. To **keep** the cord **alive**, keep the spinal needle between **L3** and **L5**.

Spinal cord and associated tracts

Legs (**L**umbosacral) are **L**ateral in **L**ateral corticospinal, spinothalamic tracts A.
Dorsal columns are organized as you are, with hands at sides. Arms outside, legs inside.

A

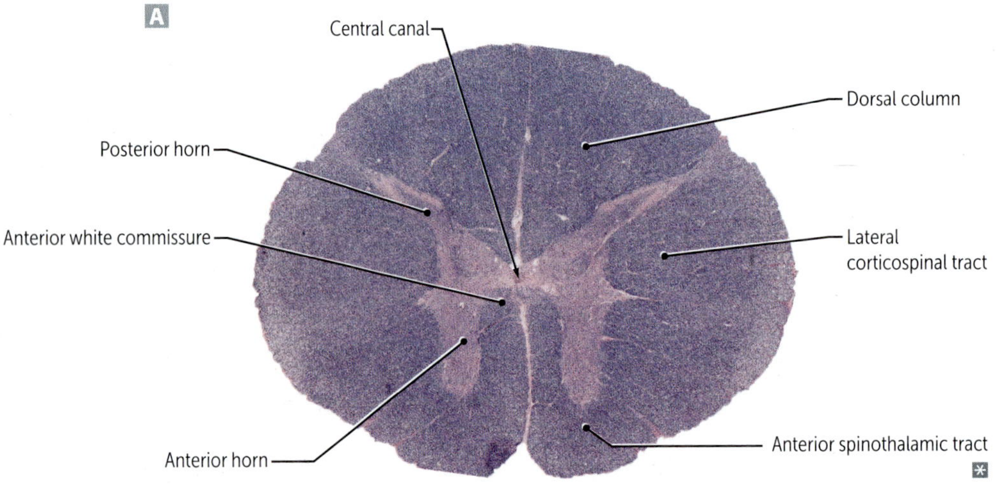

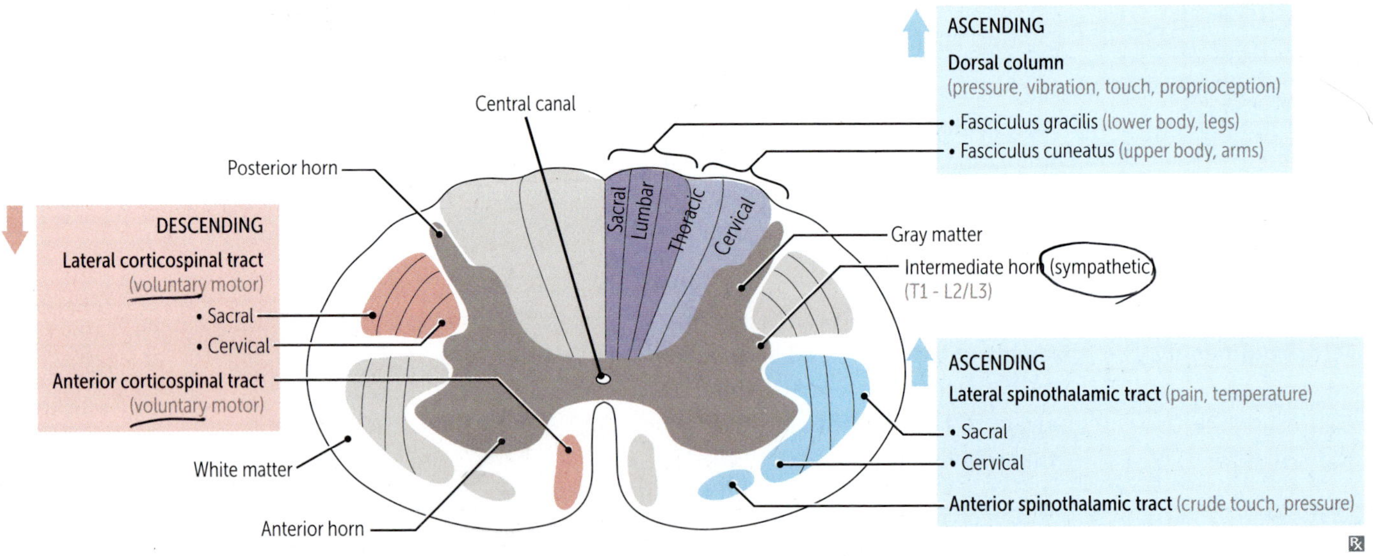

Spinal tract anatomy and functions

Remember, ascending tracts synapse and then cross.

TRACT AND FUNCTION	1ST-ORDER NEURON	SYNAPSE 1	2ND-ORDER NEURON	SYNAPSE 2	3RD-ORDER NEURON
Dorsal column Ascending: pressure, vibration, fine touch, and proprioception	Sensory nerve ending → cell body in dorsal root ganglion → enters spinal cord, ascends ipsilaterally in dorsal column	Ipsilateral nucleus cuneatus or gracilis (medulla)	Decussates in medulla → ascends contralaterally in medial lemniscus	VPL (thalamus)	Sensory cortex
Spinothalamic tract Ascending Lateral: pain, temperature Anterior: crude touch, pressure	Sensory nerve ending (Aδ and C fibers) → cell body in dorsal root ganglion → enters spinal cord	Ipsilateral gray matter (spinal cord)	Decussates at anterior white commissure → ascends contralaterally (Right at the level)	VPL (thalamus)	Sensory cortex
Lateral corticospinal tract Descending: voluntary movement of contralateral limbs	UMN: cell body in 1° motor cortex → descends ipsilaterally (through internal capsule), most fibers decussate at caudal medulla (pyramidal decussation) → descends contralaterally	Cell body of anterior horn (spinal cord) I thought first synapse was at pyr. but NO!	LMN: leaves spinal cord	NMJ	

Motor neuron signs

SIGN	UMN LESION	LMN LESION
Weakness	+	+
Atrophy	–	+
Fasciculations	–	+
Reflexes	↑	↓
Tone	↑	↓
Babinski	+	–
Spastic paralysis	+	–
Flaccid paralysis	–	+
Clasp knife spasticity	+	–

COMMENTS

Lower motor neuron = everything **lower**ed (less muscle mass, ↓ muscle tone, ↓ reflexes, downgoing toes).

Upper motor neuron = everything **up** (tone, DTRs, toes).

Fasciculations = muscle twitching.

Positive Babinski is normal in infants. bc their UMNs haven't dev- yet.

Ant horn loss = ØLMN

Spinal cord lesions

AREA AFFECTED	DISEASE	CHARACTERISTICS
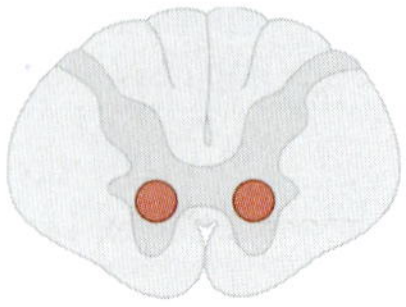	Poliomyelitis and Werdnig-Hoffmann disease	Congenital degeneration of anterior horns of spinal cord. LMN lesions only. "Floppy baby" with marked hypotonia and tongue fasciculations. Infantile type has median age of death of 7 months. Autosomal recessive inheritance. Poliomyelitis → asymmetric weakness. Werdnig-Hoffmann disease → symmetric weakness.
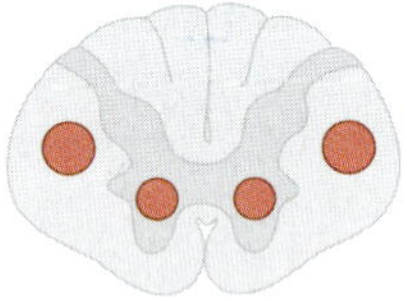	Amyotrophic lateral sclerosis	Combined UMN and LMN deficits with no sensory or bowel/bladder deficits (due to loss of cortical and spinal cord motor neurons, respectively). Can be caused by defect in superoxide dismutase 1. Commonly presents with asymmetric limb weakness (hands/feet), fasciculations, eventual atrophy. Fatal. Commonly known as Lou Gehrig disease. Treatment: riluzole.
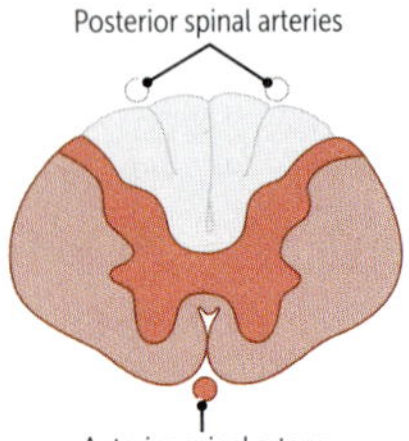	Complete occlusion of anterior spinal artery	Spares dorsal columns and Lissauer tract; upper thoracic ASA territory is watershed area, as artery of Adamkiewicz supplies ASA below ~ T8.
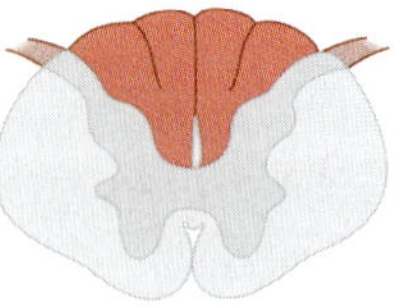	Tabes dorsalis	Caused by 3° syphilis. Results from degeneration (demyelination) of dorsal columns and roots → progressive sensory ataxia (impaired proprioception → poor coordination). Associated with Charcot joints, shooting pain, Argyll Robertson pupils. Exam will demonstrate absence of DTRs and ⊕ Romberg sign.
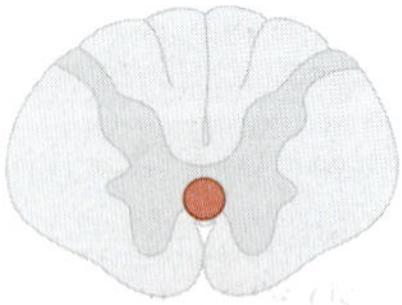	Syringomyelia	Syrinx expands and damages anterior white commissure of spinothalamic tract (2nd-order neurons) → bilateral loss of pain and temperature sensation in cape-like distribution; seen with Chiari I malformation; can expand and affect other tracts.
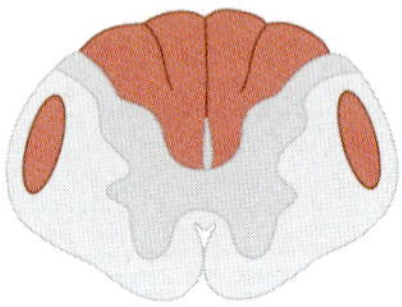	Vitamin B_{12} deficiency	Subacute combined degeneration (**SCD**)—demyelination of **S**pinocerebellar tracts, lateral **C**orticospinal tracts, and **D**orsal columns. Ataxic gait, paresthesia, impaired position/vibration sense.

Poliomyelitis

Caused by poliovirus (fecal-oral transmission). Replicates in oropharynx and small intestine before spreading via bloodstream to CNS. Infection causes destruction of cells in anterior horn of spinal cord (LMN death).

Signs of LMN lesion: weakness, hypotonia, flaccid paralysis, fasciculations, hyporeflexia, muscle atrophy. Signs of infection: malaise, headache, fever, nausea, etc.

CSF shows ↑ WBCs and slight ↑ of protein (with no change in CSF glucose). Virus recovered from stool or throat.

Friedreich ataxia

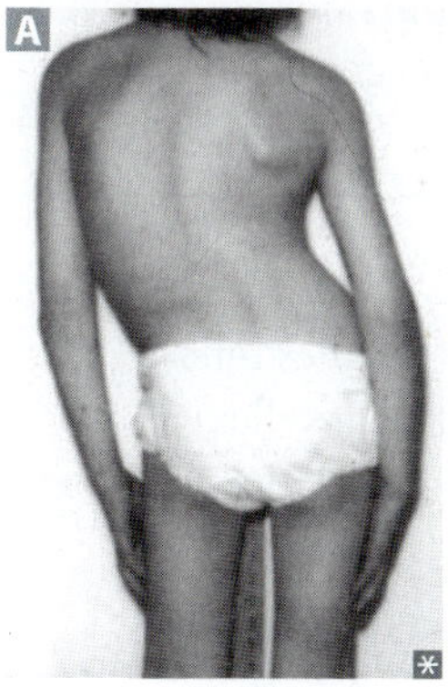

Autosomal recessive trinucleotide repeat disorder **(GAA)$_n$** on chromosome 9 in gene that encodes frataxin (iron binding protein). Leads to impairment in mitochondrial functioning. Degeneration of multiple spinal cord tracts → muscle weakness and loss of DTRs, vibratory sense, proprioception. **Staggering** gait, frequent **falling**, nystagmus, dysarthria, pes cavus, hammer toes, **diabetes** mellitus, **hypertrophic cardiomyopathy** (cause of death). Presents in childhood with kyphoscoliosis A.

Friedreich is **F**ratastic (**frataxin**): he's your favorite **frat** brother, always **staggering** and **falling** but has a **sweet**, **big heart**.

Ataxic **GAA**it.

Brown-Séquard syndrome

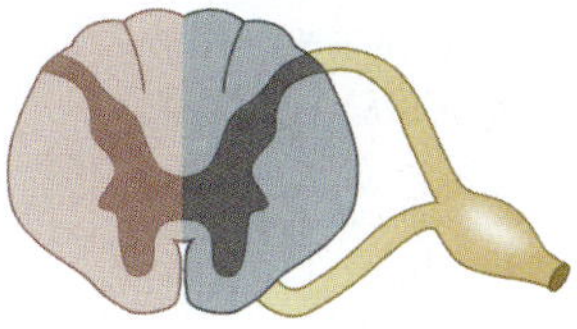

Hemisection of spinal cord. Findings:

- Ipsilateral UMN signs below level of lesion (due to corticospinal tract damage)
- Ipsilateral loss of tactile, vibration, proprioception sense below level of lesion (due to dorsal column damage)
- Contralateral pain and temperature loss below level of lesion (due to spinothalamic tract damage)
- Ipsilateral loss of all sensation at level of lesion
- Ipsilateral LMN signs (eg, flaccid paralysis) at level of lesion

If lesion occurs above T1, patient may present with ipsilateral Horner syndrome due to damage of oculosympathetic pathway.

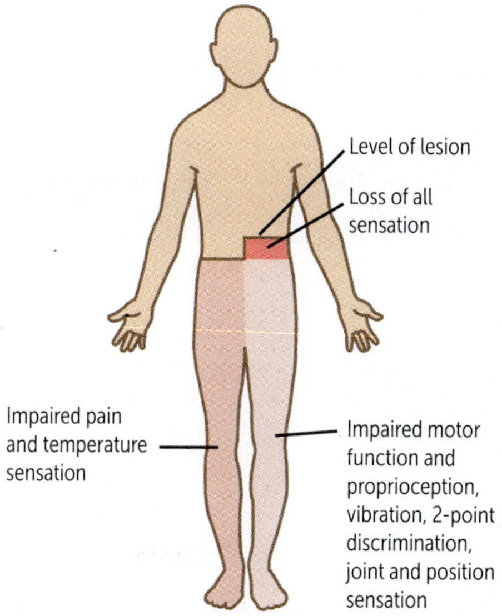

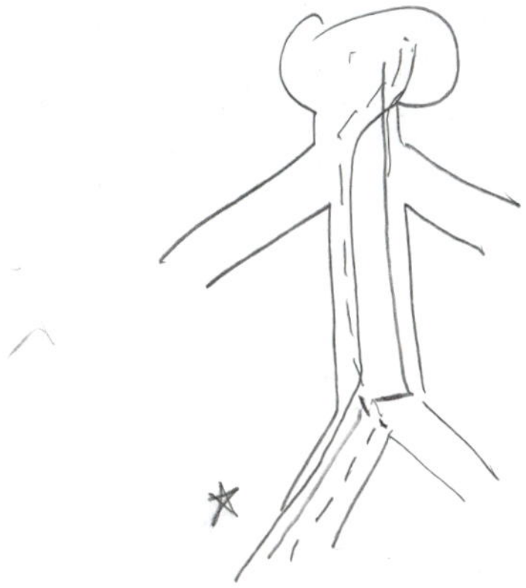

Landmark dermatomes

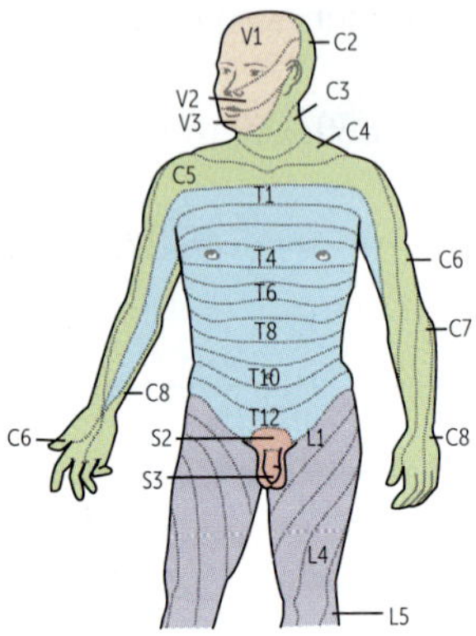

C2—posterior half of a skull "cap."
C3—high turtleneck shirt.
C4—low-collar shirt.
C6—includes thumbs.
T4—at the nipple.
T7—at the xiphoid process.
T10—at the umbilicus (important for early appendicitis pain referral).
L1—at the inguinal ligament.
L4—includes the kneecaps.
S2, S3, S4—erection and sensation of penile and anal zones.

Diaphragm and gallbladder pain referred to the right shoulder via phrenic nerve.

Thumbs up sign on left hand looks like a **six** for C**6**.
T4 at the **teat pore**.

T**10** at the belly but**ten**.

L1 is **IL** (**I**nguinal **L**igament).
Down on **ALL 4**'s (**L4**).
"**S2, 3, 4** keep the penis off the **floor**."

Clinical reflexes

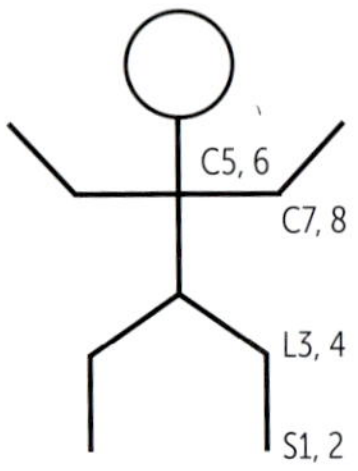

Biceps = C5 nerve root.
Triceps = C7 nerve root.
Patella = L4 nerve root.
Achilles = S1 nerve root.

Reflexes count up in order:
- S1, 2—"buckle my shoe" (Achilles reflex)
- L3, 4—"kick the door" (patellar reflex)
- C5, 6—"pick up sticks" (biceps reflex)
- C7, 8—"lay them straight" (triceps reflex)

Additional reflexes:
- L1, L2—"testicles move" (cremaster reflex)
- S3, S4—"winks galore" (anal wink reflex)

Primitive reflexes

CNS reflexes that are present in a healthy infant, but are absent in a neurologically intact adult. Normally disappear within 1st year of life. These "primitive" reflexes are inhibited by a mature/developing frontal lobe. They may reemerge in adults following frontal lobe lesions → loss of inhibition of these reflexes.

Moro reflex	"Hang on for life" reflex—abduct/extend arms when startled, and then draw together
Rooting reflex	Movement of head toward one side if cheek or mouth is stroked (nipple seeking)
Sucking reflex	Sucking response when roof of mouth is touched
Palmar reflex	Curling of fingers if palm is stroked
Plantar reflex	Dorsiflexion of large toe and fanning of other toes with plantar stimulation Babinski sign—presence of this reflex in an adult, which may signify a UMN lesion
Galant reflex	Stroking along one side of the spine while newborn is in ventral suspension (face down) causes lateral flexion of lower body toward stimulated side

Brain stem—ventral view

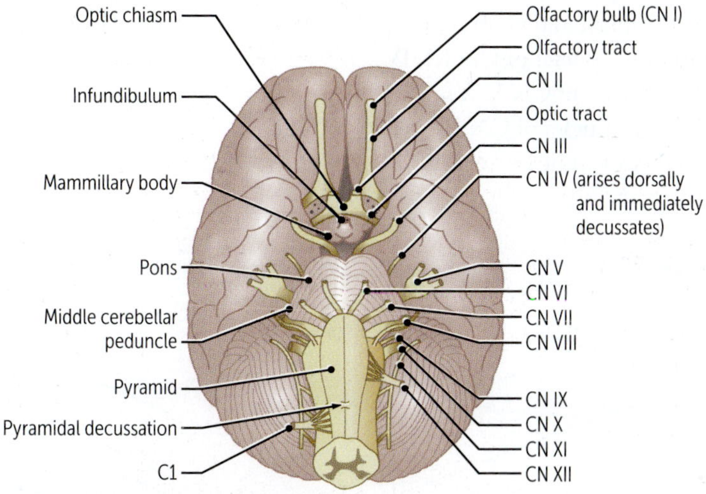

4 CN are in above pons (I, II, III, IV).
4 CN are in pons (V, VI, VII, VIII).
4 CN are in medulla (IX, X, XI, XII).
4 CN nuclei are medial (III, IV, VI, XII). "Factors of 12, except 1 and 2."

Brain stem—dorsal view (cerebellum removed)

Pineal gland—melatonin secretion, circadian rhythms.
Superior colliculi—conjugate vertical gaze center.
Inferior colliculi—auditory.
Parinaud syndrome—paralysis of conjugate vertical gaze due to lesion in superior colliculi (eg, stroke, hydrocephalus, pinealoma).

Your eyes are **above** your ears, and the superior colliculus (visual) is **above** the inferior colliculus (auditory).

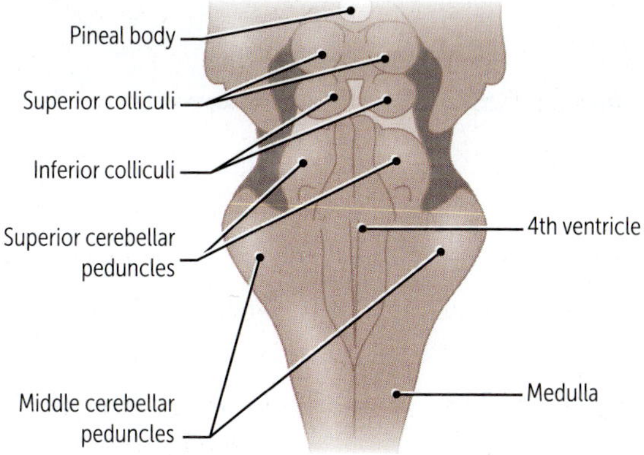

Cranial nerve nuclei	Located in tegmentum portion of brain stem (between dorsal and ventral portions): ▪ Midbrain—nuclei of CN III, IV ▪ Pons—nuclei of CN V, VI, VII, VIII ▪ Medulla—nuclei of CN IX, X, XII ▪ Spinal cord—nucleus of CN XI	**L**ateral nuclei = sensory (a**L**ar plate). —Sulcus limitans— **M**edial nuclei = **M**otor (basal plate).

Cranial nerve and vessel pathways

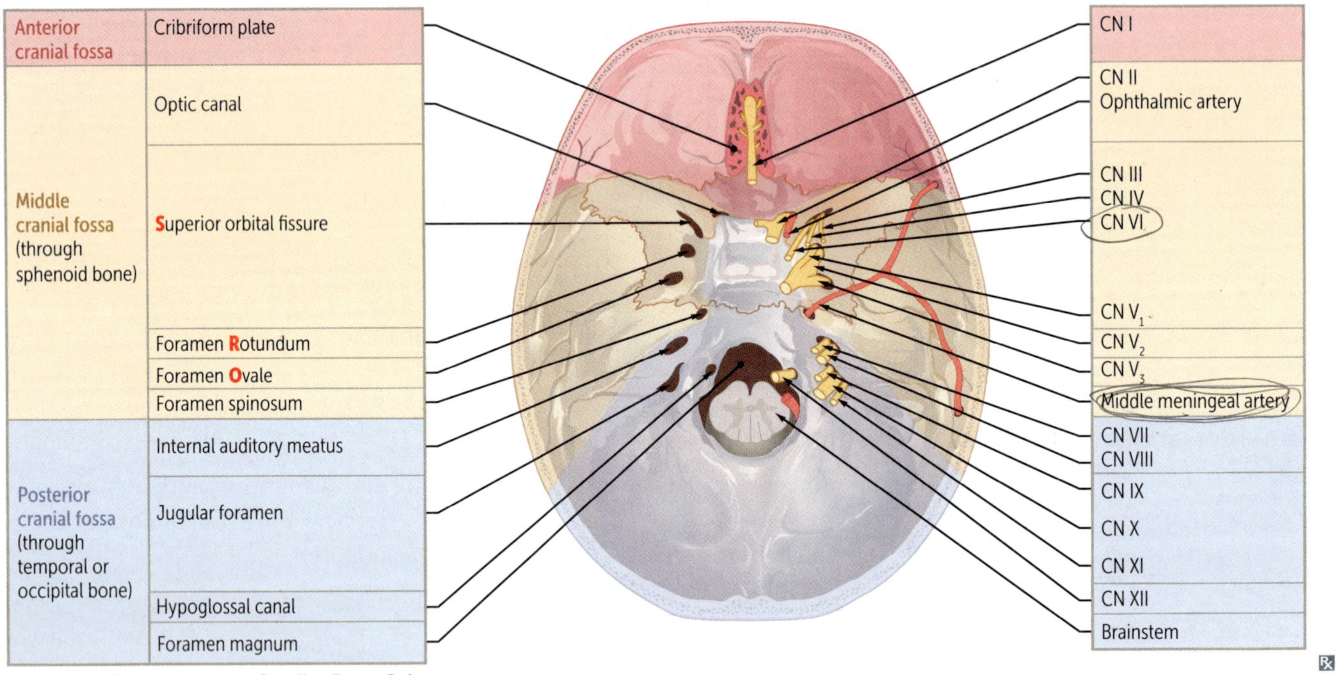

Divisions of CN V exit owing to **S**tanding **R**oom **O**nly

Cranial nerves

NERVE	CN	FUNCTION	TYPE	MNEMONIC
Olfactory	I	Smell (only CN without thalamic relay to cortex)	Sensory	Some
Optic	II	Sight	Sensory	Say
Oculomotor	III	Eye movement (SR, IR, MR, IO), pupillary constriction (sphincter pupillae: Edinger-Westphal nucleus, muscarinic receptors), accommodation, eyelid opening (levator palpebrae)	Motor	Marry
Trochlear	IV	Eye movement (SO)	Motor	Money
Trigeminal	V	Mastication, facial sensation (ophthalmic, maxillary, mandibular divisions), somatosensation from anterior 2/3 of tongue	Both	But
Abducens	VI	Eye movement (LR)	Motor	My
Facial	VII	Facial movement, taste from anterior 2/3 of tongue, lacrimation, salivation (submandibular and sublingual glands), eyelid closing (orbicularis oculi), auditory volume modulation (stapedius)	Both	Brother
Vestibulocochlear	VIII	Hearing, balance	Sensory	Says
Glossopharyngeal	IX	Taste and sensation from posterior 1/3 of tongue, swallowing, salivation (parotid gland), monitoring carotid body and sinus chemo- and baroreceptors, and elevation of pharynx/larynx (stylopharyngeus)	Both	Big
Vagus	X	Taste from supraglottic region, swallowing, soft palate elevation, midline uvula, talking, coughing, parasympathetics to thoracoabdominal viscera, monitoring aortic arch chemo- and baroreceptors	Both	Brains
Accessory	XI	Head turning, shoulder shrugging (SCM, trapezius)	Motor	Matter
Hypoglossal	XII	Tongue movement	Motor	Most

Vagal nuclei

NUCLEUS	FUNCTION	CRANIAL NERVES
Nucleus Solitarius	Visceral Sensory information (eg, taste, baroreceptors, gut distention)	VII, IX, X
Nucleus aMbiguus	Motor innervation of pharynx, larynx, upper esophagus (eg, swallowing, palate elevation)	IX, X, XI (cranial portion)
Dorsal motor nucleus	Sends autonomic (parasympathetic) fibers to heart, lungs, upper GI	X

Cranial nerve reflexes

REFLEX	AFFERENT	EFFERENT
Corneal	V_1 ophthalmic (nasociliary branch)	VII (temporal branch: orbicularis oculi)
Lacrimation	V_1 (loss of reflex does not preclude emotional tears)	VII
Jaw jerk	V_3 (sensory—muscle spindle from masseter)	V_3 (motor—masseter)
Pupillary	II	III
Gag	IX	X

Common cranial nerve lesions

CN V motor lesion	Jaw deviates **toward** side of lesion due to unopposed force from the opposite pterygoid muscle.
CN X lesion	Uvula deviates **away** from side of lesion. Weak side collapses and uvula points away.
CN XI lesion	Weakness turning head to contralateral side of lesion (SCM). Shoulder droop on side of lesion (trapezius). The left SCM contracts to help turn the head to the right.
CN XII lesion	LMN lesion. Tongue deviates **toward** side of lesion ("lick your wounds") due to weakened tongue muscles on affected side.

Mastication muscles

3 muscles close jaw: **M**asseter, te**M**poralis, **M**edial pterygoid. 1 opens: lateral pterygoid. All are innervated by trigeminal nerve (V_3).

M's **M**unch.
Lateral **L**owers (when speaking of pterygoids with respect to jaw motion).
"It takes more muscle to keep your mouth shut."

Facial nerve lesions

Upper motor neuron lesion
Destruction of motor cortex or connection between motor cortex and facial nucleus in pons → contralateral paralysis of lower muscles of facial expression. Forehead is spared due to its bilateral UMN innervation.

Lower motor neuron lesiona
Destruction of facial nucleus or CN VII anywhere along its course → ipsilateral paralysis of upper and lower muscles of facial expression A, hyperacusis, loss of taste sensation to anterior tongue.

Facial nerve palsy

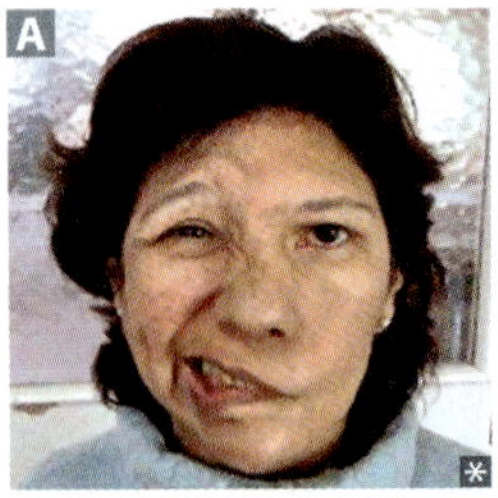

Clinical syndrome of peripheral CN VII (LMN) lesion. Depending on lesion location and severity, may cause partial or complete loss of function.
When idiopathic (most common), called Bell palsy. May also be caused by Lyme disease, herpes simplex, herpes zoster (Ramsay Hunt syndrome), sarcoidosis, tumors, diabetes mellitus. Treatment is corticosteroids, acyclovir. Most patients have gradual recovery of function.

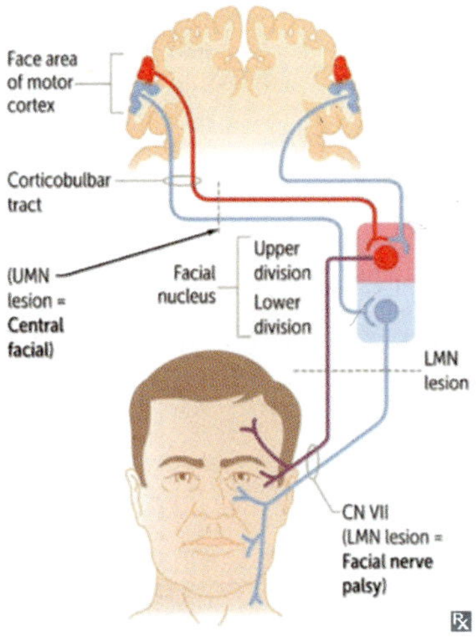

Cavernous sinus

Collection of venous sinuses on either side of pituitary. Blood from eye and superficial cortex → cavernous sinus → internal jugular vein.

CNs III, IV, V_1, VI, and occasionally V_2 plus postganglionic sympathetic pupillary fibers en route to orbit all pass through cavernous sinus. Cavernous portion of internal carotid artery is also here.

Cavernous sinus syndrome—presents with variable ophthalmoplegia, ↓ corneal sensation, Horner syndrome and occasional decreased maxillary sensation. 2° to pituitary tumor mass effect, carotid-cavernous fistula, or cavernous sinus thrombosis related to infection. CN VI is most susceptible to injury.

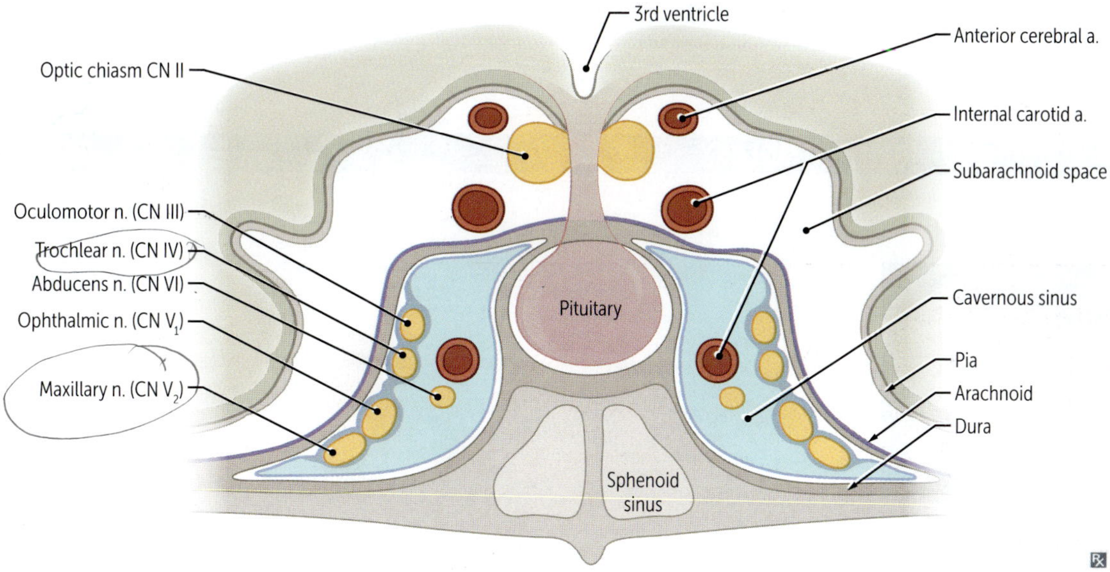

Auditory physiology

Outer ear	Visible portion of ear (pinna), includes auditory canal and eardrum. Transfers sound waves via vibration of eardrum.
Middle ear	Air-filled space with three bones called the ossicles (malleus, incus, stapes). Ossicles conduct and amplify sound from eardrum to inner ear.
Inner ear	Snail-shaped, fluid-filled cochlea. Contains basilar membrane that vibrates 2° to sound waves. Vibration transduced via specialized hair cells → auditory nerve signaling → brain stem. Each frequency leads to vibration at specific location on basilar membrane (tonotopy): ▪ Low frequency heard at apex near helicotrema (wide and flexible). ▪ High frequency heard best at base of cochlea (thin and rigid).

Hearing loss

	RINNE TEST	WEBER TEST
Conductive	Abnormal (bone > air)	Localizes to affected ear
Sensorineural	Normal (air > bone)	Localizes to unaffected ear

Noise-induced — Damage to stereociliated cells in organ of Corti; loss of high-frequency hearing 1st; sudden extremely loud noises can produce hearing loss due to tympanic membrane rupture.

Cholesteatoma

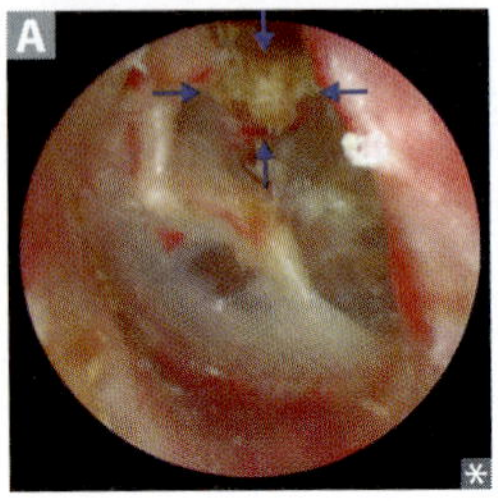

Overgrowth of desquamated keratin debris within the middle ear space (A, blue arrows); may erode ossicles, mastoid air cells → conductive hearing loss.

▶ NEUROLOGY—OPHTHALMOLOGY

Normal eye

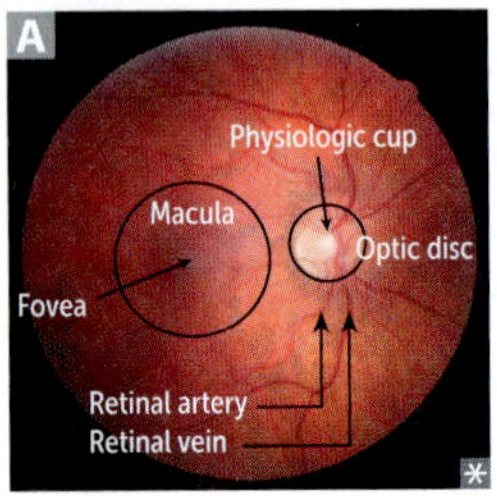

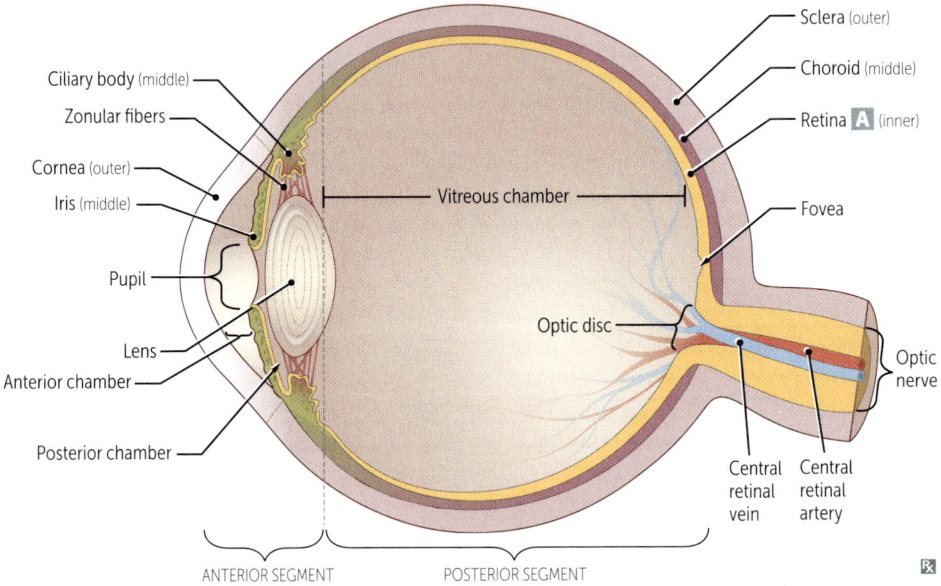

Aqueous humor pathway

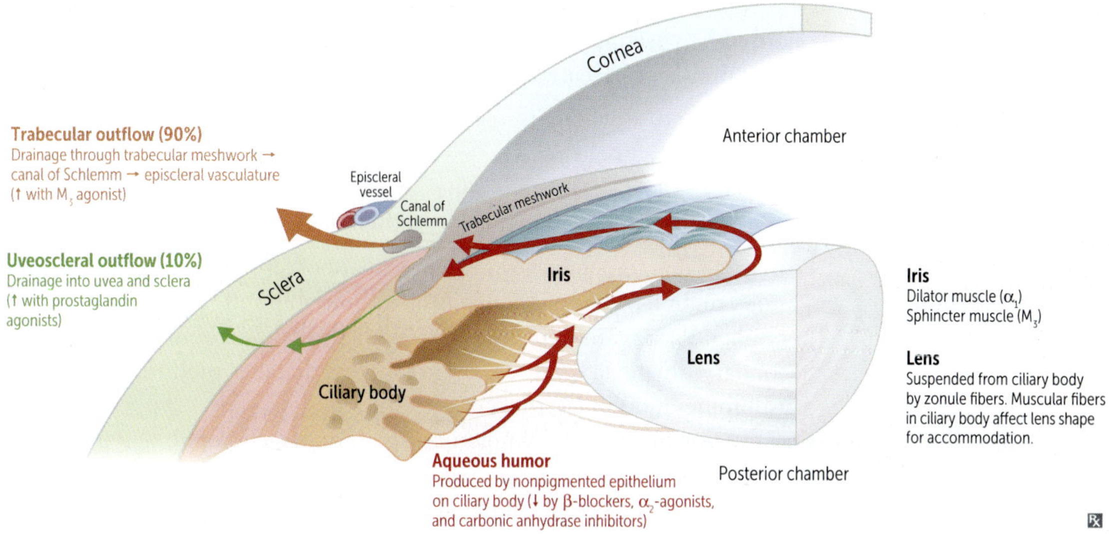

Refractive errors	Common cause of impaired vision, correctable with glasses.
Hyperopia	Eye too short for refractive power of cornea and lens → light focused behind retina.
Myopia	Eye too long for refractive power of cornea and lens → light focused in front of retina.
Astigmatism	Abnormal curvature of cornea → different refractive power at different axes.
Presbyopia	Age-related impaired accommodation (focusing on near objects), primarily due to ↓ lens elasticity. Often necessitates "reading glasses."

Cataract

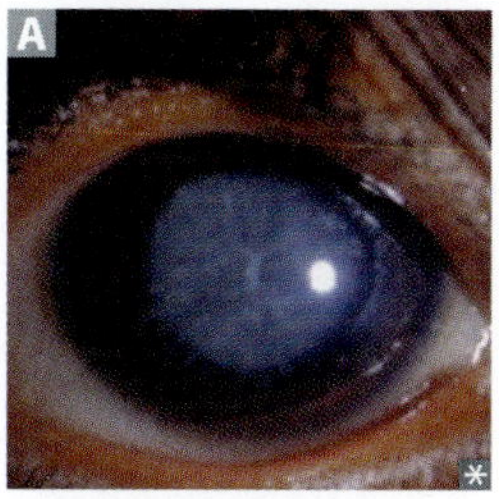

Painless, often bilateral, opacification of lens A, often resulting in ↓ vision. Acquired risk factors: ↑ age, smoking, excessive alcohol use, excessive sunlight, prolonged corticosteroid use, diabetes mellitus, trauma, infection; congenital risk factors: classic galactosemia, galactokinase deficiency, trisomies (13, 18, 21), ToRCHeS infections (eg, rubella), Marfan syndrome, Alport syndrome, myotonic dystrophy, neurofibromatosis 2.

Glaucoma

Optic disc atrophy with characteristic cupping (thinning of outer rim of optic nerve head B versus normal A), usually with elevated intraocular pressure (IOP) and progressive peripheral visual field loss if untreated. Treatment is through pharmacologic or surgical lowering of the IOP.

Open-angle glaucoma

Associated with ↑ age, African-American race, family history. Painless, more common in US.
Primary—cause unclear.
Secondary—blocked trabecular meshwork from WBCs (eg, uveitis), RBCs (eg, vitreous hemorrhage), retinal elements (eg, retinal detachment).

Closed- or narrow-angle glaucoma

Primary—enlargement or forward movement of lens against central iris (pupil margin) → obstruction of normal aqueous flow through pupil → fluid builds up behind iris, pushing peripheral iris against cornea C and impeding flow through trabecular meshwork.
Secondary—hypoxia from retinal disease (eg, diabetes mellitus, vein occlusion) induces vasoproliferation in iris that contracts angle.
Chronic closure—often asymptomatic with damage to optic nerve and peripheral vision.
Acute closure—true ophthalmic emergency. ↑ IOP pushes iris forward → angle closes abruptly. Very painful, red eye D, sudden vision loss, halos around lights, rock-hard eye, frontal headache. Do not give epinephrine because of its mydriatic effect.

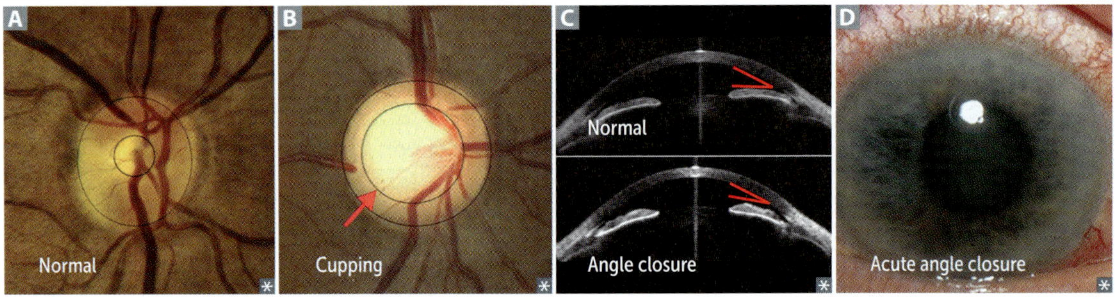

Conjunctivitis

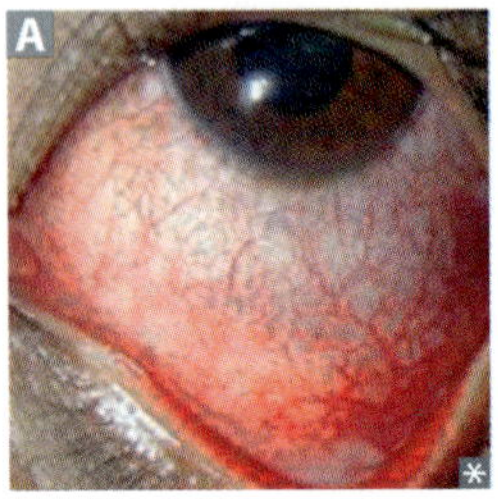

Inflammation of the conjunctiva → red eye A.
Allergic—itchy eyes, bilateral.
Bacterial—pus; treat with antibiotics.
Viral—most common, often adenovirus; sparse mucous discharge, swollen preauricular node; self-resolving.

Uveitis

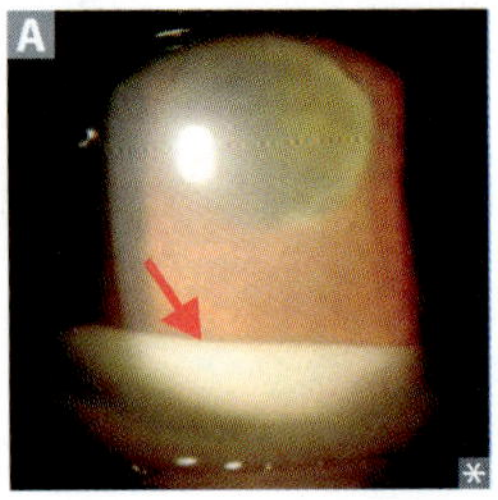

Inflammation of uvea, specific name based on location within affected eye. Anterior uveitis: iritis; intermediate uveitis: pars planitis; posterior uveitis: choroiditis and/or retinitis. May have hypopyon (accumulation of pus in anterior chamber A) or conjunctival redness. Associated with systemic inflammatory disorders (eg, sarcoidosis, rheumatoid arthritis, juvenile idiopathic arthritis, HLA-B27–associated conditions).

sclera is continu. w/ cornea.
choroid continuous w/ ciliary body & iris
- post uvea = choroid
- ant uvea = iris & CB

Age-related macular degeneration

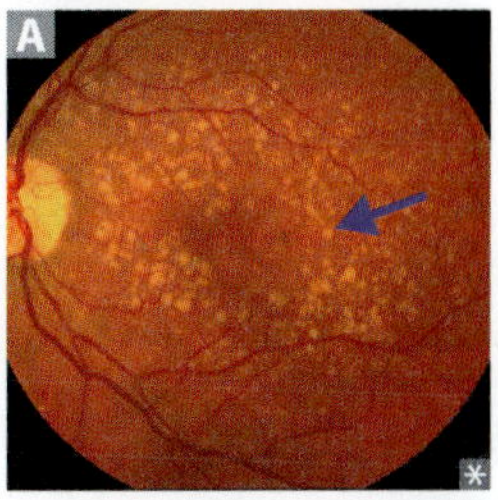

Degeneration of macula (central area of retina). Causes distortion (metamorphopsia) and eventual loss of central vision (scotomas).

- Dry (nonexudative, > 80%)—deposition of yellowish extracellular material in and between Bruch membrane and retinal pigment epithelium ("drusen") A with gradual ↓ in vision. Prevent progression with multivitamin and antioxidant supplements.
- Wet (exudative, 10–15%)—rapid loss of vision due to bleeding 2° to choroidal neovascularization. Treat with anti-VEGF (vascular endothelial growth factor) injections (eg, ranibizumab).

Diabetic retinopathy

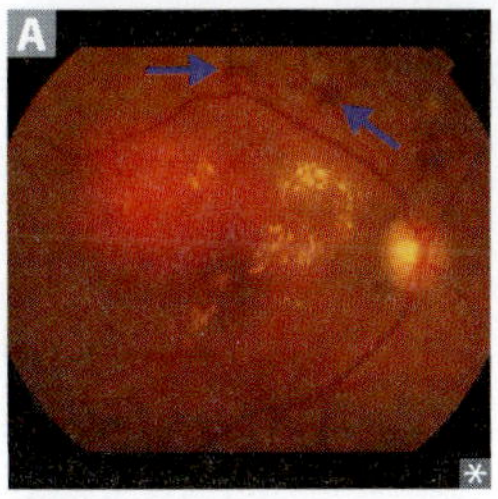

Retinal damage due to chronic hyperglycemia. Two types:

- Nonproliferative—damaged capillaries leak blood → lipids and fluid seep into retina → hemorrhages (blue arrows in A) and macular edema. Treatment: blood sugar control.
- Proliferative—chronic hypoxia results in new blood vessel formation with resultant traction on retina. Treatment: peripheral retinal photocoagulation, surgery, anti-VEGF.

Retinal vein occlusion

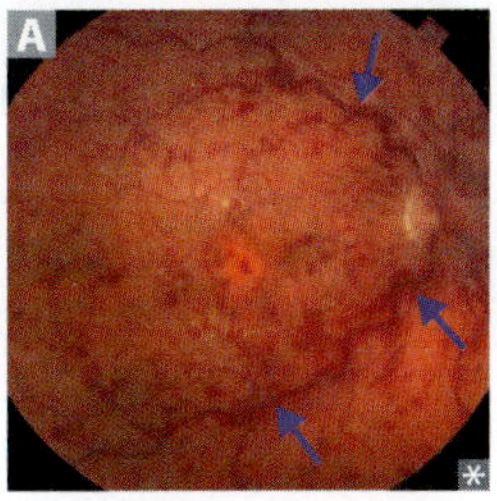

Blockage of central or branch retinal vein due to compression from nearby arterial atherosclerosis. Retinal hemorrhage and venous engorgement (blue arrows in A), edema in affected area.

Retinal detachment

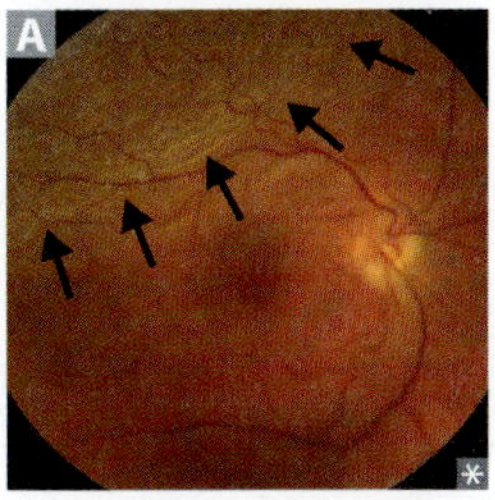

Separation of neurosensory layer of retina (photoreceptor layer with rods and cones) from outermost pigmented epithelium (normally shields excess light, supports retina) → degeneration of photoreceptors → vision loss. May be 2° to retinal breaks, diabetic traction, inflammatory effusions. Visualized on fundoscopy as crinkling of retinal tissue A and changes in vessel direction.

Breaks more common in patients with high myopia and/or history of head trauma. Often preceded by posterior vitreous detachment ("flashes" and "floaters") and eventual monocular loss of vision like a "curtain drawn down." Surgical emergency.

Central retinal artery occlusion

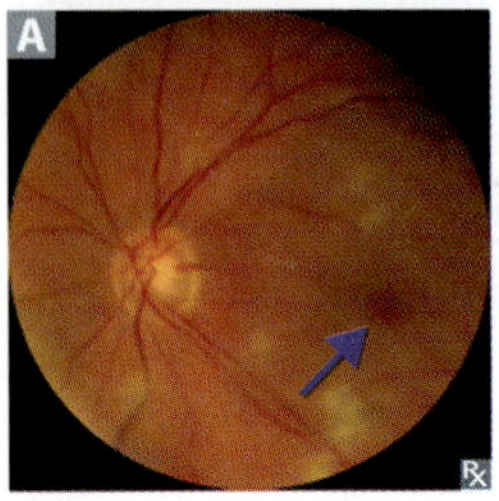

Acute, painless monocular vision loss. Retina cloudy with attenuated vessels and "cherry-red" spot at fovea (center of macula) A. Evaluate for embolic source (eg, carotid artery atherosclerosis, cardiac vegetations, patent foramen ovale).

Retinitis pigmentosa

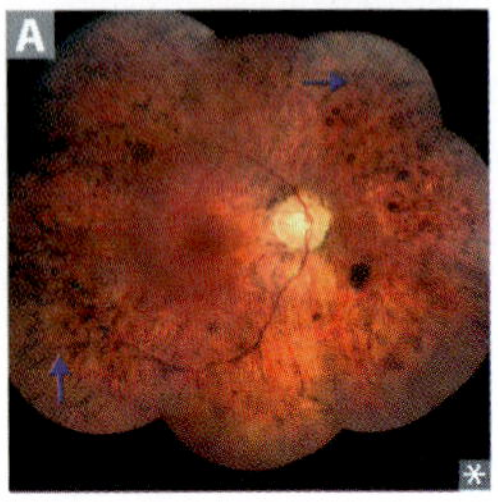

Inherited retinal degeneration. Painless, progressive vision loss beginning with night blindness (rods affected first). Bone spicule–shaped deposits around macula A.

Retinitis

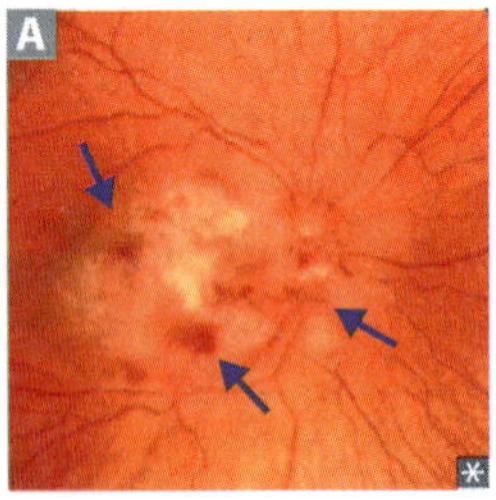

Retinal edema and necrosis (blue arrows in A) leading to scar. Often viral (CMV, HSV, VZV), but can be bacterial or parasitic. May be associated with immunosuppression.

Papilledema

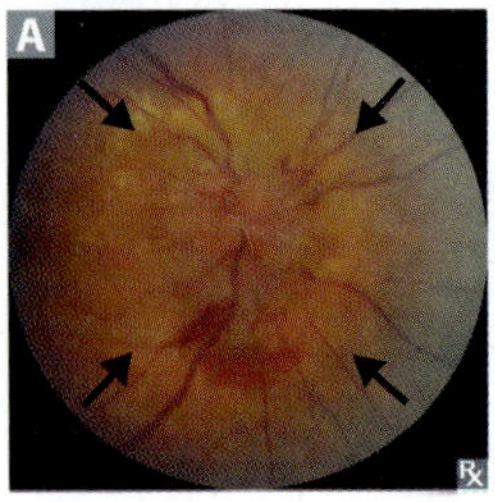

Optic disc swelling (usually bilateral) due to ↑ ICP (eg, 2° to mass effect). Enlarged blind spot and elevated optic disc with blurred margins A.

Pupillary control

Miosis

Constriction, parasympathetic:
- 1st neuron: Edinger-Westphal nucleus to ciliary ganglion via CN III
- 2nd neuron: short ciliary nerves to pupillary sphincter muscles

Pupillary light reflex

Light in either retina sends a signal via CN II to pretectal nuclei (dashed lines in image) in midbrain that activates bilateral Edinger-Westphal nuclei; pupils contract bilaterally (consensual reflex).

Result: illumination of 1 eye results in bilateral pupillary constriction.

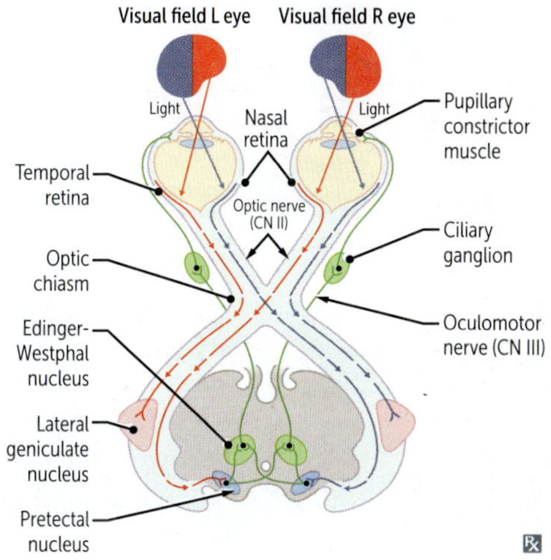

Mydriasis

Dilation, sympathetic:
- 1st neuron: hypothalamus to ciliospinal center of Budge (C8–T2)
- 2nd neuron: exit at T1 to superior cervical ganglion (travels along cervical sympathetic chain near lung apex, subclavian vessels)
- 3rd neuron: plexus along internal carotid, through cavernous sinus; enters orbit as long ciliary nerve to pupillary dilator muscles. Sympathetic fibers also innervate smooth muscle of eyelids (minor retractors) and sweat glands of forehead and face.

Marcus Gunn pupil

Afferent pupillary defect—due to optic nerve damage or severe retinal injury. ↓ bilateral pupillary constriction when light is shone in affected eye relative to unaffected eye. Tested with "swinging flashlight test."

Horner syndrome

Sympathetic denervation of face →:
- **P**tosis (slight drooping of eyelid: superior tarsal muscle)
- **A**nhidrosis (absence of sweating) and flushing of affected side of face
- **M**iosis (pupil constriction)

Associated with lesion of spinal cord above T1 (eg, Pancoast tumor, Brown-Séquard syndrome, late-stage syringomyelia).

Any interruption results in Horner syndrome.

PAM is **horn**y (Horner).
Ptosis, **anhidrosis**, and **miosis** (rhyming).

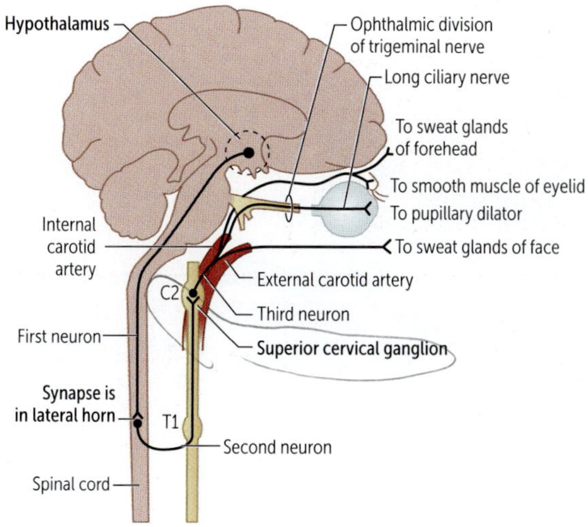

Ocular motility

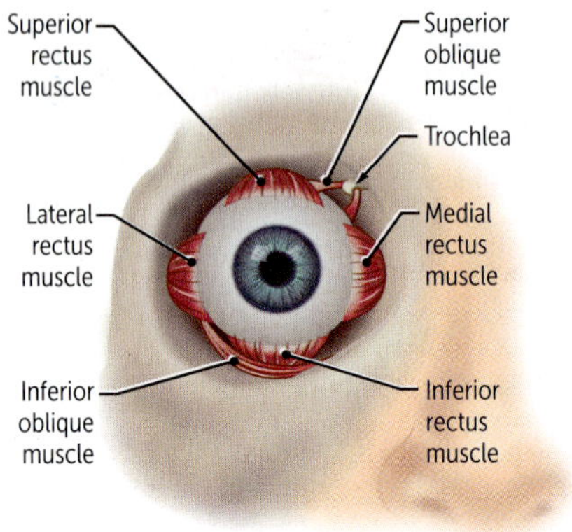

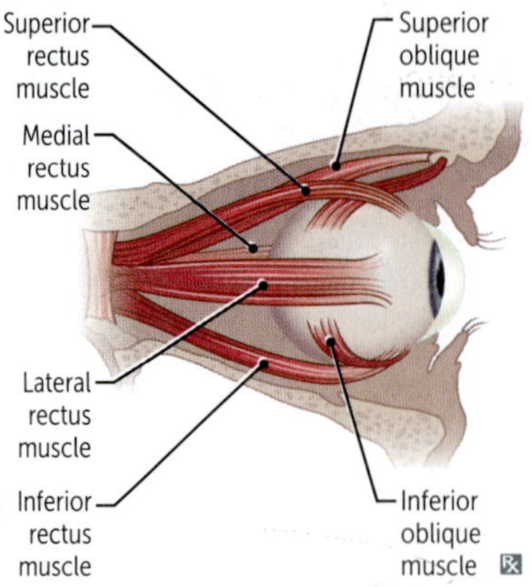

CN **VI** innervates the **L**ateral **R**ectus.
CN **IV** innervates the **S**uperior **O**blique.
CN **III** innervates the **R**est.
The "chemical formula" **$LR_6SO_4R_3$**.
The superior oblique abducts, intorts, and depresses while adducted.

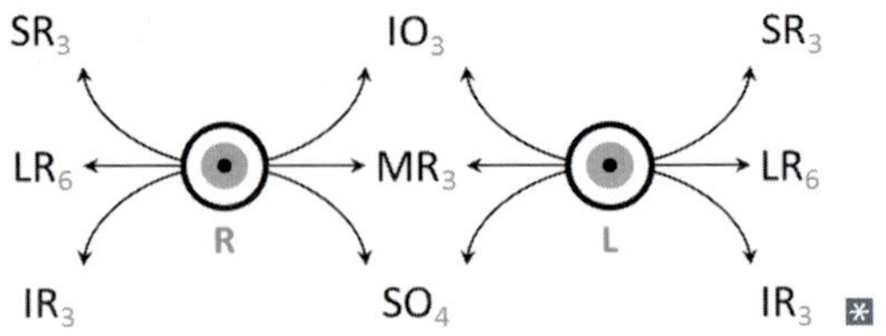

To test each muscle, ask patient to move his/her eye in the path diagrammed below, from neutral position toward the muscle being tested.

Obliques go **O**pposite (left SO and IO tested with patient looking right).
IOU: **IO** tested looking **U**p.

CN III, IV, VI palsies

CN III damage

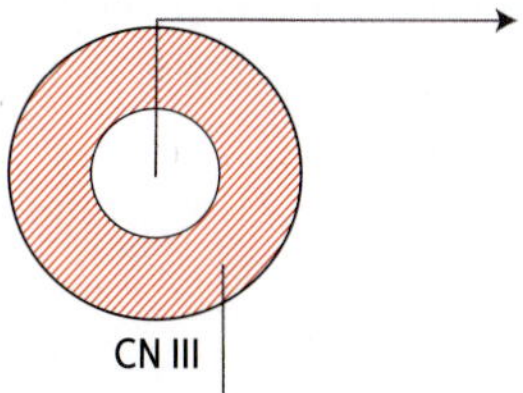

CN III has both motor (central) and parasympathetic (peripheral) components.

- Motor output to ocular muscles—affected primarily by vascular disease (eg, diabetes mellitus: glucose → sorbitol) due to ↓ diffusion of oxygen and nutrients to the interior fibers from compromised vasculature that resides on outside of nerve. Signs: ptosis, "down and out" gaze A.
- Parasympathetic output—fibers on the periphery are 1st affected by compression (eg, posterior communicating artery aneurysm, uncal herniation). Signs: diminished or absent pupillary light reflex, "blown pupil" often with "down-and-out" gaze.

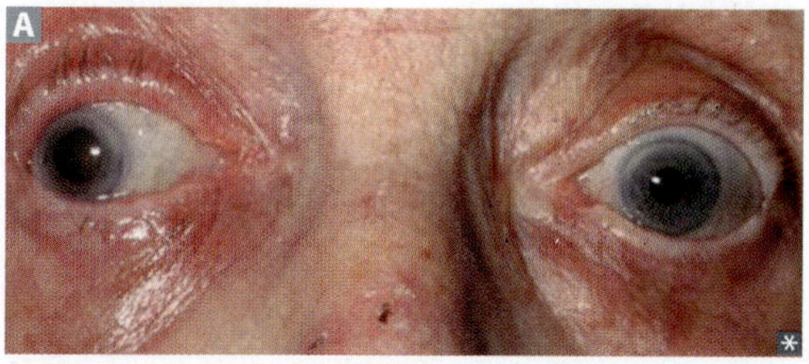

CN IV damage

Eye moves upward, particularly with contralateral gaze B and head tilt toward the side of the lesion (problems going down stairs, may present with compensatory head tilt in the opposite direction).

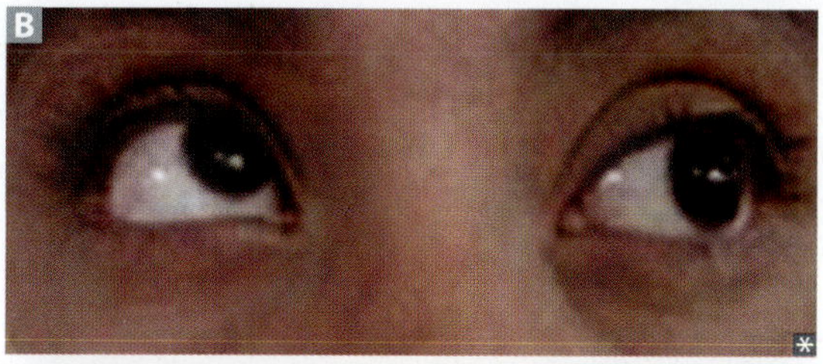

CN VI damage

Medially directed eye that cannot abduct C.

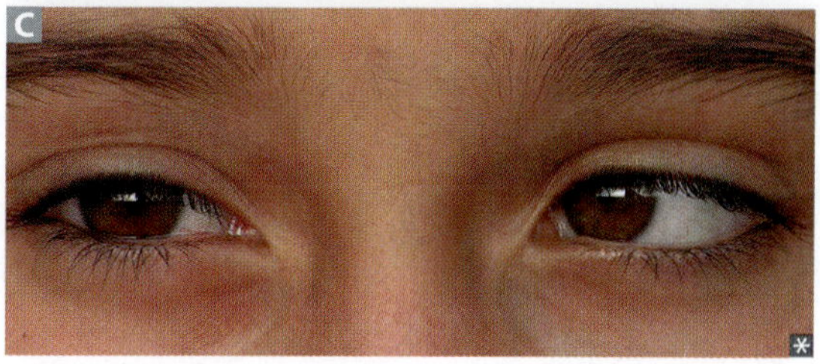

Visual field defects

1. Right anopia
2. Bitemporal hemianopia (pituitary lesion, chiasm)
3. Left homonymous hemianopia
4. Left upper quadrantic anopia (right temporal lesion, MCA)
5. Left lower quadrantic anopia (right parietal lesion, MCA)
6. Left hemianopia with macular sparing (PCA infarct)
7. Central scotoma (eg, macular degeneration)

Meyer loop—inferior retina; loops around inferior horn of lateral ventricle.
Dorsal optic radiation—superior retina; takes shortest path via internal capsule.

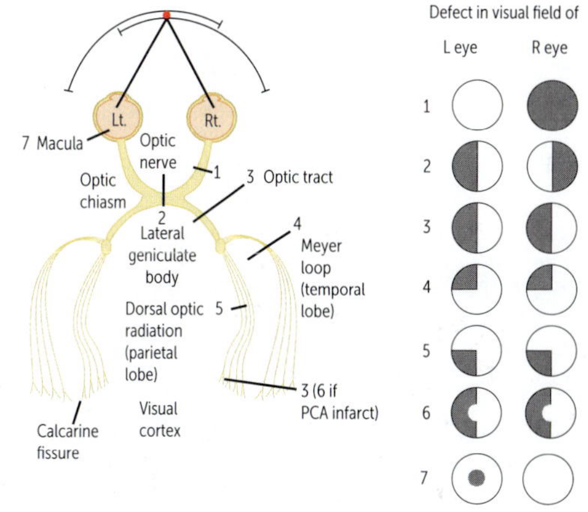

Note: When an image hits 1° visual cortex, it is upside down and left-right reversed.

Internuclear ophthalmoplegia

hence why its often affected in MS

Medial longitudinal fasciculus (MLF): pair of tracts that allows for crosstalk between CN VI and CN III nuclei. Coordinates both eyes to move in same horizontal direction. Highly myelinated (must communicate quickly so eyes move at same time). Lesions may be unilateral or bilateral (latter classically seen in multiple sclerosis).

Lesion in MLF = internuclear ophthalmoplegia (INO), a conjugate horizontal gaze palsy. Lack of communication such that when CN VI nucleus activates ipsilateral lateral rectus, contralateral CN III nucleus does not stimulate medial rectus to fire. Abducting eye gets nystagmus (CN VI overfires to stimulate CN III). Convergence normal.

MLF in MS.

When looking left, the left nucleus of CN VI fires, which contracts the left lateral rectus and stimulates the contralateral (right) nucleus of CN III via the right MLF to contract the right medial rectus.

Directional term (eg, right INO, left INO) refers to which eye is paralyzed.

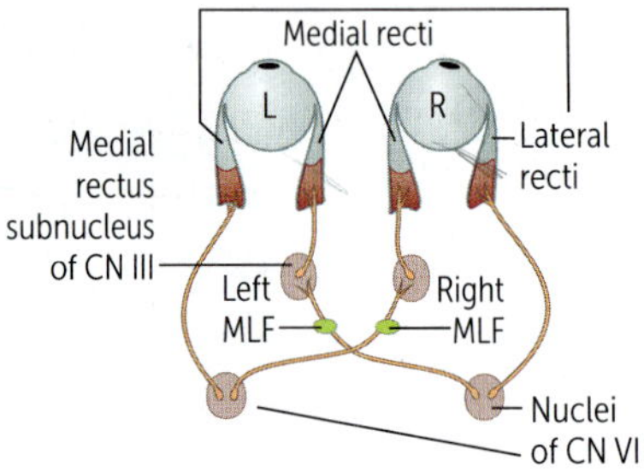

Right INO (right MLF lesion)

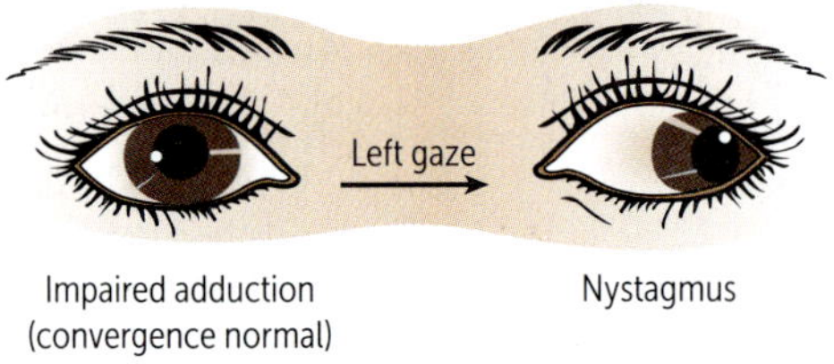

Motor cortex "look left" → R eye field → L PPRF → L CN 6 nuc

→ Left lat rectus + R CN3 med. rectus

▶ NEUROLOGY—PATHOLOGY

Dementia ↓ in cognitive ability, memory, or function with intact consciousness.

DISEASE	DESCRIPTION	HISTOLOGIC/GROSS FINDINGS
Alzheimer disease	Most common cause in elderly. Down syndrome patients have an ↑ risk of developing Alzheimer. Associated with the following altered proteins: ▪ ApoE2: ↓ risk of sporadic form ▪ ApoE4: ↑ risk of sporadic form ▪ APP, presenilin-1, presenilin-2: familial forms (10%) with earlier onset	Widespread cortical atrophy. Narrowing of gyri and widening of sulci. ↓ ACh. Senile plaques A in gray matter: extracellular β-amyloid core; may cause amyloid angiopathy → intracranial hemorrhage; Aβ (amyloid-β) synthesized by cleaving amyloid precursor protein (APP). Neurofibrillary tangles B: intracellular, hyperphosphorylated tau protein = insoluble cytoskeletal elements; number of tangles correlates with degree of dementia.
Frontotemporal dementia	Early changes in personality and behavior (behavioral variant), or aphasia (primary progressive aphasia). May have associated movement disorders (eg, parkinsonism, ALS-like UMN/LMN degeneration). Previously known as Pick disease.	Frontotemporal lobe degeneration. Inclusions of hyperphosphorylated tau (round Pick bodies; C) or ubiquitinated TDP-43.
Lewy body dementia	Initially dementia and visual hallucinations ("haLewycinations") followed by parkinsonian features.	Intracellular Lewy bodies (insoluble aggregates of α-synuclein) primarily in cortex.
Vascular dementia	Result of multiple arterial infarcts and/or chronic ischemia. Step-wise decline in cognitive ability with late-onset memory impairment. 2nd most common cause of dementia in elderly.	MRI or CT shows multiple cortical and/or subcortical infarcts.
Creutzfeldt-Jakob disease	Rapidly progressive (weeks to months) dementia with myoclonus ("startle myoclonus").	Spongiform cortex. Prions (PrP^{c} → PrP^{sc} sheet [β-pleated sheet resistant to proteases]).
Other causes	Syphilis; HIV; hypothyroidism; vitamins B_1, B_3, or B_{12} deficiency; Wilson disease; normal pressure hydrocephalus.	

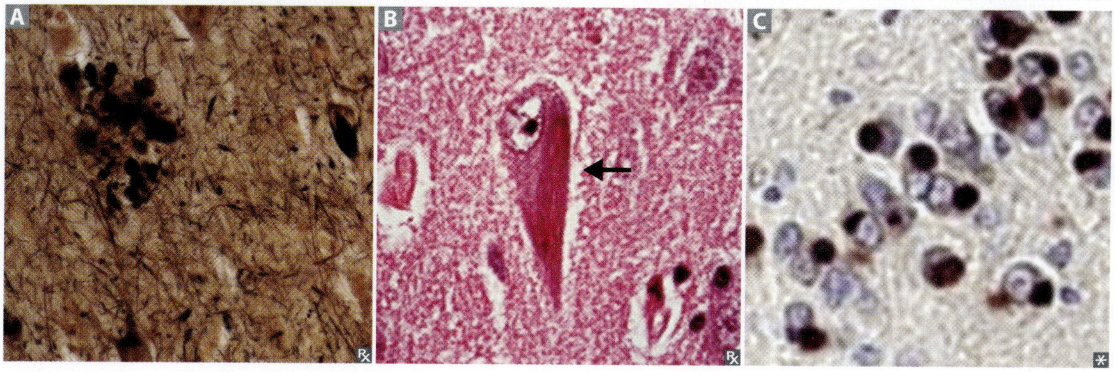

Osmotic demyelination syndrome (central pontine myelinolysis)

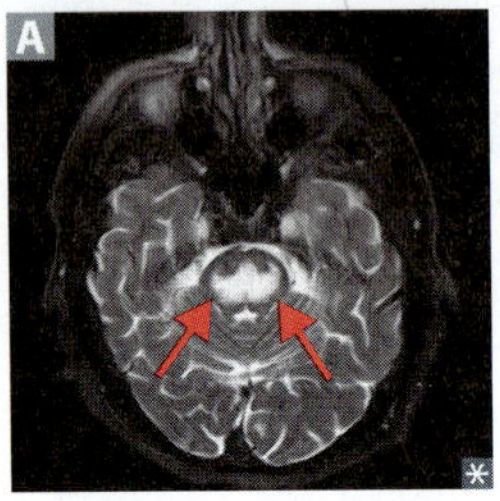

Acute paralysis, dysarthria, dysphagia, diplopia, loss of consciousness. Can cause "locked-in syndrome." Massive axonal demyelination in pontine white matter A 2° to osmotic changes. Commonly iatrogenic, caused by overly rapid correction of hyponatremia. In contrast, correcting hypernatremia too quickly results in cerebral edema/herniation.

Correcting serum Na^+ too fast:
- "From low to high, your pons will die" (osmotic demyelination syndrome)
- "From high to low, your brain will blow" (cerebral edema/herniation)

Multiple sclerosis

Autoimmune inflammation and demyelination of CNS (brain and spinal cord). Patients can present with optic neuritis (sudden loss of vision resulting in Marcus Gunn pupils), INO, hemiparesis, hemisensory symptoms, bladder/bowel dysfunction. Relapsing and remitting course. Most often affects women in their 20s and 30s; more common in whites living further from equator.

Charcot triad of MS is a **SIN**:
- **S**canning speech
- **I**ntention tremor (also **I**ncontinence and **I**nternuclear ophthalmoplegia)
- **N**ystagmus

FINDINGS

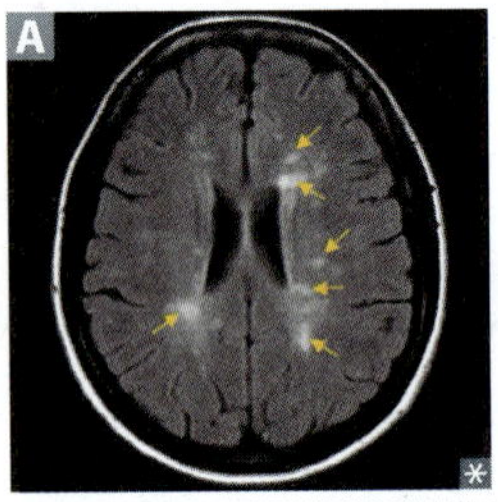

↑ IgG level and myelin basic protein in CSF. Oligoclonal bands are diagnostic. MRI is gold standard. Periventricular plaques A (areas of oligodendrocyte loss and reactive gliosis) with destruction of axons. Multiple white matter lesions separated in space and time.

TREATMENT

Slow progression with disease-modifying therapies (eg, β-interferon, glatiramer, natalizumab). Treat acute flares with IV steroids. Symptomatic treatment for neurogenic bladder (catheterization, muscarinic antagonists), spasticity (baclofen, $GABA_B$ receptor agonists), pain (opioids).

Acute inflammatory demyelinating polyradiculopathy	Most common subtype of Guillain-Barré syndrome. Autoimmune condition that destroys Schwann cells → inflammation and demyelination of peripheral nerves and motor fibers. Results in symmetric ascending muscle weakness/paralysis beginning in lower extremities. Facial paralysis in 50% of cases. May see autonomic dysregulation (eg, cardiac irregularities, hypertension, hypotension) or sensory abnormalities. Almost all patients survive; the majority recover completely after weeks to months. Findings: ↑ CSF protein with normal cell count (albuminocytologic dissociation). ↑ protein may cause papilledema.	Associated with infections (eg, *Campylobacter jejuni*, viral) → autoimmune attack of peripheral myelin due to molecular mimicry, inoculations, and stress, but no definitive link to pathogens. Respiratory support is critical until recovery. Additional treatment: plasmapheresis, IV immunoglobulins. No role for steroids.

Other demyelinating and dysmyelinating diseases

Acute disseminated (postinfectious) encephalomyelitis	Multifocal periventricular inflammation and demyelination after infection or vaccination. Presents with rapidly progressive multifocal neurologic symptoms, altered mental status.
Charcot-Marie-Tooth disease	Also known as hereditary motor and sensory neuropathy (HMSN). Group of progressive hereditary nerve disorders related to the defective production of proteins involved in the structure and function of peripheral nerves or the myelin sheath. Typically autosomal dominant inheritance pattern and associated with foot deformities (pes cavus), lower extremity weakness and sensory deficits.
Krabbe disease	Autosomal recessive lysosomal storage disease due to deficiency of galactocerebrosidase. Buildup of galactocerebroside and psychosine destroys myelin sheath. Findings: peripheral neuropathy, developmental delay, optic atrophy, globoid cells.
Metachromatic leukodystrophy	Autosomal recessive lysosomal storage disease, most commonly due to arylsulfatase A deficiency. Buildup of sulfatides → impaired production and destruction of myelin sheath. Findings: central and peripheral demyelination with ataxia, dementia.
Progressive multifocal leukoencephalopathy	Demyelination of CNS due to destruction of oligodendrocytes. Seen in 2–4% of AIDS patients (reactivation of latent JC virus infection). Rapidly progressive, usually fatal. ↑ risk associated with natalizumab, rituximab. JC = polyomavirus : small, dsDNA, naked, cytolytic. latent in kidney & BM. Ubiq but asympt. immun supp = demyelin.

Adrenoleukodystrophy	X-linked genetic disorder typically affecting males. Disrupts metabolism of very-long-chain fatty acids → excessive buildup in nervous system, adrenal gland, testes. Progressive disease that can lead to long-term coma/death and adrenal gland crisis.

Schwann cells = glia of PNS from neural crest
- small axons sit on surface of schwann (nonmyelinated)
  - they support PNS. no myelin.
- PNS w/ larger axon = myelin sheath along axon w/ nodes of ranvier
  - unlike oligoden it myelin. only ONE axon
  - literally wrapped like tape ← soma of schwann ← schwann cell memb.

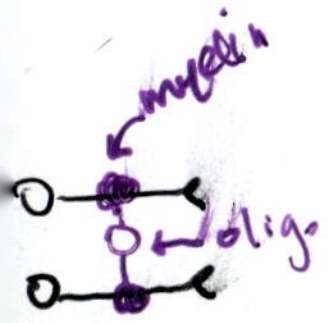

Oligodends = glia of CNS. from neural stem cells
- each oligo can create myelin for diff neurons. can have >1 oligo / neuron

→ neurons all active at the same time when they shouldn't be — ↑ Glut or ↓ GABA Tumor can ⊘ GABA recept = seiz

Seizures	Characterized by synchronized, high-frequency neuronal firing. Variety of forms.	
Partial (focal) seizures one hemisp or less	Affect single area of the brain. Most commonly originate in medial temporal lobe. Often preceded by seizure aura; can secondarily generalize. Types: ▪ Simple partial (consciousness intact)—motor, sensory, autonomic, psychic ▪ Complex partial (impaired consciousness)	Epilepsy—a disorder of recurrent seizures (febrile seizures are not epilepsy). Status epilepticus—continuous or recurring seizure(s) that may result in brain injury; defined as > 5 min. usually tonic clonic Causes of seizures by age: ▪ Children—genetic, infection (febrile), trauma, congenital, metabolic ▪ Adults—tumor, trauma, stroke, infection ▪ Elderly—stroke, tumor, trauma, metabolic, infection
Generalized seizures both hemisph	Diffuse. Types: ▪ Absence (petit mal)—3 Hz, no postictal confusion, blank stare ▪ Myoclonic—quick, repetitive jerks most → ▪ Tonic-clonic (grand mal)—alternating stiffening and movement tense (tonic) then contract & relax (clonic) ▪ Tonic—stiffening ▪ Atonic—"drop" seizures (falls to floor); commonly mistaken for fainting	Clonic = uncontrolled jerk

Headaches Pain due to irritation of structures such as the dura, cranial nerves, or extracranial structures. More common in females, except cluster headaches.

CLASSIFICATION	LOCALIZATION	DURATION	DESCRIPTION	TREATMENT
Cluster[a]	Unilateral	15 min–3 hr; repetitive	Repetitive brief headaches. Excruciating periorbital pain with lacrimation and rhinorrhea. May present with Horner syndrome.	Acute: sumatriptan, 100% O_2 Prophylaxis: verapamil
Tension	Bilateral	> 30 min (typically 4–6 hr); constant	Steady pain. No photophobia or phonophobia. No aura.	Analgesics, NSAIDs, acetaminophen; amitriptyline for chronic pain
Migraine	Unilateral	4–72 hr	Pulsating pain with nausea, photophobia, or phonophobia. May have "aura." Due to irritation of CN V, meninges, or blood vessels (release of substance P, calcitonin gene–related peptide, vasoactive peptides).	Acute: NSAIDs, triptans, dihydroergotamine Prophylaxis: lifestyle changes (eg, sleep, exercise, diet), β-blockers, calcium channel blockers, amitriptyline, topiramate, valproate. **POUND**–**P**ulsatile, **O**ne-day duration, **U**nilateral, **N**ausea, **D**isabling

Other causes of headache include subarachnoid hemorrhage ("worst headache of my life"), meningitis, hydrocephalus, neoplasia, arteritis.

[a]Compare with trigeminal neuralgia, which produces repetitive, unilateral, shooting pain in the distribution of CN V that lasts (typically) for < 1 minute.

Horner = anytime u get an eyelid droop person check pupil to see if horner

Central = sx of other brainstem lesions. Periph may be isolated vertig +/- tinnitus / hear loss

these are CN symp & brainstem

Vertigo	Sensation of spinning while actually stationary. Subtype of "dizziness," but distinct from "lightheadedness."
Peripheral vertigo 90%	More common. Inner ear etiology (eg, semicircular canal debris, vestibular nerve infection, Ménière disease). Positional testing → delayed horizontal nystagmus.
Central vertigo	Brain stem or cerebellar lesion (eg, stroke affecting vestibular nuclei or posterior fossa tumor). Findings: directional change of nystagmus, skew deviation, diplopia, dysmetria. Positional testing → immediate nystagmus in any direction; may change directions. Focal neurologic findings. MS, migraine assoc, vertebrobas insuff, drugs → pheny, carbamep or excess sedative anticonv. nystag in central unlike periph may be bidirect or vertical

Neurocutaneous disorders

Sturge-Weber syndrome (encephalotrigeminal angiomatosis)	Congenital, non-inherited (somatic), developmental anomaly of neural crest derivatives due to activating mutation of *GNAQ* gene. Affects small (capillary-sized) blood vessels → port-wine stain of the face A (nevus flammeus, a non-neoplastic "birthmark" in CN V_1/V_2 distribution); ipsilateral leptomeningeal angioma B → seizures/epilepsy; intellectual disability; and episcleral hemangioma → ↑ IOP → early-onset glaucoma. **STURGE**-Weber: **S**poradic, port-wine **S**tain; **T**ram track calcifications (opposing gyri); **U**nilateral; **R**etardation (intellectual disability); **G**laucoma; ***G**NAQ* gene; **E**pilepsy.
Tuberous sclerosis	**HAMARTOMAS**: **H**amartomas in CNS and skin; **A**ngiofibromas C; **M**itral regurgitation; **A**sh-leaf spots D; cardiac **R**habdomyoma; (**T**uberous sclerosis); autosomal d**O**minant; **M**ental retardation (intellectual disability); renal **A**ngiomyolipoma E; **S**eizures, **S**hagreen patches. ↑ incidence of subependymal astrocytomas and ungual fibromas.
Neurofibromatosis type I (von Recklinghausen disease)	Café-au-lait spots F, Lisch nodules (pigmented iris hamartomas G), cutaneous neurofibromas H, optic gliomas, pheochromocytomas. Mutated *NF1* tumor suppressor gene (neurofibromin, a negative regulator of *RAS*) on chromosome 17. Neurofibromas are derived from neural crest cells.
von Hippel-Lindau disease	Hemangioblastomas (high vascularity with hyperchromatic nuclei I) in retina, brain stem, cerebellum, spine J; angiomatosis (eg, cavernous hemangiomas in skin, mucosa, organs); bilateral renal cell carcinomas; pheochromocytomas. Blood rich areas. Blood vessel ↑

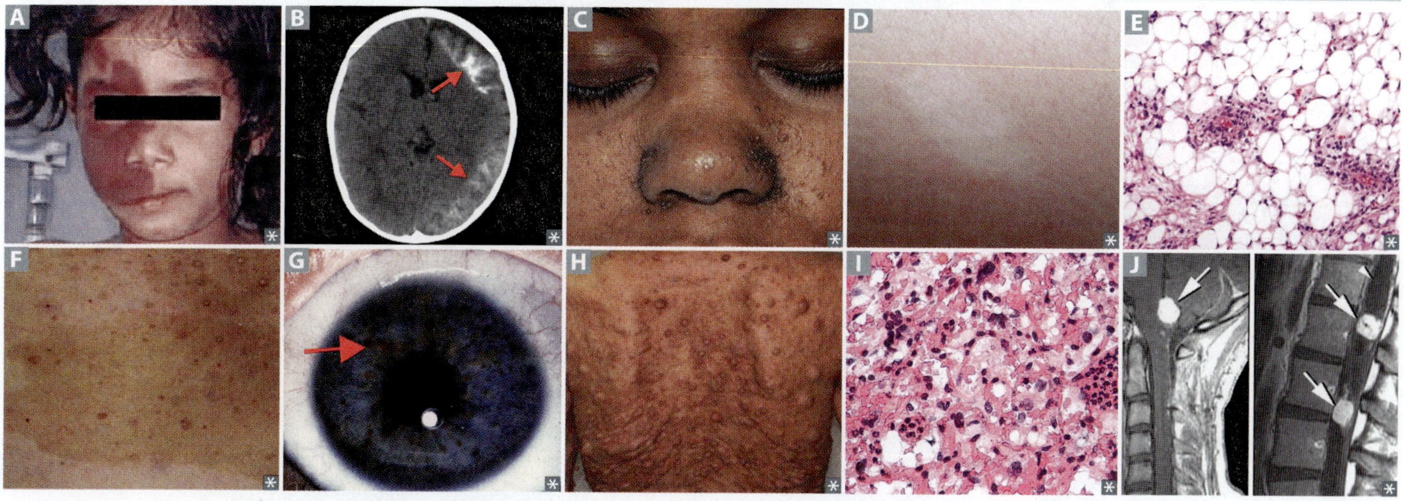

Adult primary brain tumors

Glioblastoma multiforme (grade IV astrocytoma)	Common, highly malignant 1° brain tumor with ~ 1-year median survival. Found in cerebral hemispheres A. Can cross corpus callosum ("butterfly glioma"). "Pseudopalisading" pleomorphic tumor cells B—border central areas of necrosis and hemorrhage. Stain astrocytes for GFAP.
Meningioma	Common, typically benign 1° brain tumor. Most often occurs near surfaces of brain and parasagittal region. Arises from arachnoid cells, is extra-axial (external to brain parenchyma), and may have a dural attachment ("tail" C). Often asymptomatic; may present with seizures or focal neurologic signs. Resection and/or radiosurgery. Spindle cells concentrically arranged in a whorled pattern; psammoma bodies D (laminated calcifications).
Hemangioblastoma	Most often cerebellar E. Associated with von Hippel-Lindau syndrome when found with retinal angiomas. Can produce erythropoietin → 2° polycythemia. Closely arranged, thin-walled capillaries with minimal intervening parenchyma F.
Schwannoma	Classically at the cerebellopontine angle G, but can be along any peripheral nerve. Often localized to CN VIII → vestibular schwannoma. Bilateral vestibular schwannomas found in NF-2. Resection or stereotactic radiosurgery. Schwann cell origin H, S-100 ⊕.
Oligodendroglioma	Relatively rare, slow growing. Most often in frontal lobes I. "Chicken-wire" capillary pattern. Oligodendrocytes = "fried egg" cells—round nuclei with clear cytoplasm J. Often calcified.
Pituitary adenoma	Most commonly prolactinoma K (lactotroph adenoma) or nonfunctioning adenoma. Bitemporal hemianopia due to pressure on optic chiasm (L shows normal visual field above, patient's perspective below). Hyper- or hypopituitarism are sequelae. Hyperplasia of a single type of endocrine cell found in pituitary (ie, lactotroph, gonadotroph, somatotroph, corticotroph).

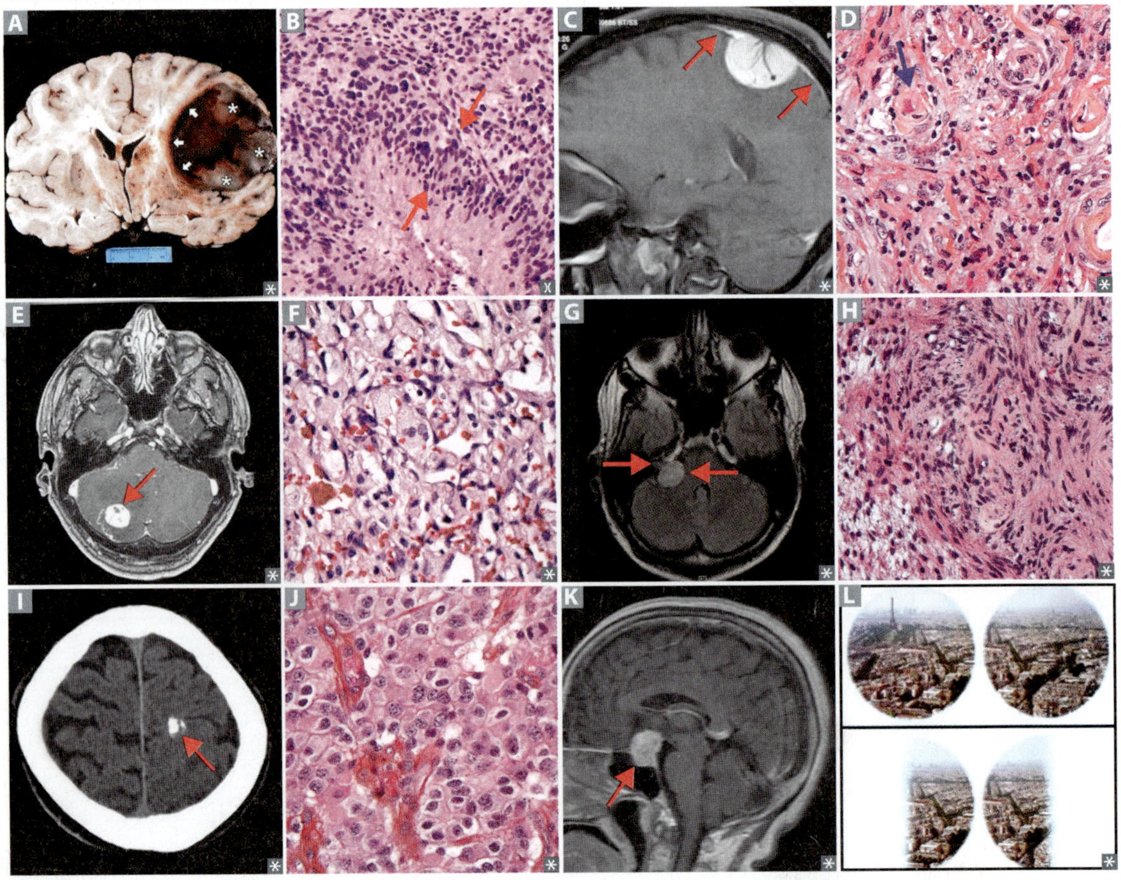

Childhood primary brain tumors

Pilocytic (low-grade) astrocytoma	Usually well circumscribed. In children, most often found in posterior fossa A (eg, cerebellum). May be supratentorial. GFAP ⊕. Benign; good prognosis. Rosenthal fibers—eosinophilic, corkscrew fibers B. Cystic + solid (gross).
Medulloblastoma	Highly malignant cerebellar tumor C. A form of primitive neuroectodermal tumor. Can compress 4th ventricle, causing noncommunicating hydrocephalus. Can send "drop metastases" to spinal cord. Homer-Wright rosettes, small blue cells D.
Ependymoma	Ependymal cell tumors most commonly found in 4th ventricle E. Can cause hydrocephalus. Poor prognosis. Characteristic perivascular rosettes F. Rod-shaped blepharoplasts (basal ciliary bodies) found near nucleus.
Craniopharyngioma	Childhood tumor, may be confused with pituitary adenoma (both can cause bitemporal hemianopia). Most common childhood supratentorial tumor. Derived from remnants of Rathke pouch. Calcification is common G H. Cholesterol crystals found in "motor oil"–like fluid within tumor.
Pinealoma	Tumor of pineal gland. Can cause Parinaud syndrome (compression of tectum → vertical gaze palsy); obstructive hydrocephalus (compression of cerebral aqueduct); precocious puberty in males (β-hCG production). Histologically similar to germ cell tumors (eg, testicular seminoma).

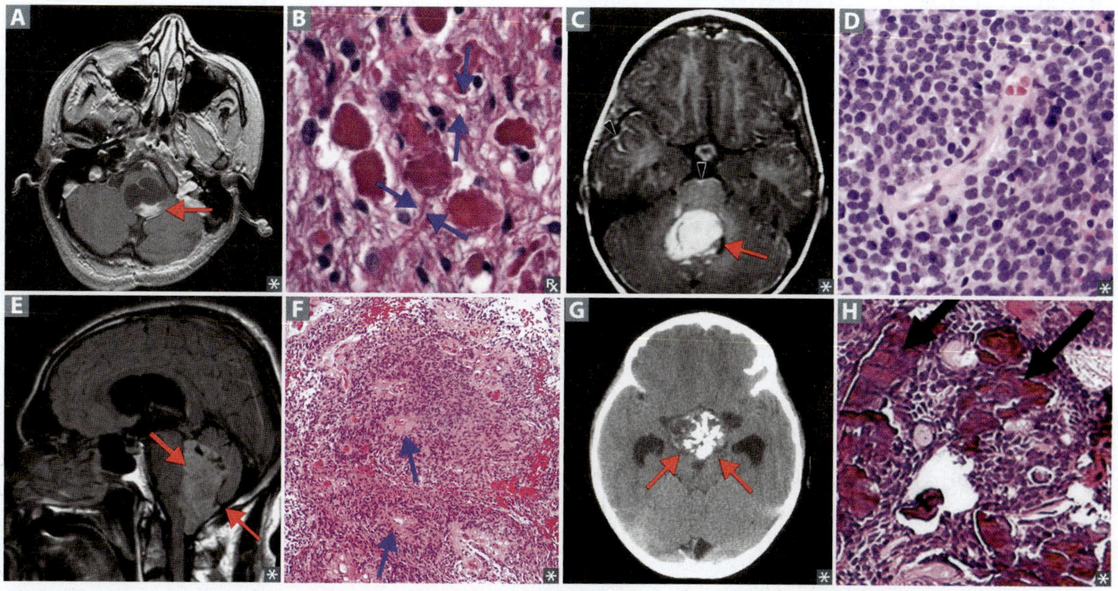

Herniation syndromes

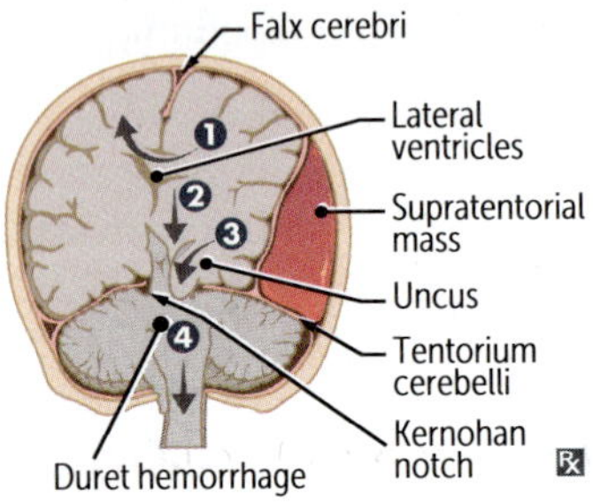

❶ Cingulate (subfalcine) herniation under falx cerebri	Can compress anterior cerebral artery.
❷ Downward transtentorial (central) herniation	Caudal displacement of brain stem → rupture of paramedian basilar artery branches → Duret hemorrhages. Usually fatal.
❸ Uncal herniation	Uncus = medial temporal lobe. Compresses ipsilateral CN III (blown pupil, "down-and-out" gaze), ipsilateral PCA (contralateral homonymous hemianopia with macular sparing), contralateral crus cerebri at the Kernohan notch (ipsilateral paresis; a "false localization" sign).
❹ Cerebellar tonsillar herniation into the foramen magnum	Coma and death result when these herniations compress the brain stem.

▸ NEUROLOGY—PHARMACOLOGY

Glaucoma drugs ↓ IOP via ↓ amount of aqueous humor (inhibit synthesis/secretion or ↑ drainage).

DRUG	MECHANISM	ADVERSE EFFECTS
α-agonists		
Epinephrine (α_1), brimonidine (α_2)	↓ aqueous humor synthesis via vasoconstriction ↓ aqueous humor synthesis	Mydriasis (α_1); do not use in closed-angle glaucoma Blurry vision, ocular hyperemia, foreign body sensation, ocular allergic reactions, ocular pruritus
β-blockers		
Timolol, betaxolol, carteolol	↓ aqueous humor synthesis	No pupillary or vision changes
Diuretics		
Acetazolamide	↓ aqueous humor synthesis via inhibition of carbonic anhydrase	No pupillary or vision changes
Cholinomimetics (M_3)		
Direct (pilocarpine, carbachol) **Indirect (physostigmine, echothiophate)**	↑ outflow of aqueous humor via contraction of ciliary muscle and opening of trabecular meshwork Use pilocarpine in emergencies—very effective at opening meshwork into canal of Schlemm	Miosis (contraction of pupillary sphincter muscles) and cyclospasm (contraction of ciliary muscle)
Prostaglandin		
Bimatoprost, latanoprost ($PGF_{2\alpha}$)	↑ outflow of aqueous humor	Darkens color of iris (browning), eyelash growth

Opioid analgesics

Morphine, fentanyl, codeine, loperamide, methadone, meperidine, dextromethorphan, diphenoxylate, pentazocine.

MECHANISM	Act as agonists at opioid receptors (μ = β-endorphin, δ = enkephalin, κ = dynorphin) to modulate synaptic transmission—open K^+ channels, close Ca^{2+} channels → ↓ synaptic transmission. Inhibit release of ACh, norepinephrine, 5-HT, glutamate, substance P.
CLINICAL USE	Pain, cough suppression (dextromethorphan), diarrhea (loperamide, diphenoxylate), acute pulmonary edema, maintenance programs for heroin addicts (methadone, buprenorphine + naloxone).
ADVERSE EFFECTS	Addiction, respiratory depression, constipation, miosis (except meperidine → mydriasis), additive CNS depression with other drugs. Tolerance does not develop to miosis and constipation. Toxicity treated with naloxone or naltrexone (opioid receptor antagonist).

Pentazocine

MECHANISM	κ-opioid receptor agonist and μ-opioid receptor antagonist.
CLINICAL USE	Analgesia for moderate to severe pain.
ADVERSE EFFECTS	Can cause opioid withdrawal symptoms if patient is also taking full opioid antagonist (competition for opioid receptors).

Butorphanol

MECHANISM	κ-opioid receptor agonist and μ-opioid receptor partial agonist; produces analgesia.
CLINICAL USE	Severe pain (eg, migraine, labor). Causes less respiratory depression than full opioid agonists.
ADVERSE EFFECTS	Can cause opioid withdrawal symptoms if patient is also taking full opioid agonist (competition for opioid receptors). Overdose not easily reversed with naloxone.

Tramadol

MECHANISM	Very weak opioid agonist; also inhibits 5-HT and norepinephrine reuptake (works on multiple neurotransmitters—"**tram it all**" in with **tramadol**).
CLINICAL USE	Chronic pain.
ADVERSE EFFECTS	Similar to opioids. Decreases seizure threshold. Serotonin syndrome.

↓ acqueus humor synthesis = α1
α2
β block
Acetozol

↑ outflow = Cholinerg (M3)
Prostagl

Epilepsy drugs

	PARTIAL (FOCAL): SIMPLE	PARTIAL (FOCAL): COMPLEX	GENERALIZED: TONIC-CLONIC	GENERALIZED: ABSENCE	GENERALIZED: STATUS EPILEPTICUS	MECHANISM	SIDE EFFECTS	NOTES
Ethosuximide				* ✓		Blocks thalamic T-type Ca^{2+} channels	GI, fatigue, headache, urticaria, Stevens-Johnson syndrome. EFGHIJ—Ethosuximide causes Fatigue, GI distress, Headache, Itching, and Stevens-Johnson syndrome	Sucks to have Silent (absence) Seizures
Benzodiazepines (eg, diazepam, lorazepam, midazolam)					** ✓	↑ $GABA_A$ action	Sedation, tolerance, dependence, respiratory depression	Also for eclampsia seizures (1st line is $MgSO_4$)
Phenobarbital	✓	✓	✓			↑ $GABA_A$ action	Sedation, tolerance, dependence, induction of cytochrome P-450, cardiorespiratory depression	1st line in neonates
Phenytoin, fosphenytoin	✓	✓	* ✓		*** ✓	Blocks Na^+ channels; zero-order kinetics	Neurologic: nystagmus, diplopia, ataxia, sedation, peripheral neuropathy. Dermatologic: hirsutism, Stevens-Johnson syndrome, gingival hyperplasia, DRESS syndrome. Musculoskeletal: osteopenia, SLE-like syndrome. Hematologic: megaloblastic anemia. Reproductive: teratogenesis (fetal hydantoin syndrome). Other: cytochrome P-450 induction	
Carbamazepine	* ✓	* ✓	✓			Blocks Na^+ channels	Diplopia, ataxia, blood dyscrasias (agranulocytosis, aplastic anemia), liver toxicity, teratogenesis, induction of cytochrome P-450, SIADH, Stevens-Johnson syndrome	1st line for trigeminal neuralgia
Valproic acid	✓	✓	* ✓	✓		↑ Na^+ channel inactivation, ↑ GABA concentration by inhibiting GABA transaminase	GI distress, rare but fatal hepatotoxicity (measure LFTs), pancreatitis, neural tube defects, tremor, weight gain, contraindicated in pregnancy	Also used for myoclonic seizures, bipolar disorder, migraine prophylaxis
Vigabatrin	✓	✓				↑ GABA by irreversibly inhibiting GABA transaminase		
Gabapentin	✓	✓				Primarily inhibits high-voltage-activated Ca^{2+} channels; designed as GABA analog	Sedation, ataxia	Also used for peripheral neuropathy, postherpetic neuralgia
Topiramate	✓	✓	✓			Blocks Na^+ channels, ↑ GABA action	Sedation, mental dulling, kidney stones, weight loss	Also used for migraine prevention
Lamotrigine	✓	✓	✓	✓		Blocks voltage-gated Na^+ channels	Stevens-Johnson syndrome (must be titrated slowly)	
Levetiracetam	✓	✓	✓			Unknown; may modulate GABA and glutamate release		
Tiagabine	✓	✓				↑ GABA by inhibiting reuptake		

* = 1st line; ** = 1st line for acute; *** = 1st line for prophylaxis.

Barbiturates	Phenobarbital, pentobarbital, thiopental, secobarbital.	
MECHANISM	Facilitate $GABA_A$ action by ↑ **duration** of Cl^- channel opening, thus ↓ neuron firing (barbi**durat**es ↑ **durat**ion). Contraindicated in porphyria.	
CLINICAL USE	Sedative for anxiety, seizures, insomnia, induction of anesthesia (thiopental).	
ADVERSE EFFECTS	Respiratory and cardiovascular depression (can be fatal); CNS depression (can be exacerbated by alcohol use); dependence; drug interactions (induces cytochrome P-450). Overdose treatment is supportive (assist respiration and maintain BP).	

Benzodiazepines	Diazepam, lorazepam, triazolam, temazepam, oxazepam, midazolam, chlordiazepoxide, alprazolam.	
MECHANISM	Facilitate $GABA_A$ action by ↑ **frequency** of Cl^- channel opening. ↓ REM sleep. Most have long half-lives and active metabolites (exceptions: **A**lprazolam, **T**riazolam, **O**xazepam, and **M**idazolam are short acting → higher addictive potential).	"**Fre**nzodiazepines" ↑ **fre**quency. Benzos, barbs, and alcohol all bind the $GABA_A$ receptor, which is a ligand-gated Cl^- channel. **ATOM**.
CLINICAL USE	Anxiety, spasticity, status epilepticus (lorazepam and diazepam), eclampsia, detoxification (especially alcohol withdrawal–DTs), night terrors, sleepwalking, general anesthetic (amnesia, muscle relaxation), hypnotic (insomnia).	
ADVERSE EFFECTS	Dependence, additive CNS depression effects with alcohol. Less risk of respiratory depression and coma than with barbiturates. Treat overdose with flumazenil (competitive antagonist at GABA benzodiazepine receptor). Can precipitate seizures by causing acute benzodiazepine withdrawal.	

Nonbenzodiazepine hypnotics	**Z**olpidem, **Z**aleplon, es**Z**opiclone. "All **ZZZ**s put you to sleep."
MECHANISM	Act via the BZ1 subtype of the GABA receptor. Effects reversed by flumazenil. Sleep cycle less affected as compared with benzodiazepine hypnotics.
CLINICAL USE	Insomnia.
ADVERSE EFFECTS	Ataxia, headaches, confusion. Short duration because of rapid metabolism by liver enzymes. Unlike older sedative-hypnotics, cause only modest day-after psychomotor depression and few amnestic effects. ↓ dependence risk than benzodiazepines.

Anesthetics—general principles	CNS drugs must be lipid soluble (cross the blood-brain barrier) or be actively transported. Drugs with ↓ solubility in blood = rapid induction and recovery times. Drugs with ↑ solubility in lipids = ↑ potency = $\frac{1}{\text{MAC}}$ MAC = Minimal Alveolar Concentration (of inhaled anesthetic) required to prevent 50% of subjects from moving in response to noxious stimulus (eg, skin incision). Examples: nitrous oxide (N_2O) has ↓ blood and lipid solubility, and thus fast induction and low potency. Halothane, in contrast, has ↑ lipid and blood solubility, and thus high potency and slow induction.

Inhaled anesthetics	Desflurane, halothane, enflurane, isoflurane, sevoflurane, methoxyflurane, N_2O.
MECHANISM	Mechanism unknown.
EFFECTS	Myocardial depression, respiratory depression, nausea/emesis, ↑ cerebral blood flow (↓ cerebral metabolic demand).
ADVERSE EFFECTS	Hepatotoxicity (halothane), nephrotoxicity (methoxyflurane), proconvulsant (enflurane), expansion of trapped gas in a body cavity (N_2O). Malignant hyperthermia—rare, life-threatening condition in which inhaled anesthetics or succinylcholine induce fever and severe muscle contractions. Susceptibility is often inherited as autosomal dominant with variable penetrance. Mutations in voltage-sensitive ryanodine receptor cause ↑ Ca^{2+} release from sarcoplasmic reticulum. Treatment: dantrolene, a ryanodine receptor antagonist.

Intravenous anesthetics	The Mighty King Proposes Foolishly to Oprah.
Barbiturates (Thiopental)	High potency, high lipid solubility, rapid entry into brain. Used for induction of anesthesia and short surgical procedures. Effect terminated by rapid redistribution into tissue and fat. ↓ cerebral blood flow.
Benzodiazepines (Midazolam)	Used for endoscopy; used adjunctively with gaseous anesthetics and narcotics. May cause severe postoperative respiratory depression, ↓ BP (treat overdose with flumazenil), anterograde amnesia.
Arylcyclohexylamines (Ketamine)	PCP analogs that act as dissociative anesthetics. Block NMDA receptors. Cardiovascular stimulants. Cause disorientation, hallucination, bad dreams. ↑ cerebral blood flow.
Propofol	Used for sedation in ICU, rapid anesthesia induction, short procedures. Less postoperative nausea than thiopental. Potentiates $GABA_A$.
Opioids	Morphine, fentanyl used with other CNS depressants during general anesthesia.

Local anesthetics

Esters—procaine, cocaine, tetracaine, benzocaine.
Amides—lIdocaIne, mepIvacaIne, bupIvacaIne (amIdes have 2 I's in name).

MECHANISM

Block Na^+ channels by binding to specific receptors on inner portion of channel. Most effective in rapidly firing neurons. 3° amine local anesthetics penetrate membrane in uncharged form, then bind to ion channels as charged form.

Can be given with vasoconstrictors (usually epinephrine) to enhance local action—↓ bleeding, ↑ anesthesia by ↓ systemic concentration.

In infected (acidic) tissue, alkaline anesthetics are charged and cannot penetrate membrane effectively → need more anesthetic.

Order of nerve blockade: small-diameter fibers > large diameter. Myelinated fibers > unmyelinated fibers. Overall, size factor predominates over myelination such that small myelinated fibers > small unmyelinated fibers > large myelinated fibers > large unmyelinated fibers.

Order of loss: (1) pain, (2) temperature, (3) touch, (4) pressure.

CLINICAL USE

Minor surgical procedures, spinal anesthesia. If allergic to esters, give amides.

ADVERSE EFFECTS

CNS excitation, severe cardiovascular toxicity (bupivacaine), hypertension, hypotension, arrhythmias (cocaine), methemoglobinemia (benzocaine).

Neuromuscular blocking drugs

Muscle paralysis in surgery or mechanical ventilation. Selective for motor (vs autonomic) nicotinic receptor.

Depolarizing

Succinylcholine—strong ACh receptor agonist; produces sustained depolarization and prevents muscle contraction.

Reversal of blockade:

- Phase I (prolonged depolarization)—no antidote. Block potentiated by cholinesterase inhibitors.
- Phase II (repolarized but blocked; ACh receptors are available, but desensitized)—may be reversed with cholinesterase inhibitors.

Complications include hypercalcemia, hyperkalemia, malignant hyperthermia.

Nondepolarizing

Tubocurarine, atracurium, mivacurium, pancuronium, vecuronium, rocuronium—competitive antagonists—compete with ACh for receptors.

Reversal of blockade—neostigmine (must be given with atropine to prevent muscarinic effects such as bradycardia), edrophonium, and other cholinesterase inhibitors.

Dantrolene

MECHANISM

Prevents release of Ca^{2+} from the sarcoplasmic reticulum of skeletal muscle by binding to the ryanodine receptor.

CLINICAL USE

Malignant hyperthermia and neuroleptic malignant syndrome (a toxicity of antipsychotic drugs).

Baclofen

MECHANISM

Activates $GABA_B$ receptors at spinal cord level, inducing skeletal muscle relaxation.

CLINICAL USE

Muscle spasms (eg, acute low back pain).

Cyclobenzaprine

MECHANISM

Centrally acting skeletal muscle relaxant. Structurally related to TCAs, similar anticholinergic side effects.

CLINICAL USE

Muscle spasms.

Parkinson disease drugs

Parkinsonism is due to loss of dopaminergic neurons and excess cholinergic activity.
Bromocriptine, **A**mantadine, **L**evodopa (with carbidopa), **S**elegiline (and COMT inhibitors), **A**ntimuscarinics—**BALSA**.

STRATEGY	AGENTS
Dopamine agonists	Ergot—**B**romocriptine Non-ergot (preferred)—pramipexole, ropinirole
↑ dopamine availability	**A**mantadine (↑ dopamine release and ↓ dopamine reuptake); toxicity = ataxia, livedo reticularis.
↑ L-DOPA availability	Agents prevent peripheral (pre-BBB) L-dopa degradation → ↑ L-DOPA entering CNS → ↑ central L-DOPA available for conversion to dopamine. ▪ **L**evodopa (L-dopa)/carbidopa—carbidopa blocks peripheral conversion of L-DOPA to dopamine by inhibiting DOPA decarboxylase. Also reduces side effects of peripheral L-dopa conversion into dopamine (eg, nausea, vomiting). ▪ Entacapone, tolcapone—prevent peripheral L-dopa degradation to 3-O-methyldopa (3-OMD) by inhibiting COMT.
Prevent dopamine breakdown	Agents act centrally (post-BBB) to inhibit breakdown of dopamine. ▪ **S**elegiline—blocks conversion of dopamine into DOPAC by selectively inhibiting MAO-B. ▪ Tolcapone—blocks conversion of dopamine to 3-OMD by inhibiting central COMT.
Curb excess cholinergic activity	**Benz**tropine (**A**ntimuscarinic; improves tremor and rigidity but has little effect on bradykinesia in **Park**inson disease). **Park** your Mercedes-**Benz**. ↳ so u can hold the wheel of ur benz

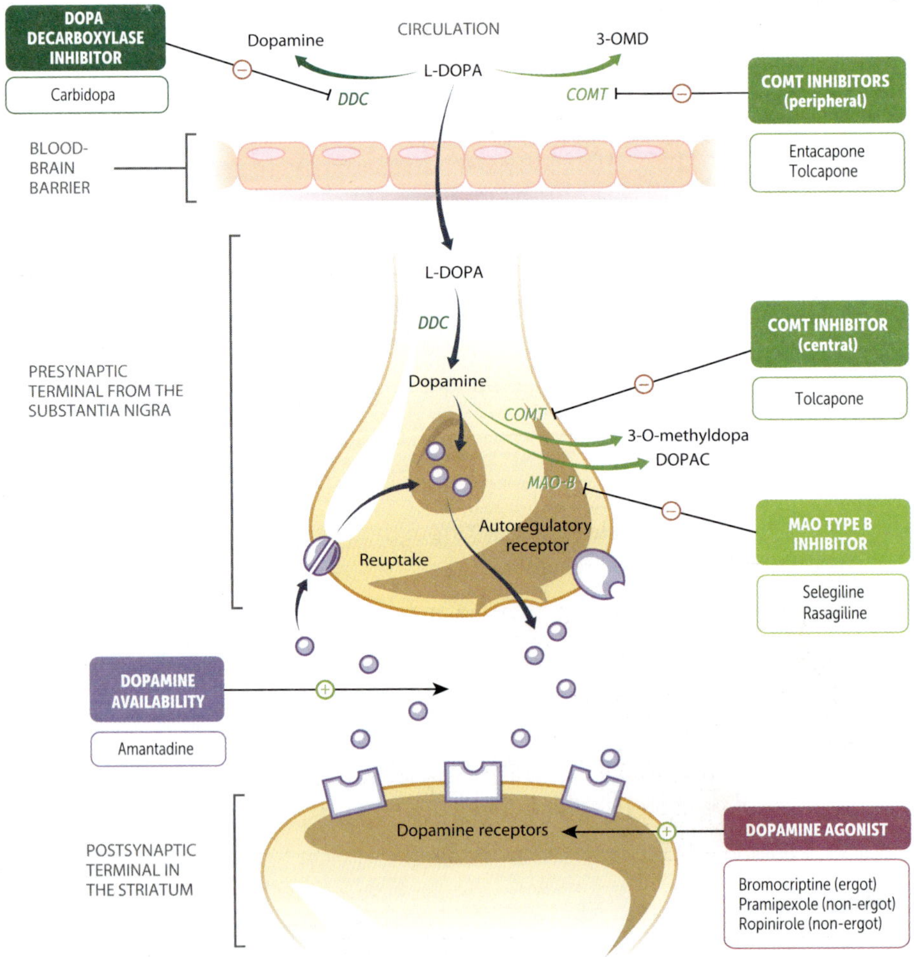

℞

L-dopa (levodopa)/carbidopa

MECHANISM	↑ level of dopamine in brain. Unlike dopamine, L-dopa can cross blood-brain barrier and is converted by dopa decarboxylase in the CNS to dopamine. Carbidopa, a peripheral DOPA decarboxylase inhibitor, is given with L-dopa to ↑ the bioavailability of L-dopa in the brain and to limit peripheral side effects.
CLINICAL USE	Parkinson disease.
ADVERSE EFFECTS	Arrhythmias from ↑ peripheral formation of catecholamines. Long-term use can lead to dyskinesia following administration ("on-off" phenomenon), akinesia between doses.

Selegiline, rasagiline

MECHANISM	Selectively inhibit MAO-B (metabolize dopamine) → ↑ dopamine availability.
CLINICAL USE	Adjunctive agent to L-dopa in treatment of Parkinson disease.
ADVERSE EFFECTS	May enhance adverse effects of L-dopa.

Alzheimer drugs

Memantine

MECHANISM	NMDA receptor antagonist; helps prevent excitotoxicity (mediated by Ca^{2+}).
ADVERSE EFFECTS	Dizziness, confusion, hallucinations.

Donepezil, galantamine, rivastigmine, tacrine

MECHANISM	AChE inhibitors.
ADVERSE EFFECTS	Nausea, dizziness, insomnia.

Huntington disease drugs

Tetrabenazine and reserpine—inhibit vesicular monoamine transporter (VMAT) → ↓ dopamine vesicle packaging and release.

Haloperidol—D_2 receptor antagonist.

Riluzole

Treatment for ALS that modestly ↑ survival by ↓ glutamate excitotoxicity via an unclear mechanism.

For **Lou** Gehrig disease, give ri**lou**zole.

Triptans

Sumatriptan

MECHANISM	$5\text{-}HT_{1B/1D}$ agonists. Inhibit trigeminal nerve activation; prevent vasoactive peptide release; induce vasoconstriction.	A **SUM**o wrestler **TRIP**s **AN**d falls on your **head**.
CLINICAL USE	Acute migraine, cluster **head**ache attacks.	
ADVERSE EFFECTS	Coronary vasospasm (contraindicated in patients with CAD or Prinzmetal angina), mild paresthesia.	

▶ NOTES

HIGH-YIELD PRINCIPLES IN

Psychiatry

"A Freudian slip is when you say one thing but mean your mother."

—Anonymous

"Men will always be mad, and those who think they can cure them are the maddest of all."

—Voltaire

"Anyone who goes to a psychiatrist ought to have his head examined."

—Samuel Goldwyn

"Words of comfort, skillfully administered, are the oldest therapy known to man."

—Louis Nizer

▸ PSYCHIATRY—PSYCHOLOGY

Classical conditioning

Learning in which a natural response (salivation) is elicited by a conditioned, or learned, stimulus (bell) that previously was presented in conjunction with an unconditioned stimulus (food).

Usually deals with **involuntary** responses. Pavlov's classical experiments with dogs—ringing the bell provoked salivation.

Operant conditioning

Learning in which a particular action is elicited because it produces a punishment or reward. Usually deals with **voluntary** responses.

Reinforcement	Target behavior (response) is followed by desired reward (positive reinforcement) or removal of aversive stimulus (negative reinforcement).
Punishment	Repeated application of aversive stimulus (positive punishment) or removal of desired reward (negative punishment) to extinguish unwanted behavior.
Extinction	Discontinuation of reinforcement (positive or negative) eventually eliminates behavior. Can occur in operant or classical conditioning.

Transference and countertransference

Transference	Patient projects feelings about formative or other important persons onto physician (eg, psychiatrist is seen as parent).
Countertransference	Doctor projects feelings about formative or other important persons onto patient (eg, patient reminds physician of younger sibling).

Ego defenses

Mental processes (unconscious or conscious) used to resolve conflict and prevent undesirable feelings (eg, anxiety, depression).

IMMATURE DEFENSES	DESCRIPTION	EXAMPLE
Acting out	Expressing unacceptable feelings and thoughts through actions.	Tantrums.
Denial	Avoiding the awareness of some painful reality.	A common reaction in newly diagnosed AIDS and cancer patients.
Displacement	Transferring avoided ideas and feelings to a neutral person or object (vs projection).	Mother yells at her child, because her husband yelled at her.
Dissociation	Temporary, drastic change in personality, memory, consciousness, or motor behavior to avoid emotional stress.	Extreme forms can result in dissociative identity disorder (multiple personality disorder).
Fixation	Partially remaining at a more childish level of development (vs regression).	Adults fixating on video games.
Idealization	Expressing extremely positive thoughts of self and others while ignoring negative thoughts.	A patient boasts about his physician and his accomplishments while ignoring any flaws.
Identification	Modeling behavior after another person who is more powerful (though not necessarily admired).	Abused child later becomes a child abuser.

Ego defenses *(continued)*

IMMATURE DEFENSES	DESCRIPTION	EXAMPLE
Intellectualization	Using facts and logic to emotionally distance oneself from a stressful situation.	In a therapy session, patient diagnosed with cancer focuses only on rates of survival.
Isolation (of affect)	Separating feelings from ideas and events.	Describing murder in graphic detail with no emotional response.
Passive aggression	Failing to meet the needs/expectations of others as an indirect show of opposition.	Disgruntled employee is repeatedly late to work.
Projection	Attributing an unacceptable internal impulse to an external source (vs displacement).	A man who wants to cheat on his wife accuses his wife of being unfaithful.
Rationalization	Proclaiming logical reasons for actions actually performed for other reasons, usually to avoid self-blame.	After getting fired, claiming that the job was not important anyway.
Reaction formation	Replacing a warded-off idea or feeling by an (unconsciously derived) emphasis on its opposite (vs sublimation).	A patient with libidinous thoughts enters a monastery.
Regression	Involuntarily turning back the maturational clock and going back to earlier modes of dealing with the world (vs fixation).	Seen in children under stress such as illness, punishment, or birth of a new sibling (eg, bedwetting in a previously toilet-trained child when hospitalized).
Repression	Involuntarily withholding an idea or feeling from conscious awareness (vs suppression).	A 20-year-old does not remember going to counseling during his parents' divorce 10 years earlier.
Splitting	Believing that people are either all good or all bad at different times due to intolerance of ambiguity. Commonly seen in borderline personality disorder.	A patient says that all the nurses are cold and insensitive but that the doctors are warm and friendly.
MATURE DEFENSES		
Sublimation	Replacing an unacceptable wish with a course of action that is similar to the wish but does not conflict with one's value system (vs reaction formation).	Teenager's aggression toward his father is redirected to perform well in sports.
Altruism	Alleviating negative feelings via unsolicited generosity.	Mafia boss makes large donation to charity.
Suppression	Intentionally withholding an idea or feeling from conscious awareness (vs repression); temporary.	Choosing to not worry about the big game until it is time to play.
Humor	Appreciating the amusing nature of an anxiety-provoking or adverse situation.	Nervous medical student jokes about the boards.
	Mature adults wear a SASH.	

▸ PSYCHIATRY—PATHOLOGY

Psychiatric genetics

Both genetic and environmental factors are involved in development of most psychiatric disorders. For example, in bipolar disorder and schizophrenia, lifetime risk in general population (~ 1%) < parent or sibling of someone affected (~ 10%) < monozygotic twin of someone affected (~ 50%).

Infant deprivation effects

Long-term deprivation of affection results in:
- Failure to thrive
- Poor language/socialization skills
- Lack of basic trust
- Reactive attachment disorder (infant withdrawn/unresponsive to comfort)

The **4 W's**: **W**eak, **W**ordless, **W**anting (socially), **W**ary.
Deprivation for > 6 months can lead to irreversible changes.
Severe deprivation can result in infant death.

Child abuse

	Physical abuse	Sexual abuse
EVIDENCE	Fractures (eg, ribs, long bone spiral, multiple in different stages of healing), bruises (eg, trunk, ear, neck; in pattern of implement), burns (eg, cigarette, buttocks/thighs), subdural hematomas, retinal hemorrhages. During exam, children often avoid eye contact.	Genital, anal, or oral trauma; STIs; UTIs.
ABUSER	Usually biological mother.	Known to victim, usually male.
EPIDEMIOLOGY	40% of deaths in children < 1 year old.	Peak incidence 9–12 years old.

Child neglect

Failure to provide a child with adequate food, shelter, supervision, education, and/or affection. Most common form of child maltreatment. Evidence: poor hygiene, malnutrition, withdrawal, impaired social/emotional development, failure to thrive.
As with child abuse, suspected child neglect must be reported to local child protective services.

Vulnerable child syndrome

Parents perceive the child as especially susceptible to illness or injury. Usually follows a serious illness or life-threatening event. Can result in missed school or overuse of medical services.

Childhood and early-onset disorders

Attention-deficit hyperactivity disorder
Onset before age 12. Limited attention span and poor impulse control. Characterized by hyperactivity, impulsivity, and/or inattention in multiple settings (school, home, places of worship, etc). Normal intelligence, but commonly coexists with difficulties in school. Continues into adulthood in as many as 50% of individuals. Treatment: stimulants (eg, methylphenidate) +/– cognitive behavioral therapy (CBT); alternatives include atomoxetine, guanfacine, clonidine.

Autism spectrum disorder
Characterized by poor social interactions, social communication deficits, repetitive/ritualized behaviors, restricted interests. Must present in early childhood. May be accompanied by intellectual disability; rarely accompanied by unusual abilities (savants). More common in boys. Associated with ↑ head/brain size.

Rett syndrome
X-linked dominant disorder seen almost exclusively in girls (affected males die in utero or shortly after birth). Symptoms usually become apparent around ages 1–4, including regression characterized by loss of development, loss of verbal abilities, intellectual disability, ataxia, stereotyped hand-wringing.

Conduct disorder
Repetitive and pervasive behavior violating the basic rights of others or societal norms (eg, aggression to people and animals, destruction of property, theft). After age 18, many of these patients will meet criteria for diagnosis of antisocial personality disorder. Treatment for both: psychotherapy such as CBT.

Oppositional defiant disorder
Enduring pattern of hostile, defiant behavior toward authority figures in the absence of serious violations of social norms. Treatment: psychotherapy such as CBT.

Separation anxiety disorder
Common onset at 7–9 years. Overwhelming fear of separation from home or loss of attachment figure. May lead to factitious physical complaints to avoid going to or staying at school. Treatment: CBT, play therapy, family therapy.

Tourette syndrome
Onset before age 18. Characterized by sudden, rapid, recurrent, nonrhythmic, stereotyped motor and vocal tics that persist for > **1 year**. Coprolalia (involuntary obscene speech) found in only 10–20% of patients. Associated with OCD and ADHD. Treatment: psychoeducation, behavioral therapy. For intractable and distressing tics, high-potency antipsychotics (eg, fluphenazine, pimozide), tetrabenazine, guanfacine, and clonidine may be used.

Neurotransmitter changes with disease

DISORDER	NEUROTRANSMITTER CHANGES
Alzheimer disease	↓ ACh ↑ glutamate
Anxiety	↑ norepinephrine ↓ GABA, ↓ 5-HT
Depression	↓ norepinephrine ↓ 5-HT, ↓ dopamine
Huntington disease	↓ GABA, ↓ ACh ↑ dopamine
Parkinson disease	↓ dopamine ↑ ACh
Schizophrenia	↑ dopamine

Understanding these changes can help guide pharmacologic treatment choice.

Orientation	Patient's ability to know who he or she is, where he or she is, and the date and time. Common causes of loss of orientation: alcohol, drugs, fluid/electrolyte imbalance, head trauma, hypoglycemia, infection, nutritional deficiencies.	Order of loss: 1st—time; 2nd—place; last—person.

Amnesias

Retrograde amnesia	Inability to remember things that occurred **before** a CNS insult.
Anterograde amnesia	Inability to remember things that occurred **a**fter a CNS insult (↓ acquisition of new memory).
Korsakoff syndrome	Amnesia (anterograde > retrograde) caused by vitamin B_1 deficiency and associated destruction of mammillary bodies. Seen in alcoholics as a late neuropsychiatric manifestation of Wernicke encephalopathy. Confabulations are characteristic.
Dissociative amnesia	Inability to recall important personal information, usually subsequent to severe trauma or stress. May be accompanied by **dissociative fugue** (abrupt travel or wandering during a period of dissociative amnesia, associated with traumatic circumstances).

Dissociative disorders

Dissociative identity disorder	Formerly known as multiple personality disorder. Presence of 2 or more distinct identities or personality states. More common in women. Associated with history of sexual abuse, PTSD, depression, substance abuse, borderline personality, somatoform conditions.
Depersonalization/derealization disorder	Persistent feelings of detachment or estrangement from one's own body, thoughts, perceptions, and actions (depersonalization) or one's environment (derealization).

Delirium	"Waxing and waning" level of consciousness with acute onset; rapid ↓ in attention span and level of arousal. Characterized by disorganized thinking, hallucinations (often visual), illusions, misperceptions, disturbance in sleep-wake cycle, cognitive dysfunction. Usually 2° to other illness (eg, CNS disease, infection, trauma, substance abuse/withdrawal, metabolic/electrolyte disturbances, hemorrhage, urinary/fecal retention). Most common presentation of altered mental status in inpatient setting. Commonly, diffuse slowing EEG. Treatment is aimed at identifying and addressing underlying condition. Haloperidol may be used as needed. Use benzodiazepines for alcohol withdrawal.	Deli**rium** = changes in senso**rium**. May be caused by medications (eg, anticholinergics), especially in the elderly. **Reversible**. **T-A-DA** approach (**T**olerate, **A**nticipate, **D**on't **A**gitate) helpful for management.

Dementia

↓ in intellectual function without affecting level of consciousness. Characterized by memory deficits, apraxia, aphasia, agnosia, loss of abstract thought, behavioral/personality changes, impaired judgment. A patient with dementia can develop delirium (eg, patient with Alzheimer disease who develops pneumonia is at ↑ risk for delirium).

Irreversible causes: Alzheimer disease, Lewy body dementia, Huntington disease, Pick disease, cerebral infarct, Creutzfeldt-Jakob disease, chronic substance abuse (due to neurotoxicity of drugs).

Reversible causes: hypothyroidism, depression, vitamin B_{12} deficiency, normal pressure hydrocephalus, neurosyphilis.

↑ incidence with age. EEG usually normal.

"Dememtia" is characterized by **mem**ory loss. Usually **irreversible**.

In elderly patients, depression and hypothyroidism may present like dementia (pseudodementia). Screen for depression and measure TSH, B_{12} levels.

- ↓ memory, ↓ intellec capacity NO change conciousness
- Alz
  - retain motor ability until later
  - goes Temporal → front / parietal
  - order = 1. mem loss 2. loss for words 3. can't copy a drawing
  - Frontal involv = emot sx, ↓ Judg
  - ↑ ventricles, Diffuse atrophy

Psychosis

Distorted perception of reality characterized by delusions, hallucinations, and/or disorganized thinking. Can occur in patients with medical illness, psychiatric illness, or both.

Delusions

Unique, false beliefs that persist despite the facts (eg, thinking aliens are communicating with you). Types include persecutory, referential, grandiose, erotomanic, somatic.

Disorganized thought

Speech may be incoherent ("word salad"), tangential, or derailed ("loose associations").

Hallucinations

Perceptions in the absence of external stimuli (eg, seeing a light that is not actually present). Contrast with illusions, misperceptions of real external stimuli. Types include:

- Visual—more commonly a feature of medical illness (eg, drug intoxication) than psychiatric illness.
- Auditory—more commonly a feature of psychiatric illness (eg, schizophrenia) than medical illness.
- Olfactory—often occur as an aura of temporal lobe epilepsy (eg, burning rubber) and in brain tumors.
- Gustatory—rare, but seen in epilepsy.
- Tactile—common in alcohol withdrawal and stimulant use (eg, cocaine, amphetamines), delusional parasitosis, "cocaine crawlies."
- ★★★ Hypnagogic—occurs while **go**ing to sleep. Sometimes seen in narcolepsy.
- Hypno**pomp**ic—occurs while waking from sleep ("**pomp**ous upon awakening"). Sometimes seen in narcolepsy.

- Thiam = Imp cofactor for 3 enz in 2 paths of carb metab.
  w/ alc = ↓ absorp, intacke, utilizat

Schizophrenia

Chronic mental disorder with periods of psychosis, disturbed behavior and thought, and decline in functioning **lasting > 6 months**. Associated with ↑ dopaminergic activity, ↓ dendritic branching.

Diagnosis requires at least 2 of the following, and at least 1 of these should include 1–3 (first 4 are "positive symptoms"):

1. Delusions
2. Hallucinations—often auditory
3. Disorganized speech
4. Disorganized or catatonic behavior
5. Negative symptoms (affective flattening, avolition, anhedonia, asociality, alogia)

Brief psychotic disorder—lasting < 1 month, usually stress related.

Schizophreniform disorder—lasting 1–6 months.

Schizoaffective disorder—> 2 weeks of hallucinations or delusions without major mood episode (major depression or mania), plus periods of concurrent major mood episode with schizophrenic symptoms.

Frequent cannabis use is associated with psychosis/schizophrenia in teens.

Lifetime prevalence—1.5% (males = females, African Americans = Caucasians). Presents earlier in men (late teens to early 20s vs late 20s to early 30s in women). Patients are at ↑ risk for suicide.

Ventriculomegaly on brain imaging.

Treatment: atypical antipsychotics (eg, risperidone) are first line.

Delusional disorder

Fixed, persistent, false belief system **lasting > 1 month**. Functioning otherwise not impaired (eg, a woman who genuinely believes she is married to a celebrity when, in fact, she is not). Can be shared by individuals in close relationships (folie à deux).

Mood disorder

Characterized by an abnormal range of moods or internal emotional states and loss of control over them. Severity of moods causes distress and impairment in social and occupational functioning. Includes major depressive disorder, bipolar disorder, dysthymic disorder, and cyclothymic disorder. Episodic superimposed psychotic features (delusions or hallucinations) may be present.

Manic episode

Distinct period of abnormally and persistently elevated, expansive, or irritable mood and abnormally and persistently ↑ activity or energy **lasting at least 1 week**. Often disturbing to patient.

Diagnosis requires hospitalization or at least 3 of the following (manics **DIG FAST**):

- **D**istractibility
- **I**rresponsibility—seeks pleasure without regard to consequences (hedonistic)
- **G**randiosity—inflated self-esteem
- **F**light of ideas—racing thoughts
- ↑ in goal-directed **A**ctivity/psychomotor **A**gitation
- ↓ need for **S**leep
- **T**alkativeness or pressured speech

Hypomanic episode	Like manic episode except mood disturbance is not severe enough to cause marked impairment in social and/or occupational functioning or to necessitate hospitalization. No psychotic features. **Lasts at least 4 consecutive days.**
Bipolar disorder (manic depression)	Bipolar I defined by presence of at least 1 manic episode +/– a hypomanic or depressive episode. Bipolar II defined by presence of a hypomanic and a depressive episode. Patient's mood and functioning usually return to normal between episodes. Use of antidepressants can precipitate mania. High suicide risk. Treatment: mood stabilizers (eg, lithium, valproic acid, carbamazepine), atypical antipsychotics. **Cyclothymic disorder**—milder form of bipolar disorder **lasting at least 2 years**, fluctuating between mild depressive and hypomanic symptoms.
Major depressive disorder	May be self-limited disorder, with major depressive episodes usually **lasting 6–12 months**. Episodes characterized by at least 5 of the following 9 symptoms for 2 or more weeks (symptoms must include patient-reported depressed mood or anhedonia). Treatment: CBT and SSRIs are first line. SNRIs, mirtazapine, bupropion can also be considered. Electroconvulsive therapy (ECT) in select patients. **Persistent depressive disorder (dysthymia)**—depression, often milder, **lasting at least 2 years**. SIG E CAPS: ▪ Depressed mood ▪ Sleep disturbance ▪ Loss of Interest (anhedonia) ▪ Guilt or feelings of worthlessness ▪ Energy loss and fatigue ▪ Concentration problems ▪ Appetite/weight changes ▪ Psychomotor retardation or agitation ▪ Suicidal ideations Patients with depression typically have the following changes in their sleep stages: ▪ ↓ slow-wave sleep ▪ ↓ REM latency ▪ ↑ REM early in sleep cycle ▪ ↑ total REM sleep ▪ Repeated nighttime awakenings ▪ Early-morning wakening (terminal insomnia)
Depression with atypical features	Differs from classical forms of depression. Characterized by mood reactivity (being able to experience improved mood in response to positive events, albeit briefly), "reversed" vegetative symptoms (hypersomnia, hyperphagia), leaden paralysis (heavy feeling in arms and legs), long-standing interpersonal rejection sensitivity. Most common subtype of depression. Treatment: CBT and SSRIs are first line. MAO inhibitors are effective but not first line because of their risk profile.

Postpartum mood disturbances	Onset within 4 weeks of delivery.
Maternal (postpartum) "blues"	50–85% incidence rate. Characterized by depressed affect, tearfulness, and fatigue starting 2–3 days after delivery. Usually resolves within 10 days. Treatment: supportive. Follow up to assess for possible postpartum depression.
Postpartum depression	10–15% incidence rate. Characterized by depressed affect, anxiety, and poor concentration. Treatment: CBT and SSRIs are first line.
Postpartum psychosis	0.1–0.2% incidence rate. Characterized by mood-congruent delusions, hallucinations, and thoughts of harming the baby or self. Risk factors include history of bipolar or psychotic disorder, first pregnancy, family history, recent discontinuation of psychotropic medication. Treatment: hospitalization and initiation of atypical antipsychotic; if insufficient, ECT may be used.

Grief

Normal grief is characterized by shock, denial, guilt, sadness, anxiety, yearning, and somatic symptoms. Hallucinations of the deceased person are common. Duration varies widely; usually < 6 months.

Pathologic grief is persistent and causes functional impairment. Can meet criteria for major depressive episode.

Electroconvulsive therapy

Used mainly for treatment-refractory depression, depression with psychotic symptoms, and acutely suicidal patients. Produces grand mal seizure in an anesthetized patient. Adverse effects include disorientation, temporary headache, partial anterograde/retrograde amnesia usually resolving in 6 months. Safe in pregnancy.

Risk factors for suicide completion

- **S**ex (male)
- **A**ge (young adult or elderly)
- **D**epression
- **P**revious attempt
- **E**thanol or drug use
- **R**ational thinking loss (psychosis)
- **S**ickness (medical illness)
- **O**rganized plan
- **N**o spouse or other social support
- **S**tated future intent

SAD PERSONS are more likely to complete suicide.

Most common method in US is firearms; access to guns ↑ risk of suicide completion.

Women try more often; men succeed more often.

Anxiety disorder

Inappropriate experience of fear/worry and its physical manifestations (anxiety) incongruent with the magnitude of the perceived stressor. Symptoms interfere with daily functioning. Includes panic disorder, phobias, generalized anxiety disorder, and selective mutism. Treatment: CBT, SSRIs, SNRIs.

Panic disorder	Defined by recurrent panic attacks (periods of intense fear and discomfort peaking in 10 minutes with at least 4 of the following): **P**alpitations, **P**aresthesias, de**P**ersonalization or derealization, **A**bdominal distress or **N**ausea, **I**ntense fear of dying, **I**ntense fear of losing control or "going crazy," l**I**ght-headedness, **C**hest pain, **C**hills, **C**hoking, **S**weating, **S**haking, **S**hortness of breath. Strong genetic component. Treatment: CBT, SSRIs, and venlafaxine are first line. Benzodiazepines occasionally used in acute setting.	**PANICS**. Diagnosis requires attack followed by 1 month (or more) of 1 (or more) of the following: ▪ Persistent concern of additional attacks ▪ Worrying about consequences of attack ▪ Behavioral change related to attacks Symptoms are the systemic manifestations of fear.
Specific phobia	Severe, persistent fear or anxiety due to presence or anticipation of a specific object or situation. Person recognizes fear is excessive. Can be treated with systematic desensitization. **Social anxiety disorder**—exaggerated fear of embarrassment in social situations (eg, public speaking, using public restrooms). Treatment: CBT, SSRIs, venlafaxine. For only occasional anxiety-inducing situations, benzodiazepine or β-blocker. **Agoraphobia**—exaggerated fear of open or enclosed places, using public transportation, being in line or in crowds, or leaving home alone. Associated with panic disorder. Treatment: CBT, SSRIs, MAO inhibitors.	
Generalized anxiety disorder	Anxiety **lasting > 6 months** unrelated to a specific person, situation, or event. Associated with restlessness, irritability, sleep disturbance, fatigue, muscle tension, difficulty concentrating. Treatment: CBT, SSRIs, SNRIs are first line. Buspirone, TCAs, benzodiazepines are second line. **Adjustment disorder**—emotional symptoms (anxiety, depression) causing impairment following an identifiable psychosocial stressor (eg, divorce, illness) and **lasting < 6 months** (> 6 months in presence of chronic stressor). Treatment: CBT, SSRIs.	
Obsessive-compulsive disorder	Recurring intrusive thoughts, feelings, or sensations (obsessions) that cause severe distress; relieved in part by the performance of repetitive actions (compulsions). Ego-dystonic: behavior inconsistent with one's own beliefs and attitudes (vs obsessive-compulsive personality disorder). Associated with Tourette syndrome. Treatment: CBT, SSRIs, and clomipramine are first line. **Body dysmorphic disorder**—preoccupation with minor or imagined defect in appearance → significant emotional distress or impaired functioning; patients often repeatedly seek cosmetic treatment. Treatment: CBT.	
Post-traumatic stress disorder	Exposure to prior trauma (eg, witnessing death, experiencing serious injury or rape) → intrusive reexperiencing of the event (nightmares, flashbacks), avoidance of associated stimuli, changes in cognition or mood (fear, horror), and persistently ↑ arousal. Disturbance **lasts > 1 month** with significant distress or impaired social-occupational functioning. Treatment: CBT, SSRIs, and venlafaxine are first line. **Acute stress disorder—lasts between 3 days and 1 month.** Treatment: CBT; pharmacotherapy is usually not indicated.	

Malingering	Patient **consciously** fakes, profoundly exaggerates, or claims to have a disorder in order to attain a specific 2° **(external) gain** (eg, avoiding work, obtaining compensation). Poor compliance with treatment or follow-up of diagnostic tests. Complaints cease after gain (vs factitious disorder).

Factitious disorders	Patient **consciously** creates physical and/or psychological symptoms in order to assume "sick role" and to get medical attention (1° [**internal**] **gain**).
Factitious disorder imposed on self (Munchausen syndrome)	**Chronic** factitious disorder with predominantly physical signs and symptoms. Characterized by a history of multiple hospital admissions and willingness to undergo invasive procedures.
Factitious disorder imposed on another (Munchausen syndrome by proxy)	Illness in a child or elderly patient is caused or fabricated by the caregiver. Motivation is to assume a sick role by proxy. Form of child/elder abuse.

Somatic symptom and related disorders	Category of disorders characterized by physical symptoms causing significant distress and impairment. Both illness production and motivation are **unconscious** drives. Symptoms not intentionally produced or feigned. More common in women.
Somatic symptom disorder	Variety of bodily complaints (eg, pain, fatigue) lasting for months to years. Associated with excessive, persistent thoughts and anxiety about symptoms. May co-occur with medical illness.
Conversion disorder (functional neurologic symptom disorder)	Loss of sensory or motor function (eg, paralysis, blindness, mutism), often following an acute stressor; patient is aware of but sometimes indifferent toward symptoms ("la belle indifférence"); more common in females, adolescents, and young adults.
Illness anxiety disorder	Excessive preoccupation with acquiring or having a serious illness, often despite medical evaluation and reassurance; minimal somatic symptoms.
Pseudocyesis	False, nondelusional belief of being pregnant. May have signs and symptoms of pregnancy but is not pregnant.

Personality	
Personality trait	An enduring, repetitive pattern of perceiving, relating to, and thinking about the environment and oneself.
Personality disorder	Inflexible, maladaptive, and rigidly pervasive pattern of behavior causing subjective distress and/or impaired functioning; person is usually not aware of problem. Usually presents by early adulthood. Three clusters, A, B, and C; remember as **Weird**, **Wild**, and **Worried** based on symptoms.

Cluster A personality disorders	Odd or eccentric; inability to develop meaningful social relationships. No psychosis; genetic association with schizophrenia.	"**Weird**" (**A**ccusatory, **A**loof, **A**wkward).
Paranoid	Pervasive distrust and suspiciousness; projection is the major defense mechanism.	
Schizoid	Voluntary social withdrawal, limited emotional expression, content with social isolation (vs avoidant).	Schizoi**d** = **d**istant.
Schizotypal	Eccentric appearance, odd beliefs or magical thinking, interpersonal awkwardness.	Schizo**t**ypal = magical **t**hinking.
Cluster B personality disorders	Dramatic, emotional, or erratic; genetic association with mood disorders and substance abuse.	"**Wild**" (**B**ad to the **B**one).
Antisocial	Disregard for and violation of rights of others, criminality, impulsivity; males > females; must be ≥ 18 years old and have history of conduct disorder before age 15. Conduct disorder if < 18 years old.	Anti**soc**ial = **soc**iopath.
Borderline	Unstable mood and interpersonal relationships, impulsivity, self-mutilation, suicidality, sense of emptiness; females > males; splitting is a major defense mechanism.	Treatment: dialectical behavior therapy.
Histrionic	Excessive emotionality and excitability, attention seeking, sexually provocative, overly concerned with appearance.	
Narcissistic	Grandiosity, sense of entitlement; lacks empathy and requires excessive admiration; often demands the "best" and reacts to criticism with rage.	
Cluster C personality disorders	Anxious or fearful; genetic association with anxiety disorders.	"**Worried**" (**C**owardly, **C**ompulsive, **C**lingy).
Avoidant	Hypersensitive to rejection, socially inhibited, timid, feelings of inadequacy, desires relationships with others (vs schizoid).	
Obsessive-compulsive	Preoccupation with order, perfectionism, and control; ego-syntonic: behavior consistent with one's own beliefs and attitudes (vs OCD).	
Dependent	Submissive and clingy, excessive need to be taken care of, low self-confidence.	Patients often get stuck in abusive relationships.

Eating disorders Most common in young females.

Anorexia nervosa Excessive dieting, exercise, or binge eating/purging with BMI < 18.5 kg/m^2; intense fear of gaining weight; and distortion or overvaluation of body image. Associated with ↓ bone density, severe weight loss, metatarsal stress fractures, amenorrhea (due to loss of pulsatile GnRH secretion), lanugo, anemia, electrolyte disturbances. Commonly coexists with depression. Psychotherapy and nutritional rehabilitation are first line. Refeeding syndrome (↑ insulin → hypophosphatemia → cardiac complications) can occur in significantly malnourished patients.

Bulimia nervosa Binge eating with recurrent inappropriate compensatory behaviors (eg, self-induced vomiting, using laxatives or diuretics, fasting, excessive exercise) occurring weekly for at least 3 months and overvaluation of body image. Body weight often maintained within normal range. Associated with parotitis, enamel erosion, electrolyte disturbances, alkalosis, dorsal hand calluses from induced vomiting (Russell sign). Treatment: psychotherapy, nutritional rehabilitation, antidepressants.

Binge eating disorder Regular episodes of excessive, uncontrollable eating without inappropriate compensatory behaviors. ↑ risk of diabetes. Treatment: psychotherapy such as CBT is first-line; SSRIs.

Gender dysphoria Strong, persistent cross-gender identification that leads to persistent discomfort with sex assigned at birth, causing significant distress and/or impaired functioning. Transgender individuals may have gender dysphoric disorder.

Transsexualism—desire to live as the opposite sex, often through surgery or hormone treatment.

Transvestism—paraphilia, not gender dysphoria. Wearing clothes (eg, vest) of the opposite sex (cross-dressing). abnormal sex desires

---

Sexual dysfunction Includes sexual desire disorders (hypoactive sexual desire or sexual aversion), sexual arousal disorders (erectile dysfunction), orgasmic disorders (anorgasmia, premature ejaculation), sexual pain disorders (dyspareunia, vaginismus).

Differential diagnosis includes:

- Drugs (eg, antihypertensives, neuroleptics, SSRIs, ethanol)
- Diseases (eg, depression, diabetes, STIs)
- Psychological (eg, performance anxiety)

Sleep terror disorder Periods of terror with screaming in the middle of the night; occurs during slow-wave/deep (stage N3) sleep. Most common in children. Occurs during non-REM sleep (no memory of arousal) as opposed to nightmares that occur during REM sleep (memory of a scary dream). Cause unknown, but triggers include emotional stress, fever, or lack of sleep. Usually self limited.

Narcolepsy

Disordered regulation of sleep-wake cycles; 1° characteristic is excessive daytime sleepiness (awaken feeling rested).

Caused by ↓ hypocretin (orexin) production in lateral hypothalamus.

Also associated with:

- Hypnagogic (just before sleep) or hypnopompic (just before awakening) hallucinations.
- Nocturnal and narcoleptic sleep episodes that start with REM sleep.
- Cataplexy (loss of all muscle tone following strong emotional stimulus, such as laughter) in some patients.

Strong genetic component. Treatment: daytime stimulants (eg, amphetamines, modafinil) and nighttime sodium oxybate (GHB).

Hypnagogic—going to sleep
Hypnopompic—"pompous upon awakening"

Substance use disorder

Maladaptive pattern of substance use defined as 2 or more of the following signs in 1 year:

- Tolerance—need more to achieve same effect
- Withdrawal
- Substance taken in larger amounts, or over longer time, than desired
- Persistent desire or unsuccessful attempts to cut down
- Significant energy spent obtaining, using, or recovering from substance
- Important social, occupational, or recreational activities reduced because of substance use
- Continued use despite knowing substance causes physical and/or psychological problems
- Craving
- Recurrent use in physically dangerous situations
- Failure to fulfill major obligations at work, school, or home due to use
- Social or interpersonal conflicts related to substance use

Stages of change in overcoming substance addiction

1. **Precontemplation**—not yet acknowledging that there is a problem
2. **Contemplation**—acknowledging that there is a problem, but not yet ready or willing to make a change
3. **Preparation/determination**—getting ready to change behaviors
4. **Action/willpower**—changing behaviors
5. **Maintenance**—maintaining the behavior changes
6. **Relapse**—returning to old behaviors and abandoning new changes

Psychoactive drug intoxication and withdrawal

DRUG	INTOXICATION	WITHDRAWAL
Depressants		
	Nonspecific: mood elevation, ↓ anxiety, sedation, behavioral disinhibition, respiratory depression.	Nonspecific: anxiety, tremor, seizures, insomnia.
Alcohol	Emotional lability, slurred speech, ataxia, coma, blackouts. Serum γ-glutamyltransferase (GGT)—sensitive indicator of alcohol use. AST value is twice ALT value.	Mild alcohol withdrawal: symptoms similar to other depressants. Severe alcohol withdrawal can cause autonomic hyperactivity and DTs (5–15% mortality rate). Treatment for DTs: benzodiazepines.
Opioids	Euphoria, respiratory and CNS depression, ↓ gag reflex, pupillary constriction (pinpoint pupils), seizures (overdose). Most common cause of drug overdose death. Treatment: naloxone, naltrexone.	Sweating, dilated pupils, piloerection ("cold turkey"), fever, rhinorrhea, yawning, nausea, stomach cramps, diarrhea ("flu-like" symptoms). Treatment: long-term support, methadone, buprenorphine.
Barbiturates	Low safety margin, marked respiratory depression. Treatment: symptom management (eg, assist respiration, ↑ BP).	Delirium, life-threatening cardiovascular collapse.
Benzodiazepines	Greater safety margin. Ataxia, minor respiratory depression. Treatment: flumazenil (benzodiazepine receptor antagonist, but rarely used as it can precipitate seizures).	Sleep disturbance, depression, rebound anxiety, seizure.
Stimulants		
	Nonspecific: mood elevation, psychomotor agitation, insomnia, cardiac arrhythmias, tachycardia, anxiety.	Nonspecific: post-use "crash," including depression, lethargy, ↑ appetite, sleep disturbance, vivid nightmares.
Amphetamines	Euphoria, grandiosity, pupillary dilation, prolonged wakefulness and attention, hypertension, tachycardia, anorexia, paranoia, fever. Severe: cardiac arrest, seizures. Treatment: benzodiazepines for agitation and seizures.	
Cocaine	Impaired judgment, pupillary dilation, hallucinations (including tactile), paranoid ideations, angina, sudden cardiac death. Treatment: α-blockers, benzodiazepines. β-blockers not recommended.	
Caffeine	Restlessness, ↑ diuresis, muscle twitching.	Headache, difficulty concentrating, flu-like symptoms.
Nicotine	Restlessness.	Irritability, anxiety, restlessness, difficulty concentrating. Treatment: nicotine patch, gum, or lozenges; bupropion/varenicline.

Psychoactive drug intoxication and withdrawal *(continued)*

DRUG	INTOXICATION	WITHDRAWAL
Hallucinogens		
Phencyclidine	Violence, impulsivity, psychomotor agitation, nystagmus, tachycardia, hypertension, analgesia, psychosis, delirium, seizures. Trauma is most common complication. Treatment: benzodiazepines, rapid-acting antipsychotic.	
Lysergic acid diethylamide	Perceptual distortion (visual, auditory), depersonalization, anxiety, paranoia, psychosis, possible flashbacks.	
Marijuana (cannabinoid)	Euphoria, anxiety, paranoid delusions, perception of slowed time, impaired judgment, social withdrawal, ↑ appetite, dry mouth, conjunctival injection, hallucinations. Pharmaceutical form is dronabinol (tetrahydrocannabinol isomer): used as antiemetic (chemotherapy) and appetite stimulant (in AIDS).	Irritability, anxiety, depression, insomnia, restlessness, ↓ appetite. Generally detectable in urine for up to 1 month.
MDMA (ecstasy)	Hallucinogenic stimulant: euphoria, disinhibition, hyperactivity. Life-threatening effects include hypertension, tachycardia, hyperthermia, hyponatremia, serotonin syndrome.	Depression, fatigue, change in appetite, difficulty concentrating, anxiety.

Heroin addiction	Users at ↑ risk for hepatitis, HIV, abscesses, bacteremia, right-heart endocarditis. Treatment is described below.
Methadone	Long-acting oral opiate used for heroin detoxification or long-term maintenance.
Naloxone + buprenorphine	Antagonist + partial agonist. Naloxone is not orally bioavailable, so withdrawal symptoms occur only if injected (lower abuse potential).
Naltrexone	Long-acting opioid antagonist used for relapse prevention once detoxified.

Alcoholism	Physiologic tolerance and dependence with symptoms of withdrawal (tremor, tachycardia, hypertension, malaise, nausea, DTs) when intake is interrupted. Complications: alcoholic cirrhosis, hepatitis, pancreatitis, peripheral neuropathy, testicular atrophy. Treatment: disulfiram (to condition the patient to abstain from alcohol use), acamprosate, naltrexone, supportive care. Support groups such as Alcoholics Anonymous are helpful in sustaining abstinence and supporting patient and family.
Wernicke-Korsakoff syndrome	Caused by vitamin B_1 (thiamine) deficiency. Triad of confusion, ophthalmoplegia, ataxia (Wernicke encephalopathy). May progress to irreversible memory loss, confabulation, personality change (Korsakoff syndrome). Associated with periventricular hemorrhage/necrosis of mammillary bodies. Treatment: IV vitamin B_1.
Mallory-Weiss syndrome	Partial thickness tear at gastroesophageal junction caused by excessive/forceful vomiting. Often presents with hematemesis and misdiagnosed as ruptured esophageal varices.

but this is painful unlike varices

Delirium tremens

Life-threatening alcohol withdrawal syndrome that peaks 2–4 days after last drink.
Characterized by autonomic hyperactivity (eg, tachycardia, tremors, anxiety, seizures). Classically occurs in hospital setting (eg, 2–4 days postsurgery) in alcoholics not able to drink as inpatients. Treatment: benzodiazepines.
Alcoholic hallucinosis is a distinct condition characterized by visual hallucinations 12–48 hours after last drink. Treatment: benzodiazepines (eg, chlordiazepoxide, lorazepam, diazepam).

▶ PSYCHIATRY—PHARMACOLOGY

Preferred medications for selected psychiatric conditions

PSYCHIATRIC CONDITION	PREFERRED DRUGS
ADHD	Stimulants (methylphenidate, amphetamines)
Alcohol withdrawal	Benzodiazepines (eg, chlordiazepoxide, lorazepam, diazepam)
Bipolar disorder	Lithium, valproic acid, atypical antipsychotics
Bulimia nervosa	SSRIs
Depression	SSRIs
Generalized anxiety disorder	SSRIs, SNRIs
Obsessive-compulsive disorder	SSRIs, venlafaxine, clomipramine
Panic disorder	SSRIs, venlafaxine, benzodiazepines
PTSD	SSRIs, venlafaxine
Schizophrenia	Atypical antipsychotics
Social anxiety disorder	SSRIs, venlafaxine Performance only: β-blockers, benzodiazepines
Tourette syndrome	Antipsychotics (eg, fluphenazine, pimozide), tetrabenazine

CNS stimulants	Methylphenidate, dextroamphetamine, methamphetamine.
MECHANISM	↑ catecholamines in the synaptic cleft, especially norepinephrine and dopamine.
CLINICAL USE	ADHD, narcolepsy, appetite control.

Antipsychotics (neuroleptics)

Haloperidol, trifluoperazine, fluphenazine, thioridazine, chlorpromazine (haloperidol + "-azines").

MECHANISM	All typical antipsychotics block dopamine D_2 receptors (↑ [cAMP]).	**High** potency: **Tri**fluoperazine, **F**luphenazine, **H**aloperidol (**Try** to **Fly High**)—neurologic side effects (eg, extrapyramidal symptoms [EPS]).
CLINICAL USE	Schizophrenia (primarily positive symptoms), psychosis, bipolar disorder, delirium, Tourette syndrome, Huntington disease, OCD.	**Low** potency: **C**hlorpromazine, **Th**ioridazine (**C**heating **Th**ieves are **low**)—non-neurologic side effects (anticholinergic, antihistamine, and α_1-blockade effects).
ADVERSE EFFECTS	Highly lipid soluble and stored in body fat; thus, very slow to be removed from body. Extrapyramidal system side effects (eg, dyskinesias). Treatment: benztropine, diphenhydramine, benzodiazepines. Endocrine side effects (eg, dopamine receptor antagonism → hyperprolactinemia → galactorrhea, oligomenorrhea, gynecomastia). * Side effects arising from blocking muscarinic (dry mouth, constipation), α_1 (orthostatic hypotension), and histamine (sedation) receptors. * Can cause QT prolongation.	**C**hlorpromazine—**C**orneal deposits; **T**hioridazine—re**T**inal deposits; haloperidol—NMS, tardive dyskinesia. Onset of EPS: **ADAPT** ▪ Hours to days: **A**cute **D**ystonia (muscle spasm, stiffness, oculogyric crisis) ▪ Days to months: **A**kathisia (restlessness) and **P**arkinsonism (bradykinesia). ▪ Months to years: **T**ardive dyskinesia
OTHER TOXICITIES	**Neuroleptic malignant syndrome (NMS)**—rigidity, myoglobinuria, autonomic instability, hyperpyrexia. Treatment: dantrolene, D_2 agonists (eg, bromocriptine). **Tardive dyskinesia**—orofacial chorea as a result of long-term antipsychotic use.	For NMS, think **FEVER**: **F**ever **E**ncephalopathy **V**itals unstable **E**nzymes ↑ **R**igidity of muscles

Atypical antipsychotics

Aripiprazole, asenapine, clozapine, iloperidone, lurasidone, olanzapine, paliperidone, quetiapine, risperidone, ziprasidone. -apine, -idone

MECHANISM	Not completely understood. Most are D_2 antagonists; aripiprazole is D_2 partial agonist. Varied effects on 5-HT_2, dopamine, and α- and H_1-receptors.	
CLINICAL USE	Schizophrenia—both positive and negative symptoms. Also used for bipolar disorder, OCD, anxiety disorder, depression, mania, Tourette syndrome.	
ADVERSE EFFECTS	All—prolonged QT interval, fewer EPS and anticholinergic side effects than typical antipsychotics. "-pines"—metabolic syndrome (weight gain, diabetes, hyperlipidemia). Clozapine—agranulocytosis (monitor WBC weekly). Risperidone—hyperprolactinemia (amenorrhea, galactorrhea, gynecomastia).	Must watch bone marrow **cloz**ely with **cloz**apine. **O**lanzapine → **O**besity

Lithium

MECHANISM	Not established; possibly related to inhibition of phosphoinositol cascade.	LMNOP—Lithium side effects: Movement (tremor) Nephrogenic diabetes insipidus HypOthyroidism Pregnancy problems
CLINICAL USE	Mood stabilizer for bipolar disorder; blocks relapse and acute manic events.	
ADVERSE EFFECTS	Tremor, hypothyroidism, polyuria (causes nephrogenic diabetes insipidus), teratogenesis. Causes Ebstein anomaly in newborn if taken by pregnant mother. Narrow therapeutic window requires close monitoring of serum levels. Almost exclusively excreted by kidneys; most is reabsorbed at PCT with Na^+. Thiazide use is implicated in lithium toxicity in bipolar patients.	

Buspirone

MECHANISM	Stimulates $5\text{-}HT_{1A}$ receptors.	I'm always anxious if the **bus** will be **on** time, so I take **buspirone**.
CLINICAL USE	Generalized anxiety disorder. Does not cause sedation, addiction, or tolerance. Takes 1–2 weeks to take effect. Does not interact with alcohol (vs barbiturates, benzodiazepines).	

Antidepressants

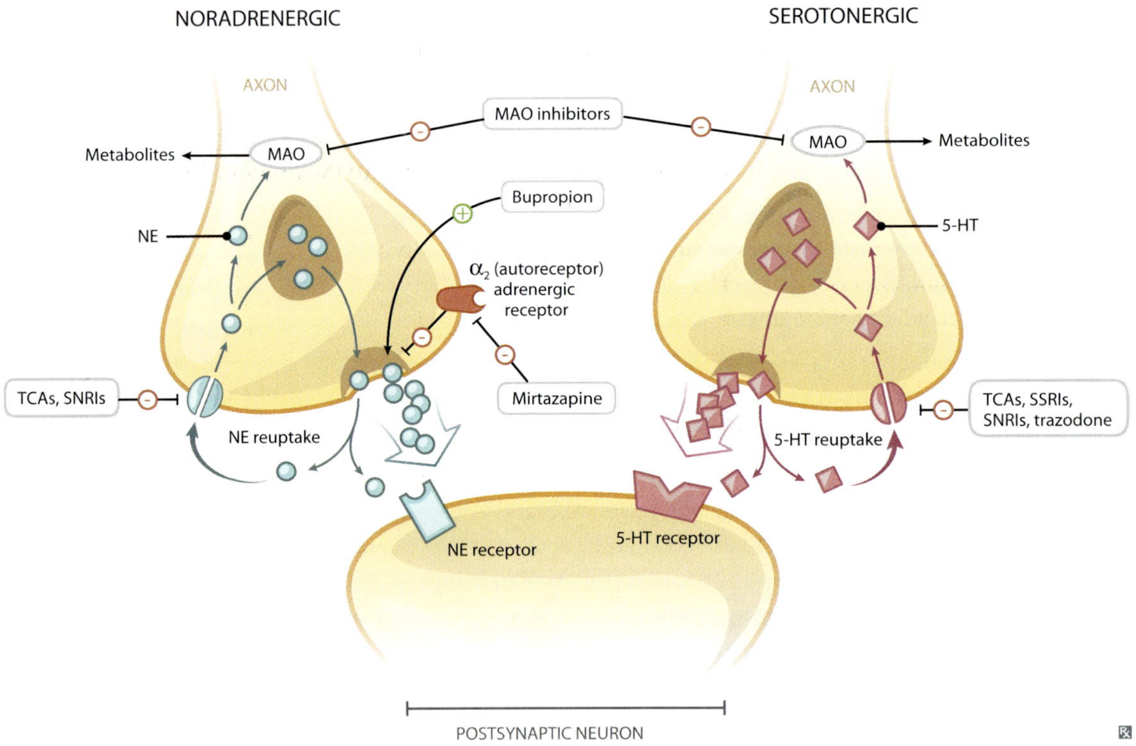

Selective serotonin reuptake inhibitors	Fluoxetine, paroxetine, sertraline, citalopram.	Flashbacks paralyze senior citizens.
MECHANISM	5-HT–specific reuptake inhibitors.	It normally takes 4–8 weeks for antidepressants to have an effect.
CLINICAL USE	Depression, generalized anxiety disorder, panic disorder, OCD, bulimia, social anxiety disorder, PTSD, premature ejaculation, premenstrual dysphoric disorder.	
ADVERSE EFFECTS	Fewer than TCAs. GI distress, SIADH, sexual dysfunction (anorgasmia, ↓ libido).	

Serotonin-norepinephrine reuptake inhibitors	Venlafaxine, desvenlafaxine, duloxetine, levomilnacipran, milnacipran.
MECHANISM	Inhibit 5-HT and norepinephrine reuptake.
CLINICAL USE	Depression, general anxiety disorder, diabetic neuropathy. Venlafaxine is also indicated for social anxiety disorder, panic disorder, PTSD, OCD.
ADVERSE EFFECTS	↑ BP most common; also stimulant effects, sedation, nausea.

Serotonin syndrome	Can occur with any drug that ↑ 5-HT (eg, MAO inhibitors, SNRIs, TCAs). Characterized by 3 A's: neuromuscular Activity (clonus, hyperreflexia, hypertonia, tremor, seizure), Autonomic stimulation (hyperthermia, diaphoresis, diarrhea), and Agitation. Treatment: cyproheptadine ($5\text{-}HT_2$ receptor antagonist).

Tricyclic antidepressants	Amitriptyline, nortriptyline, imipramine, desipramine, clomipramine, doxepin, amoxapine.
MECHANISM	Block reuptake of norepinephrine and 5-HT.
CLINICAL USE	Major depression, OCD (clomipramine), peripheral neuropathy, chronic pain, migraine prophylaxis.
ADVERSE EFFECTS	Sedation, α_1-blocking effects including postural hypotension, and atropine-like (anticholinergic) side effects (tachycardia, urinary retention, dry mouth). 3° TCAs (amitriptyline) have more anticholinergic effects than 2° TCAs (nortriptyline). Can prolong QT interval. Tri-C's: Convulsions, Coma, Cardiotoxicity (arrhythmia due to Na^+ channel inhibition); also respiratory depression, hyperpyrexia. Confusion and hallucinations in elderly due to anticholinergic side effects (use nortriptyline). Treatment: $NaHCO_3$ to prevent arrhythmia.

Monoamine oxidase inhibitors	Tranylcypromine, Phenelzine, Isocarboxazid, Selegiline (selective MAO-B inhibitor). (MAO Takes Pride In Shanghai).
MECHANISM	Nonselective MAO inhibition ↑ levels of amine neurotransmitters (norepinephrine, 5-HT, dopamine).
CLINICAL USE	Atypical depression, anxiety.
ADVERSE EFFECTS	Hypertensive crisis (most notably with ingestion of tyramine, which is found in many foods such as aged cheese and wine); CNS stimulation. Contraindicated with SSRIs, TCAs, St. John's wort, meperidine, dextromethorphan (to prevent serotonin syndrome). Wait 2 weeks after stopping MAO inhibitors before starting serotonergic drugs or stopping dietary restrictions.

Atypical antidepressants

Bupropion	↑ norepinephrine and dopamine via unknown mechanism. Also used for smoking cessation. Toxicity: stimulant effects (tachycardia, insomnia), headache, seizures in anorexic/bulimic patients. No sexual side effects.
Mirtazapine	α_2-antagonist (↑ release of NE and 5-HT), potent 5-HT_2 and 5-HT_3 receptor antagonist and H_1 antagonist. Toxicity: sedation (which may be desirable in depressed patients with insomnia), ↑ appetite, weight gain (which may be desirable in elderly or anorexic patients), dry mouth.
Trazodone	Primarily blocks 5-HT_2, α_1-adrenergic, and H_1 receptors; also weakly inhibits 5-HT reuptake. Used primarily for insomnia, as high doses are needed for antidepressant effects. Toxicity: sedation, nausea, priapism, postural hypotension. Called traZZZobone due to sedative and male-specific side effects.
Varenicline	Nicotinic ACh receptor partial agonist. Used for smoking cessation. Toxicity: sleep disturbance.

HIGH-YIELD SYSTEMS

Renal

"But I know all about love already. I know precious little still about kidneys."

—Aldous Huxley, *Antic Hay*

"This too shall pass. Just like a kidney stone."

—Hunter Madsen

"I drink too much. The last time I gave a urine sample it had an olive in it."

—Rodney Dangerfield

▶ RENAL—EMBRYOLOGY

Kidney embryology

Pronephros—week 4; then degenerates.

Mesonephros—functions as interim kidney for 1st trimester; later contributes to male genital system.

Metanephros—permanent; first appears in 5th week of gestation; nephrogenesis continues through 32–36 weeks of gestation.

- Ureteric bud—derived from caudal end of mesonephric duct; gives rise to ureter, pelvises, calyces, collecting ducts; fully canalized by 10th week
- Metanephric mesenchyme (ie, metanephric blastema)—ureteric bud interacts with this tissue; interaction induces differentiation and formation of glomerulus through to distal convoluted tubule (DCT)
- Aberrant interaction between these 2 tissues may result in several congenital malformations of the kidney

Ureteropelvic junction—last to canalize → most common site of obstruction (hydronephrosis) in fetus.

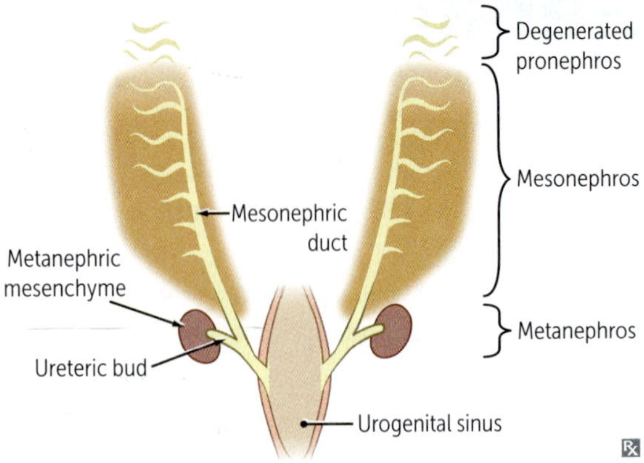

Potter sequence (syndrome)

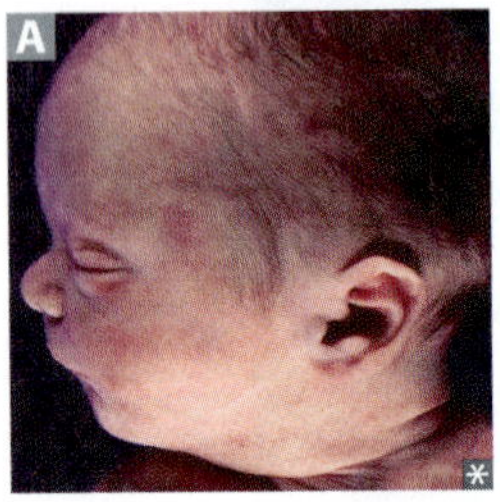

Oligohydramnios → compression of developing fetus → limb deformities, facial anomalies (eg, low-set ears and retrognathia A, flattened nose), compression of chest and lack of amniotic fluid aspiration into fetal lungs → pulmonary hypoplasia (cause of death).

Causes include ARPKD, obstructive uropathy (eg, posterior urethral valves), bilateral renal agenesis, chronic placental insufficiency.

Babies who can't "Pee" in utero develop Potter sequence.

POTTER sequence associated with:

- Pulmonary hypoplasia
- Oligohydramnios (trigger)
- Twisted face
- Twisted skin
- Extremity defects
- Renal failure (in utero)

Horseshoe kidney

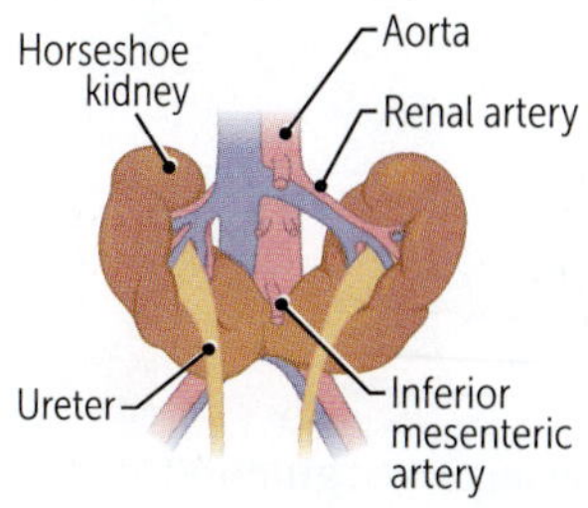

Inferior poles of both kidneys fuse abnormally A. As they ascend from pelvis during fetal development, horseshoe kidneys get trapped under inferior mesenteric artery and remain low in the abdomen. Kidneys function normally. Associated with hydronephrosis (eg, ureteropelvic junction obstruction), renal stones, infection, chromosomal aneuploidy syndromes (eg, Turner syndrome; trisomies 13, 18, 21), and rarely renal cancer.

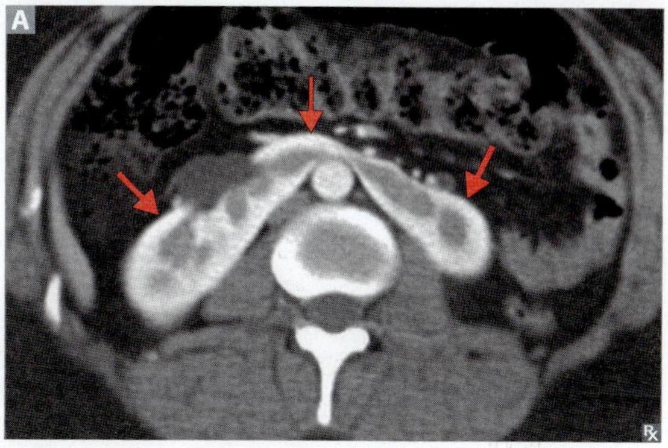

Unilateral renal agenesis

Ureteric bud fails to develop and induce differentiation of metanephric mesenchyme → complete absence of kidney and ureter. Often diagnosed prenatally via ultrasound.

Multicystic dysplastic kidney

Ureteric bud fails to induce differentiation of metanephric mesenchyme → nonfunctional kidney consisting of cysts and connective tissue. Often diagnosed prenatally via ultrasound.

Duplex collecting system

Bifurcation of ureteric bud before it enters the metanephric blastema creates a Y-shaped bifid ureter. Duplex collecting system can alternatively occur through two ureteric buds reaching and interacting with metanephric blastema. Strongly associated with vesicoureteral reflux and/or ureteral obstruction, ↑ risk for UTIs.

Congenital solitary functioning kidney

Condition of being born with only one functioning kidney. Majority asymptomatic with compensatory hypertrophy of contralateral kidney, but anomalies in contralateral kidney are common.

▶ RENAL—ANATOMY

Kidney anatomy and glomerular structure

renal a — segment — interlobar → arcuate — interlobular

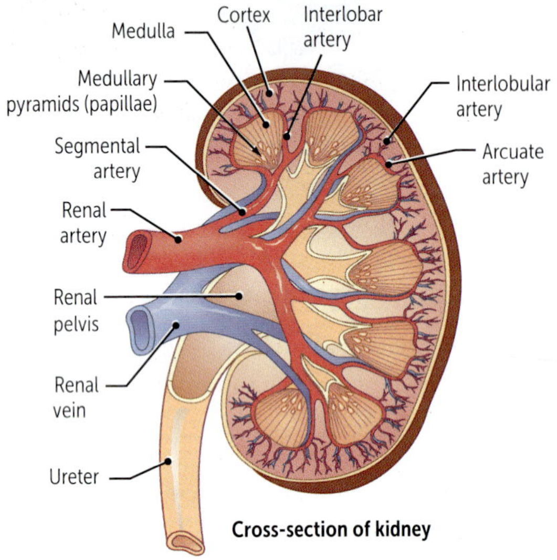

Cross-section of kidney

Left kidney is taken during donor transplantation because it has a longer renal vein.

Afferent = **A**rriving.

Efferent = **E**xiting.

Renal blood flow: renal artery → segmental artery → interlobar artery → arcuate artery → interlobular artery → afferent arteriole → glomerulus → efferent arteriole → vasa recta/ peritubular capillaries → venous outflow.

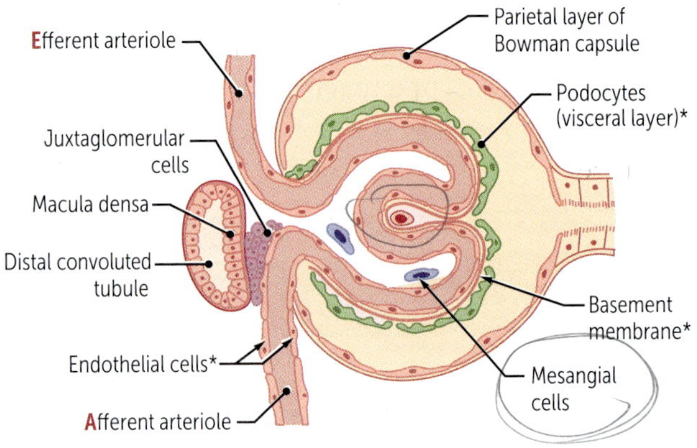

*Components of glomerular filtration barrier.

Cross-section of glomerulus A

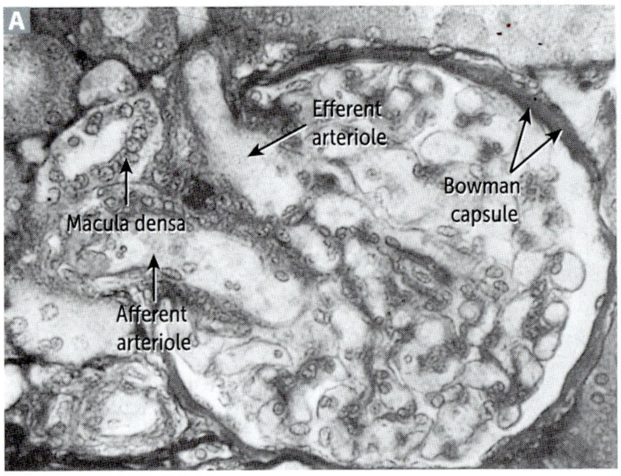

Ureters: course

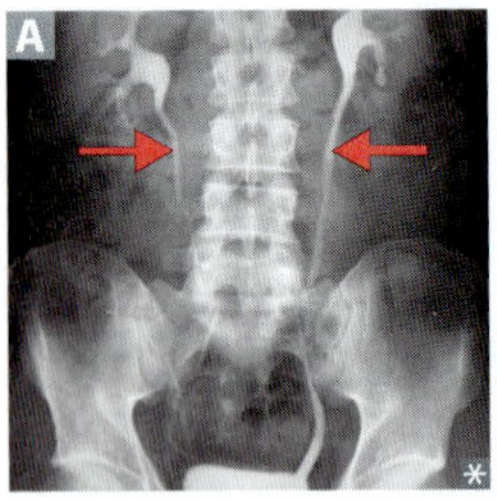

Ureters A pass **under** uterine artery or **under** vas deferens (retroperitoneal).

Gynecologic procedures (eg, ligation of uterine or ovarian vessels) may damage ureter → ureteral obstruction or leak.

"Water (ureters) **under** the bridge (uterine artery, vas deferens)."

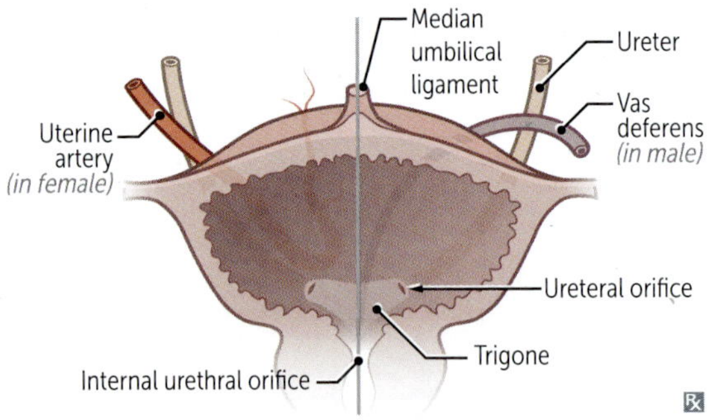

▶ RENAL—PHYSIOLOGY

Fluid compartments

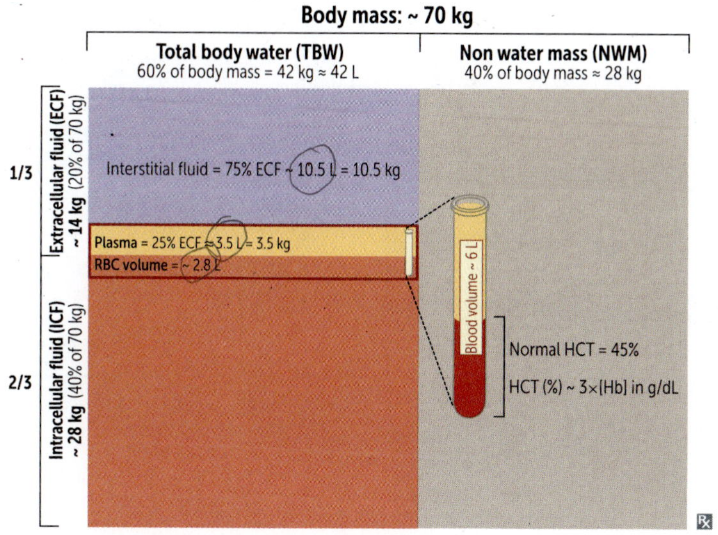

HIKIN': HIgh K^+ INtracellularly.

60–40–20 rule (% of body weight for average person):
- 60% total body water
- 40% ICF
- 20% ECF

Plasma volume can be measured by radiolabeling albumin.

Extracellular volume can be measured by inulin or mannitol.

Osmolality = 285–295 mOsm/kg H_2O.

Glomerular filtration barrier

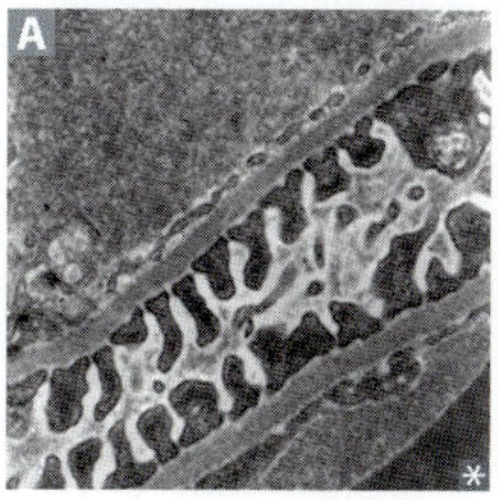

Responsible for filtration of plasma according to size and net charge.

Composed of:
- Fenestrated capillary endothelium (size barrier)
- Fused basement membrane with heparan sulfate (negative charge and size barrier)
- Epithelial layer consisting of podocyte foot processes A (negative charge barrier)

Charge barrier is lost in nephrotic syndrome → albuminuria, hypoproteinemia, generalized edema, hyperlipidemia.

Renal clearance

$C_x = U_xV/P_x$ = volume of plasma from which the substance is completely cleared per unit time.

If $C_x <$ GFR: net tubular reabsorption of X.

If $C_x >$ GFR: net tubular secretion of X.

If $C_x =$ GFR: no net secretion or reabsorption.

C_x = clearance of X (mL/min).

U_x = urine concentration of X (eg, mg/mL).

P_x = plasma concentration of X (eg, mg/mL).

V = urine flow rate (mL/min).

urine con & flow rate / what was in the plasma in the first place

Glomerular filtration rate

Inulin clearance can be used to calculate GFR because it is freely filtered and is neither reabsorbed nor secreted.

$GFR = U_{inulin} \times V/P_{inulin} = C_{inulin}$

$= K_f [(P_{GC} - P_{BS}) - (\pi_{GC} - \pi_{BS})]$

(GC = glomerular capillary; BS = Bowman space.)

π_{BS} normally equals zero; K_f = filtration constant.

Normal GFR ≈ 100 mL/min.

Creatinine clearance is an approximate measure of GFR. Slightly overestimates GFR because creatinine is moderately secreted by renal tubules.

Incremental reductions in GFR define the stages of chronic kidney disease.

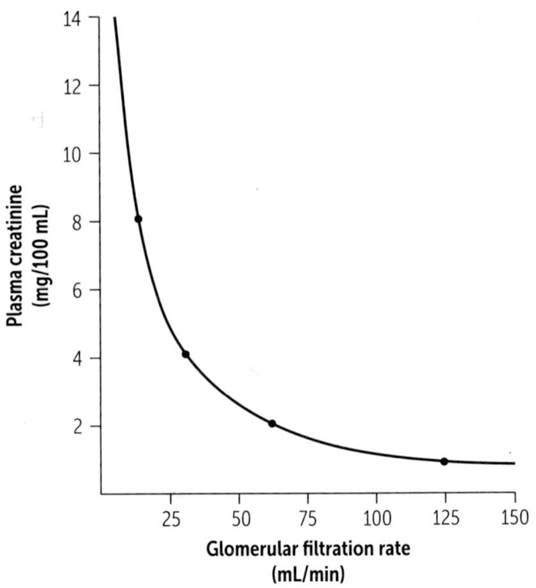

Effective renal plasma flow

Effective renal plasma flow (eRPF) can be estimated using *para*-aminohippuric acid (PAH) clearance because between filtration and secretion there is nearly 100% excretion of all PAH that enters the kidney.

$eRPF = U_{PAH} \times V/P_{PAH} = C_{PAH}$.

Renal blood flow (RBF) = RPF/(1 – Hct).

Plasma = 1 – hematocrit.

eRPF underestimates true renal plasma flow (RPF) slightly.

RBF = RPF + RBCS (plasma)

GFR = C inulin
eRPF = C PAH
renal PLASMA flow

Filtration

Filtration fraction (FF) = GFR/RPF.
Normal FF = 20%.
Filtered load (mg/min) = GFR (mL/min) × plasma concentration (mg/mL).

GFR can be estimated with creatinine clearance.
RPF is best estimated with PAH clearance.

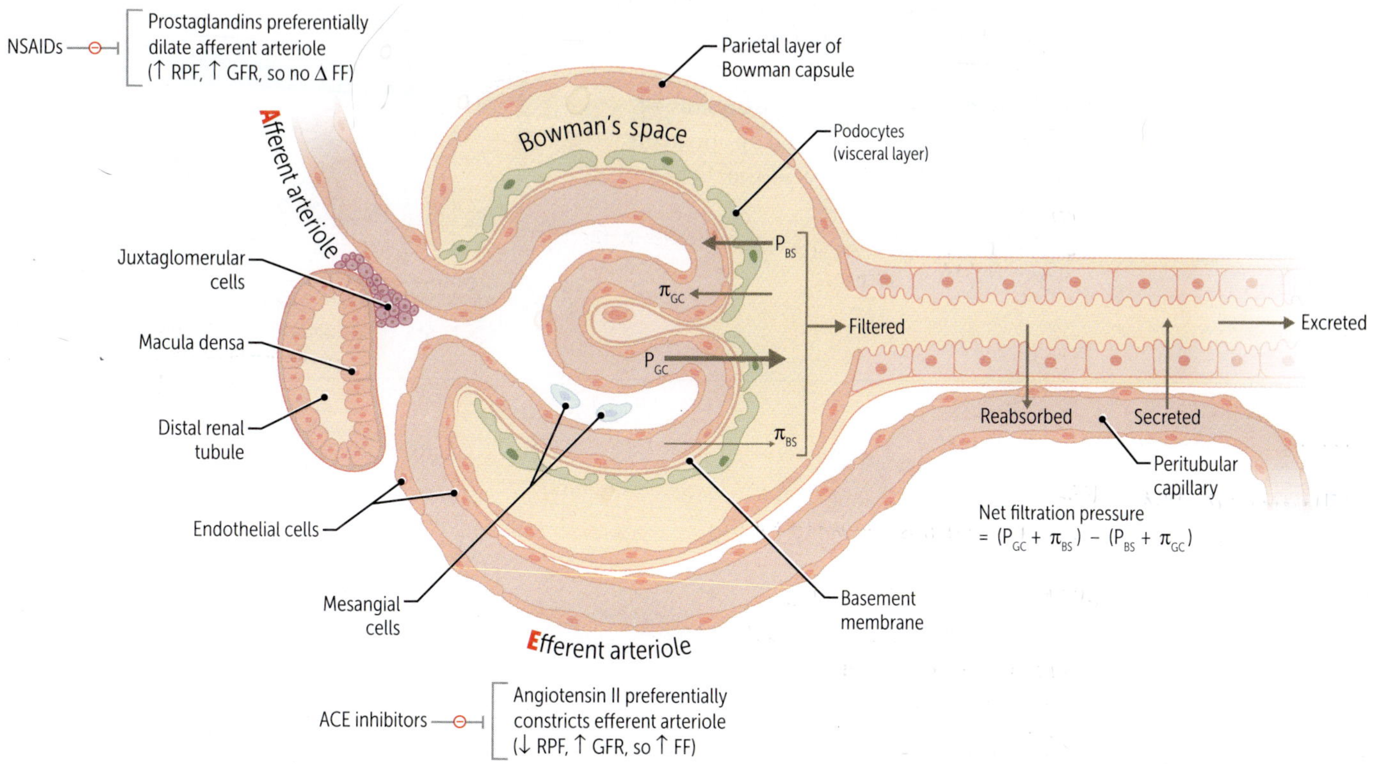

Changes in glomerular dynamics

Effect	GFR	RPF	FF (GFR/RPF)
Afferent arteriole constriction	↓	↓	—
Efferent arteriole constriction	↑	↓	↑
↑ plasma protein concentration	↓	—	↓
↓ plasma protein concentration	↑	—	↑
Constriction of ureter	↓	—	↓
Dehydration	↓	↓	↑

Calculation of reabsorption and secretion rate

Filtered load = GFR × P_x.
Excretion rate = V × U_x.
Reabsorption = filtered – excreted.
Secretion = excreted – filtered.

FE_{Na} = Na^+ excreted/Na^+ filtered = V × U_{Na}/GFR × P_{Na} (GFR = U_{Cr} × V/P_{Cr}) = P_{Cr} × U_{Na}/U_{Cr} × P_{Na}

Glucose clearance

starts showing at 200 mg/dL but all transp satur at 375

Glucose at a normal plasma level (range 60–120 mg/dL) is completely reabsorbed in proximal convoluted tubule (PCT) by Na^+/glucose cotransport. (lothin)

In adults, at plasma glucose of ~ 200 mg/dL, glucosuria begins (threshold). At rate of ~ 375 mg/min, all transporters are fully saturated (T_m).

Normal pregnancy may decrease ability of PCT to reabsorb glucose and amino acids → glucosuria and aminoaciduria.

– so don't be shocked if u see ↑gluc & AA in urine (protein NOT albumin)

Glucosuria is an important clinical clue to diabetes mellitus.

Splay is the region of substance clearance between threshold and T_m; due to the heterogeneity of nephrons.

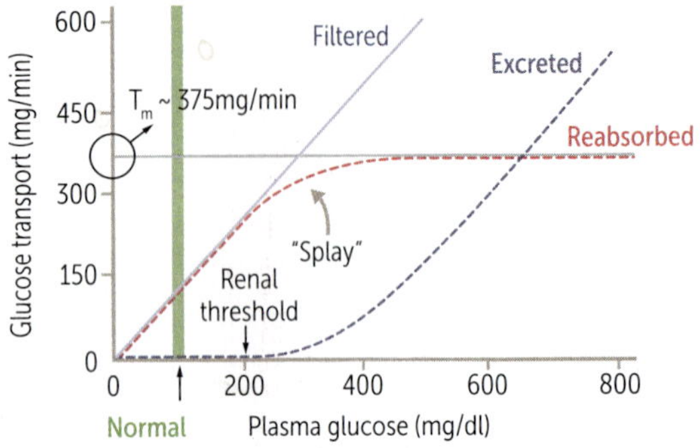

PCT

There a Na/gluc

CA turns filtered H_2CO_3 → $H_2O + CO_2$
then in cell to H + HCO_3^-

urine side = Cl in / HCO_3 out

basal = uniport HCO_3.

Nephron physiology

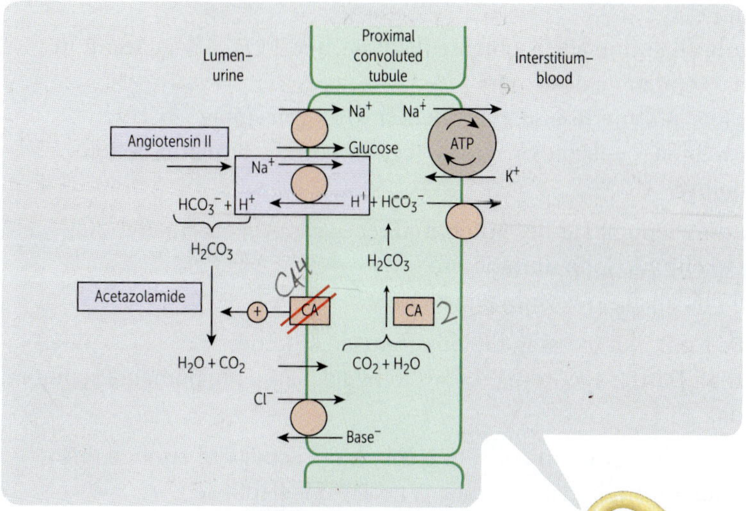

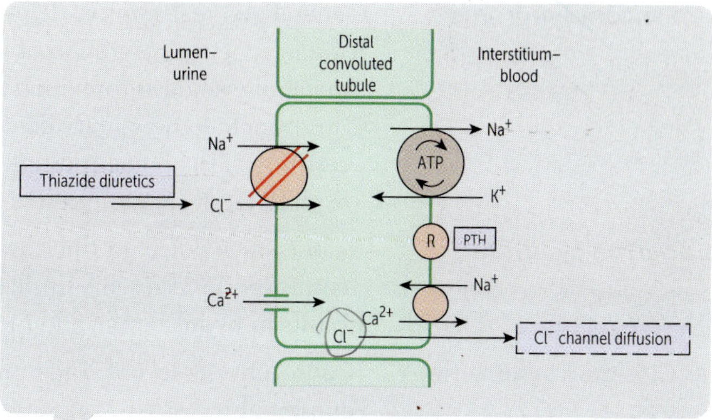

Early DCT—reabsorbs Na^+, Cl^-. Makes urine fully dilute (hypotonic).
PTH—↑ Ca^{2+}/Na^+ exchange → Ca^{2+} reabsorption.
5–10% Na^+ reabsorbed.

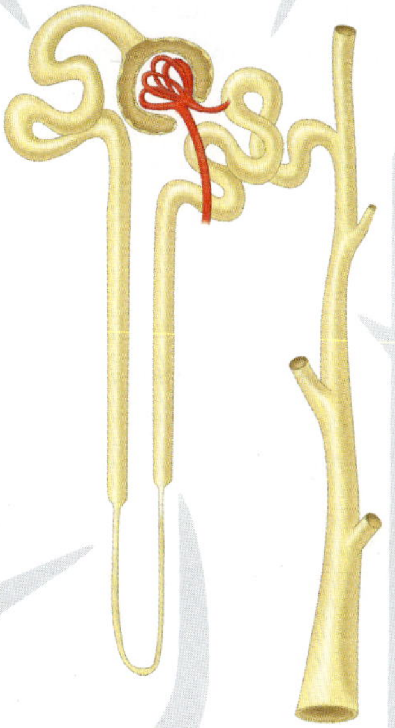

Early PCT—contains brush border. Reabsorbs all glucose and amino acids and most HCO_3^-, Na^+, Cl^-, PO_4^{3-}, K^+, H_2O, and uric acid. Isotonic absorption. Generates and secretes NH_3, which acts as a buffer for secreted H^+.
PTH—inhibits Na^+/PO_4^{3-} cotransport → PO_4^{3-} excretion.
AT II—stimulates Na^+/H^+ exchange → ↑ Na^+, H_2O, and HCO_3^- reabsorption (permitting contraction alkalosis).
65–80% Na^+ reabsorbed.

Thin descending loop of Henle—passively reabsorbs H_2O via medullary hypertonicity (impermeable to Na^+). Concentrating segment. Makes urine hypertonic.

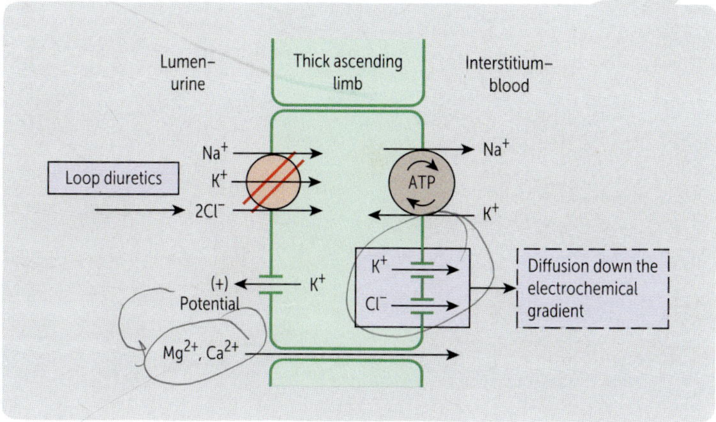

Thick ascending loop of Henle—reabsorbs Na^+, K^+, and Cl^-. Indirectly induces paracellular reabsorption of Mg^{2+} and Ca^{2+} through ⊕ lumen potential generated by K^+ backleak. Impermeable to H_2O. Makes urine less concentrated as it ascends.
10–20% Na^+ reabsorbed.

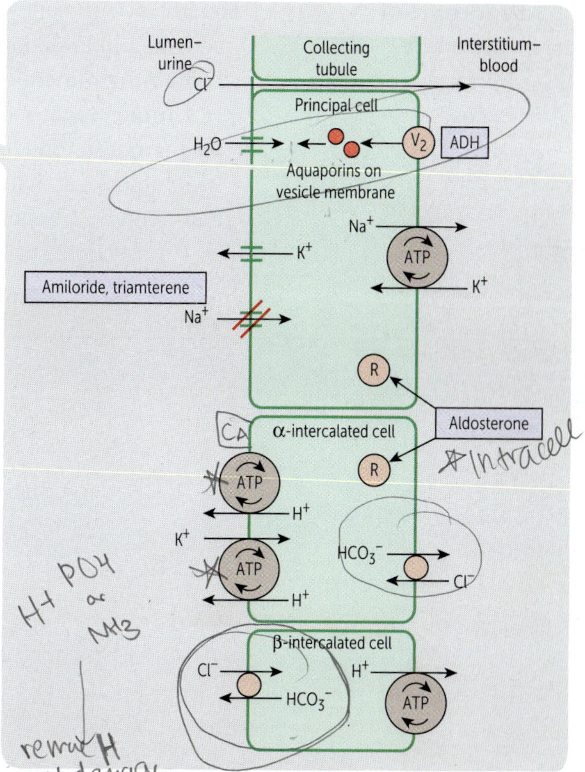

Collecting tubule—reabsorbs Na^+ in exchange for secreting K^+ and H^+ (regulated by aldosterone).
Aldosterone—acts on mineralocorticoid receptor → mRNA → protein synthesis. In principal cells: ↑ apical K^+ conductance, ↑ Na^+/K^+ pump, ↑ epithelial Na^+ channel (ENaC) activity → lumen negativity → K^+ secretion. In α-intercalated cells: lumen negativity → ↑ H^+ ATPase activity → ↑ H^+ secretion → ↑ HCO_3^-/Cl^- exchanger activity.
ADH—acts at V_2 receptor → insertion of aquaporin H_2O channels on apical side.
3–5% Na^+ reabsorbed.

Renal tubular defects	Fanconi syndrome is first (PCT), the rest are in **alphabetic** order.
Fanconi syndrome	Generalized reabsorptive defect in PCT. Associated with ↑ excretion of nearly all amino acids, glucose, HCO_3^-, and PO_4^{3-}. May result in metabolic acidosis (proximal renal tubular acidosis). Causes include hereditary defects (eg, Wilson disease, tyrosinemia, glycogen storage disease, cystinosis), ischemia, multiple myeloma, nephrotoxins/drugs (eg, ifosfamide, cisplatin, tenofovir, expired tetracyclines), lead poisoning.
Bartter syndrome AR	Reabsorptive defect in thick ascending loop of Henle. Autosomal recessive. Affects $Na^+/K^+/2Cl^-$ cotransporter. Presents similarly to chronic loop diuretic use. Results in hypokalemia and metabolic alkalosis with hypercalciuria.
Gitelman syndrome AR	Reabsorptive defect of NaCl in DCT. Similar to using lifelong thiazide diuretics. Autosomal recessive. Less severe than Bartter syndrome. Leads to hypokalemia, hypomagnesemia, metabolic alkalosis, hypocalciuria.
Liddle syndrome AD	Gain of function mutation → ↑ Na^+ reabsorption in collecting tubules (↑ activity of epithelial Na^+ channel). Presents like hyperaldosteronism, but aldosterone is nearly undetectable. Autosomal dominant. Results in hypertension, hypokalemia, metabolic alkalosis, ↓ aldosterone. Treatment: Amiloride.
Syndrome of Apparent Mineralocorticoid Excess key	Hereditary deficiency of 11β-hydroxysteroid dehydrogenase, which normally converts cortisol (can activate mineralocorticoid receptors) to cortisone (inactive on mineralocorticoid receptors) in cells containing mineralocorticoid receptors. Excess cortisol in these cells from enzyme deficiency → ↑ mineralocorticoid receptor activity → hypertension, hypokalemia, metabolic alkalosis. Low serum aldosterone levels. Can acquire disorder from glycyrrhetinic acid (present in licorice), which blocks activity of 11β-hydroxysteroid dehydrogenase. Treatment: corticosteroids (exogenous corticosteroids ↓ endogenous cortisol production → ↓ mineralocorticoid receptor activation). Cortisol tries to be the **SAME** as aldosterone.

licorice Ø 11β-OHsteroid

Relative concentrations along proximal convoluted tubules

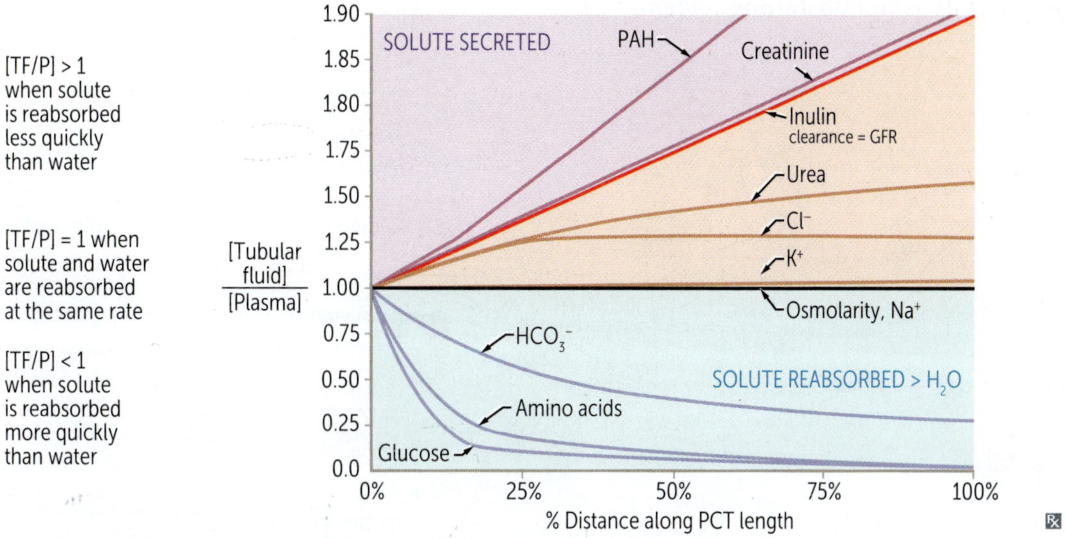

Tubular inulin ↑ in concentration (but not amount) along the PCT as a result of water reabsorption.
Cl^- reabsorption occurs at a slower rate than Na^+ in early PCT and then matches the rate of Na^+ reabsorption more distally. Thus, its relative concentration ↑ before it plateaus.

Renin-angiotensin-aldosterone system

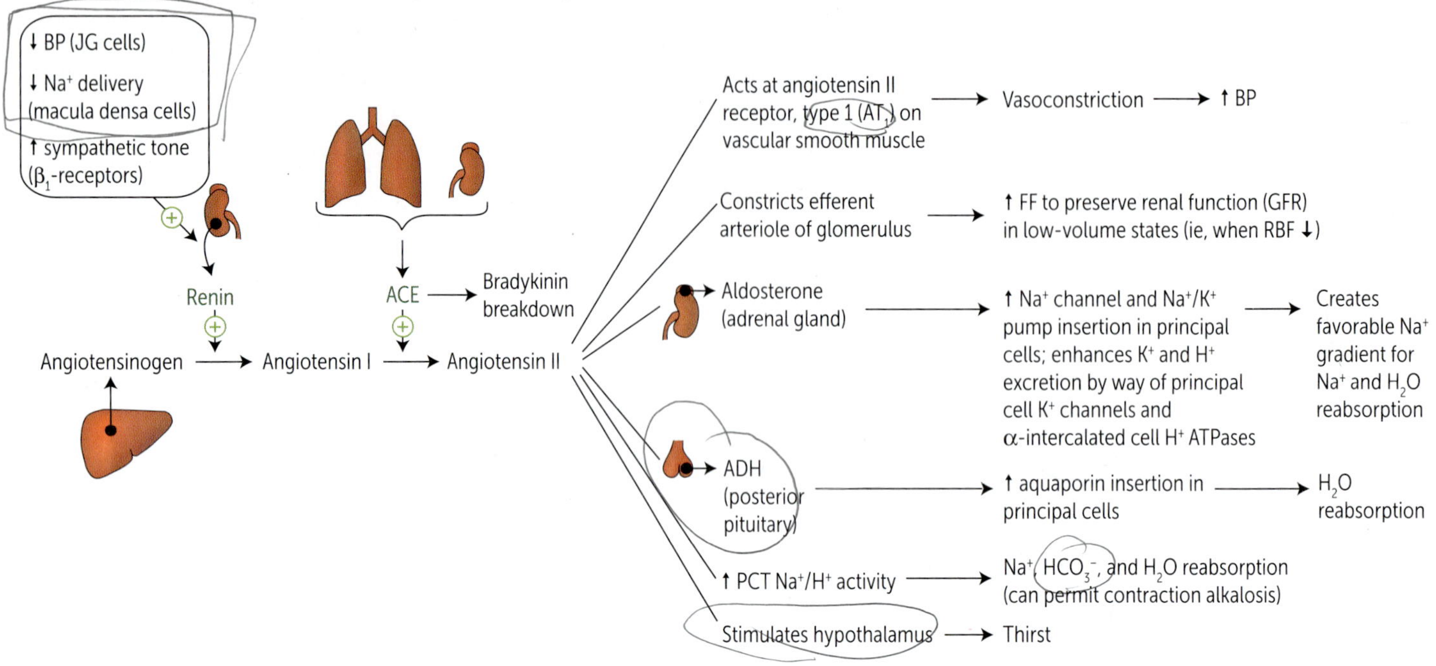

Renin	Secreted by JG cells in response to ↓ renal arterial pressure and ↑ renal sympathetic discharge (β_1 effect).
AT II	Affects baroreceptor function; limits reflex bradycardia, which would normally accompany its pressor effects. Helps maintain blood volume and blood pressure.
ANP, BNP	Released from atria (ANP) and ventricles (BNP) in response to ↑ volume; may act as a "check" on renin-angiotensin-aldosterone system; relaxes vascular smooth muscle via cGMP → ↑ GFR, ↓ renin. Dilates afferent arteriole, constricts efferent arteriole, promotes natriuresis.
ADH	Primarily regulates osmolarity; also responds to low blood volume states.
Aldosterone	Primarily regulates ECF volume and Na^+ content; responds to low blood volume states.

Juxtaglomerular apparatus

Consists of mesangial cells, JG cells (modified smooth muscle of afferent arteriole) and the macula densa (NaCl sensor, part of DCT). JG cells secrete renin in response to ↓ renal blood pressure and ↑ sympathetic tone (β_1). Macula densa cells sense ↓ NaCl delivery to DCT → ↑ renin release → efferent arteriole vasoconstriction → ↑ GFR.

JGA maintains GFR via renin-angiotensin-aldosterone system.
β-blockers can decrease BP by inhibiting β_1-receptors of the JGA → ↓ renin release.

Kidney endocrine functions

Erythropoietin	Released by interstitial cells in peritubular capillary bed in response to hypoxia.	Stimulates RBC proliferation in bone marrow. Erythropoietin often supplemented in chronic kidney disease.
Caciferol	PCT cells convert 25-OH vitamin D_3 to 1,25-$(OH)_2$ vitamin D_3 (calcitriol, active form).	25-OH D_3 → 1,25-$(OH)_2$ D_3 (1α-hydroxylase; ⊕ PTH)
Prostaglandins	Paracrine secretion vasodilates the afferent arterioles to ↑ RBF.	NSAIDs block renal-protective prostaglandin synthesis → constriction of afferent arteriole and ↓ GFR; this may result in acute renal failure in low renal blood flow states.
Dopamine	Secreted by PCT cells, promotes natriuresis. At low doses, dilates interlobular arteries, afferent arterioles, efferent arterioles → ↑ RBF, little or no change in GFR. At higher doses, acts as vasoconstrictor.	

Hormones acting on kidney

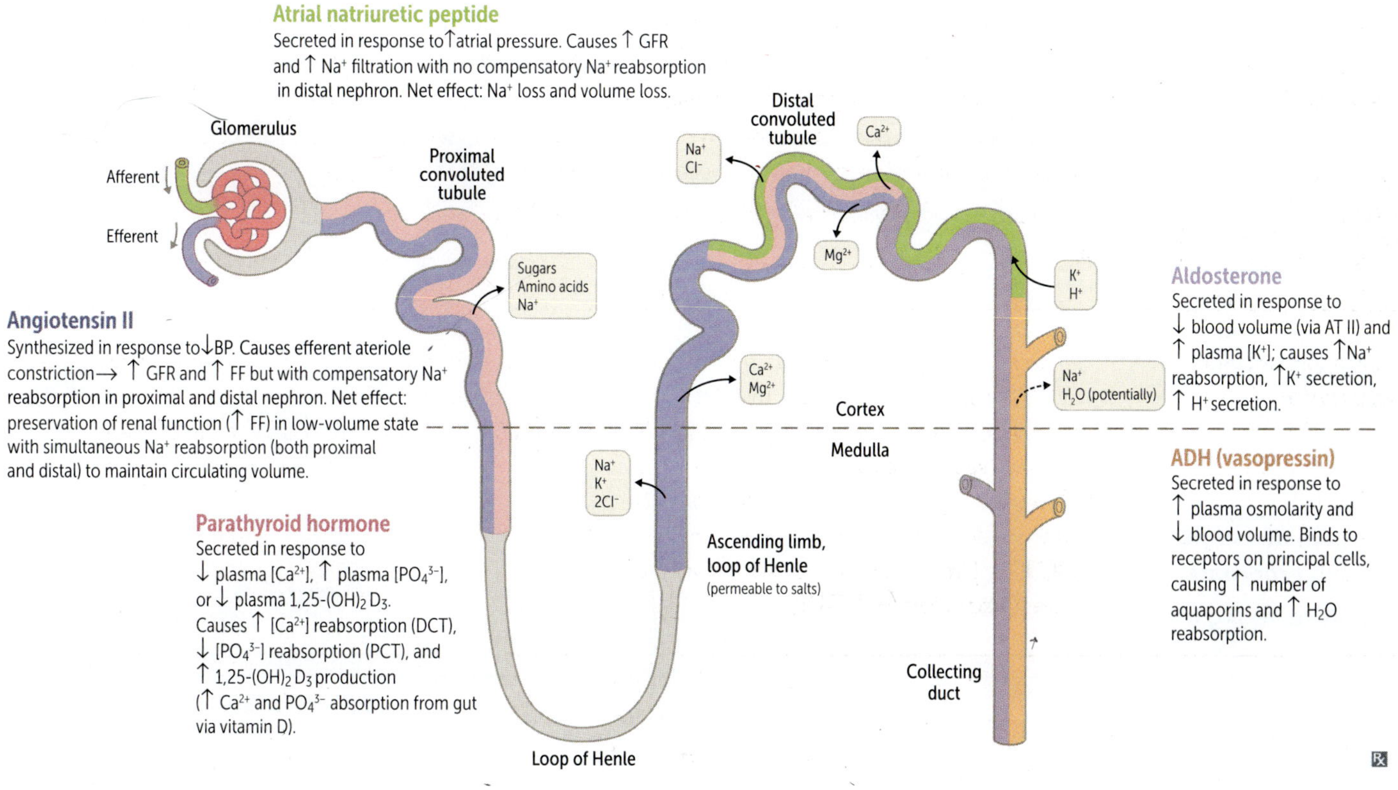

7 dehydrocholest + skin → cholecalcif —liver→ 25 OH vit D (calcidiol)
—kidney→ 1,25 OH vit D (calcitriol)
α1 OHase

Potassium shifts

SHIFTS K^+ OUT OF CELL (CAUSING HYPERKALEMIA)	SHIFTS K^+ INTO CELL (CAUSING HYPOKALEMIA)
Digitalis (blocks Na^+/K^+ ATPase)	
Hyper**O**smolarity	Hypo-osmolarity
Lysis of cells (eg, crush injury, rhabdomyolysis, tumor lysis syndrome)	
Acidosis	Alkalosis
β-blocker	β-adrenergic agonist (↑ Na^+/K^+ ATPase)
High blood **S**ugar (insulin deficiency)	Insulin (↑ Na^+/K^+ ATPase)
Patient with hyperkalemia? **DO LAβS**.	**In**sulin shifts K^+ **in**to cells

Electrolyte disturbances

ELECTROLYTE	LOW SERUM CONCENTRATION	HIGH SERUM CONCENTRATION
Na^+	Nausea and malaise, stupor, coma, seizures	Irritability, stupor, coma
K^+	U waves and flattened T waves on ECG, arrhythmias, muscle cramps, spasm, weakness	Wide QRS and peaked T waves on ECG, arrhythmias, muscle weakness
Ca^{2+}	Tetany, seizures, QT prolongation, twitching (Chvostek sign), spasm (Trousseau sign)	**Stones** (renal), **bones** (pain), **groans** (abdominal pain), **thrones** (↑ urinary frequency), **psychiatric overtones** (anxiety, altered mental status), but not necessarily calciuria
Mg^{2+}	Tetany, torsades de pointes, hypokalemia	↓ DTRs, lethargy, bradycardia, hypotension, cardiac arrest, hypocalcemia
PO_4^{3-}	Bone loss, osteomalacia (adults), rickets (children)	Renal stones, metastatic calcifications, hypocalcemia

Features of renal disorders

CONDITION	BLOOD PRESSURE	PLASMA RENIN	ALDOSTERONE	SERUM Mg^{2+}	URINE Ca^{2+}
Bartter syndrome	—	↑	↑		↑
Gitelman syndrome	—	↑	↑	↓	↓
Liddle syndrome	↑	↓	↓		
SIADH	↑	↓	↓		
Primary hyperaldosteronism (Conn syndrome)	↑	↓	↑		
Renin-secreting tumor	↑	↑	↑		

Acid-base physiology

	pH	P_{CO_2}	$[HCO_3^-]$	COMPENSATORY RESPONSE
Metabolic acidosis	↓	↓	↓	Hyperventilation (immediate)
Metabolic alkalosis	↑	↑	↑	Hypoventilation (immediate)
Respiratory acidosis	↓	↑	↑	↑ renal $[HCO_3^-]$ reabsorption (delayed)
Respiratory alkalosis	↑	↓	↓	↓ renal $[HCO_3^-]$ reabsorption (delayed)

Key: ↑ ↓ = 1° disturbance; ↓ ↑ = compensatory response.

1–2 days

Henderson-Hasselbalch equation: $pH = 6.1 + \log \frac{[HCO_3^-]}{0.03\ P_{CO_2}}$

Predicted respiratory compensation for a simple metabolic acidosis can be calculated using the Winters formula. If measured P_{CO_2} > predicted P_{CO_2} → concomitant respiratory acidosis; if measured P_{CO_2} < predicted P_{CO_2} → concomitant respiratory alkalosis:

$$P_{CO_2} = 1.5\ [HCO_3^-] + 8 \pm 2$$

Acidosis/alkalosis

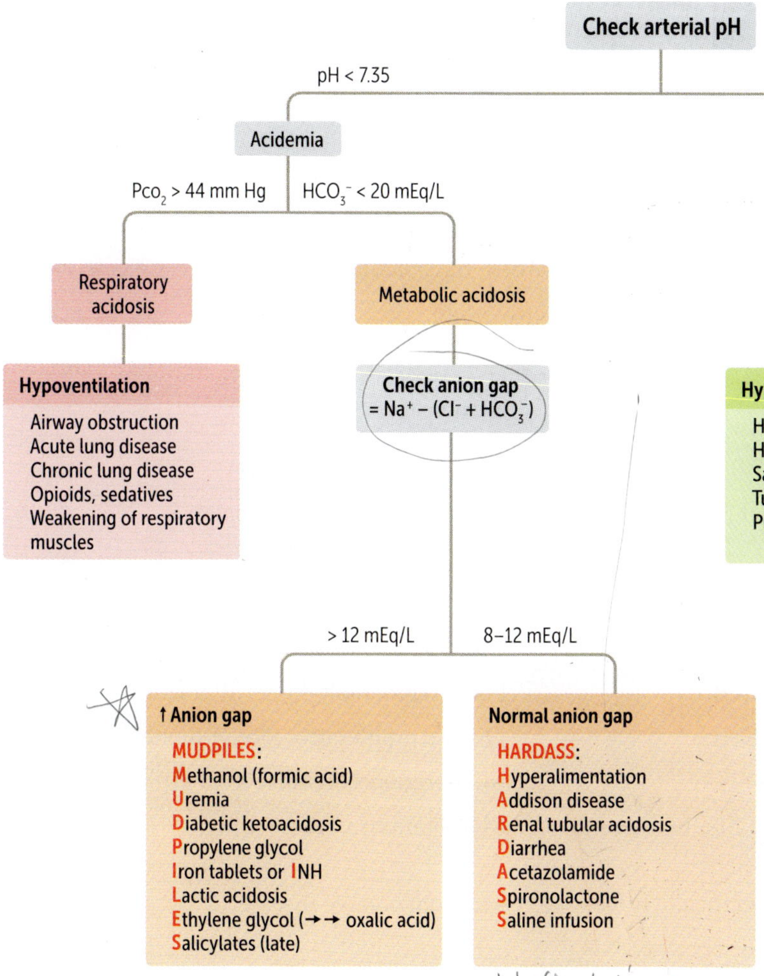

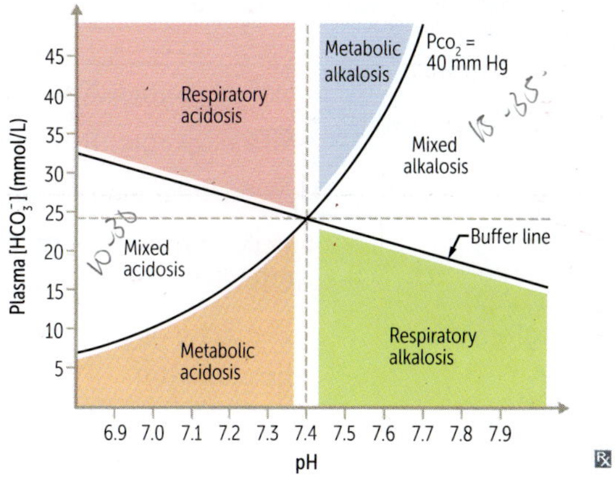

↓ HCO3 by:
– ↓ aldost
– ↓ reabs HCO3
– lose HCO3 from GI

Aspirin = 1st resp alk then metab acid

Renal tubular acidosis A disorder of the renal tubules that leads to normal anion gap (hyperchloremic) metabolic acidosis.

RTA TYPE	NOTES
Distal renal tubular acidosis (type 1)	Urine pH > 5.5. Defect in ability of α intercalated cells to secrete H^+ → no new HCO_3^- is generated → metabolic acidosis. Associated with **hypokalemia**, ↑ risk for calcium phosphate kidney stones (due to ↑ urine pH and ↑ bone turnover). Causes: amphotericin B toxicity, analgesic nephropathy, congenital anomalies (obstruction) of urinary tract.
Proximal renal tubular acidosis (type 2)	Urine pH < 5.5. Defect in PCT HCO_3^- reabsorption → ↑ excretion of HCO_3^- in urine and subsequent metabolic acidosis. Urine is acidified by α-intercalated cells in collecting tubule. Associated with **hypokalemia**, ↑ risk for hypophosphatemic rickets. Causes: Fanconi syndrome and carbonic anhydrase inhibitors.
Hyperkalemic renal tubular acidosis (type 4)	Urine pH < 5.5. Hypoaldosteronism → **hyperkalemia** → ↓ NH_3 synthesis in PCT → ↓ NH_4^+ excretion. Causes: ↓ aldosterone production (eg, diabetic hyporeninism, ACE inhibitors, ARBs, NSAIDs, heparin, cyclosporine, adrenal insufficiency) or aldosterone resistance (eg, K^+-sparing diuretics, nephropathy due to obstruction, TMP/SMX).

▸ RENAL—PATHOLOGY

Casts in urine	Presence of casts indicates that hematuria/pyuria is of glomerular or renal tubular origin. Bladder cancer, kidney stones → hematuria, no casts. Acute cystitis → pyuria, no casts.
RBC casts	Glomerulonephritis, malignant hypertension.
WBC casts	Tubulointerstitial inflammation, acute pyelonephritis, transplant rejection.
Fatty casts ("oval fat bodies")	Nephrotic syndrome. Associated with "Maltese cross" sign.
Granular ("muddy brown") casts	Acute tubular necrosis.
Waxy casts	End-stage renal disease/chronic renal failure.
Hyaline casts	Nonspecific, can be a normal finding, often seen in concentrated urine samples.

Nomenclature of glomerular disorders

TYPE	CHARACTERISTICS	EXAMPLE
Focal	< 50% of glomeruli are involved	Focal segmental glomerulosclerosis
Diffuse	> 50% of glomeruli are involved	Diffuse proliferative glomerulonephritis
Proliferative	Hypercellular glomeruli	Membranoproliferative glomerulonephritis
Membranous	Thickening of glomerular basement membrane (GBM)	Membranous nephropathy
Primary glomerular disease	A 1° disease of the kidney specifically impacting the glomeruli	Minimal change disease
Secondary glomerular disease	A systemic disease or disease of another organ system that also impacts the glomeruli	SLE, diabetic nephropathy

Glomerular diseases

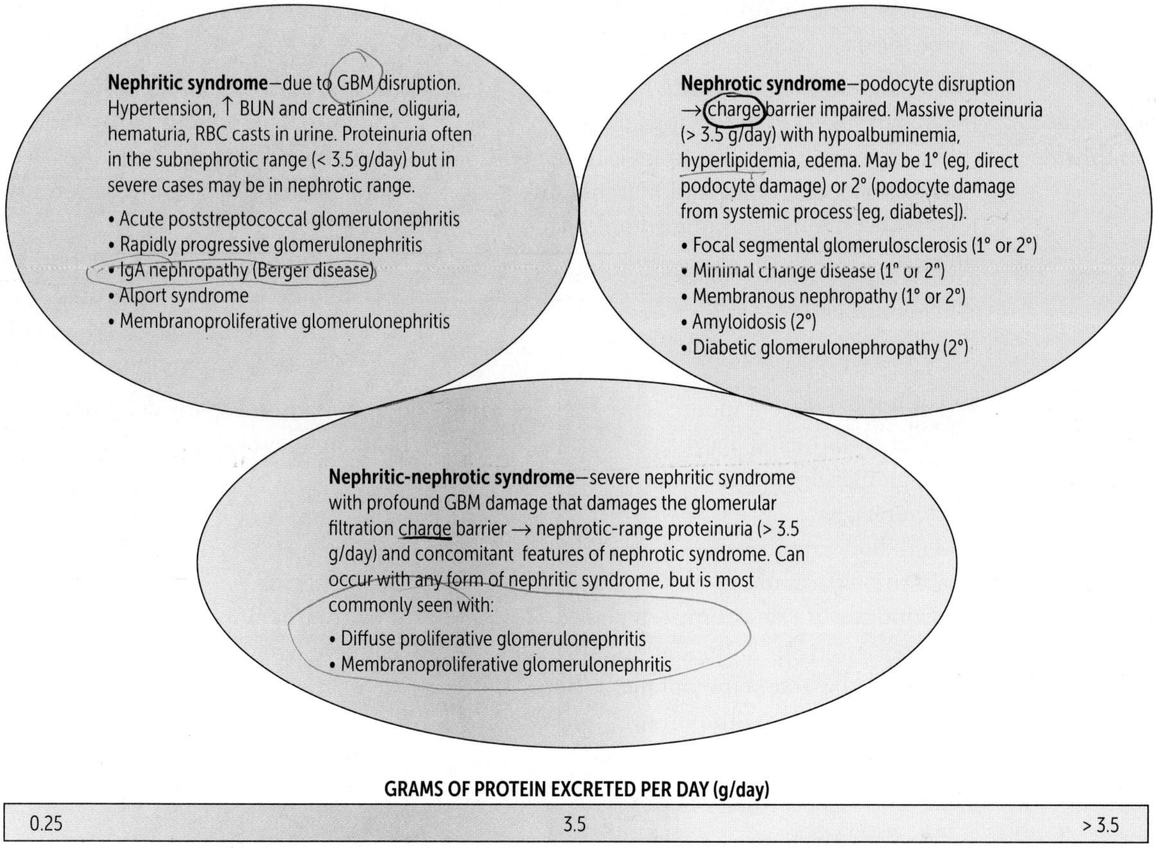

---

in α interc cells, we can reabsorb bicarb.
But, at a cost comes H so we have to secrete it
① H ATPase
② H/K ATPase
Type 1 RTA = can't excrete H. ← genetic defect or in HCO3/Cl antip or ampho/lithium making cells permeab. to H on lumen side

Type 2 = PCT can't abs. HCO3
genetic → Na/HCO3 transp.
(Distal cells can still acidify tho!)

Type 4 = ↓ Aldost or aldost resist in princip/α int
- Addis, gene - eNaC
- ↓ H ATPase = less H in lumen = ↓ NH3 excret.
↓ Na/K atpase
↓ enac

Nephritic syndrome NephrItic syndrome = Inflammatory process. When it involves glomeruli, it leads to hematuria and RBC casts in urine. Associated with azotemia, oliguria, hypertension (due to salt retention), proteinuria.

Acute poststreptococcal glomerulonephritis	LM—glomeruli enlarged and hypercellular A. IF—("starry sky") granular appearance ("lumpy-bumpy") B due to IgG, IgM, and C3 deposition along GBM and mesangium. EM—subepithelial immune complex (IC) humps.	Most frequently seen in children. Occurs ~ 2–4 weeks after group A streptococcal infection of pharynx or skin. Resolves spontaneously. Type III hypersensitivity reaction. Presents with peripheral and periorbital edema, cola-colored urine, hypertension. Positive strep titers/serologies, ↓ complement levels due to consumption.
Rapidly progressive (crescentic) glomerulonephritis	LM and IF—crescent moon shape C. Crescents consist of fibrin and plasma proteins (eg, C3b) with glomerular parietal cells, monocytes, macrophages. Several disease processes may result in this pattern, in particular:	Poor prognosis. Rapidly deteriorating renal function (days to weeks).
	▪ Goodpasture syndrome—type II hypersensitivity; antibodies to GBM and alveolar basement membrane → linear IF	Hematuria/hemoptysis. Treatment: emergent plasmapheresis.
	▪ Granulomatosis with polyangiitis (Wegener)	PR3-ANCA/c-ANCA. Pauci-immune (no Ig/C3 deposition).
	▪ Microscopic polyangiitis	MPO-ANCA/p-ANCA. Pauci-immune (no Ig/C3 deposition).
Diffuse proliferative glomerulonephritis	Due to SLE or membranoproliferative glomerulonephritis. LM—"wire looping" of capillaries. EM—subendothelial and sometimes intramembranous IgG-based ICs often with C3 deposition. IF—granular.	A common cause of death in SLE (think "wire lupus"). DPGN and MPGN often present as nephrotic syndrome and nephritic syndrome concurrently.
IgA nephropathy (Berger disease)	LM—mesangial proliferation. EM—mesangial IC deposits. IF—IgA-based IC deposits in mesangium. Renal pathology of Henoch-Schönlein purpura.	Episodic gross hematuria that occurs concurrently with respiratory or GI tract infections (IgA is secreted by mucosal linings). Not to be confused with Buerger disease (thromboangiitis obliterans).

mesAngium

Nephritic syndrome *(continued)*

Alport syndrome	Mutation in type IV collagen → thinning and splitting of glomerular basement membrane. Most commonly X-linked dominant.	Eye problems (eg, retinopathy, lens dislocation), glomerulonephritis, sensorineural deafness; "can't see, can't pee, can't hear a bee." "Basket-weave" appearance on EM.
Membrano-proliferative glomerulonephritis (MPGN)	Type I—subendothelial immune complex (IC) deposits with granular IF; "tram-track" appearance on PAS stain D and H&E stain E due to GBM splitting caused by mesangial ingrowth. Type II—also called dense deposit disease.	MPGN is a nephritic syndrome that often copresents with nephrotic syndrome. Type 1 may be 2° to hepatitis B or C infection. May also be idiopathic. Type II is associated with C3 nephritic factor (stabilizes C3 convertase → ↓ serum C3 levels).

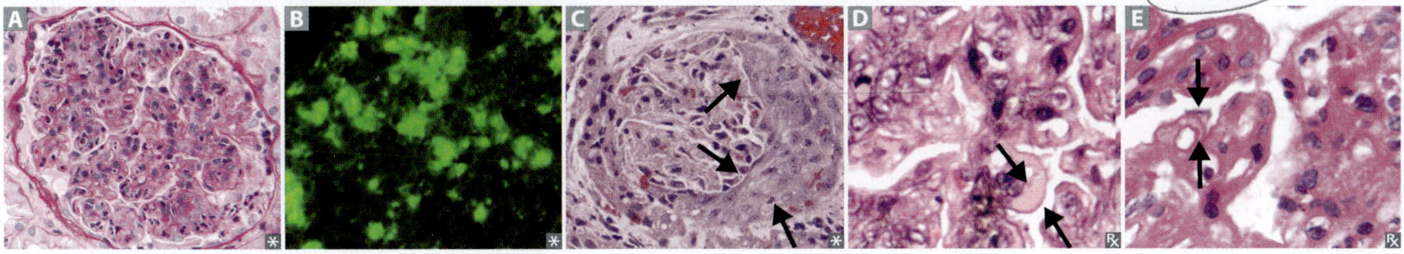

LM = light microscopy; EM = electron microscopy; IF = immunofluorescence.

Nephrotic syndrome	NephrOtic syndrome—massive prOteinuria (> 3.5 g/day) with hypoalbuminemia, resulting edema, hyperlipidemia. Frothy urine with fatty casts. Due to podocyte damage disrupting glomerular filtration charge barrier. May be 1° (eg, direct sclerosis of podocytes) or 2° (systemic process [eg, diabetes] secondarily damages podocytes). Associated with hypercoagulable state (eg, thromboembolism) due to antithrombin (AT) III loss in urine and ↑ risk of infection (due to loss of immunoglobulins in urine and soft tissue compromise by edema). Severe nephritic syndrome may present with nephrotic syndrome features (nephritic-nephrotic syndrome) if damage to GBM is severe enough to damage charge barrier.	
Minimal change disease (lipoid nephrosis)	LM—normal glomeruli (lipid may be seen in PCT cells). IF ⊖. EM—effacement of foot processes A.	Most common cause of nephrotic syndrome in children. Often 1° (idiopathic) and may be triggered by recent infection, immunization, immune stimulus. Rarely, may be 2° to lymphoma (eg, cytokine-mediated damage). 1° disease has excellent response to corticosteroids.
Focal segmental glomerulosclerosis	LM—segmental sclerosis and hyalinosis B. IF—often ⊖, but may be ⊕ for nonspecific focal deposits of IgM, C3, C1.. EM—effacement of foot process similar to minimal change disease.	Most common cause of nephrotic syndrome in African Americans and Hispanics. Can be 1° (idiopathic) or 2° to other conditions (eg, HIV infection, sickle cell disease, heroin abuse, massive obesity, interferon treatment, chronic kidney disease due to congenital malformations). 1° disease has inconsistent response to steroids. May progress to chronic renal disease.
Membranous nephropathy (membranous glomerulonephritis)	LM—diffuse capillary and GBM thickening C. IF—granular as a result of immune complex deposition. Nephrotic presentation of SLE. EM—"spike and dome" appearance with subepithelial deposits.	Most common cause of 1° nephrotic syndrome in Caucasian adults. Can be 1° (eg, antibodies to phospholipase A_2 receptor) or 2° to drugs (eg, NSAIDs, penicillamine), infections (eg, HBV, HCV), SLE, or solid tumors. 1° disease has poor response to steroids. May progress to chronic renal disease.
Amyloidosis	LM—Congo red stain shows apple-green birefringence under polarized light due to amyloid deposition in the mesangium.	Kidney is the most commonly involved organ (systemic amyloidosis). Associated with chronic conditions that predispose to amyloid deposition (eg, AL amyloid, AA amyloid).
Diabetic glomerulonephropathy	LM—mesangial expansion, GBM thickening, eosinophilic nodular glomerulosclerosis (Kimmelstiel-Wilson lesions, arrows in D).	Nonenzymatic glycosylation of GBM → ↑ permeability, thickening. Nonenzymatic glycosylation of efferent arterioles → ↑ GFR → mesangial expansion. Most common cause of end-stage renal disease in the United States.

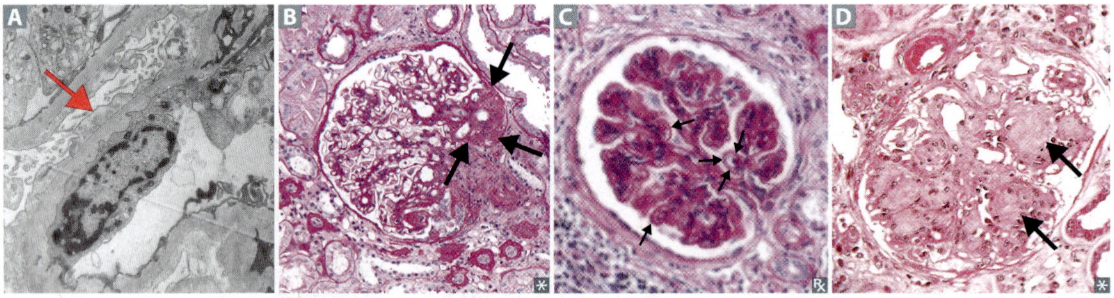

Kidney stones

Can lead to severe complications such as hydronephrosis, pyelonephritis. Presents with unilateral flank tenderness, colicky pain radiating to groin, hematuria. Treat and prevent by encouraging fluid intake.

Most common kidney stone presentation: calcium oxalate stone in patient with hypercalciuria and normocalcemia.

CONTENT	PRECIPITATES WITH	X-RAY FINDINGS	CT FINDINGS	URINE CRYSTAL	NOTES
Calcium	Calcium oxalate: hypocitraturia	Radiopaque	Radiopaque	Shaped like envelope A or dumbbell	Calcium stones most common (80%); calcium oxalate more common than calcium phosphate stones. Hypocitraturia often associated with ↓ urine pH. Can result from ethylene glycol (antifreeze) ingestion, vitamin C abuse, hypocitraturia, malabsorption (eg, Crohn disease). Treatment: thiazides, citrate, low-sodium diet.
	Calcium phosphate: ↑ pH	Radiopaque	Radiopaque	Wedge-shaped prism	Treatment: thiazides.
Ammonium magnesium phosphate	↑ pH	Radiopaque	Radiopaque	Coffin lid B	Also known as struvite; account for 15% of stones. Caused by infection with urease ⊕ bugs (eg, *Proteus mirabilis*, *Staphylococcus saprophyticus*, *Klebsiella*) that hydrolyze urea to ammonia → urine alkalinization. Commonly form staghorn calculi C. Treatment: eradication of underlying infection, surgical removal of stone.
Uric acid	↓ pH	RadiolUcent	Minimally visible	Rhomboid D or rosettes	About 5% of all stones. Risk factors: ↓ urine volume, arid climates, acidic pH. Visible on ultrasound. Strong association with hyperuricemia (eg, gout). Often seen in diseases with ↑ cell turnover, such as leukemia. Treatment: alkalinization of urine, allopurinol.
Cystine	↓ pH	Radiolucent	Sometimes visible	Hexagonal E	Hereditary (autosomal recessive) condition in which Cystine-reabsorbing PCT transporter loses function, causing cystinuria. Transporter defect also results in poor reabsorption of Ornithine, Lysine, Arginine (COLA). Cystine is poorly soluble, thus stones form in urine. Usually begins in childhood. Can form staghorn calculi. Sodium cyanide nitroprusside test ⊕. "SIXtine" stones have SIX sides. Treatment: low sodium diet, alkalinization of urine, chelating agents if refractory.

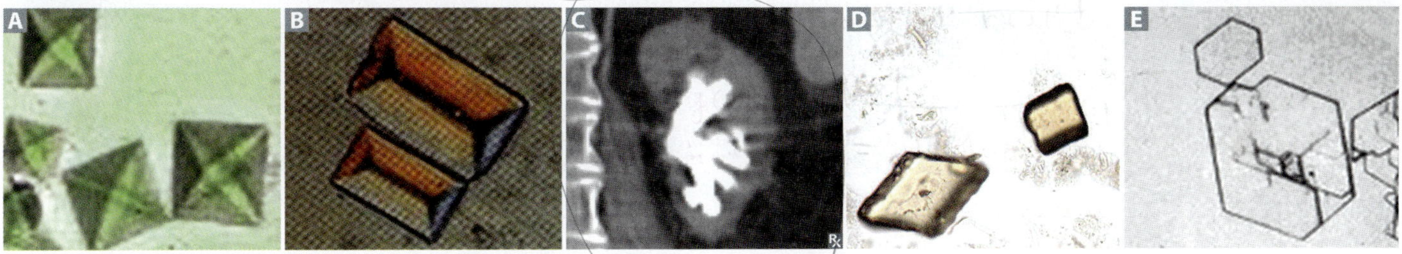

Hydronephrosis

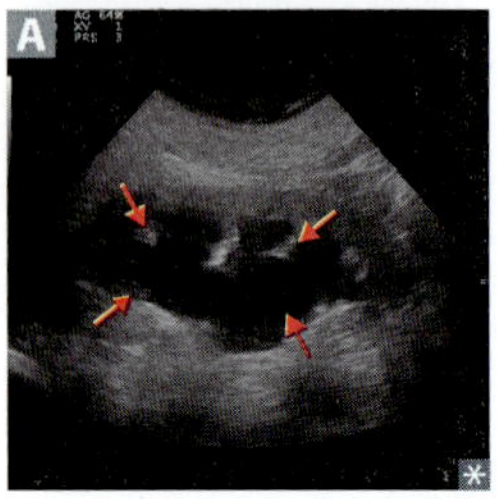

Distention/dilation of renal pelvis and calyces A. Usually caused by urinary tract obstruction (eg, renal stones, BPH, cervical cancer, injury to ureter); other causes include retroperitoneal fibrosis, vesicoureteral reflux. Dilation occurs proximal to site of pathology. Serum creatinine becomes elevated only if obstruction is bilateral or if patient has only one kidney. Leads to compression and possible atrophy of renal cortex and medulla.

Renal cell carcinoma

Originates from PCT cells → polygonal clear cells A filled with accumulated lipids and carbohydrates. Often golden-yellow B due to ↑ lipid content. Most common in men 50–70 years old. ↑ incidence with smoking and obesity. Manifests clinically with hematuria, palpable mass, 2° polycythemia, flank pain, fever, weight loss. Invades renal vein then IVC and spreads hematogenously; metastasizes to lung and bone.

Treatment: resection if localized disease. Immunotherapy (eg, aldesleukin) or targeted therapy for advanced/metastatic disease. Resistant to chemotherapy and radiation therapy.

Most common 1° renal malignancy C.

Associated with gene deletion on chromosome 3 (sporadic or inherited as von Hippel-Lindau syndrome). **RCC** = **3** letters = chromosome **3**.

Associated with paraneoplastic syndromes (eg, ectopic EPO, ACTH, PTHrP, renin).

"Silent" cancer because commonly presents as a metastatic neoplasm.

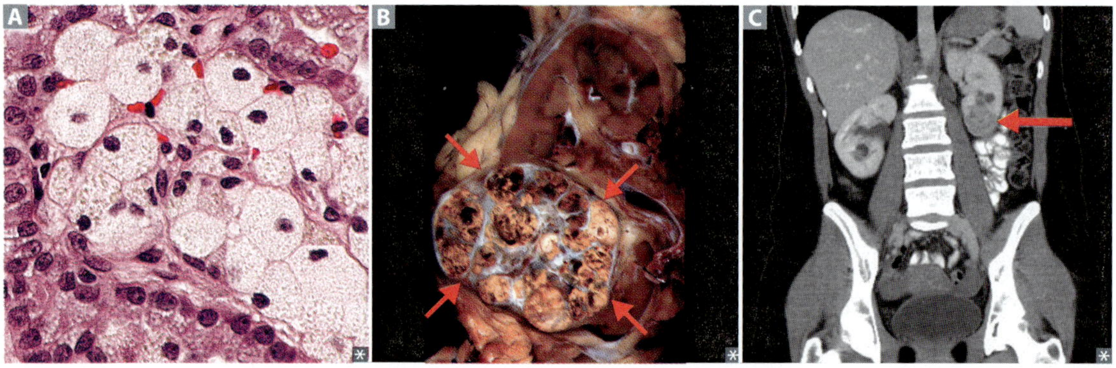

Renal oncocytoma

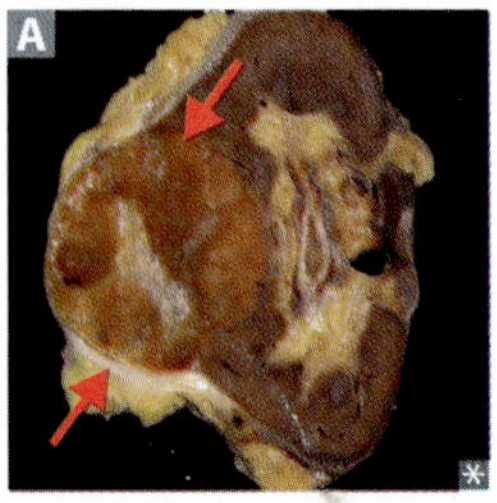

Benign epithelial cell tumor arising from collecting ducts (arrows in A point to well-circumscribed mass with central scar).

Large eosinophilic cells with abundant mitochondria without perinuclear clearing B (vs chromophobe renal cell carcinoma).

Presents with painless hematuria, flank pain, abdominal mass.

Often resected to exclude malignancy (eg, renal cell carcinoma).

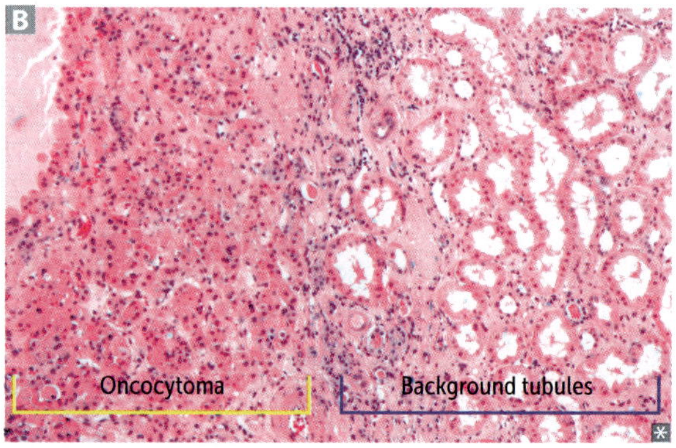

Wilms tumor (nephroblastoma)

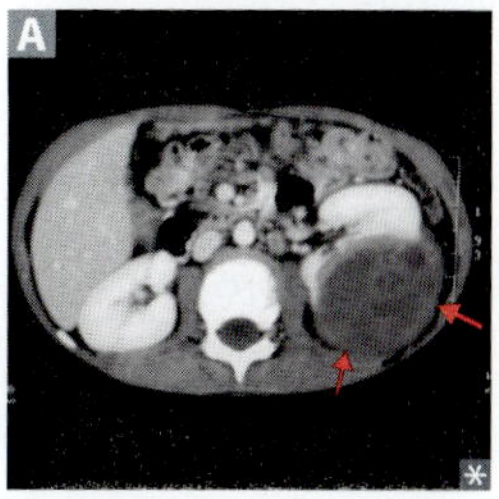

Most common renal malignancy of early childhood (ages 2–4). Contains embryonic glomerular structures. Presents with large, palpable, unilateral flank mass A and/or hematuria.

"Loss of function" mutations of tumor suppressor genes *WT1* or *WT2* on chromosome 11.

May be a part of several syndromes:

- **W**AGR complex: **W**ilms tumor, **A**niridia (absence of iris), **G**enitourinary malformations, mental **R**etardation/intellectual disability (*WT1* deletion)
- Denys-Drash: Wilms tumor, early-onset nephrotic syndrome, male pseudohermaphroditism (*WT1* mutation)
- Beckwith-Wiedemann: Wilms tumor, macroglossia, organomegaly, hemihypertrophy (*WT2* mutation)

Transitional cell carcinoma

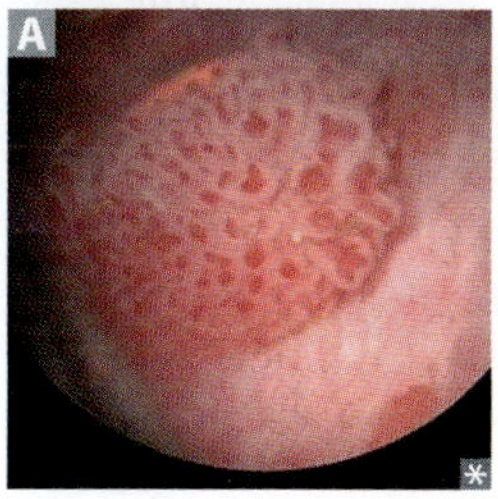

Most common tumor of urinary tract system (can occur in renal calyces, renal pelvis, ureters, and bladder) A B. Painless hematuria (no casts) suggests bladder cancer.

Associated with problems in your **P**ee **SAC**: **P**henacetin, **S**moking, **A**niline dyes, and **C**yclophosphamide.

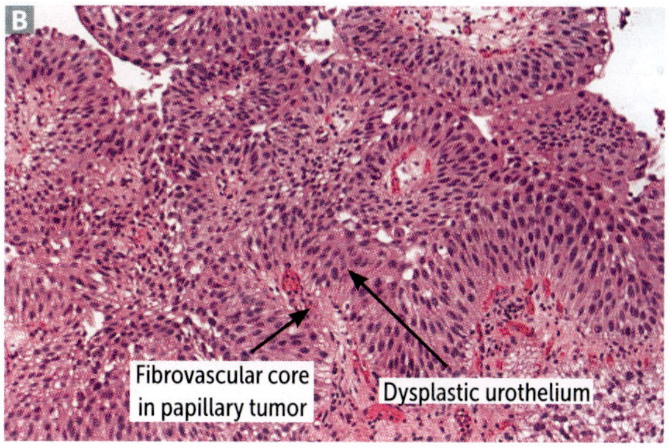

Squamous cell carcinoma of the bladder

Chronic irritation of urinary bladder → squamous metaplasia → dysplasia and squamous cell carcinoma.

Risk factors include *Schistosoma haematobium* infection (Middle East), chronic cystitis, smoking, chronic nephrolithiasis. Presents with painless hematuria.

Urinary incontinence

Stress incontinence	Outlet incompetence (urethral hypermobility or intrinsic sphincteric deficiency) → leak with ↑ intra-abdominal pressure (eg, sneezing, lifting). ↑ risk with obesity, vaginal delivery, prostate surgery. ⊕ bladder stress test (directly observed leakage from urethra upon coughing or Valsalva maneuver). Treatment: pelvic floor muscle strengthening (Kegel) exercises, weight loss, pessaries.
Urgency incontinence	Overactive bladder (detrusor instability) → leak with urge to void immediately. Treatment: Kegel exercises, bladder training (timed voiding, distraction or relaxation techniques), antimuscarinics (eg, oxybutynin).
Mixed incontinence	Features of both stress and urgency incontinence.
Overflow incontinence	Incomplete emptying (detrusor underactivity or outlet obstruction) → leak with overfilling. ↑ post-void residual (urinary retention) on catheterization or ultrasound. Treatment: catheterization, relieve obstruction (eg, α-blockers for BPH).

Urinary tract infection (acute bacterial cystitis)

Inflammation of urinary bladder. Presents as suprapubic pain, dysuria, urinary frequency, urgency. Systemic signs (eg, high fever, chills) are usually absent.

Risk factors include female gender (short urethra), sexual intercourse ("honeymoon cystitis"), indwelling catheter, diabetes mellitus, impaired bladder emptying.

Causes:

- *E coli* (most common).
- *Staphylococcus saprophyticus*—seen in sexually active young women (*E coli* is still more common in this group).
- *Klebsiella*.
- *Proteus mirabilis*—urine has ammonia scent.

Lab findings: ⊕ leukocyte esterase. ⊕ nitrites (indicate gram ⊖ organisms, especially *E coli*). Sterile pyuria and ⊖ urine cultures suggest urethritis by *Neisseria gonorrhoeae* or *Chlamydia trachomatis*.

Pyelonephritis

Acute pyelonephritis

Neutrophils infiltrate renal interstitium A. Affects cortex with relative sparing of glomeruli/vessels. Presents with fevers, flank pain (costovertebral angle tenderness), nausea/vomiting, chills.

Causes include ascending UTI (*E coli* is most common), hematogenous spread to kidney. Presents with WBCs in urine +/– WBC casts. CT would show striated parenchymal enhancement B.

Risk factors include indwelling urinary catheter, urinary tract obstruction, vesicoureteral reflux, diabetes mellitus, pregnancy.

Complications include chronic pyelonephritis, renal papillary necrosis, perinephric abscess, urosepsis.

Treatment: antibiotics.

Chronic pyelonephritis

The result of recurrent episodes of acute pyelonephritis. Typically requires predisposition to infection such as vesicoureteral reflux or chronically obstructing kidney stones.

Coarse, asymmetric corticomedullary scarring, blunted calyx. Tubules can contain eosinophilic casts resembling thyroid tissue C (thyroidization of kidney).

Xanthogranulomatous pyelonephritis—rare; characterized by widespread kidney damage due to granulomatous tissue containing foamy macrophages.

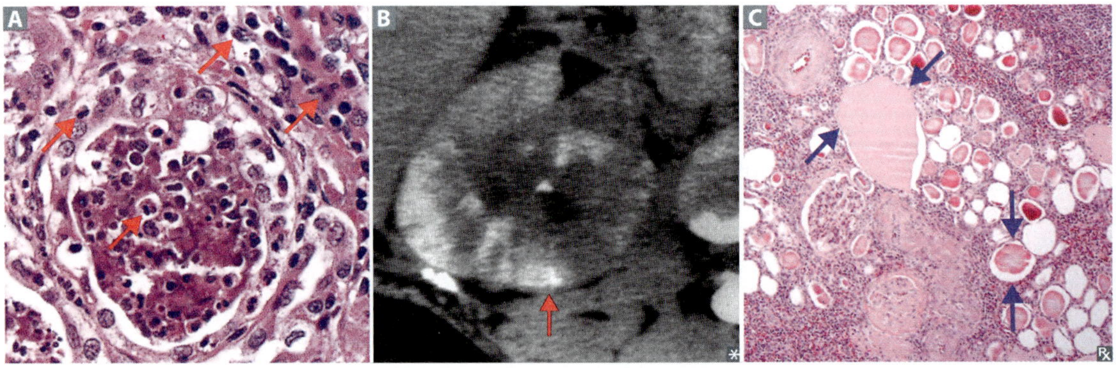

Diffuse cortical necrosis

Acute generalized cortical infarction of both kidneys. Likely due to a combination of vasospasm and DIC.

Associated with obstetric catastrophes (eg, abruptio placentae), septic shock.

Renal osteodystrophy

Hypocalcemia, hyperphosphatemia, and failure of vitamin D hydroxylation associated with chronic renal disease → 2° hyperparathyroidism. Hyperphosphatemia also independently ↓ serum Ca^{2+} by causing tissue calcifications, whereas ↓ 1,25-$(OH)_2$ D_3 → ↓ intestinal Ca^{2+} absorption. Causes subperiosteal thinning of bones.

Acute kidney injury (acute renal failure)

Acute kidney injury is defined as an abrupt decline in renal function as measured by ↑ creatinine and ↑ BUN.

Prerenal azotemia

Due to ↓ RBF (eg, hypotension) → ↓ GFR. Na^+/H_2O and BUN retained by kidney in an attempt to conserve volume → ↑ BUN/creatinine ratio (BUN is reabsorbed, creatinine is not) and ↓ FENa.

Intrinsic renal failure

Generally due to acute tubular necrosis or ischemia/toxins; less commonly due to acute glomerulonephritis (eg, RPGN, hemolytic uremic syndrome) or acute interstitial nephritis. In ATN, patchy necrosis → debris obstructing tubule and fluid backflow across necrotic tubule → ↓ GFR. Urine has epithelial/granular casts. BUN reabsorption is impaired → ↓ BUN/creatinine ratio.

Postrenal azotemia

Due to outflow obstruction (stones, BPH, neoplasia, congenital anomalies). Develops only with bilateral obstruction.

	Prerenal	Intrinsic renal	Postrenal
Urine osmolality (mOsm/kg)	> 500	< 350	< 350
Urine Na^+ (mEq/L)	< 20	> 40	> 40
FENa	< 1%	> 2%	> 1% (mild) > 2% (severe)
Serum BUN/Cr	> 20	< 15	Varies

Consequences of renal failure

Inability to make urine and excrete nitrogenous wastes.

Consequences (**MAD HUNGER**):

- **M**etabolic **A**cidosis
- **D**yslipidemia (especially ↑ triglycerides)
- **H**yperkalemia
- **U**remia—clinical syndrome marked by ↑ BUN:
  - Nausea and anorexia
  - Pericarditis
  - Asterixis
  - Encephalopathy
  - Platelet dysfunction
- **N**a^+/H_2O retention (HF, pulmonary edema, hypertension)
- **G**rowth retardation and developmental delay
- **E**rythropoietin failure (anemia)
- **R**enal osteodystrophy

2 forms of renal failure: acute (eg, ATN) and chronic (eg, hypertension, diabetes mellitus, congenital anomalies).

Acute interstitial nephritis (tubulointerstitial nephritis)

Acute interstitial renal inflammation. Pyuria (classically eosinophils) and azotemia occurring after administration of drugs that act as haptens, inducing hypersensitivity (eg, diuretics, penicillin derivatives, proton pump inhibitors, sulfonamides, rifampin, NSAIDs). Less commonly may be 2° to other processes such as systemic infections (eg, mycoplasma) or autoimmune diseases (eg, Sjögren syndrome, SLE, sarcoidosis).

Associated with fever, rash, hematuria, and costovertebral angle tenderness, but can be asymptomatic.

Remember these P's:

- Pee (diuretics)
- Pain-free (NSAIDs)
- Penicillins and cephalosporins
- Proton pump inhibitors
- RifamPin

Acute tubular necrosis

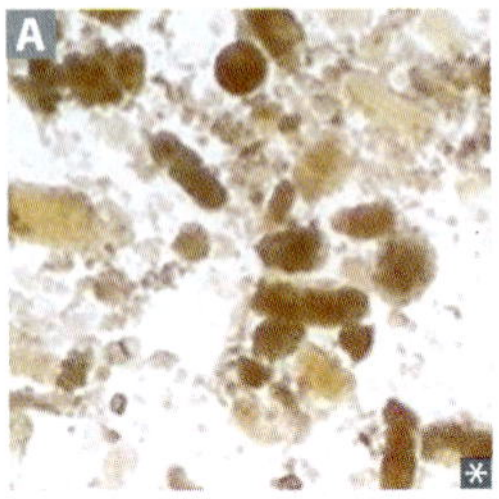

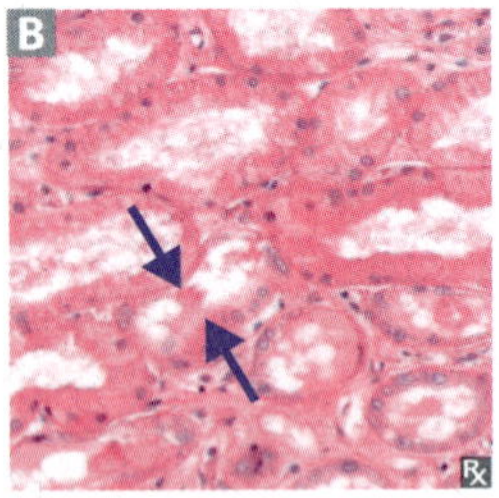

Most common cause of acute kidney injury in hospitalized patients. Spontaneously resolves in many cases. Can be fatal, especially during initial oliguric phase. ↑ FENa.

Key finding: granular ("muddy brown") casts A.

3 stages:

1. Inciting event
2. Maintenance phase—oliguric; lasts 1–3 weeks; risk of hyperkalemia, metabolic acidosis, uremia
3. Recovery phase—polyuric; BUN and serum creatinine fall; risk of hypokalemia

Can be caused by ischemic or nephrotoxic injury:

- Ischemic—2° to ↓ renal blood flow (eg, hypotension, shock, sepsis, hemorrhage, HF). Results in death of tubular cells that may slough into tubular lumen B (PCT and thick ascending limb are highly susceptible to injury).
- Nephrotoxic—2° to injury resulting from toxic substances (eg, aminoglycosides, radiocontrast agents, lead, cisplatin), crush injury (myoglobinuria), hemoglobinuria. PCT is particularly susceptible to injury.

Renal papillary necrosis

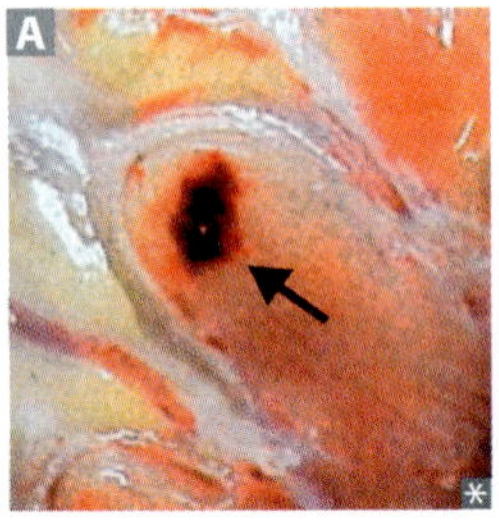

Sloughing of necrotic renal papillae A → gross hematuria and proteinuria. May be triggered by recent infection or immune stimulus. Associated with sickle cell disease or trait, acute pyelonephritis, NSAIDs, diabetes mellitus.

SAAD papa with papillary necrosis:

Sickle cell disease or trait
Acute pyelonephritis
Analgesics (NSAIDs)
Diabetes mellitus

Renal cyst disorders

Autosomal dominant polycystic kidney disease	Numerous cysts in cortex and medulla A causing bilateral enlarged kidneys ultimately destroy kidney parenchyma. Presents with flank pain, hematuria, hypertension, urinary infection, progressive renal failure in ~ 50% of individuals. Mutation in *PKD1* (85% of cases, chromosome 16) or *PKD2* (15% of cases, chromosome 4). Death from complications of chronic kidney disease or hypertension (caused by ↑ renin production). Associated with berry aneurysms, mitral valve prolapse, benign hepatic cysts. Treatment: ACE inhibitors or ARBs.
Autosomal recessive polycystic kidney disease	Cystic dilation of collecting ducts B. Often presents in infancy. Associated with congenital hepatic fibrosis. Significant oliguric renal failure in utero can lead to Potter sequence. Concerns beyond neonatal period include systemic hypertension, progressive renal insufficiency, and portal hypertension from congenital hepatic fibrosis.
Medullary cystic disease	Inherited disease causing tubulointerstitial fibrosis and progressive renal insufficiency with inability to concentrate urine. Medullary cysts usually not visualized; shrunken kidneys on ultrasound. Poor prognosis.
Simple vs complex renal cysts	Simple cysts are filled with ultrafiltrate (anechoic on ultrasound C). Very common and account for majority of all renal masses. Found incidentally and typically asymptomatic. Complex cysts, including those that are septated, enhanced, or have solid components on imaging require follow-up or removal due to risk of renal cell carcinoma.

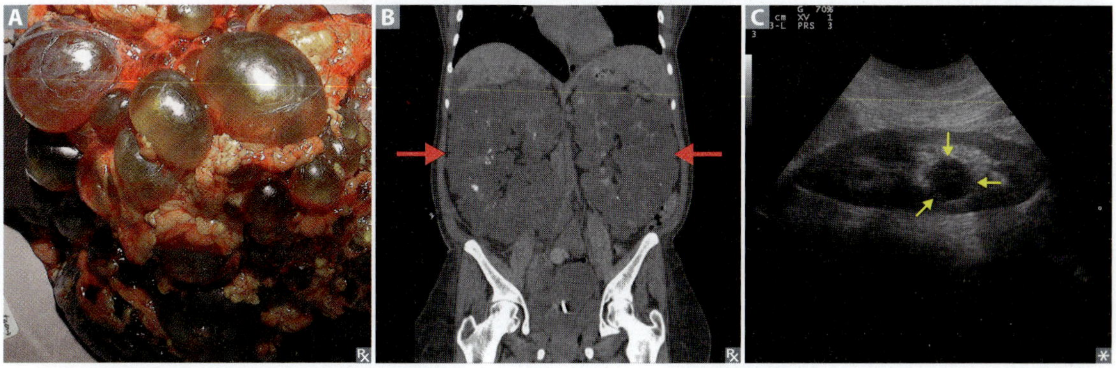

▶ RENAL—PHARMACOLOGY

Diuretics: site of action

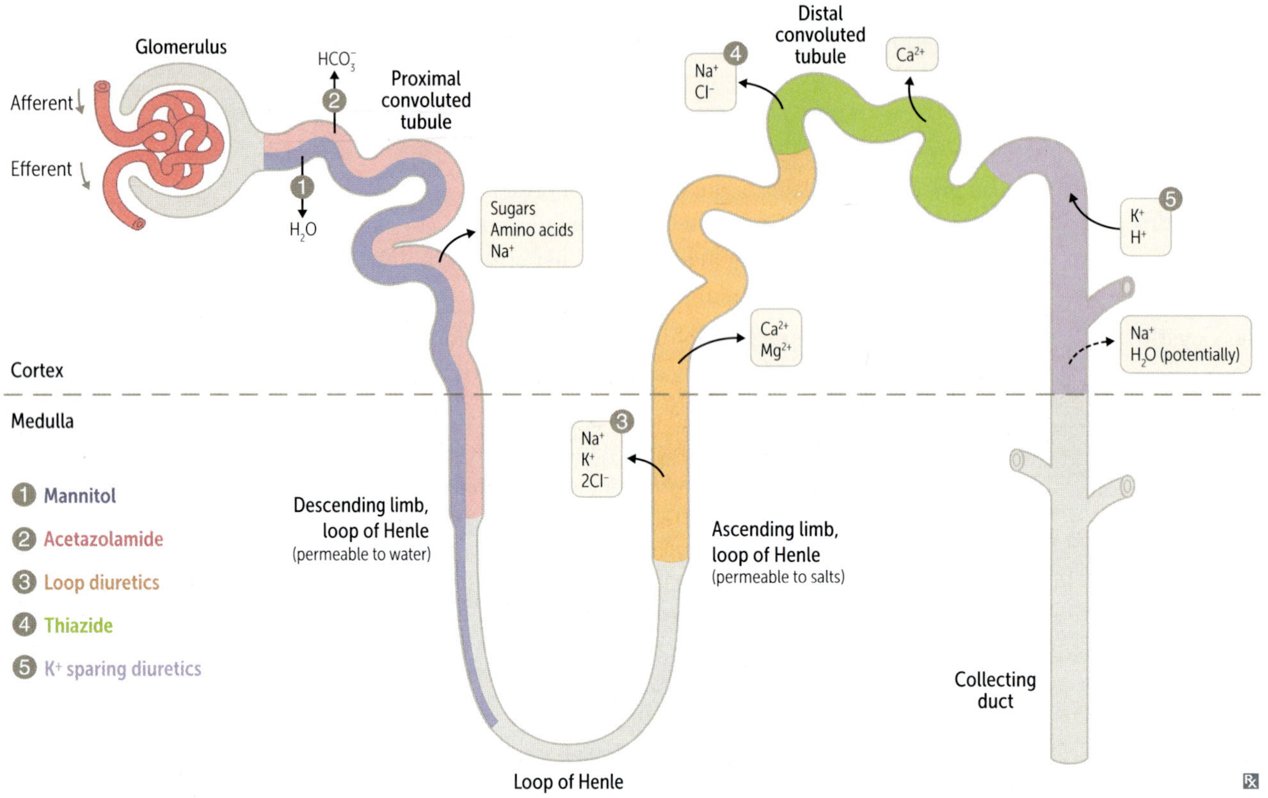

Mannitol

MECHANISM	Osmotic diuretic. ↑ tubular fluid osmolarity → ↑ urine flow, ↓ intracranial/intraocular pressure.	
CLINICAL USE	Drug overdose, elevated intracranial/intraocular pressure.	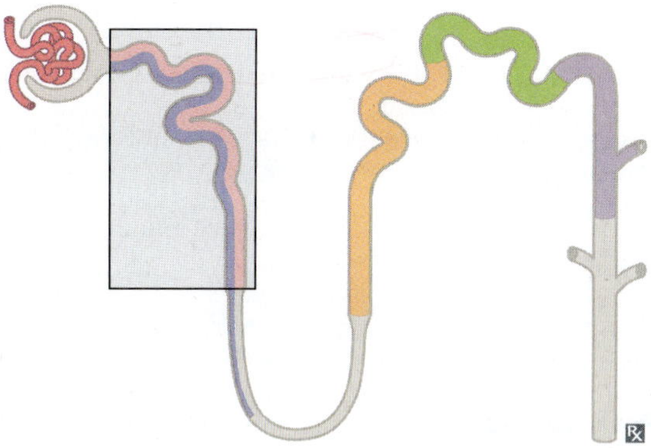
ADVERSE EFFECTS	Pulmonary edema, dehydration. Contraindicated in anuria, HF.	

Acetazolamide

MECHANISM	Carbonic anhydrase inhibitor. Causes self-limited $NaHCO_3$ diuresis and ↓ total body HCO_3^- stores.	
CLINICAL USE	Glaucoma, urinary alkalinization, metabolic alkalosis, altitude sickness, pseudotumor cerebri.	
ADVERSE EFFECTS	Proximal renal tubular acidosis, paresthesias, NH_3 toxicity, sulfa allergy.	"ACID"azolamide causes ACIDosis.

Loop diuretics

Furosemide, bumetanide, torsemide

MECHANISM	Sulfonamide loop diuretics. Inhibit cotransport system ($Na^+/K^+/2Cl^-$) of thick ascending limb of loop of Henle. Abolish hypertonicity of medulla, preventing concentration of urine. Stimulate PGE release (vasodilatory effect on afferent arteriole); inhibited by NSAIDs. ↑ Ca^{2+} excretion. Loops Lose Ca^{2+}.	
CLINICAL USE	Edematous states (HF, cirrhosis, nephrotic syndrome, pulmonary edema), hypertension, hypercalcemia.	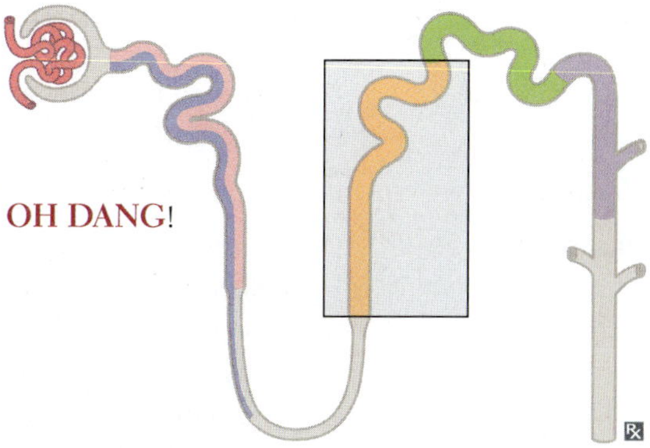
ADVERSE EFFECTS	Ototoxicity, Hypokalemia, Dehydration, Allergy (sulfa)/metabolic Alkalosis, Nephritis (interstitial), Gout.	OH DANG!

Ethacrynic acid

MECHANISM	Nonsulfonamide inhibitor of cotransport system ($Na^+/K^+/2Cl^-$) of thick ascending limb of loop of Henle.	
CLINICAL USE	Diuresis in patients allergic to sulfa drugs.	
ADVERSE EFFECTS	Similar to furosemide, but more ototoxic.	Loop earrings hurt your ears.

Thiazide diuretics — Hydrochlorothiazide, chlorthalidone, metolazone.

MECHANISM	Inhibit NaCl reabsorption in early DCT → ↓ diluting capacity of nephron. ↓ Ca^{2+} excretion.
CLINICAL USE	Hypertension, HF, idiopathic hypercalciuria, nephrogenic diabetes insipidus, osteoporosis.
ADVERSE EFFECTS	Hypokalemic metabolic alkalosis, hyponatremia, hyperGlycemia, hyperLipidemia, hyperUricemia, hyperCalcemia. Sulfa allergy.

HyperGLUC.

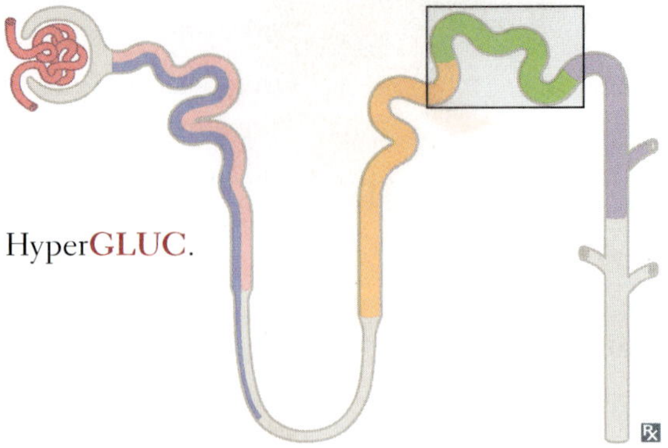

Potassium-sparing diuretics — Spironolactone and eplerenone; Triamterene, and Amiloride.

The K^+ STAys.

MECHANISM	Spironolactone and eplerenone are competitive aldosterone receptor antagonists in cortical collecting tubule. Triamterene and amiloride act at the same part of the tubule by blocking Na^+ channels in the cortical collecting tubule.
CLINICAL USE	Hyperaldosteronism, K^+ depletion, HF, hepatic ascites (spironolactone), nephrogenic DI (amiloride).
ADVERSE EFFECTS	Hyperkalemia (can lead to arrhythmias), endocrine effects with spironolactone (eg, gynecomastia, antiandrogen effects).

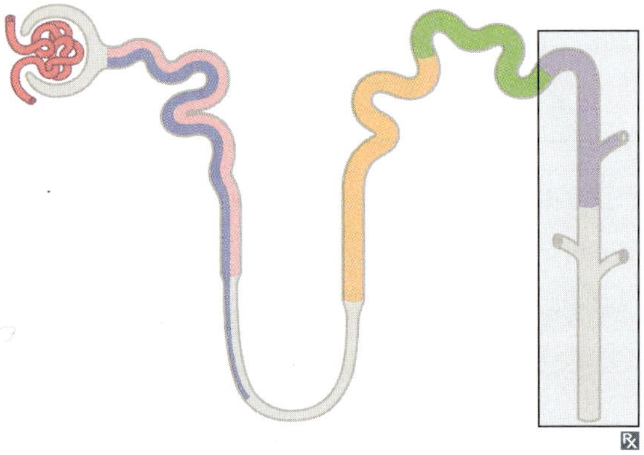

Diuretics: electrolyte changes

Urine NaCl	↑ with all diuretics (strength varies based on potency of diuretic effect). Serum NaCl may decrease as a result.
Urine K^+	↑ especially with loop and thiazide diuretics. Serum K^+ may decrease as a result.
Blood pH	↓ (**acidemia**): carbonic anhydrase inhibitors: ↓ HCO_3^- reabsorption. K^+ sparing: aldosterone blockade prevents K^+ secretion and H^+ secretion. Additionally, hyperkalemia leads to K^+ entering all cells (via H^+/K^+ exchanger) in exchange for H^+ exiting cells. ↑ (**alkalemia**): loop diuretics and thiazides cause alkalemia through several mechanisms: ▪ Volume contraction → ↑ AT II → ↑ Na^+/H^+ exchange in PCT → ↑ HCO_3^- reabsorption ("contraction alkalosis") ▪ K^+ loss leads to K^+ exiting all cells (via H^+/K^+ exchanger) in exchange for H^+ entering cells ▪ In low K^+ state, H^+ (rather than K^+) is exchanged for Na^+ in cortical collecting tubule → alkalosis and "paradoxical aciduria"
Urine Ca^{2+}	↑ with loop diuretics: ↓ paracellular Ca^{2+} reabsorption → hypocalcemia. ↓ with thiazides: enhanced Ca^{2+} reabsorption.

Angiotensin-converting enzyme inhibitors	Captopril, enalapril, lisinopril, ramipril.	
MECHANISM	Inhibit ACE → ↓ AT II → ↓ GFR by preventing constriction of efferent arterioles. ↑ renin due to loss of negative feedback. Inhibition of ACE also prevents inactivation of bradykinin, a potent vasodilator.	
CLINICAL USE	Hypertension, HF (↓ mortality), proteinuria, diabetic nephropathy. Prevent unfavorable heart remodeling as a result of chronic hypertension.	In diabetic nephropathy, ↓ intraglomerular pressure, slowing GBM thickening.
ADVERSE EFFECTS	**C**ough, **A**ngioedema (due to ↑ bradykinin; contraindicated in C1 esterase inhibitor deficiency), **T**eratogen (fetal renal malformations), ↑ **C**reatinine (↓ GFR), **H**yperkalemia, and **H**ypotension. Used with caution in bilateral renal artery stenosis, because ACE inhibitors will further ↓ GFR → renal failure.	Captopril's **CATCHH**.

Angiotensin II receptor blockers	Losartan, candesartan, valsartan.
MECHANISM	Selectively block binding of angiotensin II to AT_1 receptor. Effects similar to ACE inhibitors, but ARBs do not increase bradykinin.
CLINICAL USE	Hypertension, HF, proteinuria, or diabetic nephropathy with intolerance to ACE inhibitors (eg, cough, angioedema).
ADVERSE EFFECTS	Hyperkalemia, ↓ GFR, hypotension; teratogen.

Aliskiren	
MECHANISM	Direct renin inhibitor, blocks conversion of angiotensinogen to angiotensin I.
CLINICAL USE	Hypertension.
ADVERSE EFFECTS	Hyperkalemia, ↓ GFR, hypotension. Relatively contraindicated in patients already taking ACE inhibitors or ARBs.

▶ NOTES

Reproductive

"Artificial insemination is when the farmer does it to the cow instead of the bull."

—Student essay

"Whoever called it necking was a poor judge of anatomy."

—Groucho Marx

"See, the problem is that God gives men a brain and a penis, and only enough blood to run one at a time."

—Robin Williams

"I think you can say that life is a system in which proteins and nucleic acids interact in ways that allow the structure to grow and reproduce. It's that growth and reproduction, the ability to make more of yourself, that's important."

—Andrew H. Knloo

▶ REPRODUCTIVE—EMBRYOLOGY

Important genes of embryogenesis

Sonic hedgehog gene	Produced at base of limbs in zone of polarizing activity. Involved in patterning along anteroposterior axis and CNS development; mutation can cause holoprosencephaly.
***Wnt-7* gene**	Produced at apical ectodermal ridge (thickened ectoderm at distal end of each developing limb). Necessary for proper organization along dorsal-ventral axis.
***FGF* gene**	Produced at apical ectodermal ridge. Stimulates mitosis of underlying mesoderm, providing for lengthening of limbs.
Homeobox (Hox) genes	Involved in segmental organization of embryo in a craniocaudal direction. Code for transcription factors. Hox mutations → appendages in wrong locations.

Early fetal development

Early embryonic development

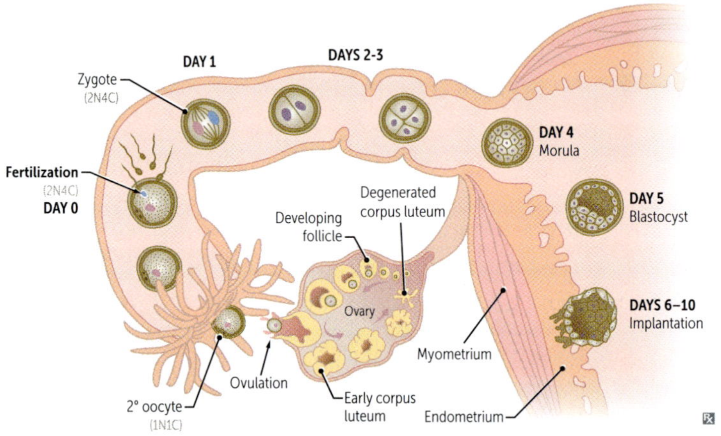

Within week 1	hCG secretion begins around the time of implantation of blastocyst.	Blastocyst "sticks" at day 6
Within week 2	Bilaminar disc (epiblast, hypoblast).	2 weeks = 2 layers.
Within week 3	Gastrulation forms trilaminar embryonic disc. Cells from epiblast invaginate → primitive streak → endoderm, mesoderm, ectoderm. Notochord arises from midline mesoderm; overlying ectoderm becomes neural plate.	3 weeks = 3 layers.
Weeks 3–8 (embryonic period)	Neural tube formed by neuroectoderm and closes by week 4. Organogenesis.	Extremely susceptible to teratogens.
Week 4	Heart begins to beat. Upper and lower limb buds begin to form.	4 weeks = 4 limbs and 4 heart chambers.
Week 6	Fetal cardiac activity visible by transvaginal ultrasound.	
Week 8	Fetal movements start.	Gait at week 8.
Week 10	Genitalia have male/female characteristics.	

Embryologic derivatives

Ectoderm		External/outer layer
Surface ectoderm	Epidermis; adenohypophysis (from Rathke pouch); lens of eye; epithelial linings of oral cavity, sensory organs of ear, and olfactory epithelium; epidermis; anal canal below the pectinate line; parotid, sweat, mammary glands.	Craniopharyngioma—benign Rathke pouch tumor with cholesterol crystals, calcifications.
Neuroectoderm	Brain (neurohypophysis, CNS neurons, oligodendrocytes, astrocytes, ependymal cells, pineal gland), retina spinal cord.	Neuroectoderm—think CNS.
Neural crest	PNS (dorsal root ganglia, cranial nerves, autonomic ganglia, Schwann cells), melanocytes, chromaffin cells of adrenal medulla, parafollicular (C) cells of thyroid, pia and arachnoid, bones of the skull, odontoblasts, aorticopulmonary septum, endocardial cushions.	Neural crest—think PNS and non-neural structures nearby.
Mesoderm	Muscle, bone, connective tissue, serous linings of body cavities (eg, peritoneum), spleen (derived from foregut mesentery), cardiovascular structures, lymphatics, blood, wall of gut tube, upper vagina, kidneys, adrenal cortex, dermis, testes, ovaries. Notochord induces ectoderm to form neuroectoderm (neural plate). Its only postnatal derivative is the nucleus pulposus of the intervertebral disc.	Middle/"meat" layer. Mesodermal defects = VACTERL: Vertebral defects Anal atresia Cardiac defects Tracheo-Esophageal fistula Renal defects Limb defects (bone and muscle)
Endoderm	Gut tube epithelium (including anal canal above the pectinate line), most of urethra and lower vagina (derived from urogenital sinus), luminal epithelial derivatives (eg, lungs, liver, gallbladder, pancreas, eustachian tube, thymus, parathyroid, thyroid follicular cells).	"Enternal" layer.

Types of errors in organ morphogenesis

Agenesis	Absent organ due to absent primordial tissue.
Aplasia	Absent organ despite presence of primordial tissue. oh
Hypoplasia	Incomplete organ development; primordial tissue present.
Disruption	2° breakdown of previously normal tissue or structure (eg, amniotic band syndrome).
Deformation	Extrinsic disruption; occurs after embryonic period.
Malformation	Intrinsic disruption; occurs during embryonic period (weeks 3–8).
Sequence	Abnormalities result from a single 1° embryologic event (eg, oligohydramnios → Potter sequence).

Teratogens Most susceptible in 3rd–8th weeks (embryonic period—organogenesis) of pregnancy. Before week 3, "all-or-none" effects. After week 8, growth and function affected.

TERATOGEN	EFFECTS ON FETUS	NOTES
Medications		
ACE inhibitors	Renal damage	
Alkylating agents	Absence of digits, multiple anomalies	
Aminoglycosides	Ototoxicity	**A mean guy** hit the baby in the ear.
Antiepileptic drugs	Neural tube defects, cardiac defects, cleft palate, skeletal abnormalities (eg, phalanx/nail hypoplasia, facial dysmorphism)	High-dose folate supplementation recommended. Most commonly valproate, carbamazepine, phenytoin, phenobarbital.
Diethylstilbestrol	Vaginal clear cell adenocarcinoma, congenital Müllerian anomalies	
Folate antagonists	Neural tube defects	Includes trimethoprim, methotrexate, antiepileptic drugs.
Isotretinoin	Multiple severe birth defects	Contraception mandatory. Iso**TERAT**inoin.
Lithium	Ebstein anomaly (apical displacement of tricuspid valve)	
Methimazole	Aplasia cutis congenita	
Tetracyclines	Discolored teeth, inhibited bone growth	"**Teeth**racyclines."
Thalidomide	Limb defects (phocomelia, micromelia—"flipper" limbs)	**Limb** defects with "tha-**limb**-domide."
Warfarin	Bone deformities, fetal hemorrhage, abortion, ophthalmologic abnormalities	Do not wage **warfar**e on the baby; keep it **hep**py with **hep**arin (does not cross placenta).
Substance abuse		
Alcohol	Common cause of birth defects and intellectual disability; fetal alcohol syndrome	
Cocaine	Low birth weight, preterm birth, IUGR, placental abruption	Cocaine → vasoconstriction.
Smoking (nicotine, CO)	Low birth weight (leading cause in developed countries), preterm labor, placental problems, IUGR, SIDS	Nicotine → vasoconstriction. CO → impaired O_2 delivery.
Other		
Iodine (lack or excess)	Congenital goiter or hypothyroidism (cretinism)	
Maternal diabetes	Caudal regression syndrome (anal atresia to sirenomelia), congenital heart defects, neural tube defects, macrosomia	
Methylmercury	Neurotoxicity	Highest in swordfish, shark, tilefish, king mackerel.
Vitamin A excess	Extremely high risk for spontaneous abortions and birth defects (cleft palate, cardiac)	
X-rays	Microcephaly, intellectual disability	Minimized by lead shielding.

Fetal alcohol syndrome

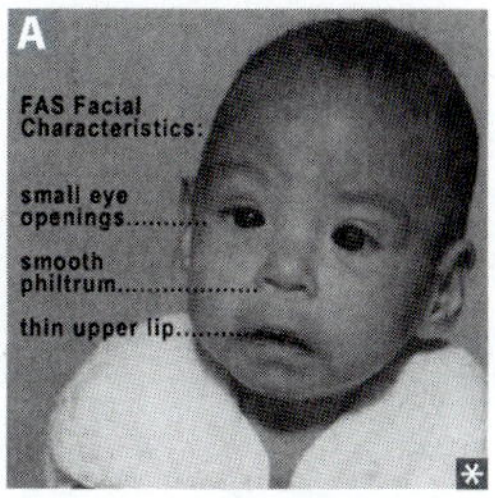

Leading cause of intellectual disability in the US. Newborns of alcohol-consuming mothers have ↑ incidence of congenital abnormalities, including pre- and postnatal developmental retardation, microcephaly, facial abnormalities A (eg, smooth philtrum, thin vermillion border [upper lip], small palpebral fissures), limb dislocation, heart defects. Heart-lung fistulas and holoprosencephaly in most severe form. Mechanism is failure of cell migration.

Twinning

Dizygotic ("fraternal") twins arise from 2 eggs that are separately fertilized by 2 different sperm (always 2 zygotes) and will have 2 separate amniotic sacs and 2 separate placentas (chorions).

Monozygotic ("identical") twins arise from 1 fertilized egg (1 egg + 1 sperm) that splits in early pregnancy. The timing of cleavage determines chorionicity (number of chorions) and amnionicity (number of amnions).

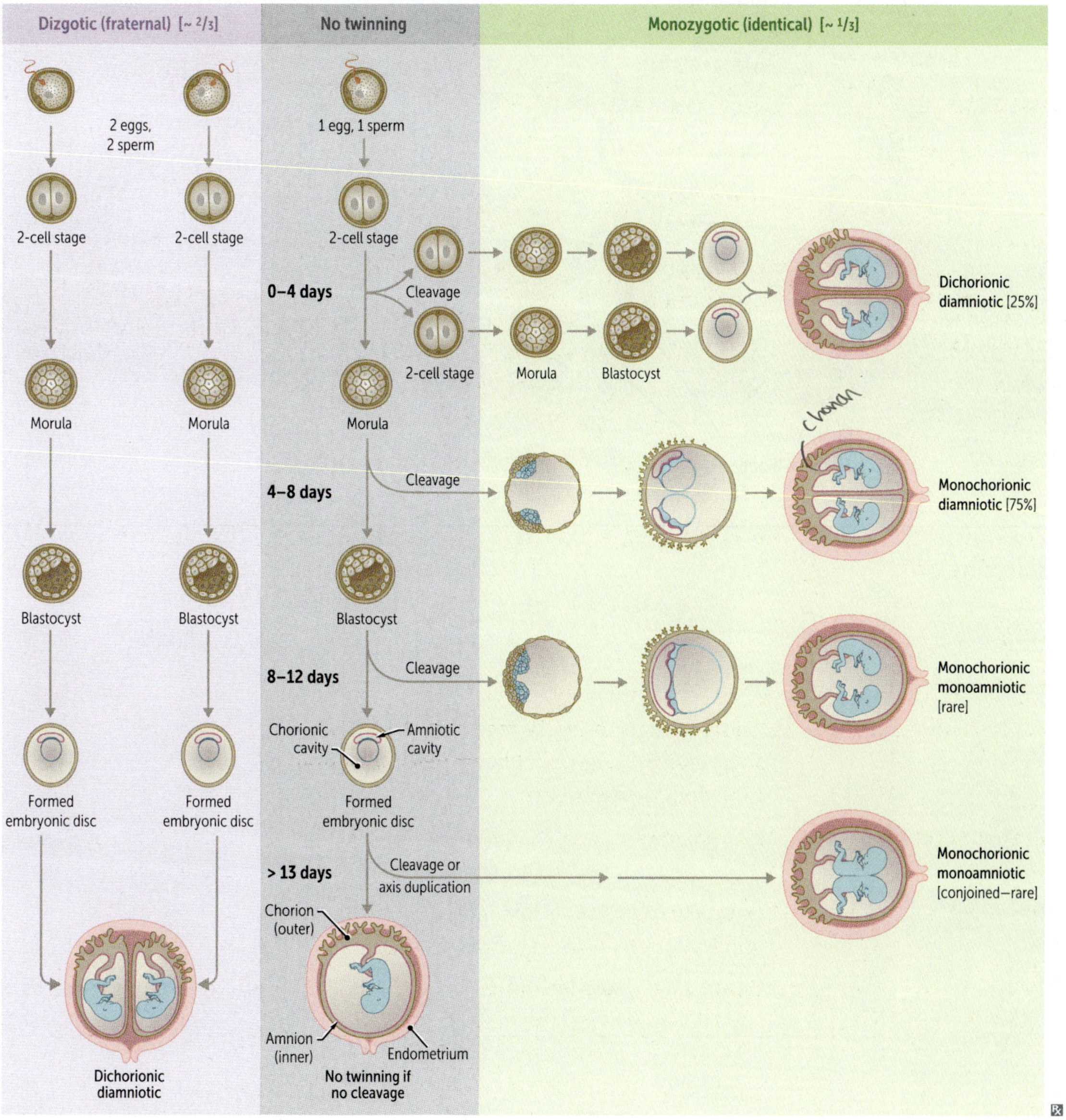

Placenta	1° site of nutrient and gas exchange between mother and fetus.	
Fetal component		
Cytotrophoblast	Inner layer of chorionic villi.	**C**ytotrophoblast makes **C**ells.
Syncytiotrophoblast	Outer layer of chorionic villi; synthesizes and secretes hormones, eg, hCG (structurally similar to LH; stimulates corpus luteum to secrete progesterone during first trimester).	**Syn**cytiotrophoblast **syn**thesizes hormones. Lacks MHC-I expression → ↓ chance of attack by maternal immune system.
Maternal component		
Decidua basalis	Derived from endometrium. Maternal blood in lacunae.	

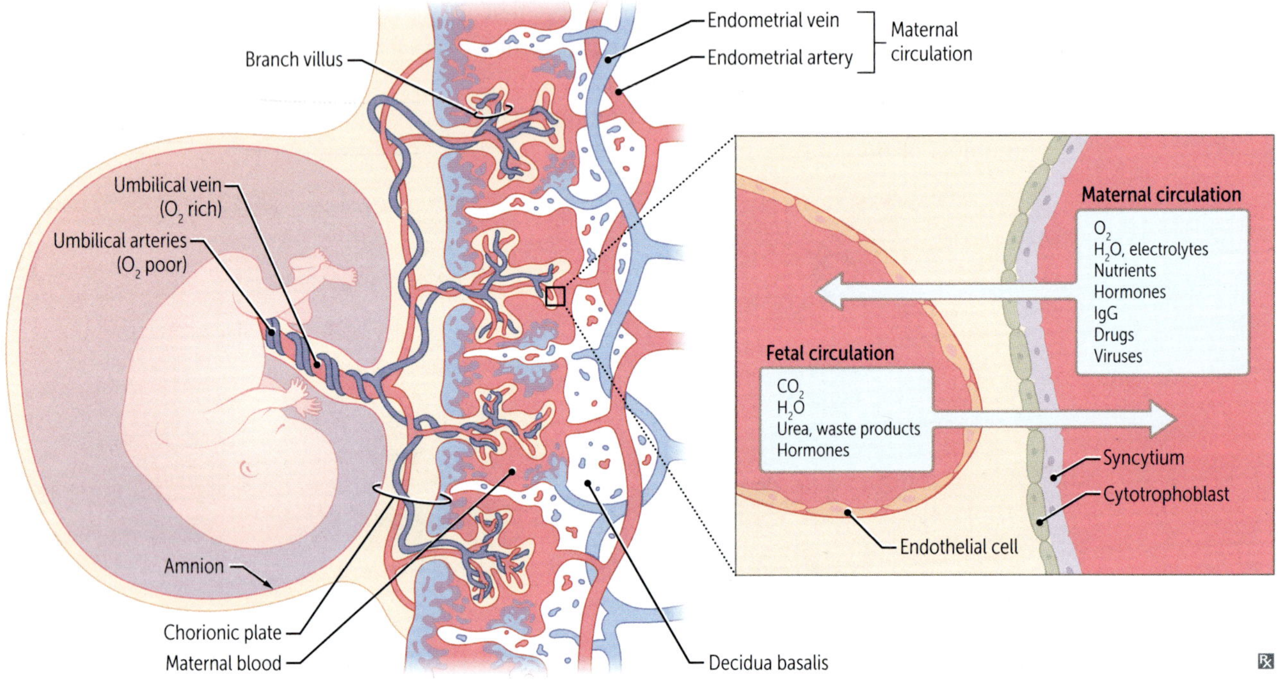

Umbilical cord

Umbilical arteries (2)—return deoxygenated blood from fetal internal iliac arteries to placenta A.
Umbilical vein (1)—supplies oxygenated blood from placenta to fetus; drains into IVC via liver or via ductus venosus.

Single umbilical artery (2-vessel cord) is associated with congenital and chromosomal anomalies.
Umbilical arteries and vein are derived from allantois.

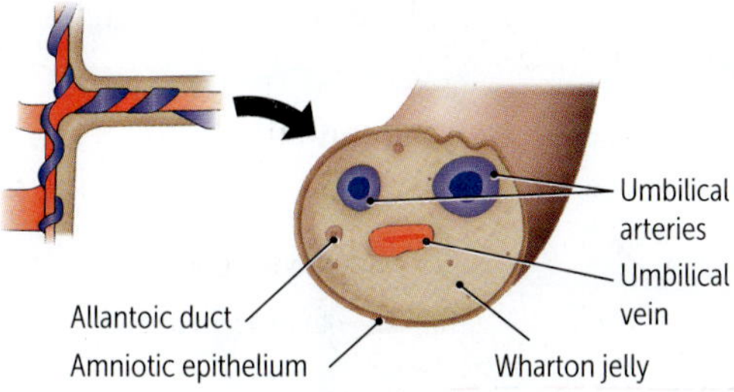

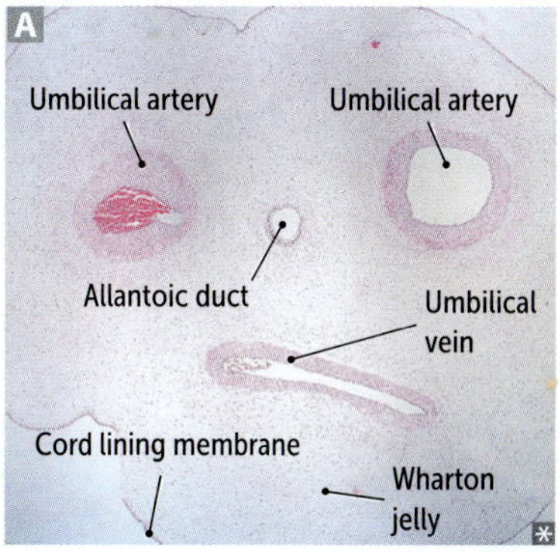

Urachus

In the 3rd week the yolk sac forms the allantois, which extends into urogenital sinus. Allantois becomes the urachus, a duct between fetal bladder and umbilicus.

Patent urachus — Total failure of urachus to obliterate → urine discharge from umbilicus.

Urachal cyst — Partial failure of urachus to obliterate; fluid-filled cavity lined with uroepithelium, between umbilicus and bladder. Can lead to infection, adenocarcinoma.

Vesicourachal diverticulum — Slight failure of urachus to obliterate → outpouching of bladder.

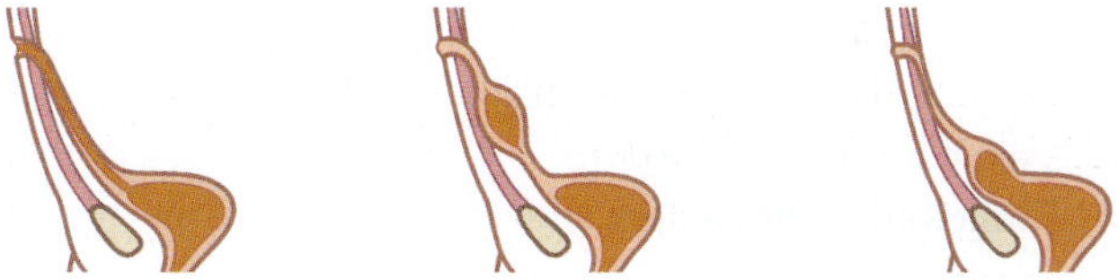

Patent urachus — Urachal cyst — Vesicourachal diverticulum

Vitelline duct

7th week—obliteration of vitelline duct (omphalo-mesenteric duct), which connects yolk sac to midgut lumen.

Vitelline fistula — Vitelline duct fails to close → meconium discharge from umbilicus.

Meckel diverticulum — Partial closure of vitelline duct, with patent portion attached to ileum (true diverticulum). May have heterotopic gastric and/or pancreatic tissue → melena, hematochezia, abdominal pain.

always remember MD when pts come in w/ these GI sx

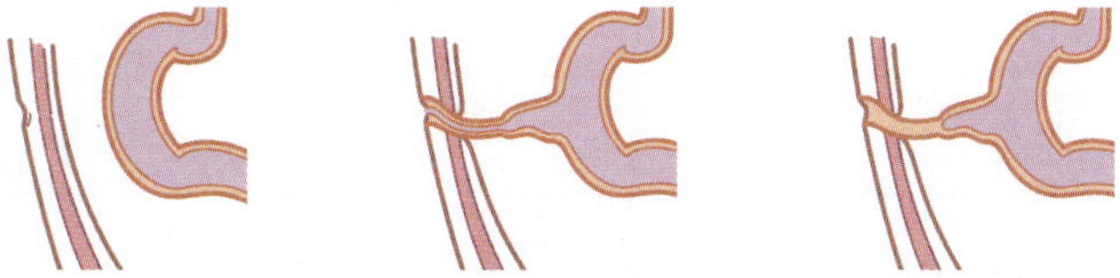

Normal — Vitelline fistula — Meckel diverticulum

look how early the poop/pee into umbil close - 3rd & 7th week

Aortic arch derivatives	Develop into arterial system.	
1st	Part of maxillary artery (branch of external carotid).	1st arch is maximal.
2nd	Stapedial artery and hyoid artery.	Second = Stapedial.
3rd	Common Carotid artery and proximal part of internal Carotid artery.	C is 3rd letter of alphabet.
4th	On left, aortic arch; on right, proximal part of right subclavian artery.	4th arch (4 limbs) = systemic.
6th	Proximal part of pulmonary arteries and (on left only) ductus arteriosus.	6th arch = pulmonary and the pulmonary-to-systemic shunt (ductus arteriosus).

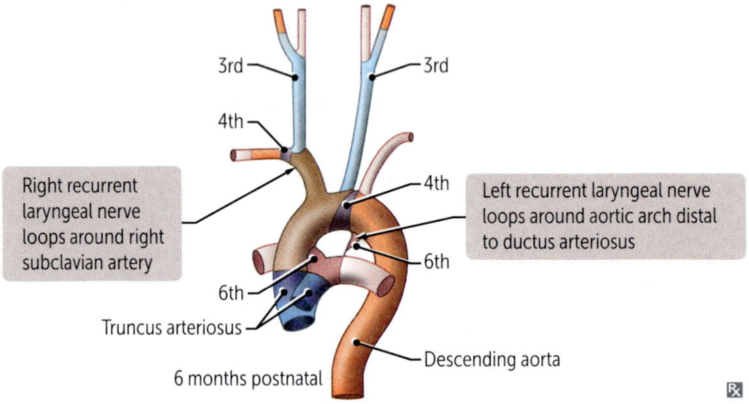

Branchial (pharyngeal) apparatus

Composed of branchial clefts, arches, pouches.
Branchial clefts—derived from ectoderm. Also called branchial grooves.
Branchial arches—derived from mesoderm (muscles, arteries) and neural crest (bones, cartilage).
Branchial pouches—derived from endoderm.

CAP covers outside to inside:
Clefts = ectoderm
Arches = mesoderm + neural crest
Pouches = endoderm

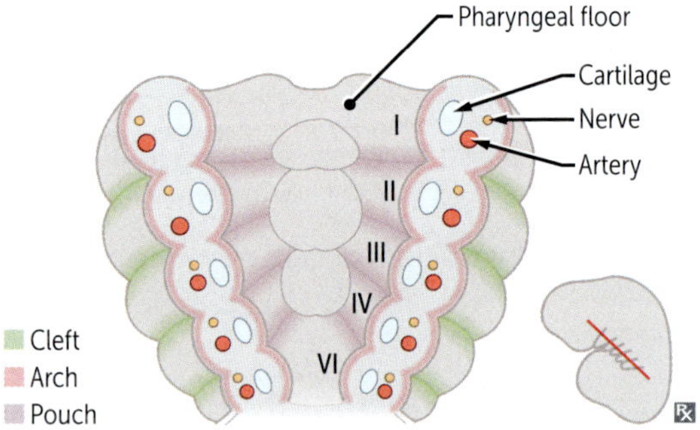

Branchial cleft derivatives

1st cleft develops into external auditory meatus.
2nd through 4th clefts form temporary cervical sinuses, which are obliterated by proliferation of 2nd arch mesenchyme.
Persistent cervical sinus → branchial cleft cyst within lateral neck, anterior to sternocleidomastoid muscle. Immobile during swallowing.

Branchial arch derivatives

ARCH	CARTILAGE	MUSCLES	NERVES[a]	ABNORMALITIES/COMMENTS
1st arch	**M**axillary process → **M**axilla, zygo**M**atic bone **M**andibular process → **M**eckel cartilage → **M**andible, **M**alleus and incus, spheno**M**andibular ligament	**M**uscles of **M**astication (temporalis, **M**asseter, lateral and **M**edial pterygoids), **M**ylohyoid, anterior belly of digastric, tensor tympani, tensor veli palatini	CN V_2 and V_3 **chew**	Pierre Robin sequence—micrognathia, glossoptosis, cleft palate, airway obstruction Treacher Collins syndrome—neural crest dysfunction → mandibular hypoplasia, facial abnormalities
2nd arch	Reichert cartilage: **S**tapes, **S**tyloid process, lesser horn of hyoid, **S**tylohyoid ligament	Muscles of facial expression, **S**tapedius, **S**tylohyoid, platy**S**ma, posterior belly of digastric	CN VII (facial expression) **smile**	
3rd arch	Greater horn of hyoid	Stylopharyngeus (think of stylo**pharyngeus** innervated by glosso**pharyngeal** nerve)	CN IX (**stylo-pharyngeus**) **swallow styl**ishly	
4th–6th arches	**A**rytenoids, **C**ricoid, **C**orniculate, **C**uneiform, **T**hyroid (used to sing and **ACCCT**)	4th arch: most pharyngeal constrictors; cricothyroid, levator veli palatini 6th arch: all intrinsic muscles of larynx except cricothyroid	4th arch: CN X (superior laryngeal branch) **simply swallow** 6th arch: CN X (recurrent laryngeal branch) **speak**	Arches 3 and 4 form posterior ⅓ of tongue; arch 5 makes no major developmental contributions

[a]These are the only CNs with both motor and sensory components (except V_2, which is sensory only).

When at the restaurant of the golden **arches**, children tend to first **chew** (1), then **smile** (2), then **swallow styl**ishly (3) or **simply swallow** (4), and then **speak** (6).

Branchial pouch derivatives

POUCH	DERIVATIVES	NOTES	MNEMONIC
1st pouch	Middle ear cavity, eustachian tube, mastoid air cells.	1st pouch contributes to endoderm-lined structures of ear.	**Ear**, **tonsils**, **bottom-to-top**: 1 (**ear**), 2 (**tonsils**), 3 dorsal (**bottom** for inferior parathyroids), 3 ventral (**to** = **t**hymus), 4 (**top** = superior parathyroids).
2nd pouch	Epithelial lining of palatine tonsil.		
3rd pouch	Dorsal wings → **inferior** parathyroids. Ventral wings → thymus.	**3**rd pouch contributes to **3** structures (thymus, left and right inferior parathyroids). 3rd-pouch structures end up **below** 4th-pouch structures.	
4th pouch	Dorsal wings → **superior** parathyroids. Ventral wings → ultimobranchial body → parafollicular (C) cells of thyroid.		

DiGeorge syndrome Chromosome 22q11 deletion. Aberrant development of 3rd and 4th pouches → T-cell deficiency (thymic aplasia) and hypocalcemia (failure of parathyroid development). Associated with cardiac defects (conotruncal anomalies).

Cleft lip and cleft palate

Cleft lip—failure of fusion of the maxillary and medial nasal processes (formation of 1° palate).

Cleft palate—failure of fusion of the two lateral palatine shelves or failure of fusion of lateral palatine shelves with the nasal septum and/or median palatine shelf (formation of 2° palate).

Cleft lip and cleft palate have distinct, multifactorial etiologies, but often occur together.

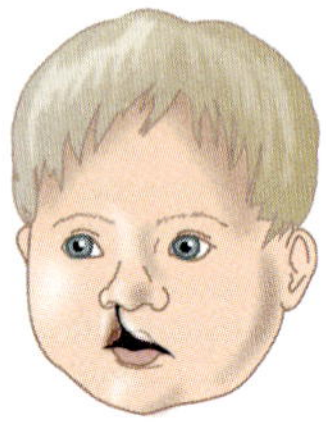

Cleft lip

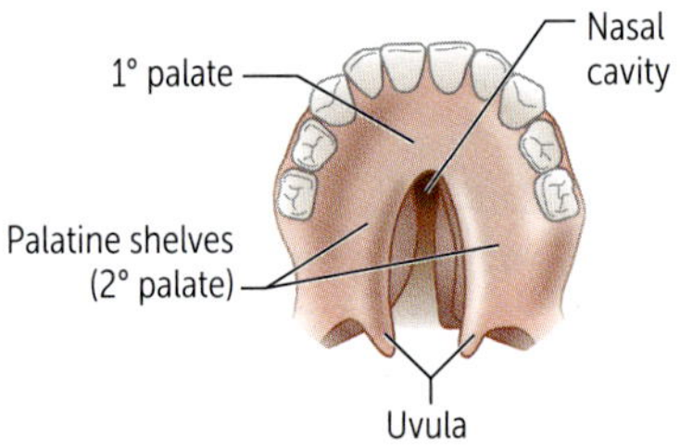

Cleft palate (partial)

Genital embryology

Female	Default development. Mesonephric duct degenerates and paramesonephric duct develops.
Male	*SRY* gene on Y chromosome—produces testis-determining factor → testes development. Sertoli cells secrete Müllerian inhibitory factor (MIF) that suppresses development of paramesonephric ducts. Leydig cells secrete androgens that stimulate development of mesonephric ducts.
Paramesonephric (Müllerian) duct	Develops into female internal structures—fallopian tubes, uterus, upper portion of vagina (lower portion from urogenital sinus). Male remnant is appendix testis. Müllerian agenesis (Mayer-Rokitansky-Küster-Hauser syndrome)—may present as 1° amenorrhea (due to a lack of uterine development) in females with fully developed 2° sexual characteristics (functional ovaries).
Mesonephric (Wolffian) duct (interim kidney for 1st TM)	Develops into male internal structures (except prostate)—**S**eminal vesicles, **E**pididymis, **E**jaculatory duct, **D**uctus deferens (**SEED**). In females, remnant of mesonephric duct → Gartner duct. – prost/penis/scrotsac = DHT

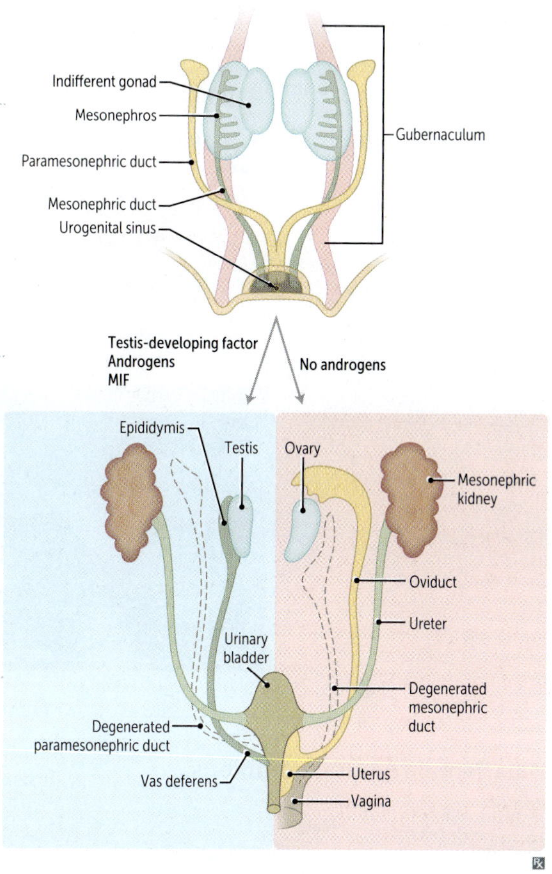

SRY gene

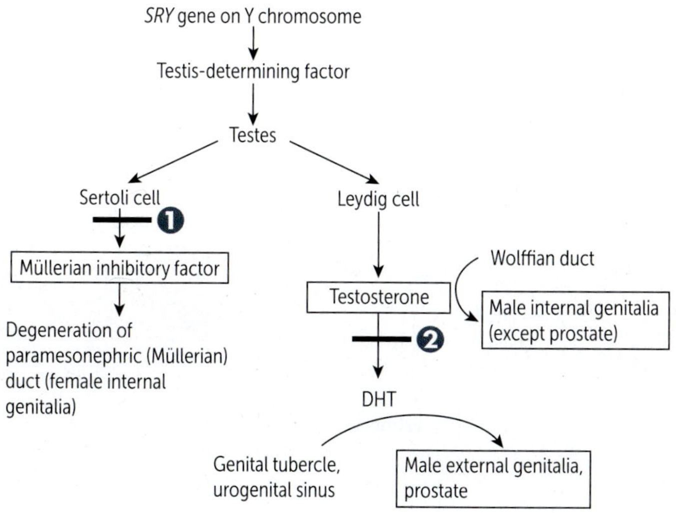

❶ No Sertoli cells or lack of Müllerian inhibitory factor → develop both male and female internal genitalia and male external genitalia

❷ 5α-reductase deficiency—inability to convert testosterone into DHT → male internal genitalia, ambiguous external genitalia until puberty (when ↑ testosterone levels cause masculinization)

Uterine (Müllerian duct) anomalies

Septate uterus	Common anomaly vs normal A uterus. Incomplete resorption of septum B. ↓ fertility. Treat with septoplasty.
Bicornuate uterus	Incomplete fusion of Müllerian ducts C. ↑ risk of complicated pregnancy.
Uterus didelphys	Complete failure of fusion → double uterus, vagina, and cervix D. Pregnancy possible.

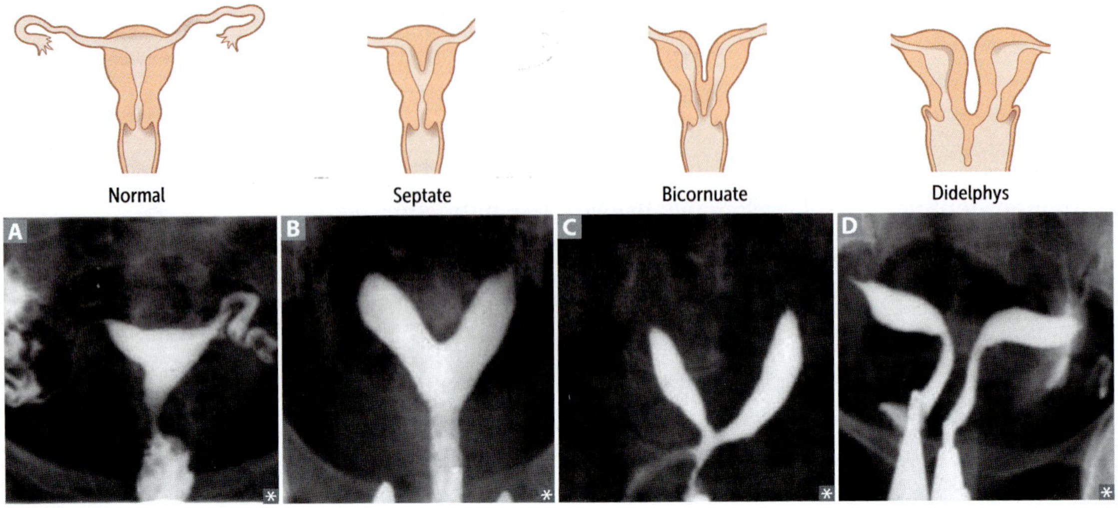

Male/female genital homologs

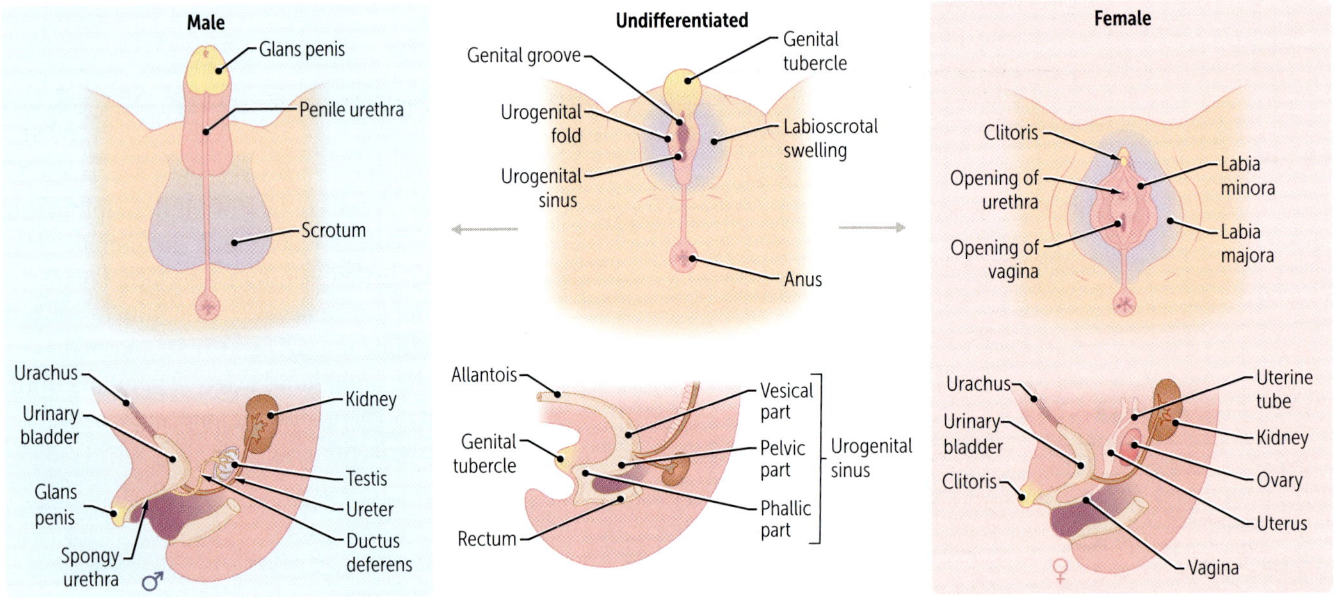

Dihydrotestosterone ←		→ Estrogen
Glans penis	Genital tubercle	Glans clitoris
Corpus cavernosum and spongiosum	Genital tubercle	Vestibular bulbs
Bulbourethral glands (of Cowper)	Urogenital sinus	Greater vestibular glands (of Bartholin)
Prostate gland	Urogenital sinus	Urethral and paraurethral glands (of Skene)
Ventral shaft of penis (penile urethra)	Urogenital folds	Labia minora
Scrotum	Labioscrotal swelling	Labia majora

Congenital penile abnormalities

Hypospadias 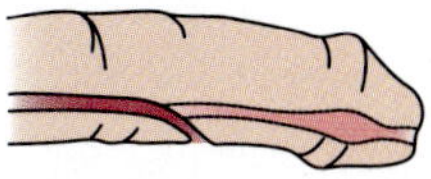	Abnormal opening of penile urethra on ventral surface of penis due to failure of urethral folds to fuse.	Hypospadias is more common than epispadias. Associated with inguinal hernia and cryptorchidism. **Hypo** is **below**.
Epispadias 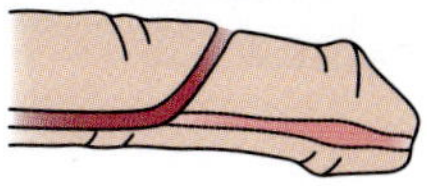	Abnormal opening of penile urethra on dorsal surface of penis due to faulty positioning of genital tubercle.	**E**xstrophy of the bladder is associated with **E**pispadias. When you have **E**pispadias, you hit your **E**ye when you p**EE**.

Descent of testes and ovaries

	MALE REMNANT	FEMALE REMNANT
Gubernaculum (band of fibrous tissue)	Anchors testes within scrotum.	Ovarian ligament + round ligament of uterus.
Processus vaginalis (evagination of peritoneum)	Forms tunica vaginalis.	Obliterated.

▶ REPRODUCTIVE—ANATOMY

Gonadal drainage

Venous drainage	Left ovary/testis → left gonadal vein → left renal vein → IVC. Right ovary/testis → right gonadal vein → IVC.	"**L**eft gonadal vein takes the **L**ongest way." Because the left spermatic vein enters the left renal vein at a 90° angle, flow is less laminar on left than on right → left venous pressure > right venous pressure → varicocele more common on the left.
Lymphatic drainage	Ovaries/testes → para-aortic lymph nodes. Body of uterus/cervix/superior bladder → external iliac nodes. Prostate/cervix/corpus cavernosum/proximal vagina → internal iliac nodes. Distal vagina/vulva/scrotum/distal anus → superficial inguinal nodes. Glans penis → deep inguinal nodes.	

Female reproductive anatomy

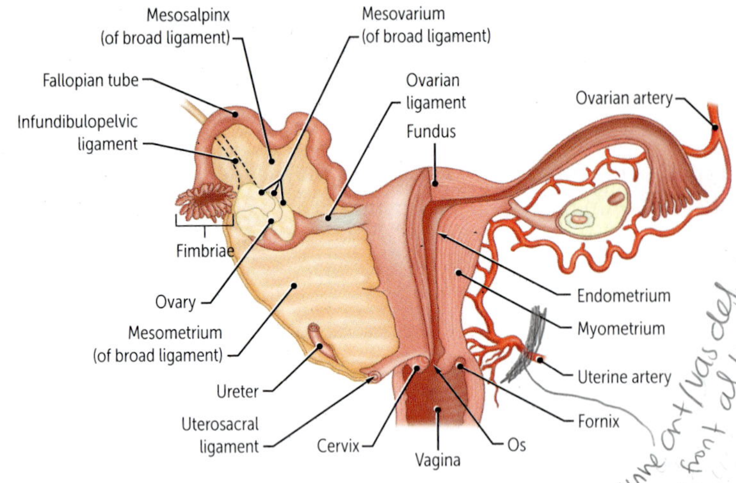

Posterior view

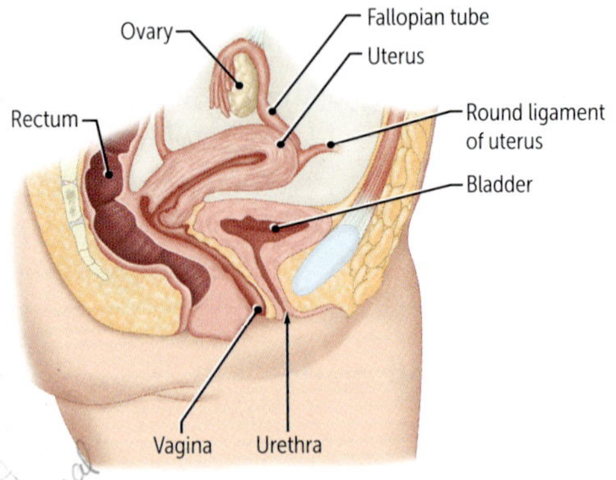

Sagittal view

LIGAMENT	CONNECTS	STRUCTURES CONTAINED	NOTES
Infundibulopelvic ligament (suspensory ligament of the ovary)	Ovaries to lateral pelvic wall	Ovarian vessels	Ligate vessels during oophorectomy to avoid bleeding. Ureter courses retroperitoneally, close to gonadal vessels → at risk of injury during ligation of ovarian vessels.
Cardinal ligament (not labeled)	Cervix to side wall of pelvis	Uterine vessels	Ureter at risk of injury during ligation of uterine vessels in hysterectomy.
Round ligament of the uterus	Uterine fundus to labia majora		Derivative of gubernaculum. Travels through **round** inguinal canal; above the artery of Sampson.
Broad ligament	Uterus, fallopian tubes, and ovaries to pelvic side wall	Ovaries, fallopian tubes, round ligaments of uterus	Fold of peritoneum that comprises the mesosalpinx, mesometrium, and mesovarium.
Ovarian ligament	Medial pole of ovary to lateral uterus	—	Derivative of gubernaculum. Ovarian **L**igament **L**atches to **L**ateral uterus.

Female reproductive epithelial histology

A

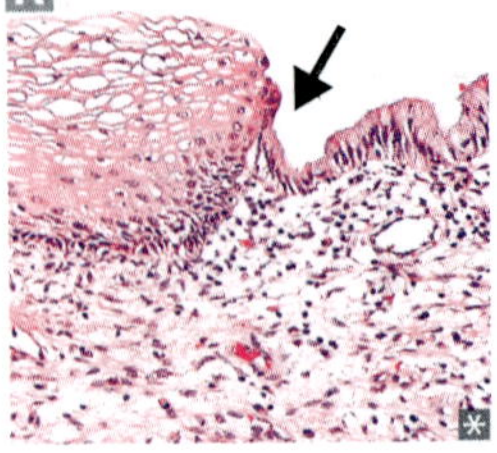

TISSUE	HISTOLOGY/NOTES
Vagina	Stratified squamous epithelium, nonkeratinized
Ectocervix	Stratified squamous epithelium, nonkeratinized
Transformation zone	Squamocolumnar junction A (most common area for cervical cancer)
Endocervix	Simple columnar epithelium
Uterus	Simple columnar epithelium with long tubular glands in proliferative phase; coiled glands in secretory phase
Fallopian tube	Simple columnar epithelium, ciliated
Ovary, outer surface	Simple cuboidal epithelium (germinal epithelium covering surface of ovary)

Male reproductive anatomy

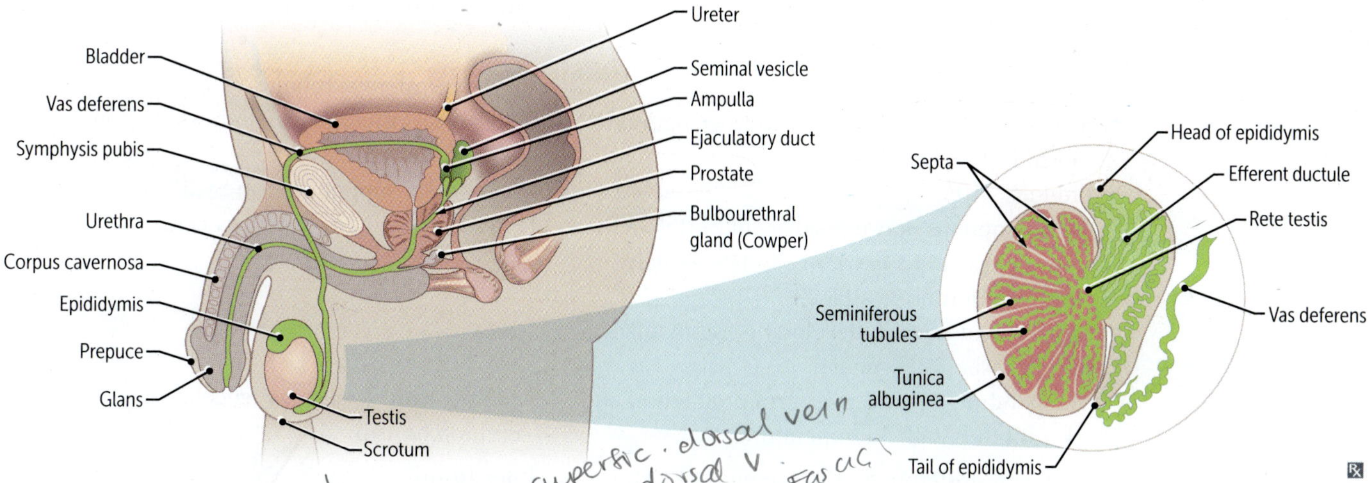

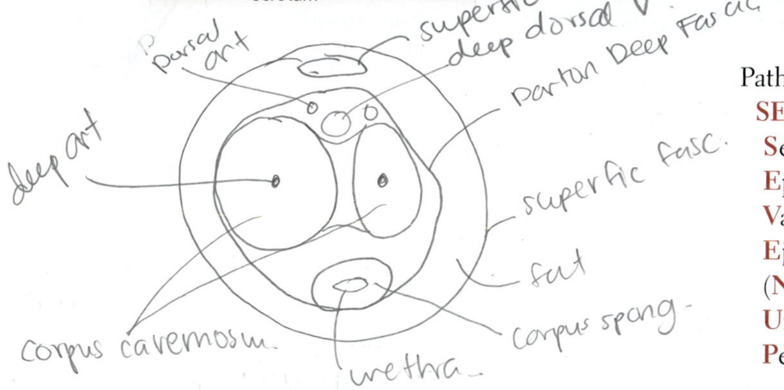

Pathway of sperm during ejaculation—
SEVEN UP:
Seminiferous tubules
Epididymis
Vas deferens
Ejaculatory ducts
(Nothing)
Urethra
Penis

Urethral injury

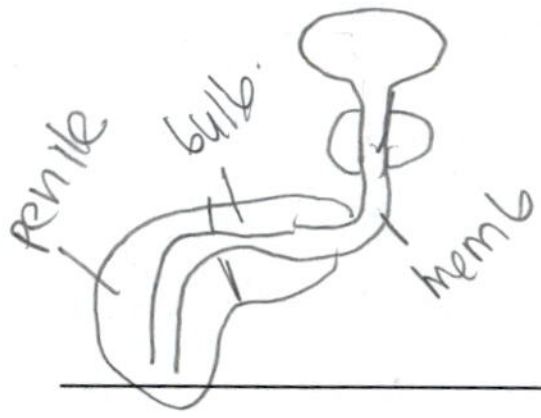

Suspect if blood seen at urethral meatus.

Posterior urethra—membranous urethra prone to injury from pelvic fracture. Injury can cause urine to leak into retropubic space.

Anterior urethra—bulbar and penile urethra at risk of damage due to perineal straddle injury. Can cause urine to leak beneath deep fascia of Buck. If fascia is torn, urine escapes into superficial perineal space.

Autonomic innervation of the male sexual response

Erection—Parasympathetic nervous system (pelvic nerve).
- NO → ↑ cGMP → smooth muscle relaxation → vasodilation → proerectile.
- Norepinephrine → ↑ $[Ca^{2+}]_{in}$ → smooth muscle contraction → vasoconstriction → antierectile.

Emission—Sympathetic nervous system (hypogastric nerve).

Ejaculation—visceral and Somatic nerves (pudendal nerve).

Point, Squeeze, and Shoot.

PDE-5 inhibitors (eg, sildenafil) ↓ cGMP breakdown.

Seminiferous tubules

CELL	FUNCTION	LOCATION/NOTES
Spermatogonia (germ cells)	Maintain germ pool and produce 1° spermatocytes.	Line seminiferous tubules A
Sertoli cells (non–germ cells)	Secrete inhibin B → inhibit FSH. Secrete androgen-binding protein → maintain local levels of testosterone. Produce MIF. Tight junctions between adjacent Sertoli cells form blood-testis barrier → isolate gametes from autoimmune attack. Support and nourish developing spermatozoa. Regulate spermatogenesis. Temperature sensitive; ↓ sperm production and ↓ inhibin B with ↑ temperature.	Line seminiferous tubules Convert testosterone and androstenedione to estrogens via aromatase Sertoli cells Support Sperm Synthesis Homolog of female granulosa cells ↑ temperature seen in varicocele, cryptorchidism
Leydig cells (endocrine cells)	Secrete testosterone in the presence of LH; testosterone production unaffected by temperature.	Interstitium Homolog of female theca interna cells

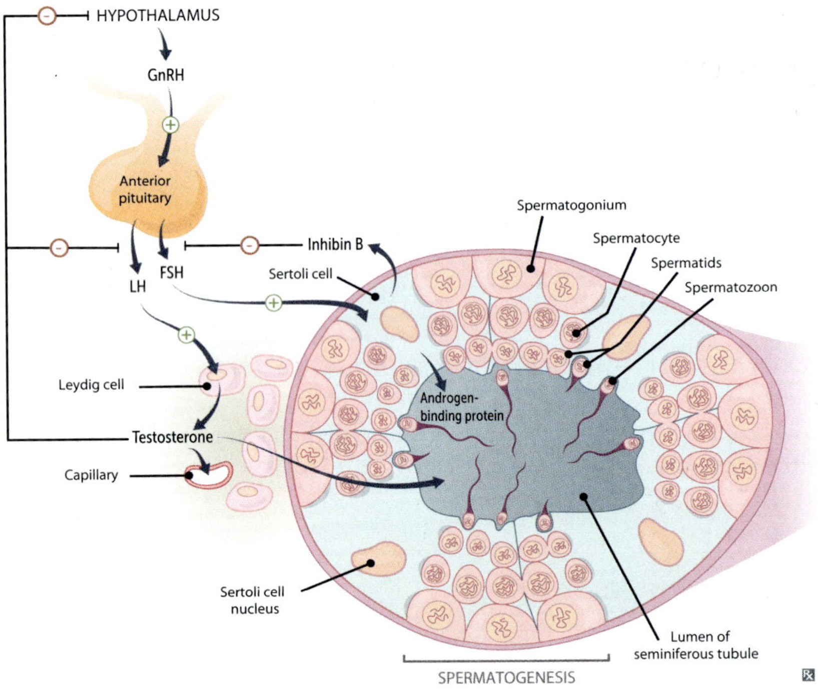

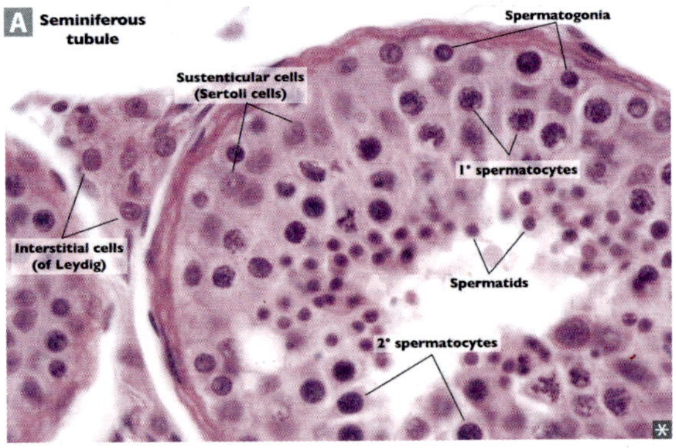

▶ REPRODUCTIVE—PHYSIOLOGY

Estrogen

SOURCE	Ovary (17β-estradiol), placenta (estriol), adipose tissue (estrone via aromatization).	Potency: estradiol > estrone > estriol
FUNCTION	Development of genitalia and breast, female fat distribution. Growth of follicle, endometrial proliferation, ↑ myometrial excitability. Upregulation of estrogen, LH, and progesterone receptors; feedback inhibition of FSH and LH, then LH surge; stimulation of prolactin secretion. ↑ transport proteins, SHBG; ↑ HDL; ↓ LDL.	Pregnancy: ▪ 50-fold ↑ in estradiol and estrone ▪ 1000-fold ↑ in estriol (indicator of fetal well-being) Trisomy 13, 18, 21 all ↓ Estrogen receptors expressed in cytoplasm; translocate to nucleus when bound by estrogen

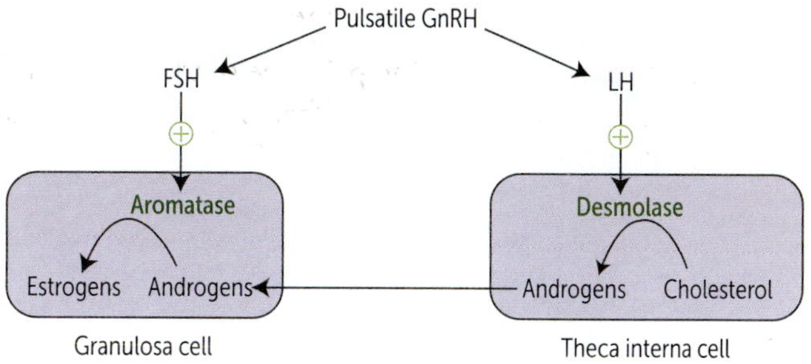

Progesterone

SOURCE	Corpus luteum, placenta, adrenal cortex, testes.	Fall in progesterone after delivery disinhibits prolactin → lactation. ↑ progesterone is indicative of ovulation. **Progesterone** is **pro-gestation**. **Prolactin** is **pro-lactation**.
FUNCTION	Stimulation of endometrial glandular secretions and spiral artery development. Maintenance of pregnancy. ↓ myometrial excitability. Production of thick cervical mucus, which inhibits sperm entry into uterus. ↑ body temperature. ← I thought w/ E the temp ↑, OH. Inhibition of gonadotropins (LH, FSH). Uterine smooth muscle relaxation (preventing contractions). ↓ estrogen receptor expression. Prevents endometrial hyperplasia.	

w/ end of preg approaching E ↑ & P ↓ & as E is high enough = contract = water break.
– w/ the ↓ P now PRL can be disinhib.

Oogenesis

1° oocytes begin meiosis I during fetal life and complete meiosis I just prior to ovulation.

Meiosis I is arrested in prOphase I for years until Ovulation (1° oocytes).

Meiosis II is arrested in **met**aphase II until fertilization (2° oocytes). "An egg **met** a sperm."

If fertilization does not occur within 1 day, the 2° oocyte degenerates.

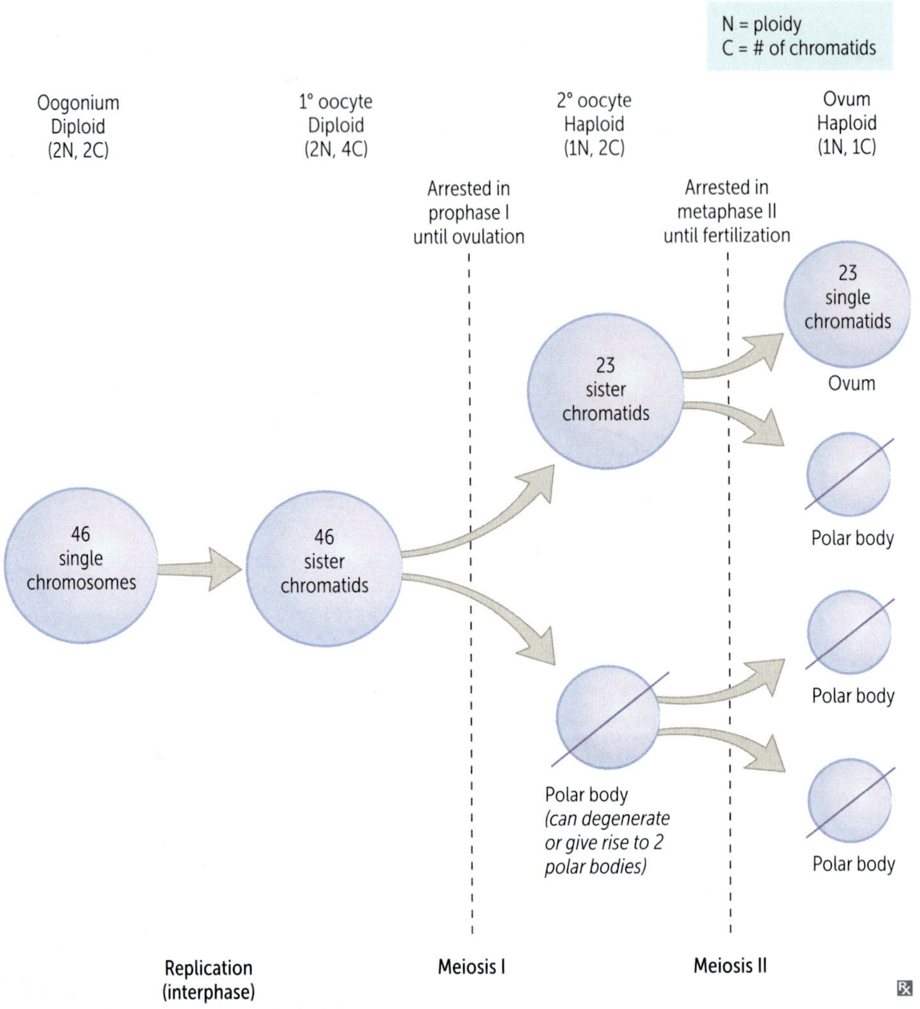

Ovulation

↑ estrogen, ↑ GnRH receptors on anterior pituitary. Estrogen surge then stimulates LH release → ovulation (rupture of follicle).

↑ temperature (progesterone induced).

Mittelschmerz—transient mid-cycle ovulatory pain ("**M**iddle hurts"); classically associated with peritoneal irritation (eg, follicular swelling/rupture, fallopian tube contraction). Can mimic appendicitis.

Menstrual cycle

Follicular phase can vary in length. Luteal phase is 14 days. Ovulation day + 14 days = menstruation.
Follicular growth is fastest during 2nd week of the follicular phase.
Estrogen stimulates endometrial proliferation.
Progesterone maintains endometrium to support implantation.
↓ progesterone → ↓ fertility.

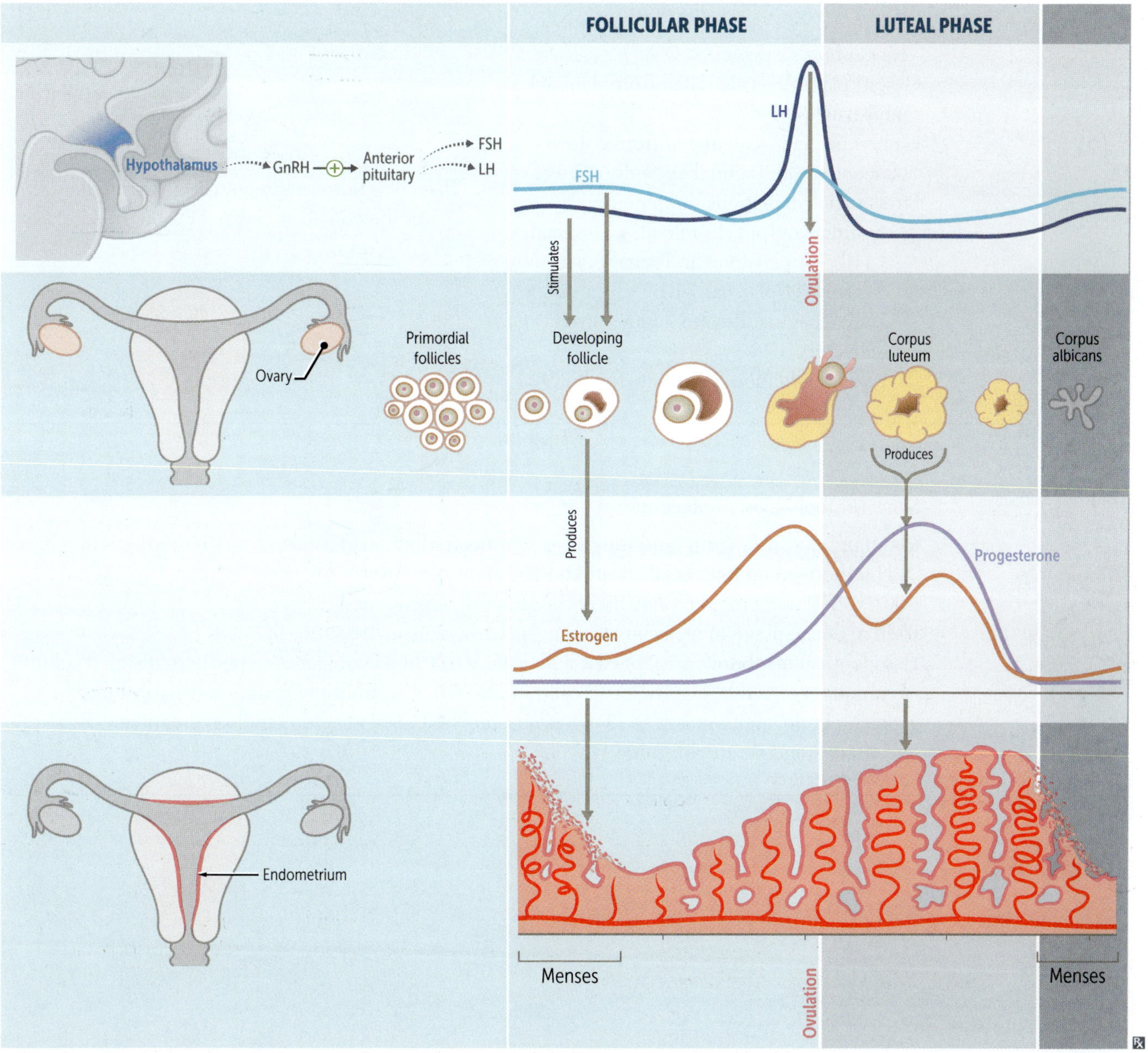

Dysmenorrhea	Pain with menses; often associated with endometriosis.
Oligomenorrhea	> 35-day cycle.
Polymenorrhea	< 21-day cycle.
Metrorrhagia	Frequent or irregular menstruation.
Menorrhagia	Heavy menstrual bleeding; > 80 mL blood loss or > 7 days of menses.
Menometrorrhagia	Heavy, irregular menstruation.

Pregnancy

Fertilization most commonly occurs in upper end of fallopian tube (the ampulla). Occurs within 1 day of ovulation.

Implantation within the wall of the uterus occurs 6 days after fertilization. Syncytiotrophoblasts secrete hCG, which is detectable in blood 1 week after conception and on home test in urine 2 weeks after conception.

Gestational age—calculated from date of last menstrual period.

Embryonic age—calculated from date of conception (gestational age minus 2 weeks).

Physiologic adaptations in pregnancy:

- ↑ cardiac output (↑ preload, ↓ afterload, ↑ HR → ↑ placental and renal perfusion)
- Anemia (↑↑ plasma, ↑ RBCs → ↓ viscosity)
- Hypercoagulability (to ↓ blood loss at delivery)
- Hyperventilation (eliminate fetal CO_2)

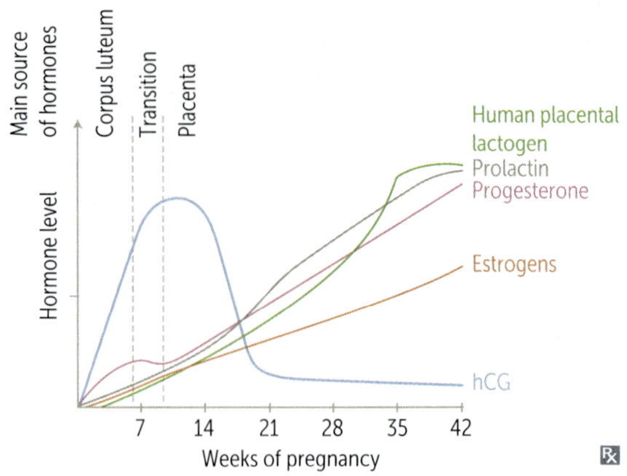

Placental hormone secretion generally increases over the course of pregnancy, but hCG peaks at 8–10 weeks.

hCG

SOURCE	Syncytiotrophoblast of placenta.
FUNCTION	Maintains corpus luteum (and thus progesterone) for first 8–10 weeks of pregnancy by acting like LH (otherwise no luteal cell stimulation → abortion). After 8–10 weeks, placenta synthesizes its own estriol and progesterone and corpus luteum degenerates. Used to detect pregnancy because it appears early in urine (see above). Has identical α subunit as LH, FSH, TSH (states of ↑ hCG can cause hyperthyroidism). β subunit is unique (pregnancy tests detect β subunit). hCG is ↑ in multiple gestations, hydatidiform moles, choriocarcinomas, and Down syndrome; hCG is ↓ in ectopic/failing pregnancy, Edward syndrome, and Patau syndrome.

C.L. is what secretes progest.
It dies in 12 days (determines luteal phase length)

Apgar score

	Score 2	Score 1	Score 0
Appearance	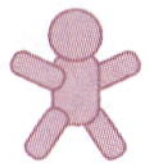 Pink	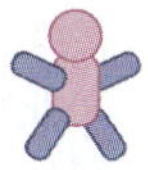 Extremities blue	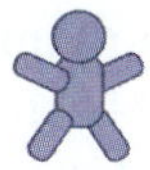 Pale or blue
Pulse	> 100 bpm	< 100 bpm	No pulse
Grimace	Cries and pulls away	Grimaces or weak cry	No response to stimulation
Activity	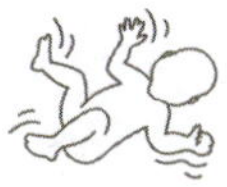 Active movement	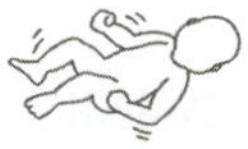 Arms, legs flexed	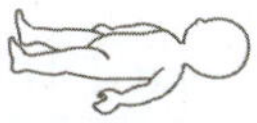 No movement
Respiration	Strong cry	Slow, irregular	No breathing

Assessment of newborn vital signs following labor via a 10-point scale evaluated at 1 minute and 5 minutes. **Apgar** score is based on **A**ppearance, **P**ulse, **G**rimace, **A**ctivity, and **R**espiration. Apgar scores < 7 require further evaluation. If Apgar score remains low at later time points, there is ↑ risk the child will develop long-term neurologic damage.

Low birth weight

Defined as < 2500 g. Caused by prematurity or intrauterine growth restriction (IUGR). Associated with ↑ risk of sudden infant death syndrome (SIDS) and with ↑ overall mortality. Other problems include impaired thermoregulation and immune function, hypoglycemia, polycythemia, and impaired neurocognitive/emotional development. Complications include infections, respiratory distress syndrome, necrotizing enterocolitis, intraventricular hemorrhage, and persistent fetal circulation.

Lactation

After labor, the ↓ in progesterone and estrogen disinhibits lactation. Suckling is required to maintain milk production, since ↑ nerve stimulation → ↑ oxytocin and prolactin.

Prolactin—induces and maintains lactation and ↓ reproductive function.

Oxytocin—assists in milk letdown; also promotes uterine contractions.

Breast milk is the ideal nutrition for infants < 6 months old. Contains maternal immunoglobulins (conferring passive immunity; mostly IgA), macrophages, lymphocytes. Breast milk reduces infant infections and is associated with ↓ risk for child to develop asthma, allergies, diabetes mellitus, and obesity. Exclusively breastfed infants require vitamin D supplementation.

Breastfeeding ↓ maternal risk of breast and ovarian cancer and facilitates mother-child bonding.

Menopause	Diagnosed by amenorrhea for 12 months. ↓ estrogen production due to age-linked decline in number of ovarian follicles. Average age at onset is 51 years (earlier in smokers). Usually preceded by 4–5 years of abnormal menstrual cycles. Source of estrogen (estrone) after menopause becomes peripheral conversion of androgens, ↑ androgens → hirsutism. ↑↑ FSH is specific for menopause (loss of negative feedback on FSH due to ↓ estrogen).	Hormonal changes: ↓ estrogen, ↑↑ FSH, ↑ LH (no surge), ↑ GnRH. Causes **HAVOCS**: **H**ot flashes, **A**trophy of the **V**agina, **O**steoporosis, **C**oronary artery disease, **S**leep disturbances. Menopause before age 40 suggests 1° ovarian insufficiency (premature ovarian failure).

Androgens	Testosterone, dihydrotestosterone (DHT), androstenedione.	
SOURCE	DHT and testosterone (testis), **A**n**D**rostenedione (**AD**renal)	Potency: DHT > testosterone > androstenedione.
FUNCTION	Testosterone: ▪ Differentiation of epididymis, vas deferens, seminal vesicles (internal genitalia, except prostate). ▪ Growth spurt: penis, seminal vesicles, sperm, muscle, RBCs. ▪ Deepening of voice. ▪ Closing of epiphyseal plates (via estrogen converted from testosterone). ▪ Libido. DHT: ▪ Early—differentiation of penis, scrotum, prostate. ▪ Late—prostate growth, balding, sebaceous gland activity.	Testosterone is converted to DHT by 5α-reductase, which is inhibited by finasteride. In the male, androgens are converted to estrogen by cytochrome P-450 aromatase (primarily in adipose tissue and testis). Aromatase is the key enzyme in conversion of androgens to estrogen. Exogenous testosterone → inhibition of hypothalamic–pituitary–gonadal axis → ↓ intratesticular testosterone → ↓ testicular size → azoospermia.

Spermatogenesis

Spermatogenesis begins at puberty with spermatogonia. Full development takes 2 months. Occurs in seminiferous tubules. Produces spermatids that undergo spermiogenesis (loss of cytoplasmic contents, gain of acrosomal cap) to form mature spermatozoon.

"**Gonium**" is **going** to be a sperm; "**Zoon**" is "**Zooming**" to egg.

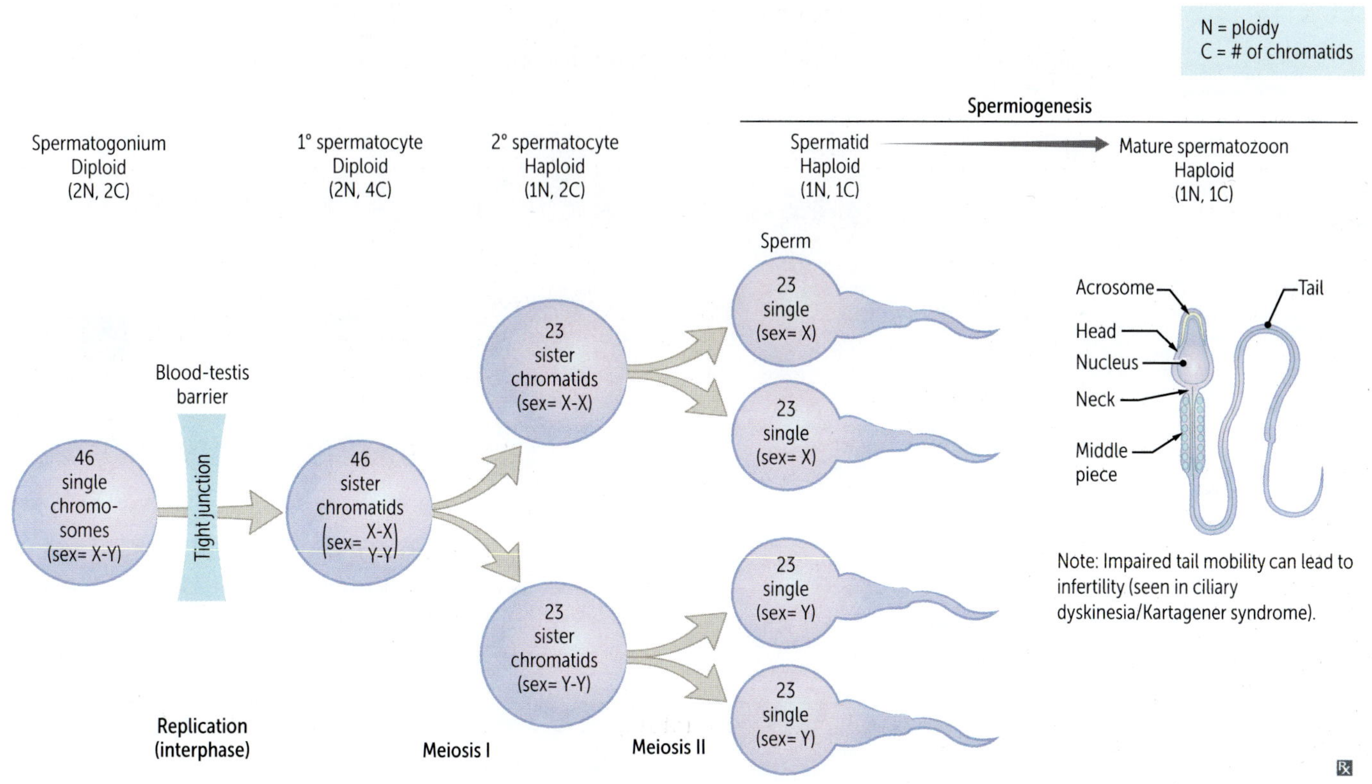

Tanner stages of sexual development

Tanner stage is assigned independently to genitalia, pubic hair, and breast (eg, a person can have Tanner stage 2 genitalia, Tanner stage 3 pubic hair).

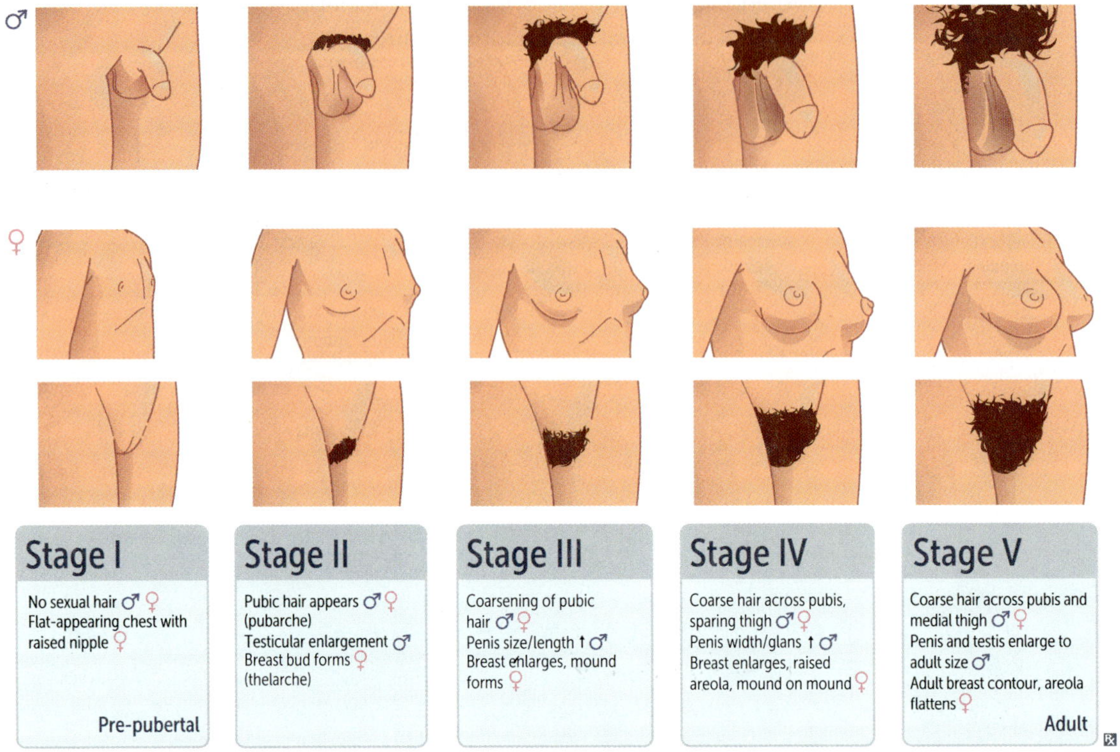

▶ REPRODUCTIVE—PATHOLOGY

Sex chromosome disorders	Aneuploidy most commonly due to meiotic nondisjunction.	
Klinefelter syndrome [male] (47,XXY) 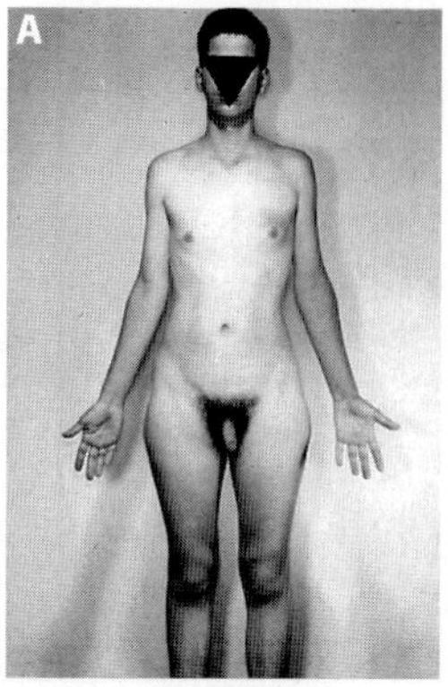	Testicular atrophy, eunuchoid body shape, tall, long extremities, gynecomastia, female hair distribution A. May present with developmental delay. Presence of inactivated X chromosome (Barr body). Common cause of hypogonadism seen in infertility work-up.	Dysgenesis of seminiferous tubules → ↓ inhibin B → ↑ FSH. Abnormal Leydig cell function → ↓ testosterone → ↑ LH → ↑ estrogen.
Turner syndrome [female] (45,XO) 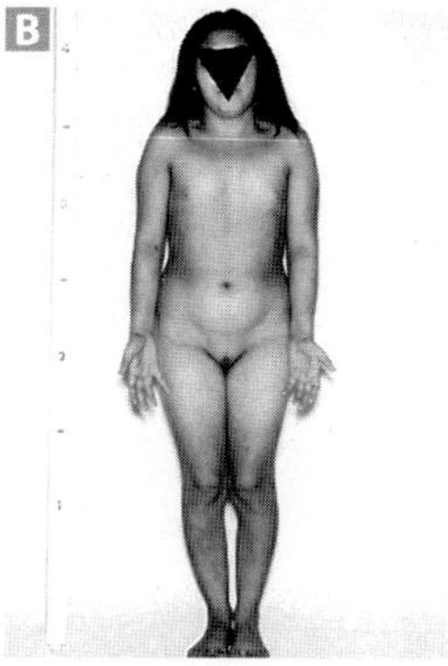	Short stature (if untreated), ovarian dysgenesis (streak ovary), shield chest, bicuspid aortic valve, coarctation (femoral < brachial pulse), lymphatic defects (result in webbed neck or cystic hygroma; lymphedema in feet, hands), horseshoe kidney B. Most common cause of 1° amenorrhea. No Barr body.	Menopause before menarche. ↓ estrogen leads to ↑ LH, FSH. Sometimes due to mitotic error → mosaicism (eg, 45,XO/46,XX). Pregnancy is possible in some cases (IVF, exogenous estradiol-17β and progesterone).
Double Y males (XYY)	Phenotypically normal (usually undiagnosed), very tall. Normal fertility. May be associated with severe acne, learning disability, autism spectrum disorders.	
Ovotesticular disorder of sex development	46,XX > 46,XY. Both ovarian and testicular tissue present (ovotestis); ambiguous genitalia. Previously called true hermaphroditism.	

Diagnosing disorders of sex hormones

Testosterone	LH	Diagnosis
↑	↑	Defective androgen receptor
↑	↓	Testosterone-secreting tumor, exogenous steroids
↓	↑	1° hypogonadism
↓	↓	Hypogonadotropic hypogonadism

Other disorders of sex development

Disagreement between the phenotypic (external genitalia) and gonadal (testes vs ovaries) sex. Include terms pseudohermaphrodite, hermaphrodite, and intersex.

46,XX DSD

Ovaries present, but external genitalia are virilized or ambiguous. Due to excessive and inappropriate exposure to androgenic steroids during early gestation (eg, congenital adrenal hyperplasia or exogenous administration of androgens during pregnancy).

46,XY DSD

Testes present, but external genitalia are female or ambiguous. Most common form is androgen insensitivity syndrome (testicular feminization).

Placental aromatase deficiency

Inability to synthesize estrogens from androgens. Masculinization of female (46,XX) infants (ambiguous genitalia), ↑ serum testosterone and androstenedione. Can present with maternal virilization during pregnancy (fetal androgens cross the placenta).

Androgen insensitivity syndrome (46,XY)

Defect in androgen receptor resulting in normal-appearing female; female external genitalia with scant sexual hair, rudimentary vagina; uterus and fallopian tubes absent. Patients develop normal functioning testes (often found in labia majora; surgically removed to prevent malignancy). ↑ testosterone, estrogen, LH (vs sex chromosome disorders).

5α-reductase deficiency

Autosomal recessive; sex limited to genetic males (46,XY). Inability to convert testosterone to DHT. Ambiguous genitalia until puberty, when ↑ testosterone causes masculinization/↑ growth of external genitalia. Testosterone/estrogen levels are normal; LH is normal or ↑. Internal genitalia are normal.

Kallmann syndrome

Failure to complete puberty; a form of hypogonadotropic hypogonadism. Defective migration of GnRH cells and formation of olfactory bulb; ↓ synthesis of GnRH in the hypothalamus; anosmia; ↓ GnRH, FSH, LH, testosterone. Infertility (low sperm count in males; amenorrhea in females).

Hydatidiform mole

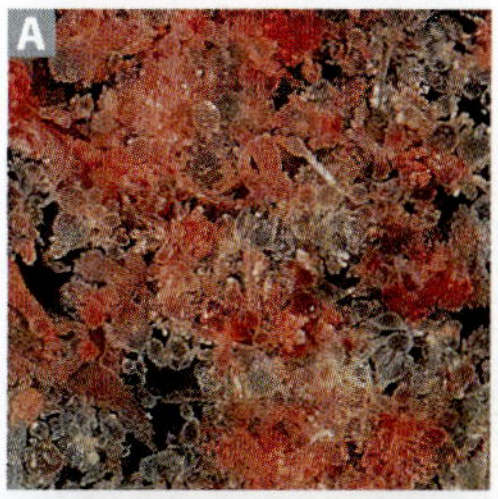

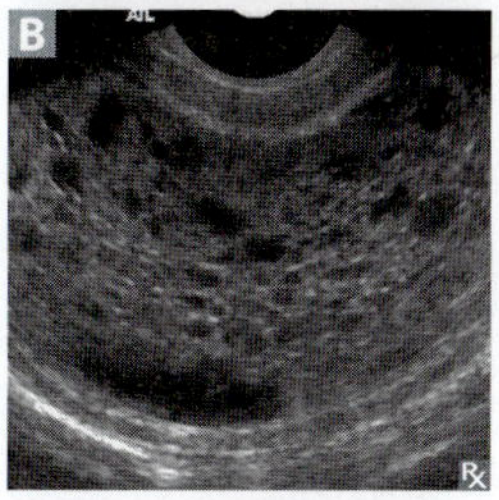

Cystic swelling of chorionic villi and proliferation of chorionic epithelium (only trophoblast).

Presents with vaginal bleeding, uterine enlargement more than expected, pelvic pressure/pain. Associated with hCG-mediated sequelae: early preeclampsia (before 20 weeks), theca-lutein cysts, hyperemesis gravidarum, hyperthyroidism.

Treatment: dilation and curettage and methotrexate. Monitor β-hCG.

	Complete mole	Partial mole
KARYOTYPE	46,XX; 46,XY	69,XXX; 69,XXY; 69,XYY
COMPONENTS	Most commonly enucleated egg + single sperm (subsequently duplicates paternal DNA)	2 sperm + 1 egg
FETAL PARTS	No	Yes (**part**ial = fetal **part**s)
UTERINE SIZE	$\uparrow$	—
hCG	$\uparrow\uparrow\uparrow\uparrow$	$\uparrow$
IMAGING	"Honeycombed" uterus or "clusters of grapes" A, "snowstorm" on ultrasound B	Fetal parts
RISK OF MALIGNANCY (GESTATIONAL TROPHOBLASTIC NEOPLASIA)	15–20%	< 5%
RISK OF CHORIOCARCINOMA	2%	Rare

Choriocarcinoma

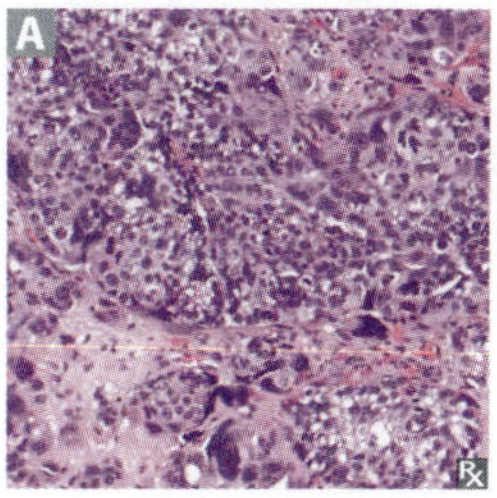

Rare; can develop during or after pregnancy in mother or baby. Malignancy of trophoblastic tissue A (cytotrophoblasts, syncytiotrophoblasts); **no** chorionic villi present. $\uparrow$ frequency of bilateral/multiple theca-lutein cysts. Presents with abnormal $\uparrow$ β-hCG, shortness of breath, hemoptysis. Hematogenous spread to lungs.

Pregnancy complications

Placental abruption (abruptio placentae)

Premature separation (partial or complete) of placenta from uterine wall before delivery of infant. Risk factors: trauma (eg, motor vehicle accident), smoking, hypertension, preeclampsia, cocaine abuse.

Presentation: **abrupt**, painful bleeding (concealed or apparent) in third trimester; possible DIC, maternal shock, fetal distress. Life threatening for mother and fetus.

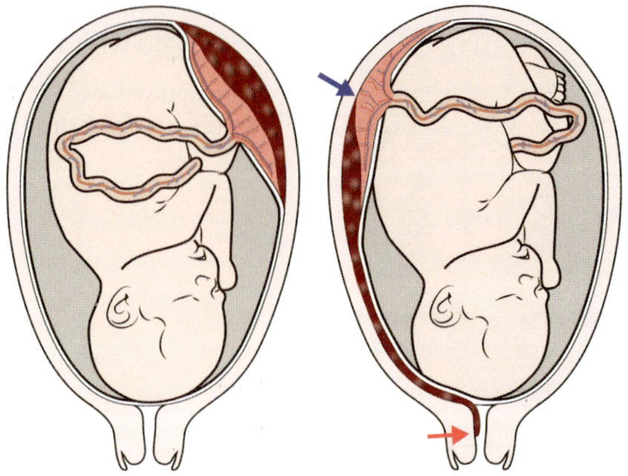

Complete abruption with concealed hemorrhage — Partial abruption with apparent hemorrhage

Placenta accreta/increta/percreta

Defective decidual layer → abnormal attachment and separation after delivery. Risk factors: prior C-section, inflammation, placenta previa. Three types distinguishable by the depth of penetration:

Placenta accreta—placenta **attaches** to myometrium without penetrating it; most common type.

Placenta increta—placenta penetrates **into** myometrium.

Placenta percreta—placenta penetrates ("**perforates**") through myometrium and into uterine serosa (invades entire uterine wall); can result in placental attachment to rectum or bladder.

Presentation: often detected on ultrasound prior to delivery. No separation of placenta after delivery → postpartum bleeding (can cause Sheehan syndrome).

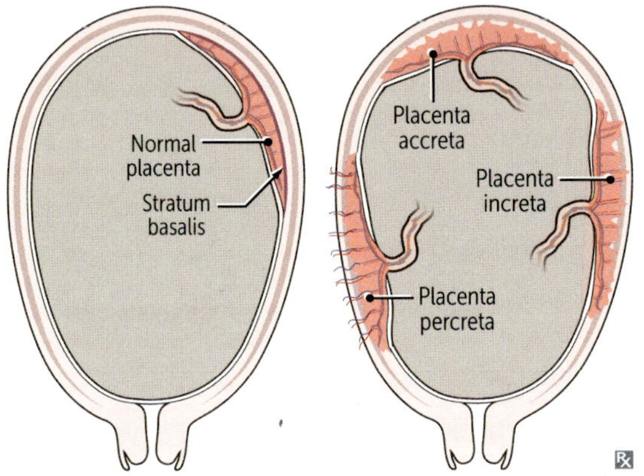

Placenta previa

Attachment of placenta to lower uterine segment over (or < 2 cm from) internal cervical os. Risk factors: multiparity, prior C-section. Associated with painless third-trimester bleeding.

ABRUPTION = PAINFUL bleed
Previa = painless

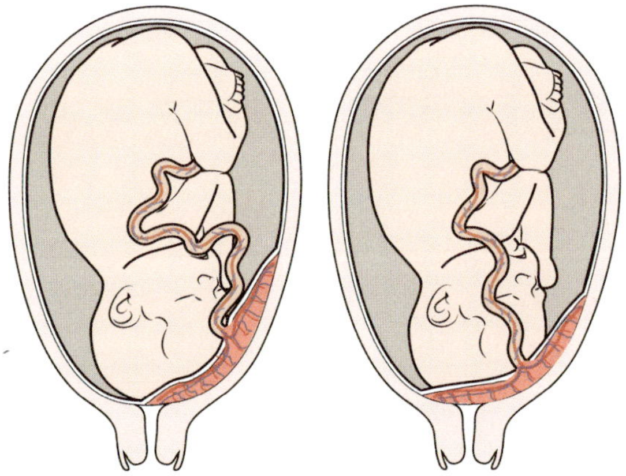

Partial placenta previa — Complete placenta previa

–same presentat as plac. previa but w/ bradycard.

Pregnancy complications *(continued)*

Vasa previa

Fetal vessels run over, or in close proximity to, cervical os. May result in vessel rupture, exsanguination, fetal death. Presents with triad of membrane rupture, painless vaginal bleeding, fetal bradycardia (< 110 beats/min). Emergency C-section usually indicated. Frequently associated with velamentous umbilical cord insertion (cord inserts in chorioamniotic membrane rather than placenta → fetal vessels travel to placenta unprotected by Wharton jelly).

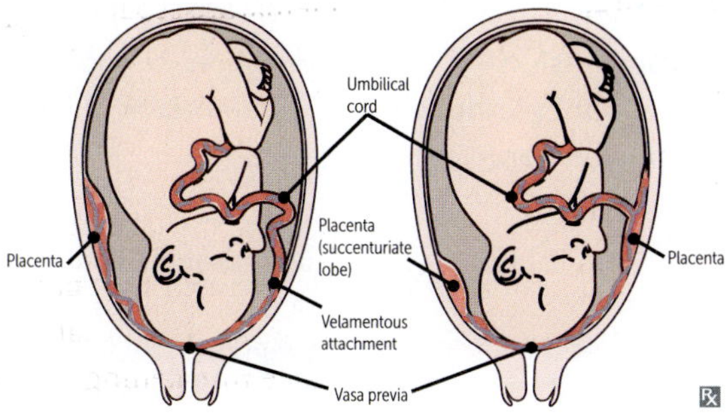

Postpartum hemorrhage

Due to 4 T's: Tone (uterine atony; most common), Trauma (lacerations, incisions, uterine rupture), Thrombin (coagulopathy), Tissue (retained products of conception).

Ectopic pregnancy

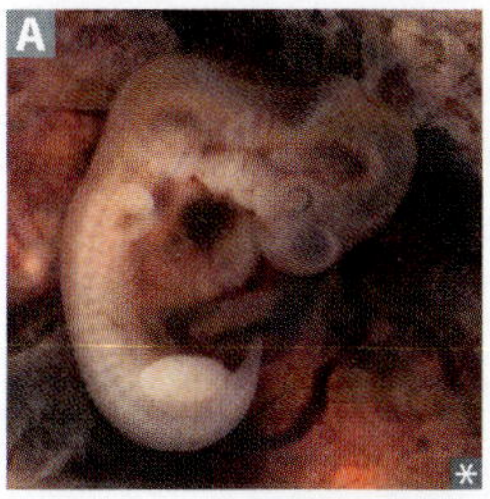

Most often in ampulla of fallopian tube (A shows 10-mm embryo in oviduct at 7 weeks of gestation). Suspect with history of amenorrhea, lower-than-expected rise in hCG based on dates, and sudden lower abdominal pain; confirm with ultrasound. Often clinically mistaken for appendicitis.

Pain +/– bleeding.
Risk factors:
- Prior ectopic pregnancy
- History of infertility
- Salpingitis (PID)
- Ruptured appendix
- Prior tubal surgery

Amniotic fluid abnormalities

Polyhydramnios

Too much amniotic fluid; associated with fetal malformations (eg, esophageal/duodenal atresia, anencephaly; both result in inability to swallow amniotic fluid), maternal diabetes, fetal anemia, multiple gestations.

Oligohydramnios

Too little amniotic fluid; associated with placental insufficiency, bilateral renal agenesis, posterior urethral valves (in males) and resultant inability to excrete urine. Any profound oligohydramnios can cause Potter sequence.

#1 cause bladder outlet obstruction in male newborns (bilat bc urethra)

Hypertension in pregnancy

Gestational hypertension (pregnancy-induced hypertension)	BP > 140/90 mm Hg after 20th week of gestation. No pre-existing hypertension. No proteinuria or end-organ damage.	Treatment: antihypertensives (**H**ydralazine, α-**M**ethyldopa, **L**abetalol, **N**ifedipine), deliver at 37–39 weeks. **H**ypertensive **M**oms **L**ove **N**ifedipine.
Preeclampsia	New-onset hypertension with either proteinuria or end-organ dysfunction after 20th week of gestation (< 20 weeks suggests molar pregnancy). May proceed to eclampsia (+ seizures) and/or HELLP syndrome. Caused by abnormal placental spiral arteries → endothelial dysfunction, vasoconstriction, ischemia. Incidence ↑ in patients with pre-existing hypertension, diabetes, chronic renal disease, autoimmune disorders. Complications: placental abruption, coagulopathy, renal failure, uteroplacental insufficiency, eclampsia.	Treatment: antihypertensives, IV magnesium sulfate (to prevent seizure); definitive is delivery of fetus.
Eclampsia	Preeclampsia + maternal seizures. Maternal death due to stroke, intracranial hemorrhage, or ARDS.	Treatment: IV magnesium sulfate, antihypertensives, immediate delivery.
HELLP syndrome	**H**emolysis, **E**levated **L**iver enzymes, **L**ow **P**latelets. A manifestation of severe preeclampsia. Blood smear shows schistocytes. Can lead to hepatic subcapsular hematomas → rupture → severe hypotension.	Treatment: immediate delivery.

Gynecologic tumor epidemiology	Incidence (US)—endometrial > ovarian > cervical; cervical cancer is more common worldwide due to lack of screening or HPV vaccination. Worst prognosis—ovarian > endometrial > cervical.

Vaginal tumors

Squamous cell carcinoma (SCC)	Usually 2° to cervical SCC; 1° vaginal carcinoma rare.
Clear cell adenocarcinoma	Affects women who had exposure to DES in utero.
Sarcoma botryoides (embryonal rhabdomyosarcoma variant)	Affects girls < 4 years old; spindle-shaped cells; desmin ⊕. Presents with clear, grape-like, polypoid mass emerging from vagina.

Cervical pathology

Dysplasia and carcinoma in situ

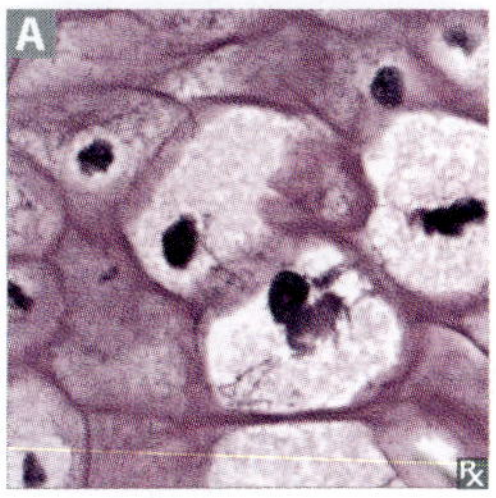

Disordered epithelial growth; begins at basal layer of squamocolumnar junction (transformation zone) and extends outward. Classified as CIN 1, CIN 2, or CIN 3 (severe dysplasia or carcinoma in situ), depending on extent of dysplasia. Associated with HPV 16 and HPV 18, which produce both the E6 gene product (inhibits *p53* suppressor gene) and E7 gene product (inhibits *RB* suppressor gene). May progress slowly to invasive carcinoma if left untreated. Typically asymptomatic (detected with Pap smear) or presents as abnormal vaginal bleeding (often postcoital).

Risk factors: multiple sexual partners (#1), smoking, starting sexual intercourse at young age, HIV infection.

Invasive carcinoma

Often squamous cell carcinoma. Pap smear can catch cervical dysplasia (koilocytes A) before it progresses to invasive carcinoma. Diagnose via colposcopy and biopsy. Lateral invasion can block ureters → renal failure.

Premature ovarian failure

Premature atresia of ovarian follicles in women of reproductive age. Patients present with signs of menopause after puberty but before age 40.

↓ estrogen, ↑ LH, ↑ FSH.

Most common causes of anovulation

Pregnancy, polycystic ovarian syndrome, obesity, HPO axis abnormalities, premature ovarian failure, hyperprolactinemia, thyroid disorders, eating disorders, competitive athletics, Cushing syndrome, adrenal insufficiency.

Polycystic ovarian syndrome (Stein-Leventhal syndrome)

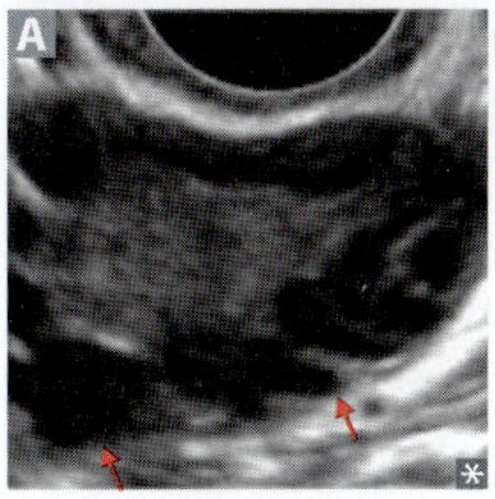

Hyperinsulinemia and/or insulin resistance hypothesized to alter hypothalamic hormonal feedback response → ↑ LH:FSH, ↑ androgens (eg, testosterone) from theca interna cells, ↓ rate of follicular maturation → unruptured follicles (cysts) + anovulation. Common cause of subfertility in women.

Enlarged, bilateral cystic ovaries A; presents with amenorrhea/oligomenorrhea, hirsutism, acne, ↓ fertility. Associated with obesity. ↑ risk of endometrial cancer 2° to unopposed estrogen from repeated anovulatory cycles.

Treatment: weight reduction, OCPs, clomiphene citrate, ketoconazole, spironolactone.

Ovarian cysts

Follicular cyst	Distention of unruptured graafian follicle. May be associated with hyperestrogenism, endometrial hyperplasia. Most common ovarian mass in young women.
Theca-lutein cyst	Often bilateral/multiple. Due to gonadotropin stimulation. Associated with choriocarcinoma and hydatidiform moles.

Ovarian neoplasms

Most common adnexal mass in women > 55 years old. Can be benign or malignant. Arise from surface epithelium, germ cells, or sex cord stromal tissue.

Majority of malignant tumors are epithelial (serous cystadenocarcinoma most common). Risk ↑ with advanced age, infertility, endometriosis, PCOS, genetic predisposition (*BRCA-1* or *BRCA-2* mutation, Lynch syndrome, strong family history). Risk ↓ with previous pregnancy, history of breastfeeding, OCPs, tubal ligation. Presents with adnexal mass, abdominal distension, bowel obstruction, pleural effusion. Monitor response to therapy/relapse by measuring CA 125 levels (not good for screening).

Benign ovarian neoplasms	
Serous cystadenoma	Most common ovarian neoplasm. Lined with fallopian tube–like epithelium. Often bilateral.
Mucinous cystadenoma	Multiloculated, large. Lined by mucus-secreting epithelium A.
Endometrioma	Endometriosis (ectopic endometrial tissue) within ovary with cyst formation. Presents with pelvic pain, dysmenorrhea, dyspareunia; symptoms may vary with menstrual cycle. "Chocolate cyst"—endometrioma filled with dark, reddish-brown blood. Complex mass on ultrasound.
Mature cystic teratoma (dermoid cyst)	Germ cell tumor, most common ovarian tumor in females 10–30 years old. Cystic mass containing elements from all 3 germ layers (eg, teeth, hair, sebum) B. Can present with pain 2° to ovarian enlargement or torsion. A monodermal form with thyroid tissue (struma ovarii) uncommonly presents with hyperthyroidism C.
Brenner tumor	Looks like bladder. Solid tumor that is pale yellow-tan and appears encapsulated. "Coffee bean" nuclei on H&E stain.
Fibromas	Bundles of spindle-shaped fibroblasts. Meigs syndrome—triad of ovarian fibroma, ascites, hydrothorax. "Pulling" sensation in groin.
Thecoma	Like granulosa cell tumors, may produce estrogen. Usually presents as abnormal uterine bleeding in a postmenopausal woman.

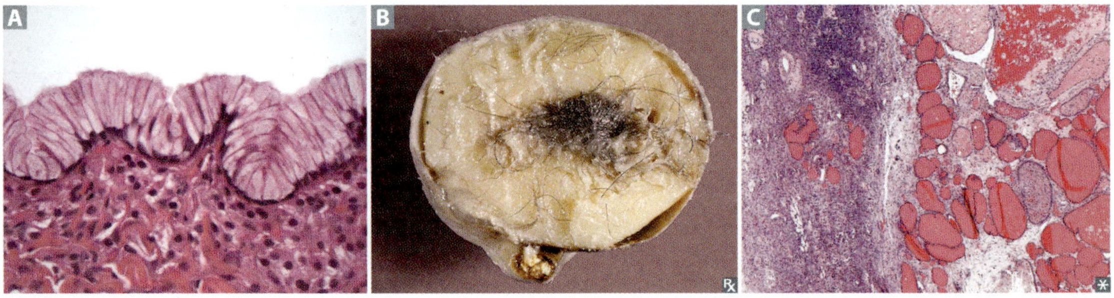

Ovarian neoplasms *(continued)*

Malignant ovarian neoplasms	
Granulosa cell tumor	Most common malignant stromal tumor. Predominantly women in their 50s. Often produces estrogen and/or progesterone and presents with postmenopausal bleeding, sexual precocity (in pre-adolescents), breast tenderness. Histology shows Call-Exner bodies D (granulosa cells arranged haphazardly around collections of eosinophilic fluid, resembling primordial follicles).
Serous cystadenocarcinoma	Most common malignant ovarian neoplasm, frequently bilateral. Psammoma bodies.
Mucinous cystadenocarcinoma	Pseudomyxoma peritonei–intraperitoneal accumulation of mucinous material from ovarian or appendiceal tumor.
Immature teratoma	Aggressive, contains fetal tissue, neuroectoderm. Commonly diagnosed after menopause. Typically represented by immature/embryonic-like neural tissue.
Dysgerminoma	Most common in adolescents. Equivalent to male seminoma but rarer. 1% of all ovarian tumors; 30% of germ cell tumors. Sheets of uniform "fried egg" cells E. hCG, LDH = tumor markers.
Yolk sac (endodermal sinus) tumor	Aggressive, in ovaries or testes (boys) and sacrococcygeal area in young children. Most common tumor in male infants. Yellow, friable (hemorrhagic), solid mass. 50% have Schiller-Duval bodies (resemble glomeruli) F. AFP = tumor marker.
Krukenberg tumor	GI malignancy that metastasizes to ovaries → mucin-secreting signet cell adenocarcinoma.

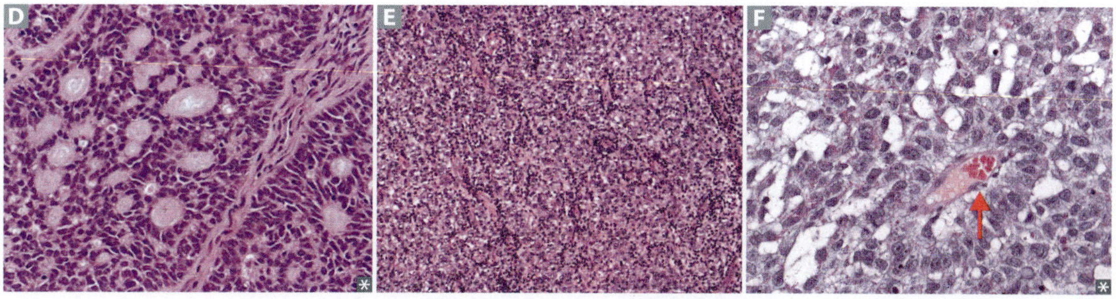

Endometrial conditions

Polyp	Well-circumscribed collection of endometrial tissue within uterine wall. May contain smooth muscle cells. Can extend into endometrial cavity in the form of a polyp. May be asymptomatic or present with painless abnormal uterine bleeding.
Adenomyosis	Extension of endometrial tissue (glandular) into uterine myometrium. Caused by hyperplasia of basal layer of endometrium. Presents with dysmenorrhea, menorrhagia, uniformly enlarged, soft, globular uterus. Treatment: GnRH agonists, hysterectomy.
Leiomyoma (fibroid)	Most common tumor in females. Often presents with multiple discrete tumors A. ↑ incidence in African Americans. Benign smooth muscle tumor; malignant transformation to leiomyosarcoma is rare. Estrogen sensitive—tumor size ↑ with pregnancy and ↓ with menopause. Peak occurrence at 20–40 years old. May be asymptomatic, cause abnormal uterine bleeding, or result in miscarriage. Severe bleeding may lead to iron deficiency anemia. Whorled pattern of smooth muscle bundles with well-demarcated borders B.
Endometrial hyperplasia	Abnormal endometrial gland proliferation C usually caused by excess estrogen stimulation. ↑ risk for endometrial carcinoma; nuclear atypia is greater risk factor than complex (vs simple) architecture. Presents as postmenopausal vaginal bleeding. Risk factors include anovulatory cycles, hormone replacement therapy, polycystic ovarian syndrome, granulosa cell tumor.
Endometrial carcinoma	Most common gynecologic malignancy D. Peak occurrence at 55–65 years old. Presents with vaginal bleeding. Typically preceded by endometrial hyperplasia. Risk factors include prolonged use of estrogen without progestins, obesity, diabetes, hypertension, nulliparity, late menopause, Lynch syndrome.
Endometritis	Inflammation of endometrium E associated with retained products of conception following delivery, miscarriage, abortion, or with foreign body (eg, IUD). Retained material in uterus promotes infection by bacterial flora from vagina or intestinal tract. Treatment: gentamicin + clindamycin +/– ampicillin.
Endometriosis	Non-neoplastic endometrial glands/stroma outside endometrial cavity F. Can be found anywhere; most common sites are ovary (frequently bilateral), pelvis, peritoneum. In ovary, appears as endometrioma (blood-filled "chocolate cyst"). May be due to retrograde flow, metaplastic transformation of multipotent cells, transportation of endometrial tissue via lymphatic system. Characterized by cyclic pelvic pain, bleeding, dysmenorrhea, dyspareunia, dyschezia (pain with defecation), infertility; normal-sized uterus. Treatment: NSAIDs, OCPs, progestins, GnRH agonists, danazol, laparoscopic removal.

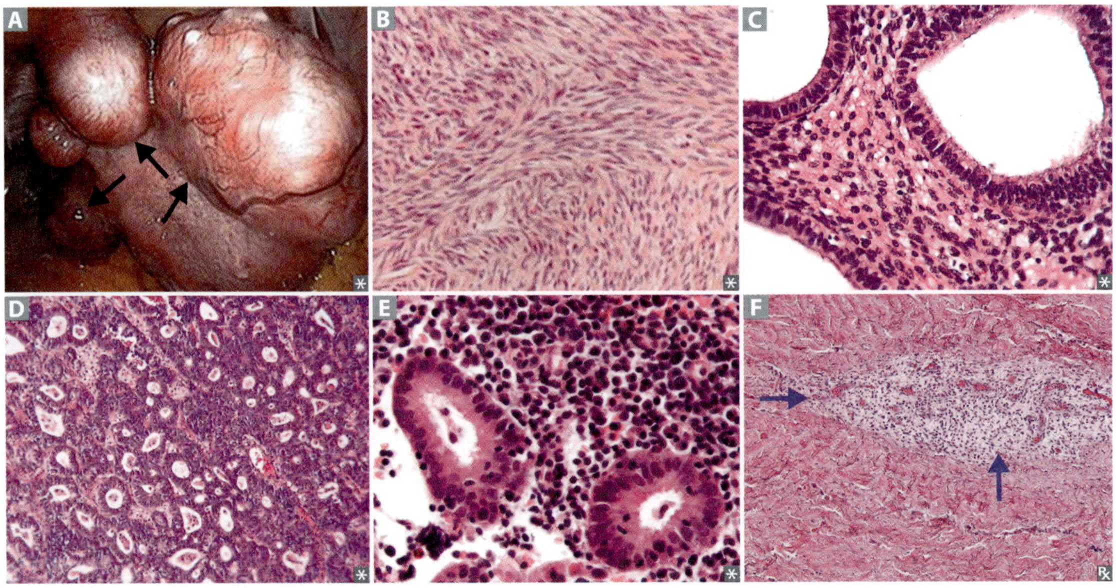

Breast pathology

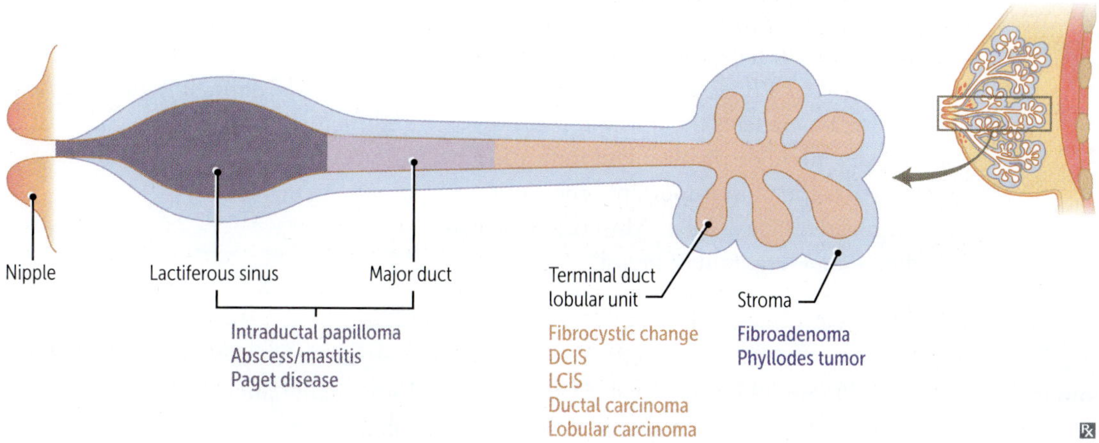

Benign breast disease

Fibroadenoma	Most common in women under 35 years. Small, well-defined, mobile mass. ↑ size and tenderness with ↑ estrogen (eg, pregnancy, prior to menstruation). Risk of cancer is usually not increased.
Fibrocystic changes	Most common in premenopausal women > 35 years. Presents with premenstrual breast pain or lumps; often bilateral and multifocal. Nonproliferative lesions include simple cysts (fluid-filled duct dilation, blue dome), papillary apocrine change/metaplasia, stromal fibrosis. Risk of cancer is usually not increased.
Sclerosing adenosis	↑ acini and stromal fibrosis, associated with calcifications. Slight (1.5–2×) ↑ risk for cancer.
Intraductal papilloma	Small papillary tumor within lactiferous ducts, typically beneath areola. Most common cause of nipple discharge (serous or bloody). Slight (1.5–2×) ↑ risk for cancer.
Epithelial hyperplasia	↑ cells in terminal ductal or lobular epithelium. ↑ risk of carcinoma with atypical cells.
Phyllodes tumor	Large mass of connective tissue and cysts with "leaf-like" lobulations. Most common in 5th decade. Some may become malignant.
Fat necrosis	Benign, usually painless, lump due to injury to breast tissue. Calcified oil cyst on mammography; necrotic fat and giant cells on biopsy. Up to 50% of patients may not report trauma.
Lactational mastitis	During breastfeeding, ↑ risk of bacterial infection through cracks in nipple. *S aureus* is most common pathogen. Treat with antibiotics and continue breastfeeding.
Gynecomastia	Breast enlargement in males due to ↑ estrogen compared with androgen activity. Physiologic (not pathologic) in newborn, pubertal, and elderly males, but may persist after puberty. Other causes include cirrhosis, hypogonadism (eg, Klinefelter syndrome), testicular tumors, and drugs (**S**pironolactone, **H**ormones, **C**imetidine, **K**etoconazole: "**S**ome **H**ormones **C**reate **K**nockers").

Malignant breast tumors

Commonly postmenopausal. Usually arise from terminal duct lobular unit. Overexpression of estrogen/progesterone receptors or *c-erbB2* (HER-2, an EGF receptor) is common; triple negative (ER ⊖, PR ⊖, and Her2/Neu ⊖) more aggressive; type affects therapy and prognosis. Axillary lymph node involvement indicating metastasis is the most important prognostic factor in early-stage disease. Most often located in upper-outer quadrant of breast.

Risk factors: ↑ estrogen exposure, ↑ total number of menstrual cycles, older age at 1st live birth, obesity (↑ estrogen exposure as adipose tissue converts androstenedione to estrone), *BRCA1* and *BRCA2* gene mutations, African American ethnicity (↑ risk for triple ⊖ breast cancer).

TYPE	CHARACTERISTICS	NOTES
Noninvasive		
Ductal carcinoma in situ	Fills ductal lumen (black arrow in A indicates neoplastic cells in duct; blue arrow shows engorged blood vessel). Arises from ductal atypia. Often seen early as microcalcifications on mammography.	Early malignancy without basement membrane penetration.
Comedocarcinoma	Ductal, central necrosis (arrow in B). Subtype of DCIS.	
Paget disease	Results from underlying DCIS or invasive breast cancer. Eczematous patches on nipple C. Paget cells = intraepithelial adenocarcinoma cells.	
Invasive		
Invasive ductal carcinoma	Firm, fibrous, "rock-hard" mass with sharp margins and small, glandular, duct-like cells D. Grossly, see classic "stellate" infiltration.	Most common (~ 75% of all breast cancers).
Invasive lobular carcinoma	Orderly row of cells ("Indian file" E), due to ↓ E-cadherin expression.	Often bilateral with multiple lesions in the same location.
Medullary carcinoma	Fleshy, cellular, lymphocytic infiltrate.	Good prognosis.
Inflammatory breast cancer	Dermal lymphatic invasion by breast carcinoma. Peau d'orange (breast skin resembles orange peel F); neoplastic cells block lymphatic drainage.	Poor prognosis (50% survival at 5 years). Often mistaken for mastitis or Paget disease.

Malignant breast tumors *(continued)*

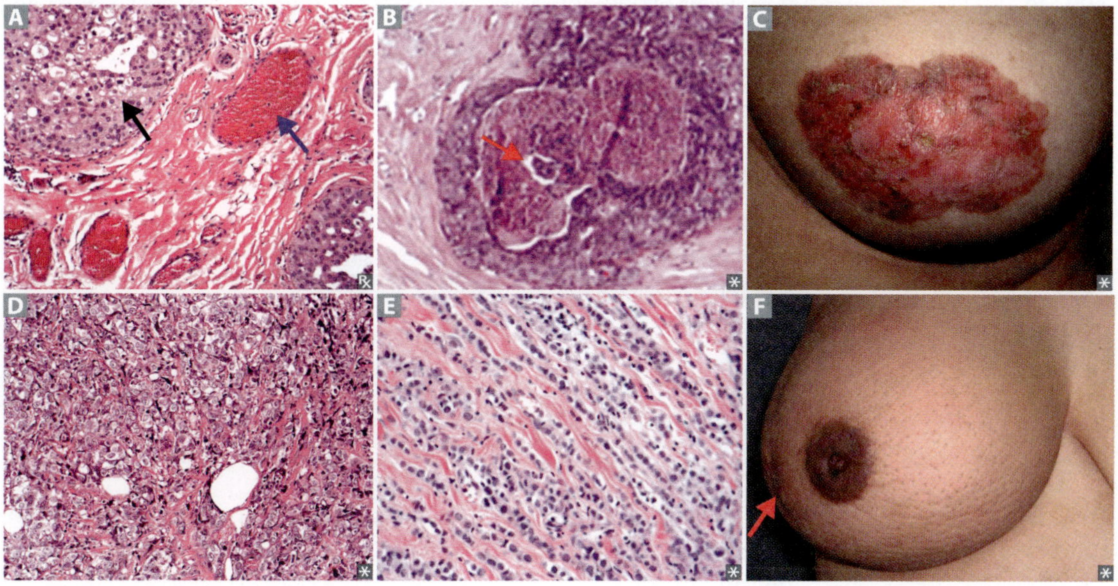

Penile pathology

Peyronie disease

Abnormal curvature of penis due to fibrous plaque within tunica albuginea. Associated with erectile dysfunction. Can cause pain, anxiety. Consider surgical repair once curvature stabilizes. Distinct from penile fracture (rupture of corpora cavernosa due to forced bending).

Ischemic priapism

Painful sustained erection lasting > 4 hours. Associated with sickle cell disease (sickled RBCs get trapped in vascular channels), medications (eg, sildenafil, trazodone). Treat immediately with corporal aspiration, intracavernosal phenylephrine, or surgical decompression to prevent ischemia.

Squamous cell carcinoma

More common in Asia, Africa, South America. Precursor in situ lesions: Bowen disease (in penile shaft, presents as leukoplakia), erythroplasia of Queyrat (cancer of glans, presents as erythroplakia), Bowenoid papulosis (carcinoma in situ of unclear malignant potential, presenting as reddish papules). Associated with HPV and lack of circumcision.

Cryptorchidism

Undescended testis (one or both); impaired spermatogenesis (since sperm develop best at temperatures < 37°C); can have normal testosterone levels (Leydig cells are unaffected by temperature); associated with ↑ risk of germ cell tumors. Prematurity ↑ risk of cryptorchidism. ↓ inhibin B, ↑ FSH, ↑ LH; testosterone ↓ in bilateral cryptorchidism, normal in unilateral.

Varicocele

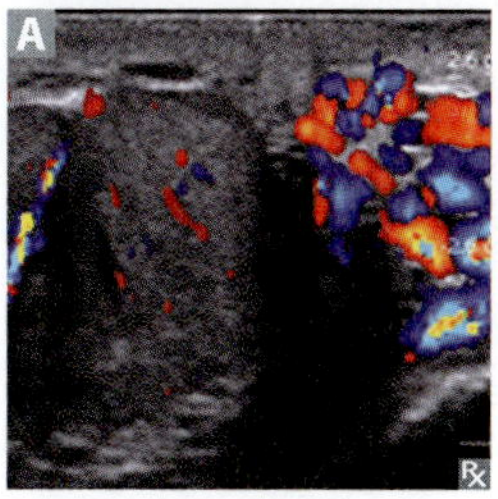

Dilated veins in pampiniform plexus due to ↑ venous pressure; most common cause of scrotal enlargement in adult males; most often on left side because of ↑ resistance to flow from left gonadal vein drainage into left renal vein; can cause infertility because of ↑ temperature; diagnosed by standing clinical exam (distension on inspection and "bag of worms" on palpation) or ultrasound with Doppler A; does not transilluminate.

Treatment: varicocelectomy, embolization.

Extragonadal germ cell tumors	Arise in midline locations. In adults, most commonly in retroperitoneum, mediastinum, pineal, and suprasellar regions. In infants and young children, sacrococcygeal teratomas are most common.	

Scrotal masses	Benign scrotal lesions present as testicular masses that can be transilluminated (vs solid testicular tumors).	
Congenital hydrocele	Common cause of scrotal swelling in infants, due to incomplete obliteration of processus vaginalis.	Transilluminating swelling.
Acquired hydrocele	Scrotal fluid collection usually 2° to infection, trauma, tumor. If bloody → hematocele.	
Spermatocele	Cyst due to dilated epididymal duct or rete testis.	Paratesticular fluctuant nodule.

Testicular germ cell tumors	~ 95% of all testicular tumors. Most often occur in young men. Risk factors: cryptorchidism, Klinefelter syndrome. Can present as a mixed germ cell tumor. Testicular mass that does not transilluminate.
Seminoma	Malignant; painless, homogenous testicular enlargement; most common testicular tumor. Does not occur in infancy. Large cells in lobules with watery cytoplasm and "fried egg" appearance. ↑ placental ALP. Radiosensitive. Late metastasis, excellent prognosis.
Yolk sac (endodermal sinus) tumor	Yellow, mucinous. Aggressive malignancy of testes, analogous to ovarian yolk sac tumor. Schiller-Duval bodies resemble primitive glomeruli. ↑ AFP is highly characteristic. Most common testicular tumor in boys < 3 years old.
Choriocarcinoma	Malignant, ↑ hCG. Disordered syncytiotrophoblastic and cytotrophoblastic elements. Hematogenous metastases to lungs and brain. May produce gynecomastia, symptoms of hyperthyroidism (hCG is structurally similar to LH, FSH, TSH).
Teratoma	Unlike in females, mature teratoma in adult males may be malignant. Benign in children.
Embryonal carcinoma	Malignant, hemorrhagic mass with necrosis; painful; worse prognosis than seminoma. Often glandular/papillary morphology. "Pure" embryonal carcinoma is rare; most commonly mixed with other tumor types. May be associated with ↑ hCG and normal AFP levels when pure (↑ AFP when mixed).

Testicular non–germ cell tumors	5% of all testicular tumors. Mostly benign.
Leydig cell	Golden brown color; contains Reinke crystals (eosinophilic cytoplasmic inclusions). Produce androgens or estrogens → gynecomastia in men, precocious puberty in boys.
Sertoli cell	Androblastoma from sex cord stroma.
Testicular lymphoma	Most common testicular cancer in older men. Not a 1° cancer; arises from metastatic lymphoma to testes. Aggressive.

Benign prostatic hyperplasia

Common in men > 50 years old. Characterized by smooth, elastic, firm nodular enlargement (hyperplasia not hypertrophy) of periurethral (lateral and middle) lobes, which compress the urethra into a vertical slit. Not premalignant.

Often presents with ↑ frequency of urination, nocturia, difficulty starting and stopping urine stream, dysuria. May lead to distention and hypertrophy of bladder, hydronephrosis, UTIs. ↑ free prostate-specific antigen (PSA).

Treatment: α_1-antagonists (terazosin, tamsulosin), which cause relaxation of smooth muscle; 5α-reductase inhibitors (eg, finasteride); tadalafil.

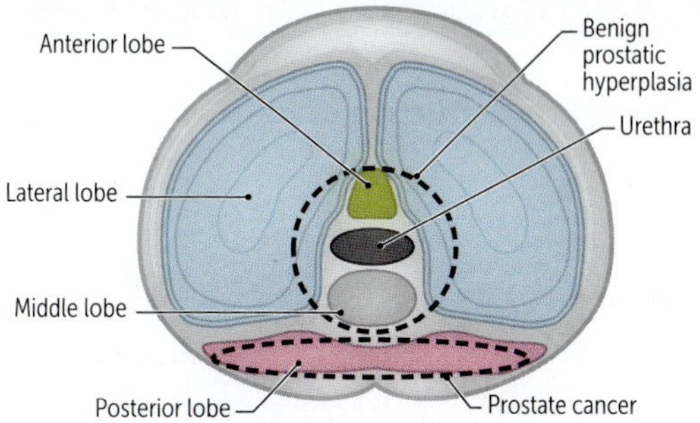

Prostatitis

Dysuria, frequency, urgency, low back pain. Warm, tender, enlarged prostate. Acute: bacterial (eg, *E coli*); chronic: bacterial or abacterial.

Prostatic adenocarcinoma

Common in men > 50 years old. Arises most often from posterior lobe (peripheral zone) of prostate gland and is most frequently diagnosed by ↑ PSA and subsequent needle core biopsies. Prostatic acid phosphatase (PAP) and PSA are useful tumor markers (↑ total PSA, with ↓ fraction of free PSA). Osteoblastic metastases in bone may develop in late stages, as indicated by lower back pain and ↑ serum ALP and PSA.

▶ REPRODUCTIVE—PHARMACOLOGY

Control of reproductive hormones

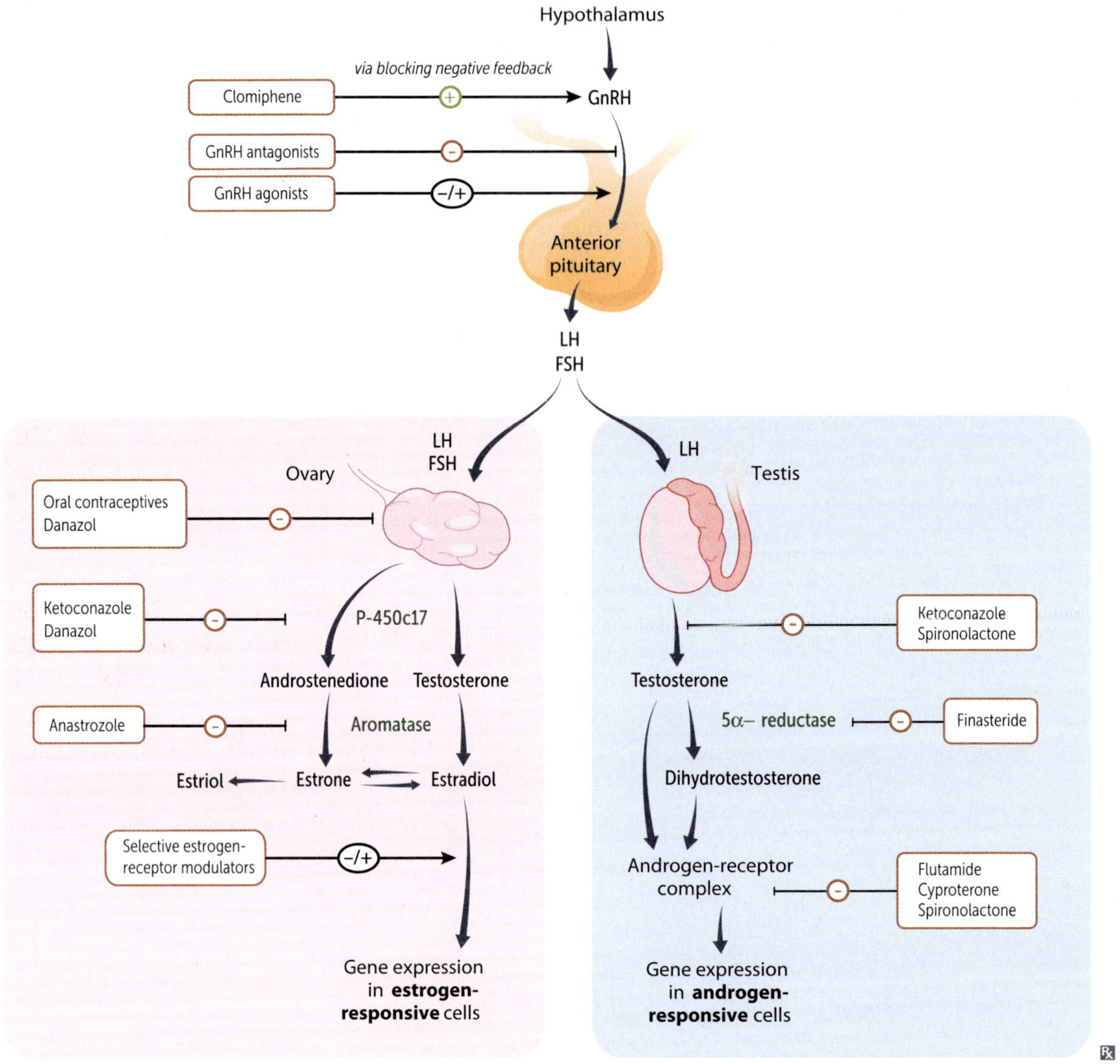

Leuprolide

MECHANISM	GnRH analog with agonist properties when used in pulsatile fashion; antagonist properties when used in continuous fashion (downregulates GnRH receptor in pituitary → ↓ FSH/LH).	Leuprolide can be used in lieu of GnRH.
CLINICAL USE	Uterine fibroids, endometriosis, precocious puberty, prostate cancer, infertility.	

Estrogens

Ethinyl estradiol, DES, mestranol.

MECHANISM	Bind estrogen receptors.
CLINICAL USE	Hypogonadism or ovarian failure, menstrual abnormalities, hormone replacement therapy in postmenopausal women; use in men with androgen-dependent prostate cancer.
ADVERSE EFFECTS	↑ risk of endometrial cancer, bleeding in postmenopausal women, clear cell adenocarcinoma of vagina in females exposed to DES in utero, ↑ risk of thrombi. Contraindications—ER ⊕ breast cancer, history of DVTs.

Selective estrogen receptor modulators

Clomiphene	Antagonist at estrogen receptors in hypothalamus. Prevents normal feedback inhibition and ↑ release of LH and FSH from pituitary, which stimulates ovulation. Used to treat infertility due to anovulation (eg, PCOS). May cause hot flashes, ovarian enlargement, multiple simultaneous pregnancies, visual disturbances.
Tamoxifen	Antagonist at breast; agonist at bone, uterus; ↑ risk of thromboembolic events and endometrial cancer. Used to treat and prevent recurrence of ER/PR ⊕ breast cancer.
Raloxifene	Antagonist at breast, uterus; agonist at bone; ↑ risk of thromboembolic events but no increased risk of endometrial cancer (vs tamoxifen); used primarily to treat osteoporosis.

Aromatase inhibitors

Anastrozole, letrozole, exemestane.

MECHANISM	Inhibit peripheral conversion of androgens to estrogen.
CLINICAL USE	ER ⊕ breast cancer in postmenopausal women.

Hormone replacement therapy

Used for relief or prevention of menopausal symptoms (eg, hot flashes, vaginal atrophy), osteoporosis (↑ estrogen, ↓ osteoclast activity).

Unopposed estrogen replacement therapy ↑ risk of endometrial cancer, so progesterone is added. Possible increased cardiovascular risk.

Progestins	Levonorgestrel, medroxyprogesterone, etonogestrel, norethindrone, megestrol, and many others when combined with estrogen.
MECHANISM	Bind progesterone receptors, ↓ growth and ↑ vascularization of endometrium, thicken cervical mucus.
CLINICAL USE	Contraception (forms include pill, intrauterine device, implant, depot injection), endometrial cancer, abnormal uterine bleeding. Progestin challenge: presence of withdrawal bleeding excludes anatomic defects (eg, Asherman syndrome) and chronic anovulation without estrogen.

Antiprogestins	Mifepristone, ulipristal.
MECHANISM	Competitive inhibitors of progestins at progesterone receptors.
CLINICAL USE	Termination of pregnancy (mifepristone with misoprostol); emergency contraception (ulipristal).

Combined contraception	Progestins and ethinyl estradiol; forms include pill, patch, vaginal ring. Estrogen and progestins inhibit LH/FSH and thus prevent estrogen surge. No estrogen surge → no LH surge → no ovulation. Progestins cause thickening of cervical mucus, thereby limiting access of sperm to uterus. Progestins also inhibit endometrial proliferation → endometrium is less suitable to the implantation of an embryo. Contraindications: smokers > 35 years old (↑ risk of cardiovascular events), patients with ↑ risk of cardiovascular disease (including history of venous thromboembolism, coronary artery disease, stroke), migraine (especially with aura), breast cancer.

Copper intrauterine device	
MECHANISM	Produces local inflammatory reaction toxic to sperm and ova, preventing fertilization and implantation; hormone free.
CLINICAL USE	Long-acting reversible contraception. Most effective emergency contraception.
ADVERSE EFFECTS	Heavier or longer menses, dysmenorrhea. Risk of PID with insertion (contraindicated in active pelvic infection).

Terbutaline, ritodrine	β_2-agonists that relax the uterus; used to ↓ contraction frequency in women during labor.

Danazol	
MECHANISM	Synthetic androgen that acts as partial agonist at androgen receptors.
CLINICAL USE	Endometriosis, hereditary angioedema.
ADVERSE EFFECTS	Weight gain, edema, acne, hirsutism, masculinization, ↓ HDL levels, hepatotoxicity.

Testosterone, methyltestosterone

MECHANISM	Agonists at androgen receptors.
CLINICAL USE	Treat hypogonadism and promote development of 2° sex characteristics; stimulate anabolism to promote recovery after burn or injury.
ADVERSE EFFECTS	Causes masculinization in females; ↓ intratesticular testosterone in males by inhibiting release of LH (via negative feedback) → gonadal atrophy. Premature closure of epiphyseal plates. ↑ LDL, ↓ HDL.

Antiandrogens

Testosterone $\xrightarrow{5\alpha\text{-reductase}}$ DHT (more potent).

Finasteride	5α-reductase inhibitor (↓ conversion of testosterone to DHT). Used for BPH and male-pattern baldness.	
Flutamide	Nonsteroidal competitive inhibitor at androgen receptors. Used for prostate carcinoma.	
Ketoconazole	Inhibits steroid synthesis (inhibits 17,20-desmolase).	Used for polycystic ovarian syndrome to reduce androgenic symptoms. Both have side effects of gynecomastia and amenorrhea.
Spironolactone	Inhibits steroid binding, 17α-hydroxylase, and 17,20-desmolase.	

Tamsulosin

α_1-antagonist used to treat BPH by inhibiting smooth muscle contraction. Selective for $\alpha_{1A,D}$ receptors (found on prostate) vs vascular α_{1B} receptors.

Phosphodiesterase type 5 inhibitors

Sildenafil, vardenafil, tadalafil.

MECHANISM	Inhibit PDE-5 → ↑ cGMP → prolonged smooth muscle relaxation in response to NO → ↑ blood flow in corpus cavernosum of penis, ↓ pulmonary vascular resistance.	Sildena**fil**, vardena**fil**, and tadala**fil** **fill** the penis.
CLINICAL USE	Erectile dysfunction, pulmonary hypertension, BPH (tadalafil only).	
ADVERSE EFFECTS	Headache, flushing, dyspepsia, cyanopia (blue-tinted vision). Risk of life-threatening hypotension in patients taking nitrates.	"**H**ot and sweaty," but then **H**eadache, **H**eartburn, **H**ypotension.

Minoxidil

MECHANISM	Direct arteriolar vasodilator.
CLINICAL USE	Androgenetic alopecia; severe refractory hypertension.

▶ NOTES

Respiratory

"There's so much pollution in the air now that if it weren't for our lungs, there'd be no place to put it all."

—Robert Orben

"Mars is essentially in the same orbit. Somewhat the same distance from the Sun, which is very important. We have seen pictures where there are canals, we believe, and water. If there is water, that means there is oxygen. If there is oxygen, that means we can breathe."

—Former Vice President Dan Quayle

"Whenever I feel blue, I start breathing again."

—L. Frank Baum

"Life is not the amount of breaths you take; it's the moments that take your breath away."

—Hitch

▶ RESPIRATORY—EMBRYOLOGY

Lung development Occurs in five periods. Initial development includes development of lung bud from distal end of respiratory diverticulum during week 4. Lung bud divides into two bronchial buds that branch off into bronchi.

STAGE	IMPORTANT TERMS	NOTES
Embryonic (weeks 4–7)	Lung bud → trachea → mainstem bronchi → secondary (lobar) bronchi → tertiary (segmental) bronchi.	Errors at this stage can lead to TE fistula.
Pseudoglandular (weeks 5–16)	Endodermal tubules → terminal bronchioles. Surrounded by modest capillary network.	Respiration impossible, incompatible with life.
Canalicular (weeks 16–26)	Terminal bronchioles → respiratory bronchioles → alveolar ducts. Surrounded by prominent capillary network.	Airways increase in diameter. Respiration capable at 25 weeks.
Saccular (weeks 26–birth)	Alveolar ducts → terminal sacs. Terminal sacs separated by 1° septae. Pneumocytes develop.	
Alveolar (weeks 32–8 years)	Terminal sacs → adult alveoli (due to 2° septation). In utero, "breathing" occurs via aspiration and expulsion of amniotic fluid → ↑ vascular resistance through gestation. At birth, fluid gets replaced with air → ↓ in pulmonary vascular resistance.	At birth: 20–70 million alveoli. By 8 years: 300–400 million alveoli.

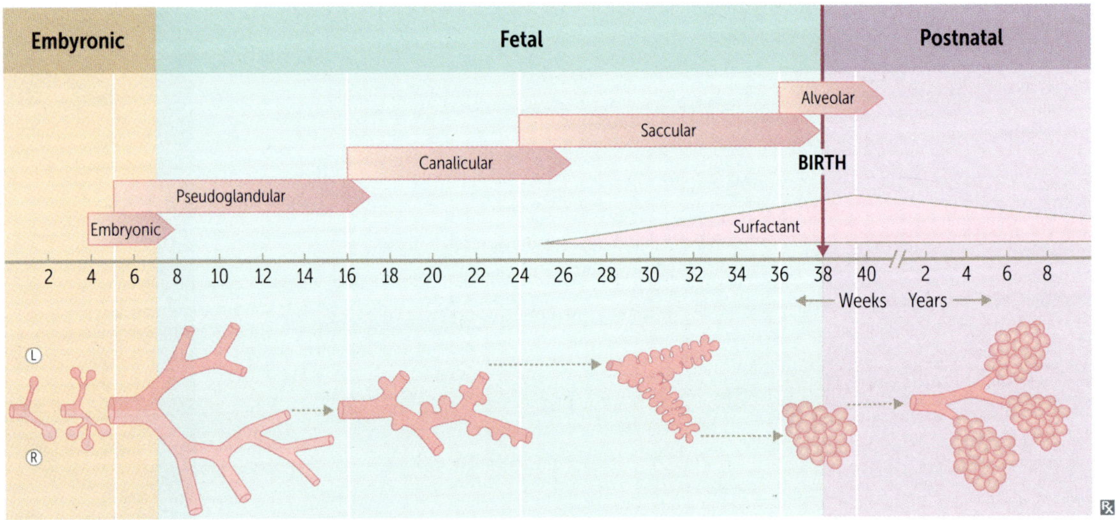

Congenital lung malformations

Pulmonary hypoplasia Poorly developed bronchial tree with abnormal histology usually involving right lung. Associated with congenital diaphragmatic hernia, bilateral renal agenesis (Potter sequence [syndrome]).

Bronchogenic cysts Caused by abnormal budding of the foregut and dilation of terminal or large bronchi. Discrete, round, sharply defined and air-filled densities on CXR. Drain poorly and cause chronic infections.

Pneumocytes

Type I cells

97% of alveolar surfaces. Line the alveoli. Squamous; thin for optimal gas diffusion.

Type II cells

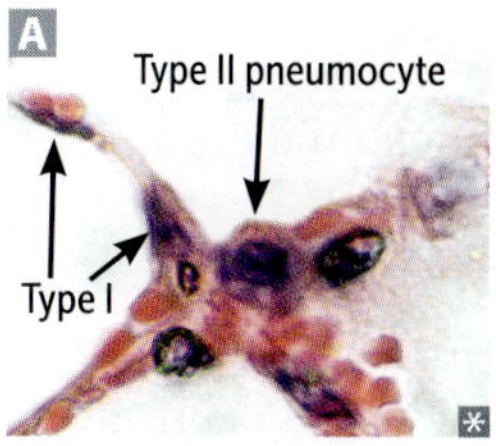

Secrete pulmonary surfactant → ↓ alveolar surface tension, prevents alveolar collapse, ↓ lung recoil, and ↑ compliance. Cuboidal and clustered A. Also serve as precursors to type I cells and other type II cells. Type II cells proliferate during lung damage.

$$\text{Collapsing pressure } (P) = \frac{2\text{ (surface tension)}}{\text{radius}}$$

Alveoli have ↑ tendency to collapse on expiration as radius ↓ (law of Laplace).

Pulmonary surfactant is a complex mix of lecithins, the most important of which is dipalmitoylphosphatidylcholine.

Surfactant synthesis begins around week 26 of gestation, but mature levels are not achieved until around week 35.

Club cells

Nonciliated; low-columnar/cuboidal with secretory granules. Secrete component of surfactant; degrade toxins; act as reserve cells.

Neonatal respiratory distress syndrome

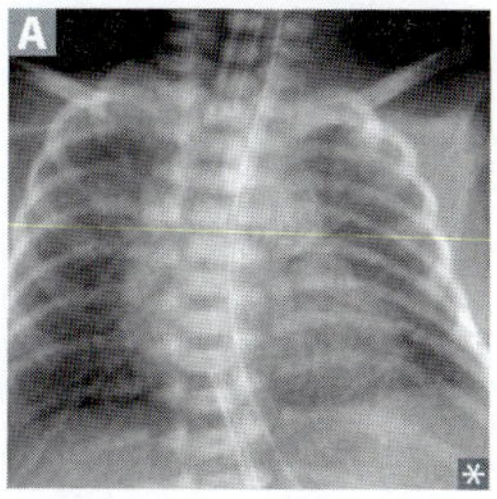

Surfactant deficiency → ↑ surface tension → alveolar collapse ("ground-glass" appearance of lung fields) A. Screening tests for fetal lung maturity: lecithin-sphingomyelin (L/S) ratio in amniotic fluid (> 2 is healthy; < 1.5 predictive of NRDS), foam stability index test, surfactant-albumin ratio. Persistently low O_2 tension → risk of PDA.

Risk factors: prematurity, maternal diabetes (due to ↑ fetal insulin), C-section delivery (↓ release of fetal glucocorticoids).

Complications: metabolic acidosis, PDA, necrotizing enterocolitis.

Treatment: maternal steroids before birth; artificial surfactant for infant.

Therapeutic supplemental O_2 can result in **R**etinopathy of prematurity, **I**ntraventricular hemorrhage, **B**ronchopulmonary dysplasia (**RIB**).

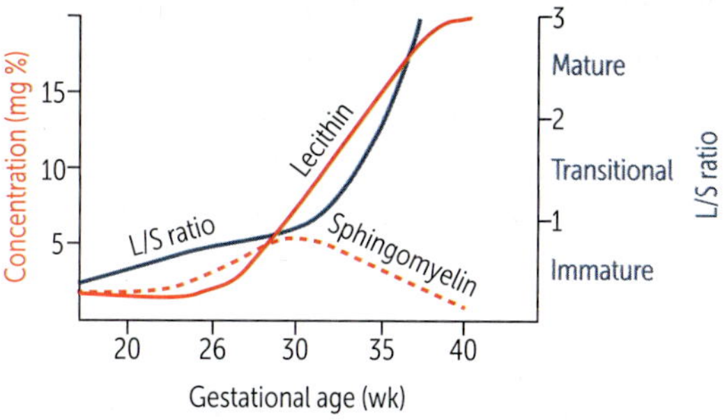

▶ RESPIRATORY—ANATOMY

Respiratory tree

Conducting zone	Large airways consist of nose, pharynx, larynx, trachea, and bronchi. Small airways consist of bronchioles that further divide into terminal bronchioles (large numbers in parallel → least airway resistance). Warms, humidifies, and filters air but does not participate in gas exchange → "anatomic dead space." Cartilage and goblet cells extend to end of bronchi. Pseudostratified ciliated columnar cells primarily make up epithelium of bronchus and extend to beginning of terminal bronchioles, then transition to cuboidal cells. Clear mucus and debris from lungs (mucociliary escalator). Airway smooth muscle cells extend to end of terminal bronchioles (sparse beyond this point).
Respiratory zone	Lung parenchyma; consists of respiratory bronchioles, alveolar ducts, and alveoli. Participates in gas exchange. Mostly cuboidal cells in respiratory bronchioles, then simple squamous cells up to alveoli. Cilia terminate in respiratory bronchioles. Alveolar macrophages clear debris and participate in immune response.

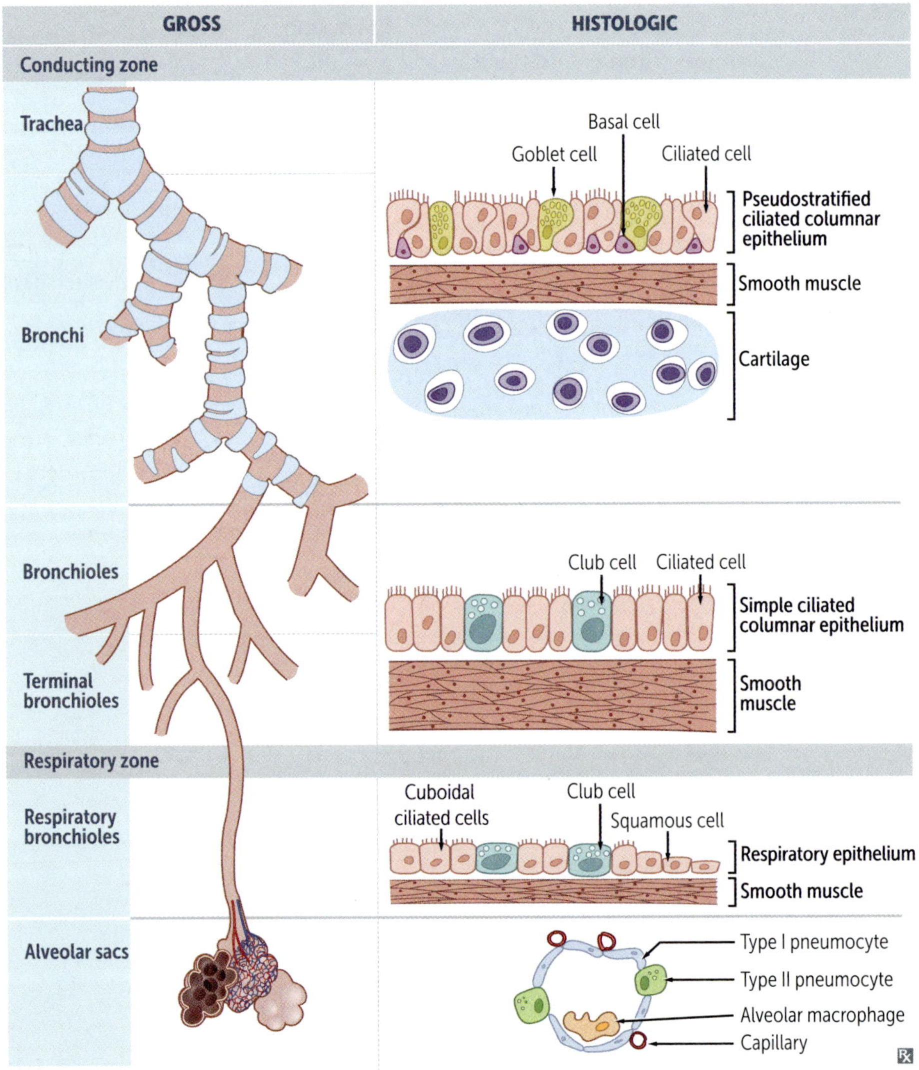

Lung relations

Right lung has 3 lobes; **L**eft has **L**ess **L**obes (2) and **L**ingula (homolog of right middle lobe). Right lung is more common site for inhaled foreign body because the right main stem bronchus is wider and more vertical than the left.

If you aspirate a peanut:
- While upright—enters inferior segment of right inferior lobe.
- While supine—enters superior segment of right inferior lobe.

Instead of a middle lobe, the left lung has a space occupied by the heart.

The relation of the pulmonary artery to the bronchus at each lung hilum is described by **RALS**—**R**ight **A**nterior; **L**eft **S**uperior.

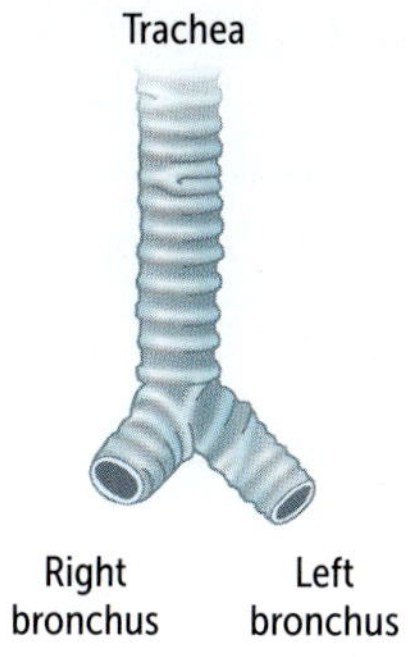

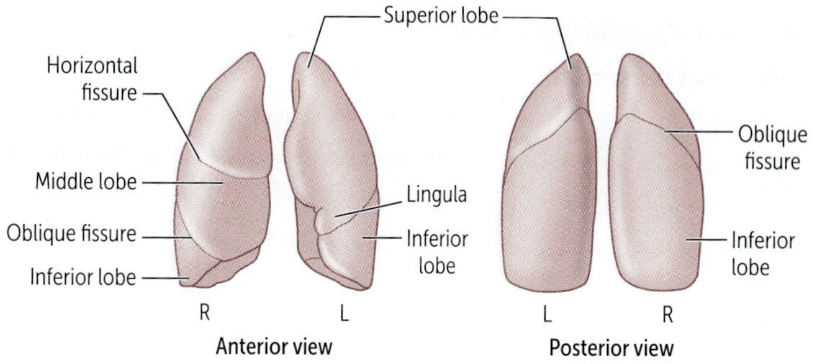

Diaphragm structures

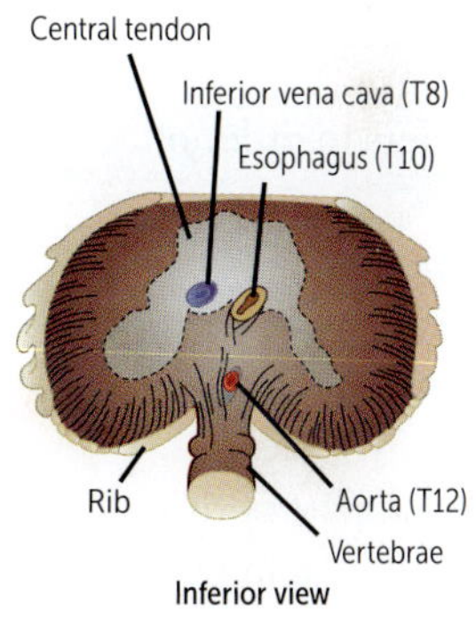

Structures perforating diaphragm:
- At T8: IVC
- At T**10**: esophagus, vagus (CN **10**; 2 trunks)
- At T12: aorta (red), thoracic duct (white), azygos vein (blue) ("At **T-1-2** it's the **red**, **white**, and **blue**")

Diaphragm is innervated by C3, 4, and 5 (phrenic nerve). Pain from diaphragm irritation (eg, air, blood, or pus in peritoneal cavity) can be referred to shoulder (C5) and trapezius ridge (C3, 4).

Number of letters = T level:
- **T8**: vena cava
- **T10**: "oesophagus"
- **T12**: aortic hiatus

I (IVC) **ate** (8) **ten** (10) **eggs** (esophagus) **at** (aorta) **twelve** (12).

C3, 4, 5 keeps the diaphragm **alive**.

Other bifurcations:
- The common carotid bi**four**cates at C**4**.
- The trachea bi**four**cates at T**4**.
- The abdominal aorta bi**four**cates at L**4**.

▶ RESPIRATORY—PHYSIOLOGY

Lung volumes

Inspiratory reserve volume	Air that can still be breathed in after normal inspiration
Tidal volume	Air that moves into lung with each quiet inspiration, typically 500 mL
Expiratory reserve volume	Air that can still be breathed out after normal expiration
Residual volume	Air in lung after maximal expiration; cannot be measured on spirometry
Inspiratory capacity	IRV + TV
Functional residual capacity	RV + ERV Volume of gas in lungs after normal expiration; includes RV, cannot be measured on spirometry
Vital capacity	TV + IRV + ERV Maximum volume of gas that can be expired after a maximal inspiration
Total lung capacity	IRV + TV + ERV + RV Volume of gas present in lungs after a maximal inspiration; includes RV, cannot be measured by spirometry

Lung volumes (LITER):

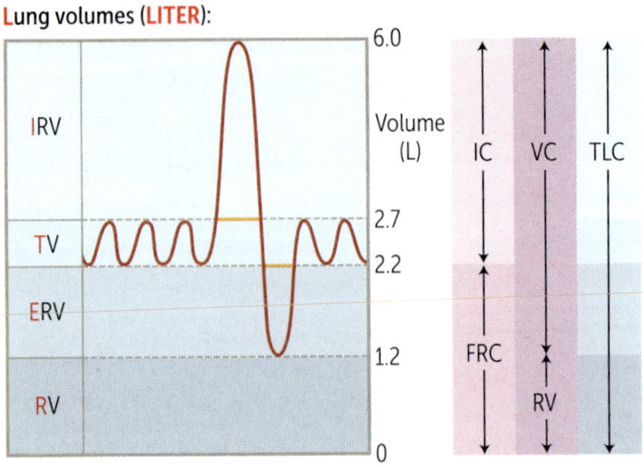

A capacity is a sum of ≥ 2 physiologic volumes.

Determination of physiologic dead space

$$V_D = V_T \times \frac{Pa_{CO_2} - Pe_{CO_2}}{Pa_{CO_2}}$$

V_D = physiologic dead space = anatomic dead space of conducting airways plus alveolar dead space; apex of healthy lung is largest contributor of alveolar dead space. Volume of inspired air that does not take part in gas exchange.

V_T = tidal volume.

Pa_{CO_2} = arterial P_{CO_2}.

Pe_{CO_2} = expired air P_{CO_2}.

Taco, Paco, PEco, Paco (refers to order of variables in equation)

Physiologic dead space—approximately equivalent to anatomic dead space in normal lungs. May be greater than anatomic dead space in lung diseases with $\dot{V}/\dot{Q}$ defects.

Pathologic dead space—when part of the respiratory zone becomes unable to perform gas exchange. Ventilated but not perfused.

Ventilation

Minute ventilation (V_E)	Total volume of gas entering lungs per minute $V_E = V_T \times RR$	Normal values: Respiratory rate (RR) = 12–20 breaths/min V_T = 500 mL/breath V_D = 150 mL/breath
Alveolar ventilation (V_A)	Volume of gas per unit time that reaches alveoli $V_A = (V_T - V_D) \times RR$	

Lung and chest wall

Elastic recoil—tendency for lungs to collapse inward and chest wall to spring outward.
At FRC, inward pull of lung is balanced by outward pull of chest wall, and system pressure is atmospheric.
Elastic properties of both chest wall and lungs determine their combined volume.
At FRC, airway and alveolar pressures are 0, and intrapleural pressure is negative (prevents pneumothorax). PVR is at minimum.
Compliance—change in lung volume for a change in pressure; expressed as $\Delta V/\Delta P$ and is inversely proportional to wall stiffness. High compliance = lung easier to fill, lower compliance = lung harder to fill. ↓ in pulmonary fibrosis, pneumonia, pulmonary edema; ↑ in emphysema, normal aging. Surfactant increases compliance.
Hysteresis—lung inflation curve follows a different curve than the lung deflation curve due to need to overcome surface tension forces in inflation.

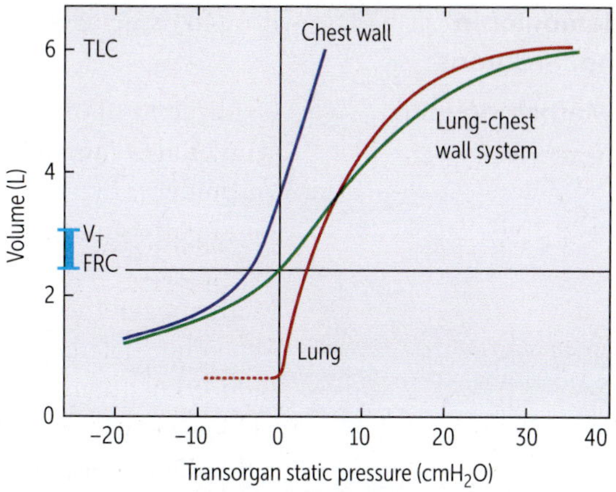

Compliant lungs **comply** (cooperate) and fill easily with air.

rememb. w/ small diam its hard to open. w/ each ↑ in radius = easier & easier to open further

---

Hemoglobin

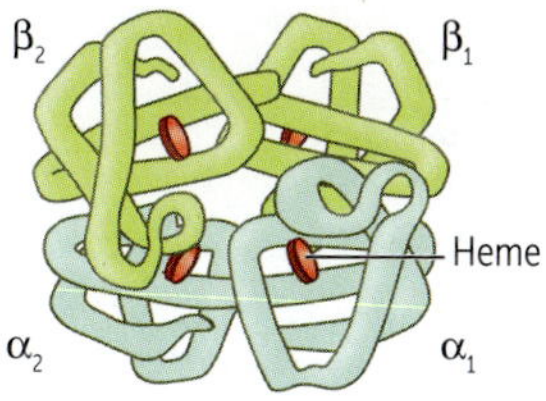

Hemoglobin (Hb) is composed of 4 polypeptide subunits (2 α and 2 β) and exists in 2 forms:

- T (taut; deoxygenated) form has low affinity for O_2, thus promoting release/unloading of O_2.
- R (relaxed; oxygenated) form has high affinity for O_2 (300×). Hb exhibits positive cooperativity and negative allostery.

↑ Cl^-, H^+, CO_2, 2,3-BPG, and temperature favor taut form over relaxed form (shifts dissociation curve right → ↑ O_2 unloading).

Fetal Hb (2α and 2γ subunits) has a higher affinity for O_2 than adult Hb, driving diffusion of oxygen across the placenta from mother to fetus. ↑ O_2 affinity results from ↓ affinity of HbF for 2,3-BPG.

Taut in **T**issues.
Relaxed in **R**espiratory area.

Hemoglobin acts as buffer for H^+ ions.

Hemoglobin modifications — Lead to tissue hypoxia from ↓ O_2 saturation and ↓ O_2 content.

Methemoglobin	Oxidized form of Hb (ferric, Fe^{3+}) that does not bind O_2 as readily, but has ↑ affinity for cyanide. Iron in Hb is normally in a reduced state (ferrous, Fe^{2+}). Methemoglobinemia may present with cyanosis and chocolate-colored blood. Induced methemoglobinemia (using nitrites, followed by thiosulfate) may be used to treat cyanide poisoning.	**Meth**emoglobinemia can be treated with **meth**ylene blue and vitamin C. Nitrites (eg, from dietary intake or polluted/high altitude H_2O) and benzocaine cause poisoning by oxidizing Fe^{2+} to Fe^{3+}. Fe^{2+} binds O_2.
Carboxyhemoglobin	Form of Hb bound to CO in place of O_2. Causes ↓ oxygen-binding capacity with left shift in oxygen-hemoglobin dissociation curve. ↓ O_2 unloading in tissues. CO binds competitively to Hb and with 200× greater affinity than O_2. Treat with 100% O_2 and hyperbaric O_2.	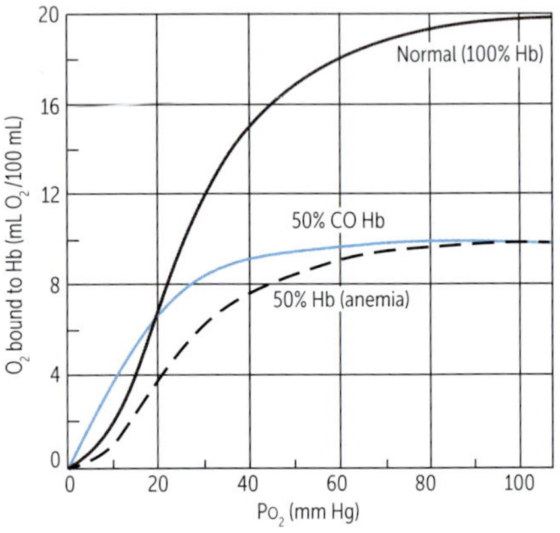

Oxygen-hemoglobin dissociation curve

Sigmoidal shape due to positive cooperativity (ie, tetrameric Hb molecule can bind 4 O_2 molecules and has higher affinity for each subsequent O_2 molecule bound). Myoglobin is monomeric and thus does not show positive cooperativity; curve lacks sigmoidal appearance.

When curve shifts to the right, ↓ affinity of Hb for O_2 (facilitates unloading of O_2 to tissue).

An ↑ in all factors (including H^+) causes a shift of the curve to the right.

A ↓ in all factors (including H^+) causes a left shift → ↓ O_2 unloading → renal hypoxia → ↑ EPO synthesis → compensatory erythrocytosis. **L**ower = **L**eft.

Fetal Hb has higher affinity for O_2 than adult Hb, so its dissociation curve is shifted left.

Right shift—**ACE BAT**s **right** handed:
- **A**cid
- **C**O_2
- **E**xercise
- 2,3-**B**PG
- **A**ltitude
- **T**emperature

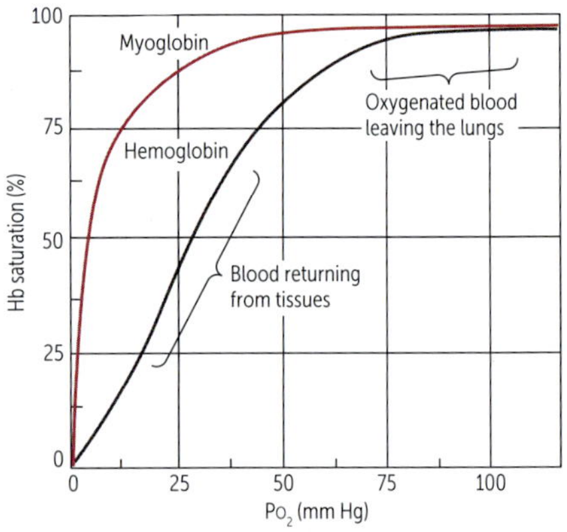

O_2 content = PaO_2 SaO_2 Hg.

Oxygen content of blood

O_2 content = $(1.34 \times Hb \times Sao_2) + (0.003 \times Pao_2)$
Hb = hemoglobin level
Sao_2 = arterial O_2 saturation
Pao_2 = partial pressure of O_2

Normally 1 g Hb can bind 1.34 mL O_2; normal Hb amount in blood is 15 g/dL.
O_2 binding capacity ≈ 20.1 mL O_2/dL blood.
With ↓ Hb there is ↓ O_2 content of arterial blood, but no change in O_2 saturation and Pao_2.
O_2 delivery to tissues = cardiac output × O_2 content of blood.

	Hb concentration	% O_2 sat of Hb	Dissolved O_2 (Pao_2)	Total O_2 content
CO poisoning	Normal	↓ (CO competes with O_2)	Normal	↓
Anemia	↓	Normal	Normal	↓
Polycythemia	↑	Normal	Normal	↑

Pulmonary circulation

Normally a low-resistance, high-compliance system. Po_2 and Pco_2 exert opposite effects on pulmonary and systemic circulation. A ↓ in P_{AO_2} causes a hypoxic vasoconstriction that shifts blood away from poorly ventilated regions of lung to well-ventilated regions of lung.

Perfusion limited—O_2 (normal health), CO_2, N_2O. Gas equilibrates early along the length of the capillary. Diffusion can be ↑ only if blood flow ↑.

Diffusion limited—O_2 (emphysema, fibrosis), CO. Gas does not equilibrate by the time blood reaches the end of the capillary.

A consequence of pulmonary hypertension is cor pulmonale and subsequent right ventricular failure (jugular venous distention, edema, hepatomegaly).

Diffusion: $\dot{V}_{gas} = A \times D_k \times \frac{P_1 - P_2}{T}$ where

A = area, T = alveolar wall thickness, $D_k(P_1 - P_2)$ ≈ difference in partial pressures:
- A ↓ in emphysema.
- T ↑ in pulmonary fibrosis.

DLCO is the extent to which oxygen passes from air sacs of lungs into blood.

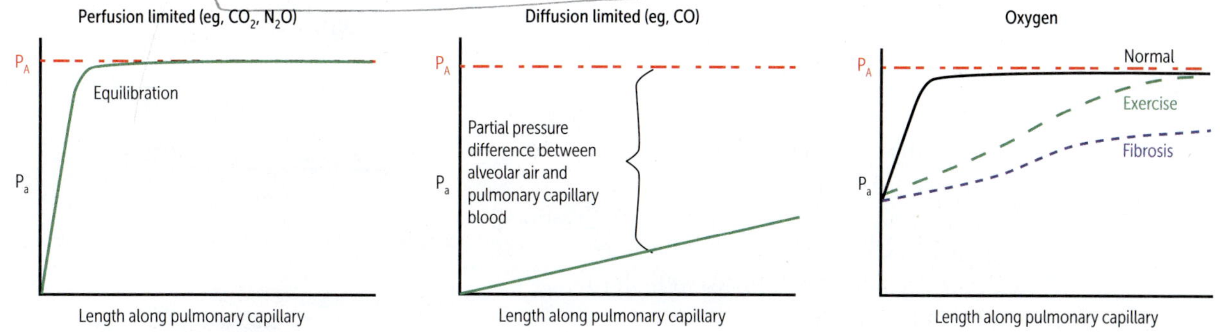

P_a = partial pressure of gas in pulmonary capillary blood
P_A = partial pressure of gas in alveolar air

Pulmonary vascular resistance

$$PVR = \frac{P_{\text{pulm artery}} - P_{\text{L atrium}}}{\text{cardiac output}}$$

R = resistance
$P_{\text{pulm artery}}$ = pressure in pulmonary artery
$P_{\text{L atrium}} \approx$ pulmonary capillary wedge pressure

Remember: $\Delta P = Q \times R$, so $R = \Delta P / Q$
$R = 8\eta l / \pi r^4$

η = viscosity of blood; l = vessel length; r = vessel radius

Alveolar gas equation

$$P_{AO_2} = P_{IO_2} - \frac{Pa_{CO_2}}{R}$$

$$\approx 150 \text{ mm Hg}^a - \frac{Pa_{CO_2}}{0.8}$$

[a] At sea level breathing room air

P_{AO_2} = alveolar P_{O_2} (mm Hg)
P_{IO_2} = P_{O_2} in inspired air (mm Hg)
Pa_{CO_2} = arterial P_{CO_2} (mm Hg)
R = respiratory quotient = CO_2 produced/O_2 consumed
A-a gradient = $P_{AO_2} - Pa_{O_2}$ = 10–15 mm Hg
↑ A-a gradient may occur in hypoxemia; causes include shunting, $\dot{V}/\dot{Q}$ mismatch, fibrosis (impairs diffusion)

Oxygen deprivation

Hypoxia (↓ O_2 delivery to tissue)	Hypoxemia (↓ Pa_{O_2})	Ischemia (loss of blood flow)
↓ cardiac output Hypoxemia Anemia CO poisoning	Normal A-a gradient ▪ High altitude ▪ Hypoventilation (eg, opioid use) ↑ A-a gradient ▪ $\dot{V}/\dot{Q}$ mismatch ▪ Diffusion limitation (eg, fibrosis) ▪ Right-to-left shunt	Impeded arterial flow ↓ venous drainage

---

$\dot{V}/\dot{Q}$ mismatch

Ideally, ventilation is matched to perfusion (ie, $\dot{V}/\dot{Q} = 1$) for adequate gas exchange.

Lung zones:
- $\dot{V}/\dot{Q}$ at apex of lung = 3 (wasted ventilation)
- $\dot{V}/\dot{Q}$ at base of lung = 0.6 (wasted perfusion)

Both ventilation and perfusion are greater at the base of the lung than at the apex of the lung.

With exercise (↑ cardiac output), there is vasodilation of apical capillaries → $\dot{V}/\dot{Q}$ ratio approaches 1.

Certain organisms that thrive in high O_2 (eg, TB) flourish in the apex.

$\dot{V}/\dot{Q} = 0$ = "oirway" obstruction (shunt). In shunt, 100% O_2 does not improve Pa_{O_2} (eg, foreign body aspiration).

$\dot{V}/\dot{Q} = \infty$ = blood flow obstruction (physiologic dead space). Assuming < 100% dead space, 100% O_2 improves Pa_{O_2} (eg, pulmonary embolus).

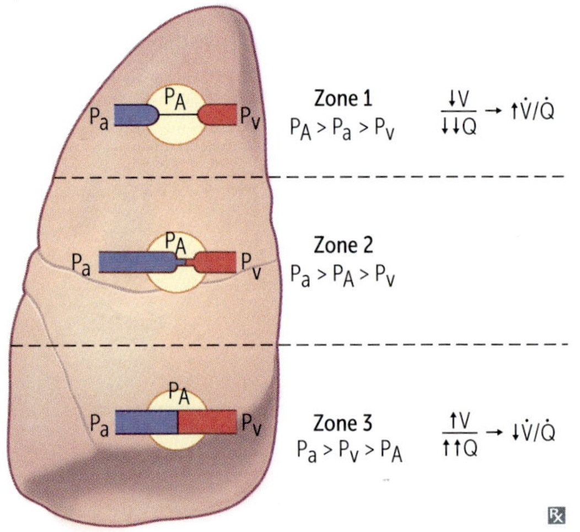

CO_2 transport

CO_2 is transported from tissues to lungs in 3 forms:

- HCO_3^- (90%).
- Carbaminohemoglobin or $HbCO_2$ (5%). CO_2 bound to Hb at N-terminus of globin (not heme). CO_2 binding favors taut form (O_2 unloaded).
- Dissolved CO_2 (5%).

In lungs, oxygenation of Hb promotes dissociation of H^+ from Hb. This shifts equilibrium toward CO_2 formation; therefore, CO_2 is released from RBCs (Haldane effect).

In peripheral tissue, ↑ H^+ from tissue metabolism shifts curve to right, unloading O_2 (Bohr effect).

Majority of blood CO_2 is carried as HCO_3^- in the plasma.

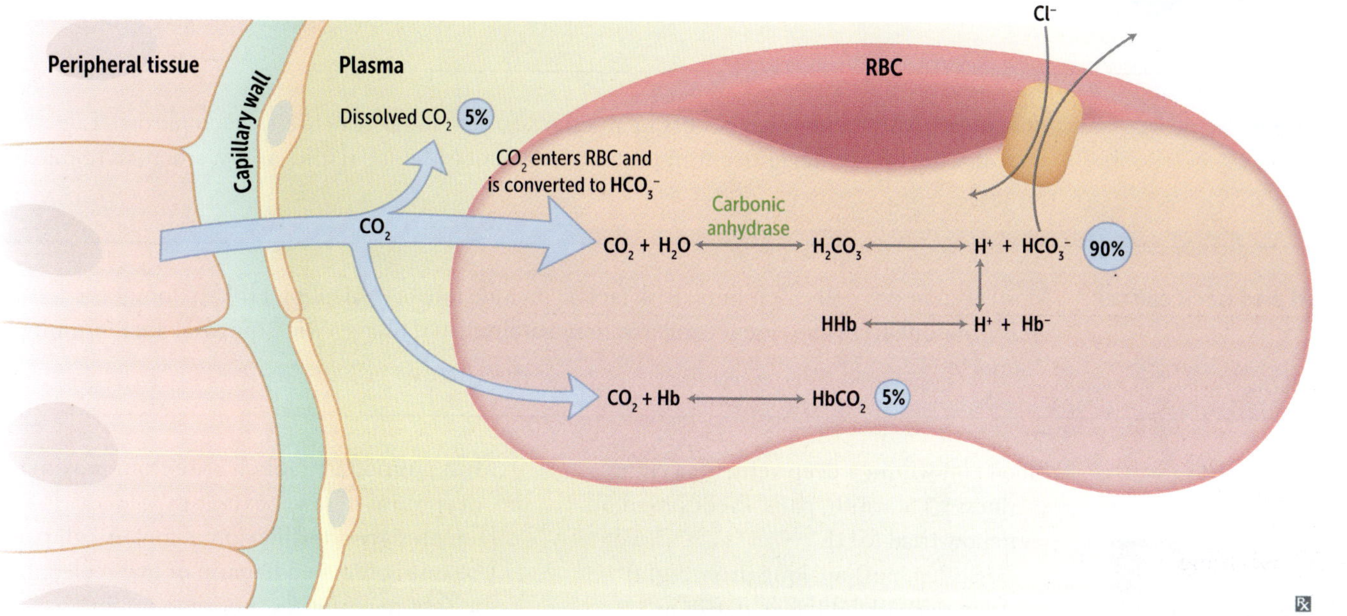

Response to high altitude

↓ atmospheric oxygen (PO_2) → ↓ Pao_2 → ↑ ventilation → ↓ $Paco_2$ → respiratory alkalosis → altitude sickness.

Chronic ↑ in ventilation.

↑ erythropoietin → ↑ hematocrit and Hb (chronic hypoxia).

↑ 2,3-BPG (binds to Hb so that Hb releases more O_2).

Cellular changes (↑ mitochondria).

↑ renal excretion of HCO_3^- to compensate for respiratory alkalosis (can augment with acetazolamide).

Chronic hypoxic pulmonary vasoconstriction results in pulmonary hypertension and RVH.

Response to exercise

↑ CO_2 production.

↑ O_2 consumption.

↑ ventilation rate to meet O_2 demand.

$\dot{V}/\dot{Q}$ ratio from apex to base becomes more uniform. b/c perfusion ↑

↑ pulmonary blood flow due to ↑ cardiac output.

↓ pH during strenuous exercise (2° to lactic acidosis).

No change in Pao_2 and $Paco_2$, but ↑ in venous CO_2 content and ↓ in venous O_2 content.

▸ RESPIRATORY—PATHOLOGY

Rhinosinusitis

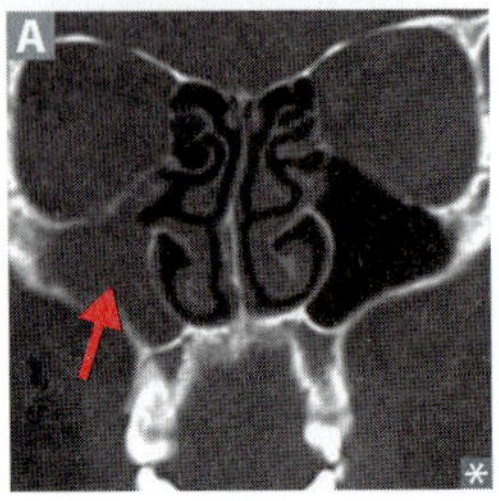

Obstruction of sinus drainage into nasal cavity → inflammation and pain over affected area (typically maxillary sinuses A, which drain into the middle meatus, in adults).

Most common acute cause is viral URI; may cause superimposed bacterial infection, most commonly *S pneumoniae, H influenzae, M catarrhalis*.

Epistaxis

Nose bleed. Most commonly occurs in anterior segment of nostril (Kiesselbach plexus). Life-threatening hemorrhages occur in posterior segment (sphenopalatine artery, a branch of maxillary artery).

Head and neck cancer

Mostly squamous cell carcinoma. Risk factors include tobacco, alcohol, HPV-16 (oropharyngeal), EBV (nasopharyngeal). Field cancerization: carcinogen damages wide mucosal area → multiple tumors.

Deep venous thrombosis

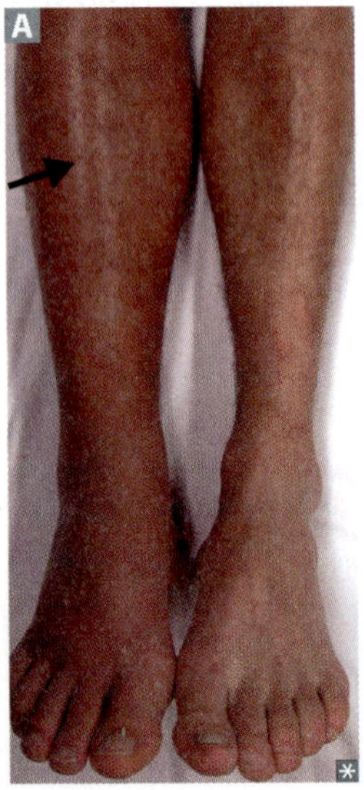

Blood clot within a deep vein → swelling, redness A, warmth, pain. Predisposed by Virchow triad (**SHE**):

- **S**tasis (eg, post-op, long drive/flight)
- **H**ypercoagulability (eg, defect in coagulation cascade proteins, such as factor V Leiden)
- **E**ndothelial damage (exposed collagen triggers clotting cascade)

D-dimer lab test used clinically to rule out DVT (high sensitivity, low specificity).

Most pulmonary emboli arise from proximal deep veins of lower extremity.

Homan sign—dorsiflexion of foot → calf pain.

Use unfractionated heparin or low-molecular-weight heparins (eg, enoxaparin) for prophylaxis and acute management.

Use oral anticoagulants (eg, warfarin, rivaroxaban) for treatment (long-term prevention).

Imaging test of choice is compression ultrasound.

Pulmonary emboli

$\dot{V}/\dot{Q}$ mismatch → hypoxemia → respiratory alkalosis. Sudden-onset dyspnea, chest pain, tachypnea, tachycardia. Large emboli or saddle embolus A may cause sudden death.

CT pulmonary angiography is imaging test of choice for PE (look for filling defects) C.

Lines of Zahn are interdigitating areas of pink (platelets, fibrin) and red (RBCs) found only in thrombi formed before death; help distinguish pre- and postmortem thrombi B.

Types: **F**at, **A**ir, **T**hrombus, **B**acteria, **A**mniotic fluid, **T**umor.

An embolus moves like a **FAT BAT**.

Fat emboli—associated with long bone fractures and liposuction; classic triad of hypoxemia, neurologic abnormalities, petechial rash.

Amniotic fluid emboli—can lead to DIC, especially postpartum.

Air emboli—nitrogen bubbles precipitate in ascending divers (caisson disease, decompression sickness); treat with hyperbaric O_2; or, can be iatrogenic 2° to invasive procedures (eg, central line placement).

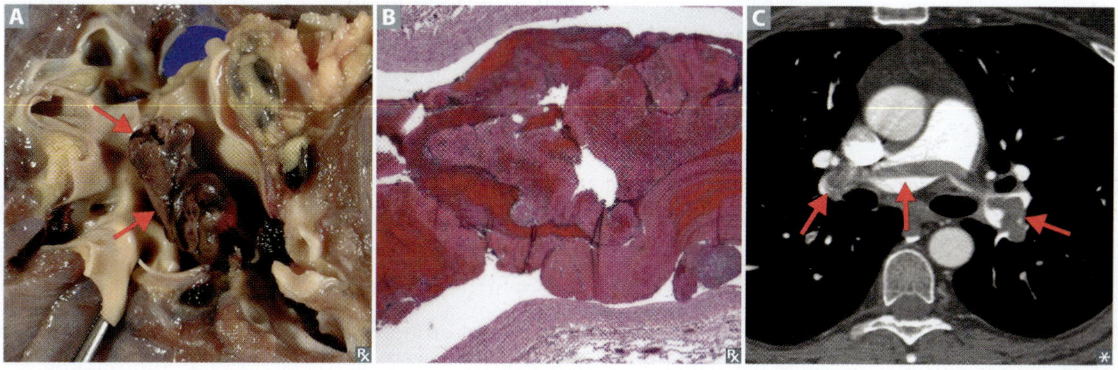

Obstructive lung diseases

Obstruction of air flow resulting in air trapping in lungs. Airways close prematurely at high lung volumes → ↑ RV and ↑ FRC, ↑ TLC. PFTs: ↓↓ FEV_1, ↓ FVC → ↓ FEV_1/FVC ratio (hallmark), $\dot{V}/\dot{Q}$ mismatch. Chronic, hypoxic pulmonary vasoconstriction can lead to cor pulmonale.

TYPE	PATHOLOGY	OTHER
Chronic bronchitis ("blue bloater")	Hyperplasia of mucus-secreting glands in bronchi → Reid index (thickness of mucosal gland layer to thickness of wall between epithelium and cartilage) > 50%.	Productive cough for > 3 (not necessarily consecutive) months per year for > 2 consecutive years. Findings: wheezing, crackles, cyanosis (early-onset hypoxemia due to shunting), late-onset dyspnea, CO_2 retention (hypercapnia), 2° polycythemia. Chronic complications: pulmonary hypertension, cor pulmonale.
Emphysema ("pink puffer")	Enlargement of air spaces, ↓ recoil, ↑ compliance, ↓ diffusing capacity for CO resulting from destruction of alveolar walls (arrow in A). Two types: ▪ Centriacinar—associated with smoking B C. Frequently in upper lobes. ▪ Panacinar—associated with α_1-antitrypsin deficiency. Frequently in lower lobes.	↑ elastase activity → loss of elastic fibers → ↑ lung compliance. Exhalation through pursed lips to ↑ airway pressure and prevent airway collapse during respiration. Barrel-shaped chest D. X-ray shows ↑ AP diameter, flattened diaphragm, ↑ lung field lucency.
Asthma	Bronchial hyperresponsiveness causes reversible bronchoconstriction. Smooth muscle hypertrophy, Curschmann spirals E (shed epithelium forms whorled mucus plugs), and Charcot-Leyden crystals (eosinophilic, hexagonal, double-pointed, needle-like crystals formed from breakdown of eosinophils in sputum).	Can be triggered by viral URIs, allergens, stress. Clinical diagnosis can be supported by spirometry and methacholine challenge. Findings: cough, wheezing, tachypnea, dyspnea, hypoxemia, ↓ inspiratory/expiratory ratio, pulsus paradoxus, mucus plugging F. Peribronchial cuffing on CXR.
Bronchiectasis	Chronic necrotizing infection of bronchi → permanently dilated airways, purulent sputum, recurrent infections, hemoptysis, digital clubbing.	Associated with bronchial obstruction, poor ciliary motility (eg, smoking, Kartagener syndrome), cystic fibrosis G, allergic bronchopulmonary aspergillosis.

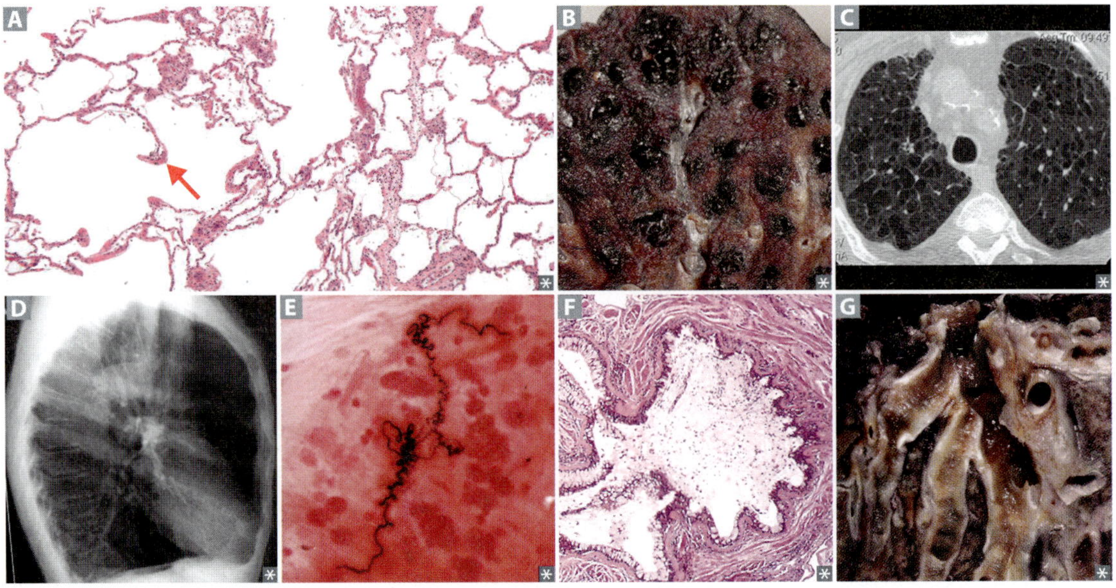

Restrictive lung diseases

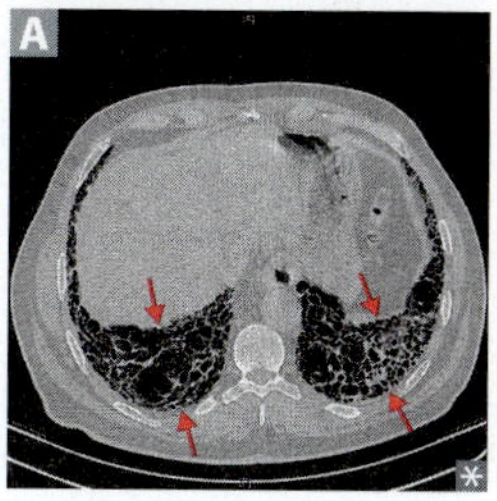

Restricted lung expansion causes ↓ lung volumes (↓ FVC and TLC). PFTs: FEV_1/FVC ratio ≥ 80%.

Types:

- Poor breathing mechanics (extrapulmonary, peripheral hypoventilation, normal A-a gradient):
  - Poor muscular effort—polio, myasthenia gravis, Guillain-Barré syndrome
  - Poor structural apparatus—scoliosis, morbid obesity
- Interstitial lung diseases (pulmonary ↓ diffusing capacity, ↑ A-a gradient):
  - Acute respiratory distress syndrome (ARDS)
  - Neonatal respiratory distress syndrome (NRDS; hyaline membrane disease)
  - Pneumoconioses (eg, anthracosis, silicosis, asbestosis)
  - Sarcoidosis: bilateral hilar lymphadenopathy, noncaseating granuloma; ↑ ACE and Ca^{2+}
  - Idiopathic pulmonary fibrosis A (repeated cycles of lung injury and wound healing with ↑ collagen deposition, "honeycomb" lung appearance and digital clubbing)
  - Goodpasture syndrome
  - Granulomatosis with polyangiitis (Wegener)
  - Pulmonary Langerhans cell histiocytosis (eosinophilic granuloma)
  - Hypersensitivity pneumonitis
  - Drug toxicity (bleomycin, busulfan, amiodarone, methotrexate)

Flow volume loops

Obstructive lung volumes > normal (↑ TLC, ↑ FRC, ↑ RV); restrictive lung volumes < normal. In both obstructive and restrictive, FEV_1 and FVC are reduced. In obstructive, however, FEV_1 is more dramatically reduced compared to FVC, resulting in a ↓ FEV_1/FVC ratio.

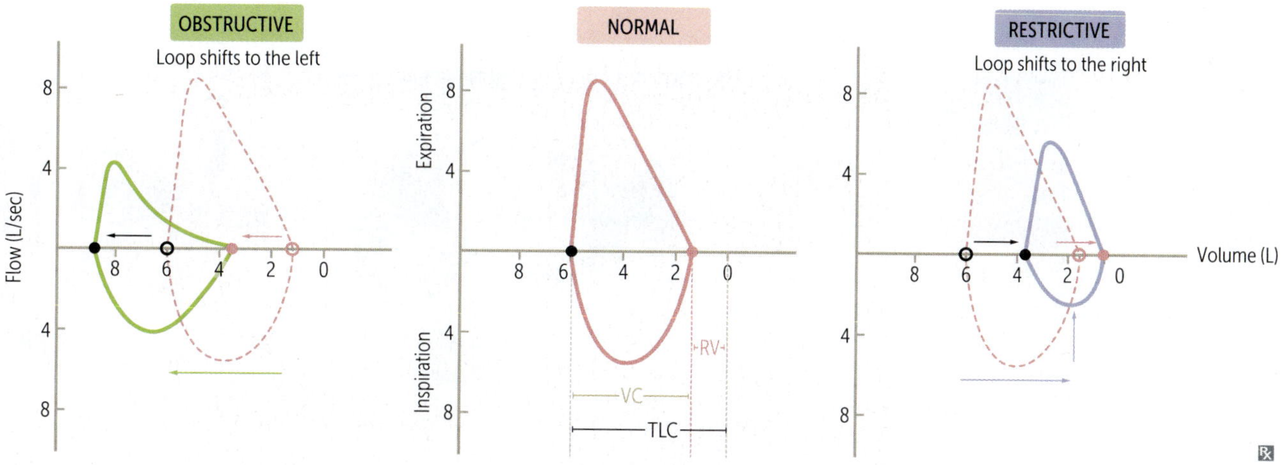

Hypersensitivity pneumonitis

Mixed type III/IV hypersensitivity reaction to environmental antigen → dyspnea, cough, chest tightness, headache. Often seen in farmers and those exposed to birds.

Pneumoconioses	Coal workers' pneumoconiosis, silicosis, and asbestosis → ↑ risk of cor pulmonale, cancer, and Caplan syndrome (rheumatoid arthritis and pneumoconioses with intrapulmonary nodules).	
Asbestosis	Associated with shipbuilding, roofing, plumbing. "Ivory white," calcified, supradiaphragmatic and pleural plaques A B are pathognomonic of asbestosis. Risk of bronchogenic carcinoma > risk of mesothelioma.	Affects lower lobes. Asbestos (ferruginous) bodies are golden-brown fusiform rods resembling dumbbells C, found in alveolar septum sputum sample, visualized using Prussian blue stain, often obtained by bronchoalveolar lavage. ↑ risk of pleural effusions.
Berylliosis	Associated with exposure to beryllium in aerospace and manufacturing industries. Granulomatous on histology and therefore occasionally responsive to steroids.	Affects upper lobes.
Coal workers' pneumoconiosis	Prolonged coal dust exposure → macrophages laden with carbon → inflammation and fibrosis. Also known as black lung disease.	Affects upper lobes. Anthracosis—asymptomatic condition found in many urban dwellers exposed to sooty air.
Silicosis	Associated with foundries, sandblasting, mines. Macrophages respond to silica and release fibrogenic factors, leading to fibrosis. It is thought that silica may disrupt phagolysosomes and impair macrophages, increasing susceptibility to TB.	Affects upper lobes. "Eggshell" calcification of hilar lymph nodes. **Asbestos** is from the **roof** (was common in insulation), but affects the **base** (lower lobes). **Silica and coal** are from the **base** (earth), but affect the **roof** (upper lobes).

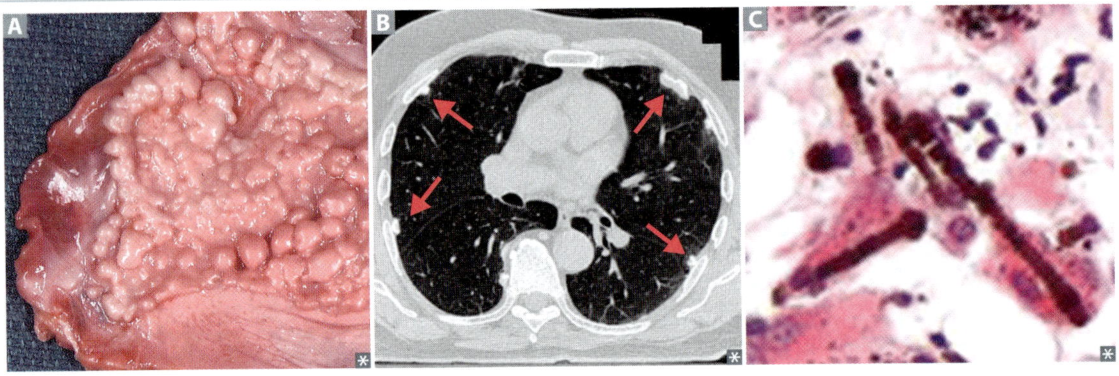

Acute respiratory distress syndrome

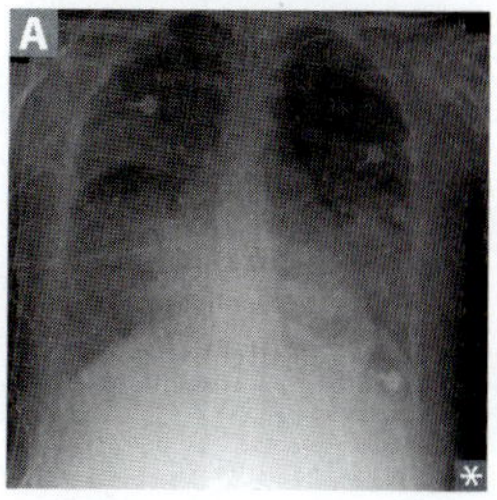

Clinical syndrome characterized by acute onset respiratory failure, bilateral lung opacities, ↓ Pa_{O_2}/F_{IO_2}, no evidence of HF/fluid overload. SPARTAS: Sepsis, Pancreatitis, Pneumonia, Aspiration, uRemia, Trauma, Amniotic fluid embolism, Shock. Endothelial damage → ↑ alveolar capillary permeability → protein-rich leakage into alveoli → diffuse alveolar damage and noncardiogenic pulmonary edema (normal PCWP) A. Results in formation of intra-alveolar hyaline membranes B. Initial damage due to release of neutrophilic substances toxic to alveolar wall, activation of coagulation cascade, and oxygen-derived free radicals.

Management: mechanical ventilation with low tidal volumes, address underlying cause.

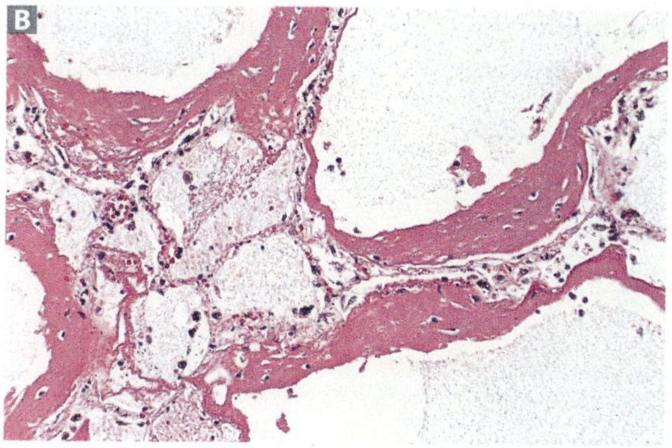

Sleep apnea	Repeated cessation of breathing > 10 seconds during sleep → disrupted sleep → daytime somnolence. Normal Pa_{O_2} during the day. Nocturnal hypoxia → systemic/pulmonary hypertension, arrhythmias (atrial fibrillation/flutter), sudden death. Hypoxia → ↑ EPO release → ↑ erythropoiesis.
Obstructive sleep apnea	Respiratory effort against airway obstruction. Associated with obesity, loud snoring. Caused by excess parapharyngeal tissue in adults, adenotonsillar hypertrophy in children. Treatment: weight loss, CPAP, surgery.
Central sleep apnea	No respiratory effort due to CNS injury/toxicity, HF, opioids.
Obesity hypoventilation syndrome	Obesity (BMI ≥ 30 kg/m^2) → hypoventilation (↓ respiratory rate) → ↓ Pa_{O_2} and ↑ Pa_{CO_2} during sleep; ↑ Pa_{CO_2} during waking hours (retention).

Pulmonary hypertension	Normal mean pulmonary artery pressure = 10–14 mm Hg; pulmonary hypertension ≥ 25 mm Hg at rest. Results in arteriosclerosis, medial hypertrophy, intimal fibrosis of pulmonary arteries. Course: severe respiratory distress → cyanosis and RVH → death from decompensated cor pulmonale.
ETIOLOGIES	
Pulmonary arterial hypertension	Idiopathic PAH. Heritable PAH—often due to an inactivating mutation in *BMPR2* gene (normally inhibits vascular smooth muscle proliferation); poor prognosis. Other causes include drugs (eg, amphetamines, cocaine), connective tissue disease, HIV infection, portal hypertension, congenital heart disease, schistosomiasis.
Left heart disease	Causes include systolic/diastolic dysfunction and valvular disease (eg, mitral lung).
Lung diseases or hypoxia	Destruction of lung parenchyma (eg, COPD), hypoxemic vasoconstriction (eg, obstructive sleep apnea, living in high altitude).
Chronic thromboembolic	Recurrent microthrombi → ↓ cross-sectional area of pulmonary vascular bed.
Multifactorial	Causes include hematologic, systemic, and metabolic disorders.

Lung—physical findings

ABNORMALITY	BREATH SOUNDS	PERCUSSION	FREMITUS	TRACHEAL DEVIATION
Pleural effusion	↓	Dull	↓	— or away from side of lesion (if large)
Atelectasis (bronchial obstruction)	↓	Dull	↓	Toward side of lesion
Simple pneumothorax	↓	Hyperresonant	↓	—
Tension pneumothorax	↓	Hyperresonant	↓	Away from side of lesion
Consolidation (lobar pneumonia, pulmonary edema)	Bronchial breath sounds; late inspiratory crackles	Dull	↑	—

Pleural effusions	Excess accumulation of fluid between pleural layers A → restricted lung expansion during inspiration. Can be treated with thoracentesis to remove fluid B.
Transudate	↓ protein content. Due to ↑ hydrostatic pressure (eg, HF) or ↓ oncotic pressure (eg, nephrotic syndrome, cirrhosis).
Exudate	↑ protein content, cloudy. Due to malignancy, pneumonia, collagen vascular disease, trauma (occurs in states of ↑ vascular permeability). Must be drained due to risk of infection.
Lymphatic	Also known as chylothorax. Due to thoracic duct injury from trauma or malignancy. Milky-appearing fluid; ↑ triglycerides.

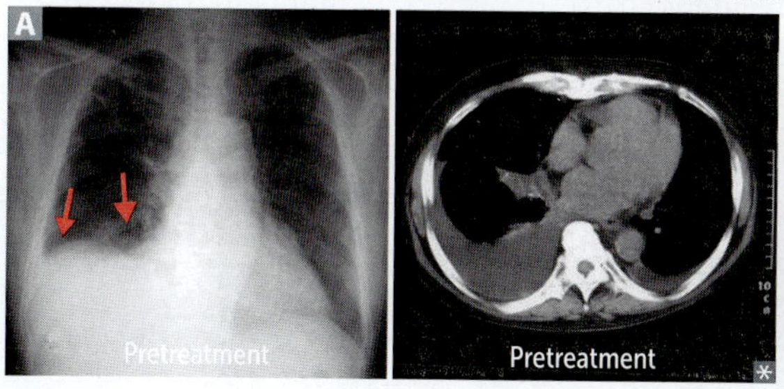

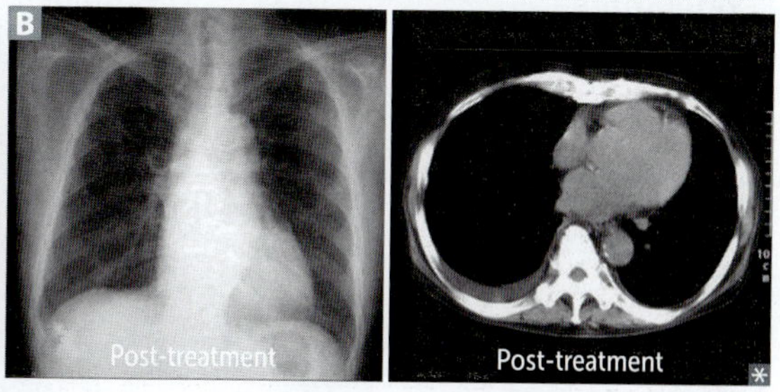

Pneumothorax	Accumulation of air in pleural space A. Unilateral chest pain and dyspnea, unilateral chest expansion, ↓ tactile fremitus, hyperresonance, diminished breath sounds, all on the affected side.
Primary spontaneous pneumothorax	Due to rupture of apical subpleural bleb or cysts. Occurs most frequently in tall, thin, young males.
Secondary spontaneous pneumothorax	Due to diseased lung (eg, bullae in emphysema, infections), mechanical ventilation with use of high pressures → barotrauma.
Traumatic pneumothorax	Caused by blunt (eg, rib fracture) or penetrating (eg, gunshot) trauma.
Tension pneumothorax	Can be any of the above. Air enters pleural space but cannot exit. Increasing trapped air → tension pneumothorax. Trachea deviates away from affected lung B. Needs immediate needle decompression and chest tube placement.

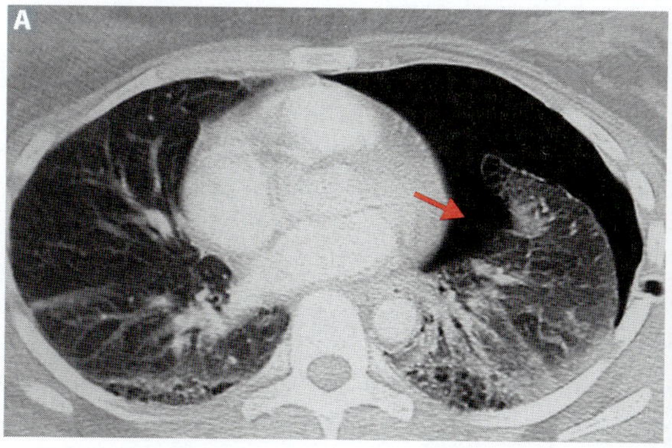

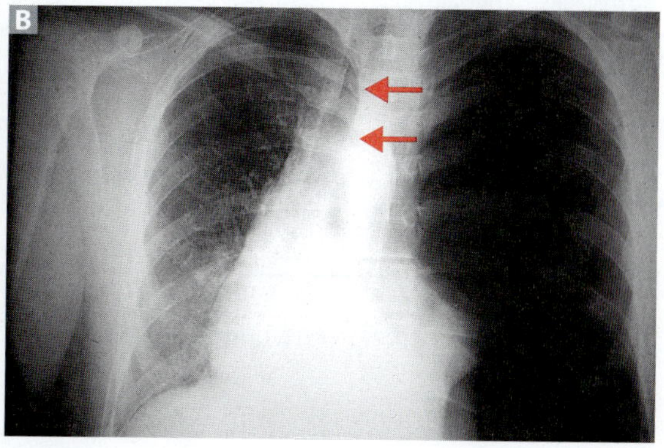

Pneumonia

TYPE	TYPICAL ORGANISMS	CHARACTERISTICS
Lobar	*S pneumoniae* most frequently, also *Legionella*, *Klebsiella*	Intra-alveolar exudate → consolidation **A**; may involve entire lobe **B** or lung.
Bronchopneumonia	*S pneumoniae*, *S aureus*, *H influenzae*, *Klebsiella*	Acute inflammatory infiltrates **C** from bronchioles into adjacent alveoli; patchy distribution involving ≥ 1 lobe **D**.
Interstitial (atypical) pneumonia	*Mycoplasma*, *Chlamydia*, *Legionella*, viruses (RSV, CMV, influenza, adenovirus)	Diffuse patchy inflammation localized to interstitial areas at alveolar walls; diffuse distribution involving ≥ 1 lobe **E**. Generally follows a more indolent course ("walking" pneumonia).

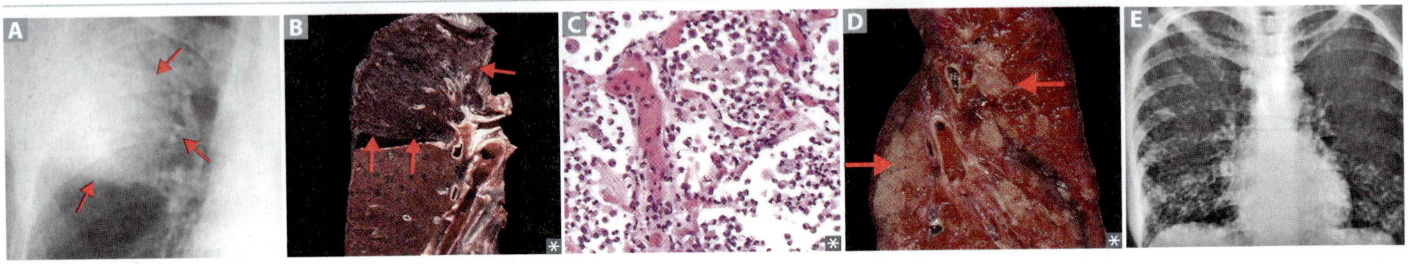

Lung abscess

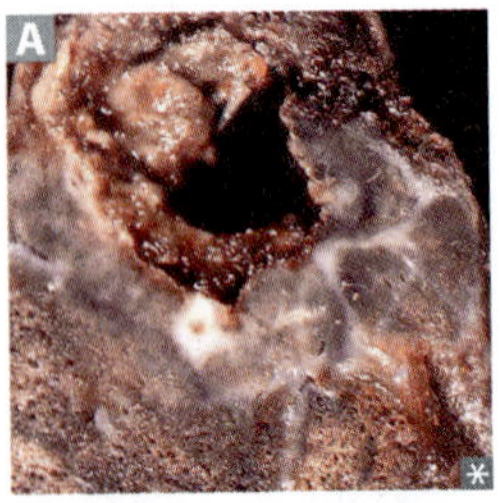

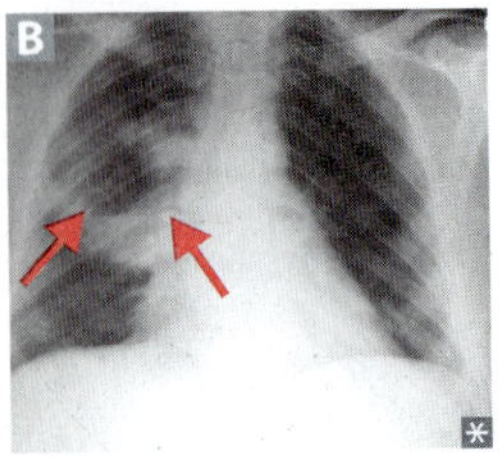

Localized collection of pus within parenchyma **A**. Caused by aspiration of oropharyngeal contents (especially in patients predisposed to loss of consciousness [eg, alcoholics, epileptics]) or bronchial obstruction (eg, cancer).

Treatment: clindamycin.

Air-fluid levels **B** often seen on CXR. Fluid levels common in cavities; presence suggests cavitation. Due to anaerobes (eg, *Bacteroides*, *Fusobacterium*, *Peptostreptococcus*) or *S aureus*.

Lung abscess 2° to aspiration is most often found in right lung. Location depends on patient's position during aspiration:

- Upright → basal segments of right lower lobe
- Supine → posterior segments of right upper lobe or superior segment of right lower lobe

Mesothelioma

Malignancy of the pleura associated with asbestosis. May result in hemorrhagic pleural effusion (exudative), pleural thickening.

Psammoma bodies seen on histology.

Cytokeratin and calretinin ⊕ in almost all mesotheliomas, ⊖ in most carcinomas.

Smoking not a risk factor.

Pancoast tumor (superior sulcus tumor)

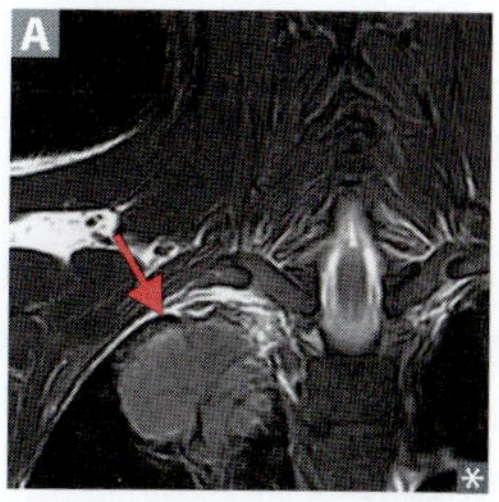

Carcinoma that occurs in the apex of lung A may cause Pancoast syndrome by invading cervical sympathetic chain.

Compression of locoregional structures may cause array of findings:

- Recurrent laryngeal nerve → hoarseness
- Superior cervical ganglion → Horner syndrome (ipsilateral ptosis, miosis, anhidrosis)
- Superior vena cava → SVC syndrome
- Sensorimotor deficit

Superior vena cava syndrome

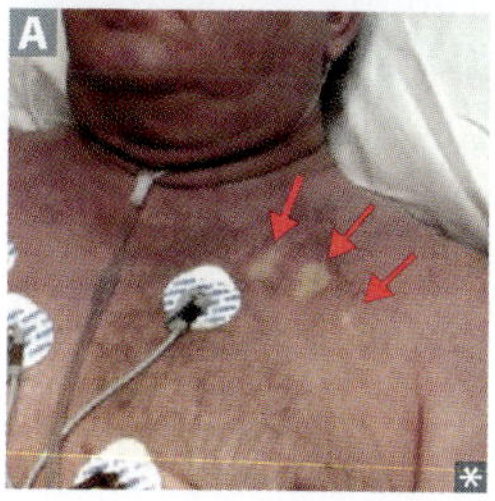

An obstruction of the SVC that impairs blood drainage from the head ("facial plethora"; note blanching after fingertip pressure in A), neck (jugular venous distention), and upper extremities (edema). Commonly caused by malignancy (eg, Pancoast tumor) and thrombosis from indwelling catheters B. Medical emergency. Can raise intracranial pressure (if obstruction is severe) → headaches, dizziness, ↑ risk of aneurysm/rupture of intracranial arteries.

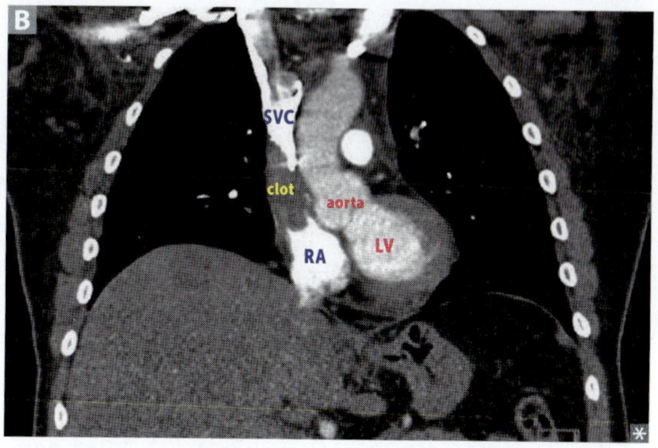

Lung cancer

Leading cause of cancer death.

Presentation: cough, hemoptysis, bronchial obstruction, wheezing, pneumonic "coin" lesion on CXR or noncalcified nodule on CT.

Sites of metastases from lung cancer: adrenals, brain, bone (pathologic fracture), liver (jaundice, hepatomegaly).

In the lung, metastases (usually multiple lesions) are more common than 1° neoplasms. Most often from breast, colon, prostate, and bladder cancer.

SPHERE of complications:
- Superior vena cava syndrome
- Pancoast tumor
- Horner syndrome
- Endocrine (paraneoplastic)
- Recurrent laryngeal nerve compression (hoarseness)
- Effusions (pleural or pericardial)

Risk factors include smoking, secondhand smoke, radon, asbestos, family history.

Squamous and Small cell carcinomas are Sentral (central) and often caused by Smoking.

TYPE	LOCATION	CHARACTERISTICS	HISTOLOGY
Small cell			
Small cell (oat cell) carcinoma	Central	Undifferentiated → very aggressive. May produce ACTH (Cushing syndrome), SIADH, or Antibodies against presynaptic Ca^{2+} channels (Lambert-Eaton myasthenic syndrome) or neurons (paraneoplastic myelitis, encephalitis, subacute cerebellar degeneration). Amplification of *myc* oncogenes common. Managed with chemotherapy +/– radiation.	Neoplasm of neuroendocrine Kulchitsky cells → small dark blue cells A. Chromogranin A $\oplus$, neuron-specific enolase $\oplus$.
Non–small cell			
Adenocarcinoma	Peripheral	Most common lung cancer in nonsmokers and overall (except for metastases). Activating mutations include *KRAS*, *EGFR*, and *ALK*. Associated with hypertrophic osteoarthropathy (clubbing). Bronchioloalveolar subtype (adenocarcinoma in situ): CXR often shows hazy infiltrates similar to pneumonia; better prognosis. Bronchial carcinoid and bronchioloalveolar cell carcinoma have lesser association with smoking.	Glandular pattern on histology, often stains mucin $\oplus$ B. Bronchioloalveolar subtype: grows along alveolar septa → apparent "thickening" of alveolar walls. Tall, columnar cells containing mucus.
Squamous cell carcinoma	Central	Hilar mass arising from bronchus C; Cavitation; Cigarettes; hyperCalcemia (produces PTHrP).	Keratin pearls D and intercellular bridges.
Large cell carcinoma	Peripheral	Highly anaplastic undifferentiated tumor; poor prognosis. Less responsive to chemotherapy; removed surgically.	Pleomorphic giant cells E. Can secrete β-hCG.
Bronchial carcinoid tumor	—	Excellent prognosis; metastasis rare. Symptoms due to mass effect or carcinoid syndrome (flushing, diarrhea, wheezing).	Nests of neuroendocrine cells; chromogranin A $\oplus$.

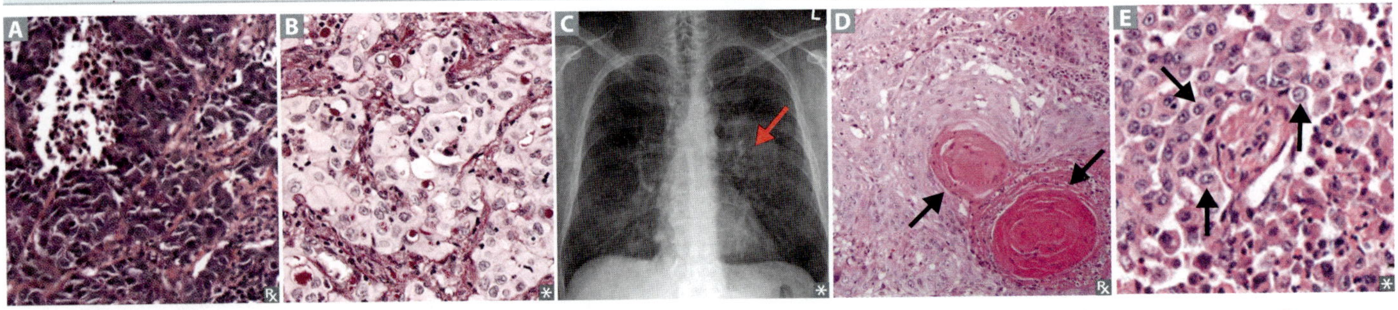

▸ RESPIRATORY—PHARMACOLOGY

Antihistamines	Reversible inhibitors of H_1 histamine receptors.	
First generation	Diphenhydramine, dimenhydrinate, chlorpheniramine.	Names contain "-en/-ine" or "-en/-ate."
CLINICAL USES	Allergy, motion sickness, sleep aid.	
ADVERSE EFFECTS	Sedation, antimuscarinic, anti-α-adrenergic.	
Second generation	Loratadine, fexofenadine, desloratadine, cetirizine.	Names usually end in "-adine."
CLINICAL USES	Allergy.	
ADVERSE EFFECTS	Far less sedating than 1st generation because of ↓ entry into CNS.	

Expectorants	
Guaifenesin	Expectorant—thins respiratory secretions; does not suppress cough reflex.
***N*-acetylcysteine**	Mucolytic—liquefies mucus in COPD patients by disrupting disulfide bonds. Also used as an antidote for acetaminophen overdose.

Dextromethorphan	Antitussive (antagonizes NMDA glutamate receptors). Synthetic codeine analog. Has mild opioid effect when used in excess. Naloxone can be given for overdose. Mild abuse potential. May cause serotonin syndrome if combined with other serotonergic agents.

Pseudoephedrine, phenylephrine	
MECHANISM	α-adrenergic agonists, used as nasal decongestants.
CLINICAL USE	Reduce hyperemia, edema, nasal congestion; open obstructed eustachian tubes. Pseudoephedrine also illicitly used to make methamphetamine.
ADVERSE EFFECTS	Hypertension. Can also cause CNS stimulation/anxiety (pseudoephedrine).

Pulmonary hypertension drugs

DRUG	MECHANISM	CLINICAL NOTES
BosENtan	Competitively antagonizes ENdothelin-1 receptors → ↓ pulmonary vascular resistance.	Hepatotoxic (monitor LFTs).
Sildenafil	Inhibits cGMP PDE-5 and prolongs vasodilatory effect of nitric oxide.	Also used to treat erectile dysfunction.
Epoprostenol, iloprost	PGI_2 (prostacyclin) with direct vasodilatory effects on pulmonary and systemic arterial vascular beds. Inhibits platelet aggregation.	Side effects: flushing, jaw pain.

Asthma drugs	Bronchoconstriction is mediated by (1) inflammatory processes and (2) parasympathetic tone; therapy is directed at these 2 pathways.
β_2-agonists	**Albuterol**—relaxes bronchial smooth muscle (short acting β_2-agonist). Used during acute exacerbation.
	Salmeterol, formoterol—long-acting agents for prophylaxis. Adverse effects are tremor and arrhythmia.
Inhaled corticosteroids	**Fluticasone, budesonide**—inhibit the synthesis of virtually all cytokines. Inactivate NF-κB, the transcription factor that induces production of TNF-α and other inflammatory agents. 1st-line therapy for chronic asthma.
Muscarinic antagonists	**Ipratropium**—competitively blocks muscarinic receptors, preventing bronchoconstriction. Also used for COPD. Tiotropium is long acting.
Antileukotrienes	**Montelukast, zafirlukast**—block leukotriene receptors (CysLT1). Especially good for aspirin-induced asthma. **Zileuton**—5-lipoxygenase pathway inhibitor. Blocks conversion of arachidonic acid to leukotrienes. Hepatotoxic. used in exerc-induced
Anti-IgE monoclonal therapy	**Omalizumab**—binds mostly unbound serum IgE and blocks binding to FcεRI. Used in allergic asthma with ↑ IgE levels resistant to inhaled steroids and long-acting β_2-agonists.
Methylxanthines	**Theophylline**—likely causes bronchodilation by inhibiting phosphodiesterase → ↑ cAMP levels due to ↓ cAMP hydrolysis. Usage is limited because of narrow therapeutic index (cardiotoxicity, neurotoxicity); metabolized by cytochrome P-450. Blocks actions of adenosine.

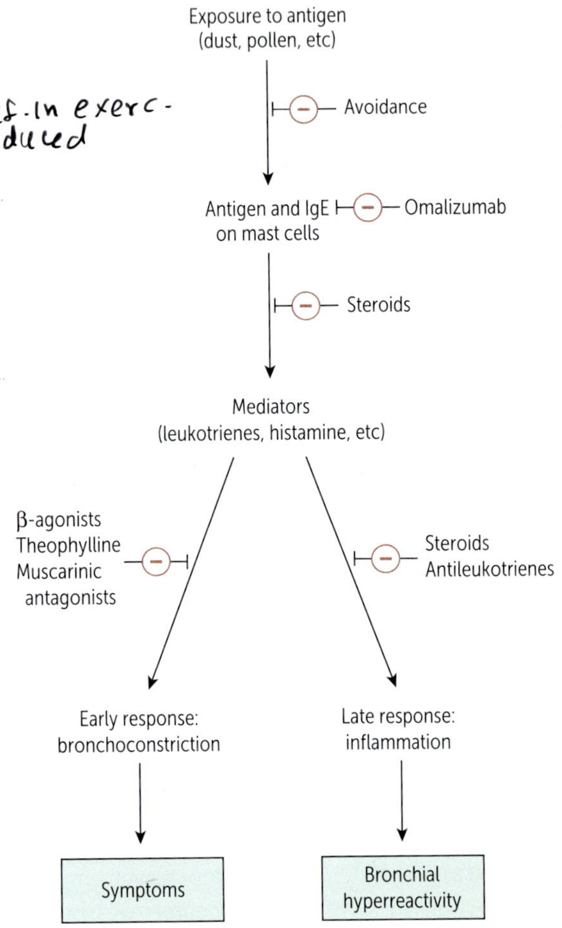

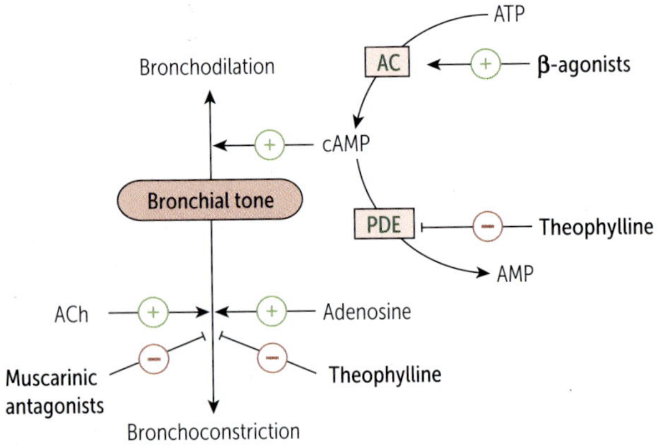

Methacholine	Muscarinic receptor (M_3) agonist. Used in bronchial challenge test to help diagnose asthma.

Rapid Review

"Study without thought is vain: thought without study is dangerous."
—Confucius

"It is better, of course, to know useless things than to know nothing."
—Lucius Annaeus Seneca

"For every complex problem there is an answer that is clear, simple, and wrong."
—H. L. Mencken

The following tables represent a collection of high-yield associations of diseases with their clinical findings, treatments, and pathophysiology. They serve as a quick review before the exam to tune your senses to commonly tested cases.

▶ CLASSIC PRESENTATIONS

CLINICAL PRESENTATION	DIAGNOSIS/DISEASE
Abdominal pain, ascites, hepatomegaly	Budd-Chiari syndrome (posthepatic venous thrombosis)
Abdominal pain, diarrhea, leukocytosis, recent antibiotic use	*Clostridium difficile* infection
Achilles tendon xanthoma	Familial hypercholesterolemia (↓ LDL receptor signaling)
Adrenal hemorrhage, hypotension, DIC	Waterhouse-Friderichsen syndrome (meningococcemia)
Anaphylaxis following blood transfusion	IgA deficiency
Anterior "drawer sign" ⊕	Anterior cruciate ligament injury
Arachnodactyly, lens dislocation (upward), aortic dissection, hyperflexible joints	Marfan syndrome (fibrillin defect)
Athlete with polycythemia	2° to erythropoietin injection
Back pain, fever, night sweats	Pott disease (vertebral TB)
Bilateral acoustic schwannomas	Neurofibromatosis type 2
Bilateral hilar adenopathy, uveitis	Sarcoidosis (noncaseating granulomas)
Black eschar on face of patient with diabetic ketoacidosis	*Mucor* or *Rhizopus* fungal infection
Blue sclera	Osteogenesis imperfecta (type I collagen defect)
Bluish line on gingiva	Burton line (lead poisoning)
Bone pain, bone enlargement, arthritis	Paget disease of bone (↑ osteoblastic and osteoclastic activity)
Bounding pulses, wide pulse pressure, diastolic heart murmur, head bobbing	Aortic regurgitation
"Butterfly" facial rash and Raynaud phenomenon in a young female	Systemic lupus erythematosus
Café-au-lait spots, Lisch nodules (iris hamartoma), cutaneous neurofibromas, pheochromocytomas, optic gliomas	Neurofibromatosis type I
Café-au-lait spots (unilateral), polyostotic fibrous dysplasia, precocious puberty, multiple endocrine abnormalities	McCune-Albright syndrome (mosaic G-protein signaling mutation)
Calf pseudohypertrophy	Muscular dystrophy (most commonly Duchenne, due to X-linked recessive frameshift mutation of dystrophin gene)
Cervical lymphadenopathy, desquamating rash, coronary aneurysms, red conjunctivae and tongue, hand-foot changes	Kawasaki disease (treat with IVIG and aspirin)
"Cherry-red spots" on macula	Tay-Sachs (ganglioside accumulation) or Niemann-Pick (sphingomyelin accumulation), central retinal artery occlusion
Chest pain on exertion	Angina (stable: with moderate exertion; unstable: with minimal exertion or at rest)
Chest pain, pericardial effusion/friction rub, persistent fever following MI	Dressler syndrome (autoimmune-mediated post-MI fibrinous pericarditis, 2 weeks to several months after acute episode)
Chest pain with ST depressions on EKG	Unstable angina (⊖ troponins) or NSTEMI (⊕ troponins)
Child uses arms to stand up from squat	Duchenne muscular dystrophy (Gowers sign)
Child with fever later develops red rash on face that spreads to body	Erythema infectiosum/fifth disease ("slapped cheeks" appearance, caused by parvovirus B19)
Chorea, dementia, caudate degeneration	Huntington disease (autosomal dominant CAG repeat expansion)
Chorioretinitis, hydrocephalus, intracranial calcifications	Congenital toxoplasmosis

CLINICAL PRESENTATION	DIAGNOSIS/DISEASE
Chronic exercise intolerance with myalgia, fatigue, painful cramps, myoglobinuria	McArdle disease (skeletal muscle glycogen phosphorylase deficiency)
Cold intolerance	Hypothyroidism
Conjugate horizontal gaze palsy, horizontal diplopia	Internuclear ophthalmoplegia (damage to MLF; may be unilateral or bilateral)
Continuous "machine-like" heart murmur	PDA (close with indomethacin; keep open with PGE analogs)
Cutaneous/dermal edema due to connective tissue deposition	Myxedema (caused by hypothyroidism, Graves disease [pretibial])
Cutaneous flushing, diarrhea, bronchospasm	Carcinoid syndrome (right-sided cardiac valvular lesions, ↑ 5-HIAA)
Dark purple skin/mouth nodules in a patient with AIDS	Kaposi sarcoma, associated with HHV-8
Deep, labored breathing/hyperventilation	Diabetic ketoacidosis (Kussmaul respirations)
Dermatitis, dementia, diarrhea	Pellagra (niacin [vitamin B_3] deficiency)
Dilated cardiomyopathy, edema, alcoholism or malnutrition	Wet beriberi (thiamine [vitamin B_1] deficiency)
Dog or cat bite resulting in infection	*Pasteurella multocida* (cellulitis at inoculation site)
Dry eyes, dry mouth, arthritis	Sjögren syndrome (autoimmune destruction of exocrine glands)
Dysphagia (esophageal webs), glossitis, iron deficiency anemia	Plummer-Vinson syndrome (may progress to esophageal squamous cell carcinoma)
Elastic skin, hypermobility of joints, ↑ bleeding tendency	Ehlers-Danlos syndrome (type V collagen defect, type III collagen defect seen in vascular subtype of ED)
Enlarged, hard left supraclavicular node	Virchow node (abdominal metastasis)
Episodic vertigo, tinnitus, hearing loss	Meniere disease
Erythroderma, lymphadenopathy, hepatosplenomegaly, atypical T cells	Mycosis fungoides (cutaneous T-cell lymphoma) or Sézary syndrome (mycosis fungoides + malignant T cells in blood)
Facial muscle spasm upon tapping	Chvostek sign (hypocalcemia)
Fat, female, forty, and fertile	Cholelithiasis (gallstones)
Fever, chills, headache, myalgia following antibiotic treatment for syphilis	Jarisch-Herxheimer reaction (rapid lysis of spirochetes results in endotoxin release)
Fever, cough, conjunctivitis, coryza, diffuse rash	Measles
Fever, night sweats, weight loss	B symptoms (staging) of lymphoma
Fibrous plaques in soft tissue of penis with abnormal curvature	Peyronie disease (connective tissue disorder)
Golden brown rings around peripheral cornea	Wilson disease (Kayser-Fleischer rings due to copper accumulation)
Gout, intellectual disability, self-mutilating behavior in a boy	Lesch-Nyhan syndrome (HGPRT deficiency, X-linked recessive)
Hamartomatous GI polyps, hyperpigmentation of mouth/feet/hands/genitalia	Peutz-Jeghers syndrome (inherited, benign polyposis can cause bowel obstruction; ↑ cancer risk, mainly GI)
Hepatosplenomegaly, pancytopenia, osteoporosis, aseptic necrosis of femoral head, bone crises	Gaucher disease (glucocerebrosidase deficiency)

CLINICAL PRESENTATION	DIAGNOSIS/DISEASE
Hereditary nephritis, sensorineural hearing loss, cataracts	Alport syndrome (mutation in collagen IV)
Hyperphagia, hypersexuality, hyperorality, hyperdocility	Klüver-Bucy syndrome (bilateral amygdala lesion)
Hyperreflexia, hypertonia, Babinski sign present	UMN damage
Hyporeflexia, hypotonia, atrophy, fasciculations	LMN damage
Hypoxemia, polycythemia, hypercapnia	Chronic bronchitis (hyperplasia of mucous cells, "blue bloater")
Indurated, ulcerated genital lesion	Nonpainful: chancre (1° syphilis, *Treponema pallidum*) Painful, with exudate: chancroid *(Haemophilus ducreyi)*
Infant with cleft lip/palate, microcephaly or holoprosencephaly, polydactyly, cutis aplasia	Patau syndrome (trisomy 13)
Infant with hypoglycemia, hepatomegaly	Cori disease (debranching enzyme deficiency) or Von Gierke disease (glucose-6-phosphatase deficiency, more severe)
Infant with microcephaly, rocker-bottom feet, clenched hands, and structural heart defect	Edwards syndrome (trisomy 18)
Jaundice, palpable distended non-tender gallbladder	Courvoisier sign (distal malignant obstruction of biliary tree)
Large rash with bull's-eye appearance	Erythema chronicum migrans from *Ixodes* tick bite (Lyme disease: *Borrelia*)
Lucid interval after traumatic brain injury	Epidural hematoma (middle meningeal artery rupture)
Male child, recurrent infections, no mature B cells	Bruton disease (X-linked agammaglobulinemia)
Mucosal bleeding and prolonged bleeding time	Glanzmann thrombasthenia (defect in platelet aggregation due to lack of GpIIb/IIIa)
Muffled heart sounds, distended neck veins, hypotension	Beck triad of cardiac tamponade
Multiple colon polyps, osteomas/soft tissue tumors, impacted/supernumerary teeth	Gardner syndrome (subtype of FAP)
Myopathy (infantile hypertrophic cardiomyopathy), exercise intolerance	Pompe disease (lysosomal α-1,4-glucosidase deficiency)
Neonate with arm paralysis following difficult birth	Erb-Duchenne palsy (superior trunk [C5–C6] brachial plexus injury: "waiter's tip")
No lactation postpartum, absent menstruation, cold intolerance	Sheehan syndrome (pituitary infarction)
Nystagmus, intention tremor, scanning speech, bilateral internuclear ophthalmoplegia	Multiple sclerosis
Painful blue fingers/toes, hemolytic anemia	Cold agglutinin disease (autoimmune hemolytic anemia caused by *Mycoplasma pneumoniae*, infectious mononucleosis, CLL)
Painful fingers/toes changing color from blue to white to red with cold or stress	Raynaud phenomenon (vasospasm in extremities)
Painful, raised red lesions on pads of fingers/toes	Osler nodes (infective endocarditis, immune complex deposition)

CLINICAL PRESENTATION	DIAGNOSIS/DISEASE
Painless erythematous lesions on palms and soles	Janeway lesions (infective endocarditis, septic emboli/ microabscesses)
Painless jaundice	Cancer of the pancreatic head obstructing bile duct
Palpable purpura on buttocks/legs, joint pain, abdominal pain (child), hematuria	Henoch-Schönlein purpura (IgA vasculitis affecting skin and kidneys)
Pancreatic, pituitary, parathyroid tumors	MEN 1 (autosomal dominant)
Periorbital and/or peripheral edema, proteinuria (> 3.5g/day), hypoalbuminemia, hypercholesterolemia	Nephrotic syndrome
Pink complexion, dyspnea, hyperventilation	Emphysema ("pink puffer," centriacinar [smoking] or panacinar [α_1-antitrypsin deficiency])
Polyuria, renal tubular acidosis type II, growth failure, electrolyte imbalances, hypophosphatemic rickets	Fanconi syndrome (multiple combined dysfunction of the proximal convoluted tubule)
Pruritic, purple, polygonal planar papules and plaques (6 P's)	Lichen planus
Ptosis, miosis, anhidrosis	Horner syndrome (sympathetic chain lesion)
Pupil accommodates but doesn't react	Neurosyphilis (Argyll Robertson pupil)
Rapidly progressive limb weakness that ascends following GI/ upper respiratory infection	Guillain-Barré syndrome (acute inflammatory demyelinating polyradiculopathy subtype)
Rash on palms and soles	Coxsackie A, 2° syphilis, Rocky Mountain spotted fever
Recurrent cold (noninflamed) abscesses, unusual eczema, high serum IgE	Hyper-IgE syndrome (Job syndrome: neutrophil chemotaxis abnormality)
Red "currant jelly" sputum in alcoholic or diabetic patients	*Klebsiella pneumoniae* pneumonia
Red "currant jelly" stools	Acute mesenteric ischemia (adults), intussusception (children)
Red, itchy, swollen rash of nipple/areola	Paget disease of the breast (sign of underlying neoplasm)
Red urine in the morning, fragile RBCs	Paroxysmal nocturnal hemoglobinuria
Renal cell carcinoma (bilateral), hemangioblastomas, angiomatosis, pheochromocytoma	von Hippel-Lindau disease (dominant tumor suppressor gene mutation)
Resting tremor, rigidity, akinesia, postural instability, shuffling gait	Parkinson disease (loss of dopaminergic neurons in substantia nigra pars compacta)
Retinal hemorrhages with pale centers	Roth spots (bacterial endocarditis)
Severe jaundice in neonate	Crigler-Najjar syndrome (congenital unconjugated hyperbilirubinemia)
Severe RLQ pain with palpation of LLQ	Rovsing sign (acute appendicitis)
Severe RLQ pain with deep tenderness	McBurney sign (acute appendicitis)
Short stature, café au lait spots, thumb/radial defects, ↑ incidence of tumors/leukemia, aplastic anemia	Fanconi anemia (genetic loss of DNA crosslink repair; often progresses to AML)
Single palmar crease	Down syndrome
Situs inversus, chronic sinusitis, bronchiectasis, infertility	Kartagener syndrome (dynein arm defect affecting cilia)
Skin hyperpigmentation, hypotension, fatigue	1° adrenocortical insufficiency (eg, Addison disease) causes ↑ ACTH and ↑ α-MSH production)
Slow, progressive muscle weakness in boys	Becker muscular dystrophy (X-linked missense mutation in dystrophin; less severe than Duchenne)

CLINICAL PRESENTATION	DIAGNOSIS/DISEASE
Small, irregular red spots on buccal/lingual mucosa with blue-white centers	Koplik spots (measles [rubeola] virus)
Smooth, moist, painless, wart-like white lesions on genitals	Condylomata lata (2° syphilis)
Splinter hemorrhages in fingernails	Bacterial endocarditis
"Strawberry tongue"	Scarlet fever, Kawasaki disease
Streak ovaries, congenital heart disease, horseshoe kidney, cystic hygroma at birth, short stature, webbed neck, lymphedema	Turner syndrome (45,XO)
Sudden swollen/painful big toe joint, tophi	Gout/podagra (hyperuricemia)
Swollen gums, mucosal bleeding, poor wound healing, petechiae	Scurvy (vitamin C deficiency: can't hydroxylate proline/lysine for collagen synthesis)
Swollen, hard, painful finger joints	Osteoarthritis (osteophytes on PIP [Bouchard nodes], DIP [Heberden nodes])
Systolic ejection murmur (crescendo-decrescendo)	Aortic stenosis
Telangiectasias, recurrent epistaxis, skin discoloration, arteriovenous malformations, GI bleeding, hematuria	Osler-Weber-Rendu syndrome
Thyroid and parathyroid tumors, pheochromocytoma	MEN 2A (autosomal dominant *RET* mutation)
Thyroid tumors, pheochromocytoma, ganglioneuromatosis	MEN 2B (autosomal dominant *RET* mutation)
Toe extension/fanning upon plantar scrape	Babinski sign (UMN lesion)
Unilateral facial drooping involving forehead	LMN facial nerve (CN VII) palsy; UMN lesions spare the forehead
Urethritis, conjunctivitis, arthritis in a male	Reactive arthritis associated with HLA-B27
Vascular birthmark (port-wine stain) of the face	Nevus flammeus (benign, but associated with Sturge-Weber syndrome)
Vomiting blood following gastroesophageal lacerations	Mallory-Weiss syndrome (alcoholic and bulimic patients)
Weight loss, diarrhea, arthritis, fever, adenopathy	Whipple disease (*Tropheryma whipplei*)
"Worst headache of my life"	Subarachnoid hemorrhage

▶ CLASSIC LABS/FINDINGS

LAB/DIAGNOSTIC FINDING	DIAGNOSIS/DISEASE
↑ AFP in amniotic fluid/maternal serum	Dating error, anencephaly, spina bifida (neural tube defects)
Anticentromere antibodies	Scleroderma (CREST)
Anti-desmoglein (anti-desmosome) antibodies	Pemphigus vulgaris (blistering)
Anti–glomerular basement membrane antibodies	Goodpasture syndrome (glomerulonephritis and hemoptysis)
Antihistone antibodies	Drug-induced SLE (eg, hydralazine, isoniazid, phenytoin, procainamide)
Anti-IgG antibodies	Rheumatoid arthritis (systemic inflammation, joint pannus, boutonnière deformity)
Antimitochondrial antibodies (AMAs)	1° biliary cirrhosis (female, cholestasis, portal hypertension)

LAB/DIAGNOSTIC FINDING	DIAGNOSIS/DISEASE
Antineutrophil cytoplasmic antibodies (ANCAs)	Microscopic polyangiitis and eosinophilic granulomatosis with polyangiitis (Churg-Strauss syndrome) (MPO-ANCA/p-ANCA); granulomatosis with polyangiitis (Wegener; PR3-ANCA/c-ANCA)
Antinuclear antibodies (ANAs: anti-Smith and anti-dsDNA)	SLE (type III hypersensitivity)
Antiplatelet antibodies	Idiopathic thrombocytopenic purpura
Anti-topoisomerase antibodies	Diffuse systemic scleroderma
Anti-transglutaminase/anti-gliadin/anti-endomysial antibodies	Celiac disease (diarrhea, weight loss)
"Apple core" lesion on barium enema x-ray	Colorectal cancer (usually left-sided)
Atypical lymphocytes	EBV
Azurophilic peroxidase ⊕ granular inclusions in granulocytes and myeloblasts	Auer rods (AML, especially the promyelocytic [M3] type)
Bacitracin response	Sensitive: *S pyogenes* (group A); resistant: *S agalactiae* (group B)
"Bamboo spine" on x-ray	Ankylosing spondylitis (chronic inflammatory arthritis: HLA-B27)
Basophilic nuclear remnants in RBCs	Howell-Jolly bodies (due to splenectomy or nonfunctional spleen)
Basophilic stippling of RBCs	Lead poisoning or sideroblastic anemia
Bloody or yellow tap on lumbar puncture	Subarachnoid hemorrhage
"Boot-shaped" heart on x-ray	Tetralogy of Fallot (due to RVH)
Branching gram ⊕ rods with sulfur granules	*Actinomyces israelii*
Bronchogenic apical lung tumor on imaging	Pancoast tumor (can compress cervical sympathetic chain and cause Horner syndrome)
"Brown" tumor of bone	Hyperparathyroidism or osteitis fibrosa cystica (deposited hemosiderin from hemorrhage gives brown color)
Cardiomegaly with apical atrophy	Chagas disease (*Trypanosoma cruzi*)
Cellular crescents in Bowman capsule	Rapidly progressive crescentic glomerulonephritis
"Chocolate cyst" of ovary	Endometriosis (frequently involves both ovaries)
Circular grouping of dark tumor cells surrounding pale neurofibrils	Homer-Wright rosettes (neuroblastoma, medulloblastoma)
Colonies of mucoid *Pseudomonas* in lungs	Cystic fibrosis (autosomal recessive mutation in *CFTR* gene → fat-soluble vitamin deficiency and mucous plugs)
↓ AFP in amniotic fluid/maternal serum	Down syndrome or other chromosomal abnormalities
Degeneration of dorsal column fibers	Tabes dorsalis (3° syphilis), subacute combined degeneration (dorsal columns, lateral corticospinal, spinocerebellar tracts affected)
"Delta wave" on EKG, short PR interval, supraventricular tachycardia	Wolff-Parkinson-White syndrome (Bundle of Kent bypasses AV node)
Depigmentation of neurons in substantia nigra	Parkinson disease (basal ganglia disorder: rigidity, resting tremor, bradykinesia)
Desquamated epithelium casts in sputum	Curschmann spirals (bronchial asthma; can result in whorled mucous plugs)

LAB/DIAGNOSTIC FINDING	DIAGNOSIS/DISEASE
Disarrayed granulosa cells arranged around collections of eosinophilic fluid	Call-Exner bodies (granulosa cell tumor of the ovary)
Dysplastic squamous cervical cells with "raisinoid" nuclei and hyperchromasia	Koilocytes (HPV: predisposes to cervical cancer)
Electrical alternans (alternating amplitude on EKG)	Pericardial tamponade
Enlarged cells with intranuclear inclusion bodies	"Owl eye" appearance of CMV
Enlarged thyroid cells with ground-glass nuclei with central clearing	"Orphan Annie" eyes nuclei (papillary carcinoma of the thyroid)
Eosinophilic cytoplasmic inclusion in liver cell	Mallory body (alcoholic liver disease)
Eosinophilic cytoplasmic inclusion in neuron	Lewy body (Parkinson disease and Lewy body dementia)
Eosinophilic globule in liver	Councilman body (viral hepatitis, yellow fever), represents hepatocyte undergoing apoptosis
Eosinophilic inclusion bodies in cytoplasm of hippocampal and cerebellar neurons	Negri bodies of rabies
Extracellular amyloid deposition in gray matter of brain	Senile plaques (Alzheimer disease)
Giant B cells with bilobed nuclei with prominent inclusions ("owl's eye")	Reed-Sternberg cells (Hodgkin lymphoma)
Glomerulus-like structure surrounding vessel in germ cells	Schiller-Duval bodies (yolk sac tumor)
"Hair on end" ("Crew-cut") appearance on x-ray	β-thalassemia, sickle cell disease (marrow expansion)
hCG elevated	Choriocarcinoma, hydatidiform mole (occurs with and without embryo, and multiple pregnancy)
Heart nodules (granulomatous)	Aschoff bodies (rheumatic fever)
Heterophile antibodies	Infectious mononucleosis (EBV)
Hexagonal, double-pointed, needle-like crystals in bronchial secretions	Bronchial asthma (Charcot-Leyden crystals: eosinophilic granules)
High level of D-dimers	DVT, PE, DIC
Hilar lymphadenopathy, peripheral granulomatous lesion in middle or lower lung lobes (can calcify)	Ghon complex (1° TB: *Mycobacterium* bacilli)
"Honeycomb lung" on x-ray or CT	Interstitial pulmonary fibrosis
Hypercoagulability (leading to migrating DVTs and vasculitis)	Trousseau syndrome (adenocarcinoma of pancreas or lung)
Hypersegmented neutrophils	Megaloblastic anemia (B_{12} deficiency: neurologic symptoms; folate deficiency: no neurologic symptoms)
Hypertension, hypokalemia, metabolic alkalosis	1° hyperaldosteronism (Conn syndrome)
Hypochromic, microcytic anemia	Iron deficiency anemia, lead poisoning, thalassemia (fetal hemoglobin sometimes present)
Intranuclear eosinophilic droplet-like bodies	Cowdry type A bodies (HSV or VZV)
Iron-containing nodules in alveolar septum	Ferruginous bodies (asbestosis: ↑ chance of mesothelioma)
Keratin pearls on a skin biopsy	Squamous cell carcinoma
Large granules in phagocytes, immunodeficiency	Chédiak-Higashi disease (congenital failure of phagolysosome formation)
"Lead pipe" appearance of colon on abdominal imaging	Ulcerative colitis (loss of haustra)
Linear appearance of IgG deposition on glomerular and alveolar basement membranes	Goodpasture syndrome

LAB/DIAGNOSTIC FINDING	DIAGNOSIS/DISEASE
Low serum ceruloplasmin	Wilson disease (hepatolenticular degeneration)
"Lumpy bumpy" appearance of glomeruli on immunofluorescence	Poststreptococcal glomerulonephritis (due to deposition of IgG, IgM, and C3)
Lytic ("punched-out") bone lesions on x-ray	Multiple myeloma
Mammary gland ("blue domed") cyst	Fibrocystic change of the breast
Monoclonal antibody spike	▪ Multiple myeloma (usually IgG or IgA) ▪ Monoclonal gammopathy of undetermined significance (MGUS consequence of aging) ▪ Waldenström (M protein = IgM) macroglobulinemia ▪ Primary amyloidosis
Mucin-filled cell with peripheral nucleus	"Signet ring" (gastric carcinoma)
Narrowing of bowel lumen on barium x-ray	"String sign" (Crohn disease)
Necrotizing vasculitis (lungs) and necrotizing glomerulonephritis	Granulomatosis with polyangiitis (Wegener; PR3-ANCA/c-ANCA) and Goodpasture syndrome (anti–basement membrane antibodies)
Needle-shaped, ⊖ birefringent crystals	Gout (monosodium urate crystals)
Nodular hyaline deposits in glomeruli	Kimmelstiel-Wilson nodules (diabetic nephropathy)
Novobiocin response	Sensitive: *S epidermidis*; resistant: *S saprophyticus*
"Nutmeg" appearance of liver	Chronic passive congestion of liver due to right heart failure or Budd-Chiari syndrome
"Onion skin" periosteal reaction	Ewing sarcoma (malignant small blue cell tumor)
Optochin response	Sensitive: *S pneumoniae*; resistant: viridans streptococci (*S mutans*, *S sanguis*)
Podocyte fusion or "effacement" on electron microscopy	Minimal change disease (child with nephrotic syndrome)
Polished, "ivory-like" appearance of bone at cartilage erosion	Eburnation (osteoarthritis resulting in bony sclerosis)
Protein aggregates in neurons from hyperphosphorylation of tau protein	Neurofibrillary tangles (Alzheimer disease) and Pick bodies (Pick disease)
Psammoma bodies	Meningiomas, papillary thyroid carcinoma, mesothelioma, papillary serous carcinoma of the endometrium and ovary
Pseudopalisading tumor cells on brain biopsy	Glioblastoma multiforme
Raised periosteum (creating a "Codman triangle")	Aggressive bone lesion (eg, osteosarcoma, Ewing sarcoma, osteomyelitis)
RBC casts in urine	Glomerulonephritis
Rectangular, crystal-like, cytoplasmic inclusions in Leydig cells	Reinke crystals (Leydig cell tumor)
Recurrent infections, eczema, thrombocytopenia	Wiskott-Aldrich syndrome
Renal epithelial casts in urine	Intrinsic renal failure (eg, ischemia or toxic injury)
Rhomboid crystals, ⊕ birefringent	Pseudogout (calcium pyrophosphate dihydrate crystals)
Rib notching (inferior surface, on x-ray)	Coarctation of the aorta
Ring-enhancing brain lesion on CT/MRI in AIDS	*Toxoplasma gondii*, CNS lymphoma
Sheets of medium-sized lymphoid cells with scattered pale, tingible body–laden macrophages ("starry sky" histology)	Burkitt lymphoma (t[8:14] c-*myc* activation, associated with EBV; "starry sky" made up of malignant cells)
Silver-staining spherical aggregation of tau proteins in neurons	Pick bodies (Pick disease: progressive dementia, changes in personality)

LAB/DIAGNOSTIC FINDING	DIAGNOSIS/DISEASE
"Soap bubble" in femur or tibia on x-ray	Giant cell tumor of bone (generally benign)
"Spikes" on basement membrane, "dome-like" subepithelial deposits	Membranous nephropathy (nephrotic syndrome)
Stacks of RBCs	Rouleaux formation (high ESR, multiple myeloma)
"Steeple" sign on frontal CXR	Croup (parainfluenza virus)
Stippled vaginal epithelial cells	"Clue cells" (*Gardnerella vaginalis*)
Streptococcus bovis bacteremia	Colon cancer
"Tennis racket"-shaped cytoplasmic organelles (EM) in Langerhans cells	Birbeck granules (Langerhans cell histiocytosis)
Thousands of polyps on colonoscopy	Familial adenomatous polyposis (autosomal dominant, mutation of APC gene)
Thrombi made of white/red layers	Lines of Zahn (arterial thrombus, layers of platelets/RBCs)
"Thumb sign" on lateral neck x-ray	Epiglottitis (*Haemophilus influenzae*)
Thyroid-like appearance of kidney	Chronic pyelonephritis (usually due to recurrent infections)
"Tram-track" appearance of capillary loops of glomerular basement membranes on light microscopy	Membranoproliferative glomerulonephritis
Triglyceride accumulation in liver cell vacuoles	Fatty liver disease (alcoholic or metabolic syndrome)
↑ uric acid levels	Gout, Lesch-Nyhan syndrome, tumor lysis syndrome, loop and thiazide diuretics
"Waxy" casts with very low urine flow	Chronic end-stage renal disease
WBC casts in urine	Acute pyelonephritis
WBCs that look "smudged"	CLL (almost always B cell)
"Wire loop" glomerular capillary appearance on light microscopy	Diffuse proliferative glomerulonephritis (usually seen with lupus)
Yellowish CSF	Xanthochromia (eg, due to subarachnoid hemorrhage)s

▶ CLASSIC/RELEVANT TREATMENTS

CONDITION	COMMON TREATMENT(S)
Absence seizures	Ethosuximide
Acute gout attack	NSAIDs, colchicine, glucocorticoids
Acute promyelocytic leukemia (M3)	All-*trans* retinoic acid
ADHD	Methylphenidate, CBT, atomoxetine, guanfacine, clonidine
Alcoholism	Disulfiram, acamprosate, naltrexone, supportive care
Alcohol withdrawal	Long-acting benzodiazepines
Anorexia	Nutrition, psychotherapy, mirtazapine
Arrhythmia in damaged cardiac tissue	Class IB antiarrhythmic (lidocaine, mexiletine)
Benign prostatic hyperplasia	α_1-antagonists, 5α-reductase inhibitors, PDE-5 inhibitors
Bipolar disorder	Mood stabilizers (eg, lithium, valproic acid, carbamazepine), atypical antipsychotics

CONDITION	COMMON TREATMENT(S)
Breast cancer in postmenopausal woman	Aromatase inhibitor (anastrozole)
Buerger disease	Smoking cessation
Bulimia nervosa	SSRIs
Candida albicans	Topical azoles (vaginitis); nystatin, fluconazole, caspofungin (oral/esophageal); fluconazole, caspofungin, amphotericin B (systemic)
Carcinoid syndrome	Octreotide
Chlamydia trachomatis	Doxycycline (+ ceftriaxone for gonorrhea coinfection), erythromycin eye drops (prophylaxis in infants)
Chronic gout	Xanthine oxidase inhibitors (eg, allopurinol, febuxostat); pegloticase; probenecid
Chronic hepatitis B or C	IFN-α (HBV and HCV); ribavirin, simeprevir, sofosbuvir (HCV)
Chronic myelogenous leukemia	Imatinib
Clostridium botulinum	Antitoxin
Clostridium difficile	Oral metronidazole; if refractory, oral vancomycin
Clostridium tetani	Antitoxin
CMV	Ganciclovir, foscarnet, cidofovir
Crohn disease	Corticosteroids, infliximab, azathioprine
Cryptococcus neoformans	Fluconazole (in AIDS patients)
Cyclophosphamide-induced hemorrhagic cystitis	Mesna
Depression	SSRIs (first-line)
Diabetes insipidus	Desmopressin (central); hydrochlorothiazide, indomethacin, amiloride (nephrogenic)
Diabetes mellitus type 1	Dietary intervention (low carbohydrate) + insulin replacement
Diabetes mellitus type 2	Dietary intervention, oral hypoglycemics, and insulin (if refractory)
Diabetic ketoacidosis	Fluids, insulin, K^+
Drug of choice for anticoagulation during pregnancy	Heparin
Enterococci	Vancomycin, aminopenicillins/cephalosporins
Erectile dysfunction	Sildenafil, tadalafil, vardenafil
ER ⊕ breast cancer	Tamoxifen
Ethylene glycol/methanol intoxication	Fomepizole (alcohol dehydrogenase inhibitor)
Haemophilus influenzae (B)	Rifampin (prophylaxis)
Generalized anxiety disorder	SSRIs, SNRIs (first line); buspirone (second line)
Granulomatosis with polyangiitis (Wegener)	Cyclophosphamide, corticosteroids
Heparin reversal	Protamine sulfate
HER2/neu ⊕ breast cancer	Trastuzumab
Hyperaldosteronism	Spironolactone

CONDITION	COMMON TREATMENT(S)
Hypercholesterolemia	Statin (first-line)
Hypertriglyceridemia	Fibrate
Immediate anticoagulation	Heparin
Infertility	Leuprolide, GnRH (pulsatile), clomiphene
Influenza	Oseltamivir, zanamivir
Kawasaki disease	IVIG, high-dose aspirin
Legionella pneumophila	Macrolides (eg, azithromycin)
Long-term anticoagulation	Warfarin, dabigatran, rivaroxaban and apixaban
Malaria	Chloroquine, mefloquine, atovaquone/proguanil (for blood schizont), primaquine (for liver hypnozoite)
Malignant hyperthermia	Dantrolene
Medical abortion	Mifepristone
Migraine	Abortive therapies (eg, sumatriptan, NSAIDs); prophylaxis (eg, propranolol, topiramate, CCBs, amitriptyline)
Multiple sclerosis	Disease-modifying therapies (eg, β-interferon, natalizumab); for acute flares, use IV steroids
Mycobacterium tuberculosis	RIPE (rifampin, isoniazid, pyrazinamide, ethambutol)
Neisseria gonorrhoeae	Ceftriaxone (add doxycycline to cover likely concurrent *C trachomatis*)
Neisseria meningitidis	Penicillin/ceftriaxone, rifampin (prophylaxis)
Neural tube defect prevention	Prenatal folic acid
Osteomalacia/rickets	Vitamin D supplementation
Osteoporosis	Calcium/vitamin D supplementation (prophylaxis); bisphosphonates, PTH analogs, SERMs, calcitonin, denosumab (treatment)
Patent ductus arteriosus	Close with indomethacin; keep open with PGE analogs
Pheochromocytoma	α-antagonists (eg, phenoxybenzamine)
Pneumocystis jirovecii	TMP-SMX (prophylaxis and treatment in immunosuppressed patients)
Prolactinoma	Cabergoline/bromocriptine (dopamine agonists)
Prostate adenocarcinoma/uterine fibroids	Leuprolide, GnRH (continuous)
Prostate adenocarcinoma	Flutamide
Pseudomonas aeruginosa	Antipseudomonal penicillins, aminoglycosides, carbapenems
Pulmonary arterial hypertension (idiopathic)	Sildenafil, bosentan, epoprostenol
Rickettsia rickettsii	Doxycycline, chloramphenicol
Schizophrenia (negative symptoms)	Atypical antipsychotics
Schizophrenia (positive symptoms)	Typical and atypical antipsychotics
SIADH	Fluid restriction, IV hypertonic saline, conivaptan/tolvaptan, demeclocycline

CONDITION	COMMON TREATMENT(S)
Sickle cell disease	Hydroxyurea (↑ fetal hemoglobin)
Sporothrix schenckii	Itraconazole, oral potassium iodide
Stable angina	Sublingual nitroglycerin
Staphylococcus aureus	MSSA: nafcillin, oxacillin, dicloxacillin (antistaphylococcal penicillins); MRSA: vancomycin, daptomycin, linezolid, ceftaroline
Streptococcus bovis	Penicillin prophylaxis; evaluation for colon cancer if linked to endocarditis
Streptococcus pneumoniae	Penicillin/cephalosporin (systemic infection, pneumonia), vancomycin (meningitis)
Streptococcus pyogenes	Penicillin prophylaxis
Temporal arteritis	High-dose steroids
Tonic-clonic seizures	Levetiracetam, phenytoin, valproate, carbamazepine
Toxoplasma gondii	Sulfadiazine + pyrimethamine
Treponema pallidum	Penicillin
Trichomonas vaginalis	Metronidazole (patient and partner)
Trigeminal neuralgia (tic douloureux)	Carbamazepine
Ulcerative colitis	5-ASA preparations (eg, mesalamine), 6-mercaptopurine, infliximab, colectomy
UTI prophylaxis	TMP-SMX
Warfarin reversal	Fresh frozen plasma (acute), vitamin K (non-acute)

▶ KEY ASSOCIATIONS

DISEASE/FINDING	MOST COMMON/IMPORTANT ASSOCIATIONS
Actinic (solar) keratosis	Precursor to squamous cell carcinoma
Acute gastric ulcer associated with CNS injury	Cushing ulcer (↑ intracranial pressure stimulates vagal gastric H^+ secretion)
Acute gastric ulcer associated with severe burns	Curling ulcer (greatly reduced plasma volume results in sloughing of gastric mucosa)
Age ranges for patient with ALL/CLL/AML/CML	ALL: child, CLL: adult > 60, AML: adult ~ 65, CML: adult 45–85
Alternating areas of transmural inflammation and normal colon	Skip lesions (Crohn disease)
Aortic aneurysm, abdominal	Atherosclerosis
Aortic aneurysm, ascending or arch	3° syphilis (syphilitic aortitis), vasa vasorum destruction
Aortic aneurysm, thoracic	Marfan syndrome (idiopathic cystic medial degeneration)
Aortic dissection	Hypertension
Atrophy of the mammillary bodies	Wernicke encephalopathy (thiamine deficiency causing ataxia, ophthalmoplegia, and confusion)

DISEASE/FINDING	MOST COMMON/IMPORTANT ASSOCIATIONS
Autosplenectomy (fibrosis and shrinkage)	Sickle cell disease (hemoglobin S)
Bacteria associated with gastritis, peptic ulcer disease, and gastric malignancies (eg, adenocarcinoma, MALToma)	*H pylori*
Bacterial meningitis (adults and elderly)	*S pneumoniae*
Bacterial meningitis (newborns and kids)	Group B streptococcus/*E coli* (newborns), *S pneumoniae*/*N meningitidis* (kids/teens)
Bilateral ovarian metastases from gastric carcinoma	Krukenberg tumor (mucin-secreting signet ring cells)
Bleeding disorder with GpIb deficiency	Bernard-Soulier syndrome (defect in platelet adhesion to von Willebrand factor)
Brain tumor (adults)	Supratentorial: metastasis, astrocytoma (including glioblastoma multiforme), meningioma, schwannoma
Brain tumor (kids)	Infratentorial: medulloblastoma (cerebellum) or supratentorial: craniopharyngioma
Breast cancer	Invasive ductal carcinoma
Breast mass	Fibrocystic change, carcinoma (in postmenopausal women)
Breast tumor (benign, young woman)	Fibroadenoma
Cardiac 1° tumor (kids)	Rhabdomyoma, often seen in tuberous sclerosis
Cardiac manifestation of lupus	Marantic/thrombotic endocarditis (nonbacterial)
Cardiac tumor (adults)	Metastasis, myxoma (90% in left atrium; "ball and valve")
Cerebellar tonsillar herniation	Chiari II malformation
Chronic arrhythmia	Atrial fibrillation (associated with high risk of emboli)
Chronic atrophic gastritis (autoimmune)	Predisposition to gastric carcinoma (can also cause pernicious anemia)
Clear cell adenocarcinoma of the vagina	DES exposure in utero
Congenital adrenal hyperplasia, hypotension	21-hydroxylase deficiency
Congenital cardiac anomaly	VSD
Congenital conjugated hyperbilirubinemia (black liver)	Dubin-Johnson syndrome (inability of hepatocytes to secrete conjugated bilirubin into bile)
Constrictive pericarditis	TB (developing world); idiopathic, viral illness (developed world)
Coronary artery involved in thrombosis	LAD > RCA > circumflex
Cretinism	Iodine deficit/congenital hypothyroidism
Cushing syndrome	▪ Iatrogenic (from corticosteroid therapy) ▪ Adrenocortical adenoma (secretes excess cortisol) ▪ ACTH-secreting pituitary adenoma (Cushing disease) ▪ Paraneoplastic (due to ACTH secretion by tumors)
Cyanosis (early; less common)	Tetralogy of Fallot, transposition of great vessels, truncus arteriosus
Death in CML	Blast crisis
Death in SLE	Lupus nephropathy

DISEASE/FINDING	MOST COMMON/IMPORTANT ASSOCIATIONS
Dementia	Alzheimer disease, multiple infarcts (vascular dementia)
Demyelinating disease in young women	Multiple sclerosis
DIC	Severe sepsis, obstetric complications, cancer, burns, trauma, major surgery, acute pancreatitis, APL
Diverticulum in pharynx	Zenker diverticulum (diagnosed by barium swallow)
Ejection click	Aortic stenosis
Esophageal cancer	Squamous cell carcinoma (worldwide); adenocarcinoma (US)
Food poisoning (exotoxin mediated)	*S aureus, B cereus*
Gastric cancer	Adenocarcinoma
Glomerulonephritis (adults)	Berger disease (IgA nephropathy)
Gynecologic malignancy	Endometrial carcinoma (most common in US); cervical carcinoma (most common worldwide)
Heart murmur, congenital	Mitral valve prolapse
Heart valve in bacterial endocarditis	Mitral > aortic (rheumatic fever), tricuspid (IV drug abuse)
Helminth infection (US)	*Enterobius vermicularis, Ascaris lumbricoides*
Hematoma—epidural	Rupture of middle meningeal artery (trauma; lentiform shaped)
Hematoma—subdural	Rupture of bridging veins (crescent shaped)
Hemochromatosis	Multiple blood transfusions or hereditary *HFE* mutation (can result in heart failure, "bronze diabetes," and ↑ risk of hepatocellular carcinoma)
Hepatocellular carcinoma	Cirrhotic liver (associated with hepatitis B and C and with alcoholism)
Hereditary bleeding disorder	von Willebrand disease
Hereditary harmless jaundice	Gilbert syndrome (benign congenital unconjugated hyperbilirubinemia)
HLA-B27	Psoriatic arthritis, ankylosing spondylitis, IBD-associated arthritis, reactive arthritis (formerly Reiter syndrome)
HLA-DR3	Diabetes mellitus type 1, SLE, Graves disease, Hashimoto thyroiditis, Addison disease
HLA-DR4	Diabetes mellitus type 1, rheumatoid arthritis, Addison disease
Holosystolic murmur	VSD, tricuspid regurgitation, mitral regurgitation
Hypercoagulability, endothelial damage, blood stasis	Virchow triad (↑ risk of thrombosis)
Hypertension, 2°	Renal artery stenosis, chronic kidney disease (eg, polycystic kidney disease, diabetic nephropathy), hyperaldosteronism
Hypoparathyroidism	Accidental excision during thyroidectomy
Hypopituitarism	Pituitary adenoma (usually benign tumor)
Infection 2° to blood transfusion	Hepatitis C
Infections in chronic granulomatous disease	*S aureus, E coli, Aspergillus* (catalase ⊕)

DISEASE/FINDING	MOST COMMON/IMPORTANT ASSOCIATIONS
Intellectual disability	Down syndrome, fragile X syndrome
Kidney stones	▪ Calcium = radiopaque ▪ Struvite (ammonium) = radiopaque (formed by urease ⊕ organisms such as *Klebsiella*, *Proteus* species, and *S saprophyticus*) ▪ Uric acid = radiolucent ▪ Cystine = radiolucent
Late cyanotic shunt (uncorrected left to right becomes right to left)	Eisenmenger syndrome (caused by ASD, VSD, PDA; results in pulmonary hypertension/polycythemia)
Liver disease	Alcoholic cirrhosis
Lysosomal storage disease	Gaucher disease
Male cancer	Prostatic carcinoma
Malignancy associated with noninfectious fever	Hodgkin lymphoma
Malignancy (kids)	ALL, medulloblastoma (cerebellum)
Metastases to bone	Prostate, breast > lung > thyroid
Metastases to brain	Lung > breast > genitourinary > melanoma > GI
Metastases to liver	Colon >> stomach, pancreas
Microcytic anemia	Iron deficiency
Mitochondrial inheritance	Disease occurs in both males and females, inherited through females only
Mitral valve stenosis	Rheumatic heart disease
Mixed (UMN and LMN) motor neuron disease	Amyotrophic lateral sclerosis
Myocarditis	Coxsackie B
Nephrotic syndrome (adults)	Focal segmental glomerulosclerosis
Nephrotic syndrome (kids)	Minimal change disease
Neuron migration failure	Kallmann syndrome (hypogonadotropic hypogonadism and anosmia)
Nosocomial pneumonia	*S aureus*, *Pseudomonas*, other enteric gram ⊖ rods
Obstruction of male urinary tract	BPH
Opening snap	Mitral stenosis
Opportunistic infection in AIDS	*Pneumocystis jirovecii* pneumonia
Osteomyelitis	*S aureus* (most common overall)
Osteomyelitis in sickle cell disease	*Salmonella*
Osteomyelitis with IV drug use	*Pseudomonas*, *Candida*, *S aureus*
Ovarian tumor (benign, bilateral)	Serous cystadenoma
Ovarian tumor (malignant)	Serous cystadenocarcinoma
Pancreatitis (acute)	Gallstones, alcohol
Pancreatitis (chronic)	Alcohol (adults), cystic fibrosis (kids)
Pelvic inflammatory disease	*C trachomatis*, *N gonorrhoeae*
Philadelphia chromosome t(9;22) (*BCR-ABL*)	CML (may sometimes be associated with ALL/AML)
Pituitary tumor	Prolactinoma, somatotropic adenoma

DISEASE/FINDING	MOST COMMON/IMPORTANT ASSOCIATIONS
1° amenorrhea	Turner syndrome (45,XO or 45,XO/46,XX mosaic)
1° bone tumor (adults)	Multiple myeloma
1° hyperaldosteronism	Adenoma of adrenal cortex
1° hyperparathyroidism	Adenomas, hyperplasia, carcinoma
1° liver cancer	Hepatocellular carcinoma (chronic hepatitis, cirrhosis, hemochromatosis, α_1-antitrypsin deficiency, Wilson disease)
Pulmonary hypertension	Idiopathic, heritable, left heart disease (eg, HF), lung disease (eg, COPD), hypoxemic vasoconstriction (eg, OSA), thromboembolic (eg, PE)
Recurrent inflammation/thrombosis of small/medium vessels in extremities	Buerger disease (strongly associated with tobacco)
Refractory peptic ulcers and high gastrin levels	Zollinger-Ellison syndrome (gastrinoma of duodenum or pancreas), associated with MEN1
Renal tumor	Renal cell carcinoma: associated with von Hippel-Lindau and cigarette smoking; paraneoplastic syndromes (EPO, renin, PTHrP, ACTH)
Right heart failure due to a pulmonary cause	Cor pulmonale
S3 heart sound	↑ ventricular filling pressure (eg, mitral regurgitation, HF), common in dilated ventricles
S4 heart sound	Stiff/hypertrophic ventricle (aortic stenosis, restrictive cardiomyopathy)
2° hyperparathyroidism	Hypocalcemia of chronic kidney disease
Sexually transmitted disease	*C trachomatis* (usually coinfected with *N gonorrhoeae*)
SIADH	Small cell carcinoma of the lung
Site of diverticula	Sigmoid colon
Sites of atherosclerosis	Abdominal aorta > coronary artery > popliteal artery > carotid artery
t(14;18)	Follicular lymphomas (*BCL-2* activation, anti-apoptotic oncogene)
t(8;14)	Burkitt lymphoma (c-*myc* fusion, transcription factor oncogene)
t(9;22)	Philadelphia chromosome, CML (*BCR-ABL* activation, tyrosine kinase oncogene)
Temporal arteritis	Risk of ipsilateral blindness due to occlusion of ophthalmic artery; polymyalgia rheumatica
Testicular tumor	Seminoma (malignant, radiosensitive), ↑ placental ALP
Thyroid cancer	Papillary carcinoma (childhood irradiation)
Tumor in women	Leiomyoma (estrogen dependent, not precancerous)
Tumor of infancy	Strawberry hemangioma (grows rapidly and regresses spontaneously by childhood)
Tumor of the adrenal medulla (adults)	Pheochromocytoma (usually benign)
Tumor of the adrenal medulla (kids)	Neuroblastoma (malignant)
Type of Hodgkin lymphoma	Nodular sclerosing (vs mixed cellularity, lymphocytic predominance, lymphocytic depletion)

DISEASE/FINDING	MOST COMMON/IMPORTANT ASSOCIATIONS
Type of non-Hodgkin lymphoma	Diffuse large B-cell lymphoma
UTI	*E coli*, *Staphylococcus saprophyticus* (young women)
Vertebral compression fracture	Osteoporosis (type I: postmenopausal woman; type II: elderly man or woman)
Viral encephalitis affecting temporal lobe	HSV-1
Vitamin deficiency (US)	Folate (pregnant women are at high risk; body stores only 3- to 4-month supply; prevents neural tube defects)

▶ EQUATION REVIEW

TOPIC	EQUATION	PAGE
Sensitivity	Sensitivity = TP / (TP + FN)	33
Specificity	Specificity = TN / (TN + FP)	33
Positive predictive value	PPV = TP / (TP + FP)	33
Negative predictive value	NPV = TN / (FN + TN)	33
Odds ratio (for case-control studies)	$OR = \frac{a/c}{b/d} = \frac{ad}{bc}$	34
Relative risk	$RR = \frac{a/(a+b)}{c/(c+d)}$	34
Attributable risk	$AR = \frac{a}{a+b} - \frac{c}{c+d}$	34
Relative risk reduction	RRR = 1 − RR	34
Absolute risk reduction	$ARR = \frac{c}{c+d} - \frac{a}{a+b}$	34
Number needed to treat	NNT = 1/ARR	34
Number needed to harm	NNH = 1/AR	34
Hardy-Weinberg equilibrium	$p^2 + 2pq + q^2 = 1$ $p + q = 1$	69
Volume of distribution	$V_d = \frac{\text{amount of drug in the body}}{\text{plasma drug concentration}}$	237
Half-life	$t_{1/2} = \frac{0.693 \times V_d}{CL}$	237
Drug clearance	$CL = \frac{\text{rate of elimination of drug}}{\text{plasma drug concentration}} = V_d \times K_e$ (elimination constant)	237
Loading dose	$LD = \frac{C_p \times V_d}{F}$	237
Maintenance dose	$D = \frac{C_p \times CL \times \tau}{F}$	237

TOPIC	EQUATION	PAGE
Cardiac output	$CO = \dfrac{\text{rate of } O_2 \text{ consumption}}{\text{arterial } O_2 \text{ content} - \text{venous } O_2 \text{ content}}$	266
	$CO = \text{stroke volume} \times \text{heart rate}$	266
Mean arterial pressure	$MAP = \text{cardiac output} \times \text{total peripheral resistance}$	266
	$MAP = \frac{2}{3}\text{ diastolic} + \frac{1}{3}\text{ systolic}$	266
Stroke volume	$SV = EDV - ESV$	266
Ejection fraction	$EF = \dfrac{SV}{EDV} = \dfrac{EDV - ESV}{EDV}$	267
Resistance	$\text{Resistance} = \dfrac{\text{driving pressure } (\Delta P)}{\text{flow } (Q)} = \dfrac{8\eta \text{ (viscosity)} \times \text{length}}{\pi r^4}$	268
Capillary fluid exchange	$J_v = \text{net fluid flow} = K_f[(P_c - P_i) - \varsigma(\pi_c - \pi_i)]$	281
Renal clearance	$C_x = U_xV/P_x$	533
Glomerular filtration rate	$GFR = U_{inulin} \times V/P_{inulin} = C_{inulin}$	534
	$GFR = K_f\,[(P_{GC} - P_{BS}) - (\pi_{GC} - \pi_{BS})]$	
Effective renal plasma flow	$eRPF = U_{PAH} \times \dfrac{V}{P_{PAH}} = C_{PAH}$	534
Renal blood flow	$RBF = \dfrac{RPF}{1 - Hct}$	534
Filtration fraction	$FF = \dfrac{GFR}{RPF}$	535
Henderson-Hasselbalch equation (for extracellular pH)	$pH = 6.1 + \log \dfrac{[HCO_3^-]}{0.03\ P_{CO_2}}$	543
Winters formula	$P_{CO_2} = 1.5\,[HCO_3^-] + 8 \pm 2$	543
Physiologic dead space	$V_D = V_T \times \dfrac{Pa_{CO_2} - P_{ECO_2}}{Pa_{CO_2}}$	610
Pulmonary vascular resistance	$PVR = \dfrac{P_{\text{pulm artery}} - P_{\text{L atrium}}}{\text{cardiac output}}$	614
Alveolar gas equation	$P_{AO_2} = P_{IO_2} - \dfrac{Pa_{CO_2}}{R}$	614

▶ NOTES

SECTION IV

Top-Rated Review Resources

"Some books are to be tasted, others to be swallowed, and some few to be chewed and digested."

—Sir Francis Bacon

"Always read something that will make you look good if you die in the middle of it."

—P.J. O'Rourke

"So many books, so little time."

—Frank Zappa

"If one cannot enjoy reading a book over and over again, there is no use in reading it at all."

—Oscar Wilde

▶ HOW TO USE THE DATABASE

This section is a database of top-rated basic science review books, sample examination books, software, websites, and apps that have been marketed to medical students studying for the USMLE Step 1. For each recommended resource, we list (where applicable) the **Title**, the **First Author** (or editor), the **Current Publisher**, the **Copyright Year**, the **Number of Pages**, the **Approximate List Price**, the **Format** of the resource, and the **Number of Test Questions**. Finally, each recommended resource receives a **Rating**. Within each section, resources are arranged first by Rating and then alphabetically by the first author within each Rating group.

For a complete list of resources, including summaries that describe their overall style and utility, go to www.firstaidteam.com/bonus.

A letter rating scale with six different grades reflects the detailed student evaluations for **Rated Resources**. Each rated resource receives a rating as follows:

A+	Excellent for boards review.
A A–	Very good for boards review; choose among the group.
B+ B	Good, but use only after exhausting better resources.
B–	Fair, but there are many better resources in the discipline; or low-yield subject material.

The Rating is meant to reflect the overall usefulness of the resource in helping medical students prepare for the USMLE Step 1. This is based on a number of factors, including:

- The cost
- The readability of the text
- The appropriateness and accuracy of the material
- The quality and number of sample questions
- The quality of written answers to sample questions
- The quality and appropriateness of the illustrations (eg, graphs, diagrams, photographs)
- The length of the text (longer is not necessarily better)
- The quality and number of other resources available in the same discipline
- The importance of the discipline for the USMLE Step 1

Please note that ratings do not reflect the quality of the resources for purposes other than reviewing for the USMLE Step 1. Many books with lower ratings are well written and informative but are not ideal for boards preparation. We have not listed or commented on general textbooks available in the basic sciences.

Evaluations are based on the cumulative results of formal and informal surveys of thousands of medical students at many medical schools across the country. The ratings represent a consensus opinion, but there may have been a broad range of opinion or limited student feedback on any particular resource.

Please note that the data listed are subject to change in that:

- Publishers' prices change frequently.
- Bookstores often charge an additional markup.
- New editions come out frequently, and the quality of updating varies.
- The same book may be reissued through another publisher.

We actively encourage medical students and faculty to submit their opinions and ratings of these basic science review materials so that we may update our database. (See p. xvii, How to Contribute.) In addition, we ask that publishers and authors submit for evaluation review copies of basic science review books, including new editions and books not included in our database. We also solicit reviews of new books or suggestions for alternate modes of study that may be useful in preparing for the examination, such as flash cards, computer software, commercial review courses, apps, and Web sites.

Disclaimer/Conflict of Interest Statement

No material in this book, including the ratings, reflects the opinion or influence of the publisher. All errors and omissions will gladly be corrected if brought to the attention of the authors through our blog at www.firstaidteam.com. Please note that USMLE-Rx and the entire *First Aid for the USMLE* series are publications by the senior authors of this book; the following ratings are based solely on recommendations from the student authors of this book as well as data from the student survey and feedback forms.

▶ TOP-RATED REVIEW RESOURCES

Question Banks

		AUTHOR	PUBLISHER	TYPE	PRICE
A+	*USMLEWorld Qbank*	USMLEWorld	www.usmleworld.com	Test/2200 q	\$129–\$399
A	*USMLE-Rx Qmax*	MedIQ Learning	www.usmle-rx.com	Test/2300 q	\$99–\$299
A−	*Kaplan Qbank*	Kaplan	www.kaplanmedical.com	Test/2200 q	\$99–\$199
B+	*USMLE Consult*	Elsevier	www.usmleconsult.com	Test/2500 q	\$75–\$395

Question Books

		AUTHOR	PUBLISHER	TYPE	PRICE
A−	*First Aid Q&A for the USMLE Step 1*	Le	McGraw-Hill, 2012, 784 pages	Test/1000 q	\$46.00
B+	*Kaplan USMLE Step 1 Qbook*	Kaplan	Kaplan, 2013, 456 pages	Test/850 q	\$44.99
B+	*PreTest Clinical Vignettes for the USMLE Step 1*	McGraw-Hill	McGraw-Hill, 2010, 318 pages	Test/322 q	\$39.00

Internet Sites

		AUTHOR	PUBLISHER	TYPE	PRICE
A	*First Aid Step 1 Express*		www.usmle-rx.com	Review/Test	\$99.00–\$249.00
B+	*Firecracker*	Firecracker Inc.	www.firecracker.me	Review/Test/1500 q	\$117–\$500
B+	*SketchyMedical*		www.SketchyMedical.com	Review	\$99–\$159
B+	*WebPath: The Internet Pathology Laboratory*		library.med.utah.edu/WebPath/	Review/Test/1300 q	Free
B	*Blue Histology*		www.lab.anhb.uwa.edu.au/mb140	Review/Test	Free
B	*Dr. Najeeb Lectures*		www.drnajeeblectures.com	Review	\$49
B	*Medical School Pathology*		www.medicalstudentpathology.com	Review	Free
B	*The Pathology Guy*	Friedlander	www.pathguy.com	Review	Free
B	*The Whole Brain Atlas*	Johnson	www.med.harvard.edu/aanlib/	Review	Free
B	*Radiopaedia.org*		www.radiopaedia.org	Cases/Test	Free
B−	*Digital Anatomist Project: Interactive Atlases*	University of Washington	www9.biostr.washington.edu/da.html	Review	Free
B−	*Picmonic*		http://www.picmonic.com	Review	\$24.99/month

Mobile Apps

		AUTHOR	PUBLISHER	TYPE	PRICE
A	*Anki*		http://ankisrs.net	Flash cards	Free/\$24.99
B+	*Cram Fighter*		www.cramfighter.com	Study plan	\$14.99/month
B	*Osmosis*		www.osmosis.org	Test	Variable

Comprehensive

		AUTHOR	PUBLISHER	TYPE	PRICE
A	*First Aid for the Basic Sciences: General Principles*	Le	McGraw-Hill, 2011, 576 pages	Review	$72.00
A	*First Aid for the Basic Sciences: Organ Systems*	Le	McGraw-Hill, 2011, 880 pages	Review	$93.00
A	*medEssentials for the USMLE Step 1*	Manley	Kaplan, 2012, 588 pages	Review	$54.99
A⁻	*USMLE Step 1 Secrets*	Brown	Elsevier, 2012, 880 pages	Review	$42.95
A⁻	*First Aid Cases for the USMLE Step 1*	Le	McGraw-Hill, 2012, 448 pages	Cases	$50.00
B⁺	*Step-Up to USMLE Step 1 2015*	Jenkins	Lippincott Williams & Wilkins, 2014, 528 pages	Review	$52.99
B⁺	*Cracking the USMLE Step 1*	Princeton Review	Princeton Review, 2013, 832 pages	Review	$44.99
B⁺	*USMLE Images for the Boards: A Comprehensive Image-Based Review*	Tully	Elsevier, 2012, 296 pages	Review	$42.95
B	*First Aid Step 1 Flash Facts*		https://www.usmle-rx.com	Flash cards	$49.00–$99.00
B	*Déjà Review: USMLE Step 1*	Naheedy	McGraw-Hill, 2010, 412 pages	Review	$24.00
B⁻	*USMLE Step 1 Made Ridiculously Simple*	Carl	MedMaster, 2014, 400 pages	Review/Test 100 q	$29.95

Anatomy, Embryology, and Neuroscience

		AUTHOR	PUBLISHER	TYPE	PRICE
A⁻	*High-Yield Embryology*	Dudek	Lippincott Williams & Wilkins, 2013, 176 pages	Review	$37.99
A⁻	*High-Yield Neuroanatomy*	Fix	Lippincott Williams & Wilkins, 2008, 160 pages	Review/ Test/50 q	$35.99
A⁻	*Anatomy—An Essential Textbook*	Gilroy	Thieme, 2013, 504 pages	Text/ Test/400 q	$44.99
A⁻	*Atlas of Anatomy*	Gilroy	Thieme, 2012, 704 pages	Text	$79.99
B⁺	*High-Yield Gross Anatomy*	Dudek	Lippincott Williams & Wilkins, 2014, 320 pages	Review	$37.99
B⁺	*Clinical Anatomy Made Ridiculously Simple*	Goldberg	MedMaster, 2012, 175 pages	Review	$29.95
B⁺	*PreTest Neuroscience*	Siegel	McGraw-Hill, 2013, 412 pages	Test/500 q	$37.00
B⁺	*Crash Course: Anatomy*	Stenhouse	Elsevier, 2015, 288 pages	Review	$44.99
B⁺	*Déjà Review: Neuroscience*	Tremblay	McGraw-Hill, 2010, 266 pages	Review	$24.00
B⁺	*USMLE Road Map: Neuroscience*	White	McGraw-Hill, 2008, 224 pages	Review/ Test/300 q	$40.00
B	*BRS Embryology*	Dudek	Lippincott Williams & Wilkins, 2014, 336 pages	Review/ Test/220 q	$50.99
B	*Anatomy Flash Cards: Anatomy on the Go*	Gilroy	Thieme, 2013, 565 flash cards	Flash cards	$59.99

Anatomy, Embryology, and Neuroscience *(continued)*

		AUTHOR	PUBLISHER	TYPE	PRICE
B	*Clinical Neuroanatomy Made Ridiculously Simple*	Goldberg	MedMaster, 2014, 90 pages + CD-ROM	Review/Test/Few q	$25.95
B	*Rapid Review: Gross and Developmental Anatomy*	Moore	Elsevier, 2010, 304 pages	Review/Test/450 q	$42.95
B	*Case Files: Anatomy*	Toy	McGraw-Hill, 2014, 402 pages	Cases	$35.00
B	*Case Files: Neuroscience*	Toy	McGraw-Hill, 2014, 418 pages	Cases	$35.00
B⁻	*Gray's Anatomy for Students Flash Cards*	Drake	Elsevier, 2015, 350 flash cards	Flash cards	$39.99
B⁻	*Netter's Anatomy Flash Cards*	Hansen	Saunders, 2014, 674 flash cards	Flash cards	$39.95

Behavioral Science

		AUTHOR	PUBLISHER	TYPE	PRICE
A	*High-Yield Behavioral Science*	Fadem	Lippincott Williams & Wilkins, 2012, 144 pages	Review	$36.99
A⁻	*BRS Behavioral Science*	Fadem	Lippincott Williams & Wilkins, 2013, 336 pages	Review/Test/700 q	$49.99
A⁻	*High-Yield Biostatistics, Epidemiology, and Public Health*	Glaser	Lippincott Williams & Wilkins, 2013, 168 pages	Review	$41.99
A⁻	*Clinical Biostatistics and Epidemiology Made Ridiculously Simple*	Weaver	MedMaster, 2011, 104 pages	Review	$22.95
B⁺	*USMLE Medical Ethics*	Fischer	Kaplan, 2012, 216 pages	Cases	$42.99
B⁺	*Jekel's Epidemiology, Biostatistics, Preventive Medicine, and Public Health*	Katz	Saunders, 2013, 420 pages	Review/Test/477 q	$59.95
B	*Déjà Review: Behavioral Science*	Quinn	McGraw-Hill, 2010, 240 pages	Review	$24.00

Biochemistry

		AUTHOR	PUBLISHER	TYPE	PRICE
A⁻	*Lange Flash Cards Biochemistry and Genetics*	Baron	McGraw-Hill, 2013, 184 flash cards	Flash cards	$38.00
A⁻	*Rapid Review: Biochemistry*	Pelley	Elsevier, 2010, 208 pages	Review/Test/350 q	$42.95
B⁺	*Lippincott's Illustrated Reviews: Biochemistry*	Ferrier	Lippincott Williams & Wilkins, 2013, 560 pages	Review/Test/500 q	$75.99
B⁺	*Déjà Review: Biochemistry*	Manzoul	McGraw-Hill, 2010, 206 pages	Review	$24.00
B⁺	*Medical Biochemistry—An Illustrated Review*	Panini	Thieme, 2013, 441 pages	Review/Test/400 q	$39.99
B⁺	*PreTest Biochemistry and Genetics*	Wilson	McGraw-Hill, 2013, 592 pages	Test/500 q	$36.00
B	*Clinical Biochemistry Made Ridiculously Simple*	Goldberg	MedMaster, 2010, 95 pages + foldout	Review	$24.95
B	*BRS Biochemistry, Molecular Biology, and Genetics*	Lieberman	Lippincott Williams & Wilkins, 2013, 432 pages	Review/Test	$49.99

Biochemistry *(continued)*

		AUTHOR	PUBLISHER	TYPE	PRICE
B⁻	*Case Files: Biochemistry*	Toy	McGraw-Hill, 2014, 480 pages	Cases	$35.00
B⁻	*High-Yield Biochemistry*	Wilcox	Lippincott Williams & Wilkins, 2009, 128 pages	Review	$40.99

Cell Biology and Histology

		AUTHOR	PUBLISHER	TYPE	PRICE
A⁻	*High-Yield Cell and Molecular Biology*	Dudek	Lippincott Williams & Wilkins, 2010, 151 pages	Review	$36.99
B	*Elsevier's Integrated Review: Genetics*	Adkison	Elsevier, 2011, 272 pages	Review	$42.95
B	*High-Yield Genetics*	Dudek	Lippincott Williams & Wilkins, 2008, 134 pages	Review	$36.99
B	*BRS Cell Biology and Histology*	Gartner	Lippincott Williams & Wilkins, 2014, 432 pages	Review/ Test/320 q	$45.99
B	*PreTest Anatomy, Histology, and Cell Biology*	Klein	McGraw-Hill, 2010, 654 pages	Test/500 q	$37.00
B	*USMLE Road Map: Genetics*	Sack	McGraw-Hill, 2008, 224 pages	Review	$40.00
B	*Déjà Review: Histology and Cell Biology*	Song	McGraw-Hill, 2010, 300 pages	Review	$24.00
B	*Crash Course: Cell Biology and Genetics*	Stubbs	Elsevier, 2015, 216 pages	Review	$46.99
B⁻	*Wheater's Functional Histology*	Young	Elsevier, 2013, 464 pages	Text	$82.95

Microbiology and Immunology

		AUTHOR	PUBLISHER	TYPE	PRICE
A	*Déjà Review: Microbiology & Immunology*	Chen	McGraw-Hill, 2010, 424 pages	Review	$24.00
A	*Clinical Microbiology Made Ridiculously Simple*	Gladwin	MedMaster, 2014, 400 pages	Review	$36.95
A	*Lange Microbiology & Infectious Diseases Flash Cards*	Somers	McGraw-Hill, 2010, 189 flash cards	Flash cards	$43.00
A⁻	*Basic Immunology*	Abbas	Elsevier, 2012, 336 pages	Review	$71.95
A⁻	*Microcards: Microbiology Flash Cards*	Harpavat	Lippincott Williams & Wilkins, 2011, 310 flash cards	Flash cards	$46.99
A⁻	*Medical Microbiology and Immunology Flash Cards*	Rosenthal	Elsevier, 2008, 324 flash cards	Flash cards	$39.95
B⁺	*Elsevier's Integrated Immunology and Microbiology*	Actor	Elsevier, 2011, 192 pages	Review	$42.95
B⁺	*Lippincott's Illustrated Reviews: Immunology*	Doan	Lippincott Williams & Wilkins, 2012, 384 pages	Review/Test/ Few q	$65.99
B⁺	*Lippincott's Illustrated Reviews: Microbiology*	Harvey	Lippincott Williams & Wilkins, 2012, 448 pages	Review/Test/ Few q	$67.99
B⁺	*Review of Medical Microbiology and Immunology*	Levinson	McGraw-Hill, 2014, 800 pages	Review/ Test/654 q	$55.00

Microbiology and Immunology *(continued)*

		AUTHOR	PUBLISHER	TYPE	PRICE
B	*The Big Picture: Medical Microbiology*	Chamberlain	McGraw-Hill, 2008, 456 pages	Review/100 q	$65.00
B	*Case Studies in Immunology: Clinical Companion*	Geha	Garland Science, 2011, 376 pages	Cases	$59.00
B	*Pretest: Microbiology*	Kettering	McGraw-Hill, 2013, 480 pages	Test/500 q	$36.00
B	*Rapid Review: Microbiology and Immunology*	Rosenthal	Elsevier, 2010, 240 pages	Review/ Test/400 q	$42.95
B	*Case Files: Microbiology*	Toy	McGraw-Hill, 2014, 401 pages	Cases	$35.00

Pathology

		AUTHOR	PUBLISHER	TYPE	PRICE
A+	*Rapid Review: Pathology*	Goljan	Elsevier, 2013, 784 pages	Review/ Test/400 q	$55.95
A+	*Pathoma: Fundamentals of Pathology*	Sattar	Pathoma, 2011, 218 pages	Review/ Lecture	$82.95
A−	*Lange Pathology Flash Cards*	Baron	McGraw-Hill, 2013, 300 flash cards	Flash cards	$39.00
A−	*Déjà Review: Pathology*	Davis	McGraw-Hill, 2010, 474 pages	Review	$24.00
A−	*Lippincott's Illustrated Q&A Review of Rubin's Pathology*	Fenderson	Lippincott Williams & Wilkins, 2010, 336 pages	Test/1000 q	$57.99
A−	*The Big Picture: Pathology*	Kemp	McGraw-Hill, 2007, 512 pages	Review/ Test/130 q	$61.00
A−	*Robbins and Cotran Review of Pathology*	Klatt	Elsevier, 2014, 504 pages	Test/1100 q	$49.95
A−	*BRS Pathology*	Schneider	Lippincott Williams & Wilkins, 2013, 480 pages	Review/ Test/450 q	$49.99
A−	*Color Atlas of Physiology*	Silbernagl	Thieme, 2015, 472 pages	Review	$49.99
A−	*Crash Course: Pathology*	Xiu	Elsevier, 2012, 356 pages	Review	$44.95
B+	*Cases & Concepts Step 1: Pathophysiology Review*	Caughey	Lippincott Williams & Wilkins, 2009, 376 pages	Cases	$48.99
B+	*Case Files: Pathology*	Toy	McGraw-Hill, 2008, 456 pages	Cases	$38.00
B	*PreTest Pathology*	Brown	McGraw-Hill, 2010, 612 pages	Test/500 q	$37.00
B	*High-Yield Histopathology*	Dudek	Lippincott Williams & Wilkins, 2011, 328 pages	Review	$36.00
B	*Pathophysiology of Disease: Introduction to Clinical Medicine*	McPhee	McGraw-Hill, 2014, 784 pages	Text	$78.00
B	*Haematology at a Glance*	Mehta	Blackwell Science, 2014, 136 pages	Review	$46.95
B	*Pocket Companion to Robbins and Cotran Pathologic Basis of Disease*	Mitchell	Elsevier, 2011, 800 pages	Review	$40.95

Pharmacology

		AUTHOR	PUBLISHER	TYPE	PRICE
A⁻	*Lange Pharmacology Flash Cards*	Baron	McGraw-Hill, 2013, 230 flash cards	Flash cards	$39.00
A⁻	*Master the Boards USMLE Step 1 Pharmacology Flashcards*	Fischer	Kaplan, 2015, 408 flash cards	Flash cards	$54.99
A⁻	*Déjà Review: Pharmacology*	Gleason	McGraw-Hill, 2010, 236 pages	Review	$24.00
A⁻	*Lippincott's Illustrated Reviews: Pharmacology*	Harvey	Lippincott Williams & Wilkins, 2014, 680 pages	Review/ Test/380 q	$69.99
A⁻	*PharmCards: Review Cards for Medical Students*	Johannsen	Lippincott Williams & Wilkins, 2010, 240 flash cards	Flash cards	$44.99
B⁺	*Crash Course: Pharmacology*	Battista	Elsevier, 2015, 236 pages	Review	$44.99
B⁺	*Pharmacology Flash Cards*	Brenner	Elsevier, 2012, 200 flash cards	Flash cards	$39.95
B⁺	*Elsevier's Integrated Pharmacology*	Kester	Elsevier, 2011, 264 pages	Review	$42.95
B⁺	*Rapid Review: Pharmacology*	Pazdernik	Elsevier, 2010, 360 pages	Review/ Test/450 q	$42.95
B⁺	*BRS Pharmacology*	Rosenfeld	Lippincott Williams & Wilkins, 2013, 384 pages	Review/ Test/200 q	$49.99
B	*PreTest Pharmacology*	Shlafer	McGraw-Hill, 2013, 567 pages	Test/500 q	$36.00
B	*Case Files: Pharmacology*	Toy	McGraw-Hill, 2013, 453 pages	Cases	$35.00
B	*Katzung & Trevor's Pharmacology: Examination and Board Review*	Trevor	McGraw-Hill, 2015, 592 pages	Review/ Test/1000 q	$54.00
B	*High-Yield Pharmacology*	Weiss	Lippincott Williams & Wilkins, 2009, 160 pages	Review	$35.99

Physiology

		AUTHOR	PUBLISHER	TYPE	PRICE
A⁺	*BRS Physiology*	Costanzo	Lippincott Williams & Wilkins, 2014, 328 pages	Review/ Test/350 q	$51.99
A	*Acid-Base, Fluids, and Electrolytes Made Ridiculously Simple*	Preston	MedMaster, 2010, 156 pages	Review	$22.95
A⁻	*Physiology*	Costanzo	Saunders, 2013, 520 pages	Text	$62.95
B⁺	*BRS Physiology Cases and Problems*	Costanzo	Lippincott Williams & Wilkins, 2012, 368 pages	Cases	$49.99
B⁺	*Déjà Review: Physiology*	Gould	McGraw-Hill, 2010, 298 pages	Review	$24.00
B⁺	*The Big Picture: Medical Physiology*	Kibble	McGraw-Hill, 2009, 448 pages	Review/ Test/108 q	$58.00
B⁺	*PreTest Physiology*	Metting	McGraw-Hill, 2013, 505 pages	Test/500 q	$36.00
B	*Rapid Review: Physiology*	Brown	Elsevier, 2011, 288 pages	Test/350 q	$42.95
B	*Vander's Renal Physiology*	Eaton	McGraw-Hill, 2013, 240 pages	Text	$45.00
B	*Endocrine Physiology*	Molina	McGraw-Hill, 2013, 320 pages	Review	$48.00
B	*Netter's Physiology Flash Cards*	Mulroney	Saunders, 2009, 200+ flash cards	Flash cards	$39.95

Physiology *(continued)*

		AUTHOR	PUBLISHER	TYPE	PRICE
B	***Case Files: Physiology***	Toy	McGraw-Hill, 2008, 456 pages	Cases	$37.00
B	***Pulmonary Pathophysiology: The Essentials***	West	Lippincott Williams & Wilkins, 2012, 208 pages	Review/Test/50 q	$51.99
B⁻	***Clinical Physiology Made Ridiculously Simple***	Goldberg	MedMaster, 2010, 160 pages	Review	$24.95

SECTION IV

Abbreviations and Symbols

ABBREVIATION	MEANING
⊕	positive
⊖	negative
1°	primary
2°	secondary
3°	tertiary
A-a	alveolar-arterial [gradient]
AA	Alcoholics Anonymous, amyloid A
AAMC	Association of American Medical Colleges
Ab	antibody
ABP	androgen-binding protein
ACA	anterior cerebral artery
Acetyl-CoA	acetyl coenzyme A
ACD	anemia of chronic disease
ACE	angiotensin-converting enzyme
ACh	acetylcholine
AChE	acetylcholinesterase
ACL	anterior cruciate ligament
ACom	anterior communicating [artery]
ACTH	adrenocorticotropic hormone
ADA	adenosine deaminase, Americans with Disabilities Act
ADH	antidiuretic hormone
ADHD	attention-deficit hyperactivity disorder
ADP	adenosine diphosphate
ADPKD	autosomal-dominant polycystic kidney disease
AFP	α-fetoprotein
Ag	antigen, silver
AICA	anterior inferior cerebellar artery
AIDS	acquired immunodeficiency syndrome
AIHA	autoimmune hemolytic anemia
AL	amyloid light [chain]
ALA	aminolevulinic acid
ALL	acute lymphoblastic (lymphocytic) leukemia
ALP	alkaline phosphatase
α_1, α_2	sympathetic receptors
ALS	amyotrophic lateral sclerosis
ALT	alanine transaminase
AMA	American Medical Association, antimitochondrial antibody
AML	acute myelogenous (myeloid) leukemia
AMP	adenosine monophosphate
ANA	antinuclear antibody
ANCA	antineutrophil cytoplasmic antibody
ANOVA	analysis of variance
ANP	atrial natriuretic peptide

ABBREVIATION	MEANING
ANS	autonomic nervous system
anti-CCP	anti-cyclic citrullinated peptide
AOA	American Osteopathic Association
AP	action potential, A & P [ribosomal binding sites]
APAF-1	apoptotic protease activating factor 1
APC	antigen-presenting cell, activated protein C
Apo	apolipoprotein
APP	amyloid precursor protein
APRT	adenine phosphoribosyltransferase
APSAC	anistreplase
aPTT	activated partial thromboplastin time
APUD	amine precursor uptake decarboxylase
AR	attributable risk, autosomal recessive, aortic regurgitation
ara-C	arabinofuranosyl cytidine (cytarabine)
ARB	angiotensin receptor blocker
ARDS	acute respiratory distress syndrome
Arg	arginine
ARMD	age-related macular degeneration
ARPKD	autosomal-recessive polycystic kidney disease
AS	aortic stenosis
ASA	anterior spinal artery
ASD	atrial septal defect
ASO	anti–streptolysin O
AST	aspartate transaminase
AT	angiotensin, antithrombin
ATCase	aspartate transcarbamoylase
ATN	acute tubular necrosis
ATP	adenosine triphosphate
ATPase	adenosine triphosphatase
ATTR	transthyretin-mediated amyloidosis
AV	atrioventricular
AZT	azidothymidine
β_1, β_2	sympathetic receptors
BAL	British anti-Lewisite [dimercaprol]
BCG	bacille Calmette-Guérin
BH_4	tetrahydrobiopterin
BIMS	Biometric Identity Management System
BM	basement membrane
BMI	body-mass index
BMR	basal metabolic rate
BP	bisphosphate, blood pressure
BPG	bisphosphoglycerate
BPH	benign prostatic hyperplasia
BT	bleeding time
BUN	blood urea nitrogen

ABBREVIATION	MEANING
Ca^{2+}	calcium ion
CAD	coronary artery disease
CAF	common application form
CALLA	common acute lymphoblastic leukemia antigen
cAMP	cyclic adenosine monophosphate
CBG	corticosteroid-binding globulin
Cbl	cobalamin
CBSE	Comprehensive Basic Science Examination
CBSSA	Comprehensive Basic Science Self-Assessment
CBT	computer-based test, cognitive behavioral therapy
CCK	cholecystokinin
CCS	computer-based case simulation
CD	cluster of differentiation
CDK	cyclin-dependent kinase
cDNA	complementary deoxyribonucleic acid
CEA	carcinoembryonic antigen
CETP	cholesteryl-ester transfer protein
CF	cystic fibrosis
CFTR	cystic fibrosis transmembrane conductance regulator
CFX	circumflex [artery]
CGD	chronic granulomatous disease
cGMP	cyclic guanosine monophosphate
CGN	*cis*-Golgi network
$C_H1–C_H3$	constant regions, heavy chain [antibody]
ChAT	choline acetyltransferase
χ^2	chi-squared
CI	confidence interval
CIN	candidate identification number, carcinoma in situ, cervical intraepithelial neoplasia
CIS	Communication and Interpersonal Skills
CK	clinical knowledge, creatine kinase
CK-MB	creatine kinase, MB fraction
C_L	constant region, light chain [antibody]
CL	clearance
Cl^-	chloride ion
CLL	chronic lymphocytic leukemia
CML	chronic myelogenous (myeloid) leukemia
CMV	cytomegalovirus
CN	cranial nerve
CN^-	cyanide ion
CNS	central nervous system
CNV	copy number variation
CO	carbon monoxide, cardiac output
CO_2	carbon dioxide
CoA	coenzyme A
COL1A1	collagen, type I, alpha 1
COL1A2	collagen, type I, alpha 2
COMT	catechol-O-methyltransferase
COOH	carboxyl group
COP	coat protein
COPD	chronic obstructive pulmonary disease
CoQ	coenzyme Q
COX	cyclooxygenase
C_p	plasma concentration
CPAP	continuous positive airway pressure

ABBREVIATION	MEANING
CPK	creatine phosphokinase
CPR	cardiopulmonary resuscitation
Cr	creatinine
CRC	colorectal cancer
CREST	calcinosis, Raynaud phenomenon, esophageal dysfunction, sclerosis, and telangiectasias [syndrome]
CRH	corticotropin-releasing hormone
CRP	C-reactive protein
CS	clinical skills
C-section	cesarean section
CSF	cerebrospinal fluid
CT	computed tomography
CTP	cytidine triphosphate
CVA	cerebrovascular accident
CVID	common variable immunodeficiency
CXR	chest x-ray
Cys	cysteine
DAF	decay-accelerating factor
DAG	diacylglycerol
dATP	deoxyadenosine triphosphate
DCIS	ductal carcinoma in situ
DCT	distal convoluted tubule
ddC	dideoxycytidine [zalcitabine]
ddI	didanosine
DES	diethylstilbestrol
DHAP	dihydroxyacetone phosphate
DHB	dihydrobiopterin
DHEA	dehydroepiandrosterone
DHF	dihydrofolic acid
DHS	Department of Homeland Security
DHT	dihydrotestosterone
DI	diabetes insipidus
DIC	disseminated intravascular coagulation
DIP	distal interphalangeal [joint]
DKA	diabetic ketoacidosis
DLCO	diffusing capacity for carbon monoxide
DM	diabetes mellitus
DNA	deoxyribonucleic acid
dNTP	deoxynucleotide triphosphate
DO	doctor of osteopathy
DPGN	diffuse proliferative glomerulonephritis
DPM	doctor of podiatric medicine
DPP-4	dipeptidyl peptidase-4
DPPC	dipalmitoylphosphatidylcholine
DS	double stranded
dsDNA	double-stranded deoxyribonucleic acid
dsRNA	double-stranded ribonucleic acid
d4T	didehydrodeoxythymidine [stavudine]
dTMP	deoxythymidine monophosphate
DTR	deep tendon reflex
DTs	delirium tremens
dUDP	deoxyuridine diphosphate
dUMP	deoxyuridine monophosphate
DVT	deep venous thrombosis
EBV	Epstein-Barr virus

ABBREVIATION	MEANING
EC	ejection click
ECF	extracellular fluid
ECFMG	Educational Commission for Foreign Medical Graduates
ECG	electrocardiogram
ECL	enterochromaffin-like [cell]
ECM	extracellular matrix
ECT	electroconvulsive therapy
ED_{50}	median effective dose
EDRF	endothelium-derived relaxing factor
EDTA	ethylenediamine tetra-acetic acid
EDV	end-diastolic volume
EEG	electroencephalogram
EF	ejection fraction
EGF	epidermal growth factor
EHEC	enterohemorrhagic *E coli*
ELISA	enzyme-linked immunosorbent assay
EM	electron micrograph/microscopy
EMB	eosin–methylene blue
Epi	epinephrine
EPO	erythropoietin
EPS	extrapyramidal system
ER	endoplasmic reticulum, estrogen receptor
ERAS	Electronic Residency Application Service
ERCP	endoscopic retrograde cholangiopancreatography
ERP	effective refractory period
eRPF	effective renal plasma flow
ERT	estrogen replacement therapy
ERV	expiratory reserve volume
ESR	erythrocyte sedimentation rate
ESRD	end-stage renal disease
ESV	end-systolic volume
ETEC	enterotoxigenic *E coli*
EtOH	ethyl alcohol
EV	esophageal vein
F	bioavailability
FA	fatty acid
Fab	fragment, antigen-binding
FAD	flavin adenine dinucleotide
FAD^+	oxidized flavin adenine dinucleotide
$FADH_2$	reduced flavin adenine dinucleotide
FAP	familial adenomatous polyposis
F1,6BP	fructose-1,6-bisphosphate
F2,6BP	fructose-2,6-bisphosphate
FBPase	fructose bisphosphatase
Fc	fragment, crystallizable
FcR	Fc receptor
5f-dUMP	5-fluorodeoxyuridine monophosphate
Fe^{2+}	ferrous ion
Fe^{3+}	ferric ion
FENa	excreted fraction of filtered sodium
FEV_1	forced expiratory volume in 1 second
FF	filtration fraction
FFA	free fatty acid
FGF	fibroblast growth factor
FGFR	fibroblast growth factor receptor

ABBREVIATION	MEANING
FISH	fluorescence in situ hybridization
FKBP	FK506 binding protein
FLAIR	fluid-attenuated inversion recovery
f-met	formylmethionine
FMG	foreign medical graduate
FMN	flavin mononucleotide
FN	false negative
FNHTR	febrile nonhemolytic transfusion reaction
FP	false positive
F1P	fructose-1-phosphate
F6P	fructose-6-phosphate
FRC	functional residual capacity
FSH	follicle-stimulating hormone
FSMB	Federation of State Medical Boards
FTA-ABS	fluorescent treponemal antibody—absorbed
5-FU	5-fluorouracil
FVC	forced vital capacity
GABA	γ-aminobutyric acid
Gal	galactose
GBM	glomerular basement membrane
GC	glomerular capillary
G-CSF	granulocyte colony-stimulating factor
GERD	gastroesophageal reflux disease
GFAP	glial fibrillary acid protein
GFR	glomerular filtration rate
GGT	γ-glutamyl transpeptidase
GH	growth hormone
GHB	γ-hydroxybutyrate
GHRH	growth hormone–releasing hormone
G_I	G protein, I polypeptide
GI	gastrointestinal
GIP	gastric inhibitory peptide
GIST	gastrointestinal stromal tumor
GLUT	glucose transporter
GM	granulocyte macrophage
GM-CSF	granulocyte-macrophage colony stimulating factor
GMP	guanosine monophosphate
GnRH	gonadotropin-releasing hormone
GP	glycoprotein
G3P	glucose-3-phosphate
G6P	glucose-6-phosphate
G6PD	glucose-6-phosphate dehydrogenase
GPe	globus pallidus externa
GPi	globus pallidus interna
GPI	glycosyl phosphatidylinositol
GRP	gastrin-releasing peptide
G_S	G protein, S polypeptide
GS	glycogen synthase
GSH	reduced glutathione
GSSG	oxidized glutathione
GTP	guanosine triphosphate
GTPase	guanosine triphosphatase
GU	genitourinary
H^+	hydrogen ion
H_1, H_2	histamine receptors

ABBREVIATION	MEANING
H_2S	hydrogen sulfide
HAART	highly active antiretroviral therapy
HAV	hepatitis A virus
HAVAb	hepatitis A antibody
Hb	hemoglobin
Hb^+	oxidized hemoglobin
Hb^-	ionized hemoglobin
HBcAb	hepatitis B core antibody
HBcAg	hepatitis B core antigen
HBeAb	hepatitis B early antibody
HBeAg	hepatitis B early antigen
HBsAb	hepatitis B surface antibody
HBsAg	hepatitis B surface antigen
$HbCO_2$	carbaminohemoglobin
HBV	hepatitis B virus
HCC	hepatocellular carcinoma
hCG	human chorionic gonadotropin
HCO_3^-	bicarbonate
Hct	hematocrit
HCTZ	hydrochlorothiazide
HCV	hepatitis C virus
HDL	high-density lipoprotein
HDV	hepatitis D virus
H&E	hematoxylin and eosin
HEV	hepatitis E virus
HF	heart failure
Hfr	high-frequency recombination [cell]
HGPRT	hypoxanthine-guanine phosphoribosyltransferase
HHb	human hemoglobin
HHV	human herpesvirus
5-HIAA	5-hydroxyindoleacetic acid
HIE	hypoxic ischemic encephalopathy
His	histidine
HIT	heparin-induced thrombocytopenia
HIV	human immunodeficiency virus
HL	hepatic lipase
HLA	human leukocyte antigen
HMG-CoA	hydroxymethylglutaryl-coenzyme A
HMP	hexose monophosphate
HMSN	hereditary motor and sensory neuropathy
HMWK	high-molecular-weight kininogen
HNPCC	hereditary nonpolyposis colorectal cancer
hnRNA	heterogeneous nuclear ribonucleic acid
H_2O	water
H_2O_2	hydrogen peroxide
HPA	hypothalamic-pituitary-adrenal [axis]
HPL	human placental lactogen
HPO	hypothalamic-pituitary-ovarian [axis]
HPV	human papillomavirus
HR	heart rate
HRE	hormone receptor element
HSV	herpes simplex virus
5-HT	5-hydroxytryptamine (serotonin)
HTLV	human T-cell leukemia virus
HTN	hypertension

ABBREVIATION	MEANING
HTR	hemolytic transfusion reaction
HUS	hemolytic-uremic syndrome
HVA	homovanillic acid
HZV	herpes zoster virus
IBD	inflammatory bowel disease
IBS	irritable bowel syndrome
IC	inspiratory capacity, immune complex
I_{Ca}	calcium current [heart]
I_f	funny current [heart]
ICA	internal carotid artery
ICAM	intracellular adhesion molecule
ICD	implantable cardioverter defibrillator
ICE	Integrated Clinical Encounter
ICF	intracellular fluid
ICP	intracranial pressure
ID	identification
ID_{50}	median infective dose
IDDM	insulin-dependent diabetes mellitus
IDL	intermediate-density lipoprotein
I/E	inspiratory/expiratory [ratio]
IF	immunofluorescence, initiation factor
IFN	interferon
Ig	immunoglobulin
IGF	insulin-like growth factor
I_K	potassium current [heart]
IL	interleukin
IM	intramuscular
IMA	inferior mesenteric artery
IMED	International Medical Education Directory
IMG	international medical graduate
IMP	inosine monophosphate
IMV	inferior mesenteric vein
I_{Na}	sodium current [heart]
INO	internuclear ophthalmoplegia
INR	International Normalized Ratio
IO	inferior oblique [muscle]
IOP	intraocular pressure
IP_3	inositol triphosphate
IPV	inactivated polio vaccine
IR	current × resistance [Ohm's law], inferior rectus [muscle]
IRV	inspiratory reserve volume
ITP	idiopathic thrombocytopenic purpura
IUD	intrauterine device
IUGR	intrauterine growth restriction
IV	intravenous
IVC	inferior vena cava
IVDU	intravenous drug use
IVIG	intravenous immunoglobulin
JAK/STAT	Janus kinase/signal transducer and activator of transcription [pathway]
JGA	juxtaglomerular apparatus
JVD	jugular venous distention
JVP	jugular venous pulse
K^+	potassium ion
KatG	catalase-peroxidase produced by *M tuberculosis*

ABBREVIATION	MEANING
K_e	elimination constant
K_f	filtration constant
KG	ketoglutarate
K_m	Michaelis-Menten constant
KOH	potassium hydroxide
L	left
LA	left atrial, left atrium
LAD	left anterior descending [artery]
LAF	left anterior fascicle
LCA	left coronary artery
LCAT	lecithin-cholesterol acyltransferase
LCFA	long-chain fatty acid
LCL	lateral collateral ligament
LCME	Liaison Committee on Medical Education
LCMV	lymphocytic choriomeningitis virus
LCX	left circumflex artery
LD	loading dose
LD_{50}	median lethal dose
LDH	lactate dehydrogenase
LDL	low-density lipoprotein
LES	lower esophageal sphincter
LFA	leukocyte function–associated antigen
LFT	liver function test
LGN	lateral geniculate nucleus
LGV	left gastric vein
LH	luteinizing hormone
LLQ	left lower quadrant
LM	light microscopy
LMN	lower motor neuron
LOS	lipooligosaccharide
LP	lumbar puncture
LPL	lipoprotein lipase
LPS	lipopolysaccharide
LR	lateral rectus [muscle]
LT	labile toxin leukotriene
LV	left ventricle, left ventricular
Lys	lysine
M_1-M_5	muscarinic (parasympathetic) ACh receptors
MAC	membrane attack complex, minimal alveolar concentration
MALT	mucosa-associated lymphoid tissue
MAO	monoamine oxidase
MAOI	monoamine oxidase inhibitor
MAP	mean arterial pressure, mitogen-activated protein
MASP	mannose-binding lectin–associated serine protease
MBL	mannose-binding lectin
MC	midsystolic click
MCA	middle cerebral artery
MCAT	Medical College Admissions Test
MCHC	mean corpuscular hemoglobin concentration
MCL	medial collateral ligament
MCP	metacarpophalangeal [joint]
MCV	mean corpuscular volume
MD	maintenance dose
MELAS syndrome	mitochondrial encephalopathy, lactic acidosis, and stroke-like episodes

ABBREVIATION	MEANING
MEN	multiple endocrine neoplasia
Mg^{2+}	magnesium ion
MGN	medial geniculate nucleus
$MgSO_4$	magnesium sulfate
MGUS	monoclonal gammopathy of undetermined significance
MHC	major histocompatibility complex
MI	myocardial infarction
MIF	müllerian inhibiting factor
MLCK	myosin light-chain kinase
MLF	medial longitudinal fasciculus
MMC	migrating motor complex
MMR	measles, mumps, rubella [vaccine]
MOPP	mechlorethamine-vincristine (Oncovin)-prednisone-procarbazine [chemotherapy]
6-MP	6-mercaptopurine
MPGN	membranoproliferative glomerulonephritis
MPO	myeloperoxidase
MPO-ANCA/p-ANCA	perinuclear antineutrophil cytoplasmic antibody
MR	medial rectus [muscle], mitral regurgitation
MRI	magnetic resonance imaging
miRNA	microribonucleic acid
mRNA	messenger ribonucleic acid
MRSA	methicillin-resistant *S aureus*
MS	mitral stenosis, multiple sclerosis
MSH	melanocyte-stimulating hormone
MSM	men who have sex with men
mtDNA	mitochondrial DNA
mtRNA	mitochondrial RNA
mTOR	mammalian target of rapamycin
MTP	metatarsophalangeal [joint]
MTX	methotrexate
MUA/P	Medically Underserved Area and Population
MVO_2	myocardial oxygen consumption
MVP	mitral valve prolapse
N/A	not applicable
Na^+	sodium ion
NAD	nicotinamide adenine dinucleotide
NAD^+	oxidized nicotinamide adenine dinucleotide
NADH	reduced nicotinamide adenine dinucleotide
$NADP^+$	oxidized nicotinamide adenine dinucleotide phosphate
NADPH	reduced nicotinamide adenine dinucleotide phosphate
NBME	National Board of Medical Examiners
NBOME	National Board of Osteopathic Medical Examiners
NBPME	National Board of Podiatric Medical Examiners
NC	no change
NE	norepinephrine
NF	neurofibromatosis
NFAT	nuclear factor of activated T-cell
NH_3	ammonia
NH_4^+	ammonium
NIDDM	non-insulin-dependent diabetes mellitus
NK	natural killer [cells]
N_M	muscarinic ACh receptor in neuromuscular junction
NMDA	N-methyl-D-aspartate
NMJ	neuromuscular junction

ABBREVIATION	MEANING
NMS	neuroleptic malignant syndrome
N_N	nicotinic ACh receptor in autonomic ganglia
NRMP	National Residency Matching Program
NNRTI	non-nucleoside reverse transcriptase inhibitor
NO	nitric oxide
N_2O	nitrous oxide
NPH	neutral protamine Hagedorn, normal pressure hydrocephalus
NPV	negative predictive value
NRI	norepinephrine receptor inhibitor
NRTI	nucleoside reverse transcriptase inhibitor
NSAID	nonsteroidal anti-inflammatory drug
NSE	neuron-specific enolase
NSTEMI	non–ST-segment elevation myocardial infarction
OAA	oxaloacetic acid
OCD	obsessive-compulsive disorder
OCP	oral contraceptive pill
OH	hydroxy
OH_2	dihydroxy
1,25-OH D_3	calcitriol (active form of vitamin D)
25-OH D_3	storage form of vitamin D
3′ OH	hydroxyl
OMT	osteopathic manipulative technique
OPV	oral polio vaccine
OR	odds ratio
OS	opening snap
OTC	ornithine transcarbamoylase
OVLT	organum vasculosum of the lamina terminalis
P-body	processing body (cytoplasmic)
P-450	cytochrome P-450 family of enzymes
PA	posteroanterior
PABA	*para*-aminobenzoic acid
$Paco_2$	arterial Pco_2
$PAco_2$	alveolar Pco_2
PAH	*para*-aminohippuric acid
PAN	polyarteritis nodosa
Pao_2	partial pressure of oxygen in arterial blood
PAo_2	partial pressure of oxygen in alveolar blood
PAP	Papanicolaou [smear], prostatic acid phosphatase
PAS	periodic acid–Schiff
PBP	penicillin-binding protein
PC	plasma colloid osmotic pressure, platelet count, pyruvate carboxylase
PCA	posterior cerebral artery
PCL	posterior cruciate ligament
Pco_2	partial pressure of carbon dioxide
PCom	posterior communicating [artery]
PCOS	polycystic ovarian syndrome
PCP	phencyclidine hydrochloride, *Pneumocystis jirovecii* pneumonia
PCR	polymerase chain reaction
PCT	proximal convoluted tubule
PCWP	pulmonary capillary wedge pressure
PD	posterior descending [artery]
PDA	patent ductus arteriosus, posterior descending artery
PDC	pyruvate dehydrogenase complex

ABBREVIATION	MEANING
PDE	phosphodiesterase
PDGF	platelet-derived growth factor
PDH	pyruvate dehydrogenase
PE	pulmonary embolism
PECAM	platelet–endothelial cell adhesion molecule
$PEco_2$	expired air Pco_2
PEP	phosphoenolpyruvate
PF	platelet factor
PFK	phosphofructokinase
PFT	pulmonary function test
PG	phosphoglycerate
P_i	plasma interstitial osmotic pressure, inorganic phosphate
PICA	posterior inferior cerebellar artery
PID	pelvic inflammatory disease
PIo_2	Po_2 in inspired air
PIP	proximal interphalangeal [joint]
PIP_2	phosphatidylinositol 4,5-bisphosphate
PKD	polycystic kidney disease
PKR	interferon-α–induced protein kinase
PKU	phenylketonuria
PLP	pyridoxal phosphate
PLS	Personalized Learning System
PML	progressive multifocal leukoencephalopathy
PMN	polymorphonuclear [leukocyte]
P_{net}	net filtration pressure
PNET	primitive neuroectodermal tumor
PNS	peripheral nervous system
Po_2	partial pressure of oxygen
PO_4	salt of phosphoric acid
PO_4^{3-}	phosphate
PPAR	peroxisome proliferator-activated receptor
PPD	purified protein derivative
PPI	proton pump inhibitor
PPV	positive predictive value
PR3-ANCA/ c-ANCA	cytoplasmic antineutrophil cytoplasmic antibody
PrP	prion protein
PRPP	phosphoribosylpyrophosphate
PSA	prostate-specific antigen
PSS	progressive systemic sclerosis
PT	prothrombin time
PTH	parathyroid hormone
PTHrP	parathyroid hormone–related protein
PTSD	post-traumatic stress disorder
PTT	partial thromboplastin time
PV	plasma volume, venous pressure
PVC	polyvinyl chloride
PVR	pulmonary vascular resistance
R	correlation coefficient, right, R variable [group]
R_3	Registration, Ranking, & Results [system]
RA	right atrium
RAAS	renin-angiotensin-aldosterone system
RANK-L	receptor activator of nuclear factor-κ B ligand
RAS	reticular activating system
RBC	red blood cell

ABBREVIATION	MEANING
RBF	renal blood flow
RCA	right coronary artery
REM	rapid eye movement
RER	rough endoplasmic reticulum
Rh	*rhesus* antigen
RLQ	right lower quadrant
RNA	ribonucleic acid
RNP	ribonucleoprotein
ROS	reactive oxygen species
RPF	renal plasma flow
RPGN	rapidly progressive glomerulonephritis
RPR	rapid plasma reagin
RR	relative risk, respiratory rate
rRNA	ribosomal ribonucleic acid
RS	Reed-Sternberg [cells]
RSV	respiratory syncytial virus
RTA	renal tubular acidosis
RUQ	right upper quadrant
RV	residual volume, right ventricle, right ventricular
RVH	right ventricular hypertrophy
Rx	medical prescription
[S]	substrate concentration
SA	sinoatrial
SAA	serum amyloid–associated [protein]
SAM	S-adenosylmethionine
SARS	severe acute respiratory syndrome
SAT	Scholastic Aptitude Test
SC	subcutaneous
SCC	squamous cell carcinoma
SCD	sudden cardiac death
SCID	severe combined immunodeficiency disease
SCJ	squamocolumnar junction
SCM	sternocleidomastoid muscle
SCN	suprachiasmatic nucleus
SD	standard deviation
SEM	standard error of the mean
SEP	Spoken English Proficiency
SER	smooth endoplasmic reticulum
SERM	selective estrogen receptor modulator
SGLT	sodium-glucose transporter
SHBG	sex hormone–binding globulin
SIADH	syndrome of inappropriate [secretion of] antidiuretic hormone
SIDS	sudden infant death syndrome
SLE	systemic lupus erythematosus
SLL	small lymphocytic lymphoma
SLT	Shiga-like toxin
SMA	superior mesenteric artery
SMX	sulfamethoxazole
SNARE	soluble NSF attachment protein receptor
SNc	substantia nigra pars compacta
SNP	single nucleotide polymorphism
SNr	substantia nigra pars reticulata
SNRI	serotonin and norepinephrine receptor inhibitor
snRNP	small nuclear ribonucleoprotein
SO	superior oblique [muscle]
SOAP	Supplemental Offer and Acceptance Program
spp.	species
SR	superior rectus [muscle]
SS	single stranded
ssDNA	single-stranded deoxyribonucleic acid
SSPE	subacute sclerosing panencephalitis
SSRI	selective serotonin reuptake inhibitor
ssRNA	single-stranded ribonucleic acid
SSSS	staphylococcal scalded-skin syndrome
ST	Shiga toxin
STEMI	ST-segment elevation myocardial infarction
STI	sexually transmitted infection
STN	subthalamic nucleus
SV	splenic vein, stroke volume
SVC	superior vena cava
SVT	supraventricular tachycardia
$t_{1/2}$	half-life
T_3	triiodothyronine
T_4	thyroxine
TAPVR	total anomalous pulmonary venous return
TB	tuberculosis
TBG	thyroxine-binding globulin
3TC	dideoxythiacytidine [lamivudine]
TCA	tricarboxylic acid [cycle], tricyclic antidepressant
Tc cell	cytotoxic T cell
TCR	T-cell receptor
TDF	tenofovir disoproxil fumarate
TdT	terminal deoxynucleotidyl transferase
TFT	thyroid function test
TG	triglyceride
TGA	*trans*-Golgi apparatus
TGF	transforming growth factor
TGN	*trans*-Golgi network
Th cell	helper T cell
THF	tetrahydrofolic acid
TI	therapeutic index
TIA	transient ischemic attack
TIBC	total iron-binding capacity
TIPS	transjugular intrahepatic portosystemic shunt
TLC	total lung capacity
T_m	maximum rate of transport
TMP	trimethoprim
TN	true negative
TNF	tumor necrosis factor
TNM	tumor, node, metastases [staging]
TOEFL	Test of English as a Foreign Language
ToRCHeS	*Toxoplasma gondii*, rubella, CMV, HIV, HSV-2, syphilis
TP	true positive
tPA	tissue plasminogen activator
TPP	thiamine pyrophosphate
TPR	total peripheral resistance
TR	tricuspid regurgitation
TRAP	tartrate-resistant acid phosphatase
TRH	thyrotropin-releasing hormone

ABBREVIATION	MEANING
tRNA	transfer ribonucleic acid
TSH	thyroid-stimulating hormone
TSI	triple sugar iron
TSS	toxic shock syndrome
TSST	toxic shock syndrome toxin
TTP	thrombotic thrombocytopenic purpura
TTR	transthyretin
TV	tidal volume
Tx	translation [factor]
TXA_2	thromboxane A_2
UCV	Underground Clinical Vignettes
UDP	uridine diphosphate
UMN	upper motor neuron
UMP	uridine monophosphate
UPD	uniparental disomy
URI	upper respiratory infection
USMLE	United States Medical Licensing Examination
UTI	urinary tract infection
UTP	uridine triphosphate
UV	ultraviolet
$\dot{V}_1$, $\dot{V}_2$	Vasopressin receptors
VA	Veterans Affairs
VC	vital capacity
V_d	volume of distribution
VD	physiologic dead space
V(D)J	heavy-chain hypervariable region [antibody]
VDRL	Venereal Disease Research Laboratory

ABBREVIATION	MEANING
VEGF	vascular endothelial growth factor
V_H	variable region, heavy chain [antibody]
VHL	von Hippel-Lindau [disease]
VIP	vasoactive intestinal peptide
VIPoma	vasoactive intestinal polypeptide-secreting tumor
VJ	light-chain hypervariable region [antibody]
VL	ventral lateral [nucleus]; variable region, light chain [antibody]
VLDL	very low density lipoprotein
VMA	vanillylmandelic acid
VMAT	vesicular monoamine transporter
V_{max}	maximum velocity
VPL	ventral posterior nucleus, lateral
VPM	ventral posterior nucleus, medial
VPN	vancomycin, polymyxin, nystatin [media]
$\dot{V}/\dot{Q}$	ventilation/perfusion [ratio]
VRE	vancomycin-resistant enterococcus
VSD	ventricular septal defect
V_T	tidal volume
vWF	von Willebrand factor
VZV	varicella-zoster virus
WBC	white blood cell
VMAT	vesicular monoamine transporter
XR	X-linked recessive
XX	normal complement of sex chromosomes for female
XY	normal complement of sex chromosomes for male
ZDV	zidovudine [formerly AZT]

SECTION IV

Image Acknowledgments

In this edition, in collaboration with MedIQ Learning, LLC, and a variety of other partners, we are pleased to include the following clinical images and diagrams for the benefit of integrative student learning.

Portions of this book identified with the symbol are listed below by page number.

This symbol refers to material that is available in the public domain.

This symbol refers to the Creative Commons Attribution license, full text at http://creativecommons.org/licenses/by/4.0/legalcode.

This symbol refers to the Creative Commons Attribution-Share Alike license, full text at: http://creativecommons.org/licenses/by-sa/4.0/legalcode.

Biochemistry

60 **Cilia structure.** Courtesy of Louisa Howard and Michael Binder. The image may have been modified by cropping, labeling, and/or captions. All rights to this adaptation by MedIQ Learning, LLC are reserved.

63 **Osteogenesis imperfecta: Image A.** Skeletal deformities in lower body of child. This image is a derivative work, adapted from the following source, available under : Vanakker OM, Hemelsoet D, De Paepe. Hereditary connective tissue diseases in young adult stroke: a comprehensive synthesis. *Stroke Res Treat* 2011;712903. doi 10.4061/2011/712903. The image may have been modified by cropping, labeling, and/or captions. All rights to this adaptation by MedIQ Learning, LLC are reserved.

63 **Osteogenesis imperfecta: Image B.** Skeletal deformities in upper extremity of child. This image is a derivative work, adapted from the following source, available under : Vanakker OM, Hemelsoet D, De Paepe. Hereditary connective tissue diseases in young adult stroke: a comprehensive synthesis. *Stroke Res Treat* 2011;712903. doi 10.4061/2011/712903. The image may have been modified by cropping, labeling, and/or captions. All rights to this adaptation by MedIQ Learning, LLC are reserved.

63 **Osteogenesis imperfecta: Image C.** Blue sclera. This image is a derivative work, adapted from the following source, available under . Courtesy of Fred H, van Dijk H. Images of memorable cases: cases 40, 41 & 42. Connexions website. December 3, 2008. Available at: http://cnx.org/content/m15020/1.3/. The image may have been modified by cropping, labeling, and/or captions. MedIQ Learning, LLC makes this image available under .

63 **Ehlers-Danlos syndrome.** Finger hypermobility. This image is a derivative work, adapted from the following source, available under . Courtesy of Piotr Dołżonek. The image may have been modified by cropping, labeling, and/or captions. MedIQ Learning, LLC makes this image available under .

68 **Obstructive lung disease: Image E.** Curschmann spirals. Courtesy of Dr. James Heilman.

73 **Muscular dystrophies.** Fibrofatty replacement of muscle. Courtesy of the US Department of Health and Human Services and Dr. Edwin P. Ewing, Jr. The image may have been modified by cropping, labeling, and/or captions. All rights to this adaptation by MedIQ Learning, LLC are reserved.

78 **Vitamin B_3 (niacin).** Pellagra. This image is a derivative work, adapted from the following source, available under : van Dijk HA, Fred H. Images of memorable cases: case 2. Connexions website. Dec 4, 2008. Available at: http://cnx.org/contents/3d3dcb2e-8e98-496f-91c2-fe94e93428a1@3@3/.

81 **Vitamin D.** X-ray of lower extremity in child with rickets. This image is a derivative work, adapted from the following source, available under . Courtesy of Dr. Michael L. Richardson. The image may have been modified by cropping, labeling, and/or captions. MedIQ Learning, LLC makes this image available under .

82 **Malnutrition.** Child with kwashiorkor. Courtesy of the US Department of Health and Human Services and Dr. Lyle Conrad.

96 **Alkaptonuria.** Pigment granules on dorsum of hand. This image is a derivative work, adapted from the following source, available under : Vasudevan B, Sawhney MPS, Radhakrishnan S. Alkaptonuria associated with degenerative collagenous palmar plaques. *Indian J Dermatol* 2009;54:299-301. doi 10.4103/0019-5154.55650.

96 **Cystinuria.** Hexagonal stones in urine. This image is a derivative work, adapted from the following source, available under : Courtesy of Cayla Devine.

100 **Lysosomal storage diseases: Image A.** Angiokeratomas. This image is a derivative work, adapted from the following source, available under : Burlina AP, Sims KB, Politei JM, et al. Early diagnosis of peripheral nervous system involvement in Fabry disease and treatment of neuropathic pain: the report of an expert panel. *BMC Neurol* 2011;11:61. doi 10.1186/1471-2377-11-61. The image may have been modified by cropping, labeling, and/or captions. All rights to this adaptation by MedIQ Learning, LLC are reserved.

100 **Lysosomal storage diseases: Image B.** Gaucher cells in Gaucher disease. This image is a derivative work, adapted from the following source, available under : Sokołowska B, Skomra D, Czartoryska B. et al. Gaucher disease diagnosed after bone marrow trephine biopsy—a report of two cases. *Folia Histochemica et Cytobiologica* 2011;49:352-356. doi 10.5603/FHC.2011.0048. The image may have been modified by cropping, labeling, and/or captions. All rights to this adaptation by MedIQ Learning, LLC are reserved.

100 **Lysosomal storage diseases: Image C.** Foam cells in Niemann-Pick disease. This image is a derivative work, adapted from the following source, available under : Hypercholesterolemia boosts joint destruction in chronic arthritis. An experimental model aggravated by foam macrophage infiltration. Prieto-Potin I, Roman-Blas JA, Martinez-Calatrava MJ, et al. *Arthritis Res Ther* 2013;15:R81. doi 10.1186/ar4261.

100 **Lysosomal storage diseases: Image D.** "Cherry-red" spot on macula in Tay-Sachs disease. This image is a derivative work, adapted from the following source, available under : Courtesy of Dr. Jonathan Trobe.

Microbiology

110 **Stains: Image A.** *Trypanosoma lewisi* on Giemsa stain. Courtesy of the US Department of Health and Human Services and Dr. Mae Melvin.

110 **Stains: Image B.** *Tropheryma whipplei* on periodic acid–schiff stain. This image is a derivative work, adapted from the following source, available under : Dr. Ed Uthman.

110 **Stains: Image C.** *Mycobacterium tuberculosis* on Ziehl-Neelsen stain. Courtesy of the US Department of Health and Human Services and Dr. George P. Kubica.

110 **Stains: Image D.** *Cryptococcus neoformans* on India ink stain. Courtesy of the US Department of Health and Human Services.

110 **Stains: Image E.** *Coccidioides immitis* on silver stain. Courtesy of the US Department of Health and Human Services and Dr. Edwin P. Ewing, Jr.

112 **Encapsulated bacteria.** Capsular swelling of *Streptococcus pneumoniae* using the Neufeld-Quellung test. Courtesy of the US Department of Health and Human Services.

112 **Catalase-positive organisms.** Oxygen bubbles released during catalase reaction. This image is a derivative work, adapted from the following source, available under . Courtesy of Stefano Nase. The image may have been modified by cropping, labeling, and/or captions. MedIQ Learning, LLC makes this image available under .

114 **Bacterial spores.** This image is a derivative work, adapted from the following source, available under :. Jones SW, Paredes CJ, Tracy B. The transcriptional program underlying the physiology of clostridial sporulation. *Genome Biol* 2008;9:R114. doi 10.1186/gb-2008-9-7-r114.

119 **α-hemolytic bacteria.** α-hemolysis. This image is a derivative work, adapted from the following source, available under . Courtesy of Y. Tambe. The image may have been modified by cropping, labeling, and/or captions. MedIQ Learning, LLC makes this image available under .

119 **β-hemolytic bacteria.** β-hemolysis. This image is a derivative work, adapted from the following source, available under . Courtesy of Y. Tambe. The image may have been modified by cropping, labeling, and/or captions. MedIQ Learning, LLC makes this image available under .

119 ***Staphylococcus aureus.*** Gram stain. Courtesy of the US Department of Health and Human Services and Dr. Richard Facklam.

120 ***Streptococcus pneumoniae.*** Courtesy of the US Department of Health and Human Services and Dr. Mike Miller.

120 ***Streptococcus pyogenes* (group A streptococci).** Gram stain. This image is a derivative work, adapted from the following source, available under . Courtesy of Y. Tambe. The image may have been modified by cropping, labeling, and/or captions. MedIQ Learning, LLC makes this image available under .

121 ***Bacillus anthracis.*** Ulcer with black eschar. Courtesy of the US Department of Health and Human Services and James H. Steele.

122 **Clostridia (with exotoxins): Image A.** Gas gangrene due to *Clostridium perfringens* infection. This image is a derivative work, adapted from the following source, available under : Courtesy of Engelbert Schröpfer, Stephan Rauthe, and Thomas Meyer.

122 **Clostridia (with exotoxins): Image B.** Pseudomembranous enterocolitis on colonoscopy. This image is a derivative work, adapted from the following source, available under . Courtesy of Klinikum Dritter Orden für die Überlassung des Bildes zur Veröffentlichu. The image may have been modified by cropping, labeling, and/or captions. MedIQ Learning, LLC makes this image available under .

123 ***Corynebacterium diphtheriae.*** Pseudomembranous pharyngitis. This image is a derivative work, adapted from the following source, available under . Courtesy of Wikimedia Commons. The image may have been modified by cropping, labeling, and/or captions. MedIQ Learning, LLC makes this image available under .

123 ***Listeria monocytogenes.*** Actin rockets. This image is a derivative work, adapted from the following source, available under : Schuppler M, Loessner MJ. The opportunistic pathogen *Listeria monocytogenes*: pathogenicity and interaction with the mucosal immune system. *Int J Inflamm* 2010;2010:704321. doi 10.4061/2010/704321. The image may have been modified by cropping, labeling, and/or captions. All rights to this adaptation by MedIQ Learning, LLC are reserved.

123 ***Nocardia* vs *Actinomyces*: Image A.** *Nocardia* on acid-fast stain. This image is a derivative work, adapted from the following source, available under : Adhikari L, Dey S, Pal R. Mycetoma due to *Nocardia farcinica*. *J Glob Infect Dis* 2010;2:194-195. doi 0.4103/0974-777X.62868.

123 ***Nocardia* vs *Actinomyces*: Image B.** *Actinomyces israelii* on Gram stain. Courtesy of the US Department of Health and Human Services.

124 **Mycobacteria.** Acid-fast stain. Courtesy of the US Department of Health and Human Services and Dr. Edwin P. Ewing, Jr.

125 **Leprosy (Hansen disease): Image A.** "Glove and stocking" distribution. This image is a derivative work, adapted from the following source, available under : Bruno Jehle.

126 ***Neisseria*: Image A.** Photomicrograph. Courtesy of the US Department of Health and Human Services and Dr. Mike Miller.

126 ***Haemophilus influenzae*: Image A.** Epiglottitis. This image is a derivative work, adapted from the following source, available under : Wikimedia Commons. The image may have been modified by cropping, labeling, and/or captions. All rights to this adaptation by MedIQ Learning, LLC are reserved.

127 ***Legionella pneumophila*.** Courtesy of the US Department of Health and Human Services and Grottola A, Forghieri F, Meacci M, et al. Severe pneumonia caused by *Legionella pneumophila* serogroup 11, Italy. *Emerg Infect Dis* 2012. doi 10.3201/eid1811.120216.

127 ***Pseudomonas aeruginosa*: Image A.** Blue-green pigment. This image is a derivative work, adapted from the following source, available under . Courtesy of Hansen. The image may have been modified by cropping, labeling, and/or captions. MedIQ Learning, LLC makes this image available under .

127 ***Pseudomonas aeruginosa*: Image B.** Ecthyma gangrenosum. This image is a derivative work, adapted from the following source, available under : Gencer S, Ozer S, Gul AE, et al. Ecthyma gangrenosum without bacteremia in a previously healthy man: a case report. *J Med Case Rep* 2008;2:14. doi 10.1186/1752-1947-2-14. The image may have been modified by cropping, labeling, and/or captions. All rights to this adaptation by MedIQ Learning, LLC are reserved.

128 ***Klebsiella*.** Courtesy of the US Department of Health and Human Services.

128 ***Campylobacter jejuni*.** Courtesy of the US Department of Health and Human Services.

129 ***Vibrio cholerae*.** This image is a derivative work, adapted from the following source, available under : Phetsouvanh R, Nakatsu M, Arakawa E, et al. Fatal bacteremia due to immotile *Vibrio cholerae* serogroup O21 in Vientiane, Laos—a case report. *Ann Clin Microbiol Antimicrob* 2008;7:10. doi 10.1186/1476-0711-7-10.

130 ***Helicobacter pylori*.** Courtesy of the US Department of Health and Human Services, Dr. Patricia Fields, and Dr. Collette Fitzgerald.

130 **Spirochetes.** Dark-field microscopic appearance. Courtesy of the US Department of Health and Human Services.

130 **Lyme disease: Image A.** *Ixodes* tick. Courtesy of the US Department of Health and Human Services and Dr. Michael L. Levin.

130 **Lyme disease: Image B.** Erythema migrans. Courtesy of the US Department of Health and Human Services and James Gathany.

131 **Syphilis: Image A.** Painless chancre in 1° syphilis. Courtesy of the US Department of Health and Human Services and M. Rein.

131 **Syphilis: Image B.** Treponeme on dark-field microscopy. Courtesy of the US Department of Health and Human Services and Renelle Woodall.

131 **Syphilis: Image D.** Rash on palms. This image is a derivative work, adapted from the following source, available under : Drahansky M, Dolezel M, Urbanek J, et al. Influence of skin diseases on fingerprint recognition. *J Biomed Biotechnol* 2012;626148. doi 10.1155/2012/626148.

131 **Syphilis: Image E.** Condyloma lata. Courtesy of the US Department of Health and Human Services and Susan Lindsley.

131 **Syphilis: Image F.** Gumma. This image is a derivative work, adapted from the following source, available under : Chakir K, Benchikhi H. Granulome centro-facial révélant une syphilis tertiaire. *Pan Afr Med J* 2013;15:82. doi 10.11604/pamj.2013.15.82.3011.

131 **Syphilis: Image G.** Congenital syphilis. Courtesy of the US Department of Health and Human Services and Dr. Norman Cole.

131 **Syphilis: Image H.** Hutchinson teeth. Courtesy of the US Department of Health and Human Services and Susan Lindsley.

132 ***Gardnerella vaginalis*.** Courtesy of the US Department of Health and Human Services and M. Rein.

133 **Rickettsial diseases and vector-borne illnesses: Image A.** Rash of Rocky Mountain spotted fever. Courtesy of the US Department of Health and Human Services.

133 **Rickettsial diseases and vector-borne illnesses: Image B.** *Ehrlichia morulae*. This image is a derivative work, adapted from the following source, available under : Dantas-Torres F. Canine vector-borne diseases in Brazil. *Parasit Vectors* 2008;1:25. doi 10.1186/1756-3305-1-25. The image may have been modified by cropping, labeling, and/or captions. All rights to this adaptation by MedIQ Learning, LLC are reserved.

133 **Rickettsial diseases and vector-borne illnesses: Image C.** *Anaplasma phagocytophilum* in neutrophil. Courtesy of the US Department of Health and Human Services and Dumler JS, Choi K, Garcia-Garcia JC, et al. Human granulocytic anaplasmosis. *Emerg Infect Dis* 2005. doi 10.3201/eid1112.050898.

134 ***Mycoplasma pneumoniae*.** This image is a derivative work, adapted from the following source, available under : Rottem S, Kosower NS, Kornspan JD. Contamination of tissue cultures by Mycoplasma. In: Ceccherini-Nelli L, ed: Biomedical tissue culture. doi 10.5772/51518.

135 **Systemic mycoses: Image A.** *Histoplasma*. Courtesy of the US Department of Health and Human Services and Dr. D.T. McClenan.

135 **Systemic mycoses: Image B.** *Blastomyces dermatitidis* undergoing broad-base budding. Courtesy of the US Department of Health and Human Services and Dr. Libero Ajello.

135 **Systemic mycoses: Image D.** "Captain's wheel" shape of *Paracoccidioides*. Courtesy of the US Department of Health and Human Services and Dr. Lucille K. Georg.

136 **Cutaneous mycoses: Image G.** Tinea versicolor. This image is a derivative work, adapted from the following source, available under . Courtesy of Sarah (Rosenau) Korf. The image may have been modified by cropping, labeling, and/or captions. MedIQ Learning, LLC makes this image available under .

137 **Opportunistic fungal infections: Image A.** Budding yeast of *Candida albicans*. This image is a derivative work, adapted from the following source, available under . Courtesy of Y. Tambe. The image may have been modified by cropping, labeling, and/or captions. MedIQ Learning, LLC makes this image available under .

137 **Opportunistic fungal infections: Image B.** Germ tubes of *Candida albicans*. This image is a derivative work, adapted from the following source, available under . Courtesy of Y. Tambe. The image may have been modified by cropping, labeling, and/or captions. MedIQ Learning, LLC makes this image available under .

137 **Opportunistic fungal infections: Image C.** Oral thrush. Courtesy of the US Department of Health and Human Services and Dr. Sol Silverman, Jr.

137 **Opportunistic fungal infections: Image E.** Conidiophores of *Aspergillus fumigatus*. Courtesy of the US Department of Health and Human Services.

137 **Opportunistic fungal infections: Image F.** *Cryptococcus neoformans*. Courtesy of the US Department of Health and Human Services and Dr. Leanor Haley.

137 **Opportunistic fungal infections: Image G.** *Cryptococcus neoformans* on mucicarmine stain. Courtesy of the US Department of Health and Human Services and Dr. Leanor Haley.

137 **Opportunistic fungal infections: Image H.** Mucor. Courtesy of the US Department of Health and Human Services and Dr. Libero Ajello.

138 ***Pneumocystis jirovecii*: Image A.** Interstitial opacities in lung. This image is a derivative work, adapted from the following source, available under : Chuang C, Zhanhong X, Yinyin G, et al. Unsuspected *Pneumocystis pneumonia* in an HIV-seronegative patient with untreated lung cancer: circa case report. *J Med Case Reports* 2007;1:15. doi 10.1186/1752-1947-1-115.

138 ***Pneumocystis jirovecii*: Image B.** Ground-glass opacities on CT. This image is a derivative work, adapted from the following source, available under : Oikonomou A and Prassopoulos P. Mimics in chest disease: interstitial opacities. *Insights Imaging* 2013; 4: 9-27. doi 0.1007/s13244-012-0207-7. The image may have been modified by cropping, labeling, and/or captions. All rights to this adaptation by MedIQ Learning, LLC are reserved.

139 **Protozoa—GI infections: Image A.** *Giardia lamblia* trophozoite. This image is a derivative work, adapted from the following source, available under : Lipoldová M. *Giardia* and Vilém Dušan Lambl. *PLoS Negl Trop Dis* 2014;8:e2686. doi 10.1371/journal.pntd.0002686.

139 **Protozoa—GI infections: Image B.** *Giardia lamblia* cyst. Courtesy of the US Department of Health and Human Services.

139 **Protozoa—GI infections: Image C.** *Entamoeba histolytica* trophozoites. Courtesy of the US Department of Health and Human Services.

139 **Protozoa—GI infections. Image D.** *Entamoeba histolytica* cyst. Courtesy of the US Department of Health and Human Services.

139 **Protozoa—GI infections: Image E.** *Cryptosporidium* oocysts. Courtesy of the US Department of Health and Human Services.

140 **Protozoa—CNS infections: Image A.** Cerebral toxoplasmosis. This image is a derivative work, adapted from the following source, available under : Adurthi S, Mahadevan A, Bantwal R, et al. Utility of molecular and serodiagnostic tools in cerebral toxoplasmosis with and without tuberculous meningitis in AIDS patients: a study from South India. *Ann Indian Acad Neurol* 2010;13:263-270. doi 10.4103/0972-2327.74197. The image may have been modified by cropping, labeling, and/or captions. All rights to this adaptation by MedIQ Learning, LLC are reserved.

140 **Protozoa—CNS infections: Image B.** *Toxoplasma gondii* tachyzoite. Courtesy of the US Department of Health and Human Services and Dr. L.L. Moore, Jr.

140 **Protozoa—CNS infections: Image C.** *Naegleria fowleri* amoebas. Courtesy of the US Department of Health and Human Services.

140 **Protozoa—CNS infections: Image D.** *Trypanosoma brucei gambiense*. Courtesy of the US Department of Health and Human Services and Dr. Mae Melvin.

141 **Protozoa—hematologic infections: Image A.** *Plasmodium* trophozoite ring form. Courtesy of the US Department of Health and Human Services.

141 **Protozoa—hematologic infections: Image B.** *Plasmodium* schizont containing merozoites. Courtesy of the US Department of Health and Human Services and Steven Glenn.

141 **Protozoa—hematologic infections: Image C.** *Babesia*. Courtesy of the US Department of Health and Human Services.

142 **Protozoa—others: Image A.** Trypanosoma cruzi. Courtesy of the US Department of Health and Human Services and Dr. Mae Melvin.

142 **Protozoa—others: Image B.** Leishmania donovani. Courtesy of the US Department of Health and Human Services and Dr. Francis W. Chandler. The image may have been modified by cropping, labeling, and/or captions. All rights to this adaptation by MedIQ Learning, LLC are reserved.

142 **Protozoa—Others: Image C.** *Trichomonas vaginalis*. Courtesy of the US Department of Health and Human Services.

143 **Nematodes (roundworms): Image A.** *Enterobius vermicularis* eggs. Courtesy of the US Department of Health and Human Services, B.G. Partin, and Dr. Moore.

143 **Nematodes (roundworms): Image B.** *Ascaris lumbricoides* egg. Courtesy of the US Department of Health and Human Services.

143 **Nematodes (roundworms): Image C.** Elephantiasis. Courtesy of the US Department of Health and Human Services.

144 **Cestodes (tapeworms): Image A.** *Taenia solium* scolex. This image is a derivative work, adapted from the following source, available under . Courtesy of Robert J. Galindo. The image may have been modified by cropping, labeling, and/or captions. MedIQ Learning, LLC makes this image available under .

144 Cestodes (tapeworms): Image B. Neurocysticercosis. This image is a derivative work, adapted from the following source, available under : Coyle CM, Tanowitz HB. Diagnosis and treatment of neurocysticercosis. *Interdiscip Perspect Infect Dis* 2009;2009:180742. doi 10.1155/2009/180742. The image may have been modified by cropping, labeling, and/or captions. All rights to this adaptation by MedIQ Learning, LLC are reserved.

144 Cestodes (tapeworms): Image C. *Echinococcus granulosus* scolex. Courtesy of the US Department of Health and Human Services and Dr. L.A.A. Moore, Jr.

144 Cestodes (tapeworms): Image D. Gross hyatid cyst of *Echinococcus granulosus*. Courtesy of the US Department of Health and Human Services and Dr. I. Kagan.

144 Cestodes (tapeworms): Image E. *Echinococcus granulosus* cyst in liver. This image is a derivative work, adapted from the following source, available under : Ma Z, Yang W, Yao Y, et al. The adventitia resection in treatment of liver hydatid cyst: a case report of a 15-year-old boy. *Case Rep Surg* 2014;2014:123149. doi 10.1155/2014/123149.

144 Trematodes (flukes): Image A. *Schistosoma mansoni* egg with lateral spine. Courtesy of the US Department of Health and Human Services.

144 Trematodes (flukes): Image B. *Schistosoma mansoni* egg with terminal spine. Courtesy of the US Department of Health and Human Services.

145 Ectoparasites: Image A. Scabies. Courtesy of the US Department of Health and Human Services and J. Pledger.

145 Ectoparasites: Image B. Lice. Courtesy of the US Department of Health and Human Services and Joe Miller.

149 Herpesviruses: Image A. Keratoconjunctivitis in HSV-1 infection. This image is a derivative work, adapted from the following source, available under : Yang HK, Han YK, Wee WR, et al. Bilateral herpetic keratitis presenting with unilateral neurotrophic keratitis in pemphigus foliaceus: a case report. *J Med Case Rep* 2011;5:328. doi 10.1186/1752-1947-5-328.

149 Herpesviruses: Image B. Herpes labialis. Courtesy of the US Department of Health and Human Services and Dr. Herrmann.

149 Herpesviruses: Image E. Shingles (varicella-zoster virus infection). This image is a derivative work, adapted from the following source, available under . Courtesy of Fisle. The image may have been modified by cropping, labeling, and/or captions. MedIQ Learning, LLC makes this image available under .

149 Herpesviruses: Image F. Lymphadenopathy in VZV infection. This image is a derivative work, adapted from the following source, available under . Courtesy of Dr. James Heilman. The image may have been modified by cropping, labeling, and/or captions. MedIQ Learning, LLC makes this image available under ..

149 Herpesviruses: Image G. Atypical lymphocytes in Epstein-Barr virus infection. This image is a derivative work, adapted from the following source, available under : Dr. Ed Uthman. The image may have been modified by cropping, labeling, and/or captions. All rights to this adaptation by MedIQ Learning, LLC are reserved.

149 Herpesviruses: Image I. Roseola. Courtesy of Emiliano Burzagli.

149 Herpesvirus: Image J. Kaposi sarcoma. Courtesy of the US Department of Health and Human Services.

150 HSV identification. Positive Tzanck smear in HSV-2 infection. This image is a derivative work, adapted from the following source, available under . Courtesy of Yale Rosen. The image may have been modified by cropping, labeling, and/or captions. MedIQ Learning, LLC makes this image available under .

152 Yellow fever virus. *Aedes aegypti* mosquito. Courtesy of the US Department of Health and Human Services and James Gathany.

152 Rotavirus. Courtesy of the US Department of Health and Human Services and Erskine Palmer.

153 Rubella virus. Rubella rash. Courtesy of the US Department of Health and Human Services.

154 Croup (acute laryngotracheobronchitis). Steeple sign. Reproduced, with permission, from Dr. Frank Gaillard and www.radiopaedia.org.

154 Measles (rubeola) virus: Image A. Koplik spots. Courtesy of the US Department of Health and Human Services. The image may have been modified by cropping, labeling, and/or captions. All rights to this adaptation by MedIQ Learning, LLC are reserved.

154 Measles (rubeola) virus: Image B. Rash of measles. Courtesy of the US Department of Health and Human Services.

155 Mumps virus. Swollen neck and parotid glands. Courtesy of the US Department of Health and Human Services.

155 Rabies virus: Image A. Transmission electron micrograph. Courtesy of the US Department of Health and Human Services Dr. Fred Murphy, and Sylvia Whitfield.

155 Rabies virus: Image B. Negri bodies. Courtesy of the US Department of Health and Human Services and Dr. Daniel P. Perl.

156 Ebola virus. Courtesy of the US Department of Health and Human Services and Cynthia Goldsmith.

161 Prions. Spongiform changes in Creutzfeld-Jacob disease. This image is a derivative work, adapted from the following source, available under . Courtesy of DRdoubleB. The image may have been modified by cropping, labeling, and/or captions. MedIQ Learning, LLC makes this image available under .

163 Osteomyelitis: Images A and B. This image is a derivative work, adapted from the following source, available under : Pandey V, Rao SP, Rao S, et al. *Burkholderia pseudomallei* musculoskeletal infections (melioidosis) in India. *Indian J Orthop* 2010;44:216-220. doi 10.4103/0019-5413.61829.

164 Common vaginal infections: Image C. *Candida* vulvovaginitis. Courtesy of Mikael Häggström.

165 ToRCHeS infections: Image A. "Blueberry muffin" rash. This image is a derivative work, adapted from the following source, available under : Benmiloud S, Elhaddou G, Belghiti ZA, et al. Blueberry muffin syndrome. *Pan Afr Med J* 2012;13:23. PMCID: PMC3527055.

165 ToRCHeS infections: Image B. Periventricular calcifications in congenital cytomegalovirus infection. This image is a derivative work, adapted from the following source, available under : Bonthius D, Perlman S. Congenital viral infections of the brain: lessons learned from lymphocytic choriomeningitis virus in the neonatal rat. *PLoS Pathog* 2007;3:e149. doi 10.1371/journal.ppat.0030149. The image may have been modified by cropping, labeling, and/or captions. All rights to this adaptation by MedIQ Learning, LLC are reserved.

166 Red rashes of childhood: Image C. Child with scarlet fever. This image is a derivative work, adapted from the following source, available under : www.badobadop.co.uk.

167 Pelvic inflammatory disease: Image A. Purulent cervical discharge. This image is a derivative work, adapted from the following source, available under . Courtesy of SOS-AIDS Amsterdam The image may have been modified by cropping, labeling, and/or captions. MedIQ Learning, LLC makes this image available under .

167 Pelvic inflammatory disease: Image B. Adhesions in Fitz-Hugh–Curtis syndrome. Courtesy of Hic et nunc.

173 Vancomycin. Red man syndrome. This image is a derivative work, adapted from the following source, available under : O'Meara P, Borici-Mazi R, Morton R, et al. DRESS with delayed onset acute interstitial nephritis and profound refractory eosinophilia secondary to vancomycin. *Allergy Asthma Clin Immunol* 2011;7:16. doi 10.1186/1710-1492-7-16.

Immunology

191 Sinusoids of spleen. Red and white pulp. This image is a derivative work, adapted from the following source, available under : Heinrichs S, Conover LF, Bueso-Ramos CE, et al. MYBL2 is a sub-haploinsufficient tumor suppressor gene in myeloid malignancy. *eLife* 2013;2:e00825. doi 10.7554/eLife.00825. The image may have been modified by cropping, labeling, and/or captions. All rights to this adaptation by MedIQ Learning, LLC are reserved.

209 Immunodeficiencies. Giant granules in granulocytes in Chédiak-Higashi syndrome. This image is a derivative work, adapted from the following source, available under : Bharti S, Bhatia P, Bansal D, et al. The accelerated phase of Chediak-Higashi syndrome: the importance of hematological evaluation. *Turk J Haematol* 2013;30:85-87. doi 10.4274/tjh.2012.0027. The image may have been modified by cropping, labeling, and/or captions. All rights to this adaptation by MedIQ Learning, LLC are reserved.

Pathology

217 Necrosis: Image A. Coagulative necrosis. Courtesy of the US Department of Health and Human Services and Dr. Steven Rosenberg.

217 Necrosis: Image B. Liquefactive necrosis. Courtesy of Daftblogger.

217 Necrosis: Image C. Caseous necrosis. This image is a derivative work, adapted from the following source, available under . Courtesy of Dr. Yale Rosen. The image may have been modified by cropping, labeling, and/or captions. MedIQ Learning, LLC makes this image available under .

217 Necrosis: Image D. Fat necrosis. This image is a derivative work, adapted from the following source, available under . Courtesy of Patho. The image may have been modified by cropping, labeling, and/or captions. MedIQ Learning, LLC makes this image available under .

217 Necrosis: Image E. Fibrinoid necrosis. This image is a derivative work, adapted from the following source, available under . Courtesy of Dr. Yale Rosen. The image may have been modified by cropping, labeling, and/or captions. MedIQ Learning, LLC makes this image available under .

217 Necrosis: Image F. Acral gangrene. Courtesy of the US Department of Health and Human Services and William Archibald.

219 Infarcts: red vs. pale: Image B. Pale infarct. Courtesy of the US Department of Health and Human Services and Armed Forces Institute of Pathology.

220 Chromatolysis. This image is a derivative work, adapted from the following source, available under . Courtesy of Nephron. The image may have been modified by cropping, labeling, and/or captions. MedIQ Learning, LLC makes this image available under .

220 Types of calcification: Image A. Dystrophic calcification. This image is a derivative work, adapted from the following source, available under : Chun J-S, Hong R, Kim J-A. Osseous metaplasia with mature bone formation of the thyroid gland: three case reports. *Oncol Lett* 2013;6:977-979. doi 10.3892/ol.2013.1475. The image may have been modified by cropping, labeling, and/or captions. All rights to this adaptation by MedIQ Learning, LLC are reserved.

220 Types of calcification: Image B. Metastatic calcification. This image is a derivative work, adapted from the following source, available under . Courtesy of Dr. Yale Rosen. The image may have been modified by cropping, labeling, and/or captions. MedIQ Learning, LLC makes this image available under .

222 Inhalational injury and sequelae. Images A (18 hours after inhalation injury) and B (11 days after injury). This image is a derivative work, adapted from the following source, available under : Bai C, Huang H, Yao X, et al. Application of flexible bronchoscopy in inhalation lung injury. *Diagn Pathol* 2013;8:174. doi 10.1186/1746-1596-8-174.

222 Scar formation: Image A. Hypertrophic scar. This image is a derivative work, adapted from the following source, available under : Baker R, Urso-Baiarda F, Linge C, et al. Cutaneous scarring: a clinical review. *Dermatol Res Pract* 2009;2009:625376. doi 10.1155/2009/625376.

222 Scar formation: Image B. Keloid scar. This image is a derivative work, adapted from the following source, available under . Courtesy of Dr. Andreas Settje. The image may have been modified by cropping, labeling, and/or captions. MedIQ Learning, LLC makes this image available under .

223 Granulomatous diseases. Granuloma. Courtesy of Sanjay Mukhopadhyay.

225 Amyloidosis: Image A. Amyloid deposits on Congo red stain. This image is a derivative work, adapted from the following source, available under [CC BY]: Dr. Ed Uthman.

225 Amyloidosis: Image B. Amyloid deposits on Congo red stain under polarized light. This image is a derivative work, adapted from the following source, available under [CC BY-SA]. Courtesy of Dr. Ed Uthman. The image may have been modified by cropping, labeling, and/or captions. MedIQ Learning, LLC makes this image available under [CC BY-SA].

225 Amyloidosis: Image C. Amyloidosis on H&E stain. This image is a derivative work, adapted from the following source, available under [CC BY]: Mendoza JM, Peev V, Ponce MA, et al. Amyloid A amyloidosis with subcutaneous drug abuse. *J Renal Inj Prev* 014;3:11-16. doi 10.12861/jrip.2014.06.

225 Lipofuscin. This image is a derivative work, adapted from the following source, available under [CC BY-SA]. Courtesy of Nephron. The image may have been modified by cropping, labeling, and/or captions. MedIQ Learning, LLC makes this image available under [CC BY-SA].

227 Neoplastic progression. Cervical tissue. This image is a derivative work, adapted from the following source, available under [CC BY]: Dr. Ed Uthman. The image may have been modified by cropping, labeling, and/or captions. All rights to this adaptation by MedIQ Learning, LLC are reserved.

232 Psammoma bodies. Psammoma body in papillary carcinoma. [Public Domain] Courtesy of the US Department of Health and Human Services and Armed Forces Institute of Pathology.

233 Common metastases: Image A. Breast cancer metastases to brain. This image is a derivative work, adapted from the following source, available under [CC BY-SA]. Courtesy of Jordi March i Nogué. The image may have been modified by cropping, labeling, and/or captions. MedIQ Learning, LLC makes this image available under [CC BY-SA].

233 Common metastases: Image B. Thyroid cancer metastasis to brain. [Public Domain] Courtesy of the US Department of Health and Human Services and Armed Forces Institute of Pathology.

233 Common metastases: Image C. Multiple metastases to liver. This image is a derivative work, adapted from the following source, available under [CC BY-SA]. Courtesy of Dr. James Heilman. The image may have been modified by cropping, labeling, and/or captions. MedIQ Learning, LLC makes this image available under [CC BY-SA].

233 Common metastases: Image D. Pancreatic metastases to liver. [Public Domain] Courtesy of J. Hayman.

233 Common metastases: Image E. Renal cell carcinoma metastases to bone. This image is a derivative work, adapted from the following source, available under [CC BY-SA]. Courtesy of Hellerhoff. The image may have been modified by cropping, labeling, and/or captions. MedIQ Learning, LLC makes this image available under [CC BY-SA].

233 Common metastases: Image F. Bone metastases. This image is a derivative work, adapted from the following source, available under [CC BY]: M. Emmanuel.

Cardiovascular

282 Congenital heart diseases: Image A. Tetralogy of Fallot. This image is a derivative work, adapted from the following source, available under [CC BY]: Rashid AKM: Heart diseases in Down syndrome. In: Dey S, ed: Down syndrome. doi 10.5772/46009. The image may have been modified by cropping, labeling, and/or captions. All rights to this adaptation by MedIQ Learning, LLC are reserved.

283 Congenital heart diseases: Image B. Atrial septal defect. This image is a derivative work, adapted from the following source, available under [CC BY]: Teo KSL, Disney PJ, Dundon BK, et al. Assessment of atrial septal defects in adults comparing cardiovascular magnetic resonance with transesophageal echocardiography. *J Cardiovasc Magnet Resonance* 2010;12:44. doi 10.1186/1532-429X-12-44. The image may have been modified by cropping, labeling, and/or captions. All rights to this adaptation by MedIQ Learning, LLC are reserved.

283 Congenital heart diseases: Image C. Patent ductus arteriosus. This image is a derivative work, adapted from the following source, available under [CC BY]: Henjes CR, Nolte I, Wesfaedt P. Multidetector-row computed tomography of thoracic aortic anomalies in dogs and cats: patent ductus arteriosus and vascular rings. *BMC Vet Res* 2011;7:57. doi 10.1186/1746-6148-7-57.

283 Congenital heart diseases: Image D. Clubbing of fingers. [Public Domain] Courtesy of Ann McGrath.

284 Hypertension: Image A. "String of beads" appearance in fibromuscular dysplasia. This image is a derivative work, adapted from the following source, available under [CC BY]: Plouin PF, Perdu J, LaBatide-Alanore A, et al. Fibromuscular dysplasia. *Orphanet J Rare Dis* 2007;7:28. doi 10.1186/1750-1172-2-28. The image may have been modified by cropping, labeling, and/or captions. All rights to this adaptation by MedIQ Learning, LLC are reserved.

284 Hypertension: Image B. Hypertensive nephropathy. This image is a derivative work, adapted from the following source, available under [CC BY-SA]. Courtesy of Nephron. The image may have been modified by cropping, labeling, and/or captions. MedIQ Learning, LLC makes this image available under [CC BY-SA].

285 Hyperlipidemia signs: Image C. Tendinous xanthoma. This image is a derivative work, adapted from the following source, available under [CC BY-SA]. Courtesy of Min.neel. The image may have been modified by cropping, labeling, and/or captions. MedIQ Learning, LLC makes this image available under [CC BY-SA].

285 Arteriosclerosis: Image A. Hyaline type. This image is a derivative work, adapted from the following source, available under [CC BY-SA]. Courtesy of Nephron. The image may have been modified by cropping, labeling, and/or captions. MedIQ Learning, LLC makes this image available under [CC BY-SA].

285 Arteriosclerosis: Image B. Hyperplastic type. This image is a derivative work, adapted from the following source, available under [CC BY-SA]. Courtesy of Paco Larosa. The image may have been modified by cropping, labeling, and/or captions. MedIQ Learning, LLC makes this image available under [CC BY-SA].

285 Arteriosclerosis: Image C. Monckeberg sclerosis (medial calcific sclerosis). This image is a derivative work, adapted from the following source, available under [CC BY]: C.E. Couri, G.A. da Silva, J.A. Martinez, F.A. Pereira, and F. de Paula. The image may have been modified by cropping, labeling, and/or captions. All rights to this adaptation by MedIQ Learning, LLC are reserved.

286 **Atherosclerosis: Image A.** Carotid plaque. This image is a derivative work, adapted from the following source, available under : Dr. Ed Uthman. The image may have been modified by cropping, labeling, and/or captions. All rights to this adaptation by MedIQ Learning, LLC are reserved.

287 **Aortic dissection.** This image is a derivative work, adapted from the following source, available under : Apostolakis EE, Baikoussis NG, Katsanos K, et al. Postoperative peri-axillary seroma following axillary artery cannulation for surgical treatment of acute type A aortic dissection: case report. *J Cardiothor Surg* 2010;5:43. doi 0.1186/1749-8090-5-43. The image may have been modified by cropping, labeling, and/or captions. All rights to this adaptation by MedIQ Learning, LLC are reserved.

290 **Myocardial infarction complications: Image A.** Papillary muscle rupture. This image is a derivative work, adapted from the following source, available under : Routy B, Huynh T, Fraser R, et al. Vascular endothelial cell function in catastrophic antiphospholipid syndrome: a case report and review of the literature. *Case Rep Hematol* 2013;2013:710365. doi 10.1155/2013/710365.

290 **Myocardial infarction complications: Image B.**Drawing of pseudoaneurysm. This image is a derivative work, adapted from the following source, available under : Patrick J. Lynch and Dr. C. Carl Jaffe.

290 **Myocardial infarction complications: Image C.** Free wall rupture of left ventricle. This image is a derivative work, adapted from the following source, available under : Zacarias ML, da Trindade H, Tsutsu J, et al. Left ventricular free wall impeding rupture in post-myocardial infarction period diagnosed by myocardial contrast echocardiography: case report. *Cardiovasc Ultrasound* 2006;4:7. doi 10.1186/1476-7120-4-7.

291 **Cardiomyopathies: Image A.** Dilated cardiomyopathy. This image is a derivative work, adapted from the following source, available under : Gho JMIH, van Es R, Stathonikos N, et al. High resolution systematic digital histological quantification of cardiac fibrosis and adipose tissue in phospholamban p.Arg14del mutation associated cardiomyopathy. *PLoS One* 2014;9:e94820. doi 10.1371/journal.pone.0094820.

292 **Heart failure.** Pedal edema. This image is a derivative work, adapted from the following source, available under . Courtesy of Dr. James Heilman. The image may have been modified by cropping, labeling, and/or captions. MedIQ Learning, LLC makes this image available under .

293 **Bacterial endocarditis: Image A.** Janeway lesions on sole. This image is a derivative work, adapted from the following source, available under : DeNanneke.

294 **Rheumatic fever.** Aschoff body and Anitschkow cells. This image is a derivative work, adapted from the following source, available under : Dr. Ed Uthman. The image may have been modified by cropping, labeling, and/or captions. All rights to this adaptation by MedIQ Learning, LLC are reserved.

294 **Acute pericarditis.** This image is a derivative work, adapted from the following source, available under : Bogaert J, Francone M. Cardiovascular magnetic resonance in pericardial diseases. *J Cardiovasc Magn Reson* 2009;11:14. doi 10.1186/1532-429X-11-14. The image may have been modified by cropping, labeling, and/or captions. All rights to this adaptation by MedIQ Learning, LLC are reserved.

294 **Cardiac tamponade.** This image is a derivative work, adapted from the following source, available under : Lin E, Boire A, Hemmige V, et al. Cardiac tamponade mimicking tuberculous pericarditis as the initial presentation of chronic lymphocytic leukemia in a 58-year-old woman: a case report. *J Med Case Rep* 2010;4:246. doi 10.1186/1752-1947-4-246. The image may have been modified by cropping, labeling, and/or captions. All rights to this adaptation by MedIQ Learning, LLC are reserved.

297 **Vasculitides: Image A.** Temporal arteritis histology. This image is a derivative work, adapted from the following source, available under . Courtesy of Marvin. The image may have been modified by cropping, labeling, and/or captions. MedIQ Learning, LLC makes this image available under .

297 **Vasculitides: Image B.** Angiogram in patient with Takayasu arteritis. Courtesy of the US Department of Health and Human Services and Justin Ly.

297 **Vasculitides: Image C.** Microaneurysms in polyarteritis nodosa. Reproduced, with permission, from Dr. Frank Gaillard and www.radiopaedia.org.

297 **Vasculitides: Image D.** Strawberry tongue in patient with Kawasaki disease. This image is a derivative work, adapted from the following source, available under : Natr.

297 **Vasculitides: Image E.** Coronary artery aneurysm in Kawasaki disease. This image is a derivative work, adapted from the following source, available under : Wikimedia Commons. The image may have been modified by cropping, labeling, and/or captions. All rights to this adaptation by MedIQ Learning, LLC are reserved.

297 **Vasculitides: Image F.** Gangrene as a consequence of Buerger disease. This image is a derivative work, adapted from the following source, available under : Afsjarfard A, Mozaffar M, Malekpour F, et al. The wound healing effects of iloprost in patients with Buerger's disease: claudication and prevention of major amputations. *Iran Red Crescent Med J* 2011;13:420-423. PMCID PMC3371931.

297 **Vasculitides: Image G.** Granulomatosis with polyangiitis (formerly Wegener) and PR3-ANCA/c-ANCA. Courtesy of M.A. Little.

297 **Vasculitides: Image H.** Microscopic polyangiitis and MPO-ANCA/p-ANCA. Courtesy of the US Department of Health and Human Services and M.A. Little.

297 **Vasculitides: Image I.** Churg-Strauss syndrome histology. This image is a derivative work, adapted from the following source, available under . Courtesy of Nephron. The image may have been modified by cropping, labeling, and/or captions. MedIQ Learning, LLC makes this image available under .

297 **Vasculitides: Image J.** Henoch-Schönlein purpura. Courtesy of Okwikikim.

Endocrine

306 **Thyroid development.** Thyroglossal duct cyst. This image is a derivative work, adapted from the following source, available under : Karlatti PD, Nagvekar S, Lekshmi TP, Kothari As. Migratory intralaryngeal thyroglossal duct cyst. *Indian J Radiol Imaging* 2010;20: 115-117. doi 10.4103/0971-3026.63053. The image may have been modified by cropping, labeling, and/or captions. All rights to this adaptation by MedIQ Learning, LLC are reserved.

306 Adrenal cortex and medulla. Courtesy of Wikimedia Commons. The image may have been modified by cropping, labeling, and/or captions. All rights to this adaptation by MedIQ Learning, LLC are reserved.

318 Adrenal insufficiency. Mucosal hyperpigmentation in 1° adrenal insufficiency. Courtesy of FlatOut. The image may have been modified by cropping, labeling, and/or captions. All rights to this adaptation by MedIQ Learning, LLC are reserved.

319 Neuroblastoma: Image A. CT scan of abdomen. This image is a derivative work, adapted from the following source, available under : Koumarianou A, Oikonomopoulou P, Baka M, et al. Implications of the incidental finding of a MYCN amplified adrenal tumor: a case report and update of a pediatric disease diagnosed in adults. *Case Rep Oncol Med* 2013;2013:393128. doi 10.1155/2013/393128. The image may have been modified by cropping, labeling, and/or captions. All rights to this adaptation by MedIQ Learning, LLC arc reserved.

319 Neuroblastoma. Image B: Homer-Wright rosettes. Image courtesy of Dr. Kristine Krafts.

320 Pheochromocytoma. This image is a derivative work, adapted from the following source, available under : Dr. Michael Feldman.

322 Hypothyroidism: Image B. Before and after treatment of congenital hypothyroidism. Courtesy of the US Department of Health and Human Services.

322 Hypothyroidism: Image C. Congenital hypothyroidism. This image is a derivative work, adapted from the following source, available under : Sadasiv Swain. The image may have been modified by cropping, labeling, and/or captions. All rights to this adaptation by MedIQ Learning, LLC are reserved.

322 Hypothyroidism: Image D. Reidel thyroiditis histology. Image courtesy of Dr. Kristine Krafts.

323 Hyperthyroidism: Image B. Scalloped colloid. Image courtesy of Dr. Kristine Krafts.

324 Thyroid adenoma. Image courtesy of Dr. Kristine Krafts.

326 Hyperparathyroidism. Multiple lytic lesions. This image is a derivative work, adapted from the following source, available under : Khaoula BA, Kaouther BA, Ines C, et al. An unusual presentation of primary hyperparathyroidism: pathological fracture. *Case Rep Orthop* 2011;2011:521578. doi 10.1155/2011/521578. The image may have been modified by cropping, labeling, and/or captions. All rights to this adaptation by MedIQ Learning, LLC are reserved.

326 Pituitary adenoma. Reproduced, with permission, from Dr. Frank Gaillard and www.radiopaedia.org.

332 Carcinoid syndrome. Carcinoid tumor histology. Courtesy of the US Department of Health and Human Services and Armed Forces Institute of Pathology.

Gastrointestinal

338 Intestinal atresia. "Double bubble" sign of duodenal atresia. This image is a derivative work, adapted from the following source, available under : Alorainy IA, Barlas NB, Al-Boukai AA. Pictorial essay: infants of diabetic mothers. *Indian J Radiol Imaging* 2010;20:174-181. doi 0.4103/0971-3026.69349.

339 Pancreas and spleen embryology. Annular pancreas. This image is a derivative work, adapted from the following source, available under : Mahdi B, Selim S, Hassen T, et al. A rare cause of proximal intestinal obstruction in adults—annular pancreas: a case report. *Pan Afr Med J* 2011;10:56. PMCID PMC3290886. The image may have been modified by cropping, labeling, and/or captions. All rights to this adaptation by MedIQ Learning, LLC are reserved.

346 Liver tissue architecture. Kupffer cells. This image is a derivative work, adapted from the following source, available under . Courtesy of Nephron. The image may have been modified by cropping, labeling, and/or captions. MedIQ Learning, LLC makes this image available under .

347 Biliary structures. Gallstones. This image is a derivative work, adapted from the following source, available under . Courtesy of J. Guntau. The image may have been modified by cropping, labeling, and/or captions. MedIQ Learning, LLC makes this image available under .

349 Hernias: Image A. Congenital diaphragmatic hernia. This image is a derivative work, adapted from the following source, available under : Tovar J. Congenital diaphragmatic hernia. *Orphanet J Rare Dis* 2012;7:1. doi 10.1186/1750-1172-7-1.

352 Peyer patches. This image is a derivative work, adapted from the following source, available under . Courtesy of Plainpaper. The image may have been modified by cropping, labeling, and/or captions. MedIQ Learning, LLC makes this image available under .

353 Salivary gland tumors: Image A. Pleomorphic adenoma histology. This image is a derivative work, adapted from the following source, available under . Courtesy of Wikimedia Commons. The image may have been modified by cropping, labeling, and/or captions. MedIQ Learning, LLC makes this image available under .

354 Achalasia. This image is a derivative work, adapted from the following source, available under : Farnoosh Farrokhi and Michael F. Vaezi. The image may have been modified by cropping, labeling, and/or captions. All rights to this adaptation by MedIQ Learning, LLC are reserved.

354 Esophageal pathologies: Image A. Pneumomediastinum in Boerhaave syndrome. This image is a derivative work, adapted from the following source, available under . Courtesy of Wikimedia Commons. The image may have been modified by cropping, labeling, and/or captions. MedIQ Learning, LLC makes this image available under .

354 Esophageal pathologies: Image B. Esophageal varices on endoscopy. This image is a derivative work, adapted from the following source, available under : Costaguta A, Alvarez F. Etiology and management of hemorrhagic complications of portal hypertension in children. *Int J Hepatol* 2012;2012:879163. doi 10.1155/2012/879163.

354 Esophageal pathologies: Image C. Esophageal varices on CT. This image is a derivative work, adapted from the following source, available under . Courtesy of Hellerhoff. The image may have been modified by cropping, labeling, and/or captions. MedIQ Learning, LLC makes this image available under .

355 **Barrett esophagus: Image A.** Endoscopy. This image is a derivative work, adapted from the following source, available under: Coda S, Thillainayagam AV. State of the art in advanced endoscopic imaging for the detection and evaluation of dysplasia and early cancer of the gastrointestinal tract. *Clin Exp Gastroenterol* 2014;7:133-150. doi 10.2147/CEG.S58157. The image may have been modified by cropping, labeling, and/or captions. All rights to this adaptation by MedIQ Learning, LLC are reserved.

355 **Barrett esophagus: Image B.** Goblet cells. This image is a derivative work, adapted from the following source, available under. Courtesy of Nephron. The image may have been modified by cropping, labeling, and/or captions. MedIQ Learning, LLC makes this image available under.

356 **Ménétriere disease.** This image is a derivative work, adapted from the following source, available under. Courtesy of Hellerhoff. The image may have been modified by cropping, labeling, and/or captions. MedIQ Learning, LLC makes this image available under.

357 **Ulcer complications.** Reproduced, with permission, from Dr. Frank Gaillard and www.radiopaedia.org.

358 **Malabsorption syndromes: Image B.** Whipple disease. This image is a derivative work, adapted from the following source, available under. Courtesy of Nephron. The image may have been modified by cropping, labeling, and/or captions. MedIQ Learning, LLC makes this image available under.

359 **Inflammatory bowel diseases: Image A.** "String sign" on barium swallow in Crohn disease. This image is a derivative work, adapted from the following source, available under: Al-Mofarreh MA, Al Mofleh IA, Al-Teimi IN, et al. Crohn's disease in a Saudi outpatient population: is it still rare? *Saudi J Gastroenterol* 2009;15:111-116. doi 10.4103/1319-3767.45357. The image may have been modified by cropping, labeling, and/or captions. All rights to this adaptation by MedIQ Learning, LLC are reserved.

359 **Inflammatory bowel diseases: Images B** (normal mucosa) **and C** (punched-out ulcers) **in ulcerative colitis.** This image is a derivative work, adapted from the following source, available under: Ishikawa D, Ando T, Watanabe O, et al. Images of colonic real-time tissue sonoelastography correlate with those of colonoscopy and may predict response to therapy in patients with ulcerative colitis. *BMC Gastroenterol* 2011;11:29. doi 10.1186/1471-230X-11-29.

360 **Appendicitis.** Fecalith. This image is a derivative work, adapted from the following source, available under. Courtesy of Dr. James Heilman. The image may have been modified by cropping, labeling, and/or captions. MedIQ Learning, LLC makes this image available under.

360 **Diverticula of the gastrointestinal tract: Image B.** Diverticulitis. This image is a derivative work, adapted from the following source, available under. Courtesy of Dr. James Heilman. The image may have been modified by cropping, labeling, and/or captions. MedIQ Learning, LLC makes this image available under.

361 **Zenker diverticulum.** This image is a derivative work, adapted from the following source, available under: Bernd Brägelmann.

362 **Volvulus.** This image is a derivative work, adapted from the following source, available under. Courtesy of herecomesdoc. The image may have been modified by cropping, labeling, and/or captions. MedIQ Learning, LLC makes this image available under.

362 **Intussusception.** This image is a derivative work, adapted from the following source, available under: Vasiliadis K, Kogopoulos E, Katsamakas M, et al. Ileoileal intussusception induced by a gastrointestinal stromal tumor. *World J Surg Oncol* 2008:6:133. doi 10.1186/1477-7819-6-133. The image may have been modified by cropping, labeling, and/or captions. All rights to this adaptation by MedIQ Learning, LLC are reserved.

363 **Colonic polyps: Image A.** Colonic polyps and cancer. This image is a derivative work, adapted from the following source, available under: Emannuelm.

364 **Colorectal cancer: Image A.** Polyp on endoscopy. This image is a derivative work, adapted from the following source, available under: Chen C-W, Hsiao K-H, Yue C-T, et al. Invasive adenocarcinoma arising from a mixed hyperplastic/adenomatous polyp and synchronous transverse colon cancer. *World J Surg Oncol* 2013;11:214. doi 10.1186/1477-7819-11-214.

365 **Cirrhosis and portal hypertension.** Splenomegaly and liver nodularity in cirrhosis. This image is a derivative work, adapted from the following source, available under. Courtesy of Inversitus. The image may have been modified by cropping, labeling, and/or captions. MedIQ Learning, LLC makes this image available under.

367 **Alcoholic liver disease: Image B.** Mallory bodies. This image is a derivative work, adapted from the following source, available under. Courtesy of Nephron. The image may have been modified by cropping, labeling, and/or captions. MedIQ Learning, LLC makes this image available under.

367 **Alcoholic liver disease: Image C.** Sclerosis in alcoholic cirrhosis. This image is a derivative work, adapted from the following source, available under. Courtesy of Nephron. The image may have been modified by cropping, labeling, and/or captions. MedIQ Learning, LLC makes this image available under.

367 **Non-alcoholic fatty liver disease.** This image is a derivative work, adapted from the following source, available under: El-Karaksy HM, El-Koofy NM, Anwar GM, et al. Predictors of non-alcoholic fatty liver disease in obese and overweight Egyptian children: single center study. *Saudi J Gastroenterol* 2011;17:40-46. doi 10.4103/1319-3767.74476.

368 **Hepatocellular carcinoma/hepatoma: Image A.** Gross specimen. Reproduced, with permission, from Jean-Christophe Fournet and Humpath.

369 **Other liver tumors.** Cavernous liver hemangioma. This image is a derivative work, adapted from the following source, available under. Courtesy of Nephron. The image may have been modified by cropping, labeling, and/or captions. MedIQ Learning, LLC makes this image available under.

369 **α_1-antitrypsin deficiency.** Liver histology. This image is a derivative work, adapted from the following source, available under. Courtesy of Dr. Jerad M. Gardner. The image may have been modified by cropping, labeling, and/or captions. MedIQ Learning, LLC makes this image available under.

369 **Jaundice.** Yellow sclera. Courtesy of the US Department of Health and Human Services and Dr. Thomas F. Sellers.

371 **Hemochromatosis.** Hemosiderin deposits. This image is a derivative work, adapted from the following source, available under : Mathew J, Leong MY, Morley N, et al. A liver fibrosis cocktail? Psoriasis, methotrexate and genetic hemochromatosis. *BMC Dermatol* 2005;5:12. doi 10.1186/1471-5945-5-12.

372 **Gallstones (cholelithiasis): Image. A** Gross specimen. This image is a derivative work, adapted from the following source, available under : M. Emmanuel.

372 **Gallstones (cholelithiasis): Image B.** Ultrasound. This image is a derivative work, adapted from the following source, available under . Courtesy of Dr. James Heilman. The image may have been modified by cropping, labeling, and/or captions. MedIQ Learning, LLC makes this image available under .

372 **Porcelain gallbladder.** This image is a derivative work, adapted from the following source, available under : Fred H, van Dijk H. Images of memorable cases: case 19. Connexions website. December 4, 2008. Available at: http://cnx.org/content/m14939/1.3/. The image may have been modified by cropping, labeling, and/or captions. All rights to this adaptation by MedIQ Learning, LLC are reserved.

373 **Acute pancreatitis: Image A.** Acute exudative pancreatitis. This image is a derivative work, adapted from the following source, available under . Courtesy of Hellerhoff. The image may have been modified by cropping, labeling, and/or captions. MedIQ Learning, LLC makes this image available under .

373 **Acute pancreatitis: Image B.** Pancreatic pseudocyst. This image is a derivative work, adapted from the following source, available under . Courtesy of Thomas Zimmerman. The image may have been modified by cropping, labeling, and/or captions. MedIQ Learning, LLC makes this image available under .

373 **Chronic pancreatitis.** This image is a derivative work, adapted from the following source, available under . Courtesy of Hellerhoff. The image may have been modified by cropping, labeling, and/or captions. MedIQ Learning, LLC makes this image available under .

373 **Pancreatic adenocarcinoma: Image A.** Histology. This image is a derivative work, adapted from the following source, available under . Courtesy of KGH. The image may have been modified by cropping, labeling, and/or captions. MedIQ Learning, LLC makes this image available under .

373 **Pancreatic adenocarcinoma: Image B.** CT scan. Courtesy of MBq. The image may have been modified by cropping, labeling, and/or captions. All rights to this adaptation by MedIQ Learning, LLC are reserved.

Hematology and Oncology

378 **Erythrocyte.** Courtesy of the US Department of Health and Human Services and Drs. Noguchi, Rodgers, and Schechter.

378 **Thrombocyte (platelet).** This image is a derivative work, adapted from the following source, available under . Courtesy of Dr. Ed Uthman. The image may have been modified by cropping, labeling, and/or captions. MedIQ Learning, LLC makes this image available under .

378 **Neutrophil.** Courtesy of the US Department of Health and Human Services B. Lennert.

379 **Monocyte.** This image is a derivative work, adapted from the following source, available under . Courtesy of Dr. Graham Beards. The image may have been modified by cropping, labeling, and/or captions. MedIQ Learning, LLC makes this image available under .

379 **Macrophage.** Courtesy of the US Department of Health and Human Services and Dr. Francis W. Chandler. The image may have been modified by cropping, labeling, and/or captions. All rights to this adaptation by MedIQ Learning, LLC are reserved.

379 **Eosinophil.** This image is a derivative work, adapted from the following source, available under : Dr. Ed Uthman.

379 **Basophil.** This image is a derivative work, adapted from the following source, available under . Courtesy of Dr. Erhabor Osaro. The image may have been modified by cropping, labeling, and/or captions. MedIQ Learning, LLC makes this image available under .

379 **Mast cell.** Courtesy of Wikimedia Commons.

380 **Dendritic cell.** This image is a derivative work, adapted from the following source, available under : Cheng J-H, Lee S-Y, Lien Y-Y, et al. Immunomodulating activity of *Nymphaea rubra* roxb. extracts: activation of rat dendritic cells and improvement of the TH1 immune response. *Int J Mol Sci* 2012;13:10722-10735. doi 10.3390/ijms130910722.

380 **Lymphocyte.** This image is a derivative work, adapted from the following source, available under . Courtesy of Wikimedia Commons. The image may have been modified by cropping, labeling, and/or captions. MedIQ Learning, LLC makes this image available under .

381 **Plasma cell.** Courtesy of the US Department of Health and Human Services and Dr. Francis W. Chandler. The image may have been modified by cropping, labeling, and/or captions. All rights to this adaptation by MedIQ Learning, LLC are reserved.

386 **Pathologic RBC forms: Image A.** Acanthocyte ("spur cell"). Image courtesy of Dr. Kristine Krafts.

386 **Pathologic RBC forms: Image B.** Basophilic stippling. This image is a derivative work, adapted from the following source, available under : van Dijk HA, Fred HL. Images of memorable cases: case 81. Connexions website. December 3, 2008. Available at http://cnx.org/contents/3196bf3e-1e1e-4c4d-a1ac-d4fc9ab65443@4@4.

386 **Pathologic RBC forms: Image C.** Dacrocyte ("teardrop cell"). Image courtesy of Dr. Kristine Krafts.

386 **Pathologic RBC forms: Image D.** Degmacyte ("bite cell"). Image courtesy of Dr. Kristine Krafts.

386 **Pathologic RBC forms: Image E.** Echinocyte ("burr cell"). Image courtesy of Dr. Kristine Krafts.

386 **Pathologic RBC forms: Image F.** Elliptocyte. Image courtesy of Dr. Kristine Krafts.

386 **Pathologic RBC forms: Image G.** Macro-ovalocyte. Image courtesy of Dr. Kristine Krafts.

387 **Pathologic RBC forms: Image H.** Ringed sideroblast. This image is a derivative work, adapted from the following source, available under . Courtesy of Paulo Henrique Orlandi Mourao. The image may have been modified by cropping, labeling, and/or captions. MedIQ Learning, LLC makes this image available under .

387 Pathologic RBC forms: Image I. Schistocyte. Image courtesy of Dr. Kristine Krafts.

387 Pathologic RBC forms: Image J. Sickle cell. Courtesy of the US Department of Health and Human Services and the Sickle Cell Foundation of Georgia, Jackie George, and Beverly Sinclair.

387 Pathologic RBC forms: Image K. Spherocyte. Image courtesy of Dr. Kristine Krafts.

387 Pathologic RBC forms: Image L. Target cell. Image courtesy of Dr. Kristine Krafts.

387 Other RBC pathologies: Image A. Heinz bodies. Image courtesy of Dr. Kristine Krafts.

387 Other RBC pathologies: Image B. Howell-Jolly body. This image is a derivative work, adapted from the following source, available under . Courtesy of Paulo Henrique Orlandi Mourao and Mikael Häggström. The image may have been modified by cropping, labeling, and/or captions. MedIQ Learning, LLC makes this image available under .

389 Microcytic (MCV < 80 fL), hypochromic anemia: Image C. β-thalassemia. Image courtesy of Dr. Kristine Krafts.

389 Microcytic (MCV < 80 fL), hypochromic anemia: Image D. Lead lines in lead poisoning. Reproduced, with permission, from Dr. Frank Gaillard and www.radiopaedia.org.

389 Microcytic (MCV < 80 fL), hypochromic anemia: Image E. Sideroblastic anemia. This image is a derivative work, adapted from the following source, available under . Courtesy of Paulo Henrique Orlandi Moura. The image may have been modified by cropping, labeling, and/or captions. MedIQ Learning, LLC makes this image available under .

390 Macrocytic (MCV > 100 fL) anemia. Megaloblastic anemia. This image is a derivative work, adapted from the following source, available under : Dr. Ed Uthman.

392 Intrinsic hemolytic anemia: Image B. Dactylitis. This image is a derivative work, adapted from the following source, available under : Pedram M, Jaseb K, Haghi S, et al. First presentation of sickle cell anemia in a 3.5-year-old girl: a case report. *Iran Red Crescent Med J* 2012;14:184-185.

393 Extrinsic hemolytic anemia: Image A. Autoimmune hemolytic anemia. Image courtesy of Dr. Kristine Krafts.

395 Heme synthesis, porphyrias, and lead poisoning. Basophilic stippling in lead poisoning. This image is a derivative work, adapted from the following source, available under : van Dijk HA, Fred HL. Images of memorable cases: case 81. Connexions website. December 3, 2008. Available at http://cnx.org/contents/3196bf3e-1e1e-4c4d-a1ac-d4fc9ab65443@4@4.

396 Coagulation disorders. Hemarthrosis. This image is a derivative work, adapted from the following source, available under : Rodriguez-Merchan EC. Prevention of the musculoskeletal complications of hemophilia. *Adv Prev Med* 2012;2012:201271. doi 10.1155/2012/201271.

400 Non-Hodgkin lymphoma: Image C. Mycosis fungoides. This image is a derivative work, adapted from the following source, available under : Chaudhary S, Bansal C, Ranga U, et al. Erythrodermic mycosis fungoides with hypereosinophilic syndrome: a rare presentation. *Ecancermedicalscience* 2013;7:337. doi 10.3332/ecancer.2013.337.

401 Multiple myeloma: Image B. RBC rouleaux formation. Image courtesy of Dr. Kristine Krafts.

401 Multiple myeloma: Image C. Plasma cells. This image is a derivative work, adapted from the following source, available under : Sharma A, Kaushal M, Chaturvedi NK, et al. Cytodiagnosis of multiple myeloma presenting as orbital involvement: a case report. *Cytojournal* 2006;3:19. doi 10.1186/1742-6413-3-19.

402 Leukemias: Image C. Hairy cell leukemia. Image courtesy of Dr. Kristine Krafts.

402 Leukemias: Image E. Chronic myelogenous leukemia. Image courtesy of Dr. Kristine Krafts.

403 Langerhans cell histiocytosis: Image A. Lytic bone lesion. This image is a derivative work, adapted from the following source, available under : Dehkordi NR, Rajabi P, Naimi A, et al. Langerhans cell histiocytosis following Hodgkin lymphoma: a case report from Iran. *J Res Med Sci* 2010;15:58-61. PMCID PMC3082786.

403 Langerhans cell histiocytosis: Image B. Birbeck granules. This image is a derivative work, adapted from the following source, available under . Courtesy of Dr. Yale Rosen. The image may have been modified by cropping, labeling, and/or captions. MedIQ Learning, LLC makes this image available under .

404 Chronic myeloproliferative disorders: Image A. Erythromelalgia in polycythemia vera. This image is a derivative work, adapted from the following source, available under : Fred H, van Dijk H. Images of memorable cases: case 151. Connexions website. December 4, 2008. Available at http://cnx.org/content/m14932/1.3/.

404 Chronic myeloproliferative disorders: Image B. Essential thrombocytosis with enlarged megakaryocytes. Image courtesy of Dr. Kristine Krafts.

404 Chronic myeloproliferative disorders: Image C. Myelofibrosis. This image is a derivative work, adapted from the following source, available under : Dr. Ed Uthman.

404 Chronic myeloproliferative disorders: Image D. Dacrocyte ("teardrop cell"). Image courtesy of Dr. Kristine Krafts.

406 Warfarin. Toxic effect. This image is a derivative work, adapted from the following source, available under : Fred H, van Dijk H. Images of memorable cases: cases 84 and 85. Connexions website. December 2, 2008. Available at http://cnx.org/content/m14932/1.3/.

Musculoskeletal, Skin, and Connective Tissue

417 Common knee conditions: Image A. ACL tear. This image is a derivative work, adapted from the following source, available under : Chang MJ, Chang CB, Choi J-Y, et al. Can magnetic resonance imaging findings predict the degree of knee joint laxity in patients undergoing anterior cruciate ligament reconstruction? *BMC Musculoskelet Disord* 2014;15:214. doi 10.1186/1471-2474-15-214. The image may have been modified by cropping, labeling, and/or captions. All rights to this adaptation by MedIQ Learning, LLC are reserved.

417 **Common knee conditions: Images B** (prepatellar bursitis) and **C** (Baker cyst). This image is a derivative work, adapted from the following source, available under : Hirji Z, Hunhun JS, Choudur HN. Imaging of the bursae. *J Clin Imaging Sci* 2011;1:22. doi 10.4103/2156-7514.80374. The image may have been modified by cropping, labeling, and/or captions. All rights to this adaptation by MedIQ Learning, LLC are reserved.

417 **Rotator cuff muscles.** Glenohumeral instability. This image is a derivative work, adapted from the following source, available under : Koike Y, Sano H, Imamura I, et al. Changes with time in skin temperature of the shoulders in healthy controls and a patient with shoulder-hand syndrome. *Ups J Med Sci* 2010;115:260-265. doi 10.3109/03009734.2010.503354. The image may have been modified by cropping, labeling, and/or captions. All rights to this adaptation by MedIQ Learning, LLC are reserved.

424 **Muscle conduction to contraction.** Human skeletal muscle. Courtesy of Louisa Howard. The image may have been modified by cropping, labeling, and/or captions. All rights to this adaptation by MedIQ Learning, LLC are reserved.

426 **Osteoporosis.** Vertebral compression fractures of spine. This image is a derivative work, adapted from the following source, available under : Sexton C, Crichlow C. Multiple myeloma: imaging evaluation of skeletal disease. *J Community Hosp Intern Med Perspect* 2013;3. doi 10.3402/jchimp.v3i2.21419.

426 **Osteopetrosis (marble bone disease).** This image is a derivative work, adapted from the following source, available under : Kant P, Sharda N, Bhowate RR. Clinical and radiological findings of autosomal dominant osteopetrosis type II: a case report. *Case Rep Dent* 2013;2013:707343. doi 10.1155/2013/707343.

427 **Osteomalacia/rickets.** This image is a derivative work, adapted from the following source, available under : Linglart A, Biosse-Duplan M, Briot K, et al. Therapeutic management of hypophosphatemic rickets from infancy to adulthood. *Endocr Connect* 2014;3:R13-R30. doi 10.1530/EC-13-0103.

427 **Paget disease of bone (osteitis deformans).** Thickened calvarium. This image is a derivative work, adapted from the following source, available under : Dawes L. Paget's disease. [Radiology Picture of the Day Website]. Published June 21, 2007. Available at http://www.radpod.org/2007/06/21/pagets-disease/.

427 **Osteonecrosis (avascular necrosis).** Bilateral necrosis of femoral head. This image is a derivative work, adapted from the following source, available under : Ding H, Chen S-B, Lin S, et al. The effect of postoperative corticosteroid administration on free vascularized fibular grafting for treating osteonecrosis of the femoral head. *Sci World J* 2013;708014. doi 10.1155/2013/708014. The image may have been modified by cropping, labeling, and/or captions. All rights to this adaptation by MedIQ Learning, LLC are reserved.

429 **Primary bone tumors: Image A.** Osteochondroma. This image is a derivative work, adapted from the following source, available under . Courtesy of Lucien Monfils. The image may have been modified by cropping, labeling, and/or captions. MedIQ Learning, LLC makes this image available under .

429 **Primary bone tumors: Image B.** Giant cell tumor. Reproduced, with permission, from Dr. Frank Gaillard and www.radiopaedia.org.

429 **Primary bone tumors: Image C.** Osteosarcoma. Reproduced, with permission, from Dr. Frank Gaillard and www.radiopaedia.org.

431 **Gout: Image B.** Uric acid crystals under polarized light. This image is a derivative work, adapted from the following source, available under . Courtesy of Robert J. Galindo. The image may have been modified by cropping, labeling, and/or captions. MedIQ Learning, LLC makes this image available under .

431 **Gout: Image C.** Podagra. This image is a derivative work, adapted from the following source, available under : Roddy E. Revisiting the pathogenesis of podagra: why does gout target the foot? *J Foot Ankle Res* 2011;4:13. doi 10.1186/1757-1146-4-13.

431 **Calcium pyrophosphate deposition disease.** Calcium phosphate crystals. Image courtesy of Medical Research Council and Drs. P. Diepke and K. Swan.

432 **Sjögren syndrome.** Lymphocytic infiltration. Courtesy of the US Department of Health and Human Services.

432 **Septic arthritis.** Joint effusion. This image is a derivative work, adapted from the following source, available under . Courtesy of Dr. James Heilman. The image may have been modified by cropping, labeling, and/or captions. MedIQ Learning, LLC makes this image available under .

433 **Seronegative spondyloarthropathies: Image C, left.** Bamboo spine. This image is a derivative work, adapted from the following source, available under . Courtesy of Stevenfruitsmaak. The image may have been modified by cropping, labeling, and/or captions. MedIQ Learning, LLC makes this image available under .

433 **Seronegative spondyloarthropathies: Image C, right.** Bamboo spine. Courtesy of Heather Hawker.

435 **Sarcoidosis: Images B** (X-ray of the chest) and **C** (CT of the chest). This image is a derivative work, adapted from the following source, available under : Lønborg J, Ward M, Gill A, et al. Utility of cardiac magnetic resonance in assessing right-sided heart failure in sarcoidosis. *BMC Med Imaging* 2013;13:2. doi 10.1186/1471-2342-13-2.

436 **Myositis ossificans.** This image is a derivative work, adapted from the following source, available under . Courtesy of T. Dvorak. The image may have been modified by cropping, labeling, and/or captions. MedIQ Learning, LLC makes this image available under .

437 **Scleroderma (systemic sclerosis): Image C.** Calcinosis. This image is a derivative work, adapted from the following source, available under . Courtesy of Dr. James Heilman. The image may have been modified by cropping, labeling, and/or captions. MedIQ Learning, LLC makes this image available under .

437 **Raynaud phenomenon.** This image is a derivative work, adapted from the following source, available under . Courtesy of Jamclaassen. The image may have been modified by cropping, labeling, and/or captions. MedIQ Learning, LLC makes this image available under .

440 **Common skin disorders: Image O.** Urticaria. This image is a derivative work, adapted from the following source, available under . Courtesy of Dr. James Heilman. The image may have been modified by cropping, labeling, and/or captions. MedIQ Learning, LLC makes this image available under .

441 **Vascular tumors: Image C.** Cystic hygroma. This image is a derivative work, adapted from the following source, available under : Sannoh S, Quezada E, Merer DM, et al. Cystic hygroma and potential airway obstruction in a newborn: a case report and review of the literature. *Cases J* 2009;2:48. doi 10.1186/1757-1626-2-48. The image may have been modified by cropping, labeling, and/or captions. All rights to this adaptation by MedIQ Learning, LLC are reserved.

442 **Skin infections: Image D.** Erysipelas. This image is a derivative work, adapted from the following source, available under : Klaus D. Peter.

443 **Blistering skin disorders: Image D.** Bullous pemphigoid on immunofluorescence. This image is a derivative work, adapted from the following source, available under : M. Emmanuel.

445 **Skin cancer: Image D.** Basal cell carcinoma histopathology. This image is a derivative work, adapted from the following source, available under . Courtesy of Wikimedia Commons. The image may have been modified by cropping, labeling, and/or captions. MedIQ Learning, LLC makes this image available under .

Neurology

451 **Posterior fossa malformations.** Dandy-Walker malformation. This image is a derivative work, adapted from the following source, available under : Krupa K, Bekiesinska-Figatowska M. Congenital and acquired abnormalities of the corpus callosum: a pictorial essay. *Biomed Res Int* 2013;2013:265619. doi 10.1155/2013/265619.

452 **Syringomyelia.** Reproduced, with permission, from Dr. Frank Gaillard and www.radiopaedia.org.

453 **Myelin.** Myelinated neuron. Courtesy of the Electron Microscopy Facility at Trinity College.

458 **Limbic system.** Brain scan. Courtesy of Kieran Maher. The image may have been modified by cropping, labeling, and/or captions. All rights to this adaptation by MedIQ Learning, LLC are reserved.

461 **Parkinson disease.** Lewy body in substantia nigra. This image is a derivative work, adapted from the following source, available under : Werner CJ, Heyny-von Haussen R, Mall G, et al. Parkinson's disease. *Proteome Sci* 2008;6:8. doi 10.1186/1477-5956-6-8. The image may have been modified by cropping, labeling, and/or captions. All rights to this adaptation by MedIQ Learning, LLC are reserved.

462 **Huntington disease.** Reproduced, with permission, from Dr. Frank Gaillard and www.radiopaedia.org.

469 **Intracranial hemorrhage: Image A.** Axial CT of brain showing epidural blood. This image is a derivative work, adapted from the following source, available under . Courtesy of Hellerhoff. The image may have been modified by cropping, labeling, and/or captions. MedIQ Learning, LLC makes this image available under .

469 **Intracranial hemorrhage: Image B.** Axial CT of brain showing skull fracture and scalp hematoma. This image is a derivative work, adapted from the following source, available under . Courtesy of Hellerhoff. The image may have been modified by cropping, labeling, and/or captions. MedIQ Learning, LLC makes this image available under .

469 **Intracranial hemorrhage: Image C.** Subdural hematoma. This image is a derivative work, adapted from the following source, available under . Courtesy of Dr. James Heilman. The image may have been modified by cropping, labeling, and/or captions. MedIQ Learning, LLC makes this image available under .

469 **Intracranial hemorrhage: Image E.** Subarachnoid hemorrhage. This image is a derivative work, adapted from the following source, available under : Hakan T, Turk CC, Celik H. Intra-operative real time intracranial subarachnoid haemorrhage during glial tumour resection: a case report. *Cases J* 2008;1:306. doi 10.1186/1757-1626-1-306. The image may have been modified by cropping, labeling, and/or captions. All rights to this adaptation by MedIQ Learning, LLC are reserved.

471 **Hydrocephalus: Image A.** Normal pressure hydrocephalus. Image courtesy of Dr. Brian Walcott.

471 **Hydrocephalus: Image B.** Communicating hydrocephalus. This image is a derivative work, adapted from the following source, available under : Torres-Martin M, Pena-Granero C, Carceller F, et al. Homozygous deletion of *TNFRSF4*, *TP73*, *PPAP2B* and *DPYD* at 1p and *PDCD5* at 19q identified by multiplex ligation-dependent probe amplification (MLPA) analysis in pediatric anaplastic glioma with questionable oligodendroglial component. *Mol Cytogenet* 2014;7:1. doi 10.1186/1755-8166-7-1.

472 **Spinal cord and associated tracts.** Spinal cord cross-section. This image is a derivative work, adapted from the following source, available under : Regents of University of Michigan Medical School.

475 **Friedreich ataxia.** Kyphoscoliosis. This image is a derivative work, adapted from the following source, available under : Axelrod FB, Gold-von Simson G. Hereditary sensory and autonomic neuropathies: types II, III, and IV. *Orphanet J Rare Dis* 2007;2:39. doi 10.1186/1750-1172-2-39.

480 **Facial nerve lesions.** This image is a derivative work, adapted from the following source, available under : Socolovsky M, Paez MD, Di Masi G, et al. Bell's palsy and partial hypoglossal to facial nerve transfer: Case presentation and literature review. *Surg Neurol Int* 2012;3:46. doi 10.4103/2152-7806.95391.

482 **Cholesteatoma.** This image is a derivative work, adapted from the following source, available under . Courtesy of Welleschik. The image may have been modified by cropping, labeling, and/or captions. MedIQ Learning, LLC makes this image available under .

482 **Normal eye.** This image is a derivative work, adapted from the following source, available under . Courtesy of Jan Kaláb. The image may have been modified by cropping, labeling, and/or captions. MedIQ Learning, LLC makes this image available under .

483 **Cataract.** Juvenile cataract. This image is a derivative work, adapted from the following source, available under : Roshan M, Vijaya PH, Lavanya GR, et al. A novel human *CRYGD* mutation in a juvenile autosomal dominant cataract. *Mol Vis* 2010;16:887-896. PMCID PMC2875257.

484 **Glaucoma: Images A (normal optic cup) and B (optic cup in glaucoma).** Image courtesy of EyeRounds.

484 Glaucoma: Image C. Closed/narrow angle glaucoma. This image is a derivative work, adapted from the following source, available under [CC BY]: Low S, Davidson AE, Holder GE, et al. Autosomal dominant Best disease with an unusual electrooculographic light rise and risk of angle-closure glaucoma: a clinical and molecular genetic study. *Mol Vis* 2011;17:2272-2282. PMCID PMC3171497. The image may have been modified by cropping, labeling, and/or captions. All rights to this adaptation by MedIQ Learning, LLC are reserved.

484 Glaucoma: Image D. Acute angle closure glaucoma. This image is a derivative work, adapted from the following source, available under [CC BY]:. CImage courtesy of Dr. Jonathan Trobe.

484 Conjunctivitis. This image is a derivative work, adapted from the following source, available under [CC BY]: Baiyeroju A, Bowman R, Gilbert C, et al. Managing eye health in young children. *Community Eye Health* 2010;23:4-11.

484 Uveitis. Image courtesy of EyeRounds.

485 Age-related macular degeneration. [Public Domain] Courtesy of the US Department of Health and Human Services.

485 Diabetic retinopathy. This image is a derivative work, adapted from the following source, available under [CC BY]: Stefanini FR, Badaró E, Falabella P, et al. Anti-VEGF for the management of diabetic macular edema. *J Immunol Res* 2014;2014:632307. doi 10.1155/2014/632307. The image may have been modified by cropping, labeling, and/or captions. All rights to this adaptation by MedIQ Learning, LLC are reserved.

485 Retinal vein occlusion. This image is a derivative work, adapted from the following source, available under [CC BY]: Alasil T, Rauser ME. Intravitreal bevacizumab in the treatment of neovascular glaucoma secondary to central retinal vein occlusion: a case report. *Cases J* 2009;2:176. doi 10.1186/1757-1626-2-176. The image may have been modified by cropping, labeling, and/or captions. All rights to this adaptation by MedIQ Learning, LLC are reserved.

485 Retinal detachment. Image courtesy of EyeRounds.

486 Retinitis pigmentosa. Image courtesy of EyeRounds.

486 Retinitis. [Public Domain] Courtesy of the US Department of Health and Human Services.

488 Ocular motility. Testing ocular muscles. This image is a derivative work, adapted from the following source, available under [CC BY-SA]. Courtesy of Au.yousef. The image may have been modified by cropping, labeling, and/or captions. MedIQ Learning, LLC makes this image available under [CC BY-SA].

489 Cranial nerve III, IV, VI palsies: Image A. Cranial nerve III damage. This image is a derivative work, adapted from the following source, available under [CC BY]: Hakim W, Sherman R, Rezk T, et al. An acute case of herpes zoster ophthalmicus with ophthalmoplegia. *Case Rep Ophthalmol Med* 1012; 2012:953910. Doi 10.1155/2012/953910.

489 Cranial nerve III, IV, VI palsies: Image B. Cranial nerve IV damage. This image is a derivative work, adapted from the following source, available under [CC BY]: Mendez JA, Arias CR, Sanchez D, et al. Painful ophthalmoplegia of the left eye in a 19-year-old female, with an emphasis in Tolosa-Hunt syndrome: a case report. *Cases J* 2009; 2: 8271. doi 10.4076/1757-1626-2-8271.

489 Cranial nerve III, IV, VI palsies: Image C. Cranial nerve VI damage. This image is a derivative work, adapted from the following source, available under [CC BY-SA]. Courtesy of Jordi March i Nogué. The image may have been modified by cropping, labeling, and/or captions. MedIQ Learning, LLC makes this image available under [CC BY-SA].

491 Dementia: Image B. Neurofibrillary tangles in Alzheimer disease. Image courtesy of Dr. Kristine Krafts.

491 Dementia: Image C. Pick bodies in frontotemporal dementia. This image is a derivative work, adapted from the following source, available under [CC BY]: Niedowicz DM, Nelson PT, Murphy MP. Alzheimer's disease: pathological mechanisms and recent insights. *Curr Neuropharmacol* 2011;9:674-684. doi 10.2174/157015911798376181.

492 Osmotic demyelination syndrome (central pontine myelinolysis). This image is a derivative work, adapted from the following source, available under [CC BY-SA]. Courtesy of Wikimedia Commons. The image may have been modified by cropping, labeling, and/or captions. MedIQ Learning, LLC makes this image available under [CC BY-SA].

492 Multiple sclerosis. Periventricular plaques. This image is a derivative work, adapted from the following source, available under [CC BY]: Buzzard KA, Broadley SA, Butzkueven H. What do effective treatments for multiple sclerosis tell us about the molecular mechanisms involved in pathogenesis? *Int J Mol Sci* 2012;13:12665-12709. doi 10.3390/ijms131012665.

495 Neurocutaneous disorders: Image A. Sturge-Weber syndrome and port wine stain. This image is a derivative work, adapted from the following source, available under [CC BY]: Babaji P, Bansal A, Krishna G, et al. Sturge-Weber syndrome with osteohypertrophy of maxilla. *Case Rep Pediatr* 2013. doi 10.1155/2013/964596.

495 Neurocutaneous disorders: Image B. Leptomeningeal angioma in Sturge-Weber syndrome. Reproduced, with permission, from Dr. Frank Gaillard and www.radiopaedia.org.

495 Neurocutaneous disorders: Image C. Tuberous sclerosis. This image is a derivative work, adapted from the following source, available under [CC BY]: Fred H, van Dijk H. Images of memorable cases: case 143. Connexions website. December 4, 2008. Available at: http://cnx.org/content/m14923/1.3/.

495 Neurocutaneous disorders: Image D. Ash leaf spots in tuberous sclerosis. This image is a derivative work, adapted from the following source, available under [CC BY]: Tonekaboni SH, Tousi P, Ebrahimi A, et al. Clinical and para clinical manifestations of tuberous sclerosis: a cross sectional study on 81 pediatric patients. *Iran J Child Neurol* 2012;6:25-31. PMCID PMC3943027.

495 Neurocutaneous disorders: Image E. Angiomyolipoma in tuberous sclerosis. This image is a derivative work, adapted from the following source, available under [CC BY-SA]. Courtesy of KGH. The image may have been modified by cropping, labeling, and/or captions. MedIQ Learning, LLC makes this image available under [CC BY-SA].

495 Neurocutaneous disorders: Image F. Café-au-lait spots in neurofibromatosis. This image is a derivative work, adapted from the following source, available under [CC BY-SA]. Courtesy of Wikimedia Commons. The image may have been modified by cropping, labeling, and/or captions. MedIQ Learning, LLC makes this image available under [CC BY-SA].

495 **Neurocutaneous disorders: Image G.** Lisch nodules in neurofibromatosis. Courtesy of the US Department of Health and Human Services.

495 **Neurocutaneous disorders: Image H.** Cutaneous neurofibromas. This image is a derivative work, adapted from the following source, available under : Kim BK, Choi YS, Gwoo S, et al. Neurofibromatosis type 1 associated with papillary thyroid carcinoma incidentally detected by thyroid ultrasonography: a case report. *J Med Case Rep* 2012;6:179. doi 10.1186/1752-1947-6-179.

495 **Neurocutaneous disorders: Image I.** Cerebellar hemangioblastoma histology. This image is a derivative work, adapted from the following source, available under . Courtesy of Nephron. The image may have been modified by cropping, labeling, and/or captions. MedIQ Learning, LLC makes this image available under .

495 **Neurocutaneous disorders: Image J.** Cerebellar hemangioblastomas imaging. This image is a derivative work, adapted from the following source, available under : Park DM, Zhuang Z, Chen L, et al. von Hippel-Lindau disease-associated hemangioblastomas are derived from embryologic multipotent cells. *PLoS Medicine* Feb. 13, 2007. doi 10.1371/journal.pmed.0040060.

496 **Adult primary brain tumors: Image A.** Glioblastoma multiforme at autopsy. Courtesy of the US Department of Health and Human Services and Armed Forces Institute of Pathology.

496 **Adult primary brain tumors: Image B.** Glioblastoma multiforme histology. This image is a derivative work, adapted from the following source, available under . Courtesy of Wikimedia Commons. The image may have been modified by cropping, labeling, and/or captions. MedIQ Learning, LLC makes this image available under .

496 **Adult primary brain tumors: Image C.** Dural tail in meningioma. Courtesy of the US Department of Health and Human Services and Armed Forces Institute of Pathology.

496 **Adult primary brain tumors: Image D.** Meningioma histology. This image is a derivative work, adapted from the following source, available under . Courtesy of Nephron. The image may have been modified by cropping, labeling, and/or captions. MedIQ Learning, LLC makes this image available under .

496 **Adult primary brain tumors: Image E.** MRI of hemangioblastoma. This image is a derivative work, adapted from the following source, available under : Park DM, Zhuang Z, Chen L, et al. von Hippel-Lindau disease-associated hemangioblastomas are derived from embryologic multipotent cells. *PLoS Med* 2007;4:e60. doi 10.1371/journal.pmed.0040060.

496 **Adult primary brain tumors: Image F.** Hemangioblastoma histology. This image is a derivative work, adapted from the following source, available under . Courtesy of Wikimedia Commons. The image may have been modified by cropping, labeling, and/or captions. MedIQ Learning, LLC makes this image available under .

496 **Adult primary brain tumors: Image G.** MRI of schwannoma. Courtesy of Wikimedia Commons.

496 **Adult primary brain tumors: Image H.** Schwannoma histology. This image is a derivative work, adapted from the following source, available under . Courtesy of Nephron. The image may have been modified by cropping, labeling, and/or captions. MedIQ Learning, LLC makes this image available under .

496 **Adult primary brain tumors: Image I.** MRI of oligodendroglioma. This image is a derivative work, adapted from the following source, available under : Celzo FG, Venstermans C, De Belder F, et al. Brain stones revisited—between a rock and a hard place. *Insights Imaging* 2013;4:625-635. doi 10.1007/s13244-013-0279-z.

496 **Adult primary brain tumors: Image J.** Oligodendroglioma histology. This image is a derivative work, adapted from the following source, available under . Courtesy of Nephron. The image may have been modified by cropping, labeling, and/or captions. MedIQ Learning, LLC makes this image available under .

496 **Adult primary brain tumors: Image K.** Prolactinoma. This image is a derivative work, adapted from the following source, available under : Wang C-S, Yeh T-C, Wu T-C, et al. Pituitary macroadenoma co-existent with supraclinoid internal carotid artery cerebral aneurysm: a case report and review of the literature. *Cases J* 2009;2:6459. doi 10.4076/1757-1626-2-6459.

496 **Adult primary brain tumors: Image L.** Field of vision in bitemporal hemianopia. This image is a derivative work, adapted from the following source, available under . Courtesy of Wikimedia Commons. The image may have been modified by cropping, labeling, and/or captions. MedIQ Learning, LLC makes this image available under .

497 **Childhood primary brain tumors: Image A.** MRI of pilocytic astrocytoma. This image is a derivative work, adapted from the following source, available under : Hafez RFA. Stereotaxic gamma knife surgery in treatment of critically located pilocytic astrocytoma: preliminary result. *World J Surg Oncol* 2007;5:39. doi 10.1186/1477-7819-5-39.

497 **Childhood primary brain tumors: Image C.** CT of medulloblastoma. Courtesy of the US Department of Health and Human Services and Armed Forces Institute of Pathology.

497 **Childhood primary brain tumors: Image D.** Medulloblastoma histology. This image is a derivative work, adapted from the following source, available under . Courtesy of KGH. The image may have been modified by cropping, labeling, and/or captions. MedIQ Learning, LLC makes this image available under .

497 **Childhood primary brain tumors: Image E.** MRI of ependymoma. This image is a derivative work, adapted from the following source, available under . Courtesy of Hellerhoff. The image may have been modified by cropping, labeling, and/or captions. MedIQ Learning, LLC makes this image available under .

497 **Childhood primary brain tumors: Image F.** Ependymoma histology. This image is a derivative work, adapted from the following source, available under . Courtesy of Nephron. The image may have been modified by cropping, labeling, and/or captions. MedIQ Learning, LLC makes this image available under .

497 **Childhood primary brain tumors: Image G.** CT of craniopharyngioma. This image is a derivative work, adapted from the following source, available under : Garnet MR, Puget S, Grill J, et al. Craniopharyngioma. *Orphanet J Rare Dis* 2007;2:18. doi 10.1186/1750-1172-2-18.

497 **Childhood primary brain tumor: Image H.** Craniopharyngioma histology. This image is a derivative work, adapted from the following source, available under . Courtesy of Nephron. The image may have been modified by cropping, labeling, and/or captions. MedIQ Learning, LLC makes this image available under .

Renal

530 **Potter sequence (syndrome).** Courtesy of the US Department of Health and Human Services and Armed Forces Institute of Pathology.

532 **Ureters: course.** This image is a derivative work, adapted from the following source, available under . Courtesy of Wikimedia Commons. The image may have been modified by cropping, labeling, and/or captions. MedIQ Learning, LLC makes this image available under .

533 **Glomerular filtration barrier.** This image is a derivative work, adapted from the following source, available under : Feng J, Wei H, Sun Y, et al. Regulation of podocalyxin expression in the kidney of streptozotocin-induced diabetic rats with Chinese herbs (Yishen capsule). *BMC Complement Altern Med* 2013;13:76. doi 10.1186/1472-6882-13-76.

547 **Nephritic syndrome: Image A.** Histology of acute poststreptococcal glomerulonephritis. This image is a derivative work, adapted from the following source, available under . Courtesy of Nephron. The image may have been modified by cropping, labeling, and/or captions. MedIQ Learning, LLC makes this image available under .

547 **Nephritic syndrome: Image B.** This image is a derivative work, adapted from the following source, available under : Immunofluorescence of acute poststreptococcal glomerulonephritis. Oda T, Yoshizawa N, Yamakami K, et al. The role of nephritis-associated plasmin receptor (naplr) in glomerulonephritis associated with streptococcal infection. *Biomed Biotechnol* 2012;2012:417675. doi 10.1155/2012/417675.

547 **Nephritic syndrome: Image C.** Histology of rapidly progressive glomerulonephritis. Courtesy of the US Department of Health and Human Services and Uniformed Services University of the Health Sciences.

548 **Nephrotic syndrome: Image B.** Histology of focal segmental glomerulosclerosis. This image is a derivative work, adapted from the following source, available under . Courtesy of Nephron. The image may have been modified by cropping, labeling, and/or captions. MedIQ Learning, LLC makes this image available under .

548 **Nephrotic syndrome: Image D.** Diabetic glomerulosclerosis with Kimmelstiel-Wilson lesions. This image is a derivative work, adapted from the following source, available under . Courtesy of Doc Mari. The image may have been modified by cropping, labeling, and/or captions. MedIQ Learning, LLC makes this image available under .

549 **Kidney stones: Image D.** Uric acid crystals. Image courtesy of Dr. Adam Weinstein.

550 **Hydronephrosis.** Ultrasound. This image is a derivative work, adapted from the following source, available under . Courtesy of Wikimedia Commons. The image may have been modified by cropping, labeling, and/or captions. MedIQ Learning, LLC makes this image available under .

550 **Renal cell carcinoma: Image A.** Histology. This image is a derivative work, adapted from the following source, available under . Courtesy of Nephron. The image may have been modified by cropping, labeling, and/or captions. MedIQ Learning, LLC makes this image available under .

550 **Renal cell carcinoma: Image B.** Gross specimen. Courtesy of Dr. Ed Uthman.

550 **Renal cell carcinoma: Image C.** CT scan. This image is a derivative work, adapted from the following source, available under : Behnes CL, Schlegel C, Shoukier M, et al. Hereditary papillary renal cell carcinoma primarily diagnosed in a cervical lymph node: a case report of a 30-year-old woman with multiple metastases. *BMC Urol* 2013;13:3. doi 10.1186/1471-2490-13-3.

550 **Renal oncocytoma: Image A.** Gross specimen. This image is a derivative work, adapted from the following source, available under : M. Emmanuel.

550 **Renal oncocytoma: Image B.** Histology. This image is a derivative work, adapted from the following source, available under . Courtesy of Nephron. The image may have been modified by cropping, labeling, and/or captions. MedIQ Learning, LLC makes this image available under .

551 **Wilms tumor.** This image is a derivative work, adapted from the following source, available under : Refaie H, Sarhan M, Hafez A. Role of CT in assessment of unresectable Wilms tumor response after preoperative chemotherapy in pediatrics. *Sci World J* 2008;8:661-669. doi 10.1100/tsw.2008.96.

551 **Transitional cell carcinoma: Image A.** This image is a derivative work, adapted from the following source, available under : Geavlete B, Stanescu F, Moldoveanu C, et al. NBI cystoscopy and bipolar electrosurgery in NMIBC management—an overview of daily practice. *J Med Life* 2013;6:140-145. PMCID PMC3725437.

552 **Pyelonephritis: Image B.** CT scan. Courtesy of the US Department of Health and Human Services and Armed Forces Institute of Pathology.

554 **Acute tubular necrosis: Image A.** Muddy brown casts. This image is a derivative work, adapted from the following source, available under . Courtesy of Dr. Serban Nicolescu.

554 **Renal papillary necrosis.** Courtesy of the US Department of Health and Human Services and William D. Craig, Dr. Brent J. Wagner, and Mark D. Travis.

555 **Renal cyst disorders: Image C.** Ultrasound of simple cyst. This image is a derivative work, adapted from the following source, available under . Courtesy of Nevit Dilmen. The image may have been modified by cropping, labeling, and/or captions. MedIQ Learning, LLC makes this image available under .

Reproductive

565 **Fetal alcohol syndrome.** Image courtesy of Teresa Kellerman.

567 **Umbilical cord.** Cross-section of normal umbilical cord. This image is a derivative work, adapted from the following source, available under . Courtesy of Dr. Ed Uthman. The image may have been modified by cropping, labeling, and/or captions. MedIQ Learning, LLC makes this image available under .

572 **Uterine (Müllerian) duct anomalies: Images A-D.** This image is a derivative work, adapted from the following source, available under : Ahmadi F, Zafarani F, Haghighi H, et al. Application of 3D ultrasonography in detection of uterine abnormalities. *Int J Fertil Sterili* 2011; 4:144-147. PMCID PMC4023499.

574 **Female reproductive epithelial histology.** Transformation zone. This image is a derivative work, adapted from the following source, available under : Dr. Ed Uthman. The image may have been modified by cropping, labeling, and/or captions. All rights to this adaptation by MedIQ Learning, LLC are reserved.

576 **Seminiferous tubules.** This image is a derivative work, adapted from the following source, available under . Courtesy of Dr. Anlt Rao. The image may have been modified by cropping, labeling, and/or captions. MedIQ Learning, LLC makes this image available under .

588 **Pregnancy complications.** Ectopic pregnancy. This image is a derivative work, adapted from the following source, available under : Dr. Ed Uthman.

591 **Polycystic ovarian syndrome (Stein-Leventhal syndrome).** This image is a derivative work, adapted from the following source, available under : Lujan ME, Chizen DR, Peppin AK, et al. Improving inter-observer variability in the evaluation of ultrasonographic features of polycystic ovaries. *Reprod Biol Endocrinol* 2008;6:30. doi 10.1186/1477-7827-6-30.

592 **Ovarian neoplasms: Image C.** Mature cystic teratoma. This image is a derivative work, adapted from the following source, available under . Courtesy of Nephron. The image may have been modified by cropping, labeling, and/or captions. MedIQ Learning, LLC makes this image available under .

593 **Ovarian neoplasms: Image D.** Call-Exner bodies. This image is a derivative work, adapted from the following source, available under : Katoh T, Yasuda M, Hasegawa K, et al. Estrogen-producing endometrioid adenocarcinoma resembling sex cord-stromal tumor of the ovary: a review of four postmenopausal cases. *Diagn Pathol* 2012;7:164. doi 10.1186/1746-1596-7-164.

593 **Ovarian neoplasms: Image F.** Yolk sac tumor. This image is a derivative work, adapted from the following source, available under . Courtesy of Jensflorian. The image may have been modified by cropping, labeling, and/or captions. MedIQ Learning, LLC makes this image available under .

594 **Endometrial conditions: Image A.** Leiomyoma (fibroid), gross specimen. This image is a derivative work, adapted from the following source, available under : Hic et nunc.

594 **Endometrial conditions: Image B.** Leiomyoma (fibroid) histology. This image is a derivative work, adapted from the following source, available under : Londero AP, Perego P, Mangioni C, et al. Locally relapsed and metastatic uterine leiomyoma: A case report. *J Med Case Rep* 2008;2:308. doi 10.1186/1752-1947-2-308. The image may have been modified by cropping, labeling, and/or captions. All rights to this adaptation by MedIQ Learning, LLC are reserved.

594 **Endometrial conditions: Images C** (endometrial hyperplasia) **and D** (endometrial carcinoma). This image is a derivative work, adapted from the following source, available under : Izadi-Mood N, Yarmohammadi M, Ahmadi SA, et al. Reproducibility determination of WHO classification of endometrial hyperplasia/well differentiated adenocarcinoma and comparison with computerized morphometric data in curettage specimens in Iran. *Diagn Pathol* 2009;4:10. doi 10.1186/1746-1596-4-10.

594 **Endometrial conditions: Image E.** Endometritis. This image is a derivative work, adapted from the following source, available under . Courtesy of Nephron. The image may have been modified by cropping, labeling, and/or captions. MedIQ Learning, LLC makes this image available under .

597 **Malignant breast tumors: Image B.** Comedocarcinoma. This image is a derivative work, adapted from the following source, available under : Costarelli L, Campagna D, Mauri M, et al. Intraductal proliferative lesions of the breast—terminology and biology matter: premalignant lesions or preinvasive cancer? *Int J Surg Oncol* 2012;501904. doi 10.1155/2012/501904. The image may have been modified by cropping, labeling, and/or captions. All rights to this adaptation by MedIQ Learning, LLC are reserved.

597 **Malignant breast tumors: Image C.** Paget disease of breast. This image is a derivative work, adapted from the following source, available under : Muttarak M, Siriya B, Kongmebhol P, et al. Paget's disease of the breast: clinical, imaging and pathologic findings: a review of 16 patients. *Biomed Imaging Interv J* 2011;7:e16. doi 10.2349/biij.7.2.e16.

597 **Malignant breast tumors: Image D.** Invasive ductal carcinoma. This image is a derivative work, adapted from the following source, available under : Zhou X-C, Zhou, Ye Y-H, et al. Invasive ductal breast cancer metastatic to the sigmoid colon. *World J Surg Oncol* 2012;10:256. doi 10.1186/1477-7819-10-256.

597 **Malignant breast tumors: Image E.** Invasive lobular carcinoma. This image is a derivative work, adapted from the following source, available under : Franceschini G, Manno A, Mule A, et al. Gastro-intestinal symptoms as clinical manifestation of peritoneal and retroperitoneal spread of an invasive lobular breast cancer: report of a case and review of the literature. *BMC Cancer* 2006;6:193. doi 10.1186/1471-2407-6-193.

597 **Malignant breast tumors: Image F.** Peau d'orange of inflammatory breast cancer. Courtesy of the US Department of Health and Human Services.

597 **Varicocele.** Dilated pampiniform veins. Image courtesy of Dr. Bruce R. GIlbert.

Respiratory

607 **Pneumocytes.** Type II pneumocyte. This image is a derivative work, adapted from the following source, available under : Courtesy of Dr. Thomas Caceci.

607 **Neonatal respiratory distress syndrome.** This image is a derivative work, adapted from the following source, available under : Aloraіny IA, Balas NB, Al-Boukai AA. Pictorial essay: infants of diabetic mothers. *Indian J Radiol Imaging* 2010;20:174-181. doi 10.4103/0971-3026.69349.

616 Rhinosinusitis. This image is a derivative work, adapted from the following source, available under : Strek P, Zagolski O, Sktadzien J. Fatty tissue within the maxillary sinus: a rare finding. *Head Face Med* 2006;2:28. doi 10.1186/1746-160X-2-28.

616 Deep venous thrombosis. This image is a derivative work, adapted from the following source, available under . Courtesy of Dr. James Heilman. The image may have been modified by cropping, labeling, and/or captions. MedIQ Learning, LLC makes this image available under .

617 Pulmonary emboli: Image C. CT scan. This image is a derivative work, adapted from the following source, available under . Courtesy of Dr. Carl Chartrand-Lefebvre. The image may have been modified by cropping, labeling, and/or captions. MedIQ Learning, LLC makes this image available under .

618 Obstructive lung diseases: Image A. Emphysema histology. This image is a derivative work, adapted from the following source, available under . Courtesy of Nephron. The image may have been modified by cropping, labeling, and/or captions. MedIQ Learning, LLC makes this image available under .

618 Obstructive lung diseases: Image B. Centriacinar emphysema, gross specimen. Courtesy of the US Department of Health and Human Services and Dr. Edwin P. Ewing, Jr.

618 Obstructive lung diseases: Image C. CT of centriacinar emphysema. This image is a derivative work, adapted from the following source, available under : Oikonomou A, Prassopoulo P. Mimics in chest disease: interstitial opacities. *Insights Imaging* 2013;4:9-27. doi 10.1007/s13244-012-0207-7.

618 Obstructive lung diseases: Image D. Barrel-shaped chest in emphysema. This image is a derivative work, adapted from the following source, available under . Courtesy of Dr. James Heilman. The image may have been modified by cropping, labeling, and/or captions. MedIQ Learning, LLC makes this image available under .

618 Obstructive lung diseases: Image F. Mucus plugs in asthma. This image is a derivative work, adapted from the following source, available under . Courtesy of Dr. Yale Rosen. The image may have been modified by cropping, labeling, and/or captions. MedIQ Learning, LLC makes this image available under .

618 Obstructive lung disease: Image G. Bronchiectasis in cystic fibrosis. This image is a derivative work, adapted from the following source, available under . Courtesy of Dr. Yale Rosen. The image may have been modified by cropping, labeling, and/or captions. MedIQ Learning, LLC makes this image available under .

619 Restrictive lung diseases. This image is a derivative work, adapted from the following source, available under . Courtesy of IPFeditor. The image may have been modified by cropping, labeling, and/or captions. MedIQ Learning, LLC makes this image available under .

620 Pneumoconioses: Image A. Pleural plaques in asbestosis. This image is a derivative work, adapted from the following source, available under . Courtesy of Dr. Yale Rosen. The image may have been modified by cropping, labeling, and/or captions. MedIQ Learning, LLC makes this image available under .

620 Pneumoconioses: Image B. CT scan of asbestosis. This image is a derivative work, adapted from the following source, available under : Miles SE, Sandrini A, Johnson AR, et al. Clinical consequences of asbestos-related diffuse pleural thickening: a review. *J Occup Med Toxicol* 2008;3:20. doi 10.1186/1745-6673-3-20.

620 Pneumoconioses: Image C. Ferruginous bodies in asbestosis. This image is a derivative work, adapted from the following source, available under . Courtesy of Nephron. The image may have been modified by cropping, labeling, and/or captions. MedIQ Learning, LLC makes this image available under .

621 Acute respiratory distress syndrome. X-ray of the lungs. This image is a derivative work, adapted from the following source, available under . Courtesy of Samir. The image may have been modified by cropping, labeling, and/or captions. MedIQ Learning, LLC makes this image available under .

623 Pleural effusions: Images A and B. This image is a derivative work, adapted from the following source, available under : Toshikazu A, Takeoka H, Nishioka K, et al. Successful management of refractory pleural effusion due to systemic immunoglobulin light chain amyloidosis by vincristine adriamycin dexamethasone chemotherapy: a case report. *Med Case Rep* 2010;4:322. doi 10.1186/1752-1947-4-322.

624 Pneumonia: Image B. Lobar pneumonia, gross specimen. This image is a derivative work, adapted from the following source, available under . Courtesy of Dr. Yale Rosen. The image may have been modified by cropping, labeling, and/or captions. MedIQ Learning, LLC makes this image available under .

624 Pneumonia: Image C. Acute inflammatory infiltrates in bronchopneumonia. This image is a derivative work, adapted from the following source, available under . Courtesy of Dr. Yale Rosen. The image may have been modified by cropping, labeling, and/or captions. MedIQ Learning, LLC makes this image available under .

624 Pneumonia: Image D. Bronchopneumonia, gross specimen. This image is a derivative work, adapted from the following source, available under . Courtesy of Dr. Yale Rosen. The image may have been modified by cropping, labeling, and/or captions. MedIQ Learning, LLC makes this image available under .

624 Lung abscess: Image A. Gross specimen. This image is a derivative work, adapted from the following source, available under . Courtesy of Dr. Yale Rosen. The image may have been modified by cropping, labeling, and/or captions. MedIQ Learning, LLC makes this image available under .

624 Lung abscess: Image B. X-ray. This image is a derivative work, adapted from the following source, available under : Dr. Yale Rosen.

625 Pancoast tumor. This image is a derivative work, adapted from the following source, available under : Manenti G, Raguso M, D'Onofrio S, et al. Pancoast tumor: the role of magnetic resonance imaging. *Case Rep Radiol* 2013; 2013:479120. doi 10.1155/2013/479120.

625 Superior vena cava syndrome: Images A (blanching of skin with pressure) **and B** (CT of chest). This image is a derivative work, adapted from the following source, available under : Shaikh I, Berg K, Kman N. Thrombogenic catheter-associated superior vena cava syndrome. *Case Rep Emerg Med* 2013; 2013: 793054. doi 10.1155/2013/793054.

626 Lung cancer: Image B. Adenocarcinoma histology. Courtesy of the US Department of Health and Human Services and Armed Forces Institute of Pathology.

626 Lung cancer: Image C. Squamous cell carcinoma. This image is a derivative work, adapted from the following source, available under . Courtesy of Dr. James Heilman. The image may have been modified by cropping, labeling, and/or captions. MedIQ Learning, LLC makes this image available under .

626 Lung cancer: Image E. Large cell lung cancer. This image is a derivative work, adapted from the following source, available under : Jala VR, Radde BN, Haribabu B, et al. Enhanced expression of G-protein coupled estrogen receptor (GPER/GPR30) in lung cancer. *BMC Cancer* 2012;12:624. doi 10.1186/1471-2407-12-624.

Index

J

K

M

N

Q

R

U

V

▶ NOTES

▶ NOTES

▶ NOTES

NOTES

▶ NOTES

▶ NOTES

▶ NOTES

▶ NOTES

About the Editors

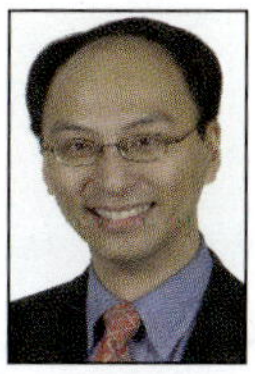

Tao Le, MD, MHS

Tao developed a passion for medical education as a medical student. He currently edits more than 15 titles in the *First Aid* series. In addition, he is the founder and editor of the *USMLE-Rx* test bank and online video series as well as a cofounder of the *Underground Clinical Vignettes* series. As a medical student, he was editor-in-chief of the University of California, San Francisco (UCSF) Synapse, a university newspaper with a weekly circulation of 9000. Tao earned his medical degree from UCSF in 1996 and completed his residency training in internal medicine at Yale University and fellowship training at Johns Hopkins University. Tao subsequently went on to cofound Medsn, a medical education technology venture, and served as its chief medical officer. He is currently conducting research in asthma education at the University of Louisville.

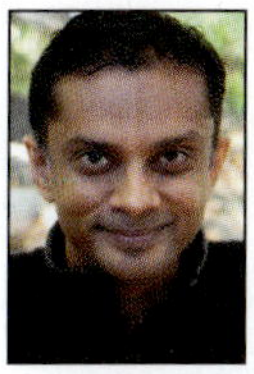

Vikas Bhushan, MD

Vikas is a writer, editor, entrepreneur, and teleradiologist on sabbatical. In 1990 he conceived and authored the original *First Aid for the USMLE Step 1*. His entrepreneurial endeavors include a student-focused medical publisher (S2S), an e-learning company (medschool.com/Medsn), and an ER teleradiology practice (24/7 Radiology). Firmly anchored to the Left Coast, Vikas completed a bachelor's degree at the University of California Berkeley; an MD with thesis at UCSF; and a diagnostic radiology residency at UCLA. His eclectic interests include technology, information design, photography, South Asian diasporic culture, and avoiding a day job. Always finding the long shortcut, Vikas is an adventurer, knowledge seeker, and occasional innovator. He enjoys novice status as a kiteboarder and single father, and strives to raise his children as global citizens.

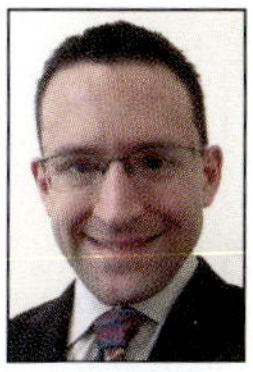

Matthew Sochat, MD

Matthew is a second-year internal medicine resident at Temple University Hospital in Philadelphia. He completed medical school in 2013 at Brown University and is a 2008 graduate of the University of Massachusetts, Amherst, where he studied biochemistry and the classics. Pastimes include skiing, cooking/baking, traveling, the company of friends/loved ones, the Spanish language, and computer/video gaming. Be warned: Matt also loves to come up with corny jokes at (in)opportune moments.

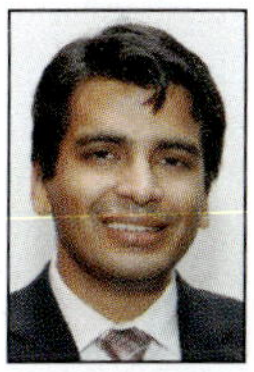

Yash Chavda, DO

Yash is an emergency medicine resident at St. Barnabas Hospital in the Bronx. He earned his medical degree from NYIT College of Osteopathic Medicine, and completed his undergraduate degrees in biology and psychology at CUNY Baruch College in 2010. Yash has many interests outside of medicine and enjoys spending time with his loved ones. He is a developing photographer, former web/graphic designer (who still dabbles), video gamer, foodie, and avid explorer who wants to travel the world (whenever he actually gets a chance). He hopes to always keep improving at everything he does.

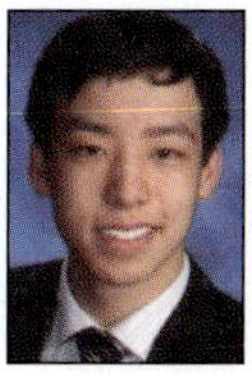

Francis Deng

Francis is a fourth-year medical student at Washington University in St. Louis, where he was elected to the Alpha Omega Alpha honor society. He earned his bachelor degree in human developmental and regenerative biology from Harvard College, graduating Phi Beta Kappa and magna cum laude. Francis serves on the Board of Directors of the National Resident Matching Program and is a Match applicant in diagnostic radiology.

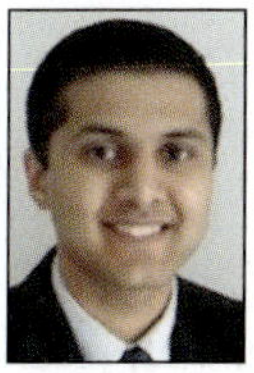

Mehboob Kalani, MD

Mehboob is a first-year internal medicine resident at Allegheny Health Network Medical Education Consortium in Pittsburgh. He was born in Karachi, Pakistan, grew up in Toronto, Canada, and pursued medicine upon completing high school. He earned his premedical and medical degrees at American University of Integrative Sciences in 2015. After residency, his interests lie in pulmonary critical care medicine, and he is researching COPD exacerbation treatment and readmission rates. In his limited leisure time, Mehboob enjoys playing or watching soccer, long drives, and family gatherings.

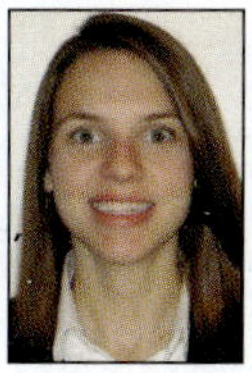

Kimberly Kallianos, MD

Originally from Atlanta, Kimberly graduated from the University of North Carolina at Chapel Hill in 2006 and from Harvard Medical School in 2011. She is a fourth-year radiology resident at the University of California, San Francisco and will complete a fellowship in cardiac and pulmonary imaging at UCSF from 2016 to 2017.

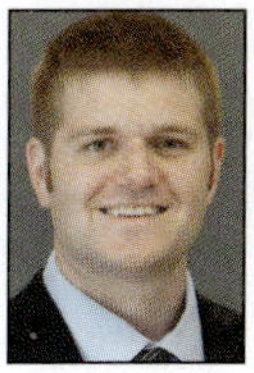

Patrick Sylvester, MD

Patrick is a resident at The Ohio State University, where he is completing a combined residency program in internal medicine and emergency medicine. Originally from Illinois, he completed his undergraduate studies at the University of Illinois at Urbana-Champaign before moving to Columbus, where he completed medical school at OSU. Outside of medicine, Patrick enjoys home improvement projects, cooking, and spending time with his infinitely patient wife and their dog, Chief.